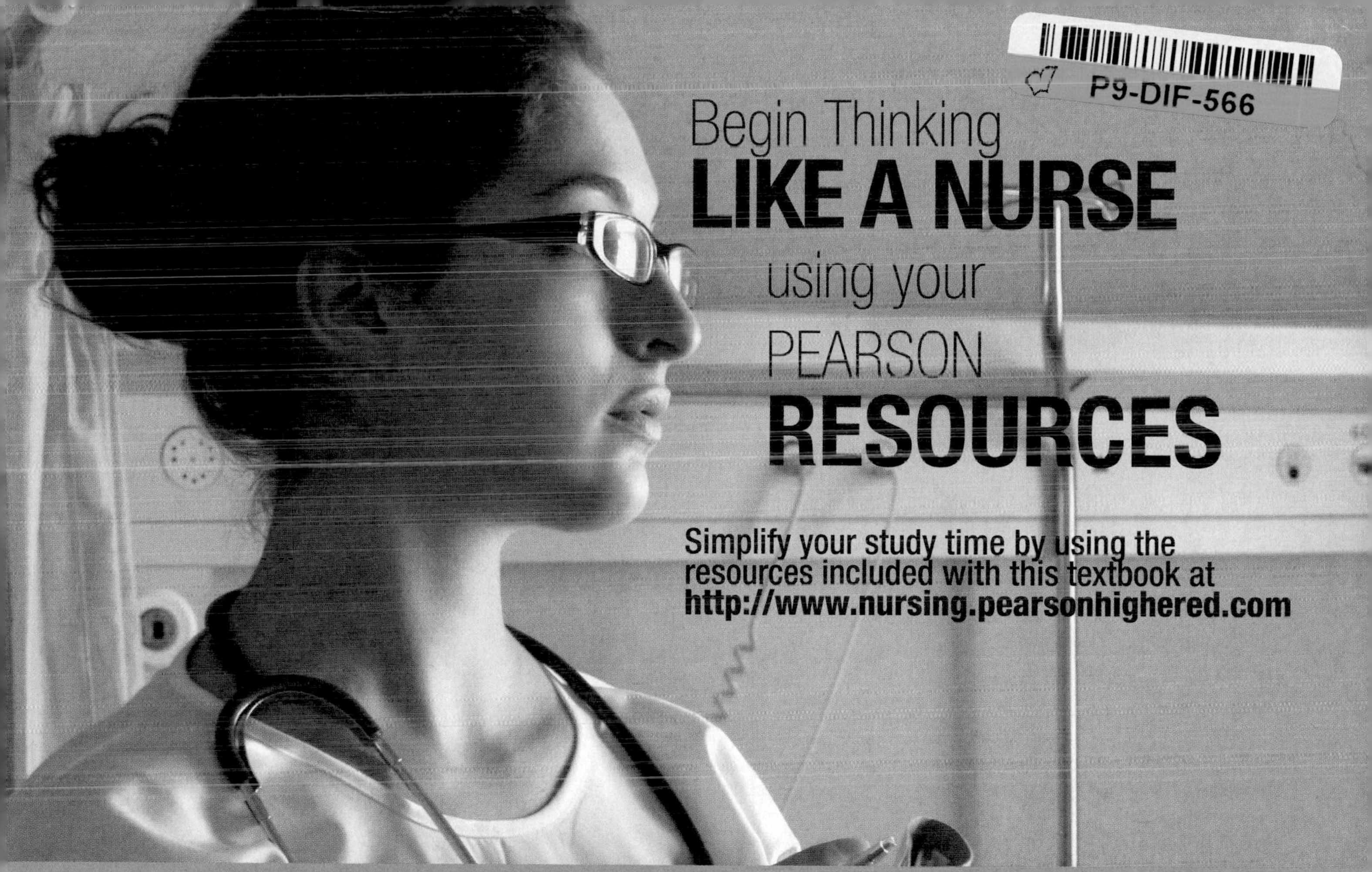

Begin Thinking **LIKE A NURSE** using your PEARSON **RESOURCES**

Simplify your study time by using the resources included with this textbook at http://www.nursing.pearsonhighered.com

Further enhance your Clinical Reasoning with the additional resources below. For more information and purchasing options visit **www.mypearsonstore.com**.

Break Through to improving results

MyNursingLab®

MyNursingLab provides a guided learning path that is proven to help students synthesize vast amounts of information, guiding them from memorization to true understanding through application.

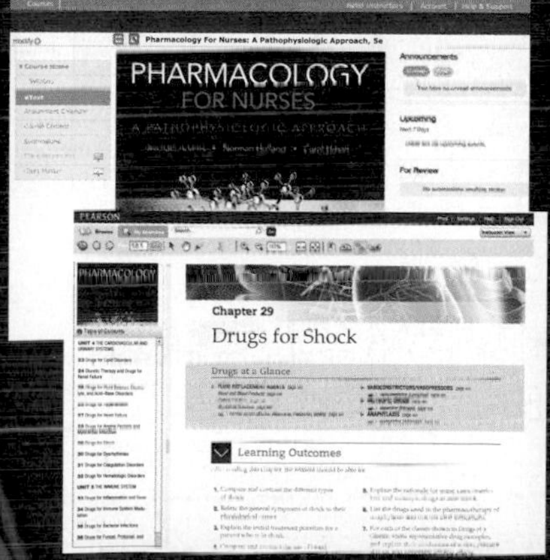

Think Like a Nurse in Clinical

Clinical references across the nursing curriculum available!

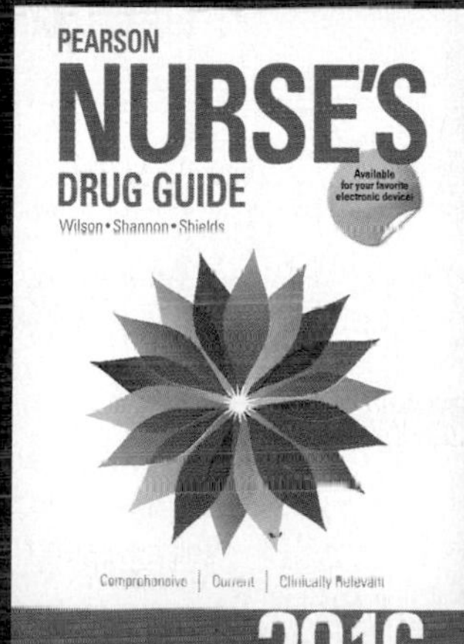

Thinking Like a Nurse for Classroom Success

Companion workbook that helps you to succeed in nursing includes review questions, calculations, case study applications, and more!

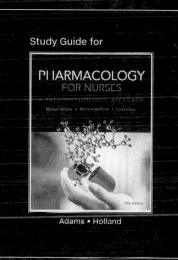

ALWAYS LEARNING

PEARSON

Pharmacology for Nurses

Pharmacology for Nurses

A Pathophysiologic Approach

FIFTH EDITION

Michael Patrick Adams
Adjunct Professor of Biological Sciences
Pasco-Hernando State College
Hillsborough Community College
Formerly Dean of Health Professions
Pasco-Hernando State College

Leland Norman Holland, Jr.
Program Manager
Hillsborough Community College
Brandon Campus, Tampa, Florida

Carol Quam Urban
Director, School of Nursing
Associate Dean, College of Health and Human Services
Associate Professor
George Mason University

PEARSON

Boston Columbus Indianapolis New York San Francisco Amsterdam
Cape Town Dubai London Madrid Milan Munich Paris Montreal Toronto Delhi
Mexico City São Paulo Sydney Hong Kong Seoul Singapore Taipei Tokyo

Publisher: Julie Levin Alexander
Publisher's Assistant: Sarah Henrich
Executive Acquisitions Editor: Pamela Fuller
Editorial Assistant: Erin Sullivan
Project Manager: Cathy O'Connell
Program Manager: Erin Rafferty
Development Editor: Teri Zak
Director, Product Management Services: Etain O'Dea
Team Lead, Program Management: Melissa Bashe
Team Lead, Project Management: Cynthia Zonneveld
Full-Service Project Manager: Mary Tindle, Cenveo Publisher Services
Manufacturing Buyer: Maura Zaldivar-Garcia
Art Director and Interior Design: Maria Guglielmo-Walsh
Cover Design: Beth Paquin
Vice President of Sales & Marketing: David Gesell
Vice President, Director of Marketing: Margaret Waples
Senior Product Marketing Manager: Phoenix Harvey
Field Marketing Manager: Deborah Doyle
Marketing Specialist: Michael Sirinides
Marketing Assistant: Amy Pfund
Media Project Manager: Lisa Rinaldi
Composition: Cenveo Publisher Services
Printer/Binder: LSC Communications/Menasha
Cover Printer: Phoenix Color/Hagerstown
Cover Image: Everythingpossible/Fotolia

Credits and acknowledgments for content borrowed from other sources and reproduced, with permission, in this textbook appear on appropriate page within text except for the following:

Unit 1 opener, chapter openers 1–5: Dimdimich/Fotolia
Unit 2 opener, chapter openers 6–11: Stockdevil/Fotolia
Unit 3 opener, chapter openers 12–22: Nerthuz/Fotolia
Unit 4 opener, chapter openers 23–32: Nerthuz/Fotolia
Unit 5 opener, chapter openers 33–38: Sebastian Kaulitzki/Fotolia
Unit 6 opener, chapter openers 39–40: Nerthuz/Fotolia
Unit 7 opener, chapter openers 41–43: Nerthuz/Fotolia
Unit 8 opener, chapter openers 44–47: Nerthuz/Fotolia
Unit 9 opener, chapter openers 48–50: Dimdimich/Fotolia

In order to make safe and effective judgments using NANDA-I nursing diagnoses it is essential that nurses refer to the definitions and defining characteristics of the diagnoses listed in this work.

Notice: Care has been taken to confirm the accuracy of information presented in this book. The authors, editors, and the publisher, however, cannot accept any responsibility for errors or omissions or for consequences from application of the information in this book and make no warranty, express or implied, with respect to its contents.

The authors and publisher have exerted every effort to ensure that drug selections and dosages set forth in this text are in accord with current recommendations and practice at the time of publication. However, in view of ongoing research, changes in government regulations, and the constant flow of information relating to drug therapy and drug reactions, the reader is urged to check the package inserts of all drugs for any change in indications of dosage and for added warnings and precautions. This is particularly important when the recommended agent is a new or infrequently employed drug.

Library of Congress Cataloging-in-Publication Data
Adams, Michael
Pharmacology for nurses: a pathophysiologic approach / Michael Patrick Adams, Leland N. Holland, Carol Quam Urban.—5th ed.
p.; cm.
Includes bibliographical references and index.
ISBN 10 0-13-425516-X
ISBN 13: 978-0-13-425516-3
I. Holland, Leland Norman, II. Urban, Carol Q. (Carol Quam) III. Title.
[DNLM: 1. Drug Therapy—Nursing. 2. Pharmacological Phenomena—Nurses' Instruction. 3. Pharmacology—Nurses' Instruction. WB 330]
LC Classification not assigned
615'.1—dc23

2012039180

5 17

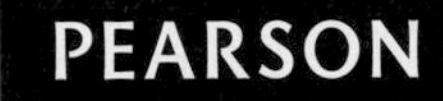

ISBN-10: 0-13-425516-X
ISBN-13: 978-0-13-425516-3

About the Authors

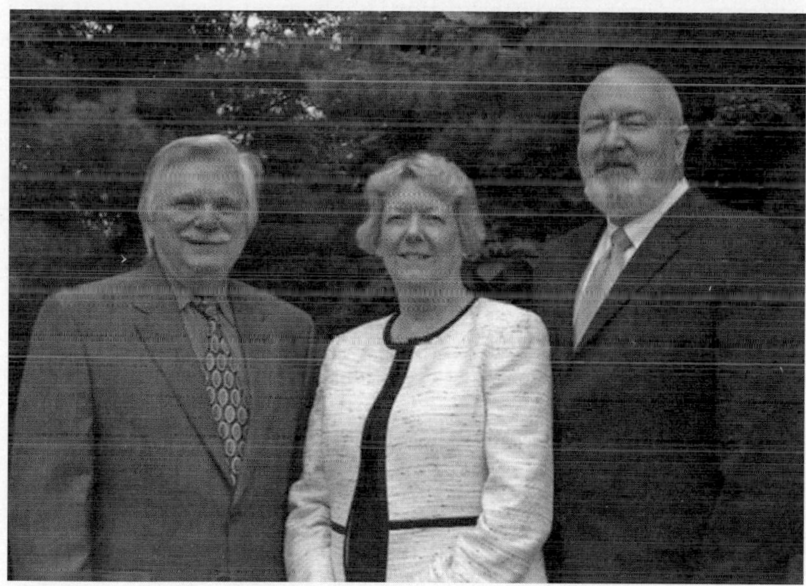

MICHAEL PATRICK ADAMS, PHD, is an accomplished educator, author, and national speaker. The National Institute for Staff and Organizational Development in Austin, Texas, named Dr. Adams a Master Teacher. He has published two other textbooks with Pearson Publishing: *Core Concepts in Pharmacology* and *Pharmacology: Connections to Nursing Practice.*

Dr. Adams obtained his master's degree in pharmacology from Michigan State University and his doctorate in education from the University of South Florida. Dr. Adams was on the faculty of Lansing Community College and St. Petersburg College, and served as Dean of Health Professions at Pasco-Hernando State College for 15 years. He is currently Adjunct Professor of Biological Sciences at Pasco-Hernando State College and Hillsborough Community College.

I dedicate this book to nursing educators, who contribute every day to making the world a better and more caring place.

—MPA

LELAND NORMAN HOLLAND, JR., PHD (NORM), over 20 years ago, started out like many scientists, planning for a career in basic science research. He was quickly drawn to the field of teaching in higher medical education, where he has spent most of his career. Among the areas where he has been particularly effective are preparatory programs in nursing, medicine, dentistry, pharmacy, and allied health. Dr. Holland is both a professor and supporter in nursing education nationwide. He brings to the profession a depth of knowledge in biology, chemistry, and medically related subjects such as microbiology, biological chemistry, and pharmacology. Dr. Holland's doctoral degree is in medical pharmacology. He has published one other textbook with Pearson Publishing: *Core Concepts in Pharmacology.* He is very much dedicated to the success of students and their preparation for careers in health care. He continues to motivate students in the lifelong pursuit of learning.

To the greatest family in the world: Karen, Alexandria, Caleb, and Joshua.

—LNHII

CAROL QUAM URBAN, PHD, RN, Associate Professor, is the Director of the School of Nursing, and an Associate Dean in the College of Health and Human Services at George Mason University in Fairfax, Virginia. She has been on the faculty at Mason and considers the study of pharmacology to be a course that truly integrates nursing knowledge, skills, and interdisciplinary teamwork. She credits her students, past and present, for providing a never-ending source of real-world stories that make learning about pharmacology enjoyable in class. She has also published the Pearson textbook *Pharmacology: Connections to Nursing Practice* with Dr. Adams.

To my daughter, Joy, who has started her own journey in nursing. And in memory of my son, Keith, the bravest and happiest soul I know.

—CQU

Thank You

Our heartfelt thanks go out to our colleagues from schools of nursing across the country who have given their time generously to help create this exciting new edition. These individuals helped us plan and shape our book and resources by reviewing chapters, art, design, and more. *Pharmacology for Nurses: A Pathophysiologic Approach,* Fifth Edition, has reaped the benefit of your collective knowledge and experience as nurses and teachers, and we have improved the materials due to your efforts, suggestions, objections, endorsements, and inspiration. Among those who gave their time generously are the following:

Beatrice Adams, PharmD
Critical Care Clinical Pharmacist
Tampa General Hospital
Department of Pharmacy
Tampa, Florida

Shannon Allen, CRNA, MSNA
Professor
New Mexico Junior College
Hobbs, New Mexico

Candyce Antley, RN, MN
Instructor
Midlands Technical College
Columbia, South Carolina

Culeta Armstrong, MSN, RN
Clinical Assistant Professor
University of Memphis
Memphis, Tennessee

Wanda Barlow, MSN, RN, FNP-BC
Instructor
Winston-Salem State University
Winston-Salem, North Carolina

Sophia Beydoun, RN, BSN, MSN, AA-AND
Professor
Henry Ford Community College
Dearborn, Michigan

Staci Boruff, PhD, RN
Assistant Academic Dean of Health Programs
Professor of Nursing
Walters State Community College
Morristown, Tennessee

Bridget Bradley, PharmD, BCPP
Assistant Professor
Pacific University
Hillsboro, Oregon

Mary M. Bridgeman, PharmD, BCPS, CGP
Clinical Assistant Professor
Rutgers University
Piscataway, New Jersey

Reamer L. Bushardt, PharmD, P.A.-C
Professor
Wake Forest Baptist Health
Winston-Salem, North Carolina

Marcus W. Campbell, PharmD, BC-ADM
Assistant Professor Pharmacy Practice
Director, Center for Drug Information & Research
LECOM School of Pharmacy
Bradenton, Florida

Rachel Choudhury, MSN, MS, RN, CNE
Associate Dean and Program Director, ABSN
Musco School of Nursing and Health Professions
Brandman University
Irvine, California

Darlene Clark, MS, RN
Senior Lecturer in Nursing
Pennsylvania State University
University Park, Pennsylvania

Janice DiFalco, RN, MSN, CNS, CMSRN, FAACVPR
Professor
San Jacinto College
Pasadena, Texas

Deepali Dixit, PharmD, BCPS
Clinical Assistant Professor
Rutgers University
Piscataway, New Jersey

Rachael Durie, PharmD, BCPS
Cardiology Clinical Pharmacist
Assistant Professor of Clinical Pharmacy
Rutgers University
Neptune, New Jersey

Deborah Dye, RN, MSN
Assistant Professor/Nursing Department Chair
Ivy Tech Community College
Lafayette, Indiana

Jacqueline Frock, RN, MSN
Professor of Nursing
Oklahoma City Community College
Oklahoma City, Oklahoma

Jasmine D. Gonzalvo, PharmD, BCPS, BC-ADM, CDE
Clinical Associate Professor
Purdue University
West Lafayette, Indiana

Adina C. Hirsch, PharmD, BCNSP
Assistant Professor of Pharmacy Practice
Philadelphia College of Osteopathic Medicine
Philadelphia, Pennsylvania

Linda Howe, PhD, RN, CNS, CNE
Associate Professor
University of Central Florida
Orlando, Florida

Anne L. Hume, PharmD, FCCP, BCPS
Professor of Pharmacy
University of Rhode Island
Kingston, Rhode Island

Ragan Johnson, DNP, APRN-BC
Assistant Professor
University of Tennessee
Memphis, Tennessee

Vinh Kieu, PharmD
Assistant Professor
George Mason University
Fairfax, Virginia

Dorothy Lee, PhD, RN, ANP-BC
Associate Professor of Nursing
Saginaw Valley State University
University Center, Michigan

Toby Ann Nishikawa, MSN, RN
Assistant Professor
Weber State University
Ogden, Utah

Dr. Diana Rangaves, PharmD, RPh
Director, Pharmacy Technology Program
Santa Rosa Junior College
Santa Rosa, California

Timothy Reilly, PharmD, BCPS, CGP, FASCP
Clinical Assistant Professor
Rutgers University
Piscataway, New Jersey

Janet Czermak Russell, MS, MA, APN-BC
Associate Professor
Essex County College
Newark, New Jersey

Pooja Shah, PharmD
Clinical Assistant Professor
Rutgers University
Piscataway, New Jersey

Samantha Smeltzer, RN
Professor of Nursing
Mount Aloysius College
Cresson, Pennsylvania

Rose Marie Smith, RN, MS, CNE
Division Dean of Nursing, Liberal Arts, Social and Behavioral Sciences
Redlands Community College
El Reno, Oklahoma

Dustin Spencer, DNP, NP-C, ENP-BC
Assistant Professor of Nursing
Saginaw Valley State University
University Center, Michigan

Dr. Jacqueline Stewart, DNP, CEN, CCRN
Associate Professor of Nursing
Wilkes University
Wilkes-Barre, Pennsylvania

Rebecca E. Sutter, DNP, APRN, BC-FNP
Assistant Professor
George Mason University
Fairfax, Virginia

Suzanne Tang, MSN, APRN, FNP-BC
Instructor
Rio Hondo College
Whittier, California

Ryan Wargo, PharmD, BCACP
Assistant Professor of Pharmacy Practice
Director of Admissions
LECOM School of Pharmacy
Bradenton, Florida

Timothy Voytilla, MSN, ARNP
Nursing Program Director
Keiser University
Tampa, Florida

Preface

When students are asked which subject in their nursing program is the most challenging, pharmacology always appears near the top of the list. The study of pharmacology demands that students apply knowledge from a wide variety of the natural and applied sciences. Successfully predicting drug action requires a thorough knowledge of anatomy, physiology, chemistry, and pathology as well as the social sciences of psychology and sociology. Lack of adequate pharmacology knowledge can result in immediate and direct harm to the patient; thus, the stakes in learning the subject are high.

Pharmacology cannot be made easy, but it can be made understandable if the proper connections are made to knowledge learned in these other disciplines. The vast majority of drugs in clinical practice are prescribed for specific diseases, yet many pharmacology textbooks fail to recognize the complex interrelationships between pharmacology and pathophysiology. When drugs are learned in isolation from their associated diseases or conditions, students have difficulty connecting pharmacotherapy to therapeutic goals and patient wellness. The pathophysiology focus of this textbook gives the student a clearer picture of the importance of pharmacology to disease and, ultimately, to patient care. The approach and rationale of this textbook focus on a holistic perspective to patient care which clearly shows the benefits and limitations of pharmacotherapy in curing or preventing illness. In addition to its pathophysiology focus, medication safety and interdisciplinary teamwork are consistently emphasized throughout the text. Although difficult and challenging, the study of pharmacology is truly a fascinating, lifelong journey.

New to This Edition

The fifth edition of *Pharmacology for Nurses: A Pathophysiologic Approach* has been thoroughly updated to reflect current pharmacotherapeutics and advances in understanding disease.

- **NEW!** Incorporation of the QSEN competencies: The QSEN competencies related to patient-centered care, teamwork and collaboration, evidence-based practice, and patient safety are incorporated throughout the features and Nursing Practice Application charts.
- **NEW!** Chapter added on Individual Variations in Drug Response that focuses on specific factors that can influence pharmacotherapeutic outcomes.
- **NEW!** Check Your Understanding questions appear throughout the drug chapters to reinforce student knowledge.
- **NEW!** Community-Oriented Practice feature provides important information that nurses need to convey to their patients to ensure that they receive effective pharmacotherapy after leaving the hospital or clinical setting.
- **NEW!** Patient-Focused Case Study
- **EXPANDED!** The chapter on autonomic drugs has been split into two chapters to reflect increased used of these drug classes in pharmacotherapeutics.
- **EXPANDED!** Includes more than 40 new drugs, drug classes, indications, and therapies that have been approved since the last edition.
- **UPDATED!** Black Box Warnings issued by the FDA are included for all appropriate drug prototypes.
- **EXPANDED!** Pharmacotherapy Illustrated diagrams help students visualize the connection between pharmacology and the patient.
- **UPDATED!** Nursing Practice Application charts have been revised to contain current applications to clinical practice with key life span and diversity considerations noted.
- **UPDATED!** End-of-chapter NCLEX-RN®-style questions now include alternative format items and complete rationales in the answers.

Organization and Structure—A Body System and Disease Approach

Pharmacology for Nurses: A Pathophysiologic Approach is organized according to body systems (units) and diseases (chapters). Each chapter provides the complete information on the drug classifications used to treat the diseases. Specially designed numbered headings describe key concepts and cue students to each drug classification discussion.

The pathophysiologic approach clearly places the drugs in context with how they are used therapeutically. The student is able to locate easily all relevant anatomy, physiology, pathology, and pharmacology in the same chapter in which the drugs are discussed. This approach provides the student with a clear view of the connection among pharmacology, pathophysiology, and the nursing care learned in other clinical courses.

The vast number of drugs available in clinical practice is staggering. To facilitate learning, this text uses drug prototypes in which the most representative drugs in each classification are introduced in detail. Students are less intimidated when they can focus their learning on one representative drug in each class.

This text uses several strategies to connect pharmacology to nursing practice. Throughout the text the student will find interesting features such as Complementary and Alternative Therapies, Treating the Diverse Patient, Community-Oriented Practice, and Lifespan Considerations that clearly place the drugs in context with their clinical applications. Evidence-Based Practice features illustrate how current medical research is used to improve patient teaching. Patient Safety illustrates potential pitfalls that can lead to medication errors. PharmFacts contain statistics and facts that are relevant to the chapter.

Prototype Drug | Physostigmine *(Antilirium)*

Therapeutic Class: Antidote for anticholinergic toxicity **Pharmacologic Class:** Acetylcholinesterase inhibitor

Actions and Uses

Physostigmine is an indirect-acting parasympathomimetic that inhibits the destruction of Ach by AchE. Its effects occur at the neuromuscular junction and at central and peripheral locations where Ach is the neurotransmitter. It reverses toxic and life-threatening delirium caused by atropine, diphenhydramine, dimenhydrinate, *Atropa belladonna* (deadly nightshade), or jimson weed. Physostigmine is usually administered as an injectable solution, IM or IV, although it is not intended as a first-line agent for anticholinergic toxicity or Parkinson's disease.

Administration Alerts

- Administer slowly over 5 minutes to avoid seizures and respiratory distress.
- Continuous infusions should never be used.
- Monitor blood pressure, pulse, and respirations, and look for hypersalivation.
- Pregnancy category C.

PHARMACOKINETICS

Onset	Peak	Duration
Less than 5 min IM/IV	20–40 min IM/IV	1–2 h IM/IV

Adverse Effects

Unfavorable effects of physostigmine are bradycardia, asystole, restlessness, nervousness, seizures, salivation, urinary frequency, muscle twitching, and respiratory paralysis.

Contraindications: Use with caution in patients with asthma, epilepsy, diabetes, cardiovascular disease, or bradycardia. Discontinue if excessive sweating, diarrhea, or frequent urination occurs. Physostigmine is not recommended in patients with known or suspected tricyclic antidepressant (TCA) intoxication.

Interactions

Drug–Drug: Drug interactions with physostigmine include increased effects from cholinergic agents and beta blockers. The levels of physostigmine may be increased by systemic corticosteroids. Physostigmine may decrease effects of neuromuscular-blocking agents.

Lab Tests: Physostigmine may cause an increase in serum alanine aminotransferase (ALT), AST, and amylase.

Herbal/Food: Toxic effects caused by physostigmine may be enhanced by ginkgo biloba.

Treatment of Overdose: Due to the possibility of hypersensitivity or cholinergic crisis, atropine should be available.

Complementary and Alternative Therapies

MELATONIN

Melatonin is a natural hormone produced during the night by the pineal gland. The secretion of melatonin is stimulated by darkness and inhibited by light. As melatonin production rises, alertness decreases and body temperature starts to fall, both of which make sleep more inviting. Melatonin production is related to age. Children manufacture more melatonin than older adults; however, melatonin production begins to drop at puberty.

Melatonin appears to help people, particularly older adults, to fall asleep faster. The National Center for Complementary and Integrative Health (NCCIH, 2014) cites evidence that melatonin also appears to be useful in people with insomnia related to disrupted circadian rhythm cycles. It is believed that melatonin helps to reset the circadian rhythm for these patients, rather than cause drowsiness. Melatonin appears to be safe for short-term use but it is not free of side effects. It may cause nausea, headache, or dizziness, and has been noted to adversely affect mood in patients with dementia (NCCIH, 2014).

Check Your Understanding 11.1

True or False? The most dangerous infectious diseases in the world are those potentially used as weapons of bioterrorism. Explain your answer. *Visit www.pearsonhighered.com/nursingresources for the answer.*

Treating the Diverse Patient: Medication Refusal for Religious or Spiritual Reasons

One of the rights of medication administration is refusal. Patients have the right to refuse their medications for religious or spiritually-related reasons. Perhaps most familiar is a refusal to accept blood or blood products by a Jehovah's Witness member because of religious beliefs. Less familiar is refusal due to the fact that the medication contains animal-derived products.

Erickson, Burcharth, and Rosenburg (2013) explored potential acceptance or refusal of animal-derived products such as porcine (pork) and bovine (beef) surgical products by members of various religious faiths, including Christian, Judaism, Buddhism, Hindu, Islam, and Sikhism. In their study, they discovered that while all tradition, beef, pork, chicken, fish, shellfish, or all meats may be refused on religious or moral grounds. They recommended that when possible, a compounding laboratory b[...] making a comparable product for the patie[...] tain the offending ingredient. That option sh[...] ternative formulations are not available for u[...] animal-derived drug such as heparin, the pr[...] the medication with the patient and explore [...]

It is important that nurses consider the [...] spiritual beliefs about medications. Patients [...] time to work through their decisions on spiri[...] [...]nsult their religious adv[...] [...]orating with and encou[...] [...]s or spiritual leader whe[...] [...]or medical product, and [...] [...]s or spiritual beliefs and [...] [...]ntain a holistic focus in m[...]

Community-Oriented Practice

DECREASING DRUG ERRORS BY FOCUSING ON HEALTH LITERACY

Limited health literacy may have profound effects on how well a patient follows instructions for medication administration. For some patients, having a clear understanding of how to take their medications is further hampered when a language other than English is spoken. Samuels-Kalow, Stack, & Porter (2013) found that overall, 30% of all patients demonstrated a medication error with acetaminophen after receiving instructions upon discharge from an emergency department, but 50% of Spanish-speaking patients had a dosing error. Even with the use of a Spanish-speaking translator, errors occurred.

Health literacy encompasses more than understanding which drugs to take and how to take them, and limited health literacy occurs across all populations in society, regardless of one's native language. Because the majority of medications are taken in a setting other than a health-care facility, to decrease errors in the patient's home or community setting, it is vital that the patient has an adequate understanding of medication administration.

The nurse can work to improve a patient's health literacy about medication administration and decrease the possibility of errors by ensuring a variety of methods are used to educate the patient. These include using printed materials that use "plain language" wording such as "take one pill in the morning and one at bedtime," rather than "take one tablet, twice a day" (Bailey, Sarkar, Chen, Schillinger, & Wolf, 2012; Smith & Wallace, 2013); using written materials that incorporate simple graphics that reinforce the material; and reviewing the material verbally with the patient (Samuels-Kalow et al., 2013) before discharging the patient from the health care setting. Because it is the nurse who most often provides patient education, understanding and addressing the effects that limited health literacy may have on their patients' safe and effective medication administration is crucial for all nurses.

Lifespan Considerations: Pediatric

The Challenges of Pediatric Drug Administration

Administering medication to infants and young children requires special knowledge and techniques. Nurses must have knowledge of growth and development patterns. When possible, the child should be given a choice regarding the use of a spoon, dropper, or syringe. A matter-of-fact attitude should be presented in giving a child medications; using threats or dishonesty is unacceptable and professionally unethical. Oral medications that must be crushed for the child to swallow can be mixed with flavored syrup, jelly, or the child's choice of food to avoid unpleasan[...] necessary [...] an unpleas[...] consume t[...] tions can b[...] ated bever[...]

Evidence-Based Practice: Informed Consent Procedures

Clinical Question: How can nurses assist in the informed consent procedures for patients considering participation in a clinical drug research trial?

Evidence: At some point in their career, the nurse may care for a patient who is enrolled in, or considering participation in, a clinical drug research trial. The publication of the Belmont Report (HHS, 1979) provided guidance and principles for obtaining informed consent from patients enrolled in clinical trials. The FDA has guidelines that include how informed consent is to be obtained from children and illiterate adults (FDA, 2014). Although providing information about the research trial is beyond the scope of nursing practice and the responsibility of the researcher and health care provider, nurses can participate by helping to ensure that any questions or concerns the patient has regarding participation are addressed before signing the informed consent document. Special populations require careful assessment of the patient's ability to understand or make informed decisions about research participation. These populations may include children, patients with cognitive or mental impairments, and patients with sensory or language barriers. Other circumstances which may make obtaining informed consent for research participation more difficult include situations in which the p[...] may be critically ill or suffering from a traumatic injury. These[...] delay obtaining consent directly from the patient and result i[...] patient's exclusion from the clinical trial. Differences in cultural b[...] ground and beliefs about what is appropriate for a patient to [...] may run counter to the established guidelines that informed co[...] must provide the patient with the information necessary to ma[...] informed decision to participate.

Nursing Implications: Ensuring that a patient, family, or guardian has the information necessary to make informed [...] sions is a potential role for the nurse when caring for patients [...] sidering or participating in a clinical research trial. Whereas pr[...] ing the information is beyond the scope of most nursing prac[...] the patient will often ask questions of the nurse, and the [...] can relay these questions to the health care provider. This i[...] pecially important when working with patients or families wh[...] have special needs, such as language or cultural differences, [...] emergency situations, in which the patient is not able to re[...] the information and a family member or legal guardian must [...] the decision.

PharmFacts

PATIENTS WITH DEPRESSIVE SYMPTOMS

- Major depression, bipolar disorder, and situational depression are common mental health challenges worldwide.
- Clinical depression affects more than 19 million Americans each year. The strongest risk factor for suicide is depression.
- For young people 15–24 years old, suicide is the second leading cause of death in the United States.
- Fewer than half of the people who suffer from depression seek medical treatment. 80% of people who seek treatment for depression are treated successfully.
- Most patients consider depression a weakness rather than an illness.
- There are no common age, sex, or ethnic factors related to depression—it can happen to anyone.

Pharmacotherapy Illustrated

4.1 | First-Pass Effect: Oral Drug Is Metabolized to an Inactive Form Before It Has an Opportunity to Reach Target Cells

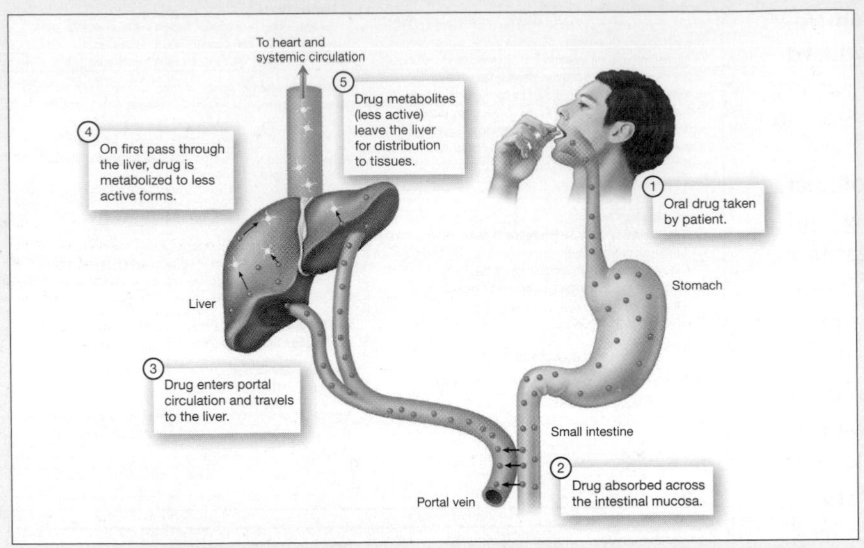

Source: Based on *Pharmacology: Connections to Nursing Practice* (3rd Ed.), by M. Adams and C. Urban, 2016. Reprinted and electronically reproduced by permission of Pearson Education, Inc., Upper Saddle River, New Jersey.

Students learn better when supplied with accurate, attractive graphics and rich media resources. *Pharmacology for Nurses: A Pathophysiologic Approach* contains a generous number of figures, with an unequaled art program. Pharmacotherapy Illustrated features appear throughout the text, breaking down complex topics into easily understood formats. Animations of drug mechanisms show the student step-by-step how drugs act.

One of the strongest components of *Pharmacology for Nurses: A Pathophysiologic Approach* is the Nursing Process Application feature. This feature clearly and concisely relates pharmacotherapy to patient assessment, nursing diagnoses, planning patient outcomes, implementing patient-centered care, and evaluating the outcomes. Student feedback has shown that these Nursing Process Application charts are a significant component of planning and implementing nursing care plans.

Nursing Practice Application

Pharmacotherapy With Adrenergic Drugs

ASSESSMENT	POTENTIAL NURSING DIAGNOSES*
Baseline assessment prior to administration: • Obtain a complete health history including cardiovascular, cerebrovascular, respiratory disease, or diabetes. Obtain a drug history including allergies, current prescription and over-the-counter (OTC) drugs, and herbal preparations. Be alert to possible drug interactions. • Evaluate appropriate laboratory findings such as hepatic or renal function studies. • Obtain baseline vital signs, weight, and urinary and cardiac output as appropriate. • Assess the nasal mucosa for excoriation or bleeding prior to beginning therapy for nasal congestion. • Assess the patient's ability to receive and understand instruction. Include the family and caregivers as needed.	• *Decreased Cardiac Output* • *Ineffective Tissue Perfusion* • *Impaired Gas Exchange* • *Ineffective Airway Clearance* • *Deficient Knowledge* (drug therapy) • *Risk for Injury,* related to adverse effects of drug therapy or administration • *Risk for Disturbed Sleep Pattern,* related to adverse effects of drug therapy
Assessment throughout administration: • Assess for desired therapeutic effects dependent on the reason for the drug (e.g., increased ease of breathing, blood pressure (BP) within normal range, nasal congestion improved). • Continue frequent and careful monitoring of vital signs and urinary and cardiac output as appropriate, especially if IV administration is used. • Assess for and promptly report adverse effects: tachycardia, hypertension, dysrhythmias, tremors, dizziness, headache, and decreased urinary output. Immediately report severe hypertension, seizures, and angina which may signal drug toxicity.	

IMPLEMENTATION	
Interventions and (Rationales)	**Patient-Centered Care**
Ensuring therapeutic effects: • Continue frequent assessments for therapeutic effects dependent on the reason the drug therapy is given. (Pulse, BP, and respiratory rate should be within normal limits or within the parameters set by the health care provider. Nasal congestion should be decreased; reddened, irritated sclera should be improved.)	• Teach the patient, family, or caregiver how to monitor the pulse and BP, as appropriate. Ensure the proper use and functioning of any home equipment obtained.
• Provide supportive nursing measures; e.g., proper positioning for dyspnea, shock, etc. (Supportive nursing measures will supplement therapeutic drug effects and optimize the outcome.)	• Teach the patient to report increasing dyspnea despite medication therapy and to not take more than the prescribed dose unless instructed otherwise by the health care provider.
Minimizing adverse effects: • Monitor for signs of excessive autonomic nervous system stimulation and notify the health care provider if the BP or pulse exceeds established parameters. Continue frequent cardiac monitoring (e.g., ECG, cardiac output) and urine output if IV adrenergics are given. (Because adrenergic drugs stimulate the heart rate and raise BP, they must be closely monitored to avoid adverse effects. **Lifespan:** The older adult may be at greater risk due to previously existing cardiovascular disease. **Diverse Patients:** Research suggests African Americans may experience an impaired [diminished] vascular response to isoproterenol, and vital signs should be monitored frequently during administration.)	• Instruct the patient to report palpitations, shortness of breath, chest pain, excessive nervousness or tremors, headache, or urinary retention immediately. • Teach the patient to limit or eliminate the use of foods and beverages that contain caffeine because these may cause excessive nervousness, insomnia, and tremors.
• Closely monitor the IV infusion site when using IV adrenergics. All IV adrenergic drips should be given via infusion pump. (Blanching at the IV site is an indicator of extravasation and the IV infusion should be immediately stopped and the provider contacted for further treatment orders. Infusion pumps allow precise dosing of the medication.)	• To allay possible anxiety, teach the patient about the rationale for all equipment used and the need for frequent monitoring.

No pharmacology text is complete unless it contains a method of self-assessment by which students may gauge their progress. *Pharmacology for Nurses: A Pathophysiologic Approach* contains an end-of-chapter review of the major concepts. NCLEX-RN®-style questions, a Patient-Focused Case Study with critical thinking questions, and an additional set of Critical Thinking questions allow students to check their retention of chapter material.

PATIENT-FOCUSED Case Study

Katisha Moore is a 68-year-old who enjoys working in her large rose garden. This morning, she noticed that insects had infested the plants. To avoid further damage, she powdered the plants with an insecticide. In her rush to finish, she accidentally contaminated herself with the insecticide and kept working for several hours before showering.

Mrs. Moore is brought into the local emergency department (ED) by her husband that afternoon. She has nausea, dizziness, sweating, excessive salivation, weepy eyes, and a runny nose. She reports intermittent twitching of her upper extremities and uncoordinated movement.

Her initial assessment reveals a 64 kg (142 lb) Caucasian female with a past medication history of hypertension diagnosed 5 years ago. She is married and has two adult children. Her vital signs are blood pressure, 158/94 mmHg; heart rate, 58; respiratory rate, 30; and temperature, 37.3°C (99.2°F). Her skin is pale and moist. She exhibits copious lacrimation and rhinorrhea. Both pupils are constricted. Crackles are heard bilaterally in all lung fields on inspiration. Since admission to the ED she has vomited twice and had one large diarrhea stool.

She is diagnosed with acute organophosphate poisoning. Mrs. Moore is started on oxygen therapy, and the nurse will observe her closely for further respiratory distress. Atropine 2 mg is administered IV every 15 minutes over the next hour.

1. What is the mechanism of action associated with atropine.
2. Why is this drug being given to Mrs. Moore?
3. What adverse effects should you expect for the patient from the administration of atropine?

REVIEW Questions

1. The nurse recognizes which of the following to be initial symptoms of inhaled anthrax? (Select all that apply.)
   1. Cramping and diarrhea
   2. Skin lesions that develop into black scabs
   3. Fever
   4. Headache
   5. Cough and dyspnea
2. Potassium iodine (KI) taken immediately following a nuclear incident can prevent 100% of radioactive iodine from entering which body organ?
   1. Brain
   2. Thyroid
   3. Kidney
   4. Liver
3. Patients who may have been exposed to nerve agents may be expected to display which of these symptoms?
   1. Convulsions and loss of consciousness
   2. Memory loss and fatigue
   3. Malaise and hemorrhaging
   4. Fever and headaches
4. Which of these medications is primarily used as a treatment of anthrax?
   1. Diphtheria vaccine
   2. Amoxicillin (Amoxil)
   3. Ciprofloxacin (Cipro)
   4. Smallpox vaccine
5. How does the Centers for Disease Control and Prevention categorize biologic threats?
   1. Based on their potential adverse effects
   2. Based on the potential impact on public health
   3. Based on their potential cost of treatment
   4. Based on the potential loss of life
6. What key roles does the nurse play in the event of a potential bioterrorist attack? (Select all that apply.)
   1. Helping to plan for emergencies and develop emergency management plans
   2. Recognizing and reporting signs and symptoms of chemical or biologic agent exposure and assisting with treatment
   3. Storing antidotes, antibiotics, vaccines, and supplies in their homes
   4. Keeping a list of resources such as health and law enforcement agencies and other contacts who would assist in the event of a bioterrorist attack
   5. Keeping up to date on emergency management protocols and volunteering to become members of a first-response team

CRITICAL THINKING Questions

1. Why would the medical community be opposed to the mass vaccination of the general public for potential bioterrorist threats such as anthrax and smallpox?
2. What is the purpose of the Strategic National Stockpile (SNS)? What is the difference between a push package and a vendor-managed inventory (VMI) package? How might the nurse be called to assist with these supplies?
3. Why do nurses play such a central role in emergency preparedness and treatment of poisonings?

Visit www.pearsonhighered.com/nursingresources for answers and rationales for all activities.

Acknowledgments

When authoring a textbook like this, many dedicated and talented professionals are needed to bring the vision to reality. Pamela Fuller, Executive Acquisitions Editor, and Erin Rafferty, Program Manager, are responsible for guiding the many details in the development and production of the fifth edition. Our Development Editor, Teri Zak, provided leadership, motivation, and expert guidance to keep everyone on track and on schedule. Her steadfast attention to detail and editorial expertise enabled an excellent outcome for this edition.

The superb design staff at Pearson, especially Maria Guglielmo Walsh and Beth Paquin, created wonderful text and cover designs. The content management and production process was guided by Project Manager Cathy O'Connell. Mary Tindle and her colleagues at Cenveo provided expert, professional guidance in all aspects of the art and production process.

Although difficult and challenging, the study of pharmacology is truly a fascinating lifelong journey. We hope we have succeeded in writing a textbook that makes that study easier and more understandable so that nursing students will be able to provide safe, effective nursing care to patients who are undergoing drug therapy. We hope students and faculty will share with us their experiences using this textbook and all its resources.

Contents

Unit 1

Core Concepts in Pharmacology

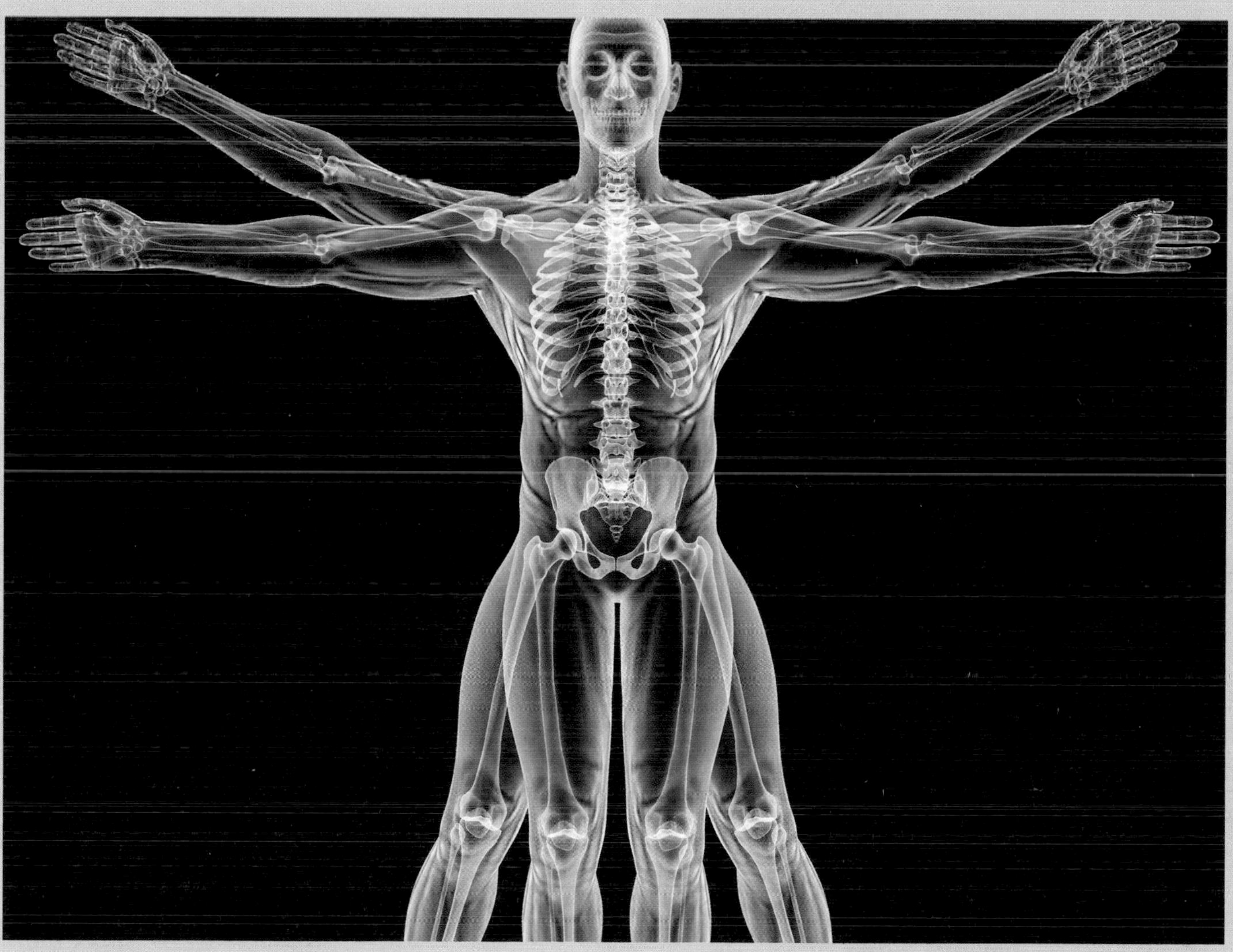

Core Concepts in Pharmacology

Chapter 1

Introduction to Pharmacology

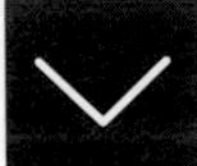

Learning Outcomes

After reading this chapter, the student should be able to:

1. Identify key events in the history of pharmacology.
2. Explain the interdisciplinary nature of pharmacology, giving an example of how knowledge from different sciences impacts the nurse's role in drug administration.
3. Compare and contrast therapeutics and pharmacology.
4. Compare and contrast traditional drugs, biologics, and complementary and alternative medicine therapies.
5. Explain the basis for placing drugs into therapeutic and pharmacologic classes.
6. Discuss the prototype approach to drug classification.
7. Describe what is meant by a drug's mechanism of action.
8. Distinguish among a drug's chemical name, generic name, and trade name.
9. Outline the major differences between prescription and over-the-counter drugs.
10. Explain the differences between trade-name drugs and their generic equivalents.
11. Describe how decisions are made relative to drug therapy among groups of patients.

When students are introduced to the topic of pharmacology, they are immediately confronted with new drug concepts and the various ways that drugs are identified. There are hundreds of drugs having specific dosages, side effects, and mechanisms of action. To prevent errors when administering drugs, the nurse must constantly check and cross-check trade names, generic equivalents, correct name spelling, adverse drug reactions, warnings, contraindications, and other important facts. Without a means of organizing this information, most students would be overwhelmed by the vast amounts of data. This chapter serves as a starting point for connecting introductory pharmacologic concepts to nursing practice. It discusses the methods for organizing drugs: by therapeutic or pharmacologic classification, by dispensing methods (prescription or over-the-counter), and whether dispensing trade name drugs or generic equivalents should be preferred. This chapter also introduces drug therapy for larger patient groups.

1.1 History of Pharmacology

The story of pharmacology is rich and exciting, filled with accidental discoveries and landmark events. Its history likely began when humans first used plants to relieve symptoms of disease. One of the oldest forms of health care, herbal medicine has been practiced in virtually every culture dating to antiquity. The Babylonians recorded the earliest surviving "prescriptions" on clay tablets in 3000 B.C. At about the same time, the Chinese recorded the *Pen Tsao* (Great Herbal), a 40-volume compendium of plant remedies dating to 2700 B.C. The Egyptians followed in 1500 B.C. by archiving their remedies on a document known as the *Eber's Papyrus*.

Little is known about pharmacology during the Dark Ages. Although it is likely that herbal medicine continued to be practiced, few historical events related to this topic were recorded. Pharmacology, and indeed medicine, could not advance until the discipline of science was eventually viewed as legitimate by the religious doctrines of the era.

The first recorded reference to the word *pharmacology* was found in a text entitled "Pharmacologia sen Manuductio and Materiam Medicum," by Samuel Dale, in 1693. Before this date, the study of herbal remedies was called "Materia Medica," a term that persisted into the early 20th century.

Modern pharmacology is thought to have begun in the early 1800s. At that time, chemists were making remarkable progress in isolating specific substances from complex mixtures. This enabled scientists to isolate the active drugs morphine, colchicine, curare, cocaine, and other early pharmacologic agents from their natural sources. Using standardized amounts, pharmacologists could then study drug effects in animals more precisely. Indeed, some of the early researchers used themselves as test subjects. Friedrich Serturner, who first isolated morphine from opium in 1805, injected himself and three friends with a huge dose (100 mg) of his new product. He and his colleagues suffered acute morphine intoxication for several days afterward.

Pharmacology as a distinct discipline was officially recognized when the first department of pharmacology was established in Estonia in 1847. John Jacob Abel, who is considered the father of American pharmacology owing to his many contributions to the field, founded the first pharmacology department in the United States at the University of Michigan in 1890.

In the 20th century, the pace of change in all areas of medicine continued exponentially. Pharmacologists no longer needed to rely on the slow, laborious process of isolating active agents from scarce natural sources; they could synthesize drugs in the laboratory. Hundreds of new drugs could be synthesized and tested in a relatively short time. More importantly, it became possible to understand how drugs produced their effects, down to their molecular mechanism of action.

The current practice of pharmacology is extremely complex and far advanced compared with its early, primitive history. The nurse who consults with a pharmacist in the use of pharmacologic substances and other health professionals who practice it must never forget its early roots: the application of products to relieve human suffering. Whether a substance is extracted from the Pacific yew tree, isolated from a fungus, or created totally in a laboratory, the central purpose of pharmacology is to focus on the patient and to improve the quality of life.

1.2 Pharmacology: The Study of Medicines

The word **pharmacology** is derived from two Greek words: *pharmakon,* which means "medicine," and *logos,* which means "study." Thus, pharmacology is most simply defined as the study of medicine. Pharmacology is an expansive subject ranging from understanding how drugs are administered, to where they travel in the body, to the actual responses produced. To learn the discipline well, nursing students must acquire a broad knowledge base from various foundation areas such as anatomy and physiology, chemistry, microbiology, and pathophysiology.

As an example, aminoglycosides are a class of antibiotics that are useful in the treatment of many infectious diseases. The mainstay of treatment for infective endocarditis is antibiotic therapy, and this is instituted as soon as possible to minimize valvular damage. Caution must be used, however, because some aminoglycosides can cause inner ear toxicity and neuromuscular impairment, especially if furosemide (a loop diuretic) is administered at the same time. You can see how, in this case, concepts from multiple science disciplines are integrated. Knowledge of chemistry would be inferred by the terms *amino* and *glyco*. Further study about "infectives" would draw information from the subject of microbiology including the use of antibiotics and sensitivities of gram-positive and gram-negative bacteria. The fields of anatomy and physiology would correlate much information with emphasis on ear anatomy and organs of the muscular, nervous, renal, and cardiovascular systems. "Endocarditis" would be the central pathophysiological focus of treatment. Most of the time pharmacology incorporates knowledge from multiple areas, which health care providers must use in making decisions about drug administration.

More than 10,000 trade-name drugs, generic drugs, and combination drugs are currently available. Each has its own characteristic set of therapeutic applications, interactions, adverse effects, and mechanisms of action. Many drugs are prescribed for more than one disease, and most produce multiple effects within the body. Drugs may elicit different responses depending on individual patient factors such as age, sex, body mass, health status, and genetics. Drug effects may be enhanced or reduced by combined factors. For example, patients with liver or renal impairment may experience enhanced responses due to reduced clearance of drugs from the body. Indeed, learning the applications of existing medications and staying current with new drugs introduced every year are among the formidable but necessary tasks for the nurse. These challenges are critical for both the patient and the health care practitioner. If applied properly, drugs can dramatically improve the quality of life. If administered improperly, drugs can produce devastating consequences.

1.3 Pharmacology and Therapeutics

It is obvious that a thorough study of pharmacology is important to health care providers who prescribe drugs on a daily basis. The nurse is often the health care provider most directly involved with patient care and is active in educating, managing, and monitoring the proper use of drugs. This applies not only to nurses in clinics, hospitals, and home health care settings but also to nurses who teach and to students entering the nursing profession. In all these cases, it is necessary that individuals have a thorough knowledge of pharmacology to perform their duties. As nursing students progress toward their chosen specialty, pharmacology is at the core of patient care and is integrated into every step of the nursing process. Learning pharmacology is a gradual, continuous process that does not end with graduation. One never completely masters every facet of drug action and application. This is one of the motivating challenges of the nursing profession.

Another important area of focus for the nurse, sometimes challenging to distinguish from pharmacology, is therapeutics. Therapeutics is slightly different from pharmacology, although the areas are closely connected. **Therapeutics** is concerned with the prevention of disease and treatment of suffering. **Pharmacotherapy,** or *pharmacotherapeutics,* is the application of drugs for the purpose of treating diseases and alleviating human suffering. Drugs are just one of many tools available to the nurse for these purposes.

1.4 Classification of Therapeutic Agents as Drugs, Biologics, and Complementary and Alternative Medicine Therapies

Substances applied for therapeutic purposes fall into one of the following three general categories:

- Drugs or medications
- Biologics
- Complementary and alternative medicine therapies.

A **drug** is a chemical agent capable of producing biologic responses within the body. These responses may be desirable (therapeutic) or undesirable (adverse). After a drug is administered, it is called a **medication.** Drugs and medications may be considered a part of the body's normal activities, from the essential gases that we breathe to the foods that we eat. Because drugs are defined so broadly, it is necessary to clearly distinguish them from other substances such as foods, household products, and cosmetics. Many agents such as antiperspirants, sunscreens, toothpaste, and shampoos may alter the body's normal activities, but they are not necessarily considered medically therapeutic, as are drugs.

Although most modern drugs are synthesized in a laboratory, **biologics** are agents naturally produced in animal cells, by microorganisms, or by the body itself. Examples of biologics include hormones, monoclonal antibodies, natural blood products and components, interferons, and vaccines. Biologics are used to treat a wide variety of illnesses and conditions.

Other therapeutic approaches include **complementary and alternative medicine (CAM) therapies.** These involve natural plant extracts, herbs, vitamins, minerals, dietary supplements, and additional techniques outside of the realm of conventional therapeutics. Such therapies include body-based practices such as physical therapy, manipulations, massage, acupuncture, hypnosis, and biofeedback. Because of their great popularity, herbal and alternative therapies are featured throughout this text wherever they show promise in treating a disease or condition. CAM therapies are presented in chapter 10.

1.5 Therapeutic and Pharmacologic Classification of Drugs

One useful method of organizing drugs is based on their therapeutic usefulness in treating particular diseases or disorders. This is referred to as a **therapeutic classification.** Drugs may also be organized by **pharmacologic classification.** A pharmacologic classification refers to the way a drug works at the molecular, tissue, or body system level. Both types of classification are widely used in categorizing the thousands of available drugs.

Table 1.1 shows the method of therapeutic classification, using cardiac care as an example. Many different types of drugs affect cardiovascular function. Some drugs influence blood clotting, whereas others lower blood cholesterol or prevent the onset of stroke. Drugs may be used to treat elevated blood pressure, heart failure, abnormal rhythm, chest pain, heart attack, or circulatory shock. Thus, drugs that treat cardiac disorders may be placed in several types of therapeutic classes, for example, anticoagulants, antihyperlipidemics, and antihypertensives.

A therapeutic classification need not be complicated. For example, it is appropriate to simply classify a medication as a "drug used for stroke" or a "drug used for shock." The key to therapeutic classification is to clearly state what a particular drug does clinically. Other examples of therapeutic classifications include antidepressants, antipsychotics, drugs for erectile dysfunction, and antineoplastics.

The pharmacologic classification addresses a drug's **mechanism of action**, or how a drug produces its physiological effect in the body. Table 1.2 shows a variety of pharmacologic classifications using hypertension as the therapeutic focus. A diuretic treats hypertension by lowering plasma volume. Calcium channel blockers treat this disorder by decreasing cardiac contractility. Other drugs block intermediates of the renin–angiotensin pathway. Notice that each example describes how hypertension is controlled. A drug's pharmacologic classification is more specific than a therapeutic classification and requires a more in depth understanding of biochemistry and physiology. In addition, pharmacologic classifications may be described with varying degrees of complexity, sometimes taking into account the drugs' chemical names.

Table 1.1 Therapeutic Classification

FOCUS: CARDIOVASCULAR FUNCTION	
Usefulness	**Drug Classification**
Influence blood clotting	Anticoagulant
Lower blood cholesterol	Antihyperlipidemic
Lower blood pressure	Antihypertensive
Restore normal cardiac rhythm	Antidysrhythmic
Treat angina	Antianginal

Table 1.2 Pharmacologic Classification

FOCUSING ON THERAPEUTIC APPLICATION: PHARMACOTHERAPY FOR HYPERTENSION	
Mechanism of Action	**Drug Classification**
Lowers plasma volume	Diuretic
Blocks heart calcium channels	Calcium channel blocker
Blocks hormonal activity	Angiotensin-converting enzyme inhibitor
Blocks physiological reactions to stress	Adrenergic antagonist
Dilates peripheral blood vessels	Vasodilator

When classifying drugs, it is common practice to select a single drug from a class and compare all other medications within this representative group. A **prototype drug** is the well-understood drug model with which other drugs in its representative class are compared. By learning the characteristics of the prototype drug, students may predict the actions and adverse effects of other drugs in the same class. For example, by knowing the effects of penicillin V, students can extend this knowledge to the other drugs in the penicillin class of antibiotics. The original drug prototype is not always the most widely used drug in its class. Newer drugs in the same class may be more effective, have a more favorable safety profile, or have a longer duration of action. These factors may sway health care providers from using the original prototype drug. Becoming familiar with the drug prototypes and keeping up with newer drugs as they are developed is an essential part of mastering drugs and drug classes.

1.6 Chemical, Generic, and Trade Names for Drugs

A major challenge in studying pharmacology is mastering the thousands of drug names. Adding to this difficulty is the fact that most drugs have multiple names. The three basic types of drug names are chemical, generic, and trade names.

A **chemical name** is assigned using standard nomenclature established by the International Union of Pure and Applied Chemistry (IUPAC). A drug has only one chemical name, which is sometimes helpful in predicting a substance's physical and chemical properties. Although chemical names convey a clear and concise meaning about the nature of a drug, they are often complicated and difficult to remember or pronounce. For example, few nurses know the chemical name for diazepam: 7-chloro-1, 3-dihydro-1-methyl-5-phenyl-2H-1,4-benzodiazepin-2-one. In only a few cases, usually when the name is brief and easily remembered, will the nurse use chemical names. Examples of useful chemical names include lithium carbonate, calcium gluconate, and sodium chloride.

More practically, drugs are sometimes classified by a portion of their chemical structure, known as the chemical group name. Examples are antibiotics such as the fluoroquinolones and cephalosporins. Other common examples include the phenothiazines, thiazides, and benzodiazepines. Although chemical group names may seem complicated when first encountered, knowing them will become invaluable as the nursing student begins to understand and communicate major drug actions and adverse side effects.

The **generic name** of a drug is assigned by the U.S. Adopted Name Council. With few exceptions, generic names are less complicated and easier to remember than chemical names. Many organizations, including the U.S. Food and Drug Administration (FDA), the U.S. Pharmacopoeia, and the World Health Organization (WHO), routinely describe a medication by its generic name. Because there is only one generic name for each drug, there is value in using this name and students generally must memorize it.

A drug's **trade name** is assigned by the company marketing the drug. The name is usually short and easy to remember. The trade name is sometimes called the proprietary, product, or brand name. The term *proprietary* suggests ownership. In the United States, a drug developer is given exclusive rights to name and market a drug for 17 years after a New Drug Application is submitted to the FDA (chapter 2). Because it takes several years for a drug to be approved, the amount of time spent in approval is usually subtracted from the 17 years. For example, if it takes 7 years for a drug to be approved, competing companies will not be allowed to market a generic equivalent drug for another 10 years. The rationale is that the developing company is allowed sufficient time to recoup the millions of dollars in research and development costs in designing the new drug. After 17 years, competing companies may sell a generic equivalent drug, sometimes using a different name, which the FDA must approve.

Trade names may be a challenge for students to learn because of the dozens of products containing similar ingredients. A **combination drug** contains more than one active generic ingredient. This poses a problem in trying to match one generic name with one product name. As an example, Table 1.3 lists the drug diphenhydramine (generic name), also called Benadryl (one of the many trade names).

Table 1.3 Examples of Trade-Name Products Containing Popular Generic Substances

Generic Substance	Trade Names
aspirin	Acuprin, Anacin, Aspergum, Bayer, Bufferin, Ecotrin, Empirin, Excedrin, Maprin, Norgesic, Salatin, Salocol, Salsprin, Supac, Talwin, Triaphen-10, Vanquish, Verin, Zorprin
diphenhydramine	Allerdryl, Benadryl, Benahist, Bendylate, Caladryl, Compoz, Diahist, Diphenadril, Eldadryl, Fenylhist, Fynex, Hydramine, Hydril, Insomnal, Noradryl, Nordryl, Nytol, Tusstat, Wehdryl
ibuprofen	Advil, Amersol, Apsifen, Brufen, Haltran, Medipren, Midol 200, Motrin, Neuvil, Novoprofen, Nuprin, Pamprin-IB, Rufen, Trendar

Diphenhydramine is an antihistamine. Low doses of diphenhydramine may be purchased over the counter (OTC); higher doses require a prescription. When looking for diphenhydramine, the nurse may find it listed under many trade names, such as Allerdryl and Compoz, or provided alone or in combination with other active ingredients. Ibuprofen and aspirin are additional drug examples with different trade names. The rule of thumb is that the active ingredients in a drug are described by their generic name. The generic name of a drug is usually lowercase, whereas the trade name is capitalized.

1.7 Prescription and Over-the-Counter Drugs

Many drugs are obtained by prescription or OTC. To obtain prescription drugs, the person must receive a written order from someone with the legal authority to write such a prescription. The advantages to requiring this authorization are numerous. The health care provider or nurse practitioner has an opportunity to examine the patient and determine a specific diagnosis. The provider can maximize therapy by ordering the proper drug for the patient's condition and by conveying the amount and frequency of drug to be dispensed. In addition, the health care provider has an opportunity to teach the patient the proper use of the drug and which adverse effects may occur. In a few instances, a high margin of safety observed over many years can prompt a change in the status of a drug from prescription to OTC.

In contrast to prescription drugs, OTC drugs do not require a health care provider's order. In most cases, patients may treat themselves safely if they carefully follow the instructions included with the medication. If patients do not follow these guidelines, OTC drugs can have serious adverse effects.

Patients prefer to take OTC drugs for many reasons. They are obtained more easily than prescription drugs. No appointment with a health care provider is required, thus saving time and money. Without the assistance of a health care provider, however, choosing the proper drug for a specific problem can be challenging for a patient. OTC drugs may react with foods, herbal products, prescription medications, or other OTC drugs. Patients may not be aware that some OTC drugs can impair their ability to function safely. Self-treatment is sometimes ineffectual, and the potential for harm may increase if the disease is allowed to progress.

1.8 Differences Between Trade-Name Drugs and Their Generic Equivalents

During its 17 years of exclusive rights to a new drug, the pharmaceutical company determines the price of the medication. Because there is no competition, the price is generally quite high. The developing company sometimes uses legal tactics to extend its exclusive rights, since this can mean hundreds of millions of dollars per year in profits for a popular medicine. Once the exclusive rights end, competing companies market the generic drug for less money, and consumer savings may be considerable. In some states, pharmacists may routinely substitute a generic drug when the prescription calls for a trade name. In other states, the pharmacist must dispense drugs directly as written by a health care provider or obtain approval from the provider before providing a generic substitute. Drugs not approved are placed on a closed formulary or a list of drugs that are not covered for reimbursement.

The companies marketing trade-name drugs often lobby aggressively against laws restricting the routine use of their trade-name products. The lobbyists claim significant differences exist between a trade-name drug and its generic equivalent and switching to the generic drug may be harmful for the patient. Patients and consumer advocates, on the other hand, argue that generic substitutions should always be permitted because of the cost savings.

Are there really differences between a trade-name drug and its generic equivalent? The answer is unclear and will depend on the situation. Despite the fact that the dosages may be identical, drug formulations are not always the same. The two drugs may have different inert ingredients. For example, if the drug is in tablet form, the active ingredients may be more tightly compressed in one of the preparations. Public information often focuses on generic drugs having the same active ingredients but different colors, flavors, and certain other filler ingredients. It is the "certain other filler ingredients" where the problem may occur. It is important that generic medications do not work differently from trade-name medications. The FDA provides electronic resources for searching out drug products by active ingredients, trade name, generic equivalents, and the manufacturer. One major source, the *Electronic Orange Book* can be searched online. Since there is a lag time before generic products appear in the *Orange Book*, first-time generic drug approvals can also be searched online at the FDA website.

The key to comparing trade-name drugs and their generic equivalents may lie in measuring the bioavailability of the two preparations. As shown in Figure 1.1, **bioavailability** is the physiological ability of the drug to reach its target cells and produce its effect. Bioavailability may indeed be affected by inert ingredients and tablet compression. Anything that affects absorption of a drug, or its distribution to the target cells, can certainly affect drug action (chapters 4 and 5). Measuring how long a drug takes to exert its effect gives pharmacologists a crude measure of bioavailability. For example, if a patient is in circulatory shock and the generic-equivalent drug takes 5 minutes longer to produce its effect, this is indeed significant; however, if a generic medication for arthritis pain relief takes 45 minutes to act, compared with the trade-name drug, which takes 40 minutes, it probably does not matter which drug is prescribed.

To address issues of bioavailability, some states have compiled a negative formulary. This negative formulary is a list of trade name drugs that pharmacists may not dispense as generic drugs. These drugs must be dispensed exactly as written on the prescription, using the trade-name drug the health care provider prescribed. In some cases, pharmacists must inform or notify patients of substitutions. Pharmaceutical companies and some health care

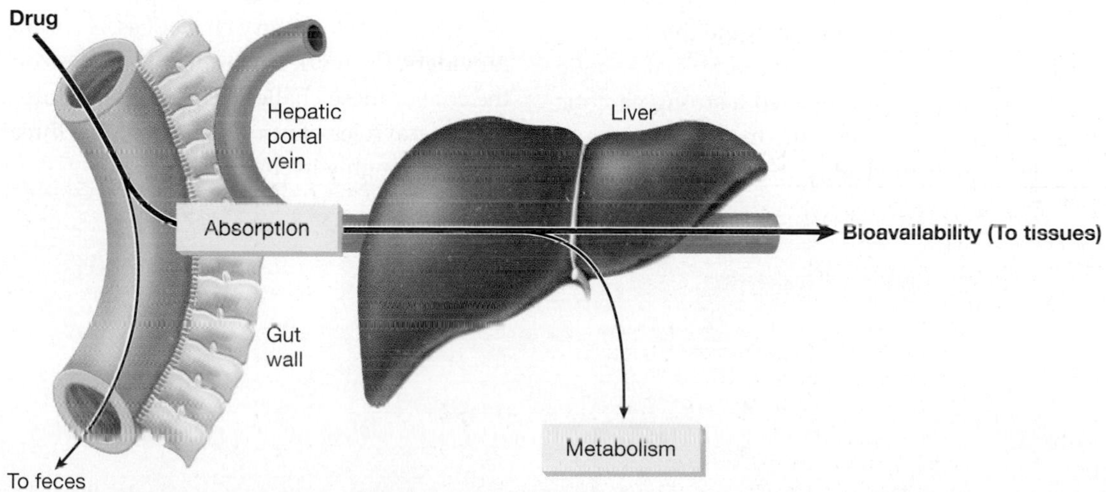

FIGURE 1.1 A drug's bioavailability will depend on the dosage form and how much will actually reach the target location

Patient Safety: Look-Alike Generic Drug Names

A student nurse is preparing medications for the patient. When checking the medication administration record against the drug found in the patient's medication cassette, the student nurse notes that hydroxyzine has been ordered for the patient, but hydralazine has been dispensed from the pharmacy. What should the student nurse do? *Answer to the Patient Safety Question can be found at www.pearsonhighered.com/nursingresources.*

practitioners have supported this action, claiming that generic drugs—even those that have small differences in bioavailability and bioequivalence—could adversely affect patient outcomes in those with critical conditions or illnesses. However, laws frequently change, and in many instances, the efforts of consumer advocacy groups have led to changes in or elimination of negative formulary lists.

1.9 Decisions Relative to Proper Drug Choices

Lawmakers, manufacturers, nurses, and patients along with family members are often placed in the position of making difficult decisions about proper drug choices. **Pharmacoeconomics,** a subdiscipline of health economics has helped in situations involving broader application of a particular type of drug therapy. For example, some groups of patients may benefit from the development of a particular class of drugs. Decisions are often based on costs (resources) and the outcomes considered, not only for patient and family groups but also for the providers, lawmakers and drug manufacturers. When making therapy- or production-related decisions, the following basic outcomes are generally considered: (1) benefit in dollars, (2) effectiveness in health improvement (e.g., variables of improved cardiovascular or nervous system function), (3) minimization in terms of the same benefit provided to other patients in a similar group, and (4) improved utility (both quantitative and qualitative benefits). You might imagine these factors being considered on a focused level, for example, if a single patient were in terrible pain and needed a strong narcotic medication. The nurse might deny the medication due to fear of possible addiction. Today most nurses would probably not be as concerned about administering a potent pain medication if the patient were in acute pain, but this has not always been the case.

More recent concerns involve groups of patients at the state and national levels debating the legalization of marijuana for the treatment of disorders such as epilepsy, amyotrophic lateral sclerosis (ALS; also called "Lou Gehrig's Disease"), multiple sclerosis, glaucoma, acquired immune deficiency syndrome (AIDS), or other select conditions. Marijuana legalization has been a passionate topic due to strong convictions among members of the U.S. population. Residents of Colorado and Washington were among the first to have marijuana approved for recreational use. In 2014, patients in 21 states and the District of Columbia had been given limited approval for marijuana therapy provided they had a doctor's recommendation. Citizens in other states have continued to submit similar requests for legalization of marijuana and these debates are expected to continue.

On a global scale the WHO, U.S. Centers for Disease Control and Prevention (CDC), and the FDA have engaged in a series of public discussions beginning with the outbreak of Ebola in March 2014. This represented the largest and most complex outbreak of the Ebola virus since it was first discovered in West Africa in 1976. The questions of how to contain the virus; how to effectively finance, develop, and distribute vaccines to the public; and how to plan appropriately for continuing drug development have been presented as emerging 21st century challenges. As primary health care providers, the work performed by nurses continues to be at the core of these challenges. Emergency preparedness and the general roles of nurses due to global threats are covered more thoroughly in chapter 11.

Chapter Review

KEY Concepts

The numbered key concepts provide a succinct summary of the important points from the corresponding numbered section within the chapter. If any of these points are not clear, refer to the numbered section within the chapter for review.

1.1 The history of pharmacology began thousands of years ago with the use of plant products to treat disease.

1.2 Pharmacology is the study of medicines. It includes the study of how drugs are administered and how the body responds.

1.3 The fields of pharmacology and therapeutics are closely connected. Pharmacotherapy is the application of drugs to treat disease and ease human suffering.

1.4 Therapeutic agents may be classified as drugs, biologics, or complementary and alternative medicine (CAM) therapies.

1.5 Drugs may be organized by their therapeutic or pharmacologic classification.

1.6 Drugs have chemical, generic, and trade names. A drug has only one chemical or generic name but may have multiple trade names.

1.7 Drugs are available by prescription or over the counter (OTC). Prescription drugs require an order from a health care provider.

1.8 Generic drugs are less expensive than trade-name drugs, but they may differ in their bioavailability which is the ability of the drug to reach its target cell and produce its action.

1.9 Group-based decisions for drug therapy center around cost benefit, effectiveness in health improvement, minimization of benefit to patients within a similar group, and improved quantitative and qualitative utility.

CRITICAL THINKING Questions

1. What is the difference between therapeutic and pharmacologic classifications? Identify the following classifications as therapeutic or pharmacologic: beta-adrenergic blocker, oral contraceptive, laxative, folic acid antagonist, and antianginal drug.
2. What is a prototype drug, and how does it differ from other drugs in the same class?
3. Explain why a patient might seek treatment from an OTC drug instead of a more effective prescription drug.
4. A generic-equivalent drug may be legally substituted for a trade-name medication unless the medication is on a negative formulary or requested by the prescriber or patient. What advantages does this substitution have for the patient? What disadvantages might be caused by the switch?

Visit www.pearsonhighered.com/nursingresources for answers and rationales for all activities.

SELECTED BIBLIOGRAPHY

Ades, A. E., Mavranezouli, I., Dias, S., Welton, N. J., Whittington, C., & Kendall, T. (2010). Network meta-analysis with competing risk outcomes. *Value in Health, 13*, 976–983. doi:10.1111/j.1524-4733.2010.00784.x

Chippaux, J. P. (2014). Outbreaks of Ebola virus disease in Africa: The beginnings of a tragic saga. *Journal of Venomous Animals and Toxins including Tropical Diseases, 20*(1), 44. doi:10.1186/1678-9199-20-44

McCormack J., & Chmelicek, J. T. (2014). Generic versus brand name: The other drug war. *Canadian Family Physician, 60*(10), 911.

McKaig D., Collins C., & Elsaid, K. A. (2014). Impact of a reengineered electronic error-reporting system on medication event reporting and care process improvements at an urban medical center. *Joint Commission Journal on Quality and Patient Safety, 40*, 398–407.

Sitler, B., & Hughes, G. (2014, February). Healthcare analytics: Patient engagement—What can we learn from other industries? *Patient Safety & Quality Healthcare.* Retrieved from http://psqh.com/january-february-2014/healthcare-analytics-patient-engagement-what-can-we-learn-from-other-industries

Sznitman, S. R., & Zolotov, Y. (2015). Cannabis for therapeutic purposes and public health and safety: A systematic and critical review. *International Journal of Drug Policy, 26*, 20–29. doi:10.1016/j.drugpo.2014.09.005

Teunissen R., Bos J., Pot, H., Pluim, M., & Kramers, C. (2013). Clinical relevance of and risk factors associated with medication administration time errors. *American Journal Health System Pharmacy, 70*, 1052–1056. doi:10.2146/ajhp120247

Chapter 2

Drug Approval and Regulation

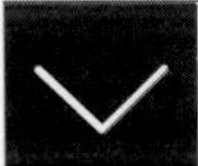

Learning Outcomes

After reading this chapter, the student should be able to:

1. Identify key U.S. drug regulations that have provided guidelines for the safe and effective use of drugs and drug therapy.
2. Discuss the role of the U.S. Food and Drug Administration (FDA) in the drug approval process.
3. Explain the four phases of approval for therapeutic and biologic drugs.
4. Discuss how the FDA has increased the speed with which new drugs reach consumers.
5. Identify the nurse's role in the drug approval process and in maintaining safety practices.
6. Explain the U.S. Controlled Substance Act of 1970 and the role of the U.S. Drug Enforcement Administration in controlling drug abuse and misuse.
7. Discuss why drugs are sometimes placed on a restrictive list, and the controversy surrounding this issue.
8. Explain the meaning of a controlled substance and teratogenic risk in pregnancy.
9. Identify the five drug schedules and give examples of drugs at each level.
10. Identify the five categories of teratogenic drug classification.

More drugs are being administered to patients than ever before. More than 3 billion prescriptions are dispensed each year in the United States. About one half of all Americans take one prescription drug regularly. One out of six persons takes at least three prescription drugs. The potential for harmful drug effects are greater than ever before. Sources of safe drug information are wide and vast, from official pharmacopoeias to compendia such as drug guides, FDA publications, pharmaceutical package inserts, and various types of web- and software-based electronic data. Data are collected through U.S. drug approval processes. Standards, schedules, and teratogenic limitations are published for general regulation purposes and enforcement. This chapter discusses the role of government in ensuring that drugs, herbals, and other natural alternatives are safe and effective for public use.

PharmFacts

CONSUMER SPENDING ON PRESCRIPTION DRUGS AND DRUG DEVELOPMENT

- Consumers in the United States spend over $1,000 per person per year on pharmaceuticals. The average number of prescription drugs taken per patient over the course of a year is about double compared to the mid-1990s.
- In 2013, 21% of adult patients did not fill or skipped prescription doses due to cost.
- Spending on prescription drugs in the U.S. accounts for about 19% of overall health spending in the world. In 2012, prescription drug spending accounted for $260.8 billion.
- Since the turn of the 21st century, the cost of drug invention in the United States has been rising dramatically, while the numbers of drugs developed have been declining.
- The Affordable Care Act of 2010 increased the number of people covered for prescription drugs. Thus, this reform will likely continue to increase the volume of prescription drugs used in the U.S.

2.1 Drug Regulations and Standards

Until the 19th century, there were few standards or guidelines in place to protect the public from drug misuse. The archives of drug regulatory agencies are filled with examples of early medicines, including rattlesnake oil for rheumatism; epilepsy treatment for spasms, hysteria, and alcoholism; and fat reducers for a slender, healthy figure. Many of these early concoctions proved ineffective, though harmless. At their worst, some contained hazardous levels of dangerous or addictive substances. Over time it became clear that drug regulations were needed to protect the public.

The first standard commonly used by pharmacists was the **formulary,** or list of drugs and drug recipes. In the United States, the first comprehensive publication of drug standards, called the *U.S. Pharmacopoeia* (USP), was established in 1820. A **pharmacopoeia** is a medical reference summarizing standards of drug purity, strength, and directions for synthesis. In 1852, a national professional society of pharmacists called the American Pharmaceutical Association (APhA) was founded. From 1852 to 1975, two major compendia maintained drug standards in the United States: the *U.S. Pharmacopoeia,* and the *National Formulary* (NF) established by the APhA. All drug products were covered in the USP; pharmaceutical ingredients were covered in the NF. In 1975, the two entities merged into a single publication, the *U.S. Pharmacopoeia–National Formulary* (USP-NF). Today, USP-NF is a resource of public pharmacopoeia standards provided in print and online. Monographs and general chapters cover public quality standards for drugs, **excipients** (inactive ingredients), and dietary supplements. The USP provides a nationwide database of documented and potential medication errors, as well as their causes. The *U.S. Pharmacopoeia Medication Errors Reporting Program* (USPMERP) provides opportunities for health care professionals to search out and report occurrences related to medication safety. Details of the USPMERP program to maximize medication safety are included in chapter 7. The USP label can be found on many medication vials verifying the purity and exact amounts of ingredients found within the container. Sample labels are illustrated in Figure 2.1.

In order to protect the public in the early 1900s, the United States began to develop and enforce tougher drug legislation. In 1902, the Biologics Control Act helped to

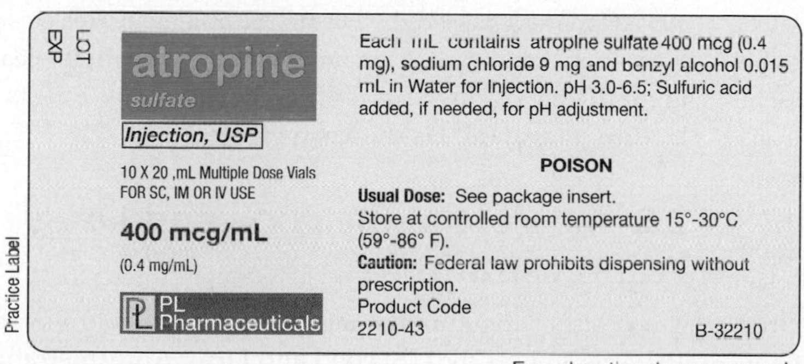

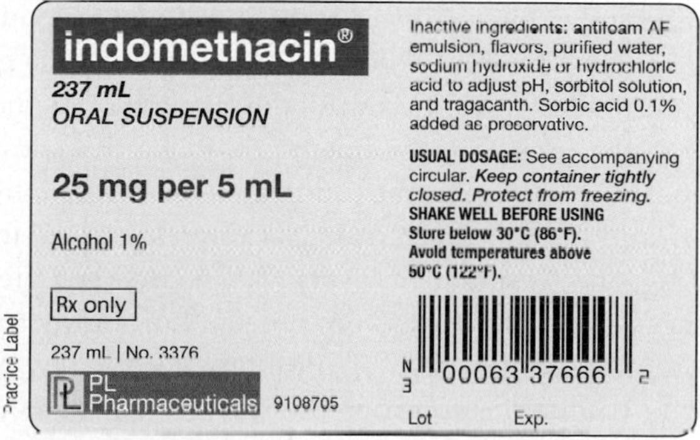

FIGURE 2.1 Medication with the USP label (left) and without USP label (right) Practice Label "for educational purposes only."

TIME LINE	REGULATORY ACTS, STANDARDS, AND ORGANIZATIONS
1820	A group of health care providers established the first comprehensive publication of drug standards called the **U.S. Pharmacopoeia (USP).**
1852	A group of pharmacists founded a national professional society called the **American Pharmaceutical Association (APhA).** The APhA then established the **National Formulary (NF),** a standardized publication focusing on pharmaceutical ingredients. The *USP* continued to catalogue all drug-related substances and products.
1862	This was the beginning of the **Federal Bureau of Chemistry,** established under the administration of President Lincoln. Over the years and with added duties, it gradually became the Food and Drug Administration (FDA).
1902	Congress passed the **Biologics Control Act** to control the quality of serums and other blood-related products.
1906	**The Pure Food and Drug Act** gave the government power to control the labeling of medicines.
1912	**The Sherley Amendment** made medicines safer by prohibiting the sale of drugs labeled with false therapeutic claims.
1938	Congress passed the **Food, Drug, and Cosmetic Act.** It was the first law preventing the marketing of drugs not thoroughly tested. This law now provides for the requirement that drug companies must submit a New Drug Application (NDA) to the FDA prior to marketing a new drug.
1944	Congress passed the **Public Health Service Act,** covering many health issues including biologic products and the control of communicable diseases.
1975	The *U.S. Pharmacopoeia* and *National Formulary* announced their union. The **USP-NF** became a single standardized publication.
1986	Congress passed the **Childhood Vaccine Act.** It authorized the FDA to acquire information about patients taking vaccines, to recall biologics, and to recommend civil penalties if guidelines regarding biologic use were not followed.
1988	The **FDA** was officially established as an agency of the **U.S. Department of Health and Human Services.**
1992	Congress passed the **Prescription Drug User Fee Act.** It required that nongeneric drug and biologic manufacturers pay fees to be used for improvements in the drug review process.
1994	Congress passed the **Dietary Supplement Health and Education Act** that requires clear labeling of dietary supplements. This act gives the FDA the power to remove supplements that cause a significant risk to the public.
1997	The **FDA Drug Modernization Act** reauthorized the Prescription Drug User Fee Act. This act represented the largest reform effort of the drug review process since 1938.
2002	The **Bioterrorism Act** implemented guidelines for registration of selected toxins that could pose a threat to human, animal, or plant safety and health.
2007	The **FDA Amendments Act** reviewed, expanded, and reaffirmed legislation to allow for additional comprehensive reviews of new drugs and medical products. This extended the reforms imposed from 1997. The **FDA's Critical Path Initiative** was a part of this reform.
2011	Provisions of the **Health Care Reform** law allowed the FDA to approve generic versions of biologic drugs. Additional drug rebates and benefits were provided to the American public. The **FDA Food Safety Modernization Act** represents the largest reform effort of food safety review since 1938.

FIGURE 2.2 A historical time line of regulatory acts, standards, and organizations

standardize the quality of serums and other blood-related products. The Pure Food and Drug Act of 1906 gave the government power to control the labeling of medicines. In 1912, the Sherley Amendment prohibited the sale of drugs labeled with false therapeutic claims that were intended to defraud the consumer. In 1938, Congress passed the Food, Drug, and Cosmetic Act. This was the first law preventing the sale of drugs that had not been thoroughly tested before marketing. Later amendments to this law required drug companies to prove the safety and efficacy of any drug before it could be sold within the United States. In reaction to the rising popularity of dietary supplements in 1994, Congress passed the Dietary Supplement Health and Education Act (DSHEA) in an attempt to control misleading industry claims. A brief time line of major events in U.S. drug regulation is shown in Figure 2.2.

2.2 The Role of the Food and Drug Administration

Much has changed in the regulation of drugs in the past 100 years. In 1988, the **U.S. Food and Drug Administration (FDA)** was officially established as an agency of the U.S. Department of Health and Human Services (HHS). The

Center for Drug Evaluation and Research (CDER), a branch of the FDA, exercises control over whether prescription and over-the-counter (OTC) drugs may be used for therapy. The CDER states its mission as facilitating the availability of safe, effective drugs; keeping unsafe or ineffective drugs off the market; improving the health of Americans; and providing clear, easily understandable drug information for safe and effective use (Brunton, Chabner, & Knollman, 2011). Any pharmaceutical laboratory, whether private, public, or academic, must solicit FDA approval before marketing a drug.

In 1997, the FDA created boxed warnings in order to regulate drugs with "special problems." At the time no precedent had been established to monitor drugs with a potential for causing death or serious injury. **Black box warnings,** named after the black box appearing around drug safety information located within package inserts, eventually became one of the primary alerts for identifying extreme adverse drug reactions discovered during and after the review process.

It would be ideal if all of the potential adverse effects were identified before a drug goes to the market. Because this is not realistic, nurses must be increasingly mindful about the standards of care necessary to promote safety, including scanning of medications, medication reconciliation, and special alerts. Black box warnings are included throughout this text for all prototype drugs.

Another branch of the FDA, the Center for Biologics Evaluation and Research (CBER), regulates the use of biologics including serums, vaccines, and blood products. One historical achievement involving biologics was the 1986 Childhood Vaccine Act. This act authorized the FDA to acquire information about patients taking vaccines, to recall biologics, and to recommend civil penalties if guidelines regarding biologics were not followed. In 1996, the Health Insurance Portability and Accountability Act (HIPAA) required health-related organizations and schools to keep private all health information including vaccinations.

The FDA oversees administration of herbal products and dietary supplements through the Center for Food Safety and Applied Nutrition (CFSAN). Herbal products and dietary supplements are regulated by the Dietary Supplement Health and Education Act of 1994. However, this act does not provide the same degree of protection for consumers as the Food, Drug, and Cosmetic Act of 1938. For example, herbal and dietary supplements can be marketed without prior approval from the FDA; however, all package inserts and information are monitored once products have gone to market. The Dietary Supplement Health and Education Act is discussed in more detail in chapter 10.

In 1998, the National Center for Complementary and Alternative Medicine (NCCAM), now called the National Center for Complementary and Integrative Health (NCCIH), was established as the federal government's lead agency for scientific research and information about complementary and alternative medicine (CAM) therapies. Its mission is to define, through rigorous scientific investigation, the usefulness and safety of complementary and integrative health interventions and their roles in improving health and health care. Among several areas of focus, this agency supports research and serves as a resource for nurses in establishing which CAM therapies are safe and effective.

2.3 Phases of Approval for Therapeutic and Biologic Drugs

The amount of time spent by the FDA in the review and approval process for a particular drug depends on several checkpoints along with a well-developed and organized plan. Therapeutic drugs and biologics are reviewed in four phases. Figure 2.3 summarizes these four phases as follows:

1. Preclinical investigation.
2. Clinical investigation.
3. Review of the New Drug Application (NDA).
4. Postmarketing surveillance.

Preclinical investigation involves extensive laboratory research. Scientists perform many tests on human and microbial cells cultured in the laboratory. Studies are performed in several species of animals to examine the drug's effectiveness at different doses and to look for adverse effects. Extensive testing on cultured cells and in animals is essential because it allows the pharmacologist to predict whether the drug will cause harm to humans. Because laboratory tests do not always reflect the way a human responds, preclinical investigation results are always inconclusive. Animal testing may overestimate or underestimate the actual risk to humans.

In January 2007, the FDA restated its concern that a number of innovative and critical medical products had decreased since the 1990s. The **FDA's Critical Path Initiative** was an effort to modernize the sciences to enhance the use of bioinformation to improve the safety, effectiveness, and manufacturability of candidate medical products. Listed areas of improvement were the fields of genomics and proteomics, imaging, and bioinformatics.

Clinical investigation, the second phase of drug testing, takes place in three different stages termed **clinical phase trials.** Clinical phase trials are the longest part of the drug approval process. Clinical pharmacologists first perform tests on volunteers to determine proper dosage and to assess for adverse effects. Large groups of selected patients with the particular disease are then given the medication. Clinical investigators from different medical specialties address concerns such as whether the drug is effective, worsens other medical conditions, interacts

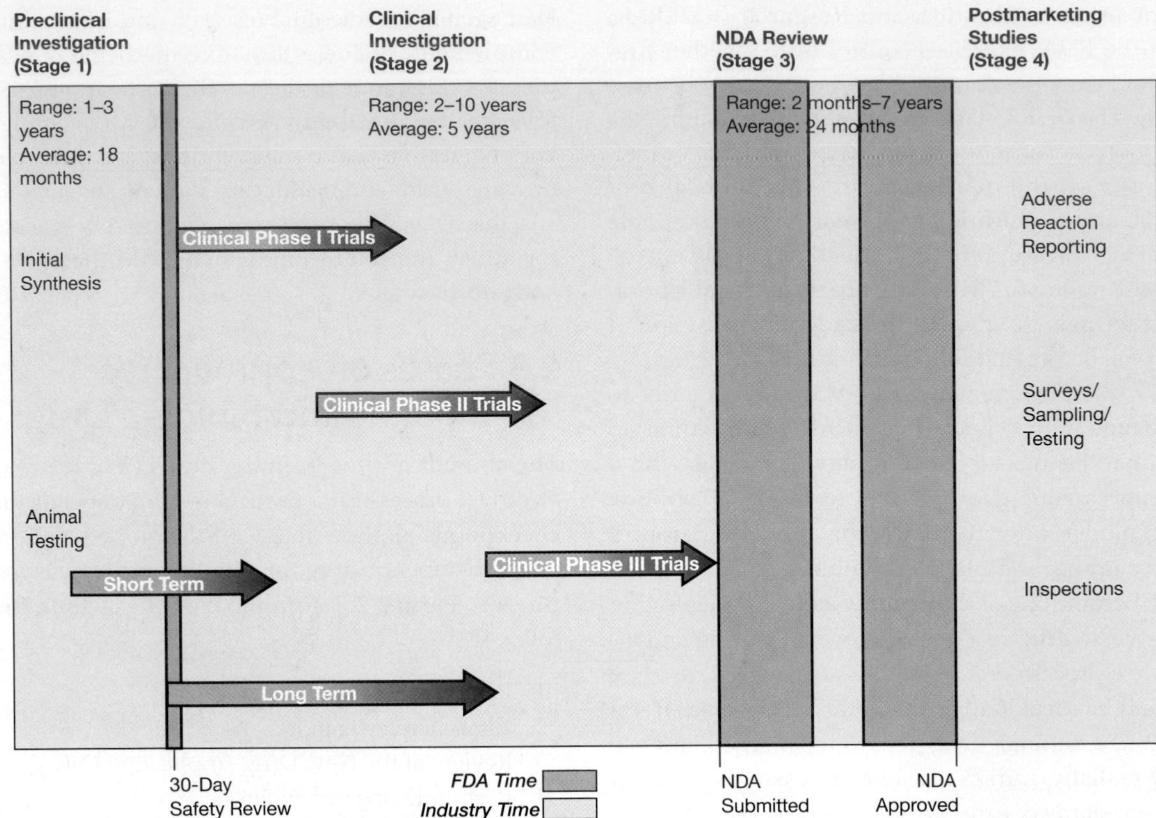

FIGURE 2.3 A new drug development time line with the four phases of drug approval

unsafely with existing medications, or affects one type of patient more than others.

Clinical phase trials are an essential component of drug evaluations due to the variability of responses among patients. If a drug appears to be effective without causing serious side effects, approval for marketing may be accelerated, or the drug may be used immediately in special cases with careful monitoring. If the drug shows promise but precautions are noted, the process is delayed until the pharmaceutical company remedies the concerns. In any case, a **New Drug Application (NDA)** must be submitted before a drug is allowed to proceed to the next phase of the approval process. An **Investigational New Drug (IND)** application may be submitted for Phase I clinical trials when it is determined that there are significant therapeutic benefits, and that the product is reasonably safe for initial use in humans. Companies usually begin developing a trade name for drugs during Phase I of the IND process.

The **New Drug Application (NDA) review** is the third phase of the drug approval process. During this phase, the drug's trade name is finalized. Clinical Phase III trials and animal testing may continue depending on the results obtained from preclinical testing. By law, the FDA is permitted 6 months to initially review an NDA. If the NDA is approved, the process continues to the final phase. If the NDA is rejected, the process is suspended until noted concerns are addressed by the pharmaceutical company. The average NDA review time for new drugs is approximately 17 to 24 months.

Postmarketing surveillance, the final phase of the drug approval process, begins after clinical trials and the NDA review have been completed. The purpose of this phase is to survey for harmful drug effects in a larger population. Some adverse effects take longer to appear and are not identified until a drug is circulated to large numbers of people. Examples of this process have been approval of the COX-2 selective nonsteroidal anti-inflammatory drugs (NSAIDs), which were evaluated by the FDA during 2004 and 2005. Manufacturers of valdecoxib (Bextra), celecoxib (Celebrex), and rofecoxib (Vioxx) were originally asked to revise their labeling due to emerging concerns that some NSAIDs exhibited extreme cardiovascular and gastrointestinal risks. In September 2004, manufacturers of rofecoxib voluntarily withdrew their product from the market due to safety concerns of heart attack and stroke. In April 2005, the FDA asked the manufacturers of valdecoxib to remove their product from the market due to similar concerns. Although celecoxib remained on the market, the FDA announced that it would continue to analyze reports to determine whether additional regulatory action would be needed. The black box warning in this instance continues to warn patients that fatal cardiovascular disease, bleeding ulceration, and serious gastrointestinal reactions may result if certain precautions are not taken.

The FDA holds annual public meetings to receive feedback from patients and professional and pharmaceutical organizations regarding the effectiveness and safety of new drug therapies. If the FDA discovers a serious problem, it will mandate that the drug be withdrawn from the market. The FDA has a free e-mail subscription service to alert the consumer regarding drugs and products withdrawn from the market. The FDA sponsors MedWatch and Drug Safety Communications, podcasts, and newsletters to alert patients, consumers, and health care providers of drug risks. They also provide safety sheets, press announcements, and other pertinent drug fact information.

2.4 Changes to the Drug Approval Process

The process of isolating or synthesizing a new drug and testing it in cells, experimental animals, and humans can take many years. The NDA can include dozens of volumes of experimental and clinical data that must be examined in the drug review process. Some NDAs contain more than 100,000 pages. Even after all experiments have been concluded and clinical data have been gathered, the FDA review process can take several years.

Expenses associated with development of a new drug can cost pharmaceutical manufacturers millions of dollars. According to the Tuft's Center for the Study of Drug Development, drug manufacturers will likely spend more than 2.5 billion dollars within the next decade in order to gain approval to sell one new prescription drug (Weisman, 2014). Drug companies are often concerned about the regulatory process and are eager to get the drug marketed to recoup their research and development expenses. The public is also eager to receive new drugs, particularly for diseases that have a high mortality rate. Although the criticisms from manufacturers and the public are certainly understandable—and sometimes justified—the fundamental priority of the FDA is to ensure that drugs are safe. Without an exhaustive review of scientific data, the public could be exposed to dangerous or ineffectual medications.

In the early 1990s, due to pressure from organized consumer groups and various drug manufacturers, government officials created a plan to speed up the drug review process. Reasons identified for delays in the FDA drug approval process included outdated guidelines, poor communication, and insufficient staff to handle the workload.

In 1992, FDA officials, members of Congress, and representatives from pharmaceutical companies negotiated the Prescription Drug User Fee Act on a 5-year trial basis. This act required drug and biologic manufacturers to provide yearly product user fees. This added income allowed the FDA to hire more employees and to restructure its organization to more efficiently handle the processing of drug applications. The result of restructuring was a resounding success. From 1992 to 1996, the FDA approved double the number of drugs while cutting some review times by as much as half. In 1997, the FDA Modernization Act reauthorized the Prescription Drug User Fee Act. Nearly 700 employees were added to the FDA's drug and biologics program, and more than $300 million was collected in user fees. The FDA Amendments Act expanded the reform effort in 2007 by allowing more U.S. resources to be used for comprehensive reviews of new drugs. In 2008, the target base revenue for new drugs was over $392 million. In 2011, the FDA expanded its reviews of drugs and legislation.

Evidence-Based Practice: Informed Consent Procedures

Clinical Question: How can nurses assist in the informed consent procedures for patients considering participation in a clinical drug research trial?

Evidence: At some point in their career, the nurse may care for a patient who is enrolled in, or considering participation in, a clinical drug research trial. The publication of the Belmont Report (HHS, 1979) provided guidance and principles for obtaining informed consent from patients enrolled in clinical trials. The FDA has guidelines that include how informed consent is to be obtained from children and illiterate adults (FDA, 2014). Although providing information about the research trial is beyond the scope of nursing practice and the responsibility of the researcher and health care provider, nurses can participate by helping to ensure that any questions or concerns the patient has regarding participation are addressed before signing the informed consent document. Special populations require careful assessment of the patient's ability to understand or make informed decisions about research participation. These populations may include children, patients with cognitive or mental impairments, and patients with sensory or language barriers. Other circumstances which may make obtaining informed consent for research participation more difficult include situations in which the patient may be critically ill or suffering from a traumatic injury. These may delay obtaining consent directly from the patient and result in the patient's exclusion from the clinical trial. Differences in cultural background and beliefs about what is appropriate for a patient to know may run counter to the established guidelines that informed consent must provide the patient with the information necessary to make an informed decision to participate.

Nursing Implications: Ensuring that a patient, family, or legal guardian has the information necessary to make informed decisions is a potential role for the nurse when caring for patients considering or participating in a clinical research trial. Whereas providing the information is beyond the scope of most nursing practice, the patient will often ask questions of the nurse, and the nurse can relay these questions to the health care provider. This is especially important when working with patients or families who may have special needs, such as language or cultural differences, or in emergency situations, in which the patient is not able to receive the information and a family member or legal guardian must make the decision.

Lifespan Considerations: Geriatric

Prescription Drug Costs and the "Doughnut Hole" for Senior Citizens

In January 2006, prescription drug coverage through Medicare Part D went into effect, in part to help protect senior citizens over age 65 from catastrophic drug expenditures. Americans older than age 65 constitute only 13% of the population but account for about 34% of all prescriptions dispensed and 40% of all OTC medications. More than 80% of all seniors take at least one prescribed medication each day. The average older adult takes more than four prescription medications, plus two OTC medications. Many of these medicines—such as those for diabetes, hypertension, and heart disease—are taken on a permanent basis.

Whereas Medicare Part D did make some substantial differences in helping seniors pay for their medications, a coverage gap occurs when drug spending totals are between approximately $2,960 and $6,400. Although the dollar amount changes year-to-year, the gap occurs when the coverage for allowable drugs paid for by the patient and the prescription plan reaches a set limit. For 2015, that limit is $2960 (Medicare.gov, n.d.). When the limit is reached, the patient bears the cost of the medications, until the upper limit is reached. This gap in coverage has been termed the "doughnut hole." Studies have suggested that seniors reaching the doughnut hole reduce spending on their medications by 14% to 40%, depending on whether they have additional insurance coverage. With most seniors taking daily medications for chronic conditions, this decrease in spending may cause seniors to forego needed medications. The one positive aspect of the doughnut hole coverage gap is that once the gap kicks in, the cost of the medications count toward the patient's deductible, more quickly assuring that coverage will re-start. Many seniors purchase gap-coverage plans through private insurers. The U.S. Affordable Care Act of 2010 includes benefits to reduce this gap in coverage for seniors with the goal of closing it completely by 2020. Nurses should include questions about the ability to afford medications as part of taking an adequate drug history, especially when working with older adult patients.

Congress passed into law the FDA Food Safety Modernization Act to give the HHS greater authority to recall certain potentially tainted products and to detect food-related illnesses and outbreaks. Although drug development has not increased in recent years, the review process continues to be critical to drug safety and effectiveness.

2.5 Nurses, the Drug Approval Process, and the Need for Effective Safety Practices

The postmarketing surveillance period (Phase 4) is when the nurse has the most opportunities to participate in the drug approval process. While the nurse working at a large, urban medical center may participate in administering medications during Phase II and III trials, *all* nurses administering medications monitor for therapeutic effects and adverse reactions from the drugs they give to their patients. Whenever a possible drug reaction is noted, the nurse is responsible for reporting the reaction to the prescriber and appropriate health care agency personnel (e.g., risk management, pharmacist). By monitoring for and reporting adverse effects, the nurse can ensure better postmarketing surveillance is achieved. Organizations like the nonprofit Institute for Safe Medication Practices (ISMP), the federal Centers for Disease Control and Prevention (CDC), and The Joint Commission accreditation/certification agency play additional roles and are resources for safety enhancement. Sentinel Event Alerts from The Joint Commission for example, describe "an unexpected occurrence involving death or serious physical or psychological injury, or the risk thereof that may or may not be directly related to administration of medications." Safety continues to be at the forefront of concerns for the nurse. The roles and responsibilities of the nurse in safe drug administration are discussed further in chapter 7.

PharmFacts

TIME LENGTH FOR NEW DRUG APPROVALS

- It takes about 11 years of research and development before a drug is submitted to the FDA for review.
- Phase I clinical trials take about 1 year and involve 20 to 80 normal, healthy volunteers.
- Phase II clinical trials last about 2 years and involve 100 to 300 volunteer patients with the disease.
- Phase III clinical trials take about 3 years and involve 1,000 to 3,000 patients in hospitals and clinic agencies.
- For every 5,000 chemicals that enter preclinical testing, only 5 make it to human testing. Of these 5 potential drugs, only 1 is finally approved.

2.6 Controlled Substances, Drug Schedules, and Teratogenic Risks

Some drugs are frequently abused or have a high potential for addiction. Technically, *addiction* refers to the overwhelming feeling that drives someone to use a drug repeatedly.

Dependence is a related term, often defined as a physiological or psychological need for a substance. *Physical dependence* refers to an altered physical condition caused by the adaptation of the nervous system to repeated drug use. In this case, when the drug is no longer available, the individual expresses physical signs of discomfort known as **withdrawal.** In contrast, when an individual is *psychologically dependent,* there are few signs of physical discomfort

Table 2.1 U.S. Drug Schedules and Examples

Drug Schedule	Abuse Potential	Potential for Physical Dependency	Potential for Psychological Dependency	Examples	Therapeutic Use
I	Highest	High	High	heroin, lysergic acid diethylamide (LSD), marijuana (cannabis), peyote, methaqualone, and 3,4-methylenedioxymethamphetamine ("ecstasy")	Limited or no therapeutic use
II	High	High	High	hydromorphone, methadone, meperidine, oxycodone, and fentanyl; amphetamine, methamphetamine, methylphenidate, cocaine, amobarbital, glutethimide, and pentobarbital	
III	Moderate	Moderate	High	combination products containing less than 15 mg of hydrocodone per dosage unit, products containing not more than 90 mg of codeine per dosage unit, buprenorphine products, benzphetamine, phendimetrazine, ketamine, and anabolic steroids	Used therapeutically with prescription; some drugs no longer used (Schedules II, III and IV)
IV	Lower	Lower	Lower	alprazolam, clonazepam, clorazepate, diazepam, lorazepam, midazolam, temazepam, and triazolam	
V	Lowest	Lowest	Lowest	cough preparations containing not more than 200 mg of codeine per 100 mL or per 100 g	Used therapeutically without prescription

when the drug is withdrawn; however, the individual feels an intense compelling desire to continue drug use. These concepts are discussed in detail in chapter 22.

In the United States, a **controlled substance** is a drug whose use is restricted by the Controlled Substances Act of 1970 and later revisions. According to this law, drugs that have a significant potential for abuse are placed into five categories called schedules. These **scheduled drugs** are classified according to their potential for abuse: Schedule I drugs have the highest potential for abuse, and Schedule V drugs have the lowest potential for abuse. Schedule I drugs are restricted for use in situations of medical necessity, if at all allowed. They have little or no therapeutic value or are only intended for research purposes. Drugs in the other four schedules may be dispensed only in cases in which therapeutic value has been determined. Schedule V is the only category in which some drugs may be dispensed without a prescription because the quantities of the controlled drug are so low that the possibility of causing dependence is extremely remote. Table 2.1 gives the five drug schedules with examples. Not all drugs with an abuse potential are regulated or placed into schedules; tobacco, alcohol, and caffeine are significant examples.

The Controlled Substances Act is also called the Comprehensive Drug Abuse Prevention and Control Act. Hospitals and pharmacies must register with the Drug Enforcement Administration (DEA) and use their assigned registration numbers to purchase scheduled drugs.

PharmFacts

EXTENT OF DRUG ABUSE

- In 2012, 23.9 percent of 18- to 20-year-olds reported using an illicit drug in the past month. There were 18.9 million users of marijuana, about 7.3 percent of people age 12 or older. Trends in drug use other than marijuana have not changed appreciably over the past decade.
- About 6.8 million Americans or 2.6 percent of people age 12 or older have reported taking psychotherapeutic drugs. More than one million Americans, (0.4 percent) have used hallucinogenic drugs (including Ecstasy and LSD).
- In 2008, over 29.8% of the U.S. population age 12 and older (70.8 million people) had smoked cigarettes during the past month. In 2012, the rate of past-month cigarette smoking among 12- to 17-year-olds had gone down by 6.6 percent. Although it is illegal in the United States to sell tobacco to under-age youths, in most cases they are still able to purchase tobacco products personally.
- From 1996 to 2009, emergency departments recorded increased use of abused substances such as gamma hydroxybutyric acid (GHB; street name *Fantasy*), ketamine (street names *jet, super acid, Special K,* among others), and MDMA (chemical name 3,4-methylenedioxymethamphetamine; street name *Ecstasy*). Use of many of these illicit drugs except for *Ecstasy* leveled off after 2009. The trend was not changed through 2012.
- Cocaine use has declined in recent years. From 2007 to 2012, the number of users age 12 or older dropped from 2.1 million to 1.7 million. Methamphetamine use has slightly declined from 530,000 current users in 2007 to 440,000 in 2012.
- In 2009, an estimated 30.2 million people (12% age 12 or older), reported driving under the influence of alcohol at least once in the past year. Alcohol use by the same age group showed a general decline from 28.8 percent to 24.3 percent between the years 2002 and 2012. Although reflecting a downward trend, alcohol abuse remains a national health concern. (National Institute of Drug Abuse, 2014)

Hospitals and pharmacies must maintain complete records of all quantities purchased and sold. Health care providers, nurse practitioners, and others with prescriptive authority must also register with the DEA and receive an assigned number before prescribing these drugs. Drugs with higher abuse potential have more restrictions. For example, in many states, a special order form must be used to obtain Schedule II drugs, and orders must be written and signed by the health care provider. Telephone orders to a pharmacy are not permitted. Refills for Schedule II drugs are not permitted: patients must visit their health care provider first. Those convicted of unlawful manufacturing, distributing, or dispensing controlled substances face severe penalties.

A teratogen is a substance that has the potential to cause a defect in an unborn child during pregnancy. A small number of drugs have been shown to be teratogenic, either in humans or in laboratory animals. Classification of **teratogenic risk** places drugs into categories A, B, C, D, and X. Category A is the safest group of drugs while Category X poses the most danger to the fetus. Birth defects are most probable in the first trimester; thus, nurses must be mindful of the various drug risks during this time. Table 2.2 outlines drug risk classification in pregnancy. Additional details on the teratogenic risk posed by medications are included in chapter 8.

Table 2.2 FDA Drug Risk Classification in Pregnancy

CATEGORY A
Controlled studies in women fail to show a risk to the fetus and the possibility of fetal harm appears unlikely.
CATEGORY B
Animal-reproduction studies have not shown a fetal risk or adverse effect. Risks have not been confirmed in controlled studies in women.
CATEGORY C
Either studies in animals have revealed adverse effects on the fetus and there are no controlled studies in women or studies in women and animals are not available.
CATEGORY D
There is confirmation of human fetal risk, but the benefits from use in pregnant women may be acceptable despite the risk (e.g., if the drug is needed in a life-threatening situation or for a serious disease for which safer drugs cannot be used).
CATEGORY X
Animal and human studies have shown fetal abnormalities. The drug is contraindicated in women who are or may become pregnant.

Chapter Review

KEY Concepts

The numbered key concepts provide a succinct summary of the important points from the corresponding numbered section within the chapter. If any of these points are not clear, refer to the numbered section within the chapter for review.

2.1 Drug regulations were created to protect the public from drug misuse and to ensure continuous evaluation of safety and effectiveness.

2.2 The regulatory agency responsible for ensuring that drugs are safe and effective is the U.S. Food and Drug Administration (FDA).

2.3 There are four phases of approval for therapeutic and biologic drugs. The phases progress from cellular and animal testing to use of the experimental drug in patients with the disease.

2.4 Once criticized for being too slow, the FDA has streamlined the process to get new drugs to market more quickly.

2.5 Nurses may participate in several phases of the drug approval process. They will have the most frequent opportunities during Phase 4, postmarketing surveillance. Medication safety is a matter of paramount importance in health care.

2.6 Drugs with a potential for abuse are restricted by the Controlled Substances Act and are categorized into schedules. Schedule I drugs are the most tightly controlled; Schedule V drugs have less potential for addiction and are less tightly controlled. Drugs are also categorized according to their teratogenic risk. Category A drugs are the safest to take during pregnancy. Category X drugs are the most dangerous to the fetus.

CRITICAL THINKING Questions

1. How does the FDA ensure the safety and effectiveness of drugs? What types of drugs does the FDA regulate or control?
2. What is a "black box warning"? Why is it important for nurses to consider these when reading drug information materials?
3. Identify opportunities the nurse has in educating about, administering, and monitoring the proper use of drugs.
4. Why are certain drugs placed in schedules? What does the nurse need to know when a scheduled drug is ordered?
5. A nurse is preparing to give a patient a medication and notes that a drug to be given is marked as a Schedule III drug. What does this information tell the nurse about this medication?

Visit www.pearsonhighered.com/nursingresources for answers and rationales for all activities.

REFERENCES

Brunton, L. L., Chabner, B.A., & Knollman, B. C. (Eds.). (2011). Drug invention & the pharmaceutical industry. In *Goodman & Gilman's The pharmacological basis of therapeutics* (12th ed., pp. 15–29). New York, NY: McGraw-Hill.

Medicare.gov. (n.d.). *Costs in the coverage gap.* Retrieved from http://www.medicare.gov/part-d/costs/coverage-gap/part-d-coverage-gap.html

National Institute of Drug Abuse. (2015). *Drug facts: Nationwide trends.* Retrieved from http://www.drugabuse.gov/publications/drugfacts/nationwide-trends

U.S. Department of Health & Human Services. (1979). *The Belmont report.* Retrieved from http://www.hhs.gov/ohrp/humansubjects/guidance/belmont.html

U.S. Food and Drug Administration. (2014). *A guide to informed consent–information sheet.* Retrieved from http://www.fda.gov/RegulatoryInformation/Guidances/ucm126431.htm

Weisman, R. (2014, November 18). Cost of bringing drug to market tops $2.5b, research finds. *Boston Globe.* Retrieved from https://www.bostonglobe.com/business/2014/11/18/cost-bringing-prescription-drug-market-tops-billion-tufts-research-center-estimates/6mPph8maRxzcvftWjr7HUN/story.html

SELECTED BIBLIOGRAPHY

Centers for Medicare & Medicaid Services, Office of the Actuary, National Health Statistics Group. (2012). *National health expenditure projections 2012–2022 forecast summary.* Retrieved from http://www.cms.gov/Research-Statistics-Data-and-Systems/Statistics-Trends-and-Reports/NationalHealthExpendData/downloads/proj2012.pdf

Consumers Union. (2009). *To err is human—to delay is deadly.* Retrieved from http://www.safepatientproject.org/safepatientproject.org/pdf/safepatientproject.org-ToDelayIsDeadly.pdf

Frank, C., Himmelstein, D. U., Woolhandler, S., Bor, D. H., Wolfe, S. M., Heymann, O., . . . Lasser, K. E. (2014). Era of faster FDA drug approval has also seen increased black-box warnings and market withdrawals. *Health Affairs. 33,* 1453–1459. doi:10.1377/hlthaff.2014.0122

Institute for Safe Medication Practices. (2009). *QuarterWatch: 2008 Quarter 2.* Retrieved from https://www.ismp.org/QuarterWatch/2008Q2.pdf

OECD. (2011). Pharmaceutical expenditure, in *Health at a Glance 2011: OECD Indicators,* OECD Publishing. doi:10.1787/health_glance-2011-63-en

OECD. (2015). *OECD health statistics.* Retrieved from http://www.oecd.org/els/health-systems/health-data.htm

Paris, V. (2014). *Why do Americans spend so much on pharmaceuticals?* Retrieved from http://www.pbs.org/newshour/updates/americans-spend-much-pharmaceuticals/

Sitler, B., & Hughes, G. (2014, February). Healthcare Analytics: Patient engagement—What can we learn from other industries? *Patient Safety & Quality Healthcare.* Retrieved from http://psqh.com/january-february-2014/healthcare-analytics-patient-engagement-what-can-we-learn-from-other-industries

Szefler, S. J., Whelan, G. J., & Leung, D. Y. (2006). "Black box" warning: Wake-up call or overreaction? *Journal of Allergy and Clinical Immunology, 117,* 26–29. doi:http://dx.doi.org/10.1016/j.jaci.2005.11.006

U.S. Food and Drug Administration. (2011). *Guidance for industry. Warnings and precautions, contraindications, and boxed warning sections of labeling for human prescription drug and biological products—content and format.* Retrieved from http://www.fda.gov/downloads/Drugs/GuidanceComplianceRegulatoryInformation/Guidances/ucm075096.pdf

U.S. Food and Drug Administration. (2014). Inside clinical trials: Testing medical products in people. Retrieved from http://www.fda.gov/Drugs/ResourcesForYou/Consumers/ucm143531.htm

Chapter 3

Principles of Drug Administration

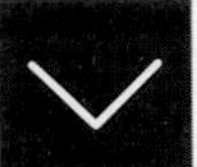

Learning Outcomes

After reading this chapter, the student should be able to:

1. Discuss drug administration as a component of safe, effective nursing care, using the nursing process.
2. Describe the roles and responsibilities of nurses regarding safe drug administration.
3. Explain how the five rights of drug administration affect patient safety.
4. Give specific examples of how nurses can increase patient compliance in taking medications.
5. Interpret drug orders that contain abbreviations.
6. Compare and contrast the three systems of measurement used in pharmacology.
7. Explain the proper methods of administering enteral, topical, and parenteral drugs.
8. Compare and contrast the advantages and disadvantages of each route of drug administration.

The primary role of the nurse in drug administration is to ensure that prescribed medications are delivered in a safe manner. Drug administration is an important component of providing comprehensive nursing care that incorporates all aspects of the nursing process. In the course of drug administration, the nurse will collaborate closely with health care providers, pharmacists, and, of course, patients. The purpose of this chapter is to introduce the roles and responsibilities of the nurse in delivering medications safely and effectively.

RESPONSIBILITIES OF THE NURSE

3.1 Medication Knowledge and Understanding

Whether administering drugs to or supervising the use of drugs by their patients, nurses are expected to understand the pharmacotherapeutic principles for all medications given to each patient. Given the large number of different drugs and the potential consequences of medication errors, this is indeed an enormous task. The nurse's responsibilities include knowledge and understanding of the following:

- What drug is ordered
- Name (generic and trade) and drug classification
- Intended or proposed use
- Effects on the body
- Contraindications
- Special considerations (e.g., how age, weight, body fat distribution, and individual pathophysiological states affect pharmacotherapeutic response)
- Side effects
- Why the medication has been prescribed for this particular patient
- How the medication is supplied by the pharmacy
- How the medication is to be administered, including dosage ranges
- What nursing process considerations related to the medication apply to this patient.

Before any drug is administered, the nurse must obtain and process pertinent information regarding the patient's medical history, physical assessment, disease processes, and learning needs and capabilities. Growth and developmental factors must always be considered. It is important to remember that a large number of variables influence a patient's response to medications. Having a firm understanding of these variables can increase the success of pharmacotherapy.

A major goal of studying pharmacology is to limit the number and severity of adverse drug events. Many adverse effects are preventable. The professional nurse can routinely avoid many unfavorable drug effects in patients by applying experience and knowledge of pharmacotherapeutics to clinical practice. Some unfavorable effects, however, are not preventable. It is vital that the nurse be prepared to recognize and respond to the potential harmful effects of medications.

An **adverse event (AE)** is any undesirable experience associated with the use of a medical product in a patient. AEs are generally described in terms of intensity (e.g., mild, moderate, severe, and life threatening). The term *serious adverse event (SAE)* is used to define threat of death or immediate risk of death. Some patients may experience AEs with a particular drug, whereas others may not.

An AE resulting from drug administration is often termed an *adverse drug event* or *adverse drug effect*. Most health professionals simply refer to an unfavorable drug reaction as an **adverse effect.** Adverse effects warrant either lowering the dosage of the drug or discontinuing the drug. They are generally perceived as negative. A *side effect* is another term often confused with adverse effect. The difference is that **side effect** describes a nontherapeutic reaction to a drug. Side effects may be transient, but this is not always the case. They may require nursing intervention, although most of the time they are perceived as tolerable. Both drug reactions have a nature and intensity that is documented and included in the published literature (e.g., drug guides, safety reports).

Allergic and anaphylactic reactions are particularly serious side effects that must be carefully monitored and prevented, when possible. An **allergic reaction** is an acquired hyperresponse of body defenses to a foreign substance (allergen). Signs of allergic reactions vary in severity and include skin rash with or without itching, edema, runny nose, or reddened eyes with tearing. On discovering that the patient is allergic to a product, it is the nurse's responsibility to alert all personnel by documenting the allergy in the medical record and by appropriately labeling patient records and the medication administration record (MAR). An appropriate, agency-approved bracelet should be placed on the patient to alert all caregivers to the specific drug allergy. Information related to a drug allergy must be communicated to the health care provider and pharmacist so the medication regimen can be evaluated for cross-sensitivity among various pharmacologic products.

Anaphylaxis is a severe type of allergic reaction that involves the massive, systemic release of histamine and other chemical mediators of inflammation that can lead to life-threatening shock. Symptoms such as acute dyspnea and the sudden appearance of hypotension or tachycardia following drug administration are indicative of anaphylaxis, which must receive immediate treatment. The pharmacotherapy of allergic reactions and anaphylaxis is covered in chapters 39 and 29, respectively.

One issue of pharmacoeconomics (chapter 1) is that some medications may be withheld due to serious adverse or

PharmFacts

POTENTIALLY FATAL DRUG REACTIONS

Toxic Epidermal Necrolysis (TEN)

- Severe and deadly drug-induced allergic reaction
- Characterized by widespread epidermal sloughing, caused by massive disintegration of the top layer of the skin and mucous membranes
- Involves multiple body systems and can cause death if not quickly diagnosed
- Occurs when the liver fails to properly break down a drug, which then cannot be excreted normally
- Associated with the use of some anticonvulsants (phenytoin [Dilantin], carbamazepine [Tegretol]), the antibiotic trimethoprim/sulfamethoxazole (Bactrim, Septra), and other drugs, but can occur with the use of any prescription or over-the-counter (OTC) preparation, including ibuprofen (Advil, Motrin)
- Risk of death decreases if the offending drug is quickly withdrawn and supportive care is maintained

Stevens–Johnson Syndrome (SJS)

- Usually prompted by the same or similar drugs as TEN, usually within 1 to 14 days of pharmacotherapy
- Start of SJS is usually signaled by nonspecific upper respiratory infection with chills, fever, and malaise
- Generalized blisterlike lesions follow within a few days, and skin sloughing may occur on 10% of the body

unfavorable health risks. In these instances, alternate drug or therapeutic treatment may be considered. Appropriate and proper health care decisions should be incorporated into the treatment plan. The boundaries for such decisions are often based on the respective policies and guidelines of the regulatory agencies, health care providers, and mutual consent given by patients and their families. In all instances of drug therapy, the major concern is safe and effective therapy for the patient and responsible evidence-based decisions made by nurses. Refer to chapters 4 and 5 for more detailed discussion of pharmacokinetic and pharmacodynamic concerns including adverse drug reactions, contraindications, drug–food interactions, and drug–drug interaction issues.

3.2 The Rights of Drug Administration

The traditional **five rights of drug administration** form the operational basis for the safe delivery of medications and are recognized by such organizations as the Institute for Safe Medication Practices (ISMP). The five rights offer simple and practical guidance for nurses to use during drug preparation, delivery, and administration, and focus on individual performance. The five rights are as follows:

1. Right patient
2. Right medication
3. Right dose
4. Right route of administration
5. Right time of delivery.

Additional rights have been added over the years, depending on particular academic curricula or agency policies. Additions to the original five rights include considerations such as the right to refuse medication, the right to receive drug education, the right preparation, and the right documentation, but deviations from the original five rights still account for the majority of medication administration errors. If a patient refuses medication, it is the responsibility of the nurse to educate the patient about drug benefits and risks, and to assess for fears and reasons why the patient might refuse the medication. The nurse should notify the health care provider and document all of the information related to these additional rights. Ethical and legal considerations regarding the five rights are discussed in chapter 7.

The **three checks of drug administration** that the nurse uses in conjunction with the five rights help to ensure patient safety and drug effectiveness. Traditionally these checks incorporate the following:

1. Checking the drug with the MAR or the medication information system when removing it from the medication drawer, refrigerator, or controlled substance locker
2. Checking the drug when preparing it, pouring it, taking it out of the unit-dose container, or connecting the IV tubing to the bag
3. Checking the drug before administering it to the patient.

Despite all attempts to provide safe drug delivery, medication errors continue to occur, some of which result in patient injury or death. Although the nurse is accountable for preparing and administering medications, the responsibility for safe and accurate administration of medications lies with multiple individuals, including prescribers, pharmacists, and other health care practitioners. The nurse who follows institutional policy and procedure when scanning is correctly checking the five rights three times. Unfortunately, when scanning is not done correctly, errors can occur. It should be noted that computerized scanning systems of medication administration do not relieve the health care provider of the responsibility to use the three checks and the five rights continuously. Factors contributing to medication errors and strategies for reducing their occurrence are presented in chapter 7.

3.3 Patient Compliance and Successful Pharmacotherapy

Compliance or adherence to a drug regimen is a major factor affecting pharmacotherapeutic success. As it relates to pharmacology, **compliance** is taking a medication in the manner

Patient Safety: Medication Errors and the Nurse's Role

Research has found that, regardless of the type of health care setting, the majority of medication errors stem from human factors (such as deficient knowledge) and prescribing or administration errors, including errors of omission (Kuo, Touchette, & Marinac, 2013; Latif, Rawat, Pustavoitau, Pronovost, & Pham, 2013). Common sources of errors include:

- Errors in patient assessment (e.g., inadequate medication history, incomplete physical assessment).
- Errors in prescribing (e.g., wrong drug, incorrect dose, miscommunication of drug orders such as inappropriate abbreviations, similar drug names).
- Administration errors (e.g., route or time of administration, omissions).
- Distracting environmental factors (e.g., interruptions during preparation for medication administration).

Many of these errors involve a breach of one of the cardinal "five rights" of medication administration: the right patient, drug, dosage, route, and time. Labeling design, changes in packaging, and problems with dispensing devices are other contributing factors.

In many settings, the nurse remains the last line of defense to prevent a medication error from occurring. Nurses must take extra caution when administering medications to avoid these key sources of error and can work proactively with the provider and health care agency to identify potential sources of error and work to prevent future occurrences.

prescribed by the health care provider, or in the case of OTC drugs, following the instructions on the label. Patient noncompliance ranges from not taking the medication at all to taking it at the wrong time or in the wrong manner.

Although the nurse may be extremely conscientious in applying all the principles of effective drug administration, these strategies are of little value unless the patient agrees that the prescribed drug regimen is personally worthwhile. Before administering the drug, the nurse should use the nursing process to formulate a personalized care plan that will best enable the patient to become an active participant in his or her care (see chapter 6). This allows the patient to accept or reject the pharmacologic course of therapy, based on accurate information that is presented in a manner that addresses individual learning styles. It is imperative to remember that a responsible, well-informed adult always has the legal option to refuse to take any medication.

In the plan of care, it is important to address essential information that the patient must know regarding the prescribed medications. This includes factors such as the name of the drug, why it has been ordered, expected drug actions, associated side effects, and potential interactions with other medications, foods, herbal supplements, or alcohol. Patients need to be reminded that they share an active role in ensuring their own medication effectiveness and safety.

Many factors can influence whether patients comply with pharmacotherapy. The drug may be too expensive or may not be approved by the patient's health insurance plan. Patients sometimes forget doses of medications, especially when they must be taken three or four times per day. Patients often discontinue the use of drugs that have annoying side effects or those that interfere with their accustomed lifestyle. Adverse effects that often prompt noncompliance are headache, dizziness, nausea, diarrhea, or impotence.

Patients often take medications in an unexpected manner, sometimes self-adjusting their doses. Some patients believe that if one tablet is good, two must be better. Others believe that they will become dependent on the medication if it is taken as prescribed; thus, they take only half the required dose. Patients are usually reluctant to admit or report noncompliance to the nurse for fear of being reprimanded or feeling embarrassed. Because the reasons for noncompliance are many and varied, the nurse must be vigilant in questioning patients about their medications. When pharmacotherapy fails to produce the expected outcomes, noncompliance should be considered a possible explanation.

Lifespan Considerations: Pediatric
The Challenges of Pediatric Drug Administration

Administering medication to infants and young children requires special knowledge and techniques. Nurses must have knowledge of growth and development patterns. When possible, the child should be given a choice regarding the use of a spoon, dropper, or syringe. A matter-of-fact attitude should be presented in giving a child medications; using threats or dishonesty is unacceptable and professionally unethical. Oral medications that must be crushed for the child to swallow can be mixed with flavored syrup, jelly, or the child's choice of food to avoid unpleasant tastes. However, care must be taken to avoid necessary food items so that the child does not develop an unpleasant association with these items and refuse to consume them in the future. To prevent nausea, medications can be preceded and followed with sips of a carbonated beverage that is poured over crushed ice.

3.4 Drug Orders and Time Schedules

Health care providers use accepted abbreviations to communicate the directions and times for drug administration. Table 3.1 lists common abbreviations that relate to universally scheduled times.

A **STAT order** refers to any medication that is needed immediately and is to be given only once. It is often associated

Table 3.1 Drug Administration Abbreviations

Abbreviation	Meaning
ac	before meals
ad lib	as desired/as directed
AM	morning
bid	twice a day
cap	capsule
gtt	drop
h or hr	hour
IM	intramuscular
IV	intravenous
no	number
pc	after meals; after eating
PO	by mouth
PM	afternoon
prn	when needed/necessary
qid	four times per day
q2h	every 2 hours (even or when first given)
q4h	every 4 hours (even)
q6h	every 6 hours (even)
q8h	every 8 hours (even)
q12h	every 12 hours
Rx	take
STAT	immediately; at once
tab	tablet
tid	three times a day

Note: The Institute for Safe Medical Practices recommends the following abbreviations be avoided because they can lead to medication errors: q: instead use "every"; qh: instead use "hourly" or "every hour"; qd: instead use "daily" or "every day"; qhs: instead use "nightly"; qod: instead use "every other day." For these and other recommendations, see the official Joint Commission "Do Not Use List" at http://www.jointcommission.org/assets/1/18/dnu_list.pdf

with emergency medications that are needed for life-threatening situations. The term *STAT* comes from *statim*, the Latin word meaning "immediately." The health care provider normally notifies the nurse of any STAT order so it can be obtained from the pharmacy and administered immediately. The time between writing the order and administering the drug should be 5 minutes or less. Although not as urgent, an **ASAP order** (as soon as possible) should be available for administration to the patient within 30 minutes of the written order.

The **single order** is for a drug that is to be given only once, and at a specific time, such as a preoperative order. A **prn order** (Latin: *pro re nata*) is administered *as required* by the patient's condition. The nurse makes judgments, based on patient assessment, as to when such a medication is to be administered. Orders not written as STAT, ASAP, NOW, or prn are called **routine orders.** These are usually carried out within 2 hours of the time the order is written by the health care provider. A **standing order** is written in advance of a situation that is to be carried out under specific circumstances. An example of a standing order is a set of postoperative prn prescriptions that are written for all patients who have undergone a specific surgical procedure. A common standing order for patients who have had a tonsillectomy is "Tylenol elixir 325 mg PO every 6 hours prn sore throat." Because of the legal implications of putting all patients into a single treatment category, standing orders are no longer permitted in some facilities.

Agency policies dictate that drug orders be reviewed by the attending health care provider within specific time frames, usually at least every 7 days. Prescriptions for narcotics and other scheduled drugs are often automatically discontinued after 72 hours, unless specifically reordered by the health care provider. Automatic stop orders do not generally apply when the number of doses or an exact period of time is specified.

Some medications must be taken at specific times. If a drug causes stomach upset, it is usually administered *with* meals to prevent epigastric pain, nausea, or vomiting. Other medications should be administered *between* meals because food interferes with absorption. Some central nervous system drugs and antihypertensives are best administered at *bedtime*, because they may cause drowsiness. Sildenafil (Viagra) is unique in that it should be taken 30 to 60 minutes prior to expected sexual intercourse to achieve an effective erection. (Note: Sildenafil is also prescribed to hospitalized patients for pulmonary hypertension.) The nurse must pay careful attention to educating patients about the timing of their medications to enhance compliance and to increase the potential for therapeutic success.

Once medications are administered, the nurse must correctly document that the medications have been given to the patient. This documentation is completed only *after* the medications have been given, not when they are prepared.

PharmFacts

GRAPEFRUIT JUICE AND DRUG INTERACTIONS

- Grapefruit juice may not be safe for people who take certain medications.
- Chemicals (most likely flavonoids) in grapefruit juice lower the activity of specific enzymes in the intestinal tract that normally break down medications. This allows a larger amount of medication to reach the bloodstream, resulting in increased drug activity.
- Drugs that may be affected by grapefruit juice include midazolam (Versed); cyclosporine (Sandimmune, Neoral); antihyperlipidemics such as lovastatin (Mevacor) and simvastatin (Zocor); calcium channel blockers including nifedipine; certain antibiotics such as erythromycin; and certain antifungals such as itraconazole (Sporanox) and ketoconazole (Nizoral).
- Grapefruit juice should be consumed at least 2 hours before or 5 hours after taking a medication that may interact with it.
- Some drinks that are flavored with fruit juice could contain grapefruit juice, even if grapefruit is not part of the name of the drink. Check the ingredients label.

It is necessary to include the drug name, dosage, time administered, any assessments, and the nurse's signature. If a medication is refused or omitted, this fact must be recorded on the appropriate form within the medical record. It is customary to document the reason when possible. Should the patient voice any concerns or adverse effects about the medication, these should also be included.

3.5 Systems of Measurement

Dosages are labeled and dispensed according to their weight or volume. Three systems of measurement are used in pharmacology: metric, apothecary, and household.

The most common system of drug measurement uses the **metric system of measurement.** The volume of a drug is expressed in terms of liters (L) or milliliters (mL). The cubic centimeter (cc) is a measurement of volume that is equivalent to 1 mL of fluid, but the *cc* abbreviation is no longer used because it can be mistaken for the abbreviation for unit (u) and cause medication errors. The metric weight of a drug is stated in kilograms (kg), grams (g), milligrams (mg), or micrograms (mcg). Note that the abbreviation *μg* should not be used for microgram, because it too can be confused with other abbreviations and cause a medication error.

The **apothecary system** and the **household system** are older systems of measurement. Although most health care providers and pharmacies use the metric system, these older systems are still encountered. In 2005, The Joint Commission, the accrediting organization for health care agencies, added "apothecary units" to its official "Do Not Use" list. However, because not all health care agencies are accredited by The Joint Commission and until the metric system totally replaces the other systems, the nurse must recognize dosages based on all three systems of measurement. Approximate equivalents among metric, apothecary, and household units of volume and weight are listed in Table 3.2.

Because Americans are very familiar with the teaspoon, tablespoon, and cup, it is important for the nurse to be able to convert between the household and metric systems of measurement. In the hospital, a glass of fluid is measured in milliliters—an 8-oz glass of water is recorded as 240 mL. If a patient being discharged is ordered to drink 2,400 mL of fluid per day, the nurse may instruct the patient to drink 10, 8-oz glasses or 10 cups of fluid per day. Likewise, when a child is to be given a drug that is administered in elixir form, the nurse should explain that 5 mL of the drug is approximately the same as 1 teaspoon. The nurse should encourage the use of accurate medical dosing devices at home, such as oral dosing syringes, oral droppers, cylindrical spoons, and medication cups. These are preferred over the traditional household measuring spoon because they are more accurate. Eating utensils that are commonly referred to as teaspoons or tablespoons often do not hold the volume that their names imply. Because of the differences in volumes among standard teaspoons, dessert spoons, tablespoons, and "salt spoons," it is recommended that a measuring spoon used for cooking be used rather than household eating utensils if a more accurate dosing device is not available. Many OTC liquid medications now come with a prepackaged medication cup to avoid under- or overdosage problems.

Table 3.2 Metric, Apothecary, and Household Approximate Measurement Equivalents

Metric	Apothecary	Household
1 mL	15–16 minims	15–16 drops
4–5 mL	1 fluid dram	1 teaspoon or 60 drops
15–16 mL	4 fluid drams	1 tablespoon or 3–4 teaspoons
30–32 mL	8 fluid drams or 1 fluid ounce	2 tablespoons
240–250 mL	8 fluid ounces (½ pint)	1 glass or cup
500 mL	1 pint	2 glasses or 2 cups
1 L	32 fluid ounces or 1 quart	4 glasses or 4 cups or 1 quart
1 mg	1/60 grain	
60–64 mg	1 grain	
300–325 mg	5 grains	
1 g	15–16 grains	
1 kg		2.2 pounds

Note: To convert grains to grams: Divide grains by 15 or 16. To convert grams to grains: Multiply grams by 15 or 16. To convert minims to milliliters: Divide minims by 15 or 16.

ROUTES OF DRUG ADMINISTRATION

The three broad categories of routes of drug administration are enteral, topical, and parenteral, and there are subsets within each of these. Each route has both advantages and disadvantages. Whereas some drugs are formulated to be given by several routes, others are specific to only one route. Pharmacokinetic considerations, such as how the route of administration affects drug absorption and distribution, are discussed in chapter 4.

Certain protocols and techniques are common to all methods of drug administration. The student should review the drug administration guidelines in the following list before proceeding to subsequent sections that discuss specific routes of administration:

- Verify the medication order and check for allergy history on the chart.
- Wash your hands and apply gloves, if indicated.
- Use aseptic technique when preparing and administering parenteral medications.
- In all cases of drug administration, identify the patient by asking the person to state his or her full name (or by asking the parent or guardian), checking the

identification band, and comparing this information with the MAR or scanner and computer. A second item of personal identification, such as asking the birth date, is also required by most health care agencies.

- Ask the patient about known allergies.
- Inform the patient of the name of the drug, the expected actions, common adverse effects, and how it will be administered.
- Position the patient for the appropriate route of administration.
- For enteral drugs, assist the patient to a sitting position.
- If the drug is prepackaged (unit dose), remove it from the packaging at the bedside.
- Unless specifically instructed to do so in the orders, do not leave drugs at the bedside.
- Document the medication administration and any pertinent patient responses on the MAR.

3.6 Enteral Drug Administration

The **enteral route** includes drugs given orally and those administered through nasogastric or gastrostomy tubes. Oral drug administration is the most common, most convenient, and usually the least costly of all routes. It is also considered the safest route because the skin barrier is not compromised. In cases of overdose, medications remaining in the stomach can be retrieved by inducing vomiting. Oral preparations are available in tablet, capsule, and liquid forms. Medications administered by the enteral route take advantage of the vast absorptive surfaces of the oral mucosa, stomach, or small intestine.

Tablets and Capsules

Tablets and capsules are the most common forms of drugs. Patients prefer tablets or capsules over other routes and forms because of their ease of use. In some cases, tablets may be scored for more individualized dosing.

Some patients, particularly children, have difficulty swallowing tablets and capsules. Crushing tablets or opening capsules and sprinkling the drug over food or mixing it with juice will make it more palatable and easier to swallow. The nurse should not crush tablets or open capsules unless the manufacturer specifically states that this is permissible. Some drugs are inactivated by crushing or opening, whereas others severely irritate the stomach mucosa and cause nausea or vomiting. Occasionally, drugs should not be crushed because they irritate the oral mucosa, are extremely bitter, or contain dyes that stain the teeth. Most drug guides provide lists of drugs that may not be crushed. Guidelines for administering tablets or capsules are given in Table 3.3 (section A).

The strongly acidic contents within the stomach can present a destructive obstacle to the absorption of some medications. To overcome this barrier, tablets may have a hard, waxy coating that enables them to resist the acidity. These **enteric-coated** tablets are designed to dissolve in the alkaline environment of the small intestine. It is important that the nurse not crush enteric-coated tablets because the medication would then be directly exposed to the stomach environment.

Studies have clearly demonstrated that compliance declines as the number of doses per day increases. With this in mind, pharmacologists have attempted to design new drugs that may be administered only once or twice daily. **Sustained-release (SR)** tablets or capsules are designed to dissolve very slowly. This releases the medication over an extended time and results in a longer duration of action for the medication. Also called extended-release (XR) or long-acting (LA) medications, these forms allow for the convenience of once- or twice-a-day dosing. Extended-release medications must not be crushed or opened.

Giving medications by the oral route has certain disadvantages. The patient must be conscious and able to swallow properly. Certain types of drugs, including proteins, are inactivated by digestive enzymes in the stomach and small intestine. Medications absorbed from the stomach and small intestine first travel to the liver, where they may be inactivated before they ever reach their target organs. This process called *first-pass metabolism,* is discussed in chapter 4. The significant variation in the motility of the gastrointestinal (GI) tract and in its ability to absorb medications can create differences in bioavailability. In addition, children and some adults have an aversion to swallowing large tablets and capsules or to taking oral medications that are distasteful.

Sublingual and Buccal Drug Administration

For sublingual and buccal administration, the tablet is not swallowed but kept in the mouth. The mucosa of the oral cavity contains a rich blood supply that provides an excellent absorptive surface for certain drugs. Medications given by this route are not subjected to destructive digestive enzymes, nor do they undergo hepatic first-pass metabolism.

For the **sublingual route,** the medication is placed under the tongue and allowed to dissolve slowly. Because of the rich blood supply in this region, the sublingual route results in a rapid onset of action. Sublingual dosage forms are most often formulated as rapidly disintegrating tablets or as soft gelatin capsules filled with liquid drug.

When multiple drugs have been ordered, the sublingual preparations should be administered after oral medications have been swallowed. The patient should be instructed not to move the drug with the tongue, nor to eat or drink anything until the medication has completely dissolved. The sublingual mucosa is not suitable for extended-release formulations because it is a relatively small area and is constantly being bathed by a substantial amount of saliva.

Table 3.3 Enteral Drug Administration

Drug Form (Example)	Administration Guidelines
A. Tablet, capsule, or liquid (Orally disintegrating tablets and soluble films are placed on the tongue and then swallowed)	1. Assess that the patient is alert and has the ability to swallow. 2. Place the tablets or capsules into a medication cup. 3. If the medication is in liquid form, shake the bottle to mix the agent, and measure the dose into the cup at eye level. 4. Hand the patient the medication cup. 5. Offer a glass of water to facilitate swallowing the medication. Milk or juice may be offered if not contraindicated. 6. Remain with the patient until all the medication is swallowed.
B. Sublingual	1. Assess that the patient is alert and has the ability to hold the medication under the tongue. 2. Place the sublingual tablet under the tongue. 3. Instruct the patient not to chew or swallow the tablet or move the tablet around with tongue. 4. Instruct the patient to allow the tablet to dissolve completely. 5. Remain with the patient to determine that all the medication has dissolved. 6. Offer a glass of water after the medication has dissolved, if the patient desires.
C. Buccal	1. Assess that the patient is alert and has the ability to hold the medication between the gums and the cheek. 2. Place the buccal tablet between the gum line and the cheek. 3. Instruct the patient not to chew or swallow the tablet or move the tablet around with tongue. 4. Instruct the patient to allow the tablet to dissolve completely. 5. Remain with the patient to determine that all of the medication has dissolved. 6. Offer a glass of water after the medication has dissolved, if the patient desires.
D. Nasogastric and gastrostomy	1. Administer liquid forms when possible to avoid clogging the tube. Contact the pharmacist or health care provider if unsure if the medication may be given through the tube. 2. If the medication is solid, crush finely into a powder and mix thoroughly with at least 30 mL of warm water until dissolved. Enteric-coated, extended-release, and other dosage types may not be crushed. Always check the drug information before crushing. 3. Assess and verify tube placement per agency protocol. 4. Turn off the enteric feeding, if applicable to the patient. 5. Aspirate stomach contents and measure the residual volume as per agency protocol. If greater than 100 mL for an adult, check agency policy. 6. Return the residual via gravity and flush with water. 7. Pour the medication into the syringe barrel and allow to flow into the tube by gravity. Give each medication separately, flushing between with water. 8. Keep the head of the bed elevated for 1 hour to prevent aspiration. 9. Reestablish continual feeding, as scheduled. Keep the head of the bed elevated 45° to prevent aspiration.

Table 3.3 (section B) and Figure 3.1a present important points regarding sublingual drug administration.

To administer by the **buccal route,** the tablet or capsule is placed in the oral cavity between the gum and the cheek. The patient must be instructed not to manipulate the medication with the tongue; otherwise, it could get displaced to the sublingual area, where it would be more rapidly absorbed, or to the back of the throat, where it could be swallowed. The buccal mucosa is less permeable to most medications than the sublingual area, providing for slower absorption. The buccal route is preferred over the sublingual route for sustained-release delivery because of the greater mucosal surface area of the former. Drugs formulated for buccal administration generally do not cause irritation and are small enough to not cause discomfort to the patient. As with the sublingual route, drugs administered by the buccal route avoid first-pass metabolism by the liver and the enzymatic processes of the stomach and

(a)
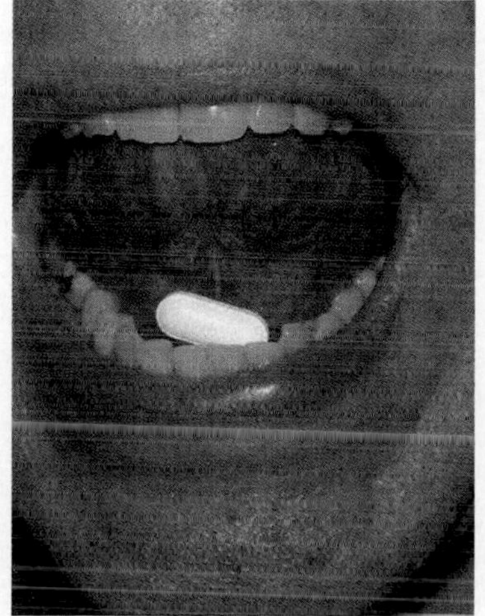

(b)
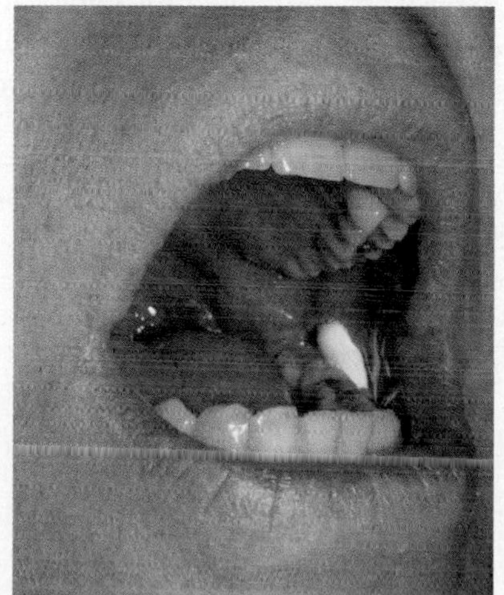

FIGURE 3.1 (a) Sublingual drug administration; (b) buccal drug administration
Pearson Education, Inc.

small intestine. Table 3.3 (section C) and Figure 3.1b provide important guidelines for buccal drug administration.

Rapid-Dissolving Tablets and Films

Orally disintegrating tablets (ODTs) and oral soluble films are newer drug delivery systems that allow for quick dissolving of medications without the need for an external source of water. Both forms are useful for children and for adults with compliance issues. These products usually contain a flavoring or sweetener to make the drug more palatable.

ODTs are designed to dissolve in less than 30 seconds after placement on the tongue. The tablet is small and disintegrates upon contact with saliva. Once dissolved, the saliva containing the drug is swallowed.

The oral soluble film drug delivery system coats the drug on a polymer about the size of a postage stamp. The soluble strip of film is flexible and dissolves very quickly when placed on or under the tongue or on the buccal surface. The first soluble film to receive FDA approval was ondansetron (Zuplenz), which is used for patients with severe nausea and vomiting. Several pediatric medications are now available by this route.

Nasogastric and Gastrostomy Drug Administration

Patients with a nasogastric tube or enteral feeding mechanism such as a gastrostomy tube may have their medications administered through these devices. A nasogastric (NG) tube is a soft, flexible tube inserted by way of the nasopharynx with the tip lying in the stomach. A gastrostomy (G) tube is surgically placed directly into the patient's stomach. Generally, the NG tube is used for short-term treatment, whereas the G tube is inserted for patients requiring long-term care. Drugs administered through these tubes are usually in liquid form. Although solid drugs can be crushed or dissolved, they tend to cause clogging within the tubes. Sustained-release drugs should not be crushed and administered through NG or G tubes. Drugs administered by this route are exposed to the same physiological processes as those given orally. Table 3.3 (section D) gives important guidelines for administering drugs through NG or G tubes.

3.7 Topical Drug Administration

Topical drugs are those applied locally to the skin or the membranous linings of the eye, ear, nose, respiratory tract, urinary tract, vagina, and rectum. These applications include the following:

- *Dermatologic preparations.* Drugs applied to the skin. The topical route is most commonly used. Formulations include creams, lotions, gels, powders, and sprays.
- *Instillations and irrigations.* Drugs applied into body cavities or orifices. These routes may include the eyes, ears, nose, urinary bladder, rectum, and vagina.
- *Inhalations.* Drugs applied to the respiratory tract by inhalers, nebulizers, or positive-pressure breathing apparatuses. The most common indication for inhaled drugs is bronchoconstriction due to bronchitis or asthma; however, a number of illegal, abused drugs are taken by this route because it provides a very rapid onset of drug action (see chapter 22). Additional details on inhalation drug administration can be found in chapter 40.

Many drugs are applied topically to produce a *local* effect. For example, antibiotics may be applied to the skin to treat skin infections. Antineoplastic agents may be instilled into the urinary bladder via catheter to treat tumors of the bladder mucosa. Corticosteroids are sprayed into the nostrils to reduce inflammation of the nasal mucosa due to allergic rhinitis. Local, topical delivery produces fewer side effects compared with oral or parenteral administration of the same drug. This is because topically applied drugs are absorbed very slowly, and amounts reaching the general circulation are minimal.

Some drugs are given topically to provide for slow release and absorption of the drug in the general circulation. These agents are administered for their *systemic* effects. For example, a nitroglycerin patch is applied to the skin not to treat a local skin condition but to treat a systemic condition, such as coronary artery disease. Likewise, prochlorperazine (Compazine) suppositories are inserted rectally not to treat a disease of the rectum but to alleviate nausea.

Treating the Diverse Patient: Religious Fasting and Compliance with Medication Administration

Religious fasting periods are a feature of many of the world's religions. During periods of religious fasting such as Ramadan or Yom Kippur, patients observing a fast may not take their prescribed medications, including non-oral medications such as eyedrops, to avoid "breaking" the fast. Different religions and religious authorities may allow the taking of required medications during the fast, but depending on the patients' compliance with personal religious beliefs, all medications may be avoided even if their religious authority allows them.

By recognizing known periods of religious fasting and discussing the observance of fasting periods with the patient, nurses can explore opportunities to develop strategies with the patient for successful medication use. For example, an alternative form of the medication may be ordered if available (e.g., a 12-hour dose that could be taken before beginning and after ending the fast, rather than an every 6-hour dose). If the patient is unable to comply with medication administration during fasting periods due to religious beliefs, the prescribing health care provider should also be notified.

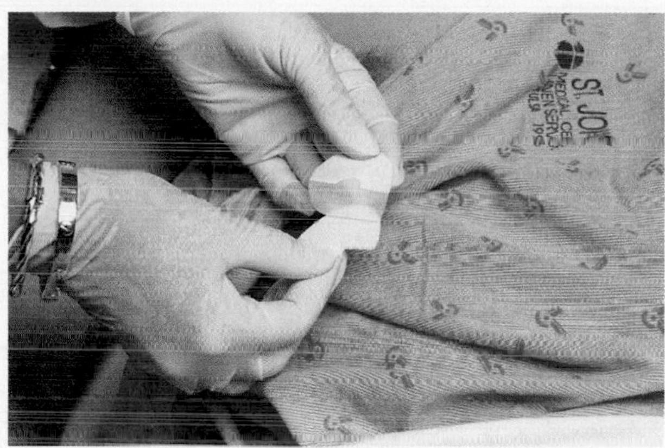

(a)

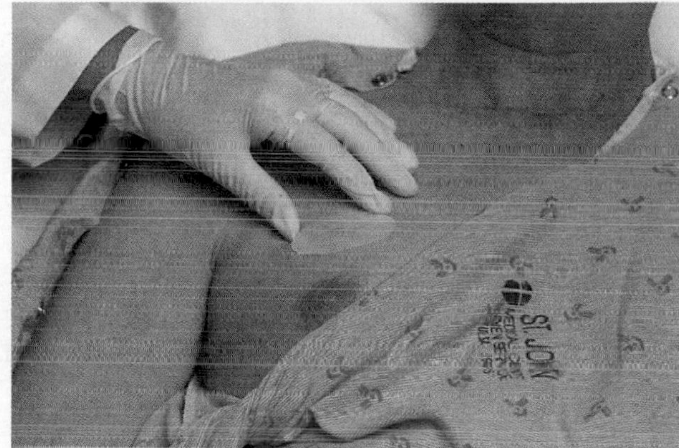

(b)

FIGURE 3.2 Transdermal patch administration: (a) protective coating removed from patch; (b) patch immediately applied to clean, dry, hairless skin and labeled with date, time, and initials
(a) Pearson Education, Inc.; (b) Ph College/Pearson Education, Inc.

The distinction between topical drugs given for local effects and those given for systemic effects is an important one for the nurse. In the case of local drugs, absorption is undesirable and may cause side effects. For systemic drugs, absorption is essential for the therapeutic action of the drug. With either type of topical agent, drugs should not be applied to abraded or denuded skin, unless directed to do so

Transdermal Delivery System

The use of transdermal patches provides an effective means of delivering certain medications. Examples include nitroglycerin for angina pectoris and scopolamine (Transderm-Scop) for motion sickness. Although transdermal patches contain a specific amount of drug, the rate of delivery and the actual dose received may be variable. Patches are changed on a regular basis, using a site rotation routine, which should be documented in the MAR. Before applying a transdermal patch, the nurse should verify that the previous patch has been removed and disposed of appropriately. Drugs to be administered by this route avoid the first-pass effect in the liver and bypass digestive enzymes. Table 3.4 (section A) and Figure 3.2 illustrate the major points of transdermal drug delivery.

Ophthalmic Administration

The ophthalmic route is used to treat local conditions of the eye and surrounding structures. Common indications include excessive dryness, infections, glaucoma, and dilation of the pupil during eye examinations. Ophthalmic drugs are available in the form of eye irrigations, drops, ointments, and medicated disks. Figure 3.3 and Table 3.4 (section B) give guidelines for adult administration. Although the procedure is the same with a child, it is advisable to enlist the help of an adult caregiver. In some cases, the infant or toddler may need to be immobilized with arms wrapped to prevent accidental injury to the eye during administration. For the young child, demonstrating the procedure using a doll facilitates cooperation and decreases anxiety.

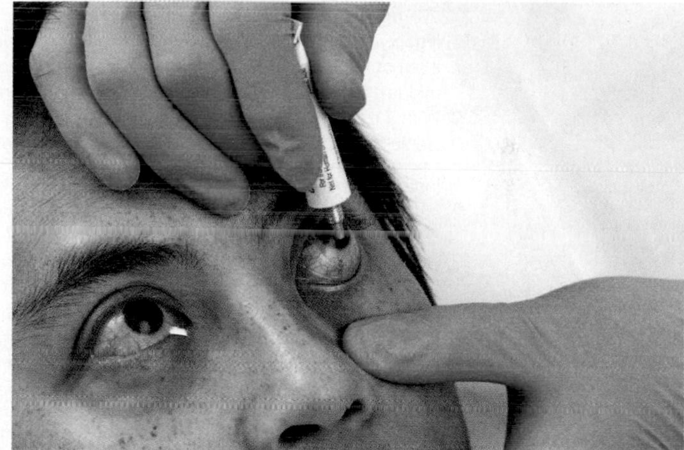

FIGURE 3.3 Instilling an eye ointment into the lower conjunctival sac
Pearson Education, Inc.

Otic Administration

The otic route is used to treat local conditions of the ear, including infections and soft blockages of the auditory canal. Otic medications include eardrops and irrigations, which are usually ordered for cleaning purposes. Administration to infants and young children must be performed carefully to avoid injury to the sensitive structures of the ear. Figure 3.4 and Table 3.4 (section C) present key points in administering otic medications.

Nasal Administration

The nasal route is used for both local and systemic drug administration. The nasal mucosa provides an excellent absorptive surface for certain medications. Advantages of this route include ease of use and avoidance of the first-pass effect and digestive enzymes. Nasal spray formulations of corticosteroids have revolutionized the treatment of allergic rhinitis owing to their high safety margin when administered by this route.

Although the nasal mucosa provides an excellent surface for drug delivery, there is the potential for damage to the cilia within the nasal cavity, and mucosal irritation is

Table 3.4 Topical Drug Administration

Drug Form (Example)	Administration Guidelines
A. Transdermal	1. Obtain the transdermal patch, and read the manufacturer's guidelines. Application site and frequency of changing differ according to the medication. 2. Apply gloves before handling to avoid absorption of the agent by the nurse. 3. Label the patch with the date, time, and the nurse's initials. 4. Remove the previous medication or patch and cleanse the area. 5. If using a transdermal ointment, apply the ordered amount of medication in an even line directly on the premeasured paper that accompanies the medication tube. 6. Press the patch or apply the medicated paper to clean, dry, and hairless skin. Many transdermal patches have pressure activated adhesive. The rate of drug release may also be altered by external factors like heat. Apply firm pressure to the patch without heat. 7. Rotate sites to prevent skin irritation.
B. Ophthalmic	1. Instruct the patient to lie supine or sit with the head slightly tilted back. 2. With the nondominant hand, pull the lower lid down gently to expose the conjunctival sac, creating a pocket. 3. Ask the patient to look upward. 4. Hold the eyedropper 1/4–1/8 inch above the conjunctival sac. Do not hold the dropper over the eye, as this may stimulate the blink reflex. 5. Instill the prescribed number of drops into the center of the pocket. Avoid touching the eye or conjunctival sac with the tip of the eye-dropper. 6. If applying ointment, apply a thin line of ointment evenly along the inner edge of the lower lid margin, from inner to outer canthus. 7. Instruct the patient to close the eye gently. Apply gentle pressure with a finger to the nasolacrimal duct at the inner canthus for 1–2 minutes to avoid overflow drainage into the nose and throat, thus minimizing the risk of absorption into the systemic circulation. 8. With a tissue, gently blot or remove excess medication around the eye. 9. Replace the dropper into the bottle if it comes separately. Do not rinse the eyedropper.
C. Otic	1. Instruct the patient to lie on the opposite side of administration or to sit with the head tilted so that the affected ear is facing up. 2. If necessary, clean the pinna of the ear and the meatus with a clean washcloth or gauze to prevent any discharge from being washed into the ear canal during the instillation of the drops. 3. Hold the dropper 1/4 inch above the ear canal, and instill the prescribed number of drops into the side of the ear canal, allowing the drops to flow downward. Avoid placing the drops directly on the tympanic membrane. 4. Gently apply intermittent pressure to the tragus of the ear three or four times. 5. Instruct the patient to remain in a side-lying position for up to 10 minutes to prevent loss of medication. 6. If a cotton ball is ordered, presoak with medication and insert it into the outermost part of the ear canal. 7. Wipe any solution that may have dripped from the ear canal with a tissue.
D. Nasal drops	1. Ask the patient to blow the nose to clear the nasal passages. 2. Draw up the correct volume of drug into the dropper. 3. Instruct the patient to open and breathe through the mouth. 4. Hold the tip of the dropper just above the nostril and, without touching the nose with the dropper, direct the solution laterally toward the midline of the superior concha of the ethmoid bone—not the base of the nasal cavity, where it will run down the throat and into the eustachian tube. 5. Ask the patient to remain in position for 5 minutes. 6. Discard any remaining solution that is in the dropper.
E. Vaginal	1. Instruct the patient to assume a supine position with knees bent and separated. 2. Place water-soluble lubricant into a medicine cup. 3. Apply gloves; open the suppository and lubricate the rounded end. 4. Expose the vaginal orifice by separating the labia with the nondominant hand. 5. Insert the rounded end of the suppository about 8–10 cm along the posterior wall of the vagina or as far as it will pass. 6. If using a cream, jelly, or foam, gently insert the applicator 5 cm along the posterior vaginal wall and slowly push the plunger until empty. Remove the applicator and place it on a paper towel. 7. Ask the patient to lower the legs and remain lying in the supine or side-lying position for 5–10 minutes following insertion. A sanitary pad may be required to prevent soiling of underclothes or bed.
F. Rectal suppositories	1. Instruct the patient to lie on the left side (Sims' position). 2. Place water-soluble lubricant into a medicine cup. 3. Apply gloves; open the suppository and lubricate the blunt end. Suppositories are designed for the rounded end to be facing out to exert less pressure on the internal anal sphincter, thereby decreasing the patient's urge to push it out. 4. Lubricate the gloved forefinger of the dominant hand with water-soluble lubricant. 5. Inform the patient when the suppository is to be inserted; instruct the patient to take slow, deep breaths and deeply exhale during insertion, to relax the anal sphincter. 6. Gently insert the lubricated end of the suppository into the rectum, beyond the anal–rectal ridge to ensure retention. 7. Instruct the patient to remain in the Sims' position or to lie supine to prevent expulsion of the suppository. 8. Instruct the patient to retain the suppository for at least 30 minutes to allow absorption to occur, unless the suppository is administered to stimulate defecation.

common. In addition, unpredictable mucus secretion among some individuals may affect drug absorption from this site.

Drops or sprays are often used for their local **astringent effect;** that is, they shrink swollen mucous membranes or loosen secretions and facilitate drainage. This brings immediate relief from the nasal congestion caused by the common cold. The nose also provides the route to reach the nasal sinuses and the eustachian tube. Proper positioning of

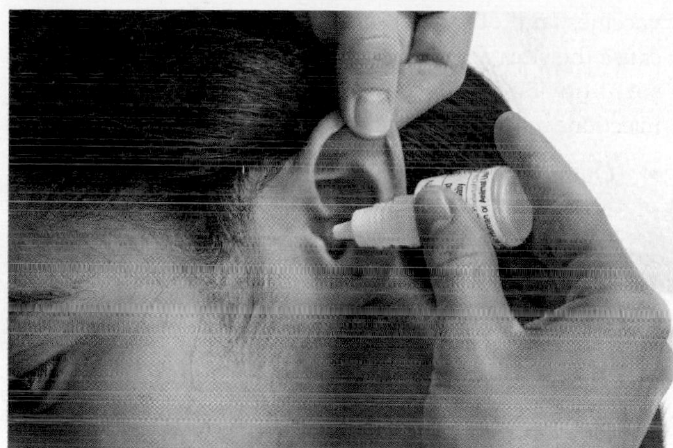

FIGURE 3.4 Instilling eardrops
Andy Crawford/DK Images.

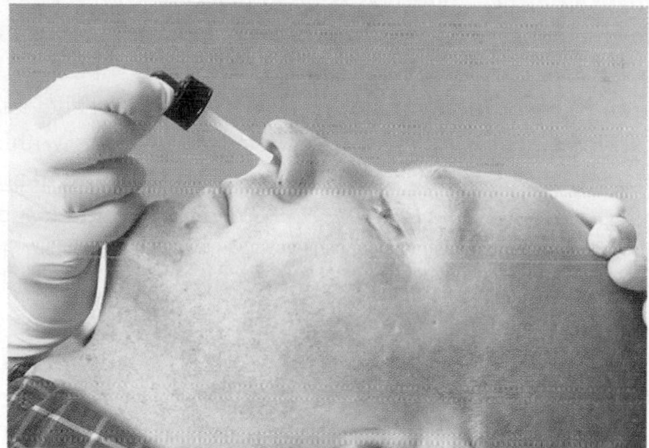

FIGURE 3.5 Nasal drug administration
Ph College/Pearson Education, Inc.

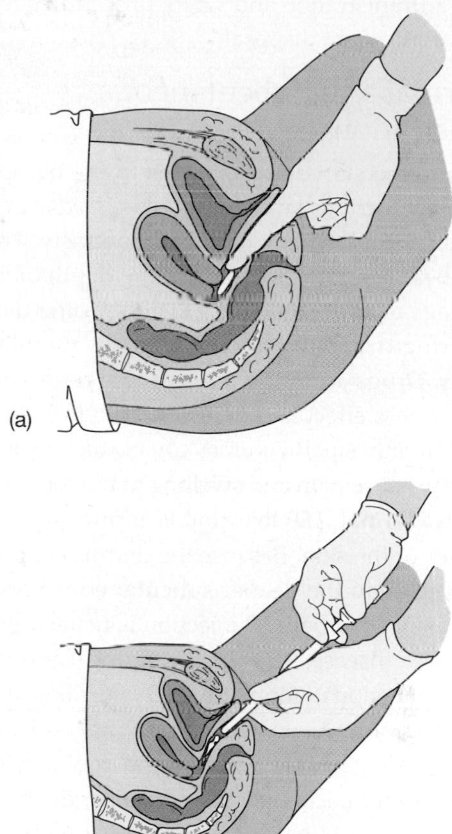

FIGURE 3.6 Vaginal drug administration: (a) instilling a vaginal suppository; (b) using an applicator to instill a vaginal cream

the patient prior to instilling nose drops for sinus disorders depends on which sinuses are being treated. The same holds true for treatment of the eustachian tube. Table 3.4 (section D) and Figure 3.5 illustrate important facts related to nasal drug administration.

Vaginal Administration

The vaginal route is used to deliver medications for treating local infections and to relieve vaginal pain and itching. Vaginal medications are inserted as suppositories, creams, jellies, or foams. It is important that the nurse explain the purpose of treatment and provide for privacy and patient dignity. Before inserting vaginal drugs, the nurse should instruct the patient to empty her bladder to lessen both the discomfort during treatment and the possibility of irritating or injuring the vaginal lining. The patient should be offered a perineal pad following administration. Table 3.4 (section E) and Figure 3.6 (a) and (b) provide guidelines regarding vaginal drug administration.

Rectal Administration

The rectal route may be used for either local or systemic drug administration. It is a safe and effective means of delivering drugs to patients who are comatose or who are experiencing nausea and vomiting. Rectal drugs are normally in suppository form, although a few laxatives and diagnostic agents are given via enema. Although absorption is slower than by other routes, it is steady and reliable provided the medication can be retained by the patient. Venous blood from the lower rectum is not transported by way of the liver; thus, the first-pass effect is avoided, as are the digestive enzymes of the upper GI tract. Table 3.4 (section F) gives selected details regarding rectal drug administration.

3.8 Parenteral Drug Administration

Parenteral administration refers to the dispensing of medications by routes other than oral or topical. The **parenteral route** delivers drugs via a needle into the skin layers, subcutaneous tissue, muscles, or veins. More advanced parenteral delivery includes administration into arteries, body cavities (such as intrathecal), and organs (such as intracardiac). Parenteral drug administration is much more invasive than topical or enteral. Because of the potential for introducing pathogenic microbes directly into the blood or body tissues, aseptic techniques must be strictly applied. The nurse is expected to identify and use appropriate materials for parenteral drug delivery, including specialized equipment and techniques involved in the preparation and administration of injectable products. The nurse must know the correct anatomic locations for parenteral administration and safety procedures regarding hazardous equipment disposal.

Intradermal and Subcutaneous Administration

Injection into the skin delivers drugs to the blood vessels that supply the various layers of the skin. Drugs may be injected either intradermally or subcutaneously. The major difference between these methods is the depth of injection. An advantage of both methods is that they offer a means of administering drugs to patients who are unable to take them orally. Drugs administered by these routes avoid the hepatic first-pass effect and digestive enzymes. Disadvantages are that only small volumes can be administered, and injections can cause pain and swelling at the injection site.

An **intradermal (ID)** injection is administered into the dermis layer of the skin. Because the dermis contains more blood vessels than the deeper subcutaneous layer, drugs are more easily absorbed. ID injection is usually employed for allergy and disease screening or for local anesthetic delivery prior to venous cannulation. ID injections are limited to very small volumes of drug, usually only 0.1 to 0.2 mL. The usual sites for ID injections are the nonhairy skin surfaces of the upper back, over the scapulae, the high upper chest, and the inner forearm. Guidelines for intradermal injections are given in Table 3.5 (section A) and Figure 3.7.

A **subcutaneous** injection is delivered to the deepest layers of the skin. Insulin, heparin, vitamins, some vaccines, and other medications are given in this area because the sites are easily accessible and provide rapid absorption. Body sites that are ideal for subcutaneous injections include the following:

- Outer aspect of the upper arms, in the area above the triceps muscle
- Middle two-thirds of the anterior thigh area
- Subscapular areas of the upper back
- Upper dorsogluteal and ventrogluteal areas
- Abdominal areas, above the iliac crest and below the diaphragm, 1.5 to 2 inches out from the umbilicus.

Subcutaneous doses are small in volume, usually ranging from 0.5 to 1 mL. The needle size varies with the patient's quantity of body fat. The length is usually half the size of a pinched/bunched skinfold that can be grasped between the thumb and forefinger. It is important to rotate injection sites in an orderly and documented manner to promote absorption, minimize tissue damage, and alleviate discomfort. For insulin, however, rotation should be within an anatomic area to promote reliable absorption and maintain consistent blood glucose levels. When performing subcutaneous injections, it is usually not necessary to aspirate prior to the injection. It depends on what is being injected and the patient's anatomy. Aspiration might prevent inadvertent administration into a vein or artery in a thin person. If the medication should not be administered directly into a vessel, aspiration is recommended. For example,

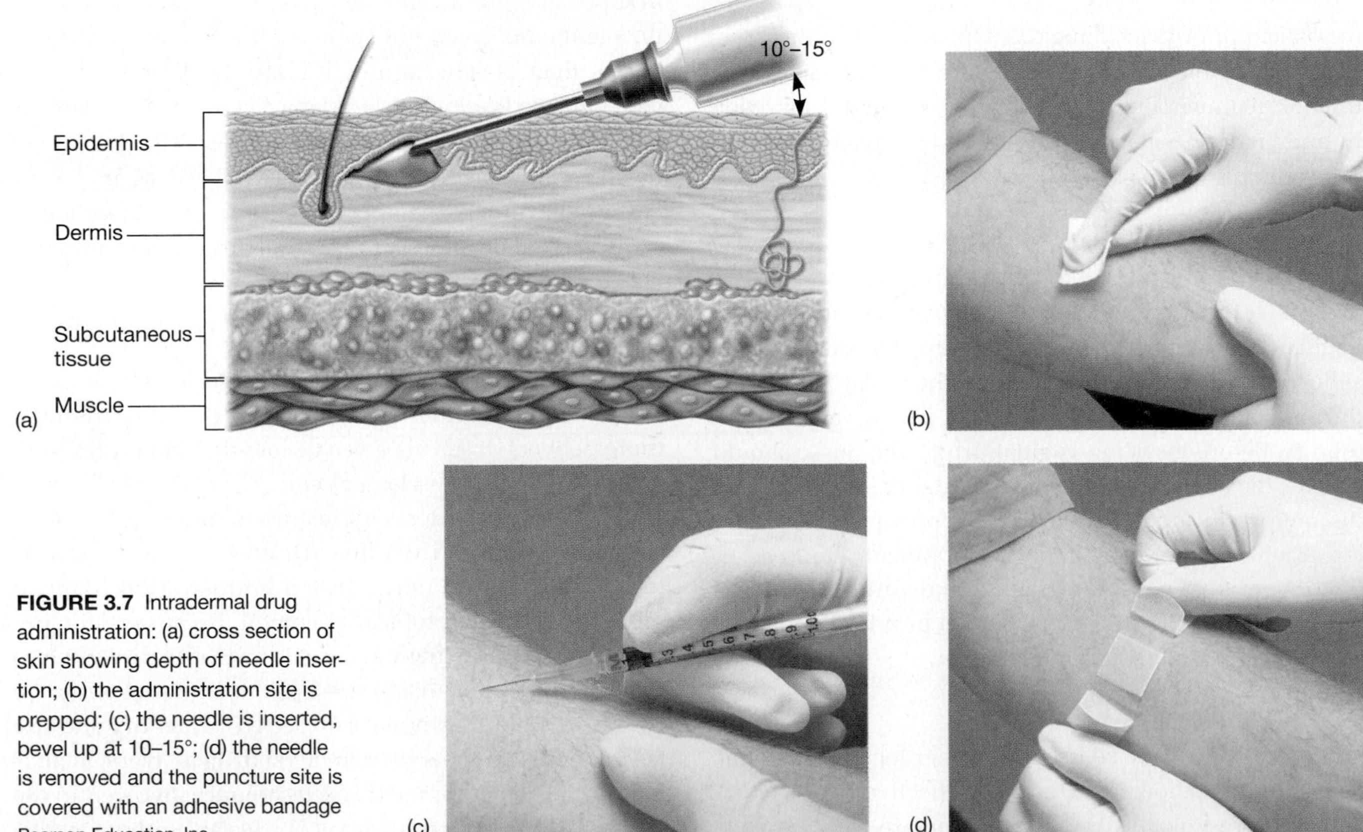

FIGURE 3.7 Intradermal drug administration: (a) cross section of skin showing depth of needle insertion; (b) the administration site is prepped; (c) the needle is inserted, bevel up at 10–15°; (d) the needle is removed and the puncture site is covered with an adhesive bandage
Pearson Education, Inc.

Table 3.5 Parenteral Drug Administration

Drug Form	Administration Guidelines
A. Intradermal route	1. Verify the order and prepare the medication in a tuberculin or 1-mL syringe with a preattached 26- to 27-gauge, 3/8- to 5/8-inch needle. 2. Apply gloves and cleanse the injection site with antiseptic swab in a circular motion. Allow to air dry. 3. With the thumb and index finger of the nondominant hand, spread the skin taut. 4. Insert the needle, with the bevel facing upward, at an angle of 10–15°. 5. Advance the needle until the entire bevel is under the skin; do not aspirate. 6. Slowly inject the medication to form a small wheal or bleb. 7. Withdraw the needle quickly, and pat the site gently with a sterile 2 × 2 gauze pad. Do not massage the area. 8. Instruct the patient not to rub or scratch the area. 9. Draw a circle around the perimeter of the injection site. Read in 48 to 72 hours.
B. Subcutaneous route	1. Verify the order and prepare the medication in a 1- to 3-mL syringe using a 23- to 25-gauge, ½- to ⅝-inch needle. For heparin, the recommended needle is ⅜ inch and 25–26 gauge. 2. Choose the site, avoiding areas of bony prominence, major nerves, and blood vessels. For heparin and other parenteral anticoagulants, check with agency policy for the preferred injection sites. 3. Check the previous rotation sites and select a new area for injection. 4. Apply gloves and cleanse the injection site with antiseptic swab in a circular motion. 5. Allow to air dry. 6. Bunch the skin between the thumb and index finger of the nondominant hand. 7. Insert the needle at a 45° or 90° angle depending on body size: 90° if obese; 45° if average weight. If the patient is very thin, gather the skin at the area of needle insertion and administer at a 90° angle. 8. Inject the medication slowly. 9. Remove the needle quickly, and gently massage the site with antiseptic swab. For heparin and other parenteral anticoagulants, do not massage the site, as this may cause increased bruising or bleeding.
C. Intramuscular route: ventrogluteal (different administration guidelines would apply to the dorsogluteal, vastus lateralis, and deltoid muscle sites)	1. Verify the order and prepare the medication using a 20- to 23-gauge, 1- to 1.5-inch needle. 2. Apply gloves and cleanse the ventrogluteal injection site with antiseptic swab in a circular motion. Allow to air dry. 3. Locate the site by placing the hand with the heel on the greater trochanter and the thumb toward the umbilicus. Point to the anterior iliac spine with the index finger, spreading the middle finger to point toward the iliac crest (forming a V). Inject the medication within the V-shaped area of the index and third finger. (Note: This is how to locate the ventrogluteal site.) 4. Insert the needle with a smooth, dartlike movement at a 90° angle within the V-shaped area. 5. Depending on agency policy and type of drug, aspirate, and observe for blood. If blood appears, withdraw the needle, discard the syringe, and prepare a new injection. 6. Inject the medication slowly and with smooth, even pressure on the plunger. 7. Remove the needle quickly. 8. Apply pressure to the site with a dry, sterile 2 × 2 gauze and massage to promote absorption of the medication into the muscle.
D. Intravenous route	1. To add a drug to an IV fluid container: 2. Verify the order and compatibility of the drug with the IV fluid. 3. Prepare the medication in a 5- to 20-mL syringe using a 1- to 1.5-inch, 19- to 21-gauge needle from the original medication vial or ampule. If a needleless system is used, use the appropriate syringe or tip required per the system in use. 4. Apply gloves and assess the injection site for signs and symptoms of inflammation or extravasation. 5. Locate the medication port on the IV fluid container and cleanse with antiseptic swab. 6. Carefully insert the needle or needleless access device into the port and inject the medication. 7. Withdraw the needle and mix the solution by rotating the container end to end. 8. Hang the container and check the infusion rate. 9. To add drug to an IV bolus (IV push) using an existing IV line or IV lock (reseal): 10. Verify the order and compatibility of the drug with the IV fluid. 11. Determine the correct rate of infusion. 12. Determine whether IV fluids are infusing at the proper rate (IV line) and that the IV site is adequate. 13. Prepare the drug in a syringe, following the procedure described above. 14. Apply gloves and assess the injection site for signs and symptoms of inflammation or extravasation. 15. Select the injection port, on tubing, closest to the insertion site (IV line). 16. Cleanse the tubing or lock port with antiseptic swab and insert the needle into the port. 17. If administering medication through an existing IV line, occlude tubing by pinching just above the injection port. 18. Slowly inject the medication over the designated time—usually not faster than 1 mL/min, unless specified. 19. Withdraw the syringe. Release the tubing and ensure proper IV infusion if using an existing IV line. 20. If using an IV lock, check agency policy for use of saline flush before and after injecting medications.

long-acting insulins should not be given IV; therefore, aspiration is justified. Heparin, on the other hand, can be safely administered IV, and so aspiration is not required. Note that tuberculin syringes and insulin syringes are not interchangeable, so the nurse should not substitute one for the other. Table 3.5 (section B) and Figure 3.8 include important information regarding subcutaneous drug administration.

Intramuscular Administration

An **intramuscular (IM)** injection delivers medication into specific muscles. Because muscle tissue has a rich blood supply, medication moves quickly into blood vessels to produce a more rapid onset of action than with oral, ID, or subcutaneous administration. The anatomic structure of muscle permits this tissue to receive a larger volume of medication than the

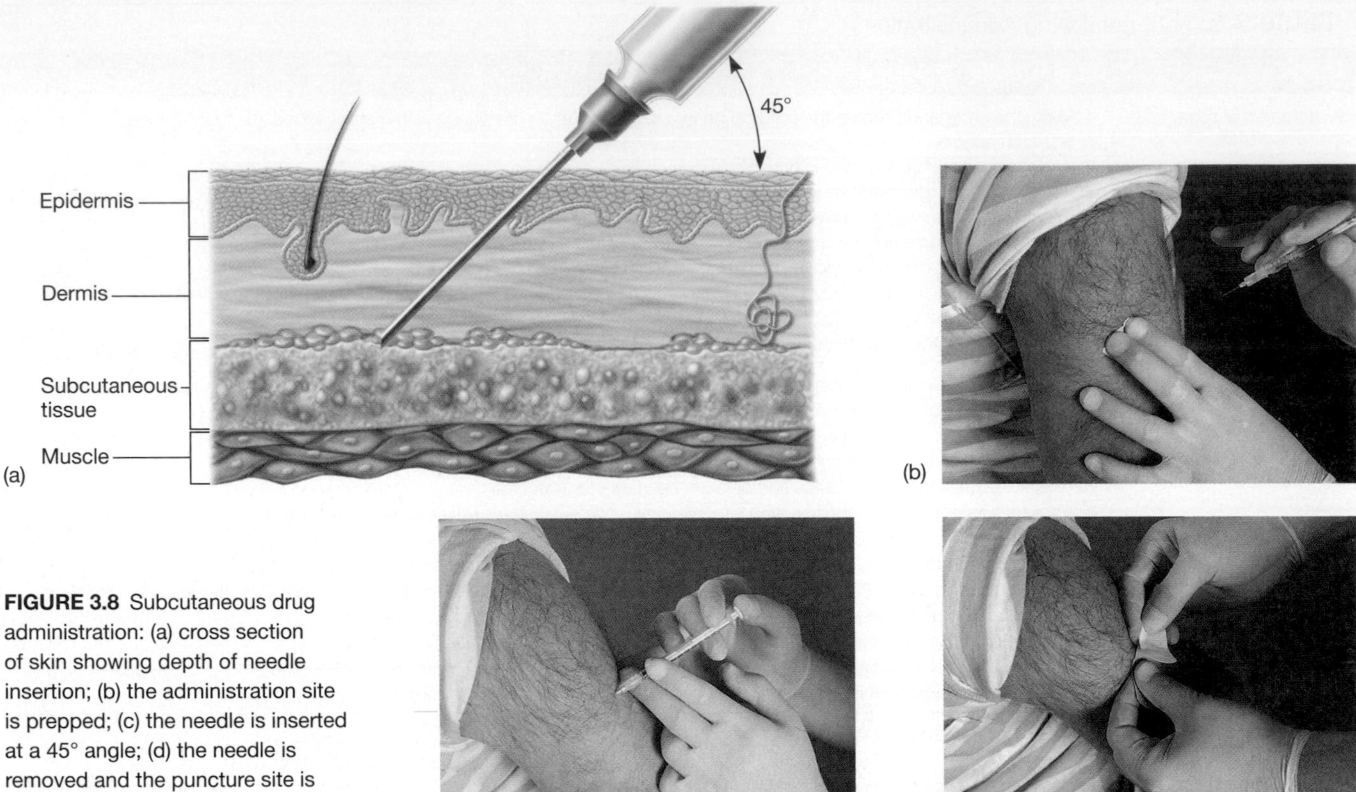

FIGURE 3.8 Subcutaneous drug administration: (a) cross section of skin showing depth of needle insertion; (b) the administration site is prepped; (c) the needle is inserted at a 45° angle; (d) the needle is removed and the puncture site is covered with an adhesive bandage
Pearson Education, Inc.

subcutaneous region. An adult with well-developed muscles can safely tolerate up to 3 mL of medication in a large muscle, although only 2 mL is recommended. The deltoid and triceps muscles should receive a maximum of 1 mL.

A major consideration for the nurse regarding IM drug administration is the selection of an appropriate injection site. Injection sites must be located away from bone, large blood vessels, and nerves. The size and length of the needle are determined by body size and muscle mass, the type of drug to be administered, the amount of adipose tissue overlying the muscle, and the age of the patient. Information regarding IM injections is given in Table 3.5 (section C) and Figure 3.9. The four common sites for intramuscular injections are as follows:

1. *Ventrogluteal site.* This is the preferred site for IM injections. This area provides the greatest thickness of gluteal muscles, contains no large blood vessels or nerves, is sealed off by bone, and contains less fat than the buttock area, thus eliminating the need to determine the depth of subcutaneous fat. It is a suitable site for children and infants over 7 months of age.
2. *Deltoid site.* This site is used in well-developed teens and adults for volumes of medication not to exceed 1 mL. Because the radial nerve lies in close proximity, the deltoid is not generally used, except for small-volume vaccines, such as for hepatitis B in adults.
3. *Dorsogluteal site.* This site is used for adults and for children who have been walking for at least 6 months. The site is rarely used due to the potential for damage to the sciatic nerve.
4. *Vastus lateralis site.* The vastus lateralis is usually thick and well developed in both adults and children. The middle third of the muscle is the site for IM injections.

Intravenous Administration

Intravenous (IV) medications and fluids are administered directly into the bloodstream and are immediately available for use by the body. The IV route is used when a very rapid onset of action is desired. As with other parenteral routes, IV medications bypass the enzymatic process of the digestive system and the first-pass effect of the liver. The three basic types of IV administration are as follows:

1. *Large-volume infusion.* This type of IV administration is for fluid maintenance, replacement, or supplementation. Compatible drugs may be mixed into a large-volume IV container with fluids such as normal saline or Ringer's lactate. Table 3.5 (section D) and Figure 3.10 illustrate this technique.
2. *Intermittent infusion.* This is a small amount of IV solution that is arranged in tandem with or piggybacked to the primary large-volume infusion (Figure 3.11). It is used to instill adjunct medications, such as antibiotics or analgesics, over a short time period.
3. *IV bolus (push) administration.* This is a concentrated dose delivered directly to the circulation via syringe to

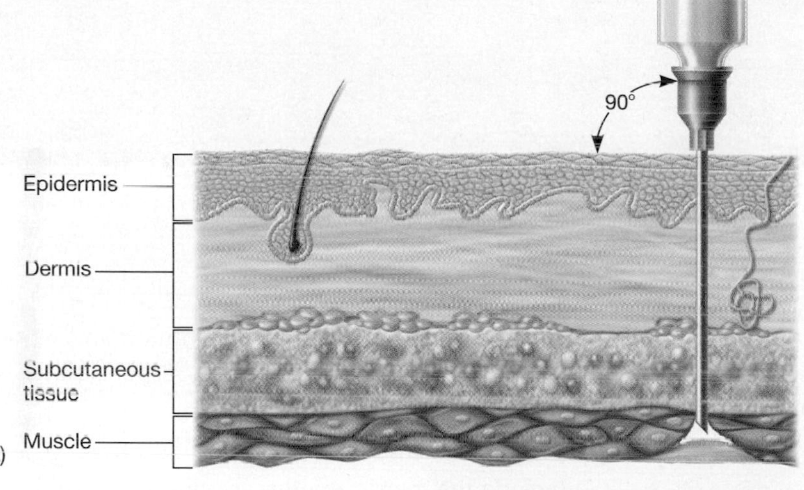

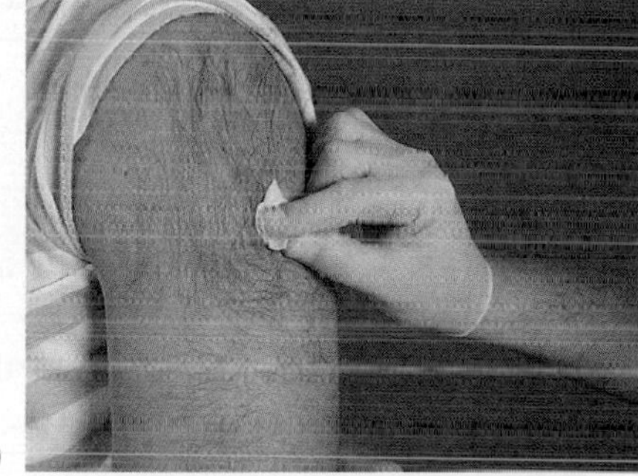

FIGURE 3.9 Intramuscular drug administration: (a) cross section of skin showing depth of needle insertion; (b) the administration site is prepped; (c) the needle is inserted at a 90° angle; (d) the needle is removed and the puncture site is covered with an adhesive bandage
Pearson Education, Inc.

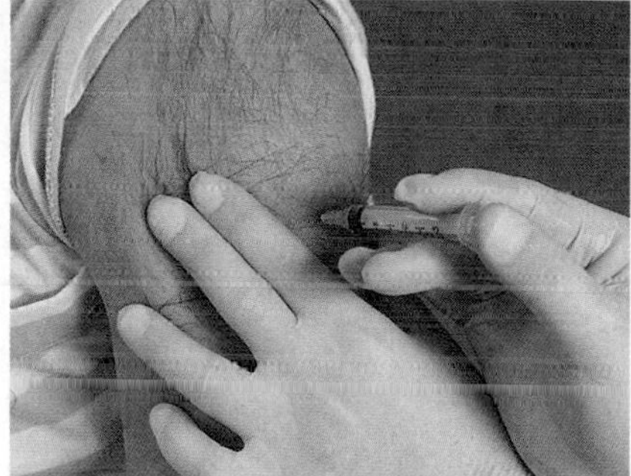

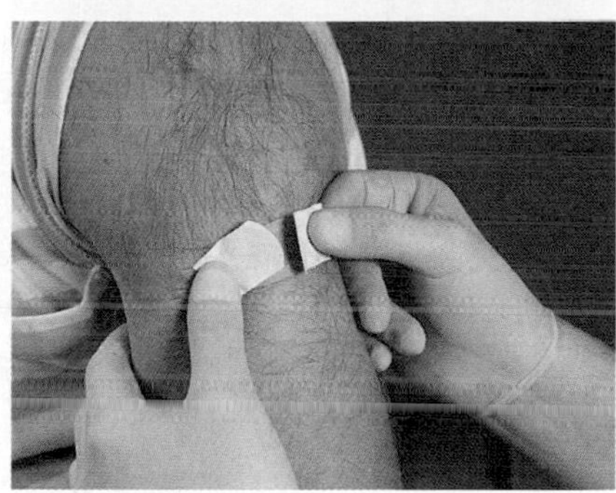

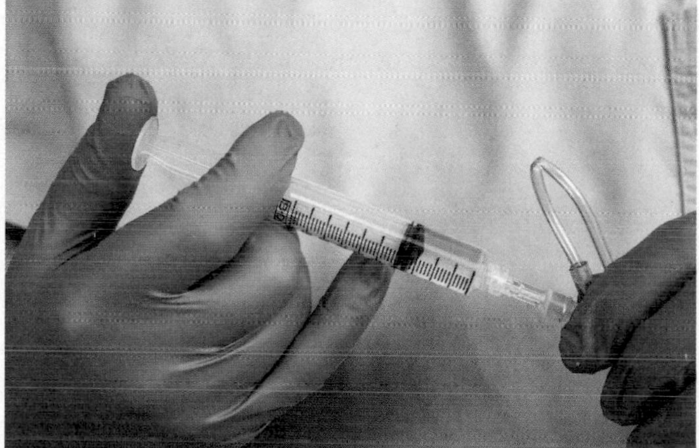

FIGURE 3.10 Injecting a medication by IV push to an existing IV using a needleless system
Pearson Education, Inc.

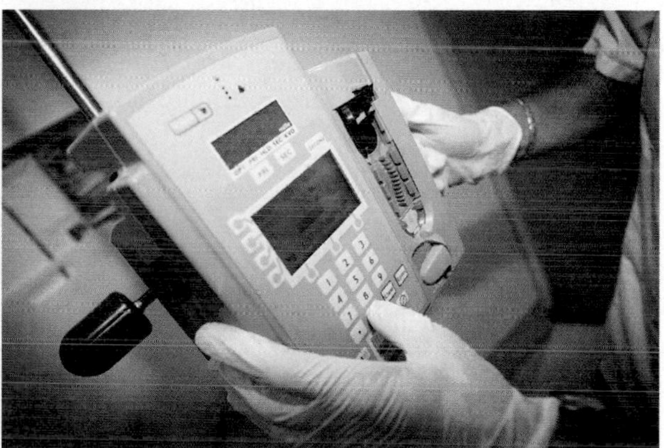

FIGURE 3.11 An infusion pump is used for both continuous and intermittent IV administration
Universal Images Group Limited/Alamy.

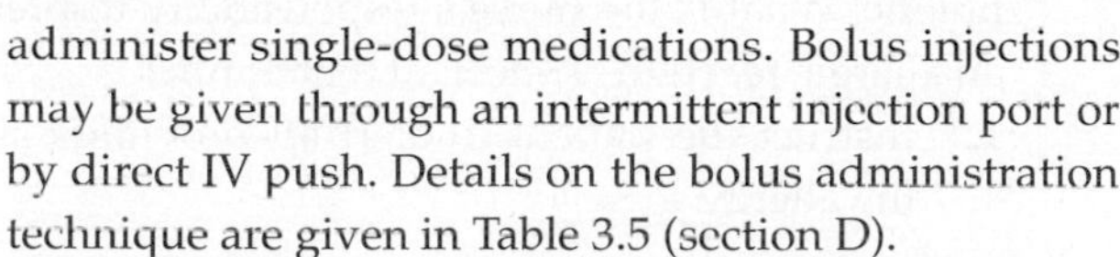

administer single-dose medications. Bolus injections may be given through an intermittent injection port or by direct IV push. Details on the bolus administration technique are given in Table 3.5 (section D).

Although the IV route offers the fastest onset of drug action, it is also the most dangerous. Once injected, the medication cannot be retrieved. If the drug solution or the needle is contaminated, pathogens have a direct route to the bloodstream and body tissues. Patients who are receiving IV injections must be closely monitored for adverse reactions. Some adverse reactions occur immediately after injection; others may take hours or days to appear. Antidotes for drugs that can cause potentially dangerous or fatal reactions must always be readily available.

Chapter Review

KEY Concepts

The numbered key concepts provide a succinct summary of the important points from the corresponding numbered section within the chapter. If any of these points are not clear, refer to the numbered section within the chapter for review.

3.1 The nurse must have a comprehensive knowledge of the actions and side effects of drugs before they are administered to limit the number and severity of adverse drug reactions.

3.2 The five rights and three checks are guidelines for safe drug administration, which is a collaborative effort among the nurse, the health care provider, and other health care professionals.

3.3 For pharmacologic compliance, the patient must understand and personally accept the value associated with the prescribed drug regimen. When pharmacotherapy fails to produce the expected outcomes, noncompliance should be considered a possible explanation.

3.4 There are established orders and time schedules by which medications are routinely administered. Documentation of drug administration and reporting of side effects are important responsibilities of the nurse.

3.5 Systems of measurement used in pharmacology include the metric, apothecary, and household systems. Although the metric system is most commonly used, the nurse must be able to convert dosages among the three systems of measurement.

3.6 The enteral route includes drugs given orally and those administered through nasogastric or gastrostomy tubes. This is the most common route of drug administration.

3.7 Topical drugs are applied locally to the skin or membranous linings of the eye, ear, nose, respiratory tract, urinary tract, vagina, and rectum.

3.8 Parenteral administration is the dispensing of medications via a needle, usually into the skin layers (ID), subcutaneous tissue, muscles (IM), or veins (IV).

REVIEW Questions

1. What is the role of the nurse in medication administration? (Select all that apply.)
   1. Ensure that medications are administered and delivered in a safe manner.
   2. Be certain that health care provider orders are accurate.
   3. Inform the patient that prescribed medications need to be taken only if the patient agrees with the treatment plan.
   4. Ensure that the patient understands the use and administration technique for all prescribed medications.
   5. Prevent adverse drug reactions by properly administering all medications.
2. Before administering drugs by the enteral route, the nurse should evaluate which of the following?
   1. Ability of the patient to lie supine
   2. Compatibility of the drug with intravenous fluid
   3. Ability of the patient to swallow
   4. Patency of the injection port
3. While the nurse takes the patient's admission history, the patient describes having a severe allergy to an antibiotic. What is the nurse's responsibility to prevent an allergic reaction? (Select all that apply.)
   1. Instruct the patient to alert all providers about the allergy.
   2. Document the allergy in the medical record.
   3. Notify the provider and the pharmacy of the allergy and type of allergic reaction.
   4. Place an allergy bracelet on the patient.
   5. Instruct the patient not to allow anyone to give the antibiotic.

4. The order reads, "Lasix 40 mg IV STAT." Which of the following actions should the nurse take?
   1. Administer the medication within 30 minutes of the order.
   2. Administer the medication within 5 minutes of the order.
   3. Administer the medication as required by the patient's condition.
   4. Assess the patient's ability to tolerate the medication before giving.
5. Which of the following medications would not be administered through a nasogastric tube? (Select all that apply.)
   1. Liquids
   2. Enteric-coated tablets
   3. Sustained-release tablets
   4. Finely crushed tablets
   5. IV medications
6. A patient with diabetes has been NPO (nothing by mouth) since midnight for surgery in the morning. He usually takes an oral type 2 antidiabetic drug to control his diabetes. What would be the best action for the nurse to take concerning the administration of his medication?
   1. Hold all medications as ordered.
   2. Give him the medication with a sip of water.
   3. Give him half the original dose.
   4. Contact the provider for further orders.

CRITICAL THINKING Questions

1. Why do errors continue to occur despite the fact that the nurse follows the five rights and three checks of drug administration?
2. What strategies can the nurse employ to ensure drug compliance for a patient who is refusing to take his or her medication?
3. Compare the oral, topical, IM, subcutaneous, and IV routes. Which has the fastest onset of drug action? Which routes avoid the hepatic first-pass effect? Which require strict aseptic technique?
4. What are the differences among a STAT order, an ASAP order, a prn order, and a standing order?

Visit www.pearsonhighered.com/nursingresources for answers and rationales for all activities.

REFERENCES

Berman, A., Snyder, S., & Frandsen, G. F. (2016). *Kozier & Erb's fundamentals of nursing: Concepts, process, and practice* (10th ed.). Hoboken, NJ: Pearson.

Kuo, G. M., Touchette, D. R., & Marinac, J. S. (2013). Drug errors and related interventions reported by United States clinical pharmacists: The American college of clinical pharmacy practice-based research network medication error detection, amelioration and prevention study. *Pharmacotherapy: The Journal of Human Pharmacology and Drug Therapy, 33*, 253–265. doi:10.1002/phar.1195

Latif, A., Rawat, N., Pustavoitau, A., Pronovost, P. J., & Pham, J. C. (2013). National study on the distribution, causes, and consequences of voluntary reported medication errors between the ICU and non-ICU settings. *Critical Care Medicine, 41*(2), 389–398. doi:10.1097/CCM.0b013e318274156a

SELECTED BIBLIOGRAPHY

Buck, M. L. (2013). *Alternative forms of oral drug delivery for pediatric patients.* Retrieved from http://www.medscape.com/viewarticle/807030_1

Giddons, J. F. (2010). *The neighborhood.* Boston, MA: Pearson. Retrieved from http://www.pearsonneighborhood.com

The Joint Commission. (2015). *Facts about the official "Do Not Use" List.* Retrieved from http://www.jointcommission.org/facts_about_do_not_use_list/

Schuster, P., & Nykolyn, L. (2010). *Communication for nurses: How to prevent harmful events and promote patient safety.* Philadelphia, PA: F.A. Davis.

Smith S. F., Duell, D. J., & Martin B., (2011). *Clinical nursing skills* (8th ed.). Upper Saddle River, NJ: Prentice Hall.

Townsend, M. C. (2014). *Essentials of psychiatric mental health nursing: Concepts of care in evidence-based practice* (6th ed.). Philadelphia, PA: F.A. Davis.

U.S. Food and Drug Administration. (2014). *Medication errors.* Retrieved from http://www.fda.gov./drugs/DrugSafety/MedicationErrors/default.htm

U.S. Food and Drug Administration. (2015). MedWatch: The FDA safety information and adverse event reporting program. Retrieved from http://www.fda.gov/Safety/MedWatch/

Chapter 4

Pharmacokinetics

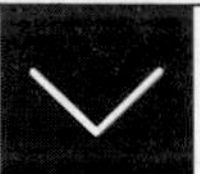

Learning Outcomes

After reading this chapter, the student should be able to:

1. Explain the applications of pharmacokinetics to clinical practice.
2. Identify the four components of pharmacokinetics.
3. Explain how substances travel across plasma membranes.
4. Discuss factors affecting drug absorption.
5. Explain the metabolism of drugs and its applications to pharmacotherapy.
6. Discuss how drugs are distributed throughout the body.
7. Describe how plasma proteins affect drug distribution.
8. Identify major processes by which drugs are excreted.
9. Explain how enterohepatic recirculation might affect drug activity.
10. Explain the applications of a drug's onset, peak, and plasma half-life ($t_{1/2}$) to duration of pharmacotherapy.
11. Explain how a drug reaches and maintains its therapeutic range in the plasma.
12. Differentiate between loading and maintenance doses.

Medications are given to achieve a desirable effect. To produce this effect, the drug must reach its target cells. For some medications, such as topical agents used to treat superficial skin conditions, this is a relatively simple task. For others, however, the process of reaching target cells in sufficient quantities to produce a physiological change may be challenging. Drugs are exposed to a myriad of different barriers and destructive processes after they enter the body. The purpose of this chapter is to examine factors that act on the drug as it travels to reach its target cells.

4.1 Pharmacokinetics: How the Body Handles Medications

The term **pharmacokinetics** is derived from the root words *pharmaco,* which means "medicine," and *kinetics,* which means "movement or motion." Pharmacokinetics is thus the study of drug movement throughout the body. In practical terms, it describes how the body deals with medications. Pharmacokinetics is a core subject in pharmacology, and a firm grasp of this topic allows the nurse to better understand and predict the actions and side effects of medications in patients.

Drugs face numerous obstacles in reaching their target cells. For most medications, the greatest barrier is crossing the many membranes that separate the drug from its target cells. A drug taken by mouth, for example, must cross the plasma membranes of the mucosal cells of the gastrointestinal (GI) tract and the capillary endothelial cells to enter the bloodstream. To leave the bloodstream, the drug must again cross capillary cells, travel through the interstitial fluid, and depending on the mechanism of action, may also need to enter target cells and cellular organelles such as the nucleus, which are surrounded by additional membranes. These are examples of just some of the barriers a drug must successfully penetrate before it can produce a response.

While moving toward target cells and passing through the various membranes, drugs are subjected to numerous physiological processes. For medications given by the enteral route, stomach acid and digestive enzymes often act to break down the drug molecules. Enzymes in the liver and other organs may chemically change the drug molecule to make it less active. If the drug is seen as foreign by the body, phagocytes may attempt to remove it, or an immune response may be triggered. The kidneys, large intestine, and other organs attempt to excrete the medication from the body.

These examples serve to illustrate pharmacokinetic processes: *how the body handles medications.* The many processes of pharmacokinetics are grouped into four categories: absorption, distribution, metabolism, and excretion, as illustrated in Figure 4.1.

4.2 The Passage of Drugs Through Plasma Membranes

Pharmacokinetic variables depend on the ability of a drug to cross plasma membranes. With few exceptions, drugs must penetrate these membranes to produce their effects. Like other chemicals, drugs primarily use two processes to cross body membranes:

1. *Active transport.* This is movement of a chemical against a concentration or electrochemical gradient; *cotransport* involves the movement of two or more chemicals across the membrane. Active transport requires expenditure of energy on the part of the cell.
2. *Diffusion or passive transport.* This is movement of a chemical from an area of higher concentration to an area of lower concentration. This type of movement occurs without any energy expenditure on the part of the cell.

Plasma membranes consist of a lipid bilayer, with proteins and other molecules interspersed in the membrane. This lipophilic membrane is relatively impermeable to large molecules, ions, and polar molecules. These physical characteristics have direct application to pharmacokinetics. For example, drug molecules that are small, nonionized, and lipid soluble will usually pass through plasma membranes by simple diffusion and more easily reach their target cells. Small water-soluble agents such as urea, alcohol, and water can enter through pores in the plasma membrane. Large molecules, ionized drugs, and water-soluble agents, however, will have more difficulty crossing plasma membranes. These agents may use other means to gain entry, such as protein carriers or active transport. Drugs may not need to enter the cell to produce their effects. Once bound to receptors, located on the plasma membrane, some drugs activate second messengers within the cell, which produce physiological changes (see chapter 5).

4.3 Absorption of Medications

Absorption is a process involving the movement of a substance from its site of administration, across body membranes, to circulating fluids. Drugs may be absorbed across the skin and associated mucous membranes, or they may move across membranes that line the GI or respiratory tract. Most drugs, with the exception of a few topical medications, intestinal anti-infectives, and some radiologic contrast agents, must be absorbed to produce an effect.

Absorption is the primary pharmacokinetic factor determining the length of time it takes a drug to produce its effect. In order for an oral drug to be absorbed it must dissolve. The rate of **dissolution** determines how quickly the drug disintegrates and disperses into simpler forms; therefore, drug formulation is an important factor of bioavailability. In

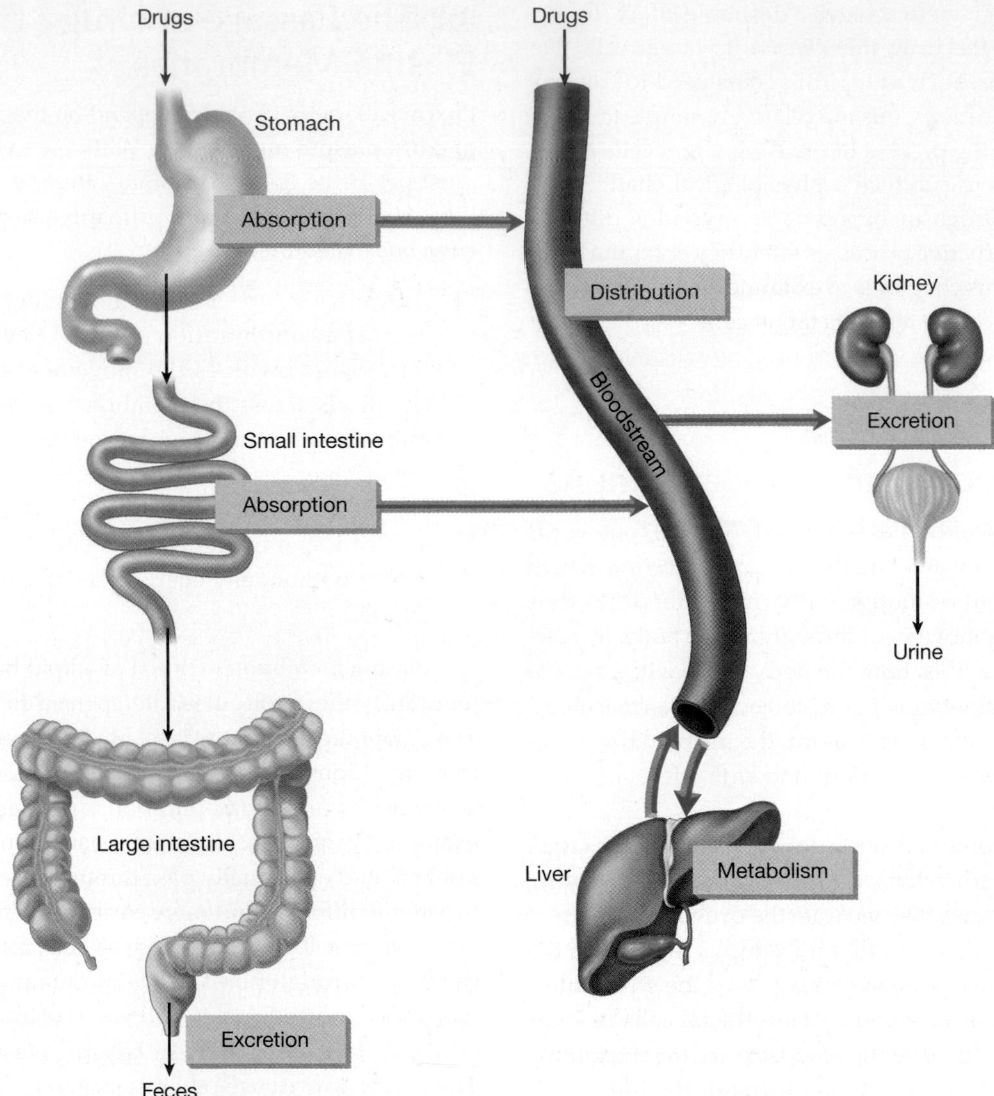

FIGURE 4.1 The four processes of pharmacokinetics: absorption, distribution, metabolism, and excretion

general, the more rapid the dissolution, the faster the drug absorption and the faster the onset of drug action. For example, famotidine (Pepcid RPD) administered as an orally disintegrating tablet dissolves within seconds and after being swallowed immediately blocks acid secretion from the stomach, thereby treating conditions of excessive acid secretion. At the other extreme, some drugs have shown good clinical response as slowly dissolving drugs. Examples are liothyronine sodium (T3) and thyroxine (T4) administered in order to reverse hypothyroid symptoms. In some instances it is advantageous for a drug to disperse rapidly. In other cases, it is better for the drug to be released slowly where the effects are more prolonged for positive therapeutic benefit.

Absorption is affected by many factors. Some general factors that influence the absorption of medications include the following:

- *Drug formulation and dose.* Liquid formulations of an oral drug are absorbed faster than tablets or capsules of the same drug.
- *Dose.* A drug administered at a high dose is generally absorbed more quickly and has a more rapid onset of action than when given in a low concentration.
- *Route of administration.* Drugs administered intravenously (IV) directly enter the bloodstream; thus, absorption to the tissues after the infusion is very rapid. Drugs administered by the oral, topical, intramuscular, and subcutaneous routes take longer to absorb.
- *Size of the drug molecule.* Larger drug molecules take longer to be absorbed than small molecules.
- *Surface area of the absorptive site.* The larger the surface area, the faster the drug will be absorbed.
- *Digestive motility.* Changes in GI motility may either speed up or slow down absorption, depending on the drug and where it is absorbed.
- *Blood flow.* Greater blood flow to the site of drug administration results in faster drug absorption.
- *Lipid solubility of the drug.* Lipid soluble drugs are absorbed more quickly than water soluble drugs.

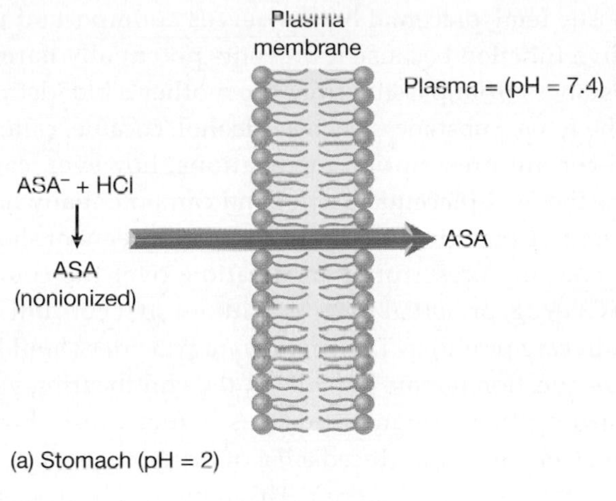

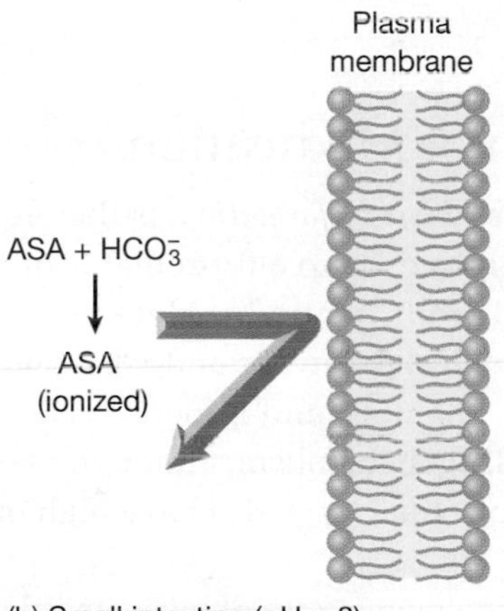

FIGURE 4.2 Effect of pH on drug absorption: (a) a weak acid such as aspirin (ASA) is in a nonionized form in an acidic environment and absorption occurs; (b) in a basic environment, aspirin is mostly in an ionized form and absorption is prevented

The degree of ionization of a drug also affects its absorption. A drug's ability to become ionized depends on the surrounding pH. Aspirin provides an excellent example of the effects of ionization on absorption, as depicted in Figure 4.2. In the acid environment of the stomach, aspirin is in its *nonionized* form and thus readily absorbed and distributed by the bloodstream. As aspirin enters the alkaline environment of the small intestine, however, it becomes *ionized*. In its ionized form, aspirin is not as likely to be absorbed and distributed to target cells. Unlike acidic drugs, medications that are weakly basic are in their nonionized form in an alkaline environment. Therefore, basic drugs are absorbed and distributed better in alkaline environments such as in the small intestine. The pH of the local environment directly influences drug absorption through its ability to ionize the drug. In simplest terms, it may help the nurse to remember that acids are absorbed in acids, and bases are absorbed in bases.

Drug–drug or food–drug interactions may influence absorption. Many examples of these interactions have been discovered. For example, administering tetracyclines with food or drugs containing calcium, iron, or magnesium can significantly delay absorption of the antibiotic. High-fat meals can slow stomach motility significantly and delay the absorption of oral medications taken with the meal. Dietary supplements may also affect absorption. Common ingredients in herbal weight-loss products such as aloe leaf, guar gum, senna, and yellow dock exert a laxative effect that may decrease intestinal transit time and reduce drug absorption. Nurses must be aware of drug interactions and advise patients to avoid known combinations of foods and medications that significantly affect drug action.

4.4 Distribution of Medications

Distribution involves the transport of drugs throughout the body. The simplest factor determining distribution is the amount of blood flow to body tissues. The heart, liver, kidneys, and brain receive the most blood supply. Skin, bone, and adipose tissue receive a lower blood supply; therefore, it is more difficult to deliver high concentrations of drugs to these areas.

The physical properties of the drug greatly influence how it moves throughout the body after administration. Lipid solubility is an important characteristic, because it determines how quickly a drug is absorbed, mixes within the bloodstream, crosses membranes, and becomes localized in body tissues. Lipid-soluble agents are not limited by the barriers that normally stop water-soluble drugs; thus, they are more completely distributed to body tissues.

Some tissues have the ability to accumulate and store drugs after absorption. The bone marrow, teeth, eyes, and adipose tissue have an especially high **affinity,** or attraction, for certain medications. Tetracycline binds to calcium salts and accumulates in the bones and teeth. It may take over a decade after bisphosphonate therapy for these drugs to decline by half in the skeletal system. Once stored, drugs may remain in the body for months to years and then slowly release back into the bloodstream.

Not all drug molecules in the plasma will reach their target cells, because many drugs bind reversibly to plasma proteins, particularly albumin, to form **drug–protein complexes.** Drug–protein complexes are too large to cross capillary membranes; thus, the drug is not available for distribution to body tissues. Drugs bound to proteins circulate in the plasma until they are released or displaced from the drug–protein complex. Only unbound (free) drugs can reach their target cells or be excreted by the kidneys. This concept is illustrated in Figure 4.3. Some drugs, such as the anticoagulant warfarin (Coumadin), are highly bound; 99% of the drug in the plasma is bound in drug–protein complexes and is unavailable to reach target cells.

Drugs and other chemicals compete with one another for plasma protein–binding sites, and some agents have a

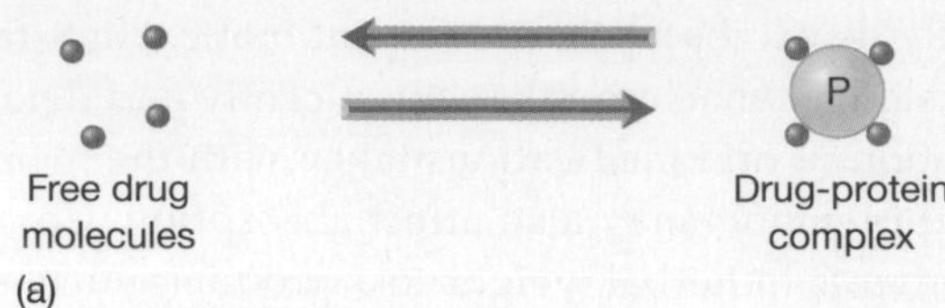

(a)

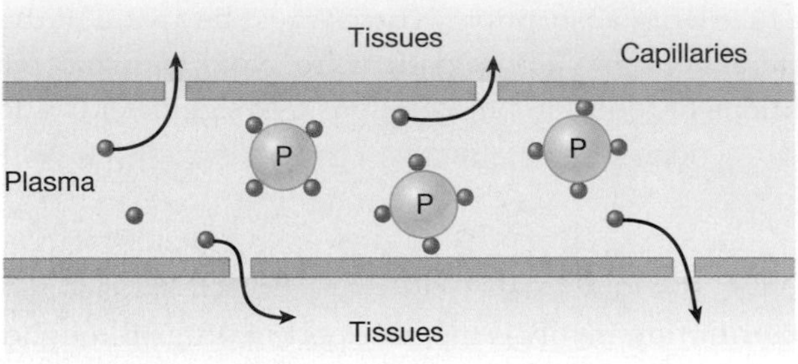

(b)

FIGURE 4.3 Plasma protein binding and drug availability: (a) drug exists in a free state or bound to plasma protein; (b) drug–protein complexes are too large to cross membranes

greater affinity for these binding sites than other agents. Drug–drug and drug–food interactions may occur when one drug displaces another from plasma proteins. The displaced medication can immediately reach high levels in the bloodstream and produce adverse effects. Valproic acid (Depakote, Depakene) or high doses of aspirin, for example, can displace warfarin (Coumadin) from the drug–protein complex, thus raising blood levels of free Coumadin and dramatically enhancing the risk of hemorrhage. Most drug guides give the percentage of medication bound to plasma proteins; when giving multiple drugs that are highly bound, the nurse should monitor the patient closely for adverse effects.

There are several types of drug–drug interactions. These include the following:

- *Addition*. The action of drugs taken together as a *total*
- *Synergism*. The action of drugs resulting in a *potentiated* (more than total) effect
- *Antagonism*. Drugs taken together with *blocked* or *opposite* effects
- *Displacement*. When drugs are taken together, one drug may shift another drug at a nonspecific protein-binding site (e.g., plasma albumin), thereby altering the desired effect.

The brain and placenta possess special anatomic barriers that prevent many chemicals and medications from entering. These barriers are referred to as the **blood–brain barrier** and the **fetal–placental barrier.** Some medications such as sedatives, antianxiety agents, and anticonvulsants readily cross the blood–brain barrier to produce actions in the central nervous system (CNS). In contrast, most antitumor medications do not easily cross this barrier, making brain cancers difficult to treat.

The fetal–placental barrier serves an important protective function because it prevents potentially harmful substances from passing from the mother's bloodstream to the fetus. Substances such as alcohol, cocaine, caffeine, and certain prescription medications, however, easily cross the fetal-placental barrier and can potentially harm the fetus. Consequently, a patient who is pregnant should not take any prescription medication, over-the-counter (OTC) drug, or herbal therapy without first consulting a health care provider. The health care provider should always question female patients in the childbearing years regarding their pregnancy status before prescribing a drug. Chapter 1 introduced a list of drug pregnancy categories for assessing fetal risk. This topic will be discussed further in chapter 8.

4.5 Metabolism of Medications

Metabolism, also called *biotransformation,* is the process of chemically converting a drug to a form that is usually more easily removed from the body. Metabolism involves complex biochemical pathways and reactions that alter drugs, nutrients, vitamins, and minerals. The liver is the primary site of drug metabolism, although the kidneys and cells of the intestinal tract also have high metabolic rates.

Medications undergo many types of biochemical reactions as they pass through the liver, including hydrolysis, oxidation, and reduction. During metabolism, the addition of side chains, known as **conjugates,** makes drugs more water soluble and more easily excreted by the kidneys.

Most metabolism in the liver is accomplished by the **hepatic microsomal enzyme system.** This enzyme complex is sometimes called the P-450 system, named after cytochrome P-450 (CYP-450), which is a key component of the system. As they relate to pharmacotherapy, the primary actions of the hepatic microsomal enzymes are to inactivate drugs and accelerate their excretion. In some cases, however, metabolism can produce a chemical alteration that makes the resulting molecule *more* active than the original. For example, the narcotic analgesic codeine undergoes biotransformation to morphine, which has significantly greater ability to relieve pain. In fact, some agents, known as **prodrugs,** have no pharmacologic activity unless they are first metabolized to their active form by the body. Examples of prodrugs include benazepril (Lotensin) and losartan (Cozaar).

Changes in the function of the hepatic microsomal enzymes can significantly affect drug metabolism. Although a large number of drugs can affect these enzymes, only a limited number have clinical importance. A few drugs have the ability to increase metabolic activity in the liver, a process called **enzyme induction.** For example, phenobarbital causes the liver to synthesize more microsomal enzymes. By doing so, phenobarbital increases the rate of its own metabolism as well as that of certain other drugs that are metabolized in the liver. In these patients, higher doses of medication may be required to achieve the optimal therapeutic effect.

Certain patients have decreased hepatic metabolic activity, which may alter drug action. Hepatic enzyme activity is generally reduced in infants and elderly patients; therefore, pediatric and geriatric patients are more sensitive to drug therapy than middle-age patients. Patients with severe liver damage, such as that caused by cirrhosis, will require reductions in drug dosage because of the decreased metabolic activity. Certain genetic disorders have been recognized in which patients lack specific metabolic enzymes; drug dosages in these patients must be adjusted accordingly. The nurse should pay careful attention to laboratory values that may indicate liver disease so that doses may be adjusted.

Awareness of genetic variations in patients can help nurses recognize which types of medications may be appropriate and why patients might not be responding as anticipated. Knowledge of **pharmacogenomics,** the study of genetic variations that influence an individual's response to drug therapy, can help inform therapeutic decisions and therefore determine the efficacy of a drug for a particular patient and even predict adverse reactions. Knowledge of pharmacogenomics can even help to predict optimal drug dose (chapter 5).

Metabolism has a number of additional therapeutic consequences. As shown in the Pharmacotherapy Illustrated feature, drugs absorbed after oral administration cross directly into the hepatic portal circulation, which carries blood to the liver before it is distributed to other body tissues. Thus, as blood passes through the liver circulation, some drugs can be completely metabolized to an inactive form before they ever reach the general circulation. This **first-pass effect** is an important mechanism, since a large number of oral drugs are rendered inactive by hepatic metabolic reactions. Alternative routes of delivery that bypass the first-pass effect (e.g., sublingual, rectal, or parenteral routes) may need consideration for these drugs.

Pharmacotherapy Illustrated

4.1 | First-Pass Effect: Oral Drug Is Metabolized to an Inactive Form Before It Has an Opportunity to Reach Target Cells

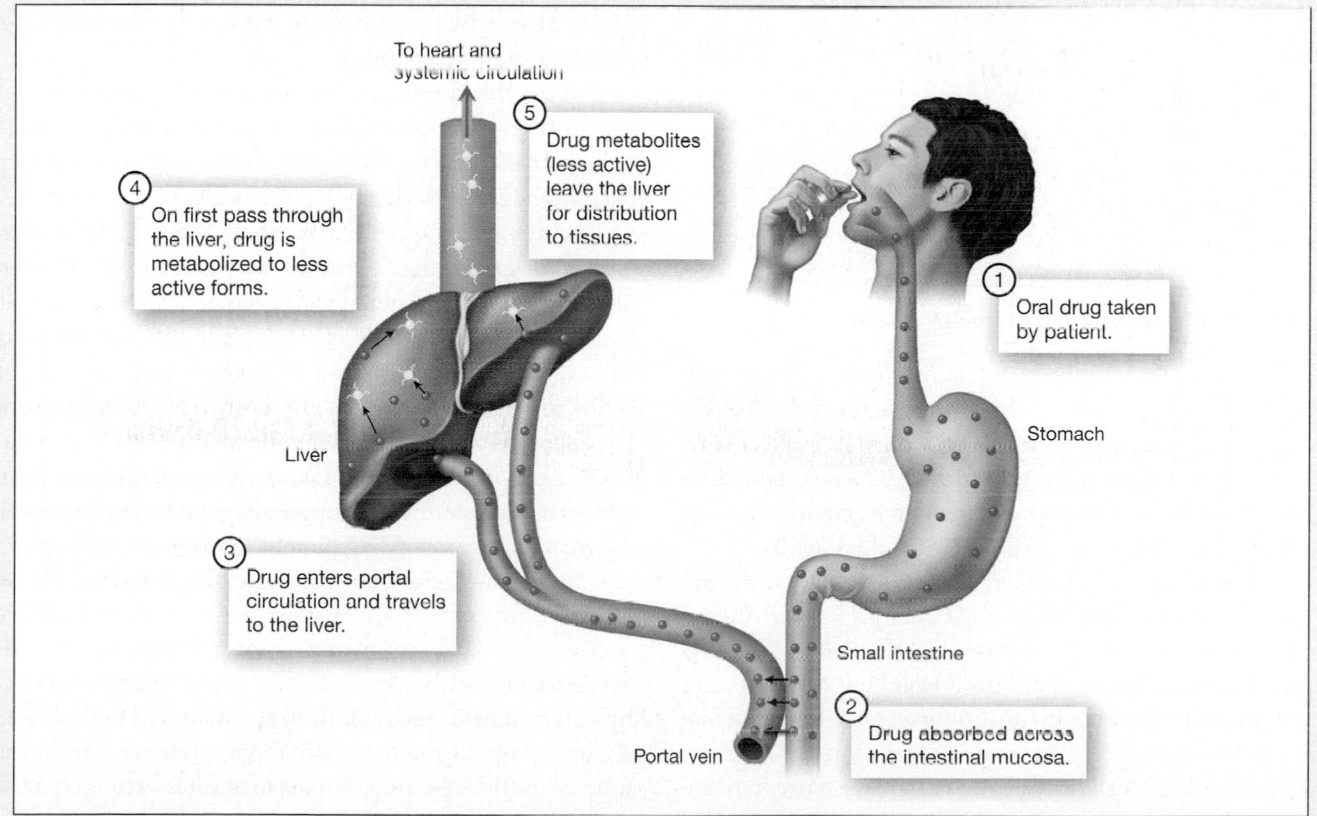

Based on *Pharmacology: Connections to Nursing Practice* (3rd Ed.), by M. Adams and C. Urban. 2016. Reprinted and electronically reproduced by permission of Pearson Education, Inc., Upper Saddle River, New Jersey.

4.6 Excretion of Medications

Drugs are removed from the body by the process of **excretion.** The rate at which medications are excreted is a primary determinant of the concentration of the drugs in the bloodstream and tissues. Excretion is important because the concentration of drugs in the bloodstream determines their duration of action. Pathologic states, such as liver disease or renal failure, often increase the duration of drug action in the body because they interfere with natural excretion mechanisms. Dosing regimens must be carefully adjusted in these patients.

Although drugs are eliminated from the body by numerous organs and tissues, the primary site of excretion is the kidney. In an average-size person, approximately 180 L of blood is filtered by the kidneys each day. Free drugs, water-soluble agents, electrolytes, and small molecules are easily filtered at the glomerulus. Proteins, blood cells, conjugates, and drug–protein complexes are not filtered because of their large size.

After filtration at the renal corpuscle, drugs are subjected to the process of reabsorption in the renal tubule. Mechanisms of reabsorption are the same as absorption elsewhere in the body. Nonionized and lipid-soluble drugs cross renal tubular membranes easily and return to the circulation; ionized and water-soluble drugs generally remain in the filtrate for excretion.

There are many factors that can affect drug excretion. These include the following:

- Liver or kidney impairment
- Blood flow
- Degree of ionization of the drug
- Lipid solubility of the drug
- Drug–protein complexes
- Metabolic activity
- Acidity or alkalinity (pH)
- Respiratory, glandular, or biliary activity.

Drug–protein complexes and substances too large to be filtered at the glomerulus are sometimes secreted into the distal tubule of the nephron. For example, only 10% of a dose of penicillin G is filtered at the glomerulus; 90% is secreted into the renal tubule. As with metabolic enzyme activity, secretion mechanisms are less active in infants and older adults.

Certain drugs may be excreted more quickly if the pH of the filtrate changes. Weak acids such as aspirin are excreted faster when the filtrate is slightly alkaline, because aspirin is ionized in an alkaline environment, and the drug will remain in the filtrate and be excreted in the urine. Weakly basic drugs such as diazepam (Valium) are excreted faster with a slightly acidic filtrate, because they are ionized in this environment. This relationship between pH and drug excretion can be used to advantage in critical care situations. To speed the renal excretion of acidic drugs such as aspirin in an overdosed patient, an order may be written to administer sodium bicarbonate. Sodium bicarbonate will make the urine more basic, which ionizes more aspirin, causing it to be excreted more readily. The excretion of diazepam, on the other hand, can be enhanced by giving ammonium chloride. This will acidify the filtrate and increase the excretion of diazepam.

Impairment of kidney function can dramatically affect pharmacokinetics. Patients with renal failure will have diminished ability to excrete medications and may retain drugs for an extended time. Doses for these patients must be reduced to avoid drug toxicity. Because small to moderate changes in renal status can cause rapid increases in serum drug levels, the nurse must constantly monitor kidney function in patients receiving drugs that may be nephrotoxic. The pharmacotherapy of renal failure is presented in chapter 24.

Drugs that can easily be changed into a gaseous form are especially suited for excretion by the respiratory system. The rate of respiratory excretion is dependent on factors that affect gas exchange, including diffusion, gas solubility, and pulmonary blood flow. The elimination of volatile anesthetics following surgery is primarily dependent on respiratory activity—the faster the respiratory rate, the greater the excretion. Conversely, the respiratory removal of water-soluble agents such as alcohol is more dependent on blood flow to the lungs—the greater the blood flow into lung capillaries, the greater the excretion. In contrast with other methods of excretion, the lungs excrete most drugs in their original nonmetabolized form.

Glandular activity is another elimination mechanism. Water-soluble drugs may be secreted into the saliva, sweat, or breast milk. The odd taste that patients sometimes experience when given IV drugs is an example of the secretion of agents into the saliva. Another example of glandular excretion is the garlic smell that can be detected when standing next to a perspiring person who has recently eaten garlic. Excretion into breast milk is of considerable importance for basic drugs such as morphine or codeine, because these can achieve high concentrations and potentially affect the nursing infant. Nursing mothers should always check with their health care provider before taking any prescription medication, OTC drug, or herbal supplement. Pharmacology of the pregnant or breast-feeding patient is discussed in chapter 8.

Some drugs are secreted in the bile, a process known as *biliary excretion.* In many cases, drugs secreted into bile will enter the duodenum and eventually leave the body in the feces. However, most bile is circulated back to the liver by **enterohepatic recirculation,** as illustrated in Figure 4.4. A percentage of the drug may be recirculated numerous times with the bile. Biliary reabsorption is extremely influential in prolonging the activity of cardiac glycosides, some antibiotics, and phenothiazines. Recirculated drugs are ultimately metabolized by the liver and excreted by the

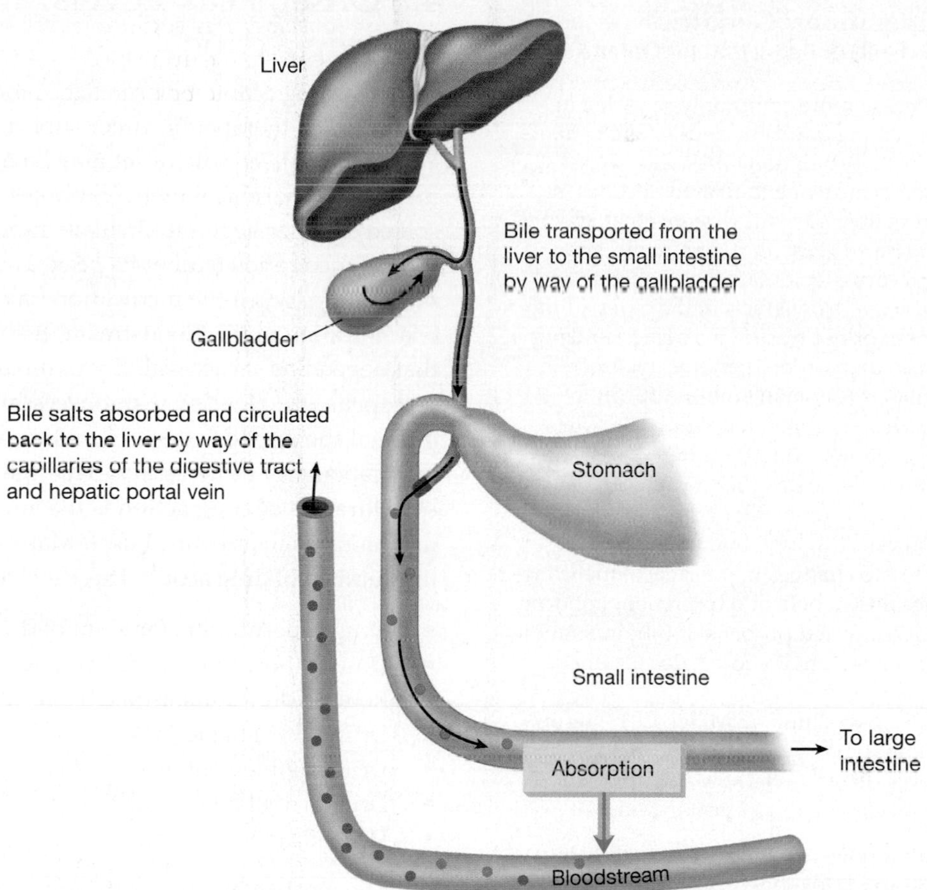

FIGURE 4.4 Enterohepatic recirculation

kidneys. Recirculation and elimination of drugs through biliary excretion may continue for several weeks after therapy has been discontinued.

4.7 Drug Plasma Concentration and Therapeutic Response

The therapeutic response of most drugs is directly related to their level in the plasma. Although the concentration of the medication at its *target tissue* is more predictive of drug action, this quantity is impossible to measure in most cases. For example, it is possible to conduct a laboratory test that measures the serum level of the drug lithium carbonate (Eskalith); it is a far different matter to measure the quantity of this drug in neurons within the CNS. Indeed, it is common practice for nurses to monitor the serum levels of certain drugs that have a low safety profile.

Several important pharmacokinetic principles can be illustrated by measuring the plasma level of a drug following a single-dose administration. These pharmacokinetic values are shown graphically in Figure 4.5. This figure demonstrates two plasma drug levels. First is the **minimum effective concentration,** the amount of drug required to produce a therapeutic effect. Second is the **toxic concentration,** the level of drug that will result in serious adverse effects. The plasma drug concentration *between* the minimum effective concentration and the toxic concentration is called the

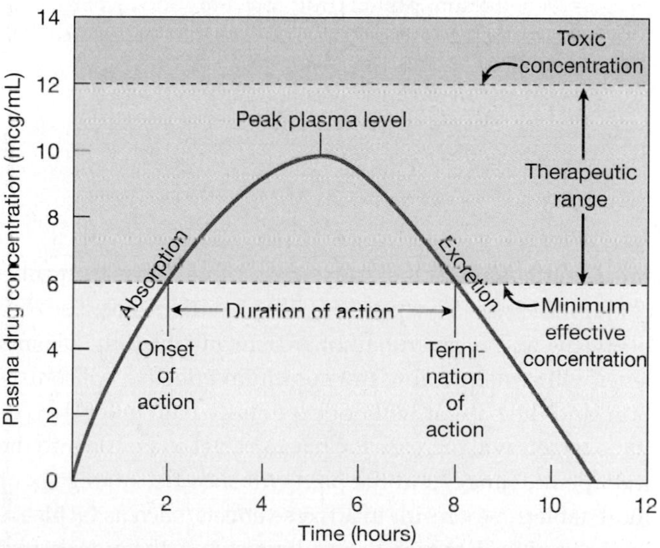

FIGURE 4.5 Single-dose drug administration: pharmacokinetic values for this drug are as follows: onset of action = 2 hours; duration of action = 6 hours; termination of action = 8 hours after administration; peak plasma concentration = 10 mcg/mL; time to peak drug effect = 5 hours; $t_{1/2}$ = 4 hours

Lifespan Considerations: Geriatrics
Adverse Drug Effects: Risk Reduction for Older Adults

Adverse drug effects are more commonly recorded in older adults than in young adults or middle-age patients, because the older adult population takes more drugs simultaneously and because of age-related declines in hepatic and renal function. Chronic diseases that affect pharmacokinetics are also present more often in older adults. However, nondrug factors may be linked to an increased risk of adverse drug effects in the older adult. Cognitive impairment or depression may lead to taking more or less of a dose than ordered; motor dysfunction may make using inhalers or small tablets difficult to manage; a complex drug regimen with multiple drugs and multiple dosages may lead to forgotten doses; and the fear of having an adverse drug reaction when new symptoms arise may lead some older adults to stop taking their medication. Although many adverse drug effects may be related to changes in pharmacokinetic factors such as decreased metabolism or excretion, nondrug factors that may have affected proper self-administration or dosing should be considered before a dosage or drug is changed.

Pretorius, Gataric, Swedlund, & Miller (2013) recommend that in addition to being aware of the factors above as a cause for adverse drug effects, strategies to reduce the risk of a possible adverse drug effect include:

- Ask about all medications the patient takes, including OTC and herbal medications.
- Evaluate medications that may have been started when the patient was younger and whether they are still needed, or whether a dose adjustment is needed.
- Evaluate whether medications given in the short-term setting (e.g., hospital) are still needed when the patient is discharged, or whether alternative medications could be used.
- When a suboptimal drug concentration level is obtained, verify with the patient that the medication has been taken as ordered.
- Review medication lists regularly and whether each drug is still needed depending on the patient's condition.

therapeutic range of the drug. These values have great clinical significance. For example, if the patient has a severe headache and is given half of an aspirin tablet, the plasma level will remain below the minimum effective concentration, and the patient will not experience pain relief. Two or three tablets will increase the plasma level of aspirin into the therapeutic range, and the pain will subside. Taking six or more tablets may result in adverse effects, such as GI bleeding or tinnitus. For each drug administered, the nurse's goal is to keep its plasma concentration in the therapeutic range. For some drugs, the therapeutic range is quite wide; for other medications, the difference between a minimum effective dose and a toxic dose may be dangerously narrow.

4.8 Onset, Peak Levels, and Duration of Drug Action

Onset of drug action represents the amount of time it takes to produce a therapeutic effect after drug administration. Factors that affect drug onset may be many, depending on numerous pharmacokinetic variables. As the drug is absorbed and then begins to circulate throughout the body, the level of medication reaches its peak. Thus, the **peak plasma level** occurs when the medication has reached its highest concentration in the bloodstream. It should be mentioned that depending on accessibility of medications to their targets, peak drug levels are not necessarily associated with optimal therapeutic effect. In addition, multiple doses of medication may be necessary to reach therapeutic drug levels. **Duration of drug action** is the amount of time a drug maintains its therapeutic effect. Many variables can affect the duration of drug action. These include the following:

- Drug concentration (amount of drug given)
- Dosage (how often a drug is given or scheduled)
- Route of drug administration (oral, parenteral, or topical)
- Drug–food interactions
- Drug–supplement interactions
- Drug–herbal interactions
- Drug–drug interactions.

The most common description of a drug's duration of action is its **plasma half-life** ($t_{½}$), defined as the length of time required for the plasma concentration of a medication to decrease by one-half after administration. Some drugs have a half-life of only a few minutes, whereas others have a half-life of several hours or days. The longer it takes a medication to be excreted, the greater the half-life. For example, a drug with a $t_{½}$ of 10 hours would take longer to be excreted and thus produce a longer effect in the body than a drug with a $t_{½}$ of 5 hours.

The plasma half-life of a drug is an essential pharmacokinetic variable with important clinical applications. Drugs with relatively short half-lives, such as aspirin ($t_{½}$ = 15 to 20 minutes), must be given every 3 to 4 hours. Drugs with longer half-lives, such as felodipine (Plendil) ($t_{½}$ = 10 hours), need to be given only once a day. If a patient has extensive renal or hepatic disease, the plasma half-life of a drug will increase, and the drug concentration may reach toxic levels. In these patients, medications must be given less frequently, or the dosages must be reduced.

4.9 Loading Doses and Maintenance Doses

Few drugs are administered as a single dose. Repeated doses result in an accumulation of drug in the bloodstream, as shown in Figure 4.6. Eventually, a plateau will be reached where the level of drug in the plasma is maintained

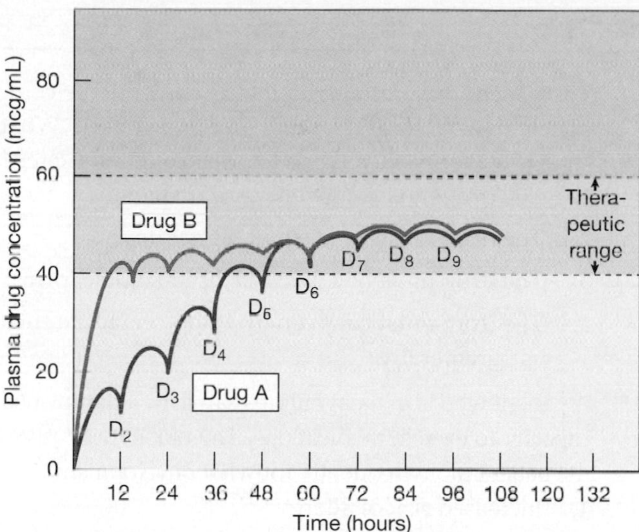

FIGURE 4.6 Multiple-dose drug administration: drug A and drug B are administered every 12 hours; drug B reaches the therapeutic range faster, because the first dose is a loading dose

continuously within the therapeutic range. At this level, the amount administered has reached equilibrium with the amount of drug being eliminated, resulting in the distribution of a continuous therapeutic level of drug to body tissues. Theoretically, it takes approximately four half-lives to reach this equilibrium. If the medication is given as a continuous infusion, the plateau can be reached quickly and be maintained with little or no fluctuation in drug plasma levels.

The plateau may be reached faster by administration of loading doses followed by regular maintenance doses. A **loading dose** is a higher amount of drug, often given only once or twice to "prime" the bloodstream with a sufficient level of drug. Before plasma levels can drop back toward zero, intermittent **maintenance doses** are given to keep the plasma drug concentration in the therapeutic range. Although blood levels of the drug fluctuate with this approach, the equilibrium state can be reached almost as rapidly as with a continuous infusion. Loading doses are particularly important for drugs with prolonged half-lives and for situations in which it is critical to raise drug plasma levels quickly, as might be the case when administering an antibiotic for a severe infection. In Figure 4.6, notice that it takes almost five doses (48 hours) before a therapeutic level is reached using a routine dosing schedule. With a loading dose, a therapeutic level is reached within 12 hours.

Chapter Review

KEY Concepts

The numbered key concepts provide a succinct summary of the important points from the corresponding numbered section within the chapter. If any of these points are not clear, refer to the numbered section within the chapter for review.

4.1 Pharmacokinetics focuses on the movement of drugs throughout the body after they are administered. The four components of pharmacokinetics are absorption, metabolism, distribution, and excretion.

4.2 The physiological properties of plasma membranes determine movement of drugs throughout the body.

4.3 Absorption is the process by which a drug moves from the site of administration to the bloodstream. Absorption depends on the size of the drug molecule, its lipid solubility, its degree of ionization, and interactions with food or other medications.

4.4 Distribution comprises the methods by which drugs are transported throughout the body. Distribution depends on the formation of drug–protein complexes and special barriers such as the placenta or brain barriers.

4.5 Metabolism is a process that changes a drug's activity and makes it more likely to be excreted. Changes in hepatic metabolism can significantly affect drug action.

4.6 Excretion processes eliminate drugs from the body. Drugs are primarily excreted by the kidneys but may be excreted into bile, by the lung, or by glandular secretions.

4.7 The therapeutic response of most drugs depends on their concentration in the plasma. The difference between the minimum effective concentration and the toxic concentration is called the therapeutic range.

4.8 Onset, peak plasma level, and plasma half-life represent the duration of action for most drugs.

4.9 Repeated dosing allows a plateau drug plasma level to be reached. Loading doses allow a therapeutic drug level to be reached rapidly.

REVIEW Questions

1. A patient has a new medication prescription and the nurse is providing education about the drug. Which statement made by the patient would indicate the need for further medication education?
   1. "I can consult my health care provider if I experience adverse effects."
   2. "If I take more, I'll have a better response."
   3. "Taking this drug with food will decrease how much drug gets into my system."
   4. "The liquid form of the drug will absorb faster than the tablets."
2. A combination of two different antihypertensive drugs in lower doses has been ordered for a patient whose hypertension has not been controlled by standard doses of either drug alone. The nursing student recognizes the interaction between these two drugs is known as what term?
   1. Addition
   2. Synergism
   3. Antagonism
   4. Displacement
3. A patient with cirrhosis of the liver has hepatic impairment. This will require what possible changes? (Select all that apply.)
   1. A reduction in the dosage of the drugs
   2. A change in the timing of medication administration
   3. An increased dose of prescribed drugs
   4. Giving all prescribed drugs by intramuscular injection
   5. More frequent monitoring for adverse drug effects
4. The patient requires a drug that is known to be completely metabolized by the first-pass effect. What change will be needed when this drug is administered?
   1. The drug must be given more frequently.
   2. The drug must be given in higher doses.
   3. The drug must be given in a lipid-soluble form.
   4. The drug must be given by a non-oral route such as parenterally.
5. A patient who is in renal failure may have a diminished capacity to excrete medications. The nurse must assess the patient more frequently for what development?
   1. Increased risk of allergy
   2. Decreased therapeutic drug effects
   3. Increased risk for drug toxicity
   4. Increased absorption of the drug from the intestines
6. What is the rationale for the administration of a loading dose of a drug?
   1. It decreases the number of doses that must be given.
   2. It results in lower dosages being required to achieve therapeutic effects.
   3. It decreases the risk of drug toxicity.
   4. It more rapidly builds plasma drug levels to a plateau level.

CRITICAL THINKING Questions

1. Describe the types of barriers drugs encounter from the time they are administered until they reach their target cells.
2. Why is a drug's plasma half-life important to nurses?
3. Describe how the excretion process of pharmacokinetics may place patients at risk for adverse drug effects.
4. Explain why drugs metabolized through the first-pass effect might need to be administered by the parenteral route.

Visit www.pearsonhighered.com/nursingresources for answers and rationales for all activities.

REFERENCES

Pretorius, R. W., Gataric, G., Swedlund, S. K., & Miller, J. R. (2013). Reducing the risk of adverse drug events in older adults. *American Family Physician, 87*, 331–336.

SELECTED BIBLIOGRAPHY

Brunton, L. L., Chabner, B. A., & Knollman, B. C. (Eds.). (2011). Pharmacokinetics: The dynamics of drug absorption, distribution, metabolism and elimination. In *Goodman & Gilman's the pharmacological basis of therapeutics* (12th ed., pp. 30–61). New York, NY: McGraw-Hill.

Chan, L. N., & Anderson, G. D. (2014) Pharmacokinetic and pharmacodynamic drug interactions with ethanol (alcohol). *Clinical Pharmacokinetics, 53*(12) 1115–1136. doi:10.1007/s40262-014-0190-x

Jain, R., Chung, S. M., Jain, L., Khurana, M., Lau, S. W., Lee, J. E., & Sahajwalla, C. G. (2011). Implications of obesity for drug therapy: Limitations and challenges. *Clinical Pharmacology and Therapeutics, 90*, 77–89. doi:10.1038/clpt.2011.104

Knadler, M. P., Lobo, E., Chappell, J., & Bergstrom, R. (2011). Duloxetine: Clinical pharmacokinetics and drug interactions. *Clinical Pharmacokinetics, 50*(5), 281–294. doi:10.2165/11539240-000000000-00000

Liles, A. M. (2011). Medication considerations for patients with chronic kidney disease who are not yet on dialysis [Review]. *Nephrology Nursing Journal, 38*(3), 263–270.

Linares, O. A., Fudin, J., Daly-Linares, A., Boston, R. C. (2015, January 23). Individualized hydrocodone therapy based on phenotype, pharmacogenetics, and pharmacokinetic dosing. *Clinical Journal of Pain*. Advance online publication.

Ma, J. D., Lee, K. C., & Kuo, G. M. (2012). Clinical application of pharmacogenomics. *Journal of Pharmacy Practice, 25*, 417–427. doi:10.1177/0897190012448309

Chapter 5

Pharmacodynamics

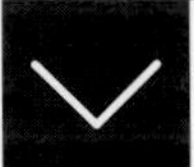

Learning Outcomes

After reading this chapter, the student should be able to:

1. Explain the applications of pharmacodynamics to nursing practice.
2. Discuss how frequency distribution curves may be used to explain how patients respond differently to medications.
3. Explain the importance of the median effective dose (ED_{50}) to nursing practice.
4. Compare and contrast median lethal dose (LD_{50}) and median toxicity dose (TD_{50}).
5. Discuss how a drug's therapeutic index is related to its margin of safety.
6. Explain the significance of the graded dose–response relationship to nursing practice.
7. Compare and contrast the terms *potency* and *efficacy*.
8. Distinguish among an agonist, a partial agonist, and an antagonist.
9. Explain the relationship between receptors and drug action.
10. Explain possible future developments in the field of pharmacogenetics.

In clinical practice, nurses quickly learn that medications do not affect all patients in the same way: A dose that produces a dramatic response in one patient may have no effect on another patient. In some cases, the differences among patients are predictable, based on the pharmacokinetic principles discussed in chapter 4. In other cases, the differences in response are not easily explained. Despite this patient variability, health care providers must choose optimal doses while avoiding unnecessary adverse effects. This is not an easy task given the wide variation of patient responses within a population. This chapter examines the mechanisms by which drugs affect patients, and how nurses can apply these principles to clinical practice.

5.1 Pharmacodynamics and Interpatient Variability

The term **pharmacodynamics** comes from the root words *pharmaco*, which means "medicine," and *dynamics*, which means "change." In simplest terms, pharmacodynamics refers to how a medicine *changes* the body. A more complete definition explains pharmacodynamics as the branch of pharmacology concerned with the mechanisms of drug action and the relationships between drug concentration at the site of action and the resulting effects in the body.

Pharmacodynamics has important nursing applications. Health care providers must be able to predict whether a drug will produce a significant change in patients. Although clinicians often begin therapy with average doses taken from a drug guide, intuitive experience often becomes the practical method for determining which doses of medications will be effective in a given patient. In addition, knowledge of therapeutic indexes, dose–response relationships, and drug–receptor interactions will help nurses provide safe and effective treatment.

Interpatient variability in responses to drugs can best be understood by examining a frequency distribution curve. A **frequency distribution curve,** shown in Figure 5.1, is a graphical representation of the number of patients responding to a drug action at different doses. Notice the wide range in doses that produced the patient responses shown on the curve. A few patients responded to the drug at very low doses. As the dose was increased, more and more patients responded. Some patients required very high doses to elicit the desired response. The peak of the curve indicates the largest number of patients responding to the drug. The curve does not show the *magnitude* of response, only whether a measurable response occurred among the patients. As an example, think of the given response to an antihypertensive drug as being a reduction of 20 mmHg in systolic blood pressure. A few patients experienced the desired 20-mm reduction at a dose of only 10 mg of drug. A 50-mg dose gave the largest number of patients a 20-mmHg reduction in blood pressure; however, a few

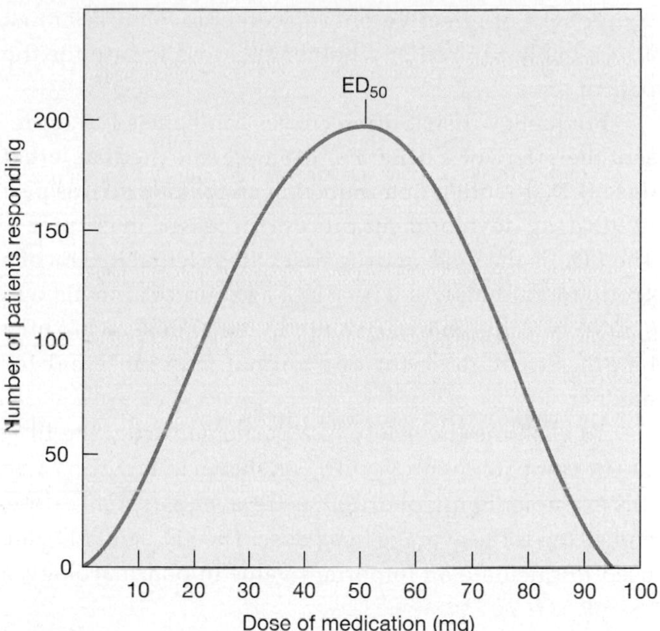

FIGURE 5.1 Frequency distribution curve: interpatient variability in drug response

patients needed as much as 90 mg of drug to produce the same amount of blood pressure reduction.

The dose in the middle of the frequency distribution curve represents the drug's **median effective dose (ED_{50}).** The ED_{50} is the dose required to produce a specific therapeutic response in 50% of a group of patients. Drug guides sometimes report the ED_{50} as the average or standard dose.

The interpatient variability shown in Figure 5.1 has important nursing implications. First, nurses should realize that the standard or average dose predicts a satisfactory therapeutic response for only *half* the population. In other words, many patients will require more or less than the average dose for optimal pharmacotherapy. Using the systolic blood pressure example, assume that a large group of patients is given the average dose of 50 mg. Some of these patients will experience toxicity at this level because they needed only 10 mg to achieve blood pressure reduction. Other patients in this group will probably have no reduction in blood pressure. By observing the patient, taking vital signs, and monitoring associated laboratory data, the nurse uses skills that are critical in determining whether the average dose is effective for the patient. It is not enough to simply memorize an average dose for a drug; the nurse must know when and how to request whether doses should be adjusted to obtain the optimal therapeutic response.

5.2 Therapeutic Index and Drug Safety

Administering a dose that produces an optimal therapeutic response for each individual patient is only one component of effective pharmacotherapy. Nurses must also be able to predict whether the dose is safe for the patient.

Frequency distribution curves can be used to represent the safety of a drug. For example, the **median lethal dose (LD_{50})** is often determined in *preclinical trials*, as part of the drug development process discussed in chapter 2. The LD_{50} is the dose of drug that will be lethal in 50% of a group of animals. As with ED_{50}, a group of animals will exhibit considerable variability in lethal dose; what may be a nontoxic dose for one animal may be lethal for another.

To examine the safety of a particular drug, the LD_{50} can be compared with the ED_{50}, as shown in Figure 5.2a. In this example, 10 mg of drug X is the average *effective* dose, and 40 mg is the average *lethal* dose. The ED_{50} and LD_{50} are used to calculate an important value in pharmacology, a drug's **therapeutic index,** the ratio of a drug's LD_{50} to its ED_{50}.

$$\text{Therapeutic index} = \frac{\text{median lethal dose } LD_{50}}{\text{median effective dose } ED_{50}}$$

The larger the difference between the two doses, the greater the therapeutic index. In Figure 5.2a, the therapeutic index is 4 (40 mg ÷ 10 mg). Essentially, this means that it would take an error in magnitude of *approximately* 4 times the average dose to be lethal. Thus, the therapeutic index is a measure of a drug's safety margin: The higher the value, the safer the drug.

As another example, the therapeutic index of a second drug is shown in Figure 5.2b. Drug Z has the same ED_{50} as drug X but shows a different LD_{50}. The therapeutic index for drug Z is only 2 (20 mg ÷ 10 mg). The difference between an effective dose and a toxic dose is very small for drug Z; thus, the drug has a narrow safety margin.

The therapeutic index offers the nurse practical information on the safety of a drug and a means to compare one drug with another. Because the LD_{50} cannot be experimentally determined in humans, the **median toxicity dose (TD_{50})** is a more practical value in a clinical setting. The TD_{50} is the dose that will produce a given toxicity in 50% of a group of patients. The TD_{50} value is usually based on adverse effects recorded in patient *clinical trials*. The median toxic dose for any study is less than the median lethal dose since it is the dose at which serious adverse effects are first observed.

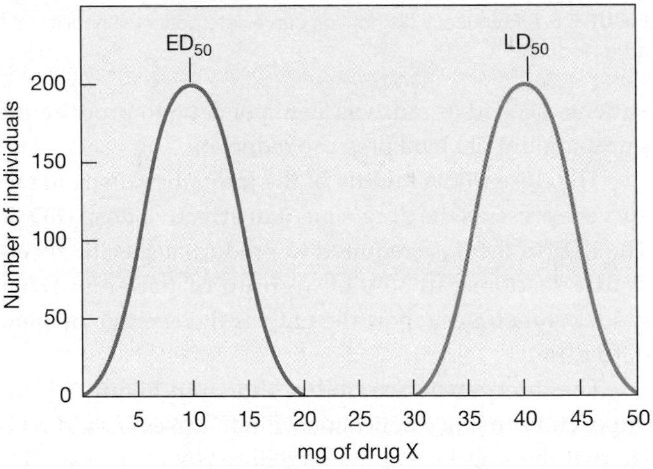

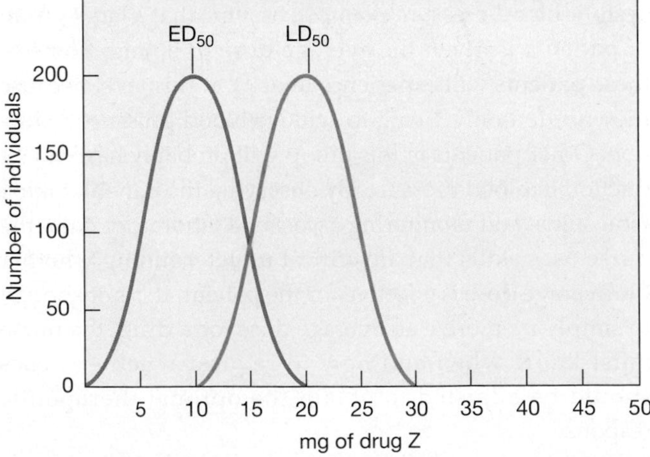

FIGURE 5.2 Therapeutic index: (a) drug X has a therapeutic index of 4; (b) drug Z has a therapeutic index of 2. In a human clinical study, LD_{50} is labeled as TD_{50}

5.3 The Graded Dose–Response Relationship and Therapeutic Response

In the previous examples, frequency distribution curves were used to graphically visualize patient differences in responses to medications in a *population*. It is also useful to visualize the variability in responses observed within a *single patient*.

The **graded dose–response** relationship is a fundamental concept in pharmacology. The graphical representation of this relationship is called a dose–response curve, as illustrated in Figure 5.3. By observing and measuring the patient's response obtained at different doses of the drug, one can explain several important clinical relationships.

The three distinct phases of a dose–response curve indicate essential pharmacodynamic principles that have relevance to nursing practice. Phase 1 occurs at the lowest doses. The flatness of this portion of the curve indicates that few target cells have been affected by the drug. Phase 2 is the straight-line portion of the curve. This portion often shows a linear relationship between the amount of drug administered and the degree of response obtained

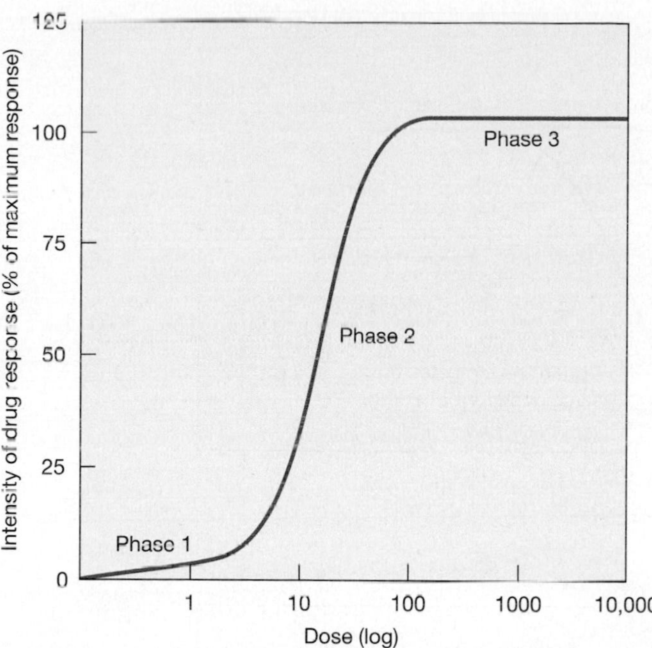

FIGURE 5.3 Dose–response relationship

from the patient. For example, if the dose is doubled, twice as much response is obtained. This is the most desirable range of doses for pharmacotherapeutics, since giving more drug results in proportionately more effect; a lower drug dose gives less effect. In phase 3, a plateau is reached in which increasing the drug dose produces no additional therapeutic response. This may occur for a number of reasons. One explanation is that all the receptors for the drug are occupied. Practically it means that the drug has brought maximal response, such as when a migraine headache has been treated to the greatest extent possible by the drug; giving higher doses produces no additional relief. In phase 3, although increasing the dose does not result in more therapeutic effect, nurses should be mindful that increasing the dose may produce toxic effects. In this instance, it would be necessary to lower the dosage of the drug or discontinue the drug in order to achieve maximal therapeutic outcomes (see chapter 4).

5.4 Potency and Efficacy

Within a pharmacologic class, not all drugs are equally effective at treating a disorder. For example, some antineoplastic drugs kill more cancer cells than others; some antihypertensive agents lower blood pressure to a greater degree than others; and some analgesics are more effective at relieving severe pain than others in the same class. Furthermore, drugs in the same class are effective at different doses; one antibiotic may be effective at a dose of 1 mg/kg, whereas another is most effective at 100 mg/kg. Nurses need a method of comparing drugs and effective drug doses in order to administer treatment effectively.

There are two fundamental ways to compare medications within therapeutic and pharmacologic classes. First is the concept of **potency.** A drug that is more potent will produce a therapeutic effect at a lower dose, compared with another drug in the same class. For example, consider two agents, drug X and drug Y, that both produce a 20-mmHg drop in blood pressure. If drug X produces this effect at a dose of 10 mg and drug Y produces it at 60 mg, then drug X is said to be more potent. Thus, potency is one way to compare the doses of two independently administered drugs in terms of how much is needed to produce a desired response. A useful way to visualize the concept of potency is by examining dose–response curves. Compare the two drugs shown in Figure 5.4a. In this example, drug A is more potent because it requires a lower dose to produce the same effect.

The second method used to compare drugs is called **efficacy,** which is the magnitude of maximal response that can be produced from a particular drug. In the example in Figure 5.4b, drug A is more efficacious because it produces a higher maximal response.

Which is more important to the success of pharmacotherapy, potency or efficacy? Perhaps the best way to understand these concepts is to use the specific example of headache pain. Two common over-the-counter (OTC) analgesics are ibuprofen (200 mg) and aspirin (650 mg). The fact that ibuprofen relieves pain at a lower dose indicates that this agent is *more potent* than aspirin. At recommended doses, however, both are equally effective at relieving headache pain; thus, they have about the *same efficacy*. If the patient is experiencing severe pain, however, neither aspirin nor ibuprofen has sufficient efficacy to bring relief. Narcotic analgesics such as morphine have a greater efficacy than aspirin or ibuprofen and can effectively treat severe pain. From a pharmacotherapeutic perspective, efficacy is almost always more important than potency. In the previous example, the average dose is unimportant to the patient, but headache relief is essential. As another comparison, the patient with cancer is much more concerned about how many cancer cells have been killed (efficacy) than what dose the nurse administered (potency). Although the nurse will often hear claims that one drug is more potent than another, a more compelling concern is whether the drug is more effective in achieving a greater therapeutic benefit (efficacy).

5.5 Cellular Receptors and Drug Action

Drugs act by modulating or changing existing physiological and biochemical processes. To exert such changes requires that drugs interact with specific molecules and chemicals normally found in the body. A cellular macromolecule to which a medication binds in order to initiate

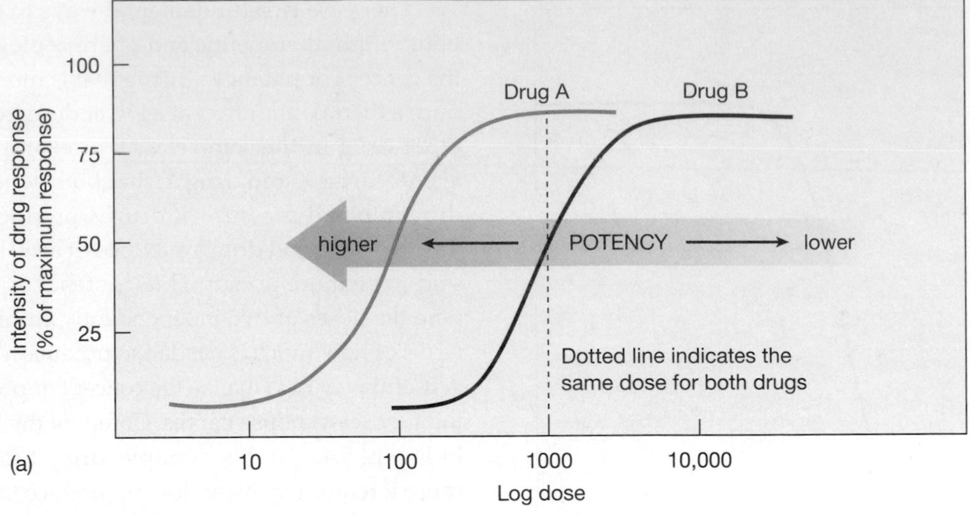

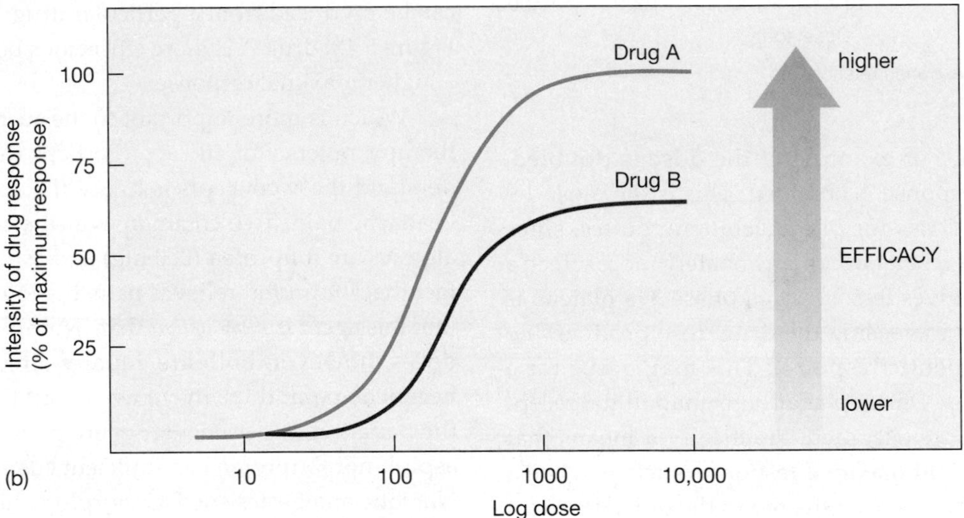

FIGURE 5.4 Potency and efficacy: (a) drug A has a higher potency than drug B; (b) drug A has a higher efficacy than drug B

its effects is called a **receptor.** The concept that a drug binds to a receptor to cause a change in body chemistry or physiology is a fundamental theory in pharmacology. *Receptor theory* explains the mechanisms by which most drugs produce their effects. It is important to understand, however, that these receptors do not exist in the body solely to bind drugs. Their normal function is to bind endogenous molecules such as hormones, neurotransmitters, and growth factors.

Although a drug receptor can be any type of macromolecule, the vast majority are proteins. As shown in Figure 5.5, a receptor is depicted as a three-dimensional protein associated with the cellular plasma membrane. The extracellular structural component of the receptor usually consists of several protein subunits arranged around a central canal or channel. Other protein segments as a part of the receptor macromolecule are inserted into the plasma membrane. Channels may be opened by changes in voltage across the membrane as when voltage-gated calcium channels are opened when electrical signals arrive at nerve endings. In this instance, an electrical signal will open channels, and calcium will rush into the nerve terminal to release vesicles containing endogenous neurotransmitters. Chemical gated channels, a second type of receptor, will be activated by neurotransmitters after they are released into the synapse. Both channel types represent ways that many drugs can produce a response by modulating receptors in the body.

A drug attaches to its receptor in a specific manner, in much the way that a thumb drive docks to a USB port in a computer (see Figures 5.5b and 5.5c). Small changes to the structure of a drug, or its receptor, may weaken or even eliminate binding (docking) between the two molecules. Once bound, drugs may trigger a series of **second messenger** events within the cell, such as the conversion of adenosine triphosphate (ATP) to cyclic adenosine monophosphate (cyclic AMP), the release of intracellular calcium, or the activation of specific G proteins and associated enzymes. This is very much like the internal actions that go on within a computer. Biochemical cascades initiate the drug's action by either stimulating or inhibiting normal activity within the cell.

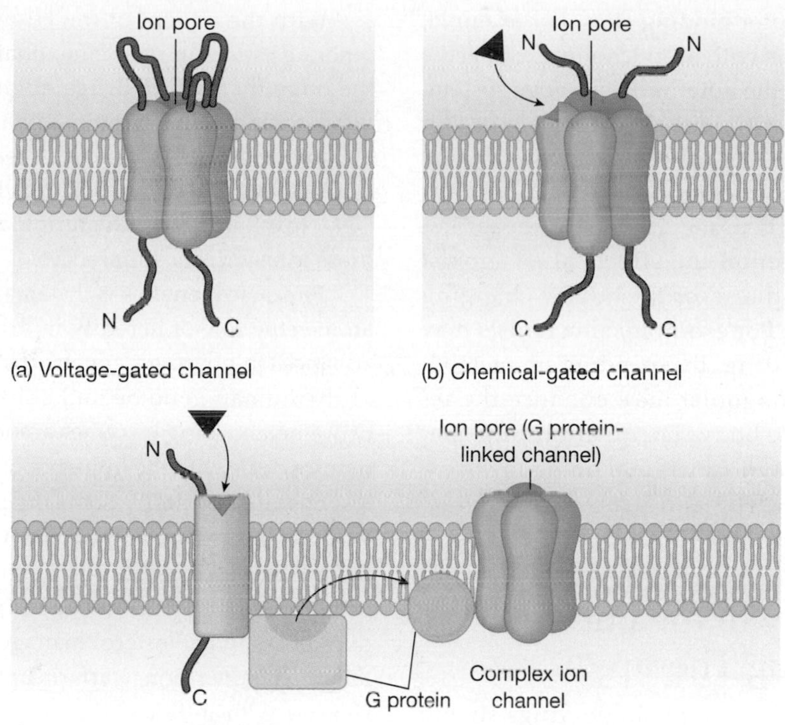

FIGURE 5.5 Cellular receptors. The red triangle represents the drug binding directly with receptors.

Not all receptors are bound to plasma membranes; some are intracellular molecules such as DNA or enzymes in the cytoplasm. By interacting with these types of receptors, medications are able to inhibit protein synthesis or regulate cellular events such as replication and metabolism. Examples of agents that bind with intracellular components include steroid medications, vitamins, and hormones.

Receptors and their associated drug mechanisms are extremely important in therapeutics. Receptor *subtypes* are being discovered, and new medications are being developed at a faster rate than at any other time in history. These subtypes permit the "fine-tuning" of pharmacology. For example, the first medications affecting the autonomic nervous system targeted all autonomic receptors. Then it was discovered that two basic receptor types existed in the body: *alpha* and *beta*. Drugs were developed to target only one receptor type. The result was more specific drug action with fewer adverse effects. Still later, several subtypes of alpha and beta receptors, including $alpha_1$, $alpha_2$, $beta_1$, $beta_2$, and $beta_3$ were discovered that allowed even more specificity in pharmacotherapy. In recent years, researchers have further divided and refined these receptor subtypes. It is likely that receptor research will continue to result in the development of new medications that activate very specific receptors and thus direct drug action to avoid unnecessary adverse effects.

Some drugs act independently of cellular receptors. These agents are associated with other mechanisms, such as changing the permeability of cellular membranes, depressing membrane excitability, or altering the activity of cellular pumps. Actions such as these are described as **nonspecific cellular responses.** Ethyl alcohol, general anesthetics, and osmotic diuretics are examples of agents that act by nonspecific mechanisms.

5.6 Types of Drug–Receptor Interactions

When a drug binds to a receptor, several therapeutic consequences can result. In simplest terms, a specific activity of the cell is either enhanced or inhibited. The actual biochemical mechanism underlying the therapeutic effect, however, may be extremely complex. In some cases, the mechanism of action may be unknown.

When a drug binds to its receptor, it produces a response that *mimics* the effect of the endogenous regulatory molecule. For example, when the drug bethanechol (Urecholine) is administered, it binds to acetylcholine receptors in the autonomic nervous system and produces the same actions as acetylcholine. A drug that produces the same type of response as the endogenous substance is called an **agonist.** Agonists sometimes produce a greater maximal response than the endogenous chemical. The term **partial agonist** or **agonist-antagonist drug** describes a medication that produces a weaker, or less efficacious, response than an agonist.

A second possibility is that a drug will occupy a receptor and *prevent* the endogenous chemical from acting. This drug is called an **antagonist.** Antagonists often compete with agonists for the receptor binding sites. For example, the drug atropine competes with acetylcholine for specific receptors associated with the autonomic nervous system. If the dose is high enough, atropine will completely inhibit the effects of acetylcholine, because acetylcholine will be blocked from binding to its receptors.

Not all antagonism is associated with receptors. *Functional* antagonists inhibit the effects of an agonist not by competing with the receptor but by changing pharmacokinetic factors. For example, antagonists may slow the absorption of a drug. By speeding up metabolism or excretion, an antagonist may enhance the removal of a drug from the body. The relationships that occur between agonists and functional antagonists explain many of the drug–drug and drug–food interactions that occur within the body.

5.7 Pharmacology of the Future: Customizing Drug Therapy

Until recently, it was thought that single drugs should provide safe and effective treatment to every patient in the same way. Unfortunately, a significant portion of the population either develops unacceptable side effects to certain drugs or is unresponsive to them. Many scientists and clinicians are now discarding the one-size-fits-all approach to drug therapy, which was designed to treat an entire population without addressing important interpatient variation.

With the advent of the Human Genome Project and other advances in medicine, pharmacologists began with the hope that future drugs might be customized for patients with specific genetic similarities. In the past, unpredictable and unexplained drug reactions have been labeled as **idiosyncratic responses.** It is hoped that performing a DNA test before administering a drug may someday address idiosyncratic differences.

Pharmacogenetics is the area of pharmacology that examines the role of heredity in drug response. The greatest advances in pharmacogenetics have been the identification of the human genome and subtle genetic differences in drug-metabolizing enzymes among patients. **Pharmacogenomics** deals with the influence of genetic variation on drug response in patients by correlating gene expression or actual variants of the human genome. Genetic differences in enzymes are responsible for a significant portion of drug-induced toxicity. Other examples have been genetic differences in cholesterol management, arrhythmias, heart failure, hypertension, warfarin anticoagulation, and responsiveness with antiplatelet agents. Further characterization of the human genome and subsequent application of pharmacogenetic information may someday allow for customized drug therapy. Imagine being able to prevent drug toxicity with a single gene test or to predict in advance whether placement of a stent will be successful. Although therapies based on a patient's genetic variability have not been cost effective, strides in both fields continue to propose new ways pharmacotherapy might be practiced in the future.

Treating the Diverse Patient: At-Home Genetics Testing for Drug Response

It is perhaps not surprising that consumers who are now familiar with researching their medical condition, drugs, or treatment plan on the Internet have an additional option, at-home or "DTC" (direct-to-consumer) pharmacogenomics testing. DTC companies have offered testing previously for paternity, genetic susceptibility to disease conditions, and ancestry testing. With the recognition that there may be potential links between a genetic variation and a person's response to, or adverse effects from a drug, companies have begun to offer pharmacogenomics testing. Only a handful of drugs are currently available for testing, including some beta blockers and anticoagulants. However, the legal, ethical, and medical issues raised are worth considering when the nurse takes a patient's medical and drug history. Has the patient sought out and had testing? What were the results? Did the patient discuss the results with their health care provider? And perhaps most important, did the patient stop taking or alter administration of the medication based on the test results? It is perhaps the last question that carries the largest concern with at-home testing. Despite disclaimer notices to "see your health care provider," consumers accustomed to finding advice on the Internet may not always do so, risking potentially dangerous consequences. Nurses should encourage patients who decide to use DTC pharmacogenomics testing services to discuss the findings with their health care provider to ensure the treatment plan remains adequate for the patient's condition.

Chapter Review

KEY Concepts

The numbered key concepts provide a succinct summary of the important points from the corresponding numbered section within the chapter. If any of these points are not clear, refer to the numbered section within the chapter for review.

5.1 Pharmacodynamics is the area of pharmacology concerned with how drugs produce change in patients and the differences in patient responses to medications.

5.2 The therapeutic index, expressed mathematically as $TD_{50} \div ED_{50}$, is a clinical value representing the margin of safety of a drug. The higher the therapeutic index, the safer is the drug.

5.3 The graded dose–response relationship describes how the therapeutic response to a drug changes as the medication dose is increased.

5.4 Potency, the dose of medication required to produce a particular response, and efficacy, the magnitude of maximal response to a drug, are means of comparing medications.

5.5 Drug–receptor theory is used to explain the mechanism of action of many medications.

5.6 Agonists, partial agonists, and antagonists are substances that compete with drugs for receptor binding and can cause drug–drug and drug–food interactions.

5.7 In the future, pharmacotherapy will likely be customized to match the genetic makeup of each patient.

REVIEW Questions

1. A patient experiences profound drowsiness when a stimulant drug is given. This is an unusual reaction for this drug, a reaction that has not been associated with this particular drug. What is the term for this type of drug reaction?
   1. Allergic reaction
   2. Idiosyncratic reaction
   3. Enzyme-specific reaction
   4. Unaltered reaction
2. The provider has ordered atropine, a drug that will prevent the patient's own chemical, acetylcholine, from causing parasympathetic effects. What type of drug would atropine be considered?
   1. An antagonist
   2. A partial agonist
   3. An agonist
   4. A protagonist
3. A nursing student reads in a pharmacology textbook that 10 mg of morphine is considered to provide the same pain relief as 200 mg of codeine. This indicates that the morphine would be considered more ____________ than codeine. (Fill in the blank.)
4. What is the term used to describe the magnitude of maximal response that can be produced from a particular drug?
   1. Efficacy
   2. Toxicity
   3. Potency
   4. Comparability
5. The nurse looks up butorphanol (Stadol) in a drug reference guide prior to administering the drug and notes that it is a partial agonist. What does this term tell the nurse about the drug?
   1. It is a drug that produces the same type of response as the endogenous substance.
   2. It is a drug that will occupy a receptor and prevent the endogenous chemical from acting.
   3. It is a drug that causes unpredictable and unexplained drug reactions.
   4. It is a drug that produces a weaker, or less efficacious, response than an agonist drug.

6. The nurse reads that the drug to be given to the patient has a "narrow therapeutic index." The nurse knows that this means that the drug has what properties?
   1. It has a narrow range of effectiveness and may not give this patient the desired therapeutic results.
   2. It has a narrow safety margin and even a small increase in dose may produce adverse or toxic effects.
   3. It has a narrow range of conditions or diseases that the drug will be expected to treat successfully.
   4. It has a narrow segment of the population for whom the drug will work as desired.

CRITICAL THINKING Questions

1. If the ED_{50} is the dose required to produce an effective response in 50% of a group of patients, what happens in the other 50% of the patients after a dose has been administered?
2. Great strides are being made in pharmacogenomics and personalized medicine. What are some of the advantages that pharmacogenomics may have for the pharmacologic treatment of patients?

Visit www.pearsonhighered.com/nursingresources for answers and rationales for all activities.

SELECTED BIBLIOGRAPHY

Blumenthal, D. K., & Garrison, J. C. (2011). Pharmacodynamics: Molecular Mechanisms of Drug Action. In L. L. Brunton, B. A. Chabner, & B. C. Knollman (Eds.). *Goodman & Gilman's the pharmacological basis of therapeutics* (12th ed., pp. 62–97). New York, NY: McGraw-Hill.

Chan, L. N., & Anderson, G. D. (2014). Pharmacokinetic and pharmacodynamic drug interactions with ethanol (alcohol). *Clinical Pharmacokinetics, 53*, 1115–1136. doi:10.1007/s40262-014-0190-x

Corbett, R. W., & Owens, L. W. (2011). Introductory pharmacology for clinical practice. *Journal of Midwifery & Women's Health, 56*, 190–197. doi:10.1111/j.1542-2011.2011.00066.x

Hoshino-Yoshino, A., Kato, M., Nakano, K., Ishigai, M., Kudo, T., & Ito, K. (2011). Bridging from preclinical to clinical studies for tyrosine kinase inhibitors based on pharmacokinetics/pharmacodynamics and toxicokinetics/toxicodynamics. *Drug Metabolism and Pharmacokinetics, 26*, 612–620. doi:10.2133/dmpk.DMPK-11-RG-043

Meechan, R., Jones, H., & Valler-Jones, T. (2011). Do medicines OSCEs improve drug administration ability? *British Journal of Nursing, 20*, 817–822.

Philip, A. K., & Philip, B. (2011). Chronopharmaceuticals: Hype or future of pharmaceutics. *Current Pharmaceutical Design, 17*, 1512–1516. doi:10.2174/138161211796197151

Roden, D. M., Johnson, J. A., Kimmel, S. E., Krauss, R. M., Medina, M. W., Shuldiner, A., & Wilke, R. A. (2011). Cardiovascular pharmacogenomics. *Circulation Research, 109*(7), 807–820. doi:10.1161/CIRCRESAHA.110.230995

Van den Anker, J. N., Schwab, M., & Kearns, G. L. (2011). Developmental pharmacokinetics. *Handbook of Experimental Pharmacology, 205*, 51–75. doi:10.1007/978-3-642-20195-0_2

Weiss, M. (2011). Functional characterization of drug uptake and metabolism in the heart. *Expert Opinion on Drug Metabolism and Toxicology, 7*, 1295–1306. doi:10.1517/17425255.2011.614233

Weiss, M., Krejcie, T. C., & Avram, M. J. (2011). A physiologically based model of hepatic ICG clearance: Interplay between sinusoidal uptake and biliary excretion. *European Journal of Pharmaceutical Sciences, 44*, 359–365. doi:10.1016/j.ejps.2011.08.018

Unit 2

Pharmacology and the Nurse–Patient Relationship

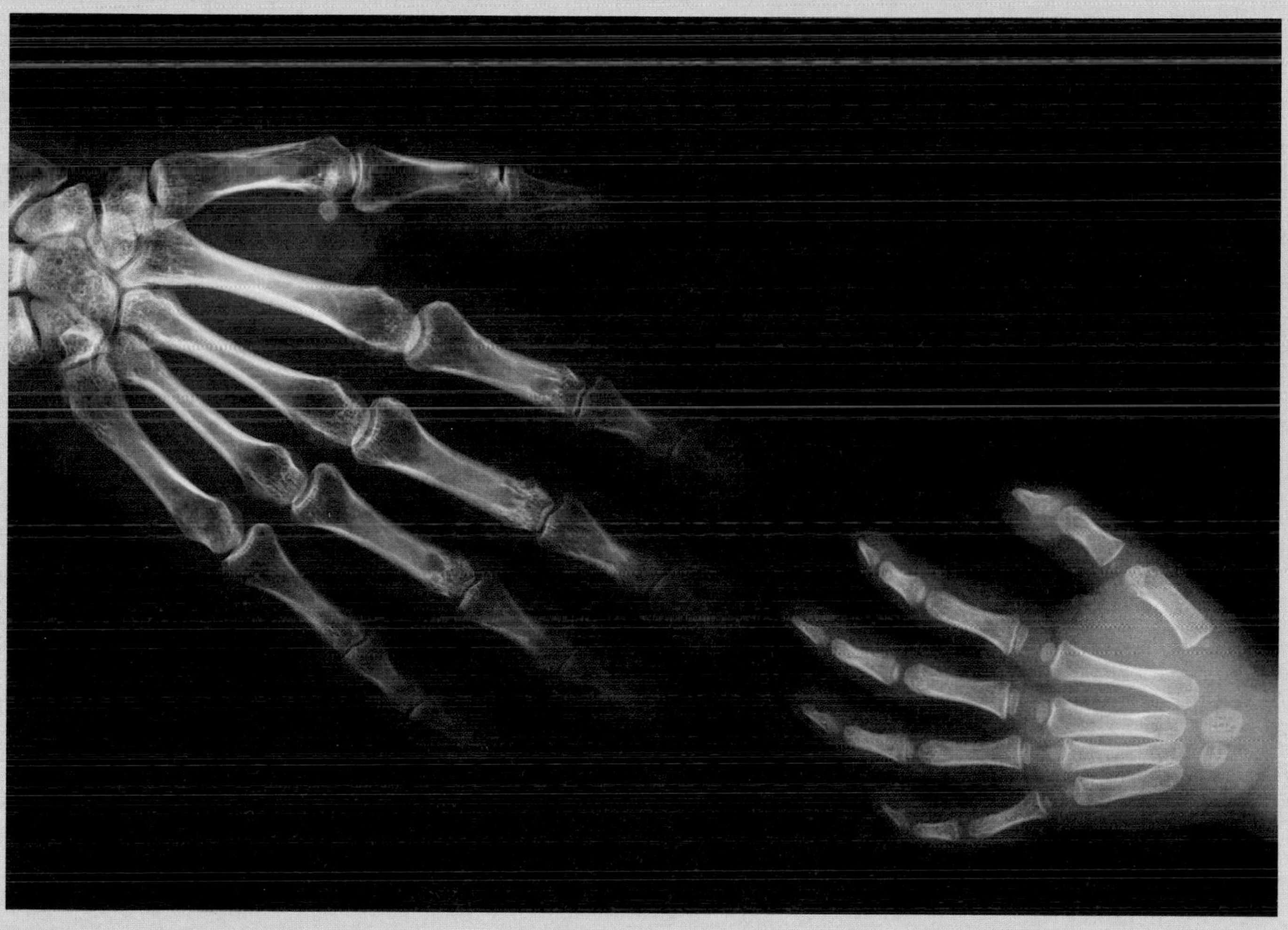

Pharmacology and the Nurse–Patient Relationship

Chapter 6

The Nursing Process in Pharmacology

Learning Outcomes

After reading this chapter, the student should be able to:

1. Compare and contrast the different steps of the nursing process.
2. Identify health history questions to ask during the assessment phase that are pertinent to medication administration.
3. Describe the areas of concern relating to pharmacotherapy that should be addressed during the diagnosis phase of the nursing process.
4. Identify the main components of the planning phase of the nursing process.
5. Discuss key nursing interventions required in the implementation phase of the nursing process for patients receiving medications.
6. Explain the importance of the evaluation phase of the nursing process as applied to pharmacotherapy.

The **nursing process** is a systematic method of problem solving that forms the foundation of nursing practice. The use of the nursing process is particularly important when working with patients who are receiving medications. By using the phases of the nursing process, the nurse can ensure that the interdisciplinary practice of pharmacology results in safe, effective, and individualized medication administration and outcomes for patients under their care.

Many nursing students enter a pharmacology course after taking a course on the fundamentals of nursing, during which the phases of the nursing process are discussed in detail. This chapter focuses on how the phases of the nursing process can be applied to pharmacotherapy. Students who are unfamiliar with the nursing process are encouraged to consult one of the many excellent fundamentals of nursing textbooks for a more detailed explanation.

6.1 Overview of the Nursing Process

The nursing process requires the nurse to use critical thinking skills to care for the patient. It is patient-centered, dynamic, and based on ongoing patient data and needs. It is also a collaborative effort between the nurse, patient, and other members of the health care team. The nurse relies on knowledge, technical and critical thinking skills, and even creativity to work through the process of gathering assessment data, establishing nursing diagnoses, planning care with the patient to meet outcomes, implementing, and, finally, evaluating care. The nursing process is cyclical and each phase is related to all the others; they are not separate entities but overlap. For example, when a nurse is evaluating whether the pain medication given to the patient has had therapeutic effects and relieved the pain, the nurse relies on assessment skills to evaluate whether the patient is pain-free or has obtained some relief from the drug. The phases of the nursing process are illustrated in Figure 6.1.

6.2 Assessment of the Patient

The **assessment phase** of the nursing process is the systematic collection, organization, validation, and documentation of patient data. Assessment is an ongoing process that begins with the nurse's initial contact with the patient and continues with every interaction thereafter.

A health history and physical assessment are completed during the initial meeting between a nurse and a patient. **Baseline data** are gathered that will be compared to information obtained from later interactions, during and following treatment. Assessment consists of gathering **subjective data,** which include what the patient says or perceives, and **objective data** gathered through physical assessment, laboratory tests, and other diagnostic sources. The accuracy of the data gathered during the assessment phase will affect the choice of nursing diagnoses, goals and outcomes determined in the planning phase, and the interventions used to meet those goals. During the assessment phase, the nurse's critical thinking skills, knowledge, and technical skills are vital to ensuring the accuracy of the assessment.

The initial **health history** is tailored to the patient's clinical condition. A complete history is the most detailed, but the nurse must consider the appropriateness of this history given the patient's condition. Often the nurse takes a problem-focused or "chief complaint" history that focuses on the symptoms that led the patient to seek care. In any history, the nurse must assess key components that could potentially affect the outcomes of drug administration. Essential questions to ask in the initial history relate to history of drug allergy; past medical history; medications currently used; personal and social history including the use of alcohol, tobacco, or caffeine; health risks such as the use of street drugs or illicit substances; and reproductive health questions such as the pregnancy status of women of childbearing age. Assessment should always include the use of over-the-counter (OTC) drugs, dietary supplements, and herbal products because these agents have the potential to affect drug therapy. Table 6.1 provides pertinent questions the nurse may ask during an initial health history that provide baseline data before medications are administered. The nurse must remember that what is *not* being said may be as important as what *is* being said. For instance, a patient may deny symptoms of pain while grimacing or guarding a certain area from being touched. The nurse must use observation skills during the history to gather such critical data.

Patient Safety: Barcodes for Patient Identification

To improve patient safety, especially during medication administration, many large health care agencies have switched to a type of patient identification band that includes a barcode. The nurse scans the barcode with a special reader before giving medication or initiating other treatments for the patient. But the barcode identification system is not foolproof; while it has improved the accuracy of medication administration and reduced patient medication errors, errors may still occur. The identification band may be placed on the wrong patient on admission, the barcode may be damaged and unreadable, or nurses and other health care providers may circumvent the system by printing out additional copies of the barcode to scan rather than using the patient's own identification band in order "to save time." It is recommended that even when a barcode band is used, the nurse continue to use two other methods of identifying the patient such as verifying the patient's name and birth date. Although the barcode identification band has significantly reduced medication errors, it is not completely fail-safe.

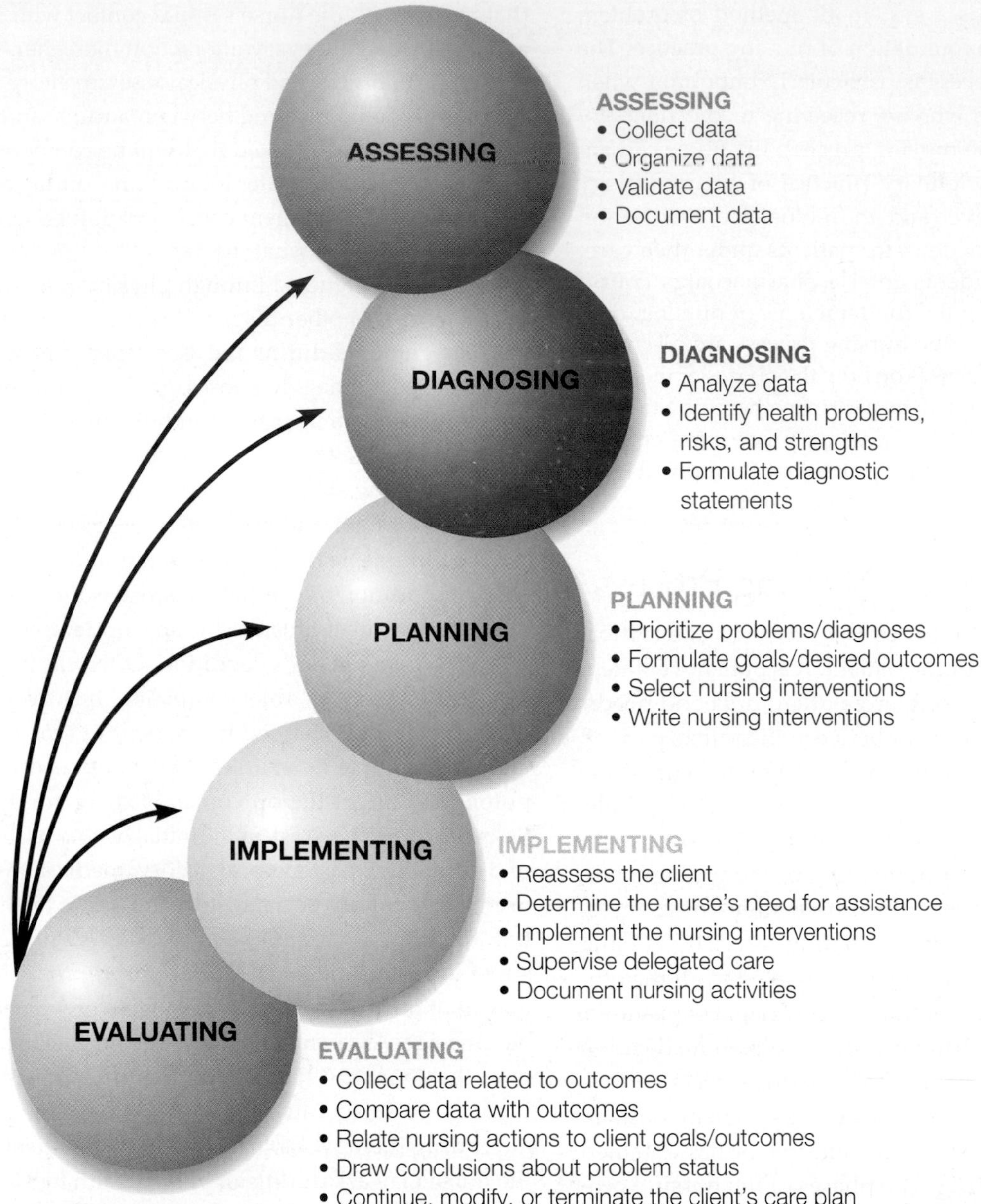
ASSESSING
ASSESSING
• Collect data
• Organize data
• Validate data
• Document data
DIAGNOSING
DIAGNOSING
• Analyze data
• Identify health problems, risks, and strengths
• Formulate diagnostic statements
PLANNING
PLANNING
• Prioritize problems/diagnoses
• Formulate goals/desired outcomes
• Select nursing interventions
• Write nursing interventions
IMPLEMENTING
IMPLEMENTING
• Reassess the client
• Determine the nurse's need for assistance
• Implement the nursing interventions
• Supervise delegated care
• Document nursing activities
EVALUATING
EVALUATING
• Collect data related to outcomes
• Compare data with outcomes
• Relate nursing actions to client goals/outcomes
• Draw conclusions about problem status
• Continue, modify, or terminate the client's care plan

FIGURE 6.1 The five overlapping phases of the nursing process. Each phase depends on the accuracy of the other phases

Source: *Kozier, & Erb's Fundamentals of Nursing: Concepts, Process, and Practice*, 10th ed., by A. Berman, S. J. Snyder, and G. Frandsen, © 2016. Reprinted and electronically reproduced by permission of Pearson Education, Inc., Hoboken, New Jersey.

Along with the health history, a physical assessment is conducted to gather objective data on the patient's condition. The nurse may obtain vital signs, height and weight, a head-to-toe physical assessment, and laboratory specimens. These provide the baseline data to compare with future assessments and guide the health care provider in deciding which medications to prescribe. Because many medications can affect the heart rate and blood pressure, the nurse should carefully document chronic conditions of the cardiovascular system. Baseline electrolyte values are important parameters to obtain, because many medications affect electrolyte balance. Renal and hepatic function tests are essential for many patients, particularly older adults and those who are critically ill, because kidney and liver disease often require adjustment in drug dosages (see chapter 4).

Once pharmacotherapy is initiated, ongoing assessments are conducted to determine the effectiveness of the medications. Assessment should first focus on determining whether the patient is experiencing the expected therapeutic benefits from the medications. For example, if a drug is given for symptoms of pain, has the pain subsided? If an antibiotic is given for an infection, have the signs of that infection improved over time? If a patient is not experiencing the therapeutic effects of the medication, then the nurse must conduct further assessment to determine possible reasons. Dosages are reviewed, and serum drug levels may be obtained.

Assessment during pharmacotherapy should also identify any adverse effects experienced by the patient. Assessment should include the patient's perceptions of the adverse

Table 6.1 Health History Assessment Questions Pertinent to Drug Administration

Health History Component Areas	Pertinent Questions
Chief complaint	• How do you feel? (Describe) • Are you having any pain? (Describe) • Are you experiencing other symptoms? (Especially pertinent to medications are nausea, vomiting, headache, itching, dizziness, shortness of breath, nervousness or anxiousness, palpitations or heart "fluttering," and weakness or fatigue.)
Allergies	• Are you allergic to any medications? • Are you allergic to any foods, environmental substances (e.g., pollen or seasonal allergies), tape, soaps, or cleansers? • What specifically happens when you experience an allergy?
Past medical history	• Do you have a history of diabetes, heart or vascular conditions, respiratory conditions, or neurologic conditions? • Do you have any dermatologic conditions? • How were these treated in the past? Currently?
Family history	• Has anyone in your family experienced difficulties with any medications? (Describe) • Does anyone in your family have any significant medical problems?
Drug history	• What prescription medications are you currently taking? (List drug name, dosage, and frequency of administration.) • What nonprescription/OTC medications are you taking? (List name, dosage, and frequency.) • What drugs, prescription or OTC, have you taken within the past month or two? • Have you ever experienced any side effects or unusual symptoms with any medications? (Describe) • What do you know, or what were you taught, about these medications? • Do you use any herbal or homeopathic remedies? Any nutritional substances or vitamins?
Health management	• Identify all the health care providers you have seen for health issues. • When was the last time you saw a health care provider? For what reason did you see this provider? • What is your normal diet? • Do you have any trouble sleeping?
Reproductive history	• Is there any possibility you are pregnant? (Ask *every* woman of child-bearing age.) • Are you breast-feeding?
Personal-social history	• Do you smoke? • What is your usual alcohol intake? • What is your usual caffeine intake? • Do you have any religious or cultural beliefs or practices concerning medications or your health that we should know about? • What is your occupation? What hours do you work? • Do you have any concerns regarding insurance or the ability to afford medications? • Have you recently traveled to another country? Which country/countries?
Health risk history	• Do you have any history of depression or other mental illness? • Do you use any street drugs or illicit substances?

effects as well as follow-up vital signs and laboratory reports. Here again, baseline data are compared with the current assessment to determine what changes have occurred since the initiation of pharmacotherapy. The Nursing Practice Application tables provided in chapters 12 through 49 illustrate key assessment data that the nurse should gather that are associated with specific medications or classes of drugs. These tables may be tailored to patient-specific data and developed as a care plan as the nurse works with patients who have been prescribed a drug in the classification covered by the table.

Finally, it is important to assess the ability of the patient to assume responsibility for self-administration of medication. Will the patient require assistance obtaining or purchasing the prescribed medications, or with taking them safely? What kind of medication storage facilities exist, and are they adequate to protect the patient, others in the home, and the efficacy of the medication? Does the patient understand the uses and effects of this medication and how it should be taken? Do assessment data suggest that the use of this medication might present a problem, such as difficulty swallowing large capsules or an inability to administer parenteral medications at home, when necessary?

After analyzing the assessment data, the nurse determines patient-specific nursing diagnoses appropriate for the drugs prescribed. These diagnoses will form the basis for the remaining steps of the nursing process.

6.3 Nursing Diagnoses

Nursing diagnoses are clinical judgments of a patient's actual or potential health problem that is within the nurse's scope of practice to address. Nursing diagnoses provide

Complementary and Alternative Therapies

MEDICATION ERRORS AND DIETARY SUPPLEMENTS

Herbal and vitamin supplements can have powerful effects on the body that may influence the effectiveness of prescription drug therapy. In some cases, OTC supplements can enhance the effects of prescription drugs; in other instances, supplements may cancel the therapeutic effects of a medication. For example, many patients with heart disease take garlic supplements in addition to warfarin (Coumadin) to prevent the potential for clots forming. Because garlic and warfarin are both anticoagulants, taking them together could result in abnormal bleeding. As another example, high doses of calcium supplements may cancel the beneficial antihypertensive effects of drugs such as nifedipine (Procardia), a calcium channel blocker.

Relatively few controlled studies have examined how concurrent use of dietary supplements affects the therapeutic effects of prescription drugs. Patients should be encouraged to report use of all OTC dietary supplements to their health care provider.

the basis for establishing goals and outcomes, planning interventions, and evaluating the effectiveness of the care given. Unlike medical diagnoses that focus on a disease or condition, nursing diagnoses focus on a patient's response to actual or potential health and life processes. NANDA International defines nursing diagnoses as:

> A clinical judgment concerning a human response to health conditions/life processes, or vulnerability for that response, by an individual, family, or community (Herdman & Kamitsuru, 2014).

Nursing diagnoses are often the most challenging part of the nursing process. Sometimes the nurse identifies what are believed to be patient problems, only to discover from further assessment that the planned goals, outcomes, and interventions have not "solved" a problem. A key point to remember is that nursing diagnoses focus on the *patient's* needs, not the nurse's needs. A primary nursing role is to enable patients to become active participants in their own care. By including the patient in identifying needs, the nurse encourages the patient to take a more active role in working toward meeting the identified goals.

When applied to pharmacotherapy, the diagnosis phase of the nursing process addresses three main areas of concern:

- Promoting therapeutic drug effects.
- Minimizing adverse drug effects and toxicity.
- Maximizing the ability of the patient for self-care, including the knowledge, skills, and resources necessary for safe and effective drug administration.

Nursing diagnoses that focus on drug administration may address actual problems, such as the treatment of pain; focus on potential problems, such as a risk for deficient fluid volume; or concentrate on maintaining the patient's current level of wellness. The diagnosis is written as a one-, two-, or three-part statement depending on whether the nurse has identified a wellness, risk, or actual problem. Actual and risk problems include the diagnostic statement and a related factor, or inferred cause. Actual diagnoses also contain a third part, the evidence gathered to support the chosen statement. There are many diagnoses appropriate to medication administration. Some are nursing specific that the nurse can manage independently, whereas other problems are multidisciplinary and require collaboration with other members of the health care team.

Two of the most common nursing diagnoses for medication administration are *Deficient Knowledge* and *Noncompliance*. A knowledge deficit may occur when the patient is given a new prescription and has no previous experience with the medication. This diagnosis may also be applicable when a patient has not received adequate education about the drugs being prescribed. When obtaining a medication history, the nurse should assess the patient's knowledge regarding the drugs currently being taken and evaluate whether the drug education was adequate. Noncompliance, sometimes called nonadherence, although that is not a recognized diagnosis in the NANDA taxonomy, assumes that the patient was properly educated about the medication but has made the decision not to take it. It is vital that the nurse assess possible factors leading to the noncompliance *before* establishing this diagnosis. Does the patient understand why the medication was prescribed? Was dosing and scheduling information explained? Are adverse effects causing the patient to refuse the medication? Are cultural, religious, or social issues impacting the decision not to take the medication? Is the noncompliance related to inadequate financial resources?

Table 6.2 provides an abbreviated list of common nursing diagnoses applicable to pharmacotherapy. This is not an exhaustive list of all NANDA-approved diagnoses, and the establishment of new diagnoses and the research and rewording of previous diagnoses is ongoing. The nurse is encouraged to consult books on nursing diagnoses for more information on establishing, writing, and researching other nursing diagnoses that may apply to drug administration. The Nursing Practice Application tables throughout the drug chapters of the text include suggested nursing diagnoses that may be applicable to patients receiving a drug in the classification covered in the table. These are common nursing diagnoses that may be related to the conditions the drug is used to treat, or to the therapeutic or adverse effects of the drug.The student is encouraged to complete a diagnostic statement, using patient-specific defining characteristics and related factors that apply to actual patients for whom the student is caring.

Table 6.2 Selected Nursing Diagnoses Applicable to Drug Administration

NANDA-Approved Nursing Diagnoses	
Activity Intolerance	Ineffective Breathing Pattern
Anxiety	Ineffective Coping
Constipation	Ineffective Health Maintenance
Decreased Cardiac Output	Ineffective Health Management
Deficient Fluid Volume	Ineffective Peripheral Tissue Perfusion
Deficient Knowledge	Nausea
Diarrhea	Noncompliance
Disturbed Sleep Pattern	Obesity
Excess Fluid Volume	Overweight
Fatigue	Pain, Acute or Chronic
Hyperthermia	Risk for Aspiration
Hypothermia	Risk for Falls
Imbalanced Nutrition: Less Than Body Requirements	Risk for Impaired Liver Function
Impaired Gas Exchange	Risk for Infection
Impaired Oral Mucous Membrane	Risk for Injury
Impaired Physical Mobility	Risk for Poisoning
Impaired Skin Integrity	Risk for Suicide
Impaired Social Interaction	Self-Care Deficit, Bathing, Dressing, Feeding
Impaired Swallowing	Sexual Dysfunction
Impaired Verbal Communication	Urinary Incontinence
Ineffective Airway Clearance	Urinary Retention

Source: Herdman, T.H. & Kamitsuru, S. (Eds.) Nursing Diagnoses: Definitions and Classification 2015–2017. Copyright © 2014, 1994–2014 NANDA International. Used by arrangement with John Wiley & Sons Limited. Companion website: www.wiley.com/go/nursingdiagnoses.

6.4 Planning: Establishing Goals and Outcomes

The **planning phase** of the nursing process prioritizes diagnoses, formulates desired outcomes, and selects nursing interventions that can assist the patient to establish an optimal level of wellness. Short- or long-term **goals** are established that focus on what the patient will be able to do or achieve, not what the nurse will do. The objective measures of those goals, or outcomes, specifically define what the patient will do, under what circumstances, and within a specified time frame. The nurse also discusses goals and outcomes with the patient or caregiver, and these are prioritized to address immediate needs first. The planning phase links the strategies, or interventions, to the established goals and outcomes.

Before administering medications, the nurse should establish clear, realistic goals and outcomes so that planned interventions ensure safe and effective use of these drugs. The nurse establishes priorities based on the assessment data and nursing diagnoses, with high-priority needs addressed before low-priority needs.

With respect to pharmacotherapy, the planning phase involves two main components: drug administration and patient teaching. The overall goal of the nursing plan of care is the safe and effective administration of medication. To achieve this, the nurse focuses on safe medication administration and monitoring of the patient's condition and planning for patient teaching needs related to the drugs prescribed. The nurse may focus on goals related to pharmacotherapy for the short term or long term, depending on the setting and situation. For example, for a patient with a thrombus in the lower extremity who is placed on anticoagulant therapy, a short-term goal may be that the patient will not experience an increase in clot size, as evidenced by improving circulation to the lower extremity distal to the clot as a result of the medication. A long-term goal might focus on teaching the patient to effectively administer parenteral anticoagulant therapy at home.

Like assessment data, pharmacotherapeutic goals should focus first on the therapeutic outcomes of medications and then on the prevention or treatment of adverse effects and patient teaching needs. For the patient on pain medication, relief of pain is a priority established before treatment of the nausea, vomiting, or dizziness caused by the medication. The nurse should remember, however, that planning for the prevention or treatment of expected adverse effects is an integral step of the planning phase.

Outcomes are the specific criteria used to measure attainment of the selected goals. They are written to include the subject (usually the patient), the actions required by that subject, under what circumstances, the expected performance, and the specific time frame in which the subject will accomplish that performance. In the example of the patient who will be taught to self-administer anticoagulant therapy at home, an outcome may be written as: "Patient will demonstrate the injection of enoxaparin (Lovenox) using the preloaded syringe provided, given subcutaneously into the anterior abdominal areas, in 2 days (1 day prior to discharge)." This outcome includes the subject (patient), actions (demonstrate injection), circumstances (using a preloaded syringe), performance (subcutaneous injection into the abdomen), and time frame (2 days from now—1 day before discharge home). Writing specific outcomes also gives the nurse a concrete time frame to work toward assisting the patient to meet the goals. In the case of children or the mentally impaired, the pharmacotherapeutic outcomes include the caregiver responsible for administering the medication in the home setting.

After goals and outcomes are identified based on the nursing diagnoses, a plan of care is written and documented in the patient's chart or electronic health record. Each agency determines whether this plan will be communicated as either nursing-centered or interdisciplinary, or both. All plans should be patient-focused and include the patient or caregiver in their development. The goals and outcomes identified in the plan of care will assist the nurse and other health care providers in implementing interventions and evaluating the effectiveness of that care.

6.5 Implementing Specific Nursing Actions

The **implementation phase** is when the nurse applies the knowledge, skills, and principles of nursing care to help move the patient toward the desired goal and optimal wellness. Implementation involves *action* on the part of the nurse or patient: administering a drug, providing patient teaching, and initiating other specific actions identified by the plan of care. When applied to pharmacotherapy, the implementation phase involves administering the medication; continuing to assess the patient and monitor drug effects; carrying out the interventions developed in the planning phase to maximize the therapeutic response and prevent adverse events; and providing patient education to ensure safe and effective home use of the medications.

Monitoring drug effects is a primary intervention that nurses perform. A thorough knowledge of the actions of each medication is necessary to carry out this monitoring process. The nurse should first monitor for the identified therapeutic effect. A lack of sufficient therapeutic effect suggests the need to reassess pharmacotherapy. Monitoring may require a reassessment of the patient's physical condition, vital signs, body weight, laboratory values, and/or serum drug levels. The patient's statements about pain relief, as well as objective data, such as a change in blood pressure, are used to monitor the therapeutic outcomes of pharmacotherapy. The nurse also monitors for side and adverse effects and attempts to prevent or limit these effects when possible.

The intervention phase includes appropriate documentation of the administration of the medication as well as any adverse effects observed or reported by the patient. The nurse may include additional objective assessment data, such as vital signs, in the documentation to provide more details about the specific drug effects. Statements from the patient can provide subjective detail to the documentation. Each health care facility determines where, when, and how to document the administration of medications and any follow-up assessment data gathered.

Patient Education

Patient teaching is a vital component of the nurse's interventions for a patient receiving medications. Knowledge deficit and noncompliance are directly related to the type and quality of medication education that a patient receives. State nurse practice acts and regulating bodies such as The Joint Commission, which accredits health care agencies, consider teaching to be a primary role for nurses, giving it the weight of law and key importance in accreditation standards. Because the goals of pharmacotherapy are the safe administration of medications with the best therapeutic outcomes possible, teaching is aimed at providing the patient with the information necessary to ensure that this occurs. Every nurse–patient interaction presents an opportunity for teaching. Small portions of education given over time are often more effective than large amounts of information given on only one occasion. Discussing medications each time they are administered is an effective way to increase the amount of education accomplished. Table 6.3 summarizes key areas of teaching and provides sample questions the nurse might ask, or observations the nurse can make, to verify that teaching was effective. The Nursing Process Applications in chapters 12 through 49 also supply information on specific drugs and drug classes that is important to include in patient teaching, both to ensure therapeutic effects and to minimize adverse effects.

Providing written material assists the patient to retain the information and review it later. Providing a small notepad or other writing material allows the patient or

Treating the Diverse Patient: Non–English-Speaking and Culturally Diverse Patients

Health care agencies are required to provide translation services for their patients. The nurse should know in advance what translation services and interpreters are available to assist with communication and how to access those services. Some agencies may have employees who are able to serve as translators, whereas others may use services provided by telephone or Internet-based providers. The nurse should use interpreter services whenever possible, validating with the interpreter that he or she is able to understand the patient. Many dialects are similar but not the same, and knowing another language is not the same as understanding the culture. Can the interpreter understand the patient's language and cultural expressions or nuances well enough for effective communication to occur?

If a family member is interpreting, the nurse should be sure that the interpreter first understands and repeats the information back to the nurse before explaining it in the patient's own language. If adult family members are not available to translate, a child relative may be called upon to act as a translator. However, this should be considered as a "last resort" if no other translator is available. The nurse should use his or her best judgment in determining whether the child is old enough or mature enough to handle the responsibility, and any information gained during this time should be validated with a reliable source such as an official translator at the earliest convenience. These are especially important points to keep in mind if the translation is a summary of what was said rather than a line-by-line translation.

Before an interpreter is available, or if one is unavailable, the use of pictures, simple drawings, nonverbal cues, and body language may be needed to communicate with the patient. The nurse should be aware of culturally-based nonverbal communication behaviors (e.g., use of personal space, eye contact, or lack of eye contact). Gender sensitivities related to culture (e.g., male nurse or health care provider for female patients) and the use of touch are often sensitive issues. In the United States, an informal and personal style is often the norm. When working with patients of other cultures, adopting a more formal style may be more appropriate.

Table 6.3 Important Areas of Teaching for a Patient Receiving Medications

Area of Teaching	Important Questions and Observations
Therapeutic use and outcomes	• Can you tell me the name of your medication and what it is used for? • What will you look for to know that the medication is effective? (How will you know that the medicine is working?)
Monitoring side and adverse effects	• Which side effects can you handle by yourself (e.g., simple nausea, diarrhea)? • Which side effects should you report to your health care provider (e.g., extreme cases of nausea or vomiting, extreme dizziness, bleeding)?
Medication administration	• Can you tell me how much of the medication you should take (milligrams, number of tablets, milliliters of liquid, etc.)? • Can you tell me how often you should take it? • What special requirements are necessary when you take this medication (e.g., take with a full glass of water, take on an empty stomach, and remain upright for 30 minutes)? • Is there a specific order in which you should take your medications (e.g., using a bronchodilator before using a corticosteroid inhaler)? • Can you show me how you will give yourself the medication (e.g., eyedrops, subcutaneous injections)? • What special monitoring is required before you take this medication (e.g., pulse rate)? Can you demonstrate this for me? Based on that monitoring, when should you *not* take the medication? • Do you know how, or where, to store this medication? • What should you do if you miss a dose?
Other monitoring and special requirements	• Are there any special tests you should have related to this medication (e.g., finger-stick glucose levels, therapeutic drug levels)? • How often should these tests be done? • What other medications should you *not* take with this medication? • Are there any foods or beverages you must not have while taking this medication?

family to keep a list of questions related to the medications that may arise at a later time. Some medications come with a self-contained teaching program that includes videotapes. The nurse should always assess whether the patient is able to read and understand the material provided. Patient educational materials are ineffective if the reading level is above what the patient can understand or is in a language unfamiliar to the patient. Even patients with low reading ability may describe their reading as "good." Providing verbal instructions along with written materials may help to clarify anything the patient cannot read. The nurse may ask the patient to summarize key points after providing the teaching to verify that the patient has understood the information.

Pediatric patients often present special challenges to patient teaching. Specialized pediatric teaching materials may assist the nurse in teaching these patients. Parents or caregivers of children must be included in the medication administration process. The nurse should base medication administration in pediatric patients on safe pediatric dosages and limiting potential adverse drug reactions. Medication research often does not include children, so data are often unclear on safe pediatric doses and potential adverse drug reactions in this population. There is also a greater risk for serious medication errors, since drug administration in children often requires drug calculations using smaller doses. The nurse must be vigilant to ensure that the dosage is correct because even small errors in drug doses have the potential to cause serious adverse effects in infants and children.

The older adult population presents the nurse with additional nursing considerations. Age-appropriate teaching materials that are repeated slowly and provided in small increments may assist the nurse in teaching these patients. It may be necessary to co-teach the patient's caregiver. Older adult patients often have chronic illnesses and age-related changes that may cause medication effects to be unpredictable. Because of chronic diseases, older adults often take multiple drugs that may cause many drug–drug interactions.

6.6 Evaluating the Effects of Medications

The **evaluation phase** compares the patient's current health status with the desired outcome. This step is important to determine if the plan of care is appropriate, if it was met, or if it needs revision. If it was met, the plan of care was appropriate, and the problem or risk was resolved. The nurse and patient can then address the next highest priority health need. If the goal was partially met, the patient is moving toward the goal; however, the nurse may need to continue interventions for a longer time, or somehow modify interventions to completely resolve the problem. The nursing process comes full circle as the nurse reassesses the patient, reviews the nursing diagnoses, makes necessary changes, reviews and rewrites goals and outcomes, and carries out further interventions to meet the stated goals and outcomes.

As it relates to pharmacotherapy, evaluation is used to determine whether the therapeutic effects of the drug were achieved as well as whether adverse effects were prevented or kept to acceptable levels. If the evaluation data show no improvement over the baseline data, the interventions may require revision. The drug dose may need to be increased, more time may be needed to achieve therapeutic drug levels, or a different or additional drug may be needed. The nurse also evaluates the effectiveness of teaching provided and notes areas where further drug education is needed.

Evaluation is not the end of the process but the beginning of another cycle as the nurse continues to work to ensure safe and effective medication use and active patient involvement in his or her care. It is a checkpoint where the nurse considers the overall goal of safe and effective administration of medications and takes the steps necessary to maximize the success of pharmacotherapy. The nursing process acts as the overall framework for working toward this success.

Chapter Review

KEY Concepts

The numbered key concepts provide a succinct summary of the important points from the corresponding numbered section within the chapter. If any of these points are not clear, refer to the numbered section within the chapter for review.

6.1 The nursing process is a systematic method of problem solving that uses a nurse's critical thinking skills to care for the patient. It is patient-centered, dynamic, and based on ongoing patient data and needs; and it is a collaborative effort between the nurse, the patient, and other members of the health care team.

6.2 Assessment is the systematic collection of patient data. Assessment of the patient receiving medications includes health history information, physical assessment data, laboratory values and other measurable data, and an assessment of medication effects, including both therapeutic and side effects.

6.3 Nursing diagnoses are written to address the patient's responses to drug administration. They are developed after an analysis of the assessment data, are focused on the patient's problems, and are verified with the patient or caregiver.

6.4 Goals and outcomes, which are developed from the nursing diagnoses, direct the interventions required by the plan of care. Goals focus on what the patient should be able to achieve, and outcomes provide the specific, measurable criteria that will be used to measure goal attainment.

6.5 The implementation phase involves administering the drug and carrying out interventions to promote a therapeutic response and minimize adverse effects of the drug. Key interventions required of the nurse in the implementation phase include monitoring drug effects, documenting medications, and patient teaching.

6.6 The evaluation phase of the nursing process compares the patient's current health status with the desired outcome. This step is important to determine if the plan of care is appropriate, if it was met, or if it needs revision. Nursing diagnoses are reviewed or rewritten, goals and outcomes are refined, and new interventions are carried out.

REVIEW Questions

1. Which of the following are correct statements regarding nursing diagnoses? (Select all that apply.)

1. They identify the medical problem experienced by the patient.
2. They are identified for the patient by the nurse.
3. They identify the patient's response to a health condition or life process.
4. They assist in determining nursing interventions.
5. They remain the same throughout the patient's health care encounter to ensure continuity of care.

2. Which of the following represents an appropriate outcome established during the planning phase?

1. The nurse will teach the patient to recognize and respond to adverse effects from the medication.
2. The patient will demonstrate self-administration of the medication, using a preloaded syringe into the subcutaneous tissue of the thigh, prior to discharge.
3. The nurse will teach the patient to accurately prepare the dose of medication.
4. The patient will be able to self-manage his disease and medications.

3. A 15-year-old adolescent with a history of diabetes is treated in the emergency department for complications related to skipping her medication for diabetes. She confides in the nurse that she deliberately skipped some of her medication doses because she did not want to gain weight and she is afraid of needle marks. Before establishing a diagnosis of "Noncompliance," what should the nurse assess?
   1. Whether the patient received adequate teaching related to her medication and expresses an understanding of that teaching
   2. Whether the patient was encouraged to skip her medication by a family member or friend
   3. Whether the patient is old enough to understand the consequences of her actions
   4. Whether the provider will write another prescription because the patient refused to take the medication the first time
4. Which factor is most important for the nurse to assess when evaluating the effectiveness of a patient's drug therapy?
   1. The patient's promise to comply with drug therapy
   2. The patient's satisfaction with the drug
   3. The cost of the medication
   4. Evidence of therapeutic benefit from the medication
5. Which method may offer the best opportunity for patient teaching?
   1. Providing detailed written information when the patient is discharged
   2. Providing the patient with Internet links to conduct research on drugs
   3. Referring the patient to external health care groups that provide patient education, such as the American Heart Association
   4. Providing education about the patient's medications each time the nurse administers the drugs
6. During the evaluation phase of drug administration, the nurse completes which responsibilities?
   1. Prepares and administers drugs correctly
   2. Establishes goals and outcome criteria related to drug therapy
   3. Monitors the patient for therapeutic and adverse effects
   4. Gathers data in a drug and dietary history

CRITICAL THINKING Questions

1. A 67-year-old patient has been diagnosed with a type of anemia that requires monthly injections of vitamin B_{12}. He is learning how to give himself the injections at home and does not have any visual or dexterity impairments. The nurse has taught and reviewed how to draw the solution out of the medication vial into the syringe and is now working on the appropriate injection technique. Write an outcome statement for this patient.
2. While evaluating the therapeutic effects of a medication prescribed for the patient with asthma, the nurse notes that the goal has been only "partially met" because the patient continues to have some wheezing, despite taking the medication for two days. What should the nurse do next?
3. A nursing student is assigned to a nurse preceptor who is administering oral medications. The student notes that the preceptor administers the drugs safely but routinely fails to offer the patient information about the drug being administered. Identify the information that the nurse should teach the patient during medication administration.

Visit www.pearsonhighered.com/nursingresources for answers and rationales for all activities.

REFERENCE

Herdman, T. H., & Kamitsuru, S. (2014). *NANDA International nursing diagnoses: Definitions and classification 2015–2017*. Oxford, United Kingdom: Wiley Blackwell.

Chapter 7

Medication Errors and Risk Reduction

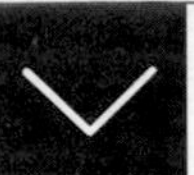

Learning Outcomes

After reading this chapter, the student should be able to:

1. Define medication error.
2. Identify factors that contribute to medication errors.
3. Explain the impact of medication errors on patients and health care agencies.
4. Describe methods for reporting and documenting medication errors.
5. Describe strategies the nurse can implement to reduce medication errors and incidents.
6. Explain how effective medication reconciliation can reduce medication errors.
7. Identify patient teaching information that can be used to reduce medication errors and incidents.
8. Explain strategies used by health care organizations to reduce the number of medication errors and incidents.
9. Identify governmental and national agencies that track medication errors and incidents and provide information to health care providers.

In clinical practice, the nurse maximizes patient safety by striving to be 100% accurate when administering medications. Drug administration, however, requires multiple complex steps by health care providers, pharmacists, nurses, and patients and can never be 100% error-free. Occasionally medication errors are made that can significantly affect treatment outcomes. The purpose of this chapter is to examine the reasons for medication errors and explore strategies the nurse can use to prevent them.

7.1 Defining Medication Errors

According to the National Coordinating Council for Medication Error Reporting and Prevention (NCC MERP), a **medication error** is defined as the following:

> any preventable event that may cause or lead to inappropriate medication use or patient harm while the medication is in the control of the health care professional, patient, or consumer. Such events may be related to professional practice, health care products, procedures, and systems, including prescribing; order communication; product labeling, packaging, and nomenclature; compounding; dispensing; distribution; administration; education; monitoring; and use (NCC MERP, 2014b).

NCC MERP has developed the **medication error index** (see Figure 7.1). This index provides a conceptual framework that places medication errors into nine categories based on the extent of harm an error can cause. For example, Category A is a medication error in which no harm occurred to the patient whereas category H is a medication error that resulted in permanent harm.

It is important to note that the NCC MERP definition of a medication error encompasses a large number of potential errors, some of which are not controlled by physicians, pharmacists, nurses, or patients. While these health professionals are certainly at the forefront of ensuring accurate medication administration, medication errors also include mistakes in product labeling, manufacturing, and distribution. This broad definition of a medication error demands collaboration of all facets of the health care industry.

7.2 Factors Contributing to Medication Errors

At its most fundamental level, accurate medication administration involves a partnership between the health care provider and the patient. This relationship is dependent on the competence of the health care provider as well as the patient's full adherence with the drug therapy regimen. This dual responsibility provides a simple, though useful, way to conceptualize medication errors as resulting from health care provider error or patient error. Clearly, the purpose of classifying and studying these errors is not to assess individual blame but to prevent future errors.

Factors contributing to medication errors by *health care providers* include, but are not limited to, the following:

- Omitting one of the rights of drug administration (see chapter 3). Common errors include giving an incorrect dose, omitting an ordered dose, and giving the wrong drug.
- Failing to perform an agency system check. The pharmacist and nurse must collaborate on checking the accuracy and appropriateness of medication orders prior to administering drugs to a patient.
- Failing to account for patient variables such as age, body size, and impairment in renal or hepatic function. The nurse should always review recent laboratory data and other information in the patient's chart before administering medications, especially for those drugs that have a narrow margin of safety.
- Giving medications based on verbal orders or phone orders, which may be misinterpreted or go undocumented. The nurse should always follow the health care agency's policy when accepting verbal or phone orders, many of which require the provider's signature within 24 hours.
- Giving medications based on an incomplete order or an illegible order when the nurse is unsure of the correct drug, dosage, or administration method. Incomplete orders should be clarified with the prescriber before the medication is administered. Written orders should avoid certain abbreviations that are frequent sources of medication errors, as listed in appendix A.
- Practicing under stressful work conditions. Studies have correlated an increased number of errors with the stress level of nurses. Studies have also indicated that the rate of medication errors may increase when individual nurses are assigned to patients who are the most acutely ill.

Patients, or their caregivers, may also contribute to medication errors by:

- Taking drugs prescribed by several practitioners without informing each of their health care providers about all prescribed medications.
- Getting their prescriptions filled at more than one pharmacy.
- Not filling or refilling their prescriptions.
- Taking medications in incorrect doses, at the wrong time of day, or otherwise not following the prescriber's instructions.
- Taking medications that may have been left over from a previous illness or prescribed for another person.

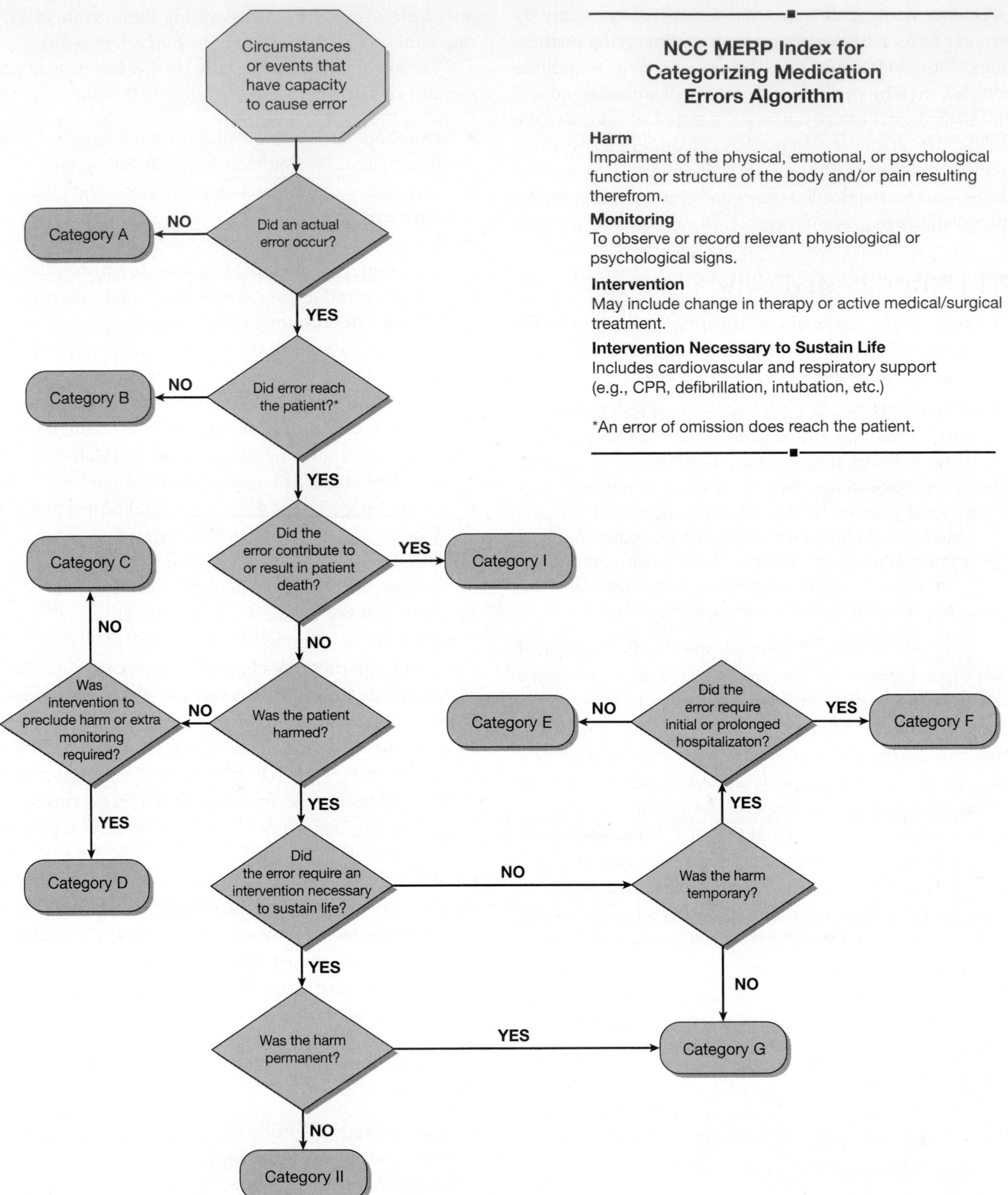

FIGURE 7.1 Index for categorizing medication errors algorithm

Source: Reprinted with the permission of the National Coordinating Council for Medication Error Reporting and Prevention, ©2001.

7.3 The Impact of Medication Errors

Medication errors are the most common cause of morbidity and preventable death within hospitals. When a medication error occurs, the repercussions can be emotionally devastating and extend beyond the particular nurse and patient involved. A medication error can lengthen the patient's hospital stay, which increases costs and the time that a patient is separated from family members. The health care provider making the medication error may suffer from self-doubt and embarrassment. If a high error rate occurs within a particular unit, the nursing unit may develop a poor reputation within the facility. If frequent medication errors or serious errors are publicized, the reputation of the facility may suffer, because it may be perceived as unsafe. Administrative personnel may also be penalized because of errors within their departments or the hospital as a whole.

NCC MERP (2008) believes there is no acceptable incidence rate for medication errors. The goal of every health care organization, however, is to continuously improve medication administration systems to keep the medication error incidence rate to its lowest possible value. All errors, whether or not they harm the patient, should be investigated with the goal of identifying ways to improve the medication administration process to prevent future errors. The investigation should occur in a nonpunitive manner that will encourage staff to report errors, thereby building a culture of safety within an organization. Analysis of error patterns can alert nurses and health care administrators that a new policy or procedure needs to be implemented to reduce or eliminate medication errors.

7.4 Reporting and Documenting Medication Errors

When a health care provider commits or observes an error, effects can be lasting and widespread. Although some errors go unreported, it is always the nurse's legal and ethical responsibility to report all occurrences. In severe cases, adverse reactions caused by medication errors may require the initiation of lifesaving interventions for the patient. After such an incident, the patient may require follow-up supervision and medical treatments.

The U.S. Food and Drug Administration (FDA) coordinates the reporting of medication errors at the federal level. The FDA Safety Information and Adverse Event Reporting Program, known as MedWatch, serves two main purposes (FDA, 2014):

- It allows health care providers and members of the public to report medication errors. The service provides a voluntary reporting form, which can be used by anyone observing or experiencing an adverse drug event. The service also provides a mandatory reporting form for health care agencies and pharmaceutical manufacturers who are required by law to report certain adverse drug events and medication errors.
- It provides up-to-date clinical information about safety issues involving medical products, including prescription and over-the-counter (OTC) drugs, biologics, medical and radiation-emitting devices, and special nutritional products. This includes public access to patient medication guides and access to current drug prescribing information

A second organization that has been established to provide assistance with medication errors is the NCC MERP. The mission of NCC MERP is "to maximize the safe use of medications and to increase awareness of medication errors through open communication, increased reporting and promotion of medication error prevention strategies" (NCC MERP, 2014a). In recent years, this organization has compiled recommendations for using barcode labels on medications, reducing medication errors in non–health settings, avoiding medication errors with drug samples, and promoting the safe use of suffixes in prescription drug names.

The federal agency responsible for reviewing all medication error reports is the FDA's Division of Medication Error Prevention and Analysis (DMEPA). Gathering and analyzing data from the MedWatch service, the NCC MERP and other patient safety organizations, the DMEPA makes recommendations such as changing product names or product labels that may be causing medication errors.

Community-Oriented Practice

DECREASING DRUG ERRORS BY FOCUSING ON HEALTH LITERACY

Limited health literacy may have profound effects on how well a patient follows instructions for medication administration. For some patients, having a clear understanding of how to take their medications is further hampered when a language other than English is spoken. Samuels-Kalow, Stack, & Porter (2013) found that overall, 30% of all patients demonstrated a medication error with acetaminophen after receiving instructions upon discharge from an emergency department, but 50% of Spanish-speaking patients had a dosing error. Even with the use of a Spanish-speaking translator, errors occurred.

Health literacy encompasses more than understanding which drugs to take and how to take them, and limited health literacy occurs across all populations in society, regardless of one's native language. Because the majority of medications are taken in a setting other than a health-care facility, to decrease errors in the patient's home or community setting, it is vital that the patient has an adequate understanding of medication administration.

The nurse can work to improve a patient's health literacy about medication administration and decrease the possibility of errors by ensuring a variety of methods are used to educate the patient. These include using printed materials that use "plain language" wording such as "take one pill in the morning and one at bedtime," rather than "take one tablet, twice a day" (Bailey, Sarkar, Chen, Schillinger, & Wolf, 2012; Smith & Wallace, 2013); using written materials that incorporate simple graphics that reinforce the material; and reviewing the material verbally with the patient (Samuels-Kalow et al., 2013) before discharging the patient from the health care setting. Because it is the nurse who most often provides patient education, understanding and addressing the effects that limited health literacy may have on their patients' safe and effective medication administration is crucial for all nurses.

Documenting in the Patient's Medical Record

All health care facilities should have clear policies and procedures for reporting medication errors. Documentation should include more than simply recording that a medical error occurred. Documentation in the medical record must include specific nursing interventions that were implemented following the error to protect patient safety, such as monitoring vital signs and assessing the patient for possible complications. Failure to report nursing actions implies either negligence (i.e., no interventions were taken) or lack of acknowledgment that the incident occurred. The nurse should also document all individuals who were notified of the error. The **medication administration record (MAR)** is another source that should contain information about what medication was given or omitted.

Reporting the Error

In addition to documenting in the patient's medical record, the nurse making or observing the medication error should complete a written report of the error. Depending on the health care agency, these reports may be called "Incident Reports," "Occurrence Reports," or similar titles. The specific details of the error should be recorded in a factual and objective manner. The report allows the nurse an opportunity to identify factors that contributed to the medication error and assists in identifying any specific performance improvement strategies that may need to be implemented. The written report is not included in the patient's medical record but is used by the agency's risk management personnel for quality improvement and assurance and may be used by nursing administration and education to identify common error occurrences and the need for performance improvement or educational intervention.

Accurate documentation in the medical record and in the error report is essential for legal reasons. These documents verify that the patient's safety was protected and serve as a tool to improve medication administration processes. Legal complications may ensue if there is an attempt to hide a mistake or delay corrective action, or if the nurse forgets to document interventions in the patient's chart.

Sentinel Events

In the context of medication safety, a **sentinel event** is one that results in an unexpected, serious, or fatal injury following the administration (or lack of administration) of a medication. The serious injury may be physical or psychological, and it may occur at the time of the drug administration or place the patient at risk to a future injury.

Not all medication errors result in sentinel events. Serious events are called sentinel because they signal the need for an immediate investigation and response. Because of the grave nature of a sentinel event, they are *always* investigated and interventions put in place to ensure that the event does not recur. Root-cause analysis is used to identify the causes and required interventions to prevent a recurrence.

7.5 Strategies for Reducing Medication Errors

The most frequent types of drug errors vary depending on the specific population (e.g., pediatrics versus geriatrics) or health care unit (e.g., intensive care versus long-term care). The most common errors usually are administering an improper dose, giving the wrong drug, and using the wrong route of administration. There is an increased risk for errors in older adults because they often take numerous medications, have multiple health care providers, and are experiencing normal age-related changes in physiology. Children are another vulnerable population because they receive medication dosages based on weight (which increases the possibility of dosage miscalculations), and the therapeutic dosages are much smaller.

What can the nurse do in the clinical setting to avoid medication errors and promote safe administration? The nurse can begin by following the steps of the nursing process:

1. *Assessment.* Ask the patient about allergies to food or medications, current health concerns, and use of OTC medications and herbal supplements. For all medications taken prior to assessment, ensure that the patient has been receiving the right dose, at the right time, and by the right route. Assess kidney, liver, and other body system functions to determine if impairments are present that could affect pharmacotherapy.
2. *Planning.* Minimize factors that contribute to medication errors: Avoid using abbreviations that can be misunderstood (see appendix A), question unclear orders, do not accept verbal orders, and follow specific facility policies and procedures related to medication administration. Ask the patient to demonstrate an understanding of the goals of therapy.
3. *Implementation.* Eliminate potential distractions during medication administration that could result in an error. Excessive noise, unrelated activity, or talking to coworkers can distract the nurse's attention and result in a medication error. In addition to following the rights of medication administration, keep the following steps in mind as well:
   - Positively verify the identity of each patient using two means (e.g., name and birth date) before administering the medication according to facility policy and procedures.
   - Use the correct procedures and techniques for all routes of administration. Use sterile materials and aseptic techniques when administering parenteral or eye medication.

- Calculate medication doses correctly and measure liquid drugs carefully. When giving medications that have a narrow safety margin, ask a colleague or a pharmacist to check the calculations to make certain the dosage is correct. Double-check all pediatric calculations prior to administration. Selected drugs that have a narrow safety margin are shown in appendix B.
- Record the medication on the MAR immediately after administration.
- Always confirm that the patient has swallowed an oral medication. Never leave the medication at the bedside unless there is a specific order that medications may be left there.
- Be alert for long-acting oral dosage forms with indicators such as *LA*, *XL*, and *XR*. Instruct the patient not to crush, chew, or break the medication in half unless instructed to do so by the health care provider because doing so could cause an overdose.
- Be alert for drugs whose names look alike and sound alike. When the names are written in a hurry or given over the phone, such drugs may be easily mistaken and cause a medication error. A selected list of look-alike and sound-alike drugs is shown in Table 7.1.

4. *Evaluation.* Assess the patient for expected outcomes and determine if any adverse effects have occurred.

The nurse must be vigilant in keeping up to date on pharmacotherapeutics and should never administer a medication without being familiar with its uses and side effects. There are many venues by which the nurse can obtain updated medication knowledge and help maintain evidence-based practice skills. Each nursing unit should have current drug references available. The nurse can also call the pharmacy to obtain information about the drug or, if available, look it up on the Internet using reliable sources. Many nurses now rely on personal digital assistants (PDAs) or smartphones to provide current information. These devices can be updated daily or weekly by downloading information that reflects current research on preventing medical errors.

Table 7.1 Look-Alike and Sound-Alike Drug Names

acetazolamide	acetohexamide
AcipHex	Aricept
Adderall	Inderal
bupropion	buspirone
carboplatin	cisplatin
Celebrex	Cerebyx
chlorpromazine	chlorpropamide
cycloserine	cyclosporine
daunorubicin	doxorubicin
dimenhydramine	diphenhydramine
Diprivan	Ditropan
dobutamine	dopamine
ephedrine	epinephrine
Humalog	Humulin
hydromorphone	morphine
infliximab	rituximab
isotretinoin	tretinoin
Kaletra	Keppra
Lamisil	Lamictal
lamivudine	lamotrigine
leucovorin	Leukeran
Lexapro	Loxitane
MS Contin	OxyContin
Neulasta	Neumega
oxycodone	OxyContin
paroxetine	fluoxetine
Retrovir	ritonavir
Seroquel	Sinequan
sumatriptan	zolmitriptan
Tiagabine	tizanidine
TobraDex	Tobrex
Tramadol	trazodone
Trental	tegretol
valacyclovir	valganciclovir
vinblastine	vincristine
Viracept	Viramune
Zantac	Zyrtec
Zestril	Zotia
Zyprexa	Celexa

7.6 Medication Reconciliation

Many geriatric patients have multiple chronic disorders, each of which may be treated by individual specialists. It is common for these patients to receive multiple prescriptions, sometimes for the same condition, that have conflicting pharmacologic actions, a condition termed **polypharmacy.** Although not unique to older adults, polypharmacy is most often seen in this age group. Keeping track of multiple medications, their doses, indications, routes, and frequency of administration is a major challenge for both patients and health care providers. Failure to properly record medication information, and to communicate that information to health care providers, is a potential cause of medication errors.

Patient Safety: Interruptions and Medication Administration Errors

Hospitals can be busy places and although that may seem self-evident, the impact of that fact may result in increased medication errors. Westbrook, Woods, Rob, Dunsmuir, and Day (2010) studied the impact of interruptions on medication administration and the risk and severity of errors. Both procedure errors (e.g., checking patient ID, using aseptic technique, co-witnessing of preparation for high-alert medications) and clinical errors (e.g., "Five Rights" of administration, extra dosages, unordered drugs) were observed during times when nurses were interrupted during medication administration as well as during uninterrupted times. While errors occurred throughout, the more interruptions that occurred, the greater the risk of errors regardless of the experience level of the nurse. An estimated risk of 2.3% for a major error was noted without interruptions during medication administration with this risk doubling to 4.7% with four interruptions. Studies conducted since that original research have not demonstrated a significant impact on error reduction when interventions aimed at decreasing interruptions were attempted (Raban & Westbrook, 2014). Nurses must be especially aware of the need to minimize distractions during medication administration in order to minimize errors.

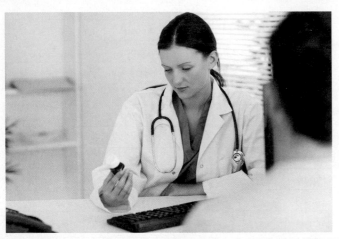

FIGURE 7.2 Medication reconciliation on admission and discharge is an important means of reducing medication errors
WavebreakmediaMicro/Fotolia.

Medication reconciliation is the process of tracking medications as the patient proceeds from one health care provider to another. Reconciliation accurately lists all medications a patient is taking in an attempt to reduce duplication, omissions, dosing errors, or drug interactions. For example, when admitted to care, the nurse records all medications the patient has been taking at home, including the dose, route, and frequency (Figure 7.2). This list is checked against admission orders and is transferred to other practitioners whenever the patient is moved to a different unit within the hospital. It is also checked at discharge. These "interfaces of care" are the most likely places that medication reconciliation errors have been found to occur.

Because lack of medication reconciliation is a major cause of medication errors, most hospitals have implemented a process for documenting a complete list of the patient's current medications upon admission. This list should include prescription and OTC medications, vitamins, and herbal products. This medication list should be communicated to the next provider of service when a patient is referred or transferred to another setting, service, health care provider, or level of care within or outside the organization. On discharge from the facility, the patient should be provided with the complete list of medications to be taken as well as instructions on how to take any newly prescribed medications.

7.7 Effective Patient Teaching for Medication Usage

An essential strategy for avoiding medication errors is to educate the patient by providing written age-appropriate handouts, audiovisual teaching aids about the medication, and contact information about whom to notify in the event of an adverse reaction. The nurse should be attentive to the patient's ability to understand the materials and to use any equipment such as medication cups appropriately. Having the patient "teach back" to the nurse to confirm that the patient has understood the content is a strategy that assists the nurse to evaluate the teaching.

To minimize the potential for medication errors, the nurse should teach the patients or home caregivers the following:

- Know the names of all medications they are taking, the uses, the doses, and when and how they should be taken.
- Know what side effects need to be reported immediately.
- Read the label prior to each drug administration and use the medication device that comes with liquid medications rather than household measuring spoons.
- Carry a list of all medications, including OTC drugs, as well as herbal and dietary supplements that are being taken. If possible, use one pharmacy for all prescriptions.
- Ask questions. Health care providers want to be partners in maintaining safe medication principles.

7.8 How the Health Care Industry Is Reducing Medication Errors

In recent years, the health care industry has implemented widespread changes in the way medications are prescribed and administered. In addition to increasing efficiency and reducing health care costs, some of these trends have resulted in a reduction in medication errors due to more accurate prescribing.

One such trend is electronic health records (EHRs), which includes **e-prescribing**, the transmission of prescription-related information through electronic transmission to a pharmacy or health care provider. Seven of ten physicians now use e-prescribing, which represents a ten-fold increase from 2008 to 2014 (Gabriel & Swain, 2014). Most electronic prescription systems check any new medications against current medications to assist the health care provider in identifying and preventing potential drug–drug interactions. Electronic prescribing also helps reduce the risk of medication error due to poorly written or misinterpreted handwritten orders.

A second important trend in health care agencies is the implementation of barcode–assisted medication administration (BCMA). BCMA is a technology used to verify and document medication administration at the point of care, usually the patient's bedside. When the nurse scans the barcode on the patient's wristband, the patient's electronic MAR opens on a bedside computer. The nurse can determine the medication and dose to be administered. Once the barcode on the medication unit-dose package is scanned and matches the patient record, the dose may be administered. An electronic alert is issued if the wrong medication is scanned, or if it is the wrong dose, or at an incorrect time of day. Studies have indicated that this technology has reduced multiple types of medication errors.

Larger health care agencies often have **risk-management** departments to examine risks and minimize the number of medication errors. Risk-management personnel investigate incidents, track data, identify problems, and provide recommendations for improvement. Nurses collaborate with the risk-management committees to seek means of reducing medication errors by modifying policies and procedures within the institution.

Through data collection, specific solutions can be created to reduce the number of medication errors. Root-cause analysis, or RCA, is being implemented in many health care organizations as a method to prevent future mistakes. By answering three basic questions—What happened? Why did it happen? and What can be done to prevent it from happening again?—RCA seeks to prevent another occurrence. Many agencies also continue RCA with the question "Has the risk of recurrence actually been reduced?" by analyzing data postoccurrence. The overall goal of reporting medication errors and conducting follow-up assessments such as RCA is safe and effective patient care and patient medication administration.

Chapter Review

KEY Concepts

The numbered key concepts provide a succinct summary of the important points from the corresponding numbered section within the chapter. If any of these points are not clear, refer to the numbered section within the chapter for review.

7.1 A medication error may be related to misinterpretations, miscalculations, misadministrations, handwriting misinterpretation, and misunderstanding of verbal or phone orders. Whether the patient is injured or not, it is still a medication error.

7.2 Numerous factors contribute to medication errors, including mistakes in the five rights of drug administration, failing to follow agency procedures or consider patient variables, giving medications based on verbal orders, not confirming orders that are illegible or incomplete, and working under stressful conditions. Patients also contribute to errors by using more than one pharmacy, not informing health care providers of all medications they are taking, or not following instructions.

7.3 The goal of every health care organization is to continuously improve medication administration systems to keep the medication error incidence rate to its lowest possible value.

7.4 The nurse is legally and ethically responsible for reporting medication errors—whether or not they cause harm to a patient—in the patient's medical record and on an incident report. The FDA and NCC MERP are two agencies that track medication errors and provide data to help institute procedures to prevent them.

7.5 The nurse can reduce medication errors by adhering to the four steps of the nursing process: assessment, planning, implementation, and evaluation. Keeping up to date on pharmacotherapeutics and knowing common error types are instrumental to safe medication administration.

7.6 Medication reconciliation is an important means of reducing medication errors. Medication reconciliation is a process of keeping track of a patient's medications as the patient proceeds from one health care provider to another.

7.7 Patient teaching includes providing age-appropriate medication handouts and encouraging patients to keep a list of all prescribed medications, OTC drugs, herbal therapies, and vitamins they are taking and to report them to all health care providers.

7.8 Facilities use electronic health records, barcode-assisted medication administration at the point of care, risk-management departments, and agency policies and procedures to decrease the incidence of medication errors.

REVIEW Questions

1. A health care provider has written an order for digoxin for the patient but the nurse cannot read whether the order is for 0.25 mg, 0.125 mg, or 125 mg because there is no "zero" and the decimal point may be a "one." What action would be the best to prevent a medication error?
   1. Check the dosage with a more experienced nurse.
   2. Consult a drug handbook and administer the normal dose.
   3. Contact the hospital pharmacist about the order.
   4. Contact the health care provider to clarify the illegible order.
2. The nurse administers a medication to the wrong patient. What are the appropriate nursing actions required? (Select all that apply.)
   1. Monitor the patient for adverse reactions.
   2. Document the error if the patient has an adverse reaction.
   3. Report the error to the health care provider.
   4. Notify the hospital legal department of the error.
   5. Document the error in a critical incident/occurrence report.
3. The nurse is teaching a postoperative patient about the medications ordered for use at home. Because this patient also has a primary care provider in addition to the surgeon, what strategy should the nurse include in this teaching session that might prevent a medication error in the home setting?
   1. Encourage the patient to consult the Internet about possible side effects.
   2. Delay taking any new medications prescribed by the surgeon until the next health visit with the primary provider.
   3. Have all prescriptions filled at one pharmacy.
   4. Insist on using only brand-name drugs because they are easier to remember than generic names.
4. As the nurse enters a room to administer medications, the patient states, "I'm in the bathroom. Just leave my pills on the table and I'll take them when I come out." What is the nurse's best response?
   1. Leave them on the table as requested and check back with the patient later to verify they were taken.
   2. Leave the medications with the patient's visitors so they can verify that they were taken.
   3. Inform the patient that the medications must be taken now; otherwise they must be documented as "refused."
   4. Inform the patient that the nurse will return in a few minutes when the patient is available to take the medications.
5. The nurse is administering medications and the patient states, "I've never seen that blue pill before." What would be the nurse's most appropriate action?
   1. Verify the order and double-check the drug label.
   2. Administer the medication in the existing form.
   3. Instruct the patient that different brands are frequently used and may account for the change of color.
   4. Recommend that the patient discuss the medication with the provider and give the medication.
6. The health care agency is implementing the use of root-cause analysis (RCA) to reduce the occurrence of medication errors. What areas does RCA analyze in order to prevent errors from recurring?
   1. Why the medication was ordered, whether it was the correct medication, and whether the patient experienced therapeutic results
   2. What happened, why it happened, and what can be done to prevent it from happening again
   3. What the cost of the medication was, whether it was the most appropriate medication to order, or whether there is a better alternative
   4. Whether the medication was documented in the provider's orders, medication administration record, and pharmacy

CRITICAL THINKING Questions

1. A nurse is teaching a young patient's mother about administering liquid medications to her child. The mother expresses concern about the ability to use the small medication cup that comes with the medicine because the printed amounts are hard to read. What might the nurse recommend as alternatives?
2. A health care provider writes an order for Tylenol PO q3–4h for mild pain. The nurse evaluates this order and is concerned that it is incomplete. Identify the probable concern and describe what the nurse should do prior to administering this medication.
3. A new nurse does not check an antibiotic dosage ordered by a health care provider for a pediatric patient and the order is for a dosage that is too high for the patient's size. The nurse subsequently overdoses a 2-year-old patient, and an experienced nurse notices the error during the evening shift change. Identify each person who is responsible for the error and how each is responsible.

Visit www.pearsonhighered.com/nursingresources for answers and rationales for all activities.

REFERENCES

Bailey, S. C., Sarkar, U., Chen, A. H., Schillinger, D., & Wolf, M. S. (2012). Evaluation of language concordant, patient-centered drug label instructions. *Journal of General Internal Medicine, 27,* 1707–1713. doi:10.1007/s11606-012-2035-3

Gabriel, M. H., & Swain, M. (2014). E-prescribing trends in the United States. *ONC Data Brief, No.18.* Office of the National Coordinator for Health Information Technology. Retrieved from http://healthit.gov/sites/default/files/oncdatabriefe-prescribingincreases2014.pdf

National Coordinating Council for Medication Error and Prevention. (2008). *Statement of medication error rates.* Retrieved from http://www.nccmerp.org/statement-medication-error-rates

National Coordinating Council for Medication Error Reporting and Prevention. (2014a). *About NCC MERP.* Retrieved from http://www.nccmerp.org/aboutNCCMERP.html

National Coordinating Council for Medication Error Reporting and Prevention. (2014b). *About medication errors: What is a medication error?* Retrieved from http://www.nccmerp.org/aboutMedErrors.html

Raban, M. Z., & Westbrook, J. I. (2014). Are interventions to reduce interruptions and errors during medication administration effective? A systematic review. *BMJ Quality & Safety, 23,* 414–421. doi:10.1136/bmjqs-2013-002118

Samuels-Kalow, M. E., Stack, A. M., & Porter, S. C. (2013). Parental language and dosing errors after discharge from the pediatric emergency department. *Pediatric Emergency Care, 29,* 982–987. doi:10.1097/PEC.0b013e3182a269ec

Smith, M. Y., & Wallace, L. S. (2013). Reducing drug self-injections errors: A randomized trial comparing a "standard" versus "plain language" version of patient instructions for use. *Research in Social & Administrative Pharmacy, 9,* 621–625. doi:10.1016/j.sapharm.2012.10.007

United States Food and Drug Administration. (2014). *Medwatch: The FDA safety information and adverse event reporting system.* Retrieved from http://www.fda.gov/Safety/MedWatch/default.htm

Westbrook, J. I., Woods, A., Rob, M. I., Dunsmuir, W. T. M., & Day, R. O. (2010). Association of interruptions with an increased risk and severity of medication administration errors. *Archives of Internal Medicine, 170,* 683–690. doi:10.1001/archinternmed.2010.65

SELECTED BIBLIOGRAPHY

Classen, D. C., Phansalkar, S., & Bates, D. W. (2011). Critical drug-drug interactions for use in electronic health records systems with computerized physician order entry: Review of leading approaches. *Journal of Patient Safety, 7,* 61–65. doi:10.1097/PTS.0b013e31821d6f6e

Dolansky, M. A., Druschel, K., Helba, M., & Courtney, K. (2013). Nursing student medication errors: A case study using root cause analysis. *Journal of Professional Nursing,* 29(2), 102–108. doi:10.1016/j.profnurs.2012.12.010

Emmerton, L. M., & Rizk, M. F. (2012). Look-alike and sound-alike medicines: Risks and 'solutions.' *International Journal of Clinical Pharmacy, 34,* 4–8. doi:10.1007/s11096-011-9595-x

Fanus, K., Huddleston, R., Wisotzkey, S., & Hempling, R. (2014). Embracing a culture of safety by decreasing medication errors. *Nursing Management, 45,* 16–19. doi:10.1097/01.NUMA.0000443940.60879.fa

Garrouste-Orgeas, M., Philippart, F., Bruel, C., Max, A., Lau, N., & Misset, B. (2012). Overview of medical errors and adverse events. *Annals of Intensive Care,* 2(1), 2. doi:10.1186/2110-5820-2-2

Getz, K. A., Stergiopoulos, S., & Kaitin, K. I. (2012). Evaluating the completeness and accuracy of MedWatch data. *American Journal of Therapeutics,* 21(6), 442–446. doi:10.1097/MJT.0b013e318262316f

The Joint Commission. (2013). *Sentinel Events.* Retrieved from http://www.jointcommission.org/assets/1/6/CAMH_2012_Update2_24_SE.pdf

Keers, R. N., Williams, S. D., Cooke, J., Walsh, T., & Ashcroft, D. M. (2014). Impact of interventions designed to reduce medication administration errors in hospitals: A systematic review. *Drug Safety, 37,* 317–332. doi:10.1007/s40264-014-0152-0

Kong, M., & Mondul, A. (2014). Medication error. In A. Agrawal (Ed.), *Patient safety: A case-based comprehensive guide* (pp. 103–114). New York, NY: Springer. doi:10.1007/978-1-4614-7419-7_7

Pham, J. C., Aswani, M. S., Rosen, M., HeeWon, L., Huddle, M., Weeks, K., & Pronovost, P. J. (2012). Reducing medical errors and adverse events. *Annual Review of Medicine, 63,* 447–463. doi:10.1146/annurev-med-061410-121352

Redley, B., & Botti, M. (2013). Reported medication errors after introducing an electronic medication management system. *Journal of Clinical Nursing,* 22(3–4), 579–589. doi:10.1111/j.1365-2702.2012.04326.x

Chapter 8

Drug Administration Throughout the Life Span

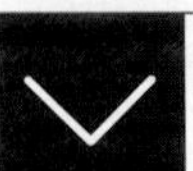

Learning Outcomes

After reading this chapter, the student should be able to:

1. Describe physiological changes during pregnancy that may affect the absorption, distribution, metabolism, and excretion of drugs.
2. Describe the placental transfer of drugs from mother to infant.
3. Identify examples of drugs that fall into the five U.S. Food and Drug Administration pregnancy risk categories.
4. Identify factors that influence the transfer of drugs into breast milk.
5. Identify techniques the breast-feeding mother can use to reduce drug exposure to the newborn.
6. Explain how differences in pharmacokinetic variables can affect drug response in pediatric patients.
7. Discuss the nursing and pharmacologic implications associated with each pediatric developmental age group.
8. Describe physiological and biochemical changes that occur in the older adult, and how these affect pharmacotherapy.
9. Develop nursing interventions that maximize pharmacotherapeutic outcomes in the older adult.

Beginning with conception, and continuing throughout the life span, organs and body systems undergo predictable physiological changes, and these changes can dramatically influence pharmacokinetics. Clearly, developmental changes in the ability to absorb, metabolize, distribute, and excrete medications can affect the outcomes of pharmacotherapy. The nurse must recognize such changes to ensure that drugs are delivered in a safe and effective manner to patients of all ages. This chapter examines how principles of developmental physiology and life span psychology apply to drug administration.

8.1 Pharmacotherapy Across the Life Span

An understanding of how pharmacology changes throughout the life span is actually an extension of the concept of holistic medicine. Indeed, each person is truly a unique individual. Other than identical twins, no two people have the exact same genetic material. Even twins experience different environmental stressors upon leaving the womb. Thus it should not be surprising that peoples' responses to and effects from medications will vary considerably from individual to individual.

As a person progresses through life, certain developmental changes are predictable. For example, an infant's liver is not fully mature and is unable to break down the same medications as an adult liver. Furthermore, as a person progresses from middle adulthood to an advanced age, liver function may diminish due to an accumulation of hepatic injury that naturally occurs throughout the life span. These are predictable changes, and ones that the nurse should expect from these populations. Indeed, failure to recognize these changes when administering drugs could result in patient harm.

There are many ways to approach individual variation in pharmacotherapeutic response. Chapter 9 will examine variations due to culture, gender, and genetics. The current chapter utilizes life span principles to look at variation in the following populations:

- Pregnant and lactating women.
- Children, including infants, toddlers, and adolescents.
- Middle-aged adults.
- Older adults.

DRUG ADMINISTRATION DURING PREGNANCY AND LACTATION

Health care providers exercise great caution when initiating pharmacotherapy during pregnancy or lactation (Figure 8.1). When possible, drug therapy is postponed until after pregnancy and lactation, or nonpharmacologic alternatives are implemented. There are some serious conditions, however, that may require pharmacotherapy in patients who are pregnant or lactating. For example, if the patient has epilepsy, hypertension, or a psychiatric disorder *prior to* the pregnancy, it would be unwise to discontinue therapy during pregnancy or lactation. Conditions such as gestational diabetes and gestational hypertension occur *during* pregnancy and must be treated for the safety of the growing fetus. Antibiotics may be necessary to treat infections during pregnancy; acute urinary tract infections and sexually transmitted infections are relatively common and can harm the fetus. In fact, it is reported that up to 90% of women take at least one medication during pregnancy, and an estimated 70% take at least one prescription medication (Centers for Disease Control and Prevention [CDC], 2014). In all cases, health care providers must weigh the therapeutic benefits of a given medication against its potential adverse effects.

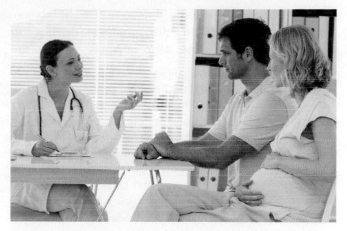

FIGURE 8.1 Teaching women about the safety of drug use during pregnancy is an essential component of nursing care.
WavebreakMediaMicro/Fotolia.

8.2 Pharmacotherapy of the Pregnant Patient

Drug therapy during pregnancy requires that the nurse consider the effects of the drug on both the mother and the growing fetus. The placental membranes separate maternal blood from fetal blood: Some substances readily pass from mother to fetus, whereas the transport of other substances is blocked. The fetal membranes contain enzymes that detoxify certain substances as they attempt to cross the membrane. For example, insulin from the mother is inactivated by placental enzymes during the early stages of pregnancy, preventing it from reaching the fetus. In general, drugs that are water soluble, ionized, or bound to plasma proteins are less likely to cross the placenta.

Physiological Changes During Pregnancy That Affect Pharmacotherapy

During pregnancy, major physiological and anatomic changes occur in the endocrine, gastrointestinal (GI), cardiovascular, circulatory, and renal systems of women. Some of these changes alter drug pharmacokinetics and pharmacodynamics and may affect the success of therapy.

Absorption. Hormonal changes as well as the pressure of the expanding uterus on the blood supply to abdominal organs may affect the absorption of drugs. Increased levels of progesterone can delay gastric emptying, thus allowing a longer time for the absorption of oral drugs. Gastric acidity is also decreased, which can affect the absorption of some drugs. Progesterone causes changes in the respiratory system during pregnancy—increased tidal volume and pulmonary vasodilation—that may cause inhaled drugs to be absorbed to a greater extent.

Distribution and Metabolism. Hemodynamic changes in the pregnant patient increase cardiac output, increase plasma volume, and alter regional blood flow. The increased blood volume in the mother causes dilution of drugs and decreases plasma protein concentrations, affecting drug distribution. Blood flow to the uterus, kidneys, and skin is increased, whereas flow to the skeletal muscles is diminished. Alterations in lipid levels may alter drug transport and distribution, especially during the third trimester. The level of drug metabolism increases for certain drugs, most notably anticonvulsants such as carbamazepine, phenytoin, and valproic acid, which may require higher doses during pregnancy. Fat-soluble drugs are distributed into the lipid-rich breast milk and may be passed to the lactating infant.

Excretion. By the third trimester of pregnancy, blood flow through the mother's kidneys increases by over 50%. This increase has a direct effect on renal plasma flow, glomerular filtration rate, and renal tubular absorption. Thus, drug excretion rates may be increased and doses of many medications may need to be adjusted.

Gestational Age and Drug Therapy

A **teratogen** is a substance, organism, or physical agent to which an embryo or fetus is exposed that produces a permanent abnormality in structure or function, causes growth retardation, or results in death. The baseline incidence of teratogenic events is approximately 3% of all pregnancies. Potential fetal consequences include intrauterine fetal death, physical malformations, growth impairment, behavioral abnormalities, and neonatal toxicity.

There are no absolute teratogens. Like other effects of drugs, there is a dose–response relationship, with risk increasing with higher doses. Because of the constant changes that occur during fetal development, the specific risk is dependent on when during gestation the drug is administered. A well-known example is the drug thalidomide, which causes fetal defects during pregnancy if it is administered day 35 to 48 after the last menstrual period. The specific malformation is linked to the time of exposure to the drug: 35 to 37 days, no ears; 39 to 41 days, no arms; 41 to 43 days, no uterus; 45 to 47 days, no tibia; and 47 to 49 days, triphalangeal thumbs.

Preimplantation period. Weeks 1 to 2 of the first trimester are known as the **preimplantation period.** Before implantation, the developing embryo has not yet established a physical connection to the mother. This is sometimes called the "all-or-none" period because exposure to a teratogen either causes death of the embryo or has no effect. Drugs are less likely to cause congenital malformations during this period because the baby's organ systems have not yet begun to form. Drugs such as nicotine, however, can create a negative environment for the embryo and potentially cause intrauterine growth retardation.

Embryonic period. During the **embryonic period,** from 3 to 8 weeks postconception, there is rapid development of internal structures. This is the period of maximum sensitivity to teratogens. Teratogenic agents taken during this phase can lead to structural malformation and spontaneous abortion. The specific abnormality depends on which organ is forming at the time of exposure.

Fetal period. The **fetal period** is from 9 to 40 weeks postconception or until birth. During this time, there is continued growth and maturation of the fetus's organ systems. Blood flow to the placenta increases and placental vascular membranes become thinner. Such alterations maximize the transfer of substances from the maternal circulation to the fetal blood. As a result, the fetus may receive larger doses of medications and other substances taken by the mother. Because the fetus lacks mature metabolic enzymes and efficient excretion mechanisms, medications will have a prolonged duration of action within the unborn child. Exposure to teratogens during the fetal period is more likely to produce slowed growth or impaired organ function, rather than gross structural malformations.

Pregnancy Drug Categories

Fortunately, the number of prescription drugs that are strongly suspected or known to be teratogenic is small. In addition, for most clinical conditions, there are alternative drugs that can be given with relative safety. New or infrequently used drugs for which there is inadequate safety information should not be given to pregnant women unless the benefits of drug therapy clearly outweigh potential fetal risks.

The U.S. Food and Drug Administration (FDA) has developed drug pregnancy categories that classify medications according to their risks during pregnancy. These were presented in chapter 2. Table 8.1 gives a more detailed explanation of the five pregnancy categories that guide the health care team and the patient in selecting drugs that are least hazardous for the fetus. Examples of prescription drugs that are associated with teratogenic effects are shown in the table. In addition to prescription medications, alcohol, nicotine, and illicit drugs such as cocaine will affect the unborn child.

Table 8.1 Current FDA Pregnancy Category Ratings with Examples

Risk Category	Interpretation	Drugs
A	Adequate, well-controlled studies in pregnant women have not shown an increased risk of fetal abnormalities to the fetus in any trimester of pregnancy.	Prenatal multivitamins, insulin, thyroxine, folic acid
B	Animal studies have revealed no evidence of harm to the fetus; however, there are no adequate and well-controlled studies in pregnant women. OR Animal studies have shown an adverse effect, but adequate and well-controlled studies in pregnant women have failed to demonstrate risk to the fetus in any trimester.	Penicillins, cephalosporins, azithromycin, acetaminophen, ibuprofen in the first and second trimesters
C	Animal studies have shown an adverse effect and there are no adequate and well-controlled studies in pregnant women. OR No animal studies have been conducted and there are no adequate and well-controlled studies in pregnant women.	Most prescription medicines; antimicrobials such as clarithromycin, fluoroquinolones, and Bactrim; selective serotonin reuptake inhibitors (SSRIs); corticosteroids; and most antihypertensives
D	Adequate well-controlled or observational studies in pregnant women have demonstrated a risk to the fetus. However, the benefits of therapy may outweigh the potential risk. For example, the drug may be acceptable if needed in a life-threatening situation or serious disease for which safer drugs cannot be used or are ineffective.	Alcohol, ACE inhibitors, angiotensin receptor blockers (ARBs) in the second and third trimesters, gentamicin, carbamazepine, cyclophosphamide, lithium carbonate, methimazole, mitomycin, nicotine, nonsteroidal anti-inflammatory drugs (NSAIDs) in the third trimester, phenytoin, propylthiouracil, streptomycin, tetracyclines, valproic acid
X	Adequate well-controlled or observational studies in animals or pregnant women have demonstrated positive evidence of fetal abnormalities or risks. The use of the product is contraindicated in women who are or may become pregnant. There is no indication for use in pregnancy.	Clomiphene, fluorouracil, isotretinoin, leuprolide, menotropins, methotrexate, misoprostol, nafarelin, oral contraceptives, raloxifene, ribavirin, statins, temazepam, testosterone and thalido mide, and warfarin

Testing drugs in human subjects to determine their teratogenicity is unethical and prohibited by law. Although drugs are tested in pregnant laboratory animals, the structure of the human placenta is unique. The FDA pregnancy drug categories are extrapolated from these animal data and may only be crude approximations of the risk to a human fetus. The actual risk to a human fetus may be much less, or magnitudes greater, than that predicted from animal data. In a few cases, human data are available to show pregnancy risks. The following statement bears repeating: *No prescription drug, over-the-counter (OTC) medication, herbal product, or dietary supplement should be taken during pregnancy unless the health care provider verifies that the therapeutic benefits to the mother clearly outweigh the potential risks for the unborn.*

The current A, B, C, D, and X pregnancy labeling system is simplistic and gives no *specific* clinical information to help guide the nurse or the patient about a medication's true safety. The system does not indicate how the dose should be adjusted during pregnancy or lactation. Most drugs are category C because very high doses in laboratory animals often produce teratogenic effects. All category D and X drugs should be avoided during pregnancy due to their potential for causing serious birth defects. Because a woman may obtain a prescription before she knows she is pregnant, it is crucial that the nurse ask *all* women of child-bearing age if there is the possibility of pregnancy as part of the routine teaching that accompanies giving a patient the prescription.

Pregnancy Registries

Pregnancy registries help identify medications that are safe to be taken during pregnancy. These registries gather information from women who took medications during pregnancy. Information on babies born to women not taking the medication is then compared with data on babies born while the medication was taken during pregnancy. The effects of the medication taken during pregnancy are then evaluated. Registries may be maintained by drug companies, governmental agencies, or special-interest groups. A list of pregnancy registries is available from the FDA.

8.3 Pharmacotherapy of the Lactating Patient

A large number of drugs are secreted into breast milk. Fortunately, there are relatively few instances in which drugs secreted into breast milk have been found to cause injury to infants. For the few drugs that are absolutely contraindicated during lactation, equally effective and safer alternatives are usually available. Although most medications probably cause no harm to the breast-feeding baby, their effects have not been fully studied. Selected medications that have been shown to cause serious harm to the breast-feeding infant are shown in Table 8.2.

It is important to understand factors that influence the amount of drug secreted into breast milk. This allows the nurse to counsel the patient in making responsible choices

Table 8.2 Selected Drugs Associated with Serious Adverse Effects During Breast-Feeding

Drug	Reported Effect or Reasons for Concern
atenolol (Tenormin)	Cyanosis, bradycardia, hypotension
ciprofloxacin	Pseudomembranous colitis
codeine	Death, bradycardia, neonatal apnea
dapsone (Aczone)	Hemolytic anemia
doxepin (Sinequan)	Sedation and respiratory arrest
erythromycin	Pyloric stenosis
fluoxetine (Prozac)	Sedation, lethargy, poor feeding
indomethacin (Indocin)	Seizures
lithium (Eskalith)	T-wave abnormalities
naproxen (Naprosyn, others)	Prolonged bleeding, hemorrhage, anemia
paroxetine (Paxel)	Hyponatremia
phenytoin (Dilantin)	Methemoglobinemia
sulfasalazine (Azulfidine)	Bloody diarrhea
valproic acid (Depakene, Depakote)	Thrombocytopenic purpura, anemia

Data from: "Safety During Breastfeeding: Drugs, Foods, Environmental Chemicals, and Maternal Infections," by C. M. Berlin and J. N. van den Anker, 2013, *Seminars in Fetal & Neonatal Medicine, 18*, pp. 13–18; and "Safe Use of Medications in Breastfeeding Mothers," by E. Grant, and P. Golightly, 2010, *Prescriber, 21*, pp. 70–73.

regarding lactation and in reducing exposure of her newborn to potentially harmful substances (Figure 8.2). The same guidelines for drug use apply during the breast-feeding period as during pregnancy—drugs should be taken only when the risk of not treating the mother's medical condition clearly outweighs the potential risks to the breastfed infant (Amir, Ryan, & Jordan, 2014).

When considering the potential effects of drugs on the breast-feeding infant, the *amount* of drug that actually reaches the infant's tissues must be considered. Some medications produce no adverse effects because they are destroyed in the infant's GI system or cannot be absorbed across the GI tract. Thus, although many drugs are secreted in breast milk, some are present in such small amounts that they cause no noticeable harm.

The final key factor concerning the effect of drugs during lactation relates to the infant's ability to metabolize small amounts of drugs. Premature, neonatal, and seriously ill infants may be at greater risk for adverse effects because they lack drug metabolizing enzymes.

General recommendations regarding pharmacotherapy during lactation are as follows:

- When feasible, pharmacotherapy should be postponed until the baby is weaned. The nurse can help the patient to identify nonpharmacologic therapies, if available, such as massage for pain or calming music for anxiety.

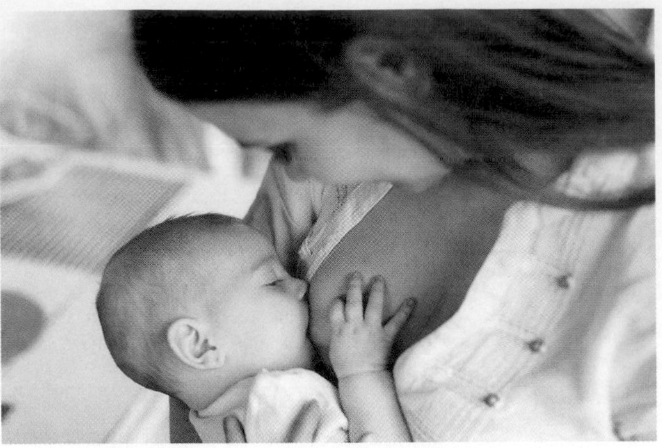

FIGURE 8.2 Nurses should teach lactating women to avoid all drugs, herbal products, and dietary supplements unless approved by their health care provider.
Halfpoint/Fotolia.

- If possible, administer the drug immediately after breast-feeding, or when the infant will be sleeping for an extended period, so that some time elapses before the next feeding. This will usually reduce the concentration of active drug in the mother's milk when she later breast-feeds her infant.
- The nurse should assist the mother in protecting the child's safety by teaching her to avoid illicit drugs, alcohol, and tobacco products during the lactation period.
- Drugs with a shorter half-life are preferable. Peak levels are rapidly reached and the drug is quickly cleared from the maternal plasma, which reduces the amount of drug exposure to the infant. The mother should avoid breast-feeding while the drug is at its peak level.
- Drugs that have long half-lives (or active metabolites) should be avoided because they can accumulate in the infant's plasma.
- Whenever possible, drugs with high protein-binding ability should be selected because they are not secreted as readily to the milk.
- OTC herbal products and dietary supplements should be avoided during lactation, unless specifically prescribed by the health care provider because the safety of most of these products to the infant has not been determined.

DRUG ADMINISTRATION DURING CHILDHOOD

As a child develops, physical growth and physiological changes require adjustments in the administration of medications. Although children often receive similar drugs via the same routes as adults, the nursing management for children is very different from that for adults. Normal physiological changes during growth and development can markedly affect pharmacokinetics and pharmacodynamics. Factors for

PharmFacts

FETAL EFFECTS CAUSED BY TOBACCO USE DURING PREGNANCY

Tobacco use has many effects on the mother and baby. These include the following:

- Difficulty in getting pregnant.
- Increased incidence of miscarriage.
- Increased risk of premature delivery.
- Increased risk for sudden infant death syndrome (SIDS).
- Increased risk for certain birth defects such as cleft lip or cleft palate.

the nurse to consider include physiological variations, maturity of body systems, and greater fluid distribution in children. Drug dosages are vastly different in children.

For the purposes of medication administration, the pediatric patient is defined as being any age from birth to 16 years and weighing less than 50 kg. Additionally, children may be classified as neonates, infants, toddlers, preschool, school age, and adolescent.

8.4 Pharmacotherapy of Infants

Infancy is the period from birth to 12 months of age (Figure 8.3). The first 28 days of life are referred to as the neonatal period. During this time, nursing care and pharmacotherapy are directed toward safety of the infant, accurate dosing of prescribed drugs, and teaching parents how to administer medications properly. A primary goal is to have the child ingest the entire dose of medication without spitting it out because it is difficult to estimate the amount lost. If the child vomits immediately after taking the drug, the dose may be reordered. The following nursing interventions and parental teaching points are important for this age group:

- The infant should be held and cuddled while medications are being administered, and a pacifier should be offered if the infant is on fluid restrictions caused by vomiting or diarrhea.
- Medications are often administered to infants via droppers into the eyes, ears, nose, or mouth. Oral medications should be directed to the inner cheek and the child given time to swallow the drug to avoid aspiration. If rectal suppositories are administered, the buttocks should be held together for 5 to 10 minutes to prevent expulsion of the drug before absorption has occurred.
- In very young infants, the medication may be given via a nipple. Some believe this is controversial because the infant may associate the nipple with medication and refuse feedings.
- Special considerations must be observed when administering intramuscular (IM) or intravenous (IV) injections to infants. Unlike adults, infants lack well-developed muscle masses, so the smallest needle appropriate for the drug should be used. For volumes less than 1 mL, a tuberculin syringe is appropriate. The vastus lateralis is a preferred site for IM injections, because it has few nerves and is relatively well developed in infants. The gluteal site is usually contraindicated because of potential damage to the sciatic nerve, injury to which may result in permanent disability.
- Because of the lack of choices for injection sites, the nurse must rotate injection sites from one leg to the next to avoid overuse and to prevent inflammation and excessive pain.
- For IV medications, the feet and scalp veins may provide more easily accessible and preferred venous access sites.

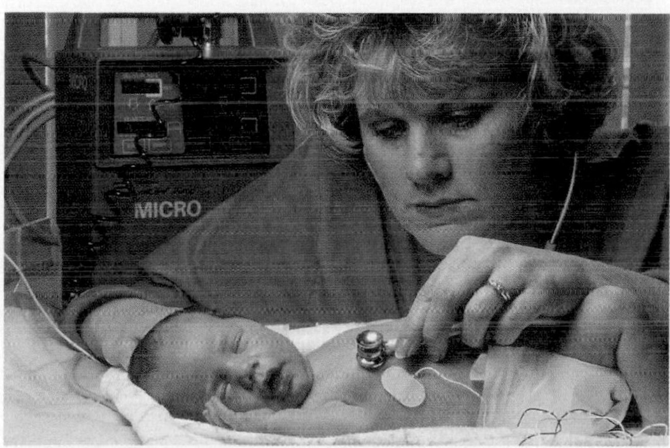

FIGURE 8.3 Treating the infant
Pearson Education, Inc.

8.5 Pharmacotherapy of Toddlers

Toddlerhood is the age period from 1 to 3 years. During this time, a toddler begins to explore, wants to try new things, and tends to place everything in the mouth. This becomes a major concern for medication and household product safety. The nurse must be instrumental in teaching parents that poisons come in all shapes, sizes, and forms and include medicines, cosmetics, cleaning supplies, arts and crafts materials, plants, and food products that are improperly stored. Parents should be instructed to request child-resistant containers from the pharmacist and to stow all medications in secure cabinets.

Toddlers can swallow liquids and may be able to chew solid medications. When prescription drugs are supplied as flavored elixirs, it is important to stress that the child not be given access to the medications. Drugs must never be left at the bedside or within easy reach of the child. A child who has access to a bottle of cherry-flavored acetaminophen (Tylenol) may ingest a fatal overdose of the tasty liquid. The nurse should educate parents about the following means of protecting their children from poisoning:

- Read and carefully follow directions on the label before using drugs and OTC products.

Evidence-Based Practice: Parents' Medication Errors with Dosing Devices

Clinical Question: Do parents accurately administer liquid drug doses to their children in the home setting using available dosing devices (medicine cups, teaspoons, droppers, syringes)?

Evidence: When given a prescription for a liquid medication or instructed to use an OTC liquid drug, parents are cautioned not to use household measuring devices such as kitchen teaspoons or tablespoons and are encouraged to obtain a medication dosing device such as a medicine cup (if one does not come with the drug itself), medicine spoon, dropper, or syringe. But do parents accurately administer the correct dose using these devices?

In a study of parents using a dosing cup, dropper, dosing spoon, or syringe, Yin et al. (2010) found that parents made dosing errors more frequently with a medicine cup, regardless of whether the dosing indicator marks were printed or etched into the cup. When using a cup, parents were confused about the difference between teaspoon and tablespoon, assumed the cup was the entire unit of measurement, or made dosing errors related to not verifying the amount of liquid dose at eye level. The level of health literacy also played a role, with parents scoring lower on a brief health literacy test having greater difficulty with accurate dosing. But even parents who scored significantly higher had more difficulty using medication cups accurately. Droppers and dosing spoons resulted in more accurate dosing and medication syringes resulted in the highest rates of accurate dose. In a follow-up study, Yin et al. (2014) determined that when a dosing device was included, along with patient education that included teach-back and show-back, errors were significantly reduced, but few parents reported receiving a device.

Nursing Implications: Teaching the family about medications ordered and the proper dose and administration of the drug is a nursing role. While the nurse may teach the parents about the reason for the child's medication, how often to give it, and any adverse effects to observe for, it is important that the nurse also teach how to appropriately use medication devices such as cups, spoons, droppers, or syringes to ensure accurate dosing. This becomes even more critical if the parents' health literacy is a barrier to accurate dosing. Whenever possible, a dosing syringe or other device should be given to the parent, although a syringe for parenteral medications should not be given to the parents because the calibration is different than a syringe designed for oral use. Dosing spoons or droppers are the next most accurate devices and may also be given if a dosing syringe is not appropriate for the age of the child. If a dosing cup must be used, the nurse should help the parent measure out several doses of water to ensure that the correct amount is being measured accurately. When providing the parent with any dosing device, adequate time for practice and teach-back or show-back should be factored into the patient teaching session.

- Store all drugs and harmful agents out of the reach of children and in locked cabinets.
- Keep all household products and drugs in their original containers. Never put chemicals in empty food or drink containers.
- Always ask the pharmacist to place the medications for everyone in the household in child-resistant containers.
- Never tell children that medicine is candy.
- Keep the Poison Control Center number near phones, and call immediately if poisoning is suspected.
- Never leave medication unattended in a child's room or in areas where the child plays.

Administration of medications to toddlers can be challenging. At this stage, the child is rapidly developing increased motor ability and learning to assert independence, but has extremely limited ability to reason or understand the relationship of medicines to health. Giving long, detailed explanations to the toddler will prolong the procedure and create additional anxiety. Short, concrete explanations followed by immediate drug administration are best for this age group. Physical comfort in the form of touching, hugging, or verbal praise following drug administration is important.

Oral medications that taste bad should be mixed with a vehicle such as jam, syrup, or fruit puree, if possible. Encourage parents to mix the medication in the smallest amount possible to ensure that the toddler receives all of it. The medication may be followed with a carbonated beverage or a beverage the child enjoys. The nurse should teach parents to avoid placing medicine in milk, orange juice, or cereals, because the child may associate these healthful foods with bad-tasting medications. Pharmaceutical companies often formulate pediatric medicines in sweet syrups to increase the ease of drug administration.

IM injections for toddlers should be given into the vastus lateralis muscle. IV injections may use scalp or feet veins; additional peripheral site options become available in late toddlerhood. The toddler presents additional safety issues to the nurse who is administering IV medications. The nurse must firmly secure the IV and then educate the parents about the dangers of the toddler trying to pull away too quickly from the IV pump. It is often helpful to put longer tubing on a toddler's IV to give the child more play room. Suppositories may be difficult to administer because of the child's resistance. For any of these invasive administration procedures, having a parent in close proximity will usually reduce the toddler's anxiety and increase cooperation, but ask the parent prior to the procedure if he or she would like to assist. The nurse should take at least one helper into the room for assistance in restraining the toddler if necessary.

8.6 Pharmacotherapy of Preschoolers and School-Age Children

The **preschool child** ranges in age from 3 to 5 years. During this period, the child begins to refine gross and fine motor skills and develop language abilities. The child initiates new activities and becomes more socially involved with other children.

Preschoolers can sometimes comprehend the difference between health and illness and that medications are administered to help them feel better. Nonetheless, medications and other potentially dangerous products must still be safely stowed out of the child's reach.

In general, principles of medication administration that pertain to the toddler also apply to this age group. Preschoolers cooperate in taking oral medications if they are crushed or mixed with food or flavored beverages. After a child has walked for about a year, the ventrogluteal site may be used for IM injections, because it causes less pain than the vastus lateralis site. The scalp veins can no longer be used for IV access; peripheral veins are used for IV injections.

Like toddlers, preschoolers often physically resist medication administration, and a long, detailed explanation of the procedure will likely promote anxiety. A brief explanation followed quickly by medication administration is usually the best method. Uncooperative children may need to be restrained, and patients older than 4 years may require two adults to administer the medication. Before and after medication procedures, the child may benefit from opportunities to play-act troubling experiences with dolls. When the child plays the role of doctor or nurse by giving a "sick" doll a pill or injection, comforting the doll, and explaining that the doll will now feel better, the little actor feels safer and more in control of the situation.

The **school-age child** is between 6 and 12 years of age. Some refer to this period as the *middle childhood* years. This is the time in a child's life when rapid physical, mental, and social development occur, and early ethical–moral development begins to take shape. Thinking processes become progressively more logical and consistent.

During this time, most children remain relatively healthy. Respiratory infections and GI upset are the most common complaints. Because the child feels well most of the time, there is little concept of illness or the risks involved with ingesting a harmful substance offered to the child by a peer or older person.

The nurse is usually able to gain considerable cooperation from school-age children. More detailed explanations may be of value, because the child has developed some reasoning ability and can understand the relationship between the medicine and feeling better. When children are old enough to welcome choices, they can be offered limited dosing alternatives to provide a sense of control and to encourage cooperation. The option of taking one medication before another or the chance to choose which drink will follow a chewable tablet helps distract children from the issue of whether they will take the medication at all. It also makes an otherwise strange or unpleasant experience a little more enjoyable. Making children feel that they are willing participants in medication administration, rather than victims, is an important foundation for compliance. Praise for cooperation is appropriate for any pediatric patient and sets the stage for successful medication administration in the future (Figure 8.4).

Lifespan Considerations
Iron Poisoning

One of the leading causes of poisonings in children under the age of 6 is iron poisoning. Iron is often found in vitamins of all kinds: prenatal, pediatric, and adult vitamins. Pediatric vitamins may be particularly tempting and may have the taste and appearance of candy that the child is familiar with. Prenatal vitamins may hold a particular danger due to the increased amounts of iron and other components. And vitamins are not always considered "medicine" or locked away with other prescription medications. Older children may open the bottle, a young child may outwit a "child-resistant" top, or a bottle is left within the child's reach. Depending on the age of the child, as few as five iron-containing tablets are known to cause iron poisoning.

Symptoms of iron poisoning include nausea, vomiting, diarrhea, and gastrointestinal bleeding and can progress to coma and death. Even if iron poisoning is only suspected, the child should be taken for medical evaluation because symptoms may be delayed. Parents should be encouraged to be certain that all medication, including OTC drugs such as vitamins, are locked away and medicine bottle tops are secured. And when visiting another home or having a visitor within the home, be sure all medication is out of a child's reach and availability, even vitamins.

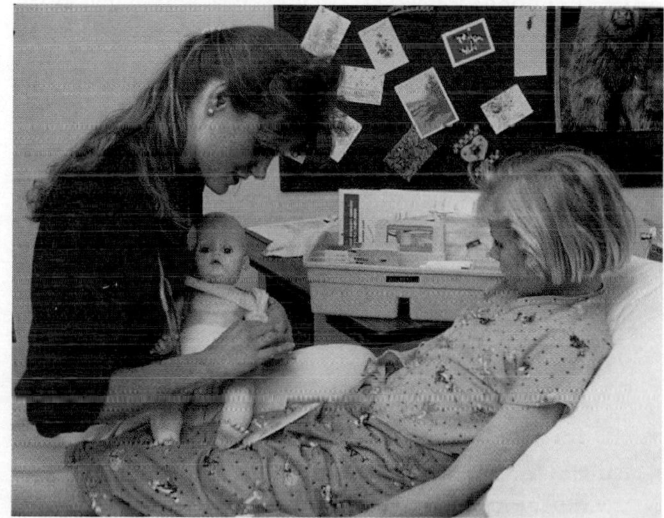

FIGURE 8.4 Treating the younger school-age child
George Dodson/Pearson Education, Inc.

PharmFacts

POISONING

According to the Global Children's Fund (n.d.):

- About 800,000 children are treated in emergency departments each year due to accidental poisoning. About 100,000 of these are due to children ingesting their grandparents' medicine.
- About 70% of non-fatal poisonings occur in children aged 1-2.
- About 5,700 children are treated in emergency departments each year due to medication overdoses given by their caregivers.
- For some adult medications, a single pill may be enough to kill or cause serious injury to a small child.

School-age children can safely take chewable tablets and may even be able to swallow tablets or capsules. Because many still resist injections, it is best to have help available for these procedures. The child should never be told that he or she is "too old" to cry and resist. The ventrogluteal site is preferred for IM injections, although the muscles of older children are developed enough for the nurse to use other sites.

8.7 Pharmacotherapy of Adolescents

Adolescence occurs between ages 13 and 16 years. Rapid physical growth and psychological maturation have a great impact on personality development. The adolescent strongly relates to peers, wanting and needing their support, approval, and presence. The strong sense of independence leads some teens to self-medicate, either with or without their parents' knowledge. Treatment objectives for the nurse should include teaching parents to keep their medications safely stowed out of sight from inquisitive, experiment-minded adolescents. Parents should also be taught the signs and symptoms of drugs commonly abused by teens such as marijuana, inhalants, and methamphetamine.

The most common needs for the pharmacotherapy of teens are for skin problems, headaches, menstrual symptoms, eating disorders, contraception, alcohol and tobacco use, and sports-related injuries.

- Of primary concern to the adolescent is the initiation of sexual intercourse and the avoidance of pregnancy and sexually transmitted infections. The nurse must be prepared to address a variety of topics related to sexuality, including the importance of responsible sexual practices, condom use, and other contraceptive methods.
- Eating disorders commonly occur in this population; therefore, the nurse should carefully question adolescents about their eating habits and their use of OTC appetite suppressants or laxatives that may be contributing to bulimia or anorexia.
- Alcohol use, tobacco use, and illicit drug experimentation are common in this population. Teenage athletes may use amphetamines to delay the onset of fatigue as well as anabolic steroids to enhance performance. The nurse assumes a key role in educating adolescent patients about the hazards of tobacco use and illicit drugs.
- The adolescent has a need for privacy and control in drug administration. The nurse should communicate with the teen more in the manner of an adult than as a child. Teens usually appreciate thorough explanations of their treatment, and ample time should be allowed for them to ask questions.
- Despite the adolescent's need for confidentiality and privacy, confidentiality laws differ from state to state. The nurse working with the adolescent population needs to be familiar with the state laws affecting confidentiality and informed consent.
- Despite their need to have independence and the desire to self-medicate, teens have a very poor understanding of medication information. Adolescents are reluctant to admit their lack of knowledge, so the nurse should carefully explain important information regarding their medications and expected side effects, even if the patient claims to understand.

DRUG ADMINISTRATION DURING ADULTHOOD

When considering adult health, it is customary to divide this period of life into three stages: **young adulthood** (18 to 40 years of age), **middle adulthood** (40 to 65 years of age), and **older adulthood** (over 65 years of age). Within each of these divisions are similar biophysical, psychosocial, and spiritual characteristics that affect nursing and pharmacotherapy.

8.8 Pharmacotherapy of Young and Middle-Aged Adults

The health status of younger adults is generally good; absorption, metabolic, and excretion mechanisms are at their peaks. There is minimal need for prescription drugs unless chronic diseases such as diabetes or immune-related conditions exist. The use of vitamins, minerals, and herbal remedies is prevalent in young adulthood. Prescription drugs are usually related to contraception or agents needed during pregnancy and delivery. Medication compliance is positive within this age range because there is clear comprehension of benefit in terms of longevity and feeling well.

Substance abuse is a cause for concern in the 18 to 24 age group, with alcohol, tobacco products, amphetamines, and illicit drugs a problem. For young adults who are sexually active, with multiple partners, prescription medications

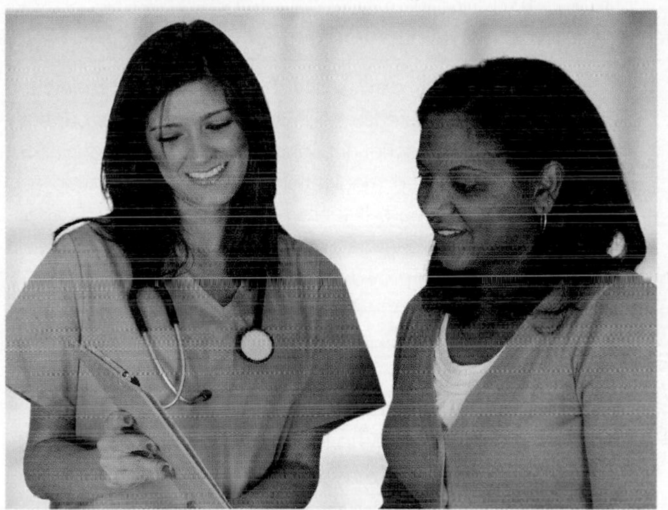

FIGURE 8.5 Treating the middle-aged adult
Rob/Fotolia.

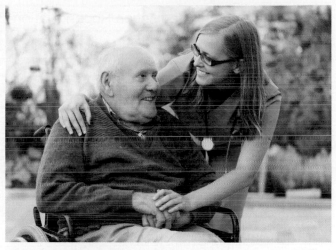

FIGURE 8.6 Treating the older adult
Barabas Attila/Fotolia.

for the treatment of herpes, gonorrhea, syphilis, and HIV infections may be necessary.

The physical status of the middle-aged adult is on a par with that of the young adult until about 45 years of age. During this period of life, numerous transitions occur that often result in excessive stress. Middle-aged adults are sometimes referred to as the "sandwich generation" because they are often caring for aging parents as well as children and grandchildren. Because of the pressures of work and family, middle-aged adults often take medication to control health alterations that could best be treated with positive lifestyle modifications. The nurse must emphasize the importance of overall health of lifestyle choices, such as limiting lipid intake, maintaining optimal weight, and exercising (Figure 8.5).

Health impairments related to cardiovascular disease, hypertension, obesity, arthritis, cancer, and anxiety begin to surface in late middle age. The use of drugs to treat hypertension, hyperlipidemia, digestive disorders, erectile dysfunction, and arthritis are common. Respiratory disorders related to lifelong tobacco use or exposure to secondhand smoke and environmental toxins may develop that require drug therapies. Adult-onset diabetes mellitus often emerges during this time of life. The use of antidepressants and antianxiety agents is prominent in the population older than age 50.

8.9 Pharmacotherapy of Older Adults

During the 20th century, an improved quality of life and the ability to effectively treat many chronic diseases contributed to increased longevity. The age-related changes in older adults, however, can influence the patient's response to drugs, altering both the therapeutic and adverse effects, and creating special needs and risks. As a consequence of aging, patients experience an increasing number of chronic health disorders, and more drugs are prescribed to treat them.

The taking of multiple drugs concurrently, known as **polypharmacy,** has become commonplace among older adults. Patients who visit multiple health care providers and use different pharmacies may experience polypharmacy because each doctor or pharmacist may not be aware of all the drugs ordered by other practitioners. Polypharmacy dramatically increases the risk for drug interactions and side effects. The nurse should urge patients to report all prescription and OTC products on each office visit and teach the patients to use one pharmacy for their prescription needs.

Although predictable physiological and psychosocial changes occur with aging, significant variability exists among patients. For example, although cognitive decline and memory loss certainly occur along the aging continuum, there is a great variation in older adults. Some older individuals do not experience cognitive impairment at all. The nurse should avoid preconceived notions that older adults will have physical or cognitive impairment simply because they have reached a certain age. Careful assessment is always necessary (Figure 8.6).

When administering medications to older adults, the nurse should offer patients the same degree of independence and dignity that would be afforded middle-aged adults, unless otherwise indicated. Like their younger counterparts, older patients have a need to understand why they are receiving a drug and what outcomes are expected. Accommodations must be made for older adults who have certain impairments. Visual and auditory changes make it important for the nurse to provide drug instructions in large type and to obtain patient feedback to be certain that medication instructions are understood. Older patients with cognitive decline and memory loss can benefit from aids such as alarmed pill containers, medicine management boxes, and clearly written instructions. During assessment, the nurse should determine if the patient is capable of self-administering medications in a consistent, safe, and effective

Patient Safety: Medication Reconciliation Before Home Discharge for the Older Adult

Medication reconciliation is the process of comparing a patient's current medication orders to all of the medications that the patient has been taking to avoid duplications, omissions, dosage differences, or drug interactions. Because the older adult may be taking multiple medications prescribed by different providers, it is especially important that the nurse perform a medication reconciliation before discharging the patient from an acute-care setting to the patient's home or other care facility. The nurse should review the patient's medications listed on admission, the patient's currently ordered medication prescriptions, and any special notations about which previously ordered medications should be continued and which should be stopped. If there are any discrepancies, omissions, duplications, or change in dosage noted, the nurse should contact the health care provider to verify the order.

manner. As long as small children are not present in the household, older patients with arthritis should be encouraged to ask the pharmacist for regular screw-cap medication bottles for ease of opening.

Older adults experience more adverse effects from drug therapy than other age groups. Although some of these effects are due to polypharmacy, many of the adverse events are predictable based on normal physiological processes that occur during aging. The principal complications of drug therapy in the older adult population are due to degeneration of organ systems, multiple and severe illness, polypharmacy, and unreliable compliance. By understanding these changes, the nurse can avoid many adverse drug effects in older patients.

In older adults, the functioning ability of all major organ systems progressively declines. For this reason, all phases of pharmacokinetics are affected, and appropriate adjustments in therapy need to be implemented. Although most of the pharmacokinetic changes are due to reduced hepatic and renal drug elimination, other systems may also initiate a variety of changes. For example, immune system function diminishes with aging, so autoimmune diseases and infections occur more frequently in older patients. Thus, there is an increased need for influenza and pneumonia vaccinations. Normal physiological changes that affect pharmacotherapy of the older adult are summarized as follows:

Absorption. In general, absorption of drugs is slower in the older adult due to diminished gastric motility and decreased blood flow to digestive organs. Because of increased gastric pH, oral tablets and capsules that require high levels of acid for absorption may take longer to dissolve and, therefore, take longer to become available to the tissues.

Distribution. Increased body fat in the older patient provides a larger storage compartment for lipid-soluble drugs and vitamins. Plasma levels are reduced, and the therapeutic response is diminished. Older adults have less body water, making the effects of dehydration more dramatic and increasing the risk for drug toxicity. For example, older patients who have reduced body fluid experience more orthostatic hypotension. The decline in lean body mass and total body water leads to an increased concentration of water-soluble drugs, because the drug is distributed in a smaller volume of water. The aging liver produces less albumin, resulting in decreased plasma protein-binding ability and increased levels of free drug in the bloodstream, thereby increasing the potential for drug–drug interactions. The aging cardiovascular system has decreased cardiac output and less efficient blood circulation, which slow drug distribution. This makes it important to initiate pharmacotherapy with smaller dosages and slowly increase the amount to a safe, effective level.

Metabolism. Enzyme production in the liver decreases and the visceral blood flow is diminished, resulting in reduced hepatic drug metabolism. This change leads to an increase in the half-life of many drugs, which prolongs and intensifies drug response. The decline in hepatic function reduces first-pass metabolism. (Recall that first-pass metabolism relates to the amount of a drug that is removed from the bloodstream during the first circulation through the liver after the drug is absorbed by the intestinal tract.) Thus, plasma levels are elevated, and tissue concentrations are increased for the particular drug. This change alters the standard dosage, the interval between doses, and the duration of side effects.

Excretion. Older adults have reduced renal blood flow, glomerular filtration rate, active tubular secretion, and nephron function. This decreases drug excretion for drugs that are eliminated by the kidneys. When excretion is reduced, serum drug levels and the potential for toxicity markedly increase. Administration schedules and dosage amounts may need to be altered in many older adults due to these changes in kidney function. Keep in mind that the most common etiology of adverse drug reactions in older adults is caused by the accumulation of toxic amounts of drugs secondary to impaired renal excretion.

Treating the Diverse Patient: Patients with Speaking, Visual, or Hearing Impairments

Health care agencies are required to assess a patient for any sensory or other impairments that may prove to be barriers to successful communication. Appropriate services are also required to ensure effective communication between the patient and the health care team. Because these services may not always be immediately available, there are several things the nurse can do to help improve communication with patients who have speaking, visual, or hearing impairments. Adequate communication between the nurse and the patient is crucial to the process of safe medication administration.

Verbal communication disorders such as those that often occur after a stroke may make obtaining responses from the patient difficult. Communication may be facilitated by having the patient write or draw responses. The nurse should clarify by paraphrasing the response back to the patient. Use of gestures, body language, and yes/no questions may be helpful if writing or drawing is difficult. It is important to allow adequate time for responses. The nurse should be especially aware of nonverbal clues, such as grimacing, when performing interventions that may cause discomfort or pain, and be aware that these may help the nurse to determine the need for pain medication.

Adequate lighting should be provided for patients with visual impairments, and the nurse should be aware of how the phrasing of verbal communication affects the message conveyed. The nonverbal cues involved in communication such as gestures may be missed by the patient. Paraphrasing responses back to patients can help ensure that they understood the message in the absence of nonverbal cues. The nurse should explain interventions in detail before implementing procedures or activities with the patient.

Patients with hearing impairments benefit from communication that is spoken clearly and slowly. The nurse should sit near the patient and avoid speaking loudly or shouting, especially if hearing devices are used, and limit the amount of background noise when possible. Writing or drawing may help to clarify verbal communication, and nonverbal gestures and body language often aid communication. It is important to allow adequate time for communication and responses. The nurse should alert other members of the health care team that the patient has a hearing impairment and may not hear a verbal answer to the nurse's call light given over an intercom system. Written materials may be preferred when providing teaching about the patient's medications.

Chapter Review

KEY Concepts

The numbered key concepts provide a succinct summary of the important points from the corresponding numbered section within the chapter. If any of these points are not clear, refer to the numbered section within the chapter for review.

8.1 To contribute to safe and effective pharmacotherapy, it is essential for the nurse to apply fundamental concepts of growth and development across the life span.

8.2 The effects of drugs on a growing embryo or fetus depend on the gestational stage and the amount of drug received. Pharmacotherapy during pregnancy should be conducted only when the benefits to the mother outweigh the potential risks to the unborn child. Pregnancy categories guide the health care provider in prescribing drugs for these patients.

8.3 Breast-feeding women must be aware that many drugs can appear in milk and cause adverse effects to the infant.

8.4 During infancy, pharmacotherapy is directed toward the safety of the child and teaching the parents how to properly administer medications and care for the infant.

8.5 Drug administration to toddlers can be challenging; short, concrete explanations followed by immediate drug administration are usually best for the toddler.

8.6 Preschool and younger school-age children can begin to assist with medication administration.

8.7 Pharmacologic compliance in the adolescent is dependent on an understanding of and respect for the uniqueness of the person in this stage of growth and development.

8.8 Young adults constitute the healthiest age group and generally need few prescription medications. Middle-aged adults begin to experience stress-related illnesses such as hypertension that require pharmacotherapy.

8.9 Older adults take more medications and experience more adverse drug events than any other age group. For drug therapy to be successful, the nurse must make accommodations for age-related changes in physiological and biochemical functions.

REVIEW Questions

1. A 16-year-old adolescent is 6 weeks pregnant. The pregnancy has exacerbated her acne. She asks the nurse if she can resume taking her isotretinoin prescription, a category X drug. What is the most appropriate response by the nurse?
   1. "Since you have a prescription for isotretinoin, it is safe to resume using it."
   2. "You should check with your health care provider at your next visit."
   3. "Isotretinoin is known to cause birth defects and should never be taken during pregnancy."
   4. "You should reduce the isotretinoin dosage by half during pregnancy."
2. To reduce the effect of a prescribed medication on the infant of a breast-feeding mother, how should the nurse teach the mother to take the medication?
   1. At night
   2. Immediately before the next feeding
   3. In divided doses at regular intervals around the clock
   4. Immediately after breast-feeding
3. An older adult patient has arthritis in her hands and takes several prescription drugs. Which statement by this patient requires further assessment by the nurse?
   1. "My pharmacist puts my pills in screw-top bottles to make it easier for me to take them."
   2. "I fill my prescriptions once per month."
   3. "I care for my 2-year-old grandson twice a week."
   4. "My arthritis medicine helps my stiff hands."
4. A nurse is administering a liquid medication to a 15-month-old child. What is the most appropriate approach to medication administration by the nurse? (Select all that apply.)
   1. Tell the child that the medication tastes just like candy.
   2. Mix the medication in 8 oz of orange juice.
   3. Ask the child if she would like to take her medication now.
   4. Sit the child up, hold the medicine cup to her lips, and kindly instruct her to drink.
   5. Offer the child a choice of cup in which to take the medicine.
5. The nurse is preparing to give an oral medication to a 6-month-old infant. How should this drug be administered?
   1. By placing the medication in the next bottle of formula
   2. By mixing the medication with juice in a bottle
   3. By placing the medicine dropper in the inner cheek, allowing time for the infant to swallow
   4. By placing the medication toward the back of the mouth to avoid having the infant immediately spit out the medication
6. To reduce the chance of duplicate medication orders for the older adult returning home after surgery, what actions should the nurse take? (Select all that apply.)
   1. Call in all prescriptions to the patient's pharmacies rather than relying on paper copies of prescriptions.
   2. Give all prescriptions to the patient's family member.
   3. Take a medication history, including all OTC and prescription medications and a pharmacy history with each patient visit.
   4. Work with the patient's health care provider to limit the number of prescriptions.
   5. Perform a medication reconciliation before sending the patient home.

CRITICAL THINKING Questions

1. A 22-year-old pregnant patient is diagnosed with a kidney infection, and an antibiotic is prescribed. The patient asks the nurse whether the antibiotic is safe to take. What factors are considered when a drug is prescribed for a patient who is pregnant?
2. An 86-year-old male patient who lives with his son and daughter-in-law at home is confused and anxious and an antianxiety drug has been ordered. What concerns might the nurse have about pharmacotherapy for this patient?
3. An 8-month-old child is prescribed acetaminophen (Tylenol) elixir for management of fever. She is recovering from gastroenteritis and is still having several loose stools each day. The child spits some of the elixir on her shirt. Should the nurse repeat the dose? What are the implications of this child's age and physical condition for oral drug administration?

Visit www.pearsonhighered.com/nursingresources for answers and rationales for all activities.

REFERENCES

Amir, L. H., Ryan, K. M., & Jordan, S. E. (2012). Avoiding risk at what cost? Putting use of medicines for breastfeeding women in perspective. *International Breastfeeding Journal, 7,* 14. doi:10.1186/1746-4358-7-14

Berlin, C. M., & van den Anker, J. N. (2013). Safety during breastfeeding: Drugs, foods, environmental chemicals, and maternal infections. *Seminars in Fetal and Neonatal Medicine, 18,* 13–18. doi:10.1016/j.siny.2012.09.003

Centers for Disease Control and Prevention (2014). *Treating for two.* Retrieved from http://www.cdc.gov/pregnancy/meds/treatingfortwo/data.html

Global Children's Fund (n.d.). *Child poisoning facts and statistics.* Retrieved from http://www.keepyourchildsafe.org/child-safety-book/child-poisoning-facts-and-statistics.html

Grant, E., & Golightly, P. (2010). Safe use of medications in breastfeeding mothers. *Prescriber, 21*(19), 70–73. doi:10.1002/psb.681

Yin, H. S., Mendelsohn, A. L., Wolf, M. S., Parker, R. M., Fierman, A., van Schaick, L., . . . Dreyer, B. P. (2010). Parents' medication administration errors. *Archives of Pediatric & Adolescent Medicine, 164,* 181–186. doi:10.1001/archpediatrics.2009.269

Yin, H. S., Dreyer, B. P., Moreira, H. A., van Schaick, L., Rodriguez, L., Boettger, S., & Mendelsohn, A. L. (2014). Liquid medication dosing errors in children: Role of provider counseling strategies. *Academic Pediatrics, 14,* 262–270. doi:10.1016/j.acap.2014.01.003

SELECTED BIBLIOGRAPHY

The Academy of Breastfeeding Medicine Protocol Committee. (2011). ABM Clinical Protocol #9: Use of galactogogues in initiating or augmenting the rate of maternal milk secretion (First Revision January 2011). *Breastfeeding Medicine, 6,* 41–49. doi:10.1089/bfm.2011.9998

Briggs, G. G., Freeman, R. K., & Yaffe, S. J. (2011). *Drugs in pregnancy and lactation* (9th ed.). Philadelphia: Lippincott Williams & Wilkins.

Budzynska, K., Gardner, Z. E., Dugoua, J. J., Low Dog, T., & Gardiner, P. (2012). Systematic review of breastfeeding and herbs. *Breastfeeding Medicine, 7,* 489–503. doi:10.1089/bfm.2011.0122

Cabbage, L. A., & Neal, J. L. (2011). Over-the counter medications and pregnancy: An integrative review. *Nurse Practitioner 36*(6), 22–28. doi:10.1097/01.NPR.0000397910.59950.71

Centers for Disease Control and Prevention. (2014). *Tobacco use and pregnancy.* Retrieved from http://www.cdc.gov/reproductivehealth/tobaccousepregnancy/

Hale, T. (2014). *Medications and mother's milk* (16th ed.). Amarillo, TX: Hale.

Hutchison, L. C., & Sleeper, R. B. (2015. *Fundamentals of geriatric pharmacotherapy,* 2nd ed. Bethesda, MD: American Society of Health-Systems Pharmacists.

Meeks, T. W., Culberson, J. W., & Horton, M. S. (2011). Medications in long-term care: When less is more. *Clinics in Geriatric Medicine 27,* 177–191. doi:10.1016/j.cger.2011.01.003

Mitchell, A. A., Gilboa, S. M., Werler, M. M., Kelley, K. E., Louik, C., & Hernandez-Diaz, S. (2011). Medication use during pregnancy, with particular focus on prescription drugs: 1976–2008. *American Journal of Obstetrics and Gynecology, 205*(1), 51.e1-51.e8. doi:10.1016/j.ajog.2011.02.029

Peters, S. L., Lind, J. N., Humphrey, J. R., Friedman, J. M., Honein, M. A., Tassinari, M. S., …Broussard, C. S. (2013). Safe lists for medications in pregnancy: Inadequate evidence base and inconsistent guidance from Web-based information, 2011. *Pharmacoepidemiology and Drug Safety, 22,* 324–328. doi:10.1002/pds.3410

Rowe, H., Baker, T., & Hale, T. W. (2013). Maternal medication, drug use, and breastfeeding. *Pediatric Clinics of North America, 60,* 275–294. doi:10.1016/j.pcl.2012.10.009

Thorpe, P. G., Gilboa, S. M., Hernandez-Diaz, S., Lind, J., Cragan, J. D., Briggs, G.,… Honein, M. A. (2013). Medications in the first trimester of pregnancy: Most common exposures and critical gaps in understanding fetal risk. *Pharmacoepidemiology and Drug Safety, 22,* 1013–1018. doi:10.1002/pds.3495

Chapter 9

Individual Variations in Drug Response

Learning Outcomes

After reading this chapter, the student should be able to:

1. Describe fundamental concepts underlying a holistic approach to patient care and their importance to pharmacotherapy.
2. Identify psychosocial factors that can affect pharmacotherapeutics.
3. Explain how culture and ethnicity can affect pharmacotherapeutic outcomes.
4. Explain how community and environmental factors can affect health care outcomes.
5. Convey how genetic polymorphisms can influence pharmacotherapy.
6. Relate the implications of gender to the actions of certain drugs.

It is convenient for a nurse to memorize an average drug dose, administer the medication, and expect all patients to achieve the same outcomes. Unfortunately, this is rarely the case. For pharmacotherapy to be successful, the nurse must assess and evaluate the needs of each individual patient. In chapter 4, variables such as absorption, metabolism, plasma protein binding, and excretion mechanisms were examined to help explain how these modify patient responses to drugs. In chapter 5, variability among patient responses was explained in terms of differences in drug-receptor interactions. Chapter 8 examined how pharmacokinetic and pharmacodynamic factors change patient responses to drugs throughout the life span. This chapter examines additional psychosocial, cultural, environmental, and biologic variables that are responsible for producing individual variation in drug response.

9.1 The Concept of Holistic Pharmacotherapy

To deliver the highest quality of care, the nurse must fully recognize the individuality and totality of the patient. Simply stated, the recipient of care must be regarded in a **holistic** context so that the nurse can better understand how established risk factors such as age, genetics, biologic characteristics, personal habits, lifestyle, and environment increase a person's likelihood of acquiring specific diseases. Pharmacology has taken the study of these characteristics one step further—to examine and explain how they influence pharmacotherapeutic outcomes.

Figure 9.1 illustrates variables that can affect individual variation in response to pharmacotherapy. This model provides a useful approach to addressing the nursing and pharmacologic needs of patients receiving medications. Because all levels of the model may contribute to pharmacotherapeutic outcomes, they should be considered when developing a patient's treatment plan. For example, when given a medication for the treatment of hypertension, a Caucasian man may experience greater effects from the medication than an African American man. In addition, cultural or ethnic differences may result in a difference in the extent to which an individual metabolizes certain drugs.

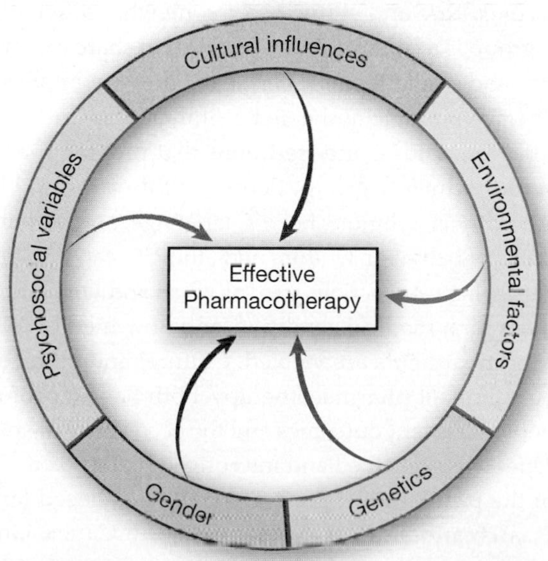

FIGURE 9.1 Holistic model of pharmacotherapy: For pharmacotherapy to be successful, the nurse must consider psychosocial, cultural, environmental, and biologic variables that could affect drug response.

By its very nature, modern (Western) medicine as it is practiced in the United States is seemingly incompatible with holistic medicine. Western medicine focuses on specific diseases, their causes, and treatments. Disease is viewed as a malfunction of a specific organ or system. Sometimes, the disease is viewed even more specifically and categorized as a change in DNA structure or a malfunction of one enzyme. Sophisticated technology is used to identify, image, measure, and classify the specific structural or functional abnormality. Somehow, the total patient is lost in this focus of categorizing disease. Too often, it does not matter how or why the patient developed cancer, diabetes, or hypertension or how he or she feels about it; the environmental, psychosocial and cultural dimensions are lost. Yet, these dimensions can have a profound impact on the success of pharmacotherapy. To be most effective at achieving positive patient outcomes, the nurse must consciously direct care toward a *holistic* treatment of each individual patient.

9.2 Psychosocial Influences on Pharmacotherapy

The term **psychosocial** is often used in health care to describe one's psychological development in the context of one's social environment. This involves both the social and psychological aspects of a person's life. Health impairments related to an individual's psychosocial situation often require a blending of individualized nursing care and therapeutic drugs in conjunction with psychotherapeutic counseling. When illness imposes threats to health, the patient commonly presents with psychosocial issues along with physical symptoms. Patients face concerns related to ill health, suffering, loneliness, despair, and death and at the same time look for meaning, value, and hope in their situation. Such issues can have a great impact on wellness and preferred methods of medical treatment, nursing care, and pharmacotherapy.

The psychosocial history of the patient is an essential component of the initial interview and assessment. This history delves into the personal life of the patient with inquiries directed toward lifestyle preferences, religious beliefs, sexual practices, alcohol intake, and tobacco and nonprescription drug use. The nurse must demonstrate

Treating the Diverse Patient: Medication Refusal for Religious or Spiritual Reasons

One of the rights of medication administration is refusal. Patients have the right to refuse their medications for religious or spiritually-related reasons. Perhaps most familiar is a refusal to accept blood or blood products by a Jehovah's Witness member because of religious beliefs. Less familiar is refusal due to the fact that the medication contains animal-derived products.

Erickson, Burcharth, and Rosenburg (2013) explored potential acceptance or refusal of animal-derived products such as porcine (pork) and bovine (beef) surgical products by members of various religious faiths, including Christian, Judaism, Buddhism, Hindu, Islam, and Sikhism. In their study, they discovered that while all religions may permit the use of animal-derived drugs or products in an emergency situation where no other alternative was possible, many religions had some restrictions on the use of such drugs or products for routine use.

In an earlier study, Hoesli and Smith (2011) found that more than 1,000 medications contain animal-based products, including inactive ingredients such as gelatin. Depending on the religious tradition, beef, pork, chicken, fish, shellfish, or all meats may be refused on religious or moral grounds. They recommended that, when possible, a compounding laboratory be approached about making a comparable product for the patient that does not contain the offending ingredient. That option should be explored if alternative formulations are not available for use. In the case of an animal-derived drug such as heparin, the provider should discuss the medication with the patient and explore alternative therapies.

It is important that nurses consider the patient's religious and spiritual beliefs about medications. Patients may also wish to have time to work through their decisions on spiritual, religious, or moral grounds, and consult their religious advisers before deciding on treatment. Collaborating with and encouraging the patient to consult their religious or spiritual leader when there are questions about a medication or medical product, and maintaining sensitivity to a patient's religious or spiritual beliefs and traditions should assist the nurse to maintain a holistic focus in medication administration and patient care.

sensitivity when gathering these types of data. If a trusting nurse–patient relationship is not quickly established, the patient will be reluctant to share important personal data that could affect nursing care.

The psychological dimension can influence the success of pharmacotherapy. Patients who are convinced that their treatment is important and beneficial to their well-being will demonstrate better compliance with drug therapy. The nurse must ascertain the patient's goals in seeking treatment and determine whether drug therapy is compatible with those goals. Past health care experiences may lead a patient to distrust medications. Drugs may not be acceptable for the social environment of the patient. For example, having to take drugs at school or in the workplace may cause embarrassment; patients may fear that they will be viewed as weak, unhealthy, or dependent. Some patients may believe that certain medications, such as antidepressants or antiseizure medications, carry a social stigma, and, therefore, they will resist using them.

Patients who display positive attitudes toward their personal health and have high expectations regarding the results of their pharmacotherapy are more likely to achieve positive outcomes. The nurse plays a pivotal role in encouraging the patient's positive expectations. The nurse must always be forthright in explaining drug actions and potential side effects. Trivializing the limitations of pharmacotherapy or minimizing potential adverse effects can cause the patient to have unrealistic expectations regarding treatment. The nurse–patient relationship may be jeopardized, and the patient may acquire an attitude of distrust.

Psychosocial interventions should be viewed as complementary to pharmacotherapy. For example, psychosocial stress increases the secretion of corticosteroids, which in turn may increase susceptibility to certain infections and suppress immune cell function. These conditions certainly have the potential to alter the course of pharmacotherapy. In addition, patients with anxiety and depressive disorders may benefit greatly from psychotherapy, self-help instruction, physical exercise, or improved sleep hygiene. Psychosocial interventions may lead to improved compliance with drug therapy.

9.3 Cultural and Ethnic Influences on Pharmacotherapy

Although the terms are often used interchangeably, the definitions of culture and ethnicity are somewhat different. An ethnic group is a community of people that share a common ancestry and similar genetic heritage. **Ethnicity** implies that people have biologic and genetic similarities. **Culture** is a set of beliefs, values, and traditions that provide meaning for an individual or group. People within a culture have common rituals, religious beliefs, language, and certain expectations of behavior. Culture and ethnicity can influence a patient's beliefs and actions such as when and where to seek treatment for a medical condition, and how medical conditions and treatments are viewed. Cultural and ethnic variables can impact pharmacotherapy. Both have a profound influence on patient outcomes and the occurrence of specific drug effects as perceived and interpreted by the user.

In the past, clinical pharmacology was based largely on research and clinical experiences with Caucasian patients. As research began to reveal the large amount of individual variation in people belonging to different cultures and ethnic groups, the makeup of the research groups began to change. Whenever feasible, modern clinical trials include people of different ethnicities and varied ages.

Evidence-Based Practice: Promoting Medication Compliance

Clinical Question: How can the nurse promote medication compliance in patients managing complex health problems with drug therapy?

Evidence: Poor compliance with a prescribed medication has become known as America's "other drug problem" but one that has health and financial consequences even greater than substance abuse. It is estimated that approximately 50% of patients with chronic illnesses do not take their medications as prescribed, leading to increased complications, death, and additional costs estimated at between $100 and $300 billion per year (Benjamin, 2012; Iagu & McGuire, 2014). The medically underserved population, those Americans of all ethnic backgrounds who are poor, lack health insurance, or have inadequate access to health care, is one of the groups most at risk. There are many reasons for medication noncompliance, such as low health literacy, complex medication routines that are overwhelming for the patient to understand and difficult to comply with, medication cost or the time involved to access and obtain medications, negative attitudes about the provider, and persistent food insecurity where choices between meals or medications must be made (Chisholm-Burns & Spivey, 2012; Craig & Wright, 2012; Sattler & Lee, 2013). With over one-third of health care spending concentrated on chronic disease management for conditions such as diabetes, cancer, respiratory conditions, mental health, and pain, the cost of noncompliance is significant (IMS Institute for Healthcare Informatics, 2014).

Research has demonstrated that the use of multiple strategies may increase medication compliance, including simplification of treatment; education given verbally, written, or by audio-visual material; providing feedback to patients on their dosing history based on electronic records such as prescriptions; and coordinating arrangements to assist with cost when possible (Demonceau et al., 2013; Giannetti & Kamal, 2014). Educating patients about their medication and providing feedback on medication use were among the most effective techniques to increase adherence (Demonceau et al., 2013).

Nursing Implications: The nurse serves a vital role in increasing medication compliance, both because of the trustful relationship nurses establish with their patients and because the nurse is often the main source of medication education for the patient and family. Knowing that patients often feel overwhelmed with the amount of information provided, or have concerns about the perceived cost of a drug, the nurse can discuss the prescription routine with the patient and ask questions such as: Will the patient be able to fill the prescription, or are there concerns about the cost and how it might impact the purchase of other necessities such as food? Does the patient understand the disease process and how this medication will be part of the treatment plan? How will it fit into the patient's usual routine or with other medications, and what strategies does the patient think might help maintain compliance? When teaching about the medications, the nurse should provide simple drug information to help the patient understand why a medication is required, when and how it should be taken, and when to call the health care provider. This is vital information that helps increase medication compliance. With each successive health care visit, the nurse can go over the medication history and ask questions about the prescribed medications. Being alert to reports that the patient is not taking, or incorrectly taking, the prescribed drugs may suggest an overwhelming, complex medication routine that needs to be reassessed if it is to be successful. Finally, being sensitive to concerns about cost, and working with the provider and the patient to find workable solutions, may be necessary to ensure compliance.

Although it is impossible to have complete knowledge about the many cultural variations among patients, the nurse can strive to understand the significance of the cultural traditions and their potential impact on the patient's care.

Cultural competence is the ability of health care providers to provide care to people with diverse values, beliefs, and behaviors, including the ability to adapt delivery of care to meet the needs of these patients. In the context of pharmacotherapy, culturally competent care is the ability to customize the delivery of medications to meet patients' diverse cultural values, beliefs, and traditions for the purpose of optimizing care and positive outcomes. The nurse should keep in mind the following variables when treating patients from different ethnic groups.

- *Dietary considerations.* Cultures vary in their dietary preferences and practices. Diets that include (or exclude) certain foods have the potential to increase or decrease the effectiveness of a medication. Certain spices and herbs important to a patient's culture may affect pharmacotherapy. For example, some cultures include a diet with abundant amounts of cheese, pickled fish, or wine that can interact with medications. Certain herbs can affect antidepressants, anticoagulants, and beta blockers. Assessing the primary foods of a patient's culture is an important component of the patient's psychosocial history.
- *Alternative therapies.* Various cultural groups believe in using alternative therapies, such as vitamins, herbs, or acupuncture, either along with or in place of modern medicines. Some folk remedies and traditional treatments have existed for thousands of years and helped form the foundation for modern medical practice. For example, Chinese patients may consult with herbalists to treat diseases, whereas Native Americans may collect, store, and use herbs to treat and prevent disease. Certain Hispanic cultures use spices and herbs to maintain a balance of hot and cold to promote wellness. The nurse can assess the treatments used and interpret the effect of these herbal and alternative therapies on the prescribed medications to maximize

positive outcomes. The nurse can explain that certain herbs or supplements may cause potential health risks when combined with prescribed drugs.

- *Beliefs about health and disease.* Cultures view health and illness in different ways. Individuals may seek assistance from people in their own community whom they believe have healing powers. Native Americans may consult with a tribal medicine man, whereas Hispanics seek a folk healer. African Americans sometimes practice healing through the gift of laying-on-of-hands. The nurse's understanding of the patient's trust in alternative healers is important. The more the nurse knows about cultural beliefs, the better able the nurse will be to provide support and guidance to patients.

Although culture and ethnicity are important variables to consider when treating patients, the nurse must be aware that not every individual within a well-prescribed cultural group will have identical values and traditions. Failure to recognize that individual variation exists within a group can lead to negative stereotyping of a patient.

9.4 Community and Environmental Influences on Pharmacotherapy

A number of community and environmental factors have been identified that influence disease and its subsequent treatment. Population growth, complex technologic advances, and evolving globalization patterns have all affected health care. Communities vary significantly in regard to population density, age distributions, socioeconomic levels, occupational patterns, and industrial growth. In much of the world, people live in areas lacking adequate sanitation and potable water supplies. All these community and environmental factors have the potential to affect health and access to pharmacotherapy.

Access to health care is perhaps the most obvious community-related influence on pharmacotherapy. There are many potential barriers to obtaining appropriate health care. Approximately 15% of all persons in the United States lack health insurance coverage (Centers for Disease Control and Prevention [CDC], 2013b). This number rises to about 30% in persons of age 25–34 and for Hispanics. Without an adequate health insurance plan, some people are reluctant to seek health care for fear of bankrupting the family unit. Older adults fear losing their retirement savings or being placed in a nursing home for the remainder of their lives. Families living in rural areas may have to travel great distances to obtain necessary treatment. Once treatment is rendered, the cost of prescription drugs may be too high for patients on limited incomes. This is especially troublesome for chronic disorders such as hypertension and diabetes. These disorders require lifetime therapy, but patients do not have noticeable symptoms early in the course of the disease. Therefore, the patient may not feel a need for pharmacotherapy. The nurse must be aware of these variables and have knowledge of social agencies in the local community that can assist in improving health care access.

Literacy is another community-related variable that can affect health care. A significant percentage of English-speaking patients do not have functional literacy—a basic ability to read, understand, and act on health information. The functional illiteracy rate is even higher in certain populations, particularly non–English-speaking individuals and older patients. The nurse must be aware that these patients may not be able to read drug labels, understand written treatment instructions, or read brochures describing their disease or therapy. Functional illiteracy can result in a lack of understanding about the importance of pharmacotherapy and can lead to poor compliance. The nurse should identify these patients and provide them with brochures, instructions, and educational materials that can be understood. For non–English-speaking patients or those for whom English is their second language, the nurse should have proper materials in the patient's primary language, or provide an interpreter who can help with accurate translations (Figure 9.2). The patient should be asked to repeat important instructions to ensure comprehension. The use of graphic-rich materials is appropriate for certain therapies.

PharmFacts

HEALTH DISPARITIES AND INEQUALITIES

- The rate of premature death due to stroke and coronary heart disease is higher among non-Hispanic Blacks than among non-Hispanic Whites.
- Rates for drug-induced death (from both legal and illegal drugs) is highest among American Indian, Alaskan Natives, and non-Hispanic Whites.
- The infant mortality rate for non-Hispanic black women is more than double that for non-Hispanic White women.
- Rates of blood pressure control among adults with hypertension are lowest among Mexican-Americans
- Diabetes is highest among non-Hispanic Blacks, Hispanics, persons with less than high school education, and those who are poor.

Source: *CDC Health Disparities and Inequalities Report-U S, 2013a: Disparities and Analytics, CHDIR 2013 Fact Sheet*, Centers for Disease Control, (2013a). Retrieved from http://www.cdc.gov/minorityhealth/CHDIReport.html

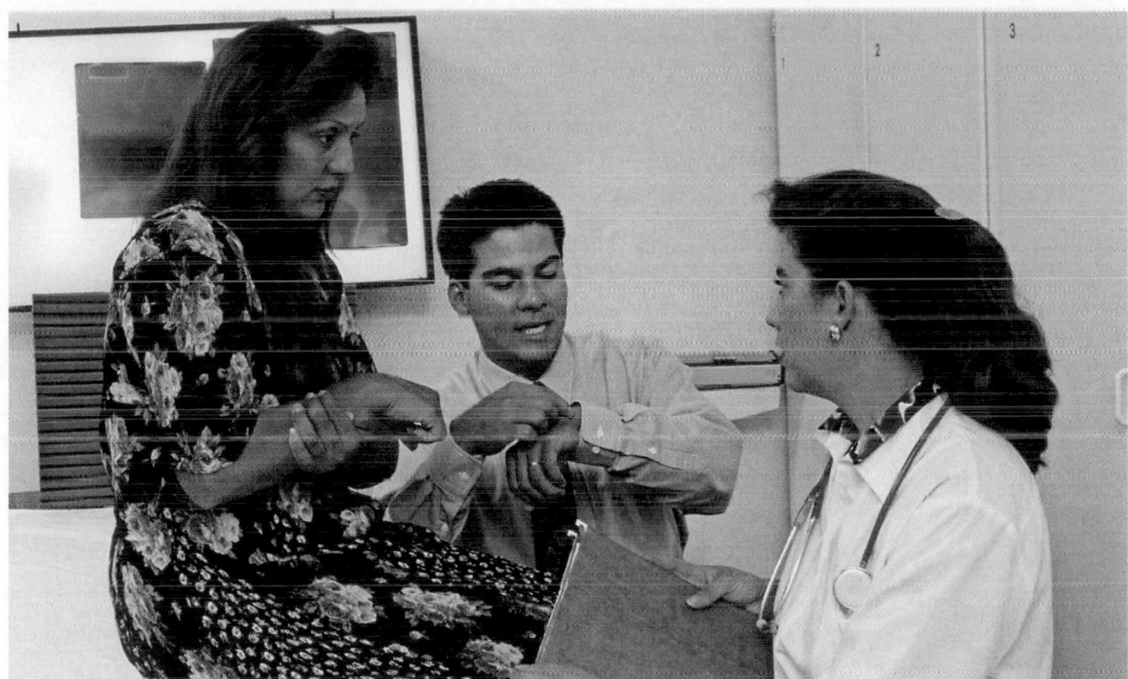

FIGURE 9.2 A nurse communicates with her non–English-speaking patient through an interpreter

Tony Freeman/PhotoEdit, Inc.

9.5 Genetic Influences on Pharmacotherapy

Although 99.8% of human DNA sequences are alike, the remaining 0.2% may result in significant differences in patients' ability to handle certain medications. Some of these differences are created when a mutation occurs in the portion of DNA responsible for encoding a certain metabolic enzyme. A single base mutation in DNA may result in an amino acid change in the enzyme, which alters its function. This creates a **genetic polymorphism**—two or more versions of the same enzyme. The best characterized genetic polymorphisms have been discovered in enzymes that metabolize drugs (CYP 450 enzymes) and in proteins that serve as receptors for drugs. **Pharmacogenetics** is the study of genetic variations that give rise to differences in drug response.

Genetic polymorphisms of CYP 450 enzymes are often identified in specific ethnic groups, because people in an ethnic group have been located in the same geographic area and have married others within the same group for hundreds of generations. Although genetic polymorphisms are generally rare in the overall population, specific ethnic groups can sometimes express a very high incidence of these defects. Some polymorphisms result in changes in drug metabolism, with patients being classified as either poor, intermediate, extensive, or ultrarapid metabolizers.

The relationship between genetic makeup and drug response has been documented for decades. One of the first polymorphisms was discovered in acetyltransferase, an enzyme that metabolizes isoniazid (INH), a drug prescribed for tuberculosis. The metabolic process, known as *acetylation*, occurs abnormally slowly in certain Caucasians. The reduced hepatic metabolism and subsequent clearance by the kidney can cause the drug to build to toxic levels in these patients, who are known as *slow acetylators* (poor metabolizers). The opposite effect, fast acetylation (extensive metabolizers), is found in many patients of Japanese descent.

Other enzyme polymorphisms have also been identified. Asian Americans are less able to metabolize codeine to morphine due to a genetic absence of the enzyme CYP2D6, a defect that interferes with the analgesic properties of codeine. Some persons of African American descent have decreased effects from beta-adrenergic antagonist drugs such as propranolol (Inderal), because of genetic variances in plasma renin levels. Another set of oxidation enzyme polymorphisms have been found that alter the response to warfarin (Coumadin) and diazepam (Valium). Table 9.1 summarizes the most common polymorphisms that impact pharmacotherapy. Expanding knowledge about the physiological impact of heredity on pharmacotherapy may someday allow for personalization of the treatment process.

9.6 Gender Influences on Pharmacotherapy

There are well-documented differences in the patterns of disease between males and females. For example, women tend to pay more attention to changes in health patterns and seek health care earlier than their male counterparts. However, many women do not seek medical attention for

Table 9.1 Genetic Polymorphisms of Drug-Metabolizing Enzymes

Enzyme	Result of Polymorphism	Drugs Using This Metabolic Enzyme or Pathway
Acetyltrans-ferase	Slow acetylation in Scandinavians, Jews, North African Caucasians; fast acetylation in Japanese	caffeine, hydralazine, isoniazid, procainamide
CYP2A6	Reduced metabolism	nicotine: may influence nicotine dependence, smoking cessation response, and risk of lung cancer
CYP2B6	Increased or decreased metabolism (depending on subtype)	bupropion, efavirenz, cyclophosphamide, nevirapine
CYP2C9	Reduced metabolism	warfarin, sulfonylurea hypoglycemics, NSAIDs
CYP2C19	Poorly metabolized in Asians and African Americans	amitriptyline, citalopram, clopidogrel, diazepam, imipramine, omeprazole, proguanil, voriconazole, warfarin
CYP2D6	Poorly metabolized in Asians and African Americans	amitriptyline, beta blockers, opioids, haloperidol, imipramine, morphine, perphenazine, tamoxifen

potential cardiac symptoms, because heart disease has traditionally been considered to be a "man's disease." Alzheimer's disease affects both men and women, but studies in various populations have shown that between 1.5 and 3 times as many women suffer from the disease. Alzheimer's disease is becoming recognized as a major "women's health issue," along with osteoporosis, breast cancer, and fertility disorders.

Compliance with the prescribed medication regimen may be influenced by gender because the side effects are specific to either males or females. A common example is certain antihypertensive agents that have the potential to cause or worsen male impotence. Several drugs can cause gynecomastia, an increase in breast size, which can be embarrassing for males. Similarly, certain drugs can cause masculine side effects such as increased hair growth, which can be a cause of noncompliance in women taking these medications. Also in females, the estrogen contained in oral contraceptives causes an elevated risk of thromboembolic disorders. With effective communication, gender-specific concerns regarding drug adverse effects can be brought into the open so alternative drug therapies can be considered. As with so many areas of health care, appropriate patient teaching by the nurse is a key aspect in preventing or alleviating drug-related health problems.

Local and systemic responses to some medications can differ between genders. These response differences may be based on differences in body composition such as the fat-to-muscle ratio. In addition, cerebral blood flow variances between males and females may alter the response to certain analgesics. An example is the benzodiazepines given for anxiety; women experience slower elimination rates and this difference becomes more significant if the woman is taking oral contraceptives.

In the past, the majority of drug research studies were conducted using only male subjects. It was wrongly assumed that the conclusions of these studies applied in the same manner to women. The U.S. Food and Drug administration (FDA) now has formal policies that require the inclusion of subjects of both genders during drug development. This includes analyses of clinical data by gender, assessment of potential pharmacokinetic and pharmacodynamic differences between genders, and, when appropriate, conducting additional studies specific to women's health.

Chapter Review

KEY Concepts

The numbered key concepts provide a succinct summary of the important points from the corresponding numbered section within the chapter. If any of these points are not clear, refer to the numbered section within the chapter for review.

9.1 To deliver effective treatment, the nurse must consider the total patient in a holistic context.

9.2 The psychosocial domain must be considered when delivering holistic care. Positive attitudes and high expectations toward therapeutic outcomes in the patient may influence the success of pharmacotherapy.

9.3 Culture and ethnicity are two interconnected perspectives that can affect pharmacotherapy. Differences in diet, use of alternative therapies, and beliefs about health and disease can influence patient drug response.

9.4 Community and environmental factors affect health and the public's access to health care and pharmacotherapy. Inadequate access to health care resources and an inability to read or understand instructions may compromise treatment outcomes.

9.5 Genetic differences in metabolic enzymes that occur among different ethnic groups must be considered for effective pharmacotherapy. Differences in the structure of enzymes, called polymorphisms, can result in profound changes in drug response.

9.6 Gender can influence many aspects of health maintenance, promotion, and treatment, as well as medication response.

REVIEW Questions

1. The patient informs the nurse that he uses herbal compounds given by a family member to treat his hypertension. What is the most appropriate action by the nurse?
    1. Inform the patient that the herbal treatments will be ineffective.
    2. Obtain more information and determine whether the herbs are compatible with prescribed medications.
    3. Notify the health care provider immediately.
    4. Inform the patient that the health care provider will not treat him if he does not accept the use of conventional medicine only.
2. The nurse provides teaching about a drug to an older adult couple. To ensure that the instructions are understood, which of the following actions would be most appropriate for the nurse to take?
    1. Provide detailed written material about the drug.
    2. Provide labels and instructions in large print.
    3. Assess the patients' reading levels and have the patients "teach back" the instructions to determine understanding.
    4. Provide instructions only when family members are present.
3. The nurse understands that gender issues also influence pharmacotherapy. What are some important considerations for the nurse to remember about these differences?
    1. Men seek health care earlier than women.
    2. Women may not seek treatment for cardiac conditions as quickly as men.
    3. Women are more likely to stop taking medications because of side effects.
    4. All drug trials are conducted on male subjects.
4. The patient informs the nurse that she will decide whether she will accept treatment after she prays with her family and minister. What is the role of spirituality in drug therapy for this client?
    1. Irrelevant because medications act on scientific principles
    2. Important to the patient's acceptance of medical treatment and response to treatment
    3. Harmless if it makes the patient feel better
    4. Harmful, especially if treatment is delayed
5. Patients characterized as slow acetylators may experience what effects related to drug therapy?
    1. They are more prone to drug toxicity.
    2. They require more time to absorb enteral medications.
    3. They must be given liquid medications only.
    4. They should be advised to decrease protein intake.
6. A patient undergoing treatment for cancer complains about nausea and fatigue. In approaching this patient problem holistically, what actions would the nurse take? (Select all that apply.)
    1. Give an antinausea drug as ordered and place the patient on bed rest.
    2. Observe for specific instances of nausea or fatigue and report them to the oncologist.
    3. Take a medication history on the patient, noting specific medication or food triggers.
    4. Talk to the patient about the symptoms, the impact they have on daily activities, and techniques that have helped lessen the problem.
    5. Encourage the patient to use alternative therapies such as herbal products.

CRITICAL THINKING Questions

1. A 72-year-old African American patient with heart disease who has been treated for atrial flutter, a type of cardiac dysrhythmia, is taking the anticoagulant, warfarin (Coumadin). The health care provider suspects that the patient has a genetic polymorphism that causes the drug to be poorly metabolized. What could the nurse do to assist in monitoring for this effect?
2. A 52-year-old female patient is admitted to the emergency department. She developed chest pressure, shortness of breath, anxiety, and nausea approximately four hours ago and now has chest pain. She tells the nurse that she "thought she had just overexerted herself gardening." How might her gender have influenced her decision to seek treatment?
3. A 19-year-old male patient of Latin American descent presents to a health clinic for migrant farm workers. In broken English, he describes severe pain in his lower jaw. An assessment reveals two abscessed molars and other oral health problems. Discuss the possible reasons for this patient's condition.

Visit www.pearsonhighered.com/nursingresources for answers and rationales for all activities.

REFERENCES

Benjamin, R. M. (2012). Medication adherence: Helping patients take their medicines as directed. *Public Health Reports, 127*(1), 2–3.

Centers for Disease Control. (2013a). *CDC health disparities and inequalities report-U S, 2013: Disparities and analytics, CHDIR 2013 fact sheet*. Retrieved from http://www.cdc.gov/minorityhealth/CHDIReport.html

Centers for Disease Control. (2013b). *Early release of selected estimates based on data from the 2012 National Health Interview Survey*. Retrieved from http://www.cdc.gov/nchs/nhis/released201306.htm#1

Chisholm-Burns, M. A., & Spivey, C. A. (2012). The 'cost' of medication nonadherence: Consequences we cannot afford to accept. *Journal of the American Pharmacists Association, 52*, 823–826. doi:10.1331/JAPhA.2012.11088

Craig, H., & Wright, B. (2012). Nonadherence to prophylactic–negative attitudes toward doctors a strong predictor. *Australian Family Physician, 41*, 815–818

Demonceau, J., Ruppar, T., Kristanto, P., Hughes, D. A., Fargher, E., Kardas, P., . . . Vrijens, B. (2013). Identification and assessment of adherence-enhancing interventions in studies assessing medication adherence through electronically compiled drug dosing histories: A systematic literature review and meta-analysis. *Drugs, 73*, 545–562. doi:10.1007/s40265-013-0041-3

Eriksson, A., Burcharth, J., & Rosenberg, J. (2013). Animal derived products may conflict with religious patients' beliefs. *BMC Medical Ethics, 14*, 48. doi:10.1186/1472-6939-14-48

Giannetti, V. J., & Kamal, K. M. (2014). Adherence with therapeutic regimens: Behavioral and pharmacoeconomic perspectives. *Journal of Pharmacy Practice*. Advance online publication. doi:10.1177/0897190014549840

Hoesli, T. M., & Smith, K. M. (2011). Effects of religious and personal beliefs on medication regimen design. *Orthopedics, 34*(4), 292. doi:10.3928/01477447-20110228-17

Iagu, A. O., & McGuire, M. J. (2014). Adherence and health care costs. *Risk Management and Healthcare Policy, 7*, 35–44. doi:10.2147/RMHP.S19801

IMS Institute for Healthcare Informatics. (2014). *Medicine use and shifting costs of healthcare: A review of the use of medicines in the U.S. in 2013*. Retrieved from http://www.imshealth.com/portal/site/imshealth/menuitem.762a961826aad98f53c753c71ad8c22a/?vgnextoid=2684d47626745410VgnVCM10000076192ca2RCRD

Sattler, E. L., & Lee, J. S. (2013). Persistent food insecurity is associated with higher levels of cost-related medication nonadherence in low-income older adults. *Journal of Nutrition in Gerontology and Geriatrics, 32*, 41–58. doi:10.1080/21551197.2012.722888

SELECTED BIBLIOGRAPHY

Chen, L. S., Bloom, A. J., Baker, T. B., Smith, S. S., Piper, M. E., Martinez, M., . . . Bierut, L. (2014). Pharmacotherapy effects on smoking cessation vary with nicotine metabolism gene (CYP2A6). *Addiction, 109*(1), 128–137. doi:10.1111/add.12353

Daly, A. K., & Cascorbi, I. (2014). Opportunities and limitations: The value of pharmacogenetics in clinical practice. *British Journal of Clinical Pharmacology, 77*(4), 583–586. doi:10.1111/bcp.12354

Du, H., Chen, X., Fang, Y., Yan, O., Xu, H., Li, L., . . . Huang, W. (2013). Slow N-acetyltransferase 2 genotype contributes to anti-tuberculosis drug-induced hepatotoxicity: A meta-analysis. *Molecular Biology Reports, 40*, 3591–3596. doi:10.1007/s11033-012-2433-y

Côté, D. (2013). Intercultural communication in health care: Challenges and solutions in work rehabilitation practices and training: a comprehensive review. *Disability and Rehabilitation, 35*, 153–163. doi:10.3109/09638288.2012.687034

Enoch, M. A. (2013). Genetic influences on response to alcohol and response to pharmacotherapies for alcoholism. *Pharmacology Biochemistry and Behavior, 123*, 17–24. doi:10.1016/j.pbb.2013.11.001

Mendrek, A., & Stip, E. (2011). Sexual dimorphism in schizophrenia: Is there a need for gender-based protocols? *Expert Review of Neurotherapeutics, 11*(7), 951–959. doi:10.1586/ern.11.78

National Center for Health Statistics. (2013). *Health, United States, 2013: With special feature on prescription drugs*. Retrieved from http://www.cdc.gov/nchs/data/hus/hus13.pdf#074

Ortega, V. E., & Meyers, D. A. (2014). Pharmacogenetics: Implications of race and ethnicity on defining genetic profiles for personalized medicine. *Journal of Allergy and Clinical Immunology, 133*, 16–26. doi:10.1016/j.jaci.2013.10.040

Sim, S. C., Kacevska, M., & Ingelman-Sundberg, M. (2012). Pharmacogenomics of drug-metabolizing enzymes: A recent update on clinical implications and endogenous effects. *The Pharmacogenomics Journal, 13*, 1–11. doi:10.1038/tpj.2012.45

Zanger, U. M., & Schwab, M. (2013). Cytochrome P450 enzymes in drug metabolism: Regulation of gene expression, enzyme activities, and impact of genetic variation. *Pharmacology & Therapeutics, 138*, 103–141. doi:10.1016/j.pharmthera.2012.12.007

Chapter 10

The Role of Complementary and Alternative Therapies in Pharmacology

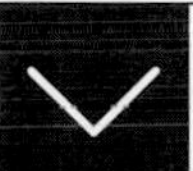

Learning Outcomes

After reading this chapter, the student should be able to:

1. Explain the role of complementary and alternative medicine in promoting patient wellness.
2. Analyze reasons why complementary and alternative therapies have increased in popularity.
3. Identify the parts of an herb that may contain active ingredients and the types of formulations made from these parts.
4. Analyze the strengths and weaknesses of legislation regulating herbal and dietary supplements.
5. Describe the pharmacologic actions and safety of herbal and dietary supplements.
6. Identify common specialty supplements taken by patients.
7. Discuss the role of the nurse in teaching patients about complementary and alternative therapies.

More than 158 million consumers use herbal supplements and alternative therapies annually in the United States. Despite the fact that these therapies have not been subjected to the same scientific scrutiny as prescription medications, consumers turn to these treatments for a variety of reasons. Many people have the impression that natural substances have more healing power than synthetic medications. The ready availability of herbal supplements at a reasonable cost, combined with effective marketing strategies, has convinced many consumers to try them.

It is important for the nurse to assess for the use of herbal products and dietary supplements in patients. In some cases, patients are using these products instead of more effective therapies, thus potentially delaying effective treatment. Drug–herb interactions have been documented that may either increase the toxicity of the prescription drug or reduce its effectiveness. This chapter examines the use of herbal therapies and dietary supplements in the prevention and treatment of disease.

10.1 Complementary and Alternative Medicine

Complementary and alternative medicine (CAM) comprises an extremely diverse set of therapies and healing systems that are considered to be outside mainstream health care. Although diverse, the major CAM systems have common characteristics, including:

- Focus on treating each person as an individual.
- Consider the health of the whole person.
- Emphasize the integration of mind and body.
- Promote disease prevention, self-care, and self-healing.
- Recognize the role of spirituality in health and healing.

Because of the widespread use of CAM, scientific attention has begun to focus on examining the effectiveness, or lack of effectiveness, of these therapies. Although some research has been conducted, few CAM therapies have been subjected to rigorous clinical and scientific study. It is likely that some of these therapies will be found ineffective, whereas others will become mainstream treatments. The line between what is defined as an alternative therapy and what is considered mainstream is constantly changing. Increasing numbers of health care providers are now recommending CAM therapies to their patients. Table 10.1 lists some of these therapies.

Nurses have long respected the value of CAM in preventing and treating certain conditions. For example, prayer, meditation, massage, and yoga have been used for centuries to treat both body and mind. From a pharmacology perspective, much of the value of CAM therapies lies in their ability to reduce the need for medications. For instance, if a patient can find anxiety relief through herbal products, massage, or biofeedback therapy, then the use of antianxiety drugs may be reduced or eliminated. Reduction of drug dose leads to fewer adverse effects and improved compliance with the therapeutic regimen. If used appropriately, pharmacotherapy and alternative therapies can serve complementary and essential roles in the healing of the total patient.

Table 10.1 Complementary and Alternative Therapies

Healing Method	Examples
Alternative health care systems	Naturopathy
	Homeopathy
	Chiropractic
	Native American medicine (e.g., sweat lodges, medicine wheel)
	Chinese traditional medicine (e.g., acupuncture, Chinese herbs)
Biologic-based therapies	Herbal therapies
	Nutritional supplements
	Special diets
Manual healing	Massage
	Physical therapy
	Pressure-point therapies
	Hand-mediated biofield therapies
Mind–body interventions	Yoga
	Meditation
	Hypnotherapy
	Guided imagery
	Biofeedback
	Movement-oriented therapies (e.g., music, dance)
Spiritual	Shamans
	Faith and prayer
Others	Bioelectromagnetics
	Detoxifying therapies
	Animal-assisted therapy

10.2 Brief History of Herbal Therapies

An **herb** is technically a **botanical** that does not contain any woody tissue such as stems or bark. Over time, the terms *botanical* and *herb* have come to be used interchangeably to refer to any plant product with some useful application either as a food enhancer, such as flavoring, or as a medicine.

The use of botanicals has been documented for thousands of years. One of the earliest recorded uses of plant products was a prescription for garlic in 3000 B.C. Eastern and Western medicine have recorded thousands of herbs and herb combinations reputed to have therapeutic value.

Table 10.2 Popular Herbal Supplements

Herb	Medicinal Part	Primary Use(s)	Herb Feature (Chapter)
Acai	Berries	Vitamin and mineral supplement, antioxidant, possible weight loss	—
Aloe vera	Leaves	Topical application for minor skin irritations and burns	49
Bilberry	Berries and leaves	Terminate diarrhea, improve and protect vision, antioxidant	50
Black cohosh	Roots	Relief of menopausal symptoms	46
Chlorophyll/chlorella	Leaves	Improve digestion, vitamin and mineral supplement	—
Cranberry	Berries/juice	Prevent urinary tract infection	24
Echinacea	Entire plant	Enhance immune system, treat the common cold	34
Elderberry	Berries and flowers	Congestion in respiratory system due to colds and flu	—
Evening primrose	Oil extracted from seeds	Source of essential fatty acids, relief of premenstrual or menopausal symptoms, relief of rheumatoid arthritis and other inflammatory symptoms	—
Flaxseed (ground) and/or oil	Seeds and oil	Reduce blood cholesterol, laxative	—
Garlic	Bulbs	Reduce blood cholesterol, reduce blood pressure, anticoagulation	31
Ginger	Root	Antiemetic, antithrombotic, diuretic, promote gastric secretions, anti-inflammatory, increase blood glucose, stimulation of peripheral circulation	41
Ginkgo	Leaves and seeds	Improve memory, reduce dizziness	20
Ginseng	Root	Relieve stress, enhance immune system, decrease fatigue	28
Grape seed	Seeds/oil	Source of essential fatty acids, antioxidant, restore microcirculation to tissues	26
Green tea	Leaves	Antioxidant; lower LDL cholesterol; prevent cancer; relieve stomach problems, nausea, vomiting	—
Horny goat weed	Leaves and roots	Enhance sexual function	—
Milk thistle	Seeds	Antitoxin, protection against liver disease	22
Red rice yeast extract	Dried in capsules	Reduce blood cholesterol	—
Saw palmetto	Berries	Treatment of benign prostatic hyperplasia	47
Soy	Beans	Source of protein, vitamins, and minerals; relief of menopausal symptoms, prevent cardiovascular disease, anticancer	—
Stevia	Leaves	Natural sweetener	—
St. John's wort	Flowers, leaves, stems	Reduce depression, reduce anxiety, anti-inflammatory	16
Valerian	Roots	Relieve stress, promote sleep	—
Wheat or barley grass	Leaves	Improve digestion, vitamin and mineral supplement	—

The most popular current herbal supplements and their claimed applications are listed in Table 10.2.

With the birth of the pharmaceutical industry in the late 1800s, interest in herbal medicines began to wane. Synthetic drugs could be standardized, produced, and distributed more cheaply than natural herbal products. When regulatory agencies eventually required that consumer products be safe and labeled accurately, many products were removed from the market. The focus of health care was on diagnosing and treating specific diseases, rather than on promoting wellness and holistic care. Most alternative therapies were no longer taught in medical or nursing schools; these healing techniques were criticized as being unscientific relics of the past.

Beginning in the 1970s and continuing to the present, alternative therapies and herbal medicines have experienced a remarkable resurgence, such that the majority of adult Americans are currently taking botanicals on a regular basis or have taken them in the past. This increase in popularity is due to factors such as increased availability of herbal products, aggressive marketing by the herbal industry, increased attention to natural alternatives, and a renewed interest in preventive medicine. The gradual aging of the population has led to an increase in patients seeking therapeutic alternatives for chronic conditions such as pain, arthritis, decreases in hormones such as occurs in menopause, and prostate enlargement. In addition, the high cost of prescription medicines has driven patients to seek less expensive alternatives. Nurses have been instrumental in promoting self-care and recommending CAM therapies for patients, when applicable.

PharmFacts

COMPLEMENTARY AND ALTERNATIVE MEDICINE IN PEOPLE AGED 50 AND OLDER

In a survey of over a thousand people aged 50 and older, the American Association of Retired People (AARP) and the National Center for Complementary and Alternative Medicine (NCCAM) (AARP & NCCAM, 2011) found the following:

- Almost half reported the use of CAM during the previous 12 months.
- Women and those with higher educational levels were most likely to use CAM.
- The most frequently used CAM were herbal products, followed by massage therapy, chiropractic, and mind-body practices.
- The most frequent reasons for using CAM were to prevent illness, promote general body wellness, and to reduce pain (17%).

10.3 Herbal Product Formulations

The pharmacologically active substances in an herbal product may be present in only one specific part of the plant or in all parts. For example, the active chemicals in chamomile are in the above-ground portion that includes the leaves, stems, and flowers. With other herbs, such as ginger, the underground rhizomes and roots are used for their healing properties. When using fresh herbs or collecting herbs for home use, it is essential to know which portion of the plant contains the active chemicals.

Most modern drugs contain only one active ingredient. This chemical is standardized, accurately measured, and delivered to the patient in precise amounts. It is a common misconception that herbs also contain one active ingredient, which can be extracted and delivered to patients in precise doses, like drugs. Herbs actually may contain dozens of active chemicals, many of which have not yet been isolated, studied, or even identified. It is possible that some of these substances work together synergistically and may not have the same activity if isolated. Furthermore, the potency of an herbal preparation may vary depending on where it was grown and how it was collected and stored.

To achieve consistency, scientists have attempted to standardize the strength or dose of herbal products, using marker substances such as the percent flavones in ginkgo or the percent lactones in kava kava. Some of these standardizations are listed in Table 10.3. It should be noted that science has not yet determined exactly which substance in an herb is therapeutic or its optimal dose. Until science can better characterize these substances, it is best to conceptualize the active ingredient of an herb as being the whole herb and not just a single chemical. An example of the ingredients and standardization of ginkgo biloba is shown in Figure 10.1.

Lifespan Considerations: Pediatric
CAM for Children With ADHD and ASD

Attention-deficit /hyperactivity disorder (ADHD) and autism spectrum disorders (ASD) are frustrating developmental conditions for families, in part because there are limited proven treatments, and for those traditional medications that exist, a fairly high incidence of adverse effects. Huang, Seshadri, Matthews, & Ostfeld (2013) found that while parents of children with ADHD and ASD used traditional therapies such as medications and behavioral therapies, they also turned to CAM such as dietary supplements (vitamin B_6, magnesium, flaxseed and omega-3) and nonmedicinal therapies such as sensory integration. The use of CAM was higher for ASD than for ADHD (82% for ASD compared to 19.5% for ADHD). Parents seeking alternative therapies were well-educated with more than half holding advanced degrees, and most expressed interest in knowing more about research into the use of CAM for ADHD and ASD. Parents also felt that their physician was not a knowledgeable resource for CAM.

Because of the current scarcity of proven traditional therapies, parents may turn to CAM, particularly for ASD. Other CAM strategies used for ASD include gluten and casein-free diets, secretin, melatonin, hyperbaric oxygen therapy, and immune therapies (Whitehouse, 2013). As many as 50% of parents of children with ASD are estimated to use some form of CAM (Valicenti-McDermott et al., 2014). Recognizing that these families may not always disclose their use of CAM, nurses and other health care providers should ensure that they ask about the use of CAM, and its effectiveness or adverse effects, with each health care encounter. Becoming more knowledgeable about CAM for ADHD and ASD will also help providers become a more informed resource for parents of children with these disorders.

Table 10.3 Standardization of Selected Herb Extracts

Herb	Standardization	Percent
Black cohosh rhizome	Triterpene glycosides	2.5
Cascara sagrada bark	Anthocyanides	25
Echinacea purpurea, whole herb	Echinacosides	4
Ginger rhizome	Pungent compounds	Greater than 10
Ginkgo leaf	Flavone glycosides	24–25
	Lactones	6
Ginseng root	Ginsenosides	5–15
Kava kava rhizome	Kavalactones	40–45
Milk thistle root	Silymarin	80
Saw palmetto fruit	Fatty acids and sterols	80–90
St. John's wort	Hypericins	0.3–0.5
	Hyperforin	3–5

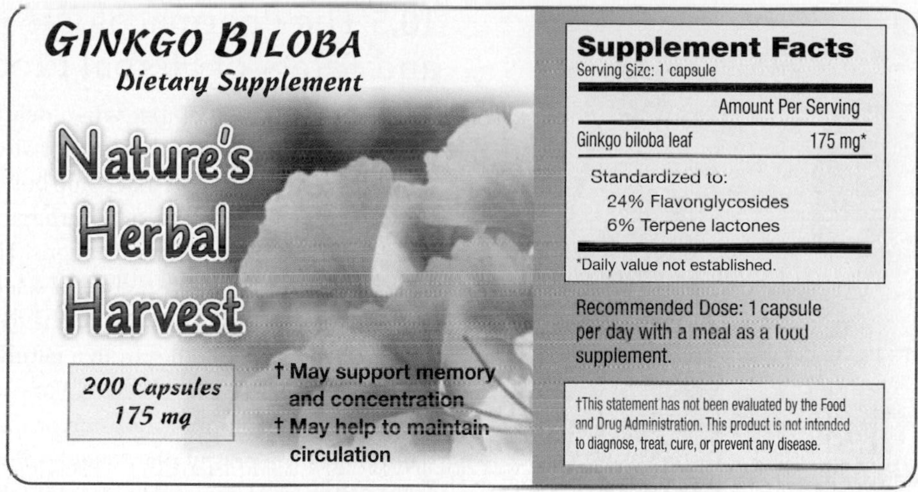

FIGURE 10.1 Ginkgo Biloba label. The label indicates the product is standardized to percentages of the two active ingredients, flavonglycosides and terpenes that are found in the ginkgo leaf. Also note the health claims on the label, which have not been evaluated by the FDA.
Source: *Pharmacology: Connections to Nursing Practice* (3rd Ed.), by M. Adams and C. Urban, 2016. Reprinted and electronically reproduced by permission of Pearson Education, Inc., Upper Saddle River, New Jersey.

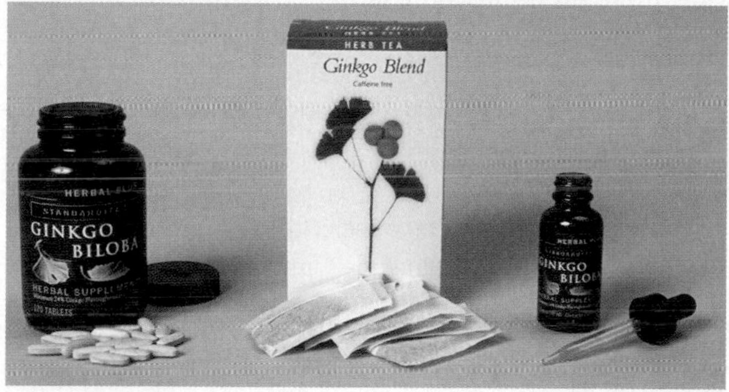

FIGURE 10.2 Three different ginkgo formulations: tablets, tea bags, and liquid extract
Al Dodge/Pearson Education, Inc.

The two basic formulations of herbal products are solid and liquid. Solid products include pills, tablets, and capsules made from the dried herbs. Other solid products are salves and ointments that are administered topically. Liquid formulations are made by extracting the active chemicals from the plant using solvents such as water, alcohol, or glycerol. The liquids are then concentrated in various strengths and ingested as extracts, infusions, teas, or tinctures. Figure 10.2 illustrates different formulations of the popular herb ginkgo biloba.

10.4 Regulation of Herbal Products and Dietary Supplements

Since the passage of the Food, Drug, and Cosmetic Act in 1936, Americans have come to expect that all approved prescription and over-the-counter (OTC) drugs have passed rigid standards of safety prior to being marketed. Furthermore, it is expected that these drugs have been tested for effectiveness and that they truly provide the medical benefits claimed by the manufacturer.

For herbal products and dietary supplements, however, Americans cannot and should not expect the same quality standards. These products are regulated by a far less rigorous law, the **Dietary Supplement Health and Education Act (DSHEA) of 1994.** The DSHEA specifically exempts dietary supplements from regulation by the Food, Drug, and Cosmetic Act.

Dietary supplements are defined as products intended to enhance or supplement the diet, such as botanicals, vitamins, minerals, or other extracts or metabolites that are not already approved as drugs by the U.S. Food and Drug Administration (FDA). A major strength of the legislation is that it gives the FDA the power to remove from the market any product that poses a "significant or unreasonable" risk to the public. It also requires these products to be clearly labeled by the manufacturer as "dietary supplements." An example of an herbal label for L-carnitine is shown in Figure 10.3.

The DSHEA contained several significant flaws that led to a lack of standardization in the dietary supplement industry and to less protection for the consumer such as:

- Effectiveness does not have to be demonstrated by the manufacturer prior to marketing.
- The manufacturer does not have to prove the safety of the dietary supplement. To be removed from the market, the government has the burden of proof to show that the supplement is unsafe.
- Dietary supplement labels must state that the product is not intended to diagnose, treat, cure, or prevent any disease; however, the label may make claims about the product's effect on body structure and function, such as the following:
  - Helps promote healthy immune systems.
  - Reduces anxiety and stress.
  - Helps maintain cardiovascular function.
  - May reduce pain and inflammation.
- The DSHEA does not regulate the accuracy of the label; the product may or may not contain the ingredients listed in the amounts claimed.

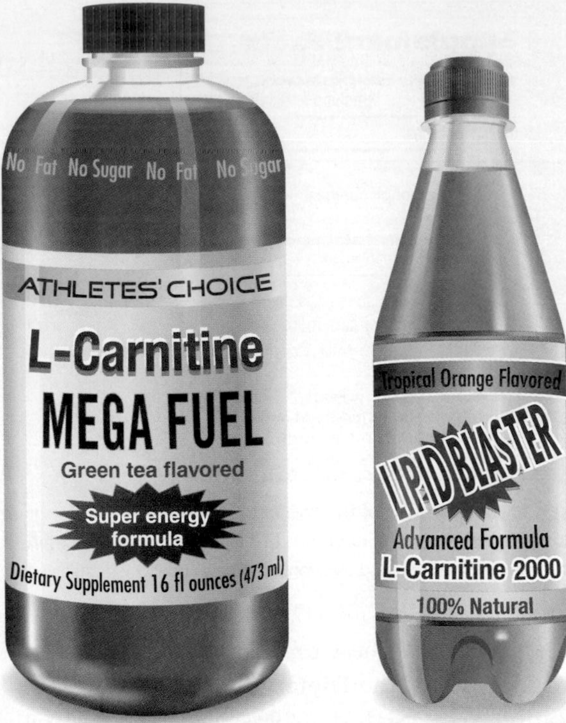

FIGURE 10.3 L-carnitine is a popular dietary supplement. Notice the claims of improving athletic performance and weight loss, neither of which has been supported by the scientific literature.

Several steps have been taken to address the lack of purity and mislabeling of herbal and dietary supplements. In an attempt to protect consumers, Congress passed the **Dietary Supplement and Nonprescription Drug Consumer Protection Act,** which took effect in 2007. Companies that market herbal and dietary supplements are now required to include contact information (address and phone number) on the product labels for consumers to use in reporting adverse effects. Companies must notify the FDA of any serious adverse event reports within 15 days of receiving such reports. Under this act, a "serious adverse event" is defined as any adverse reaction resulting in death, a life-threatening experience, inpatient hospitalization, a persistent or significant disability or incapacity, or a congenital anomaly or birth defect, as well as any event requiring a medical or surgical intervention to prevent one of these conditions, based on reasonable medical judgment. Companies must keep records of such events for at least six years, and the records are subject to inspection by the FDA.

Also in 2007, the FDA announced a final rule that requires the manufacturers of dietary supplements to evaluate the identity, purity, potency, and composition of their products. The labels must accurately reflect what is in the product, which must be free of contaminants such as pesticides, toxins, glass, or heavy metals.

10.5 The Pharmacologic Actions and Safety of Herbal Products

A key concept to remember when dealing with alternative therapies is that "natural" does not always mean better or safe. There is no question that some botanicals contain active substances as powerful as, and perhaps more effective than, some currently approved medications. Thousands of years of experience, combined with current scientific research, have shown that some herbal remedies have therapeutic actions. Because a substance comes from a natural product, however, does not make it safe or effective. For example, poison ivy is natural, but it certainly is not safe or therapeutic. The dried seedpods of the poppy plant yield opium, which has therapeutic effects but can also be fatal if taken inappropriately. Natural products may not offer an improvement over conventional therapy in treating certain disorders and, indeed, may be of no value whatsoever. Furthermore, a patient who substitutes an unproven alternative therapy for an established, effective medical treatment may delay healing, suffer harmful effects, and endanger health. Of all the herbal products available, only a few have received the level of scientific scrutiny needed to achieve a consensus recommendation from the medical community. Examples of herbal products that have received sufficient scientific evidence to suggest therapeutic effectiveness include Ginkgo biloba to treat circulatory disorders and improve memory, St. John's wort to treat mild to moderate depression, and valerian to induce relaxation or sleep (Penn State University, 2013). Disorders along with their herbal therapies, are listed in Table 10.4.

Most herbal products are safe; when taken in low to moderate doses little acute toxicity has been reported. Because these products are generally not prescribed or monitored by a health care provider, it is likely that adverse effects

Table 10.4 Diseases for Which Medical Consensus Exists That Herbal Therapies May Be Useful

Disease	Herbal Therapy
Chronic venous insufficiency	Horse chestnut seed extract
Claudication	Ginkgo biloba
Depression	St. John's wort
Hypercholesterolemia	Garlic
Hyperlipidemia	Plant sterols and stanols
Hypertension	Hawthorn
Insomnia	Valerian
Low back pain	Devil's claw, white willow bark
Memory impairment	Ginkgo biloba
Menopausal symptoms	Black cohosh, St. John's wort
Migraine prophylaxis	Butterbur
Nausea and vomiting	Ginger
Rheumatoid arthritis	Evening primrose oil, black currant seed oil

Table 10.5 Documented Herb–Drug Interactions

Herb	Interacts With	Effect(s)
Echinacea	Amiodarone, anabolic steroids, ketoconazole, methotrexate	Possible increased hepatotoxicity
Feverfew	Aspirin and other nonsteroidal anti-inflammatory drugs (NSAIDs), heparin, warfarin (Coumadin)	Increased bleeding risk
Garlic	Aspirin and other NSAIDs, warfarin (Coumadin), insulin, oral antidiabetic drugs	Increased bleeding risk Additive hypoglycemic effects
Ginger	Aspirin and other NSAIDs, heparin, warfarin	Increased bleeding risk
Ginkgo	Anticonvulsants	Possible decreased anticonvulsant effectiveness
	Aspirin, NSAIDs, heparin and warfarin (Coumadin)	Increased bleeding potential
	Tricyclic antidepressants	Possible decreased seizure threshold
Ginseng	CNS depressants	Increased sedation
	Digoxin (Lanoxin)	Increased toxicity
	Diuretics	Possible decreased diuretic effects
	Insulin and oral hypoglycemic agents	Increased hypoglycemic effects
	Warfarin (Coumadin)	Decreased anticoagulant effects
Goldenseal	Diuretics	May decrease diuretic effects
St. John's wort	CNS depressants and opioid analgesics	Increased sedation
	Cyclosporine (Sanimmune)	May decrease cyclosporine levels
	Efavirenz, indinavir, protease inhibitors	Decreased antiretroviral activity
	Oral contraceptives	Decreased drug effectiveness
	Selective serotonin reuptake inhibitors (SSRIs), tricyclic antidepressants	Possible serotonin syndrome*
	Warfarin	Decreased anticoagulant effects
Valerian	Barbiturates, benzodiazepines, and other central nervous system (CNS) depressants	Increased sedation

*Serotonin syndrome: headache, dizziness, sweating, agitation.

are underreported by patients. Those that are reported in the scientific literature occur as case studies involving only a single patient and it is impossible to generalize these types of effects to large populations. Only a few adverse events, such as hepatotoxicity caused by kava and inhibition of platelet aggregation by ginkgo biloba, are well documented.

Because they have active ingredients, herbal products do have the potential to interact with prescription and OTC medications. Herb–drug interactions are more likely to occur with prescription medications that have a narrow safety margin, such as anticoagulants, antiseizure agents, or antidysrhythmics. In addition the potential for any drug interaction increases in older adults, especially those with hepatic or renal impairment. Drug interactions with selected herbs are listed in Table 10.5. Herbal–drug interactions are noted, where applicable, in the prototype drug features throughout this text.

10.6 Specialty Supplements

Specialty supplements are nonherbal dietary products used to enhance a wide variety of body functions. These supplements form a diverse group of substances obtained from plant and animal sources. They are more specific in their action than herbal products and are generally targeted for one or a smaller number of conditions. Examples of popular specialty supplements are listed in Table 10.6.

Table 10.6 Selected Specialty Supplements

Name	Primary Uses	Supplement Feature (Chapter)
Amino acids	Build protein, muscle strength, and endurance	—
Carnitine	Enhances energy and sports performance, heart health, memory, immune function, and male fertility	27
Coenzyme Q10	Prevents heart disease, provides antioxidant therapy	23
DHEA	Boosts immune functions and memory	—
Fish oil	Reduces cholesterol levels, enhances brain function, increases visual acuity (due to presence of omega-3 fatty acids)	33
Glucosamine and chondroitin	Reduces symptoms of arthritis and other joint problems	48
Lactobacillus acidophilus	Maintains intestinal health	—
Selenium	Reduces the risk of certain types of cancer	—
Vitamin C	Prevents colds	—

In general, specialty supplements have a legitimate rationale for their use. For example, chondroitin and glucosamine are natural substances in the body necessary for cartilage growth and maintenance. Amino acids are natural building blocks of muscle protein. Flaxseed and fish oils contain omega fatty acids that have been shown to reduce the risk of heart disease in certain patients.

As with herbal products, the link between most specialty supplements and their claimed benefits is unclear. In most cases, a normal diet supplies sufficient quantities of the substance to maintain good health, and taking additional amounts may provide no benefit. In other cases, the product is marketed for conditions for which the supplement has no proven effect. The good news is that these substances are generally not harmful unless taken in large amounts. The bad news, however, is that they can give patients false hopes of an easy cure for chronic conditions such as heart disease or the pain of arthritis. As with herbal products, the nurse should advise patients to be skeptical about the health claims made for the use of these supplements.

10.7 Patient Teaching Regarding CAM

The nurse has an obligation to seek the latest medical information on herbal products because there is a good possibility that patients are using them to supplement traditional medicines. The health care provider will often need to educate patients on the role of CAM therapies in the treatment of their disorders and discuss which treatment or combination of treatments will best meet their health goals.

The nurse should be sensitive to the patient's need for alternative treatment and not be judgmental. Both advantages and limitations of CAM therapies must be presented to patients so they may make rational and informed decisions about their treatment. The following teaching points are important when assessing patients' use of these therapies:

1. Include questions on the use of CAM when obtaining medical histories. Be aware that many patients may be reluctant to report their use of herbal products due to fear of ridicule from their health care provider.
2. Ask patients why they are taking the herbal product and to articulate what benefits they are receiving (or expect to receive) from the therapy.
3. Advise patients who are taking medications with potentially serious adverse effects such as insulin, warfarin (Coumadin), or digoxin (Lanoxin) to never take any herbal product or dietary supplement without first discussing their needs with a health care provider.
4. Advise pregnant or lactating women to never take these products without approval of their health care provider.
5. Be aware that older adults are more likely to have chronic ailments such as renal, cardiac, or hepatic disease that could increase the risk for a drug–herb interaction.
6. Advise caution for all patients with serious allergies who wish to take herbal products. Most herbal products contain a mixture of ingredients and contain dozens of different chemicals. Patients who have known allergies to certain foods or medicines should seek medical advice before taking a new herbal product.
7. Advise patients to be skeptical of advertised claims for CAM and to seek health information from reputable sources.
8. Advise patients to not take more than the dose recommended on the product label. It is always wise to take the smallest amount possible when starting herbal therapy, even less than the recommended dose, to see if allergies or other adverse effects occur.

Chapter Review

KEY Concepts

The numbered key concepts provide a succinct summary of the important points from the corresponding numbered section within the chapter. If any of these points are not clear, refer to the numbered section within the chapter for review.

10.1 Complementary and alternative medicine is a set of diverse therapies and healing systems used by many people to prevent disease and promote wellness.

10.2 Natural products obtained from plants have been used as medicines for thousands of years. Recent years have seen resurgence in the popularity of these products as patients seek alternatives to conventional therapies and expensive prescription medications.

10.3 Herbal products are available in a variety of formulations; some contain standardized extracts, and others contain whole herbs.

10.4 Herbal products and dietary supplements are regulated by the Dietary Supplement Health and Education Act of 1994, which does not require safety or efficacy testing prior to marketing. More recent laws have been passed to safeguard consumer safety regarding dietary supplements.

10.5 Natural products may have pharmacologic actions and result in adverse effects, including significant interactions with prescription medications.

10.6 Specialty supplements are nonherbal dietary products used to enhance a wide variety of body functions. Like herbal products, most have not been subjected to controlled, scientific testing.

10.7 Teaching regarding the appropriate use of CAM is an essential part of the nurse–patient interaction. Patients who are pregnant, have known allergies to certain foods and medicines, or have significant organ impairment should be advised not to take herbal or specialty supplements without the approval of their health care provider.

REVIEW Questions

1. The nurse obtains information during the admission interview that the patient is taking herbal supplements in addition to prescribed medications. What is the nurse's primary concern for this patient?
   1. Herbal products are natural and pose no risk to the patient but may be costly.
   2. Herbal products are a welcome supplement to conventional medications but do not always come with instructions.
   3. The patient may be at risk for allergic reactions.
   4. The herbal products may interact with prescribed medications and affect drug action.

2. Appropriate teaching to provide safety for a patient who is planning to use herbal products should include which of the following?
   1. Take the smallest amount possible when starting herbal therapy, even less than the recommended dose, to see if allergies or other adverse effects occur.
   2. Read the labels to determine composition of the product.
   3. Research the clinical trials before using the products.
   4. Consult the Internet or herbal store staff to determine the safest dose and length of time the dose should be taken.

3. The patient states that he has been using the herbal product saw palmetto. The nurse recognizes that this supplement is often used to treat which condition?
   1. Insomnia
   2. Urinary problems associated with prostate enlargement
   3. Symptoms of menopause
   4. Urinary tract infection

4. An older adult patient tells the nurse that she has been using several herbal products recommended by a friend. Why would the nurse be concerned with this statement, given the age of the patient?
   1. The older adult patient may have difficulty reading labels and opening bottles and confuse medications.
   2. The older adult patient may have difficulty paying for additional medications and stop using prescribed drugs.
   3. The older adult patient may be more prone to allergic reactions from herbal products.
   4. The older adult patient may have other disease conditions that could increase the risk for a drug reaction.

5. Which of the following patients may be most at-risk for adverse effects related to specialty supplements? (Select all that apply.)
   1. Adolescents
   2. Pregnant women
   3. School-age children
   4. Older adult patients
   5. Patients taking prescription medication

6. What is the difference between an herbal product and a specialty supplement?
   1. An herbal product is safer to use than a specialty supplement.
   2. A specialty supplement tends to be more expensive than an herbal product.
   3. A specialty supplement is a nonherbal dietary product used to enhance a variety of body functions.
   4. There are less adverse effects or risk of allergy with specialty supplements than there are with herbal products.

CRITICAL THINKING Questions

1. A 44-year-old breast cancer survivor is placed on tamoxifen (Nolvadex), a drug that may prevent recurrence of the cancer. Since receiving chemotherapy, the patient has not had a menstrual cycle. She is concerned about being menopausal and wonders about the possibility of using a soy-based product as a form of natural hormone replacement. How should the nurse advise the patient?
2. A 62-year-old male patient is recuperating from a myocardial infarction. He is on the anticoagulant warfarin (Coumadin) and antidysrhythmic digoxin (Lanoxin). He talks to his wife about starting to take garlic, to help lower his blood lipid levels, and ginseng, because he has heard it helps in coronary artery disease. Discuss the potential concerns about the use of garlic and ginseng by this patient.
3. The patient has been taking St. John's wort for symptoms of depression. He is now scheduled for an elective surgery. What important preoperative teaching should be included?

Visit www.pearsonhighered.com/nursingresources for answers and rationales for all activities.

REFERENCES

The American Association of Retired Persons and the National Center for Complementary and Alternative Medicine. (2011). *Complementary and alternative medicine.* Retrieved from http://nccam.nih.gov/sites/nccam.nih.gov/files/news/camstats/2010/NCCAM_aarp_survey.pdf

Huang, A., Seshadri, K., Matthews, T. A., & Ostfeld, B. M. (2013). Parental perspectives on use, benefits, and physician knowledge of complementary and alternative medicine in children with autistic disorder and attention-deficit/hyperactivity disorder. *Journal of Alternative and Complementary Medicine, 19,* 746–750. doi:10.1089/acm.2012.0640

Penn State University. (2013). *Herbal medicine.* Retrieved from http://pennstatehershey.adam.com/content.aspx?productId=107&pid=33&gid=000351

Valicenti-McDermott, M., Burrows, B., Bernstein, L., Hottinger, K., Lawson, K., Seijo, R., . . . Shinnar, S. (2014). Use of complementary and alternative medicine in children with autism and other developmental disabilities: Associations with ethnicity, child comorbid symptoms, and parental stress. *Journal of Child Neurology, 29,* 360–370. doi:10.1177/0883073812474489

Whitehouse, A. J. O. (2013). Complementary and alternative medicine for autism spectrum disorders: Rationale, safety and efficacy. *Journal of Paediatrics and Child Health, 49*(9), E438–442. doi:10.1111/jpc.12242

SELECTED BIBLIOGRAPHY

American Botanical Council. (2014). *Herbal dietary supplement retail sales up 7.9% in 2013.* Retrieved from http://cms.herbalgram.org/press/2014/2013_Herb_Market_Report.html

Anastasi, J. K., Chang, M., & Capilli, B. (2011). Herbal supplements: Talking with your patients. *The Journal for Nurse Practitioners, 7,* 29–35. doi:10.1016/j.nurpra.2010.06.004

Arkowitz, H., & Lilienfeld, S. O. (2013). Can herbs ease anxiety and depression? *Scientific American Mind, 24,* 72–73. doi:10.1038/scientificamericanmind0713-72

Brantley, S. J., Argikar, A. A., Lin, Y. S., Nagar, S., & Paine, M. F. (2014). Herb–drug interactions: Challenges and opportunities for improved predictions. *Drug Metabolism and Disposition, 42*(3), 301–317. doi:10.1124/dmd.113.055236

Dante, G., Bellei, G., Neri, I., & Facchinetti, F. (2014). Herbal therapies in pregnancy: What works? *Current Opinion in Obstetrics and Gynecology, 26*(2), 83–91. doi:10.1097/GCO.0000000000000052

Fasinu, P. S., Bouic, P. J., & Rosenkranz, B. (2012). An overview of the evidence and mechanisms of herb–drug interactions. *Frontiers in Pharmacology, 3, 69.* doi:10.3389/fphar.2012.00069

Kunle, O. F., Egharevba, H. O., & Ahmadu, P. O. (2012). Standardization of herbal medicines—A review. *International Journal of Biodiversity and Conservation, 4*(3), 101–112. doi:10.5897/IJBC11.163

Lindquist, R., Snyder, M., & Tracy, M. F. (Eds.). (2013). *Complementary & alternative therapies in nursing.* New York, NY: Springer.

Posadzki, P., Watson, L. K., & Ernst, E. (2013). Adverse effects of herbal medicines: An overview of systematic reviews. *Clinical Medicine, 13*(1), 7–12.

Prasad, K., Sharma, V., Lackore, K., Jenkins, S. M., Prasad, A., & Sood, A. (2013). Use of complementary therapies in cardiovascular disease. *The American Journal of Cardiology, 111,* 339–345. doi:10.1016/j.amjcard.2012.10.010

Ravindran, A. V., & da Silva, T. L. (2013). Complementary and alternative therapies as add-on to pharmacotherapy for mood and anxiety disorders: A systematic review. *Journal of Affective Disorders, 150,* 707–719. doi:10.1016/j.jad.2013.05.042

Shen, J., & Oraka, E. (2012). Complementary and alternative medicine (CAM) use among children with current asthma. *Preventive Medicine, 54,* 27–31. doi:10.1016/j.ypmed.2011.10.007

Chapter 11

Emergency Preparedness and Poisonings

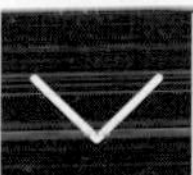

Learning Outcomes

After reading this chapter, the student should be able to:

1. Explain why drugs are important in the context of emergency preparedness.
2. Discuss the role of the nurse in preparing for and responding to worldwide epidemics and bioterrorist activity.
3. Identify the purpose and components of the Strategic National Stockpile (SNS).
4. Identify specific agents that would likely be used in a bioterrorist attack.
5. Explain the threat of anthrax contamination and how anthrax is transmitted.
6. Discuss the clinical manifestations and treatment of anthrax exposure.
7. Provide examples of treatments that might be applied during a bioterrorism incident.
8. Explain the advantages and disadvantages of vaccination as a means of preventing illness due to bioterrorist threats.
9. Describe the symptoms of acute radiation exposure and the role of potassium iodide (KI) in preventing thyroid cancer.
10. List top substances that represent human poison exposures.
11. Explain fundamental elements of toxicity treatment provided by the nurse.
12. Describe specific antidotes used to treat common overdosed substances and toxins.

It is important that the nurse understands the role drugs play in preventing and controlling the global spread of diseases and toxic outbreaks. Drugs are the most powerful tools the medical community has in order to counter large-scale biologic threats. If medical personnel were not able to identify, isolate, and treat the causes of diseases, a major incident might easily overwhelm health care resources and produce a catastrophic loss of life. In the case of bioterrorist threats, drugs are a major component of emergency preparedness planning. Drugs serve as antidotes to counteract the specific effects of a biologic, chemical, or nuclear attack. This chapter discusses the role of pharmacology in the prevention and treatment of diseases or conditions that might develop from pandemic events and bioterrorist activity. This chapter also covers how poisonings are generally managed in a clinical setting.

EMERGENCY PREPAREDNESS

11.1 The Nature of Worldwide Epidemics and Bioterrorist Threats

Prior to the September 11, 2001, terrorist attacks on the United States, the attention of health care providers mainly focused on the spread of traditional infectious diseases. Disease outbreaks included influenza, tuberculosis, cholera, and AIDS. Table 11.1 lists examples of deadly diseases that have occurred over the course of human history.

In 2009, HIV/AIDS, severe acute respiratory syndrome (SARS), and H1N1 avian influenza caused international alarm due to documented worldwide fatalities. Population growth, environmental disruption, and factors transcending time, place, and human progress were purported as reasons for emerging threats. In 2010, the Centers for Disease Control and Prevention (CDC) suggested a framework for intervention of these and other challenges. Strategies focused on impact levels of public health intervention including education and counseling, direct clinical care, long-term care, attention to select population groups, and emphasis on socioeconomic issues.

Later events would cause the CDC to redirect its efforts. An Ebola outbreak in West Africa was first reported in March 2014, and rapidly became an area of concern for citizens in the United States. Three important cases were initially discovered: one death from a man who had traveled to West Africa, and two locally-acquired cases where healthcare workers had cared for an Ebola patient in Dallas, Texas. After treatment, the health care workers recovered and were discharged from the hospital. Later a medical aid worker, who had volunteered in Guinea, would be diagnosed positive for Ebola and hospitalized in New York City. After a monitoring period, the patient recovered and was released from the hospital. Following these incidents, the CDC issued updated advice to state and local officials. When treating patients with infectious disease, public health officials reminded health care providers to use meticulous infection control procedures.They also recommended a 21-day monitoring period. "Standard, Contact,

Table 11.1 Deadly Diseases in Human History

Disease/Event	Cause	Target
Acquired immune deficiency syndrome (AIDS)	Human immunodeficiency virus (HIV)	Immune response
Bubonic plague	*Yersinia pestis,* flea and rodent vectors	Immune response and respiratory system
Cholera	*Vibrio cholerae*	Digestive tract
Dengue fever and yellow fever	Flavivirus	Entire body (fever)
Ebola	*Zaire ebolavirus* (filovirus)	Immune response and cardiovascular system
Hepatitis B	Hepatitis B virus (HBV)	Liver
Influenza (flu)	*Haemophilus influenza,* avian and swine vectors	Respiratory system
Leprosy	*Mycobacterium leprae*	Skin, nervous system, muscular system
Malaria	*Plasmodium falciparum,* female Anopheles mosquito vector	Blood disorder
Measles	Rubeola virus	Lungs and meninges
SARS (severe acute respiratory syndrome)	SARS coronavirus (SARS CoV)	Respiratory system
Smallpox	Variola virus	Skin, mucosa, lymphoid tissue
Syphilis	*Treponema pallidum*	Genitalia, mucous membranes, central nervous system
Tetanus (lockjaw)	Clostridium tetani	Entire body (infections)
Tuberculosis	Mycobacterium tuberculosis	Lungs
Whooping cough	*Bordetella pertussis*	Respiratory system

PharmFacts

POTENTIAL INFECTIOUS, BIOLOGIC, AND CHEMICAL THREATS

- In December 2014, there were 17,942 reported cases of Ebola virus disease (EVD) in five affected countries (Guinea, Liberia, Mali, Sierra Leone, and the United States of America) with 6,388 reported deaths.
- Ebola viruses are found in west and central Africa. Although the source of the viruses in nature remains unknown, monkeys (like humans) appear to be susceptible to infection and can serve as transmission sources or vectors of the virus.
- The Ebola virus causes death by hemorrhagic fever in up to 90% of the patients who show clinical symptoms of infection.
- Chemicals used in bioterrorist acts need not be sophisticated or difficult to obtain: Toxic industrial chemicals such as chlorine, phosgene, and hydrogen cyanide are used in commercial manufacturing and are readily available.
- Twenty-two confirmed or suspect cases of anthrax infection have resulted from *Bacillus anthracis* sent via the U.S. Postal Service. Eleven of these have been inhalational cases, of whom 5 have died; 11 have been cutaneous cases (see Table 11.3).
- Widespread public smallpox vaccinations ceased in the United States in 1972. Stockpiles of smallpox have been kept for research purposes in case of reinfection or biologic attack.
- It is estimated that 7 to 8 million doses of smallpox vaccine are in storage at the Centers for Disease Control and Prevention. This stock cannot be easily replenished, because all vaccine production facilities were dismantled after 1980, and now vaccine production requires 24 to 36 months.
- Most nerve agents were originally produced in a search for insecticides, but because of their toxicity, they were evaluated for military use.

and Droplet Precautions" were provided for U.S. hospital workers to follow. Eleven recommendations were given (CDC, 2014b).

Hospitals should make sure nurses and other health care workers:

- Maintain strict control and records of who comes into contact with the infected patient.
- Use personal protective equipment (PPE).
- Make sure hospital equipment is dedicated and cleaned.
- Limit the use of needles and other sharps.
- Limit or avoid aerosol generating procedures.
- Practice proper hand hygiene.
- Practice safe environmental infection control techniques.
- Adhere to safe injection practices.
- Take proper infection control precautions.
- Manage exposure to support staff at the hospital.
- Monitor, manage, and train visitors about the Ebola virus.

Pandemic events or diseases of epidemic proportion that spread across human populations are one threat. Unfortunately, terrorist attacks have prompted the health care community to expand its awareness of outbreaks and interventions to include bioterrorism and the deleterious effects of biologic and chemical weapons. **Bioterrorism** may be defined as the intentional use of infectious biologic agents, chemical substances, or radiation to cause widespread harm or illness. The public has become more aware of the threat of bioterrorism because federal agencies, such as the CDC and the U.S. Department of Defense, have stepped up efforts to inform, educate, and prepare the public for disease outbreaks of a less traditional nature.

The goals of a bioterrorist are to create widespread public panic and to cause as many casualties as possible. There is no shortage of agents that can be used for this purpose. Indeed, some of these agents are easily obtainable and require little or no specialized knowledge to disseminate. Areas of greatest concern include acutely infectious diseases such as anthrax, smallpox, plague, and hemorrhagic viruses; incapacitating chemicals such as nerve gas, cyanide, and chlorinated agents; and nuclear and radiation emergencies. The CDC has categorized the biologic threats, based on their potential impact on public health, as shown in Table 11.2.

11.2 Role of the Nurse in Emergency Preparedness

Emergency preparedness is not a new concept for the nurse and hospitals. For more than 30 years, The Joint Commission, formerly the Joint Commission on Accreditation of Healthcare Organizations (JCAHO), required accredited hospitals to develop disaster plans and to conduct periodic emergency drills to determine readiness. Prior to the late 1990s, disaster plans and training focused on natural disasters such as tornadoes, hurricanes, floods, or accidents such as explosions that could cause multiple casualties. In the late 1990s, The Joint Commission standards added the possibility of bioterrorism and virulent infectious organisms as rare, though possible, scenarios in disaster preparedness.

Roles in emergency preparedness often transfer based on current events. In 2001, The Joint Commission issued standards that shifted the focus from disaster preparedness to emergency management. The newer standards included more than just responding to the immediate casualties caused by a disaster; they also considered how an agency's health care delivery system might change during a crisis, and how it might return to normal operations following the incident. The expanded focus also included how the individual health care agency would coordinate its efforts with community resources, such as other hospitals and public health agencies. State and federal agencies revised their emergency preparedness guidelines in an attempt to plan more rationally for a range of disasters including possible bioterrorist acts.

Table 11.2 Categories of Infectious Agents

Category	Description	Examples
A	Agents that can easily be disseminated or transmitted person to person; cause high mortality, with potential for major public health impact; might cause public panic and social disruption; or require special action for public health preparedness	*Bacillus anthracis* (anthrax) *Clostridium botulinum* toxin (botulism) *Francisella tularensis* (tularemia) Variola major (smallpox) Viral hemorrhagic fevers such as Marburg and Ebola *Yersinia pestis* (plague)
B	Agents that are moderately easy to disseminate; cause moderate morbidity and low mortality; or require specific enhancements of the CDC's diagnostic capacity and enhanced disease surveillance	*Brucella* species (brucellosis) *Burkholderia mallei* (glanders) *Burkholderia pseudomallei* (melioidosis) *Chlamydia psittaci* (psittacosis) *Coxiella burnetii* (Q fever) Epsilon toxin of *Clostridium perfringens* Food safety threats such as *Salmonella* and *E. coli* Ricin toxin from *Ricinus communis* *Staphylococcus* enterotoxin B Viral encephalitis Water safety threats such as *Vibrio cholerae* and *Cryptosporidium parvum*
C	Emerging pathogens that could be engineered for mass dissemination because of their availability, ease of production and dissemination, and potential for high morbidity and mortality rates and major health impacts	Hantaviruses Multidrug-resistant tuberculosis Nipah virus (NiV) Tick-borne encephalitis viruses Yellow fever

Source: *Emergency Preparedness & Response: Bioterrorism Agents/Diseases*, Centers for Disease Control and Prevention, 2014. Retrieved from http://www.bt.cdc.gov/agent/agentlist-category.asp

Today, planning for bioterrorist acts requires close cooperation among all the different health care professionals. Nurses are central to the effort. Because a bioterrorist incident may occur in any community without warning, the nurse must be prepared to respond immediately. The following elements underscore the key roles of the nurse in meeting the challenges of a potential bioterrorist event:

- *Education.* The nurse should maintain a current knowledge and understanding of emergency management relating to bioterrorist activities. The nurse can assist the public by providing current and accurate information about potential or real threats to public health and correcting misinformation about these topics.
- *Resources.* The nurse should maintain a current listing of health and law enforcement contacts and resources in the local communities who would assist in the event of bioterrorist activity. When appropriate, the nurse may participate in local, hospital-related, or regional first-responder teams as a resource to the community.
- *Diagnosis and treatment.* The nurse should be aware of the early signs and symptoms of chemical and biologic agents and their immediate treatment and should report the findings to the appropriate authorities.
- *Planning.* The nurse should be involved in developing emergency management plans for families, assisting neighbors and the community to develop such plans, and participating through health care agencies in disaster preparedness drills.

11.3 Strategic National Stockpile

Should a chemical or biologic attack occur, it would likely be rapid and unexpected and would produce multiple casualties. Although planning for such an event is an important part of disaster preparedness, individual health care agencies and local communities could easily be caught unaware by such a crisis. Shortages of needed drugs, medical equipment, and supplies would be potential challenges.

The **Strategic National Stockpile (SNS)**, formerly called the National Pharmaceutical Stockpile, is a program designed to ensure the immediate deployment of essential medical materials to a community in the event of a large-scale chemical or biologic attack. Managed by the CDC, the stockpile consists of the following materials:

- Antibiotics
- Vaccines
- Medical, surgical, and patient support supplies such as bandages, airway supplies, and intravenous (IV) equipment

Community-Oriented Practice

CARING FOR THE LONG-TERM CARE AND SPECIAL-NEEDS POPULATIONS IN TIMES OF PUBLIC HEALTH EMERGENCIES

Residents living in long term care (LTC) facilities, as well as older adults and adults with special needs who are living in the community, comprise a population that is particularly vulnerable to a public health emergency, whether from bioterrorism or natural disasters. In the event of a mass casualty event, health care providers will need to be skilled in responding to the event and take into account the special health needs of these populations.

Similar to younger counterparts, community-dwelling older adults and those with special needs may be inclined to shelter-in-place and stay where they are. However, this population has unique needs that increase their vulnerability. Behr and Diaz (2013) cite the lack of transportation, cognitive impairment, physical limitations to mobility, and the increased presence of chronic conditions, as having an impact on the adult's ability to evacuate or be evacuated quickly. There are additional considerations that public health workers must consider in planning for disasters. Patients with dementia and those on life-support or life-sustaining equipment such as ventilators, tube-feedings, or special air mattresses, increase the challenge in preparing for, or executing an evacuation (Claver, Dobalian, Fickel, Ricci, & Mallers, 2013). Will the facility used to shelter these residents be secure for the adult with dementia? How will the ventilated patient be evacuated if the shelter is a considerable distance from the area at-risk? And if members of the community are preparing for their own safety, who is available to assist the most vulnerable?

After a disaster, additional health needs may arise. Needs that are not usually considered in disaster planning include an increased risk of deep vein thrombosis from dehydration, pneumonia from inhalation of substances released in the disaster, increased risk of pressure ulcers as special beds are not available or not working, and post-traumatic stress disorder (Aoyagi et al., 2013; Kun, Tong, Liu, Pei, & Luo, 2013; Sato & Ichioka, 2012).

In times of disaster, nurses will be a source of information and care for their communities. Participating in disaster preparedness programs, well in advance of any potential occurrence, will help ensure that a coordinated effort is available to the community and will include the most vulnerable populations in those efforts.

The SNS has two components. The first is called a *push package*, which consists of a preassembled set of supplies and pharmaceuticals designed to provide a response to an unknown biologic or chemical threat. There are eight fully stocked 50-ton push packages stored in climate-controlled warehouses throughout the United States. They are in locations where they can reach any community in the United States within 12 hours after an attack. The decision to deploy the push package is based on an assessment of the situation by federal government officials.

The second SNS component consists of a **vendor-managed inventory (VMI)** package. VMI packages are shipped, if necessary, after the chemical or biologic threat has more clearly been identified. The materials consist of supplies and pharmaceuticals more specific to the chemical or biologic agent used in the attack. VMI packages are designed to arrive within 24 to 36 hours.

The stockpiling of antibiotics and vaccines by local hospitals, clinics, or individuals for the purpose of preparing for a bioterrorist act is not recommended. Pharmaceuticals have a finite expiration date, and keeping large stores of drugs can be costly. Furthermore, stockpiling could cause drug shortages and prevent the delivery of these pharmaceuticals to communities where they may be needed most.

AGENTS USED IN BIOTERRORISM ACTS

Bioterrorists could potentially use any biologic, chemical, or physical agent to cause widespread panic and serious illness. Knowing which agents are most likely to be used in an incident helps the nurse plan and implement emergency preparedness policies.

11.4 Anthrax

One of the first threats following the terrorist attacks on the World Trade Center in 2001, was **anthrax.** Anthrax is caused by the bacterium *Bacillus anthracis*, which normally affects domestic and wild animals. A wide variety of hoofed animals are affected by the disease, including cattle, sheep, goats, horses, donkeys, pigs, American bison, antelopes, and elephants. If transmitted to humans by exposure to an open wound, through contaminated food, or by inhalation, *B. anthracis* can cause serious damage to body tissues. Symptoms of anthrax infection usually appear 1 to 6 days after exposure. Depending on how the bacterium is transmitted, specific types of anthrax "poisoning" may be observed, each characterized by hallmark symptoms. Clinical manifestations of anthrax are summarized in Table 11.3.

B. anthracis causes disease by the emission of two types of toxins, *edema toxin* and *lethal toxin*. These toxins cause necrosis and accumulation of exudate, which produces pain, swelling, and restriction of activity, the general symptoms associated with almost every form of anthrax. Another component, the *anthrax binding receptor*, allows the bacterium to bind to human cells and act as a "doorway" for both types of toxins to enter.

Further ensuring its chance for spreading, *B. anthracis* is spore forming. Anthrax spores can remain viable in soil for hundreds, and perhaps thousands, of years. Anthrax spores are resistant to drying, heat, and some harsh chemicals. These spores are the main cause for public health concern because they are responsible for producing inhalation anthrax, the most dangerous form of the disease. After entry into the lungs, *B. anthracis* spores are ingested by macrophages and carried to lymphoid tissue, resulting in tissue necrosis, swelling, and hemorrhage. One of the main

Table 11.3 Clinical Manifestations of Anthrax

Type	Description	Symptoms
Cutaneous anthrax	Most common but least complicated form of anthrax; almost always curable if treated within the first few weeks of exposure; results from direct contact of contaminated products with an open wound or cut	Small skin lesions develop and turn into black scabs; inoculation takes less than 1 week; cannot be spread by person-to-person contact
Gastrointestinal anthrax	Rare form of anthrax; without treatment, can be lethal in up to 50% of cases; results from eating anthrax-contaminated food, usually meat	Sore throat, difficulty swallowing, cramping diarrhea, and abdominal swelling
Inhalation anthrax	Least common but the most dangerous form of anthrax; can be successfully treated if identified within the first few days after exposure; results from inhaling anthrax spores	Initially, fatigue and fever for several days, followed by persistent cough and shortness of breath; without treatment, death can result within 4–6 days

body areas affected is the mediastinum, which is a potential site for tissue injury and fluid accumulation. Meningitis is also a common pathology. If treatment is delayed, inhalation anthrax is lethal in almost every case.

B. anthracis is found in contaminated animal products such as wool, hair, dander, and bonemeal, but it can also be packaged in other forms, making it transmissible through the air or by direct contact. Terrorists have delivered it in the form of a fine powder, making it less obvious to detect. The powder can be inconspicuously spread on virtually any surface, making it a serious concern for public safety.

The antibiotic ciprofloxacin (Cipro) has traditionally been used for anthrax prophylaxis and treatment. For prophylaxis, the usual dosage is 500 mg PO (by mouth), every 12 hours for 60 days. If exposure has been confirmed, ciprofloxacin should immediately be administered at a usual dose of 400 mg IV (intravenously) every 12 hours. Other antibiotics are also effective against anthrax, including penicillin, vancomycin, ampicillin, erythromycin, tetracycline, and doxycycline. In the case of inhalation anthrax, the U.S. Food and Drug Administration (FDA) has approved the use of ciprofloxacin and doxycycline in combination for treatment.

Should an anthrax threat re-emerge, some concerned members of the public may ask their health care provider to provide them with ciprofloxacin. The public should be discouraged from seeking the prophylactic use of antibiotics in cases where anthrax exposure has not been confirmed. Indiscriminate, unnecessary use of antibiotics can be expensive, can cause significant side effects, and can promote the development of resistant bacterial strains. The student should refer to chapter 35 to review the precautions and guidelines regarding the appropriate use of antibiotics.

Although anthrax immunization (vaccination) has been licensed by the FDA for about 40 years, it has not been widely used because of the extremely low incidence of this disease in the United States. The **vaccine** is prepared from proteins from the anthrax bacteria, dubbed "protective antigens." Anthrax vaccine works the same way as other vaccines: by causing the body to make protective antibodies and thus preventing the onset of disease and symptoms. Immunization for anthrax consists of three subcutaneous injections given 2 weeks apart, followed by three additional subcutaneous injections given at 6, 12, and 18 months. Annual booster injections of the vaccine are recommended. The CDC recommends vaccination for only select populations: laboratory personnel who work with anthrax, military personnel deployed to high-risk areas, and those who deal with animal products imported from areas with a high incidence of the disease. Vaccines and the immune response are discussed in more detail in chapter 34.

11.5 Viruses

In 2002, the public was astounded as researchers announced that they had "built" a poliovirus, a threat U.S. health officials thought had essentially been eradicated in 1994. Although virtually eliminated in the Western Hemisphere, polio was reported in at least 27 countries as late as 1998. The infection persists among infants and children in areas with contaminated drinking water or food, mainly in underdeveloped regions of India, Pakistan, Afghanistan, western and central Africa, and the Dominican Republic. In the United States, polio remains a potential threat in 1 of 300,000 to 500,000 patients who were vaccinated with the oral poliovirus vaccine.

A bioterrorist could culture the poliovirus and release it into regions where people have not been vaccinated. An even more dangerous threat is that a mutated strain, for which there was no effective vaccine, might be developed. Because the genetic code of the poliovirus is small, it can be manufactured in a relatively simple laboratory. Once the virus is isolated, hundreds of different mutant strains can be produced in a very short time.

In 2014, due to the threat of viral contamination, national security experts and researchers asked, "What about Ebola?" The concern is that bioterrorists have easy access to the Ebola virus, and there are multiple ways to spread an infection. Many believe that U.S. hospitals and agencies are also woefully unprepared for an Ebola attack.

Ebola has a 21-day incubation period, enough time for terrorists to infect themselves and then enter the United States with the virus. Terrorists could also collect samples of infected body fluids, and place them in strategic places, allowing Ebola to spread quietly before officials even realize a biological attack has taken place. As of 2014, there were no proven vaccines for Ebola, although there were efforts to ramp up production of promising experimental treatments. Today, there is no stockpile of Ebola vaccine. Many believe however, that even if experimental treatments are proven effective, they will not be able to address an outbreak quickly enough. The following are examples of possible responses to an Ebola outbreak:

- Brincidofovir was given to one of the first patients infected with Ebola in the U.S. without success. Consenting patients have been monitored around the world by various research teams.
- Favipiravir was approved in Japan for treatment of the influenza virus and was tested with Ebola patients in Gueckedou, Guinea.
- ZMapp attracted attention during the 2014 outbreak. Two U.S. aid workers recovered after taking ZMapp, but others patients in Europe and Africa died. This treatment is a mixture of three synthetic antibodies to the Ebola virus.
- TKM-Ebola was used after ZMapp was exhausted during the 2014 Ebola incidents. This antiviral drug is undergoing FDA phase one clinical trials in the United States.
- Convalescent serum contains Ebola-fighting antibodies that might be given in response to an infected patient who has survived an Ebola incident.
- AVI-7537 is an experimental ebola antiviral drug developed by the Sarepta drug company under acontract with the U.S. Department of Defense.The antiviral works by targeting the protein responsible for replicating the Ebola virus in the host.
- BCX4430, an antiviral drug from Biocryst Pharmaceuticals, could be used to treat different kinds of hemorrhagic fever including Ebola. The drug attempts to halt the virus by targeting a key enzyme in the virus.

In addition to polio and Ebola, smallpox is considered a potential threat. Once thought to have been eradicated from the planet in the 1970s, the variola virus that causes this disease has been harbored in research laboratories in several countries. Much of its genetic code has been sequenced and is public information. The disease is spread from person to person as an aerosol, bydroplets, or by contact with contaminated objects such as clothing or bedding. Only a few viral particles are needed to cause infection. If the virus is released into an unvaccinated population, as many as one in three people could die.

There are a few effective therapies for treating patients infected by viruses that could be used in a bioterrorist attack. Complications involve rare but serious problems, for example, postvaccinal encephalitis. In the case of smallpox, a stockpile of vaccines exists in enough quantity to administer to every person in the United States. The variola vaccine provides a high level of protection if given prior to exposure, or up to 3 days after exposure. Protection may last from 3 to 5 years. The following are general contraindications to receiving the smallpox vaccine, unless the individual has confirmed face-to-face contact with an infected patient:

- Persons with active (or a history of) atopic dermatitis or eczema
- Persons with acute, active, or exfoliative skin conditions
- Persons with altered immune states (e.g., HIV, AIDS, leukemia, lymphoma, immunosuppressive drugs)
- Pregnant and breast-feeding women
- Children younger than 1 year
- Persons who have a serious allergy to any component of the vaccine.

It has been suggested that multiple vaccines be created, mass produced, and stockpiled to meet the overall challenges of a terrorist attack. Another suggestion has called for mass vaccination of the public, or at least those health care providers and law enforcement employees who might be exposed to infected patients.

Vaccines have side effects, some of which are quite serious. In the case of smallpox vaccination, for example, it is estimated that there might be as many as 250 deaths for every million people inoculated. If the smallpox vaccine was given to every person in the United States (approximately 300 million), possible deaths from vaccination could exceed 75,000. In addition, terrorists having some knowledge of genetic structure could create a modified strain of the virus that renders existing vaccines totally ineffective. It appears, then, that mass vaccination is not an appropriate solution until research can produce safer and more effective vaccines.

11.6 Toxic Chemicals

Although chemical warfare agents have been available since World War I, medicine has produced few drug antidotes. Many treatments provide minimal help other than to relieve some symptoms and provide comfort following exposure. Most chemical agents used in warfare were created to cause mass casualties; others were designed to cause so much discomfort that soldiers would be too weak to continue fighting. Potential chemicals that could be used in a terrorist act include nerve gases, blood agents, choking and vomiting agents, and those that cause severe blistering. Table 11.4 provides a summary of selected chemical agents and known antidotes for chemical warfare and first-aid treatments.

The chemical category of main pharmacologic significance is **nerve agents.** Exposure to these acutely toxic chemicals can cause convulsions and loss of consciousness within seconds and respiratory failure within minutes. Almost all

12.5 Classification and Naming of Drugs Affecting the Parasympathetic Nervous System

Actions of drugs affecting the parasympathetic nervous system are classified based on two possible actions.

1. *Stimulation of the parasympathetic nervous system.* These drugs are called cholinergic or **parasympathomimetics,** and they produce the characteristic symptoms of the rest-and-digest response.
2. *Inhibition of the parasympathetic nervous system.* These drugs are called cholinergic-blocking drugs or **anticholinergics.** Less used terms are parasympatholytics and muscarinic blockers. These drugs produce actions *opposite* those of the cholinergic drugs.

Students beginning their study of pharmacology often have difficulty understanding the terminology and actions of autonomic drugs. Examination of drug classes, however, makes it evident that one group needs to be learned well, because the others are logical extensions of the first. If the rest-and-digest actions of the parasympathomimetics are learned, other groups of autonomic drugs can be deduced. For example, both the cholinergic drugs and the adrenergic-blocking drugs (chapter 13) reduce heart rate and constrict the pupils. The other group, the cholinergic-blocking drugs and the adrenergic drugs, have the opposite effects—elevating heart rate and dilating the pupils. Although this is an oversimplification and exceptions do exist, it is a time-saving means of learning the basic actions and adverse effects of dozens of drugs affecting the ANS.

CHOLINERGIC DRUGS

Parasympathomimetics are drugs that mimic action of the parasympathetic nervous system. These cholinergic drugs induce the rest-and-digest response.

12.6 Clinical Applications of Cholinergic Drugs

The classic parasympathomimetic is Ach, the endogenous neurotransmitter at cholinergic synapses in the ANS. Ach, however, has almost no therapeutic use because it is rapidly destroyed after administration. Recall that Ach is the neurotransmitter at the ganglia in both the parasympathetic and sympathetic divisions, at the neuroeffector junctions in the parasympathetic nervous system, as well as in skeletal muscle. Thus, it is not surprising that administration of Ach or drugs that mimic Ach will have widespread and varied effects within the body.

Parasympathomimetics are divided into two subclasses, direct acting and indirect acting, based on their mechanism of action (Table 12.1). Direct-acting agents, such as bethanechol (Urecholine), bind to cholinergic receptors to produce the rest-and-digest response. Because direct-acting parasympathomimetics are relatively resistant to the destructive effects of the enzyme AchE, they have a longer duration of action than the natural neurotransmitter Ach. Cholinergic drugs are poorly absorbed across the gastrointestinal (GI) tract and generally do not cross the blood–brain barrier. They have little effect on Ach receptors in the ganglia. Because they are moderately selective to muscarinic receptors when used at therapeutic doses, direct-acting parasympathomimetics are also described as *muscarinic agonists*.

Table 12.1 Cholinergic Drugs

Type	Drug	Primary Uses
Direct acting (muscarinic receptor agonists)	bethanechol (Urecholine)	Stimulate urination Treatment of dry mouth
	cevimeline (Evoxac)	Glaucoma, treatment of dry mouth
	pilocarpine (Isopto Carpine, Salagen)	
Cholinesterase inhibitors (indirect inhibitors of AchE enzyme)	donepezil (Aricept)	Alzheimer's disease
	edrophonium (Tensilon)	Diagnosis of myasthenia gravis
	galantamine (Razadyne)	Alzheimer's disease
	neostigmine (Prostigmin)	Myasthenia gravis, postoperative urinary retention
	physostigmine (Antilirium)	Treatment of severe anticholinergic toxicity
	pyridostigmine (Mestinon, Regonol)	Myasthenia gravis
	rivastigmine (Exelon)	Alzheimer's disease

The indirect-acting parasympathomimetics, such as neostigmine (Prostigmin), inhibit the action of AchE. This inhibition allows endogenous Ach to avoid rapid destruction and bind with cholinergic receptors for a longer time, thus prolonging its action. These drugs are called *cholinesterase inhibitors*. Unlike the direct-acting agents, the cholinesterase inhibitors are nonselective and affect all Ach sites: autonomic ganglia, muscarinic receptors, skeletal muscle, and Ach sites in the CNS.

One of the first drugs discovered in this class, physostigmine (Antilirium), was obtained from the dried ripe seeds of *Physostigma venenosum*, a plant found in West Africa. The bean of this plant was used in tribal rituals. As research continued under secrecy during World War II, similar compounds were synthesized that produced potent neurologic effects that could be used during chemical warfare. This class of agents now includes organophosphate insecticides, such as malathion and parathion, and toxic nerve gases such as Sarin. The nurse who works in an agricultural area may become quite familiar with the symptoms of acute poisoning with organophosphates. Poisoning results in intense stimulation of the parasympathetic nervous system, which may result in death, if untreated.

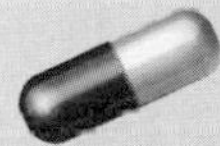

Prototype Drug | Bethanechol *(Urecholine)*

Therapeutic Class: Nonobstructive urinary retention drug **Pharmacologic Class:** Muscarinic cholinergic receptor drug

Actions and Uses

Bethanechol is a direct-acting parasympathomimetic that interacts with muscarinic receptors to cause actions typical of parasympathetic stimulation. Its effects are most noted in the digestive and urinary tracts, where it stimulates smooth-muscle contraction. These actions are useful in increasing smooth muscle tone and muscular contractions in the GI tract following general anesthesia. In addition, it is used to treat nonobstructive urinary retention in patients with atony (lack of muscle tone) of the bladder. Although poorly absorbed from the GI tract, it may be administered orally or by subcutaneous injection.

Administration Alerts

- Never administer IM or IV.
- Oral and subcutaneous doses are *not* interchangeable.
- Monitor blood pressure, pulse, and respirations before administration and for at least 1 hour after subcutaneous administration.
- Pregnancy category C.

PHARMACOKINETICS

Onset	Peak	Duration
30–90 min PO; 5–15 min subcutaneous	60 min PO; 15–30 min subcutaneous	6 h PO; 120 min subcutaneous

Adverse Effects

The side effects of bethanechol are predicted from its parasympathetic actions. It should be used with extreme caution in patients with disorders that could be aggravated by increased contractions of the digestive tract, such as suspected obstruction, active ulcer, or inflammatory disease. The same caution should be exercised in patients with suspected urinary obstruction or COPD. Side effects include increased salivation, sweating, abdominal cramping, and hypotension that could lead to fainting.

Contraindications: Patients with asthma, epilepsy, parkinsonism, hyperthyroidism, peptic ulcer disease, or bradycardia should not use this drug. Safety in pregnancy and lactation and in children younger than 8 years is not established.

Interactions

Drug–Drug: Drug interactions with bethanechol include increased cholinergic effects from cholinesterase inhibitors and decreased cholinergic effects from procainamide, quinidine, atropine, and epinephrine.

Lab Tests: Bethanechol may cause an increase in serum aspartate aminotransferase (AST), amylase, and lipase.

Herbal/Food: Cholinergic effects caused by bethanechol may be antagonized by angel's trumpet, jimson weed, or scopalia.

Treatment of Overdose: Atropine sulfate is a specific antidote. Subcutaneous injection of atropine is preferred except in emergencies when the IV route may be used.

Because of their high potential for serious adverse effects, few parasympathomimetics are widely used in pharmacotherapy. Some have clinical applications in ophthalmology, because they reduce intraocular pressure in patients with glaucoma (see chapter 50). Others are used for their stimulatory effects on the smooth muscle of the bowel or urinary tract.

Several drugs in this class are used for their effects on Ach receptors in skeletal muscle or in the CNS, rather than for their parasympathetic action. **Myasthenia gravis** is a disease characterized by destruction of nicotinic receptors in skeletal muscles. Administration of pyridostigmine (Mestinon, Regonol) or neostigmine (Prostigmin) stimulates skeletal muscle contraction and helps reverse the severe muscle weakness characteristic of this disease. In addition, donepezil (Aricept) is often useful in treating Alzheimer's disease because of its ability to increase the amount of Ach binding to receptors located within the CNS (see chapter 20).

When given too much cholinergic medication, patients sometimes develop **cholinergic crisis**, signs which include hypersalivation, small pupils, muscle twitching, unusual paleness, sweating, muscle weakness, and difficulty breathing. It can be extremely difficult to distinguish between worsening symptoms of myasthenia gravis or excessive anticholinergic medication when a patient with known myasthenia gravis presents with rapidly increasing muscular weakness, with or without respiratory difficulty. Intravenous administration of the reversible cholinesterase inhibitor, edrophonium as a test dose will often improve muscular weakness with myasthenic crisis whereas muscular symptoms will be aggravated with cholinergic medication overdose. Once diagnosed, a cholinergic crisis is immediately treated with atropine, which will reverse most symptoms.

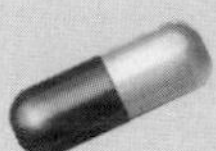

Prototype Drug | Physostigmine *(Antilirium)*

Therapeutic Class: Antidote for anticholinergic toxicity **Pharmacologic Class:** Acetylcholinesterase inhibitor

Actions and Uses

Physostigmine is an indirect-acting parasympathomimetic that inhibits the destruction of Ach by AchE. Its effects occur at the neuromuscular junction and at central and peripheral locations where Ach is the neurotransmitter. It reverses toxic and life-threatening delirium caused by atropine, diphenhydramine, dimenhydrinate, *Atropa belladonna* (deadly nightshade), or jimson weed. Physostigmine is usually administered as an injectable solution, IM or IV, although it is not intended as a first-line agent for anticholinergic toxicity or Parkinson's disease.

Administration Alerts

- Administer slowly over 5 minutes to avoid seizures and respiratory distress.
- Continuous infusions should never be used.
- Monitor blood pressure, pulse, and respirations, and look for hypersalivation.
- Pregnancy category C.

PHARMACOKINETICS

Onset	Peak	Duration
Less than 5 min IM/IV	20–40 min IM/IV	1–2 h IM/IV

Adverse Effects

Unfavorable effects of physostigmine are bradycardia, asystole, restlessness, nervousness, seizures, salivation, urinary frequency, muscle twitching, and respiratory paralysis.

Contraindications: Use with caution in patients with asthma, epilepsy, diabetes, cardiovascular disease, or bradycardia. Discontinue if excessive sweating, diarrhea, or frequent urination occurs. Physostigmine is not recommended in patients with known or suspected tricyclic antidepressant (TCA) intoxication.

Interactions

Drug–Drug: Drug interactions with physostigmine include increased effects from cholinergic agents and beta blockers. The levels of physostigmine may be increased by systemic corticosteroids. Physostigmine may decrease effects of neuromuscular-blocking agents.

Lab Tests: Physostigmine may cause an increase in serum alanine aminotransferase (ALT), AST, and amylase.

Herbal/Food: Toxic effects caused by physostigmine may be enhanced by ginkgo biloba.

Treatment of Overdose: Due to the possibility of hypersensitivity or cholinergic crisis, atropine should be available.

CHOLINERGIC-BLOCKING DRUGS (ANTICHOLINERGICS)

Cholinergic-blocking agents are drugs that inhibit parasympathetic impulses. Suppressing the parasympathetic division induces symptoms of the fight-or-flight response.

12.7 Clinical Applications of Anticholinergics

Drugs that block the action of Ach are known by various names, including anticholinergics, cholinergic blockers, muscarinic antagonists, and parasympatholytics. Although the term *anticholinergic* is most commonly used, the most accurate term for this class of drugs is *muscarinic antagonists*, because at therapeutic doses, these drugs are selective for Ach muscarinic receptors and thus have little effect on Ach nicotinic receptors.

Anticholinergics act by competing with Ach for binding with muscarinic receptors (Table 12.2). When anticholinergics occupy these receptors, cholinergic responses are blocked at the effector organs. Suppressing the effects of Ach causes sympathetic nervous system actions to predominate. Most therapeutic uses of anticholinergics are predictable extensions of their parasympathetic-blocking effects: dilation of the pupils (mydriasis), increase in heart rate, drying of glandular secretions, and relaxation of the bronchi (asthma treatment). Note that these are also effects of sympathetic activation (fight-or-flight response).

Historically, anticholinergics have been widely used for many different disorders. References to these agents, which are extracted from the deadly nightshade plant, *Atropa belladonna,* date to the ancient Hindus, the Roman Empire, and the Middle Ages. Because of the plant's extreme toxicity, extracts of belladonna were sometimes used for intentional poisoning, including suicide, as well as in religious and beautification rituals. The name *belladonna* is Latin for "pretty woman." Roman women applied extracts of belladonna to the face to create the preferred female attributes of the time—pink cheeks and dilated, doe-like eyes.

Therapeutic uses of anticholinergics include the following:

Table 12.2 Cholinergic-Blocking Drugs (Anticholinergics)

Drug	Primary Use
aclidinium (Tudorza Pressair)	Chronic obstructive pulmonary disease (COPD)
atropine (AtroPen)	Poisoning with anticholinesterase agents, to increase heart rate, dilate pupils
benztropine (Cogentin)	Parkinson's disease, neuroleptic side effects
cyclopentolate (Cyclogyl)	To dilate pupils
darifenacin (Enablex)	Overactive bladder
dicyclomine (Bentyl)	Irritable bowel syndrome
donepezil (Aricept)	Alzheimer's disease
fesoterodine (Toviaz)	To prevent urgent, frequent, or uncontrolled urination
glycopyrrolate (Cuvposa, Robinul)	To produce a dry field prior to anesthesia, reduce salivation, peptic ulcers
ipratropium (Atrovent) (see page 663 for the Prototype Drug box)	Asthma and COPD
methscopolamine (Pamine)	peptic ulcers
oxybutynin (Ditropan, Oxytrol)	Incontinence
propantheline (Pro-Banthine)	Irritable bowel syndrome, peptic ulcer
scopolamine (Transderm-Scop)	Motion sickness, irritable bowel syndrome, adjunct to anesthesia
solifenacin (Vesicare)	Overactive bladder
tiotropium (Spiriva)	Asthma and COPD
tolterodine (Detrol)	Overactive bladder with symptoms of urge urinary incontinence, urgency, and frequency
trihexyphenidyl	Parkinson's disease
tropicamide (Mydiracyl, Tropicacyl)	Mydriasis and cycloplegia for diagnostic procedures
trospium (Sanctura)	Overactive bladder

- *GI disorders.* These agents decrease the secretion of gastric acid in peptic ulcer disease (see chapter 41). They also slow intestinal motility and may be useful for reducing the cramping and diarrhea associated with irritable bowel syndrome (see chapter 42).
- *Ophthalmic procedures.* Anticholinergics may be used to cause mydriasis or cycloplegia during eye procedures (see chapter 50).
- *Cardiac rhythm abnormalities.* Anticholinergics can be used to accelerate the heart rate in patients experiencing bradycardia (see chapter 30).
- *Anesthesia adjuncts.* When combined with other agents, anticholinergics can decrease excessive respiratory secretions and reverse the bradycardia caused by general anesthetics (see chapter 19).
- *Asthma and COPD.* Several medications, such as ipratropium (Atrovent), are useful in treating asthma and brochospasms associated with chronic bronchitis and emphysema, because of their ability to dilate the bronchi (see chapter 40).
- *Overactive bladder.* Anticholinergics such as oxybutynin (Ditropan, Oxytrol) treat overactive bladder, a condition in which the patient experiences a sudden urge to urinate, resulting in an involuntary loss of urine (incontinence).
- *Parkinson's disease.* Anticholinergics such as benztropine (Cogentin) are used to treat patients who have Parkinson's disease and whose main symptom is tremor (see chapter 20).

Check Your Understanding:

What are the symptoms of a cholinergic crisis and what are the drugs of choice for reversing this condition? *Visit www.pearsonhighered.com/nursingresources for answers.*

Nursing Practice Application

Pharmacotherapy With Cholinergic Drugs

ASSESSMENT	POTENTIAL NURSING DIAGNOSES*
Baseline assessment prior to administration: • Obtain a complete health history including cardiovascular, cerebrovascular, respiratory, musculoskeletal or thyroid diseases, GI or genitourinary obstruction, or diabetes. Obtain a drug history including allergies, current prescription and OTC drugs, and herbal preparations. Be alert to possible drug interactions. • Evaluate appropriate laboratory findings such as hepatic or renal function studies. • Obtain baseline vital signs, bowel sounds, urinary output, muscle strength, and mental status as appropriate. Assess the patient's ability to swallow. • Assess the patient's ability to receive and understand instruction. Include the family and caregivers as needed.	• *Ineffective Airway Clearance* • *Impaired Physical Mobility* • *Urinary Retention or Impaired Urinary Elimination* • *Deficient Knowledge (drug therapy)* • *Risk for Injury,* related to adverse effects of drug therapy *NANDA I © 2014

continued

Nursing Practice Application *continued*

ASSESSMENT	POTENTIAL NURSING DIAGNOSES*
Assessment throughout administration: • Assess for desired therapeutic effects dependent on the reason for the drug (e.g., increased ease of urination, muscle strength and coordination improved, lessened ptosis, improved swallowing). • Continue frequent and careful monitoring of vital signs, mental status, bowel sounds, urinary output, and musculoskeletal function, including swallowing ability, as appropriate. • Assess for and promptly report adverse effects: bradycardia, hypotension, dysrhythmias, tremors, dizziness, headache, dyspnea, decreased urinary output, abdominal pain, or changes in mental status.	

IMPLEMENTATION

Interventions and (Rationales)	Patient-Centered Care
Ensuring therapeutic effects: • Continue frequent assessments as described earlier for therapeutic effects dependent on the reason the drug therapy is given. (Ability to carry out activities of daily living [ADLs] has improved; urinary elimination and output is improved; musculoskeletal weakness, ptosis, diplopia, and chewing and swallowing are improved. For patients with myasthenia gravis, a larger percentage of the dose may be needed at times of greater fatigue such as late afternoon and at mealtimes or during periods of increased stress. A decrease in dosage during remission may be needed.)	• Encourage the patient, family, or caregiver to practice supportive measures along with drug therapy to maximize therapeutic effects (e.g., adequate rest periods in myasthenia gravis). • **Safety:** Instruct the patient not to self-regulate the dosage to avoid overdosage or underdosage. If periods of weakness occur, the provider will adjust the dosage after determining the cause (e.g., under- vs. overdosage).
• Continue monitoring musculoskeletal strength, improvement in ptosis or diplopia, and improved chewing and swallowing. (Improvement demonstrates that therapeutic effects have been achieved.)	• Teach the patient, family, or caregiver the importance of keeping a "symptom diary," noting even subtle changes, and the timing of doses taken.
• Continue frequent monitoring of bowel sounds and urine output if drugs are given postoperatively or postpartum. (Assessments will detect early signs of adverse effects as well as therapeutic action. Drug onset is in approximately 60 min with increased urination and peristalsis following. Drugs are not given if a mechanical obstruction is known or suspected. **Lifespan:** Be aware that the older adult male with an enlarged prostate is at higher-risk for mechanical obstruction.)	• **Safety:** Instruct the patient to have bathroom facilities nearby after taking the drug. The patient may need assistance to the toilet or commode if dizziness occurs.
• Provide supportive nursing measures; e.g., regular toileting schedule, safety measures. (Nursing measures such as assisting the patient to normal voiding position will supplement therapeutic drug effects and optimize outcomes. **Lifespan & Safety:** A home assessment is especially important for the older adult. The presence of throw rugs and other hazards that obstruct mobility increase the risk for falls.)	• Assess ability of the patient, family, or caregiver to perform ADLs at home, and explore the need for additional health care referrals. Evaluate home safety needs.
• Schedule activities and allow for adequate periods of rest to avoid fatigue. (Excess fatigue can lead to either a cholinergic or a myasthenic crisis in patients with myasthenial gravis.)	• Instruct the patient to plan activities according to muscle strength and fatigue and to allow for frequent and adequate rest periods. • Instruct the patient to report extreme fatigue immediately.
Minimizing adverse effects: • Monitor for signs of excessive ANS stimulation and notify the health care provider if the pulse is less than 60 beats/min or blood pressure (BP) is below established parameters. (Cholinergic drugs decrease the heart rate and BP. Atropine may be ordered to counteract drug effects.)	• Instruct the patient to promptly report tremors, palpitations, changes in BP, dizziness, urinary retention, abdominal pain, or changes in behavior (e.g., confusion, depression, drowsiness). • Instruct the patient to immediately report dyspnea, salivation, sweating, or extreme fatigue, because these are signs of a potential overdose.
• Help the patient to rise from lying or sitting to standing until drug effects are assessed. (Direct-acting cholinergic drugs may cause significant orthostatic hypotension. **Lifespan:** Be aware that dizziness may increase the risk of falls in the older adult.)	• **Safety:** Instruct the patient to rise from lying or sitting to standing slowly, and to avoid prolonged standing in one place to avoid dizziness or falls. If dizziness occurs, the patient should sit or lie down and not attempt to stand or walk, until the sensation passes.

Nursing Practice Application *continued*

IMPLEMENTATION	
Interventions and (Rationales)	**Patient-Centered Care**
• Report periods of muscle weakness and association to dosage time to the provider promptly. (Muscle weakness occurring within 1 h of dose may indicate overdosage or cholinergic crisis. Weakness occurring 3 h or longer after dose may indicate underdosage, drug resistance, or myasthenic crisis.) • **Lifespan:** Assess for subtle changes in muscle strength, voice quality, or slurred speech in the older adult. (Subtle changes that occur during the day, especially if timed around drug peaks or troughs, may indicate underdosage rather than age-related changes.)	• Instruct the patient to report any severe muscle weakness that occurs 1 h or 3 or more h after taking the medication. • Instruct the patient, family, or caregiver to record variations in muscle strength, particularly periods of weakness, and associated dose times to assist the provider in appropriate dosage. • Teach the patient, family, or caregiver to notify the health care provider if shortness of breath, extreme fatigue, or difficulty with chewing or swallowing occurs or is worsening.
• Continue to monitor hepatic function laboratory work. (Cholinergic drugs may cause liver toxicity, and liver enzymes may be monitored weekly for up to 6 weeks.)	• Teach the patient, family, or caregiver about the importance of returning for follow-up laboratory studies.
• Provide for eye comfort such as an adequately lighted room and appropriate safety measures. (Cholinergic drugs can cause miosis with difficulty seeing in low light conditions and blurred vision.)	• **Safety:** Caution the patient about driving in low-light conditions, at night, or if vision is blurred. Nightlight use at home and safety measures may be needed to prevent falls.
• Carefully calculate and monitor doses. (Careful calculation will avoid overdosage.)	• Ensure that the patient, family, or caregiver is administering the correct dose by observing teach-back.
Patient understanding of drug therapy: • Use opportunities during administration of medications and during assessments to provide patient education. (Using time during nursing care helps to optimize and reinforce key teaching areas.)	• The patient, family, or caregiver should be able to state the reason for the drug; appropriate dose and scheduling; what adverse effects to observe for and when to report; equipment needed as appropriate and how to use that equipment; and the required length of medication therapy needed with any special instructions regarding renewing or continuing prescription as appropriate. • A medic-alert bracelet or other device describing the disease and the medications used should be worn.
Patient self-administration of drug therapy: • When administering the medications, instruct the patient, family, or caregiver in the proper self-administration of drugs and ophthalmic drops. (Using time during nurse administration of these drugs helps to reinforce teaching.) • Follow appropriate administration techniques for ophthalmic doses. • Sustained release tablets should not be crushed or chewed. Check drug reference material on administration with or without food. Administer the drug with food, milk, or small snack unless contraindicated. Sustained released tablets must be swallowed whole and a change of dosage form may be needed if dysphagia is present.)	• Instruct the patient in proper administration techniques, followed by teach-back. • The patient, family, or caregiver is able to discuss appropriate dosing and administration needs. • Have the patient report any difficulty in swallowing if sustained release tablets are used.

Treating the Diverse Patient: Impact of Anticholinergics on Male Sexual Function

A functioning ANS is essential for normal male sexual health. The parasympathetic nervous system is necessary for erections, whereas the sympathetic division is responsible for the process of ejaculation. Anticholinergic drugs block transmission of parasympathetic impulses and may interfere with normal erections. Adrenergic antagonists can interfere with the smooth-muscle contractions in the seminal vesicles and penis, resulting in an inability to ejaculate.

For male patients receiving autonomic medications, the nurse should include questions about sexual activity during the assessment process. For patients who are not sexually active, these side effects may be unimportant. For patients who are sexually active, however, drug-induced sexual dysfunction may be a major cause of nonadherence. The patient should be informed to expect such side effects and to promptly report them to the health care provider. In most cases, alternative medications may be available that do not affect sexual function, or a change in the scheduling of the dose may help to alleviate the problem.

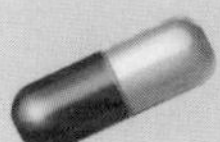

Prototype Drug | Atropine *(Atro-Pen)*

Therapeutic Class: Antidote for anticholinesterase poisoning **Pharmacologic Class:** Muscarinic cholinergic receptor blocker

Actions and Uses

By occupying muscarinic receptors, atropine blocks the parasympathetic actions of Ach and induces symptoms of the fight-or-flight response. Most prominent are increased heart rate, bronchodilation, decreased motility in the GI tract, mydriasis, and decreased secretions from glands. At therapeutic doses, atropine has no effect on nicotinic receptors in ganglia or on skeletal muscle.

Although atropine has been used for centuries for a variety of purposes, its use has declined in recent decades because of the development of safer and more effective medications. Atropine may be used to treat hypermotility diseases of the GI tract such as irritable bowel syndrome, to suppress secretions during surgical procedures, to increase the heart rate in patients with bradycardia, and to dilate the pupil during eye examinations. Once widely used to cause bronchodilation in patients with asthma, atropine is now rarely prescribed for this disorder. Atropine therapy is useful for the treatment of reflexive bradycardia in infants and infantile hypertrophic pyloric stenosis.

Administration Alerts

- Oral and subcutaneous doses are *not* interchangeable.
- Monitor blood pressure, pulse, and respirations before administration and for at least 1 hour after subcutaneous administration.
- Pregnancy category C.

PHARMACOKINETICS

Onset	Peak	Duration
30 min PO; 5–15 min subcutaneously	60–90 min PO; 15–30 min subcutaneously	6 h PO; 4 h subcutaneously

Adverse Effects

The side effects of atropine limit its therapeutic usefulness and are predictable extensions of its autonomic actions. Expected side effects include dry mouth, constipation, urinary retention, and an increased heart rate. Initial CNS excitement may progress to delirium and even coma.

Contraindications: Atropine is contraindicated in patients with glaucoma, because the drug may increase pressure within the eye. Atropine should not be administered to patients with obstructive disorders of the GI tract, paralytic ileus, bladder neck obstruction, benign prostatic hyperplasia, myasthenia gravis, cardiac insufficiency, or acute hemorrhage.

Interactions

Drug–Drug: Drug interactions with atropine include an increased effect with antihistamines, TCAs, quinidine, and procainamide. Atropine decreases effects of levodopa.

Lab Tests: Unknown.

Herbal/Food: Use with caution with herbal supplements, such as aloe, *Serona repens* (saw palmetto), buckthorn, and cascara sagrada (the name means *sacred bark* in Spanish), which may increase atropine's effect, particularly with chronic use of these herbs.

Treatment of Overdose: Accidental poisoning has occurred in children who eat the colorful, purple berries of the deadly nightshade, mistaking them for cherries. Symptoms of poisoning are those of intense parasympathetic stimulation. Overdose may cause CNS stimulation or depression. A short-acting barbiturate or diazepam (Valium) may be administered to control convulsions. Physostigmine is an antidote for atropine poisoning that quickly reverses the coma caused by large doses of atropine.

The prototype drug, atropine, is used for several additional medical conditions due to its effective muscarinic receptor blockade. These applications include reversal of adverse muscarinic effects and treatment of cholinergic agent poisoning, including that caused by overdose of bethanechol (Urecholine), cholinesterase inhibitors, or accidental ingestion of certain types of mushrooms or organophosphate pesticides.

Some of the anticholinergics are used for their effects on the CNS, rather than their autonomic actions. Scopolamine (Transderm-Scop) is used to produce sedation and prevent motion sickness (see chapter 42); benztropine (Cogentin) is prescribed to reduce the muscular tremor and rigidity associated with Parkinson's disease; and donepezil (Aricept) has a slight memory enhancement effect in patients with Alzheimer's disease (see chapter 20).

Anticholinergics exhibit a relatively high incidence of side effects. Important adverse effects that limit their usefulness include tachycardia, CNS stimulation, and the tendency to cause urinary retention in men with prostate disorders. Adverse effects such as dry mouth and dry eyes occur due to blockade of muscarinic receptors on salivary glands and lacrimal glands, respectively. Blockade of muscarinic receptors on sweat glands can inhibit sweating, which may lead to hyperthermia. Photophobia can occur because the pupil is unable to constrict in response to

Nursing Practice Application

Pharmacotherapy With Anticholinergic Drugs

ASSESSMENT	POTENTIAL NURSING DIAGNOSES*
Baseline assessment prior to administration: • Obtain a complete health history including cardiovascular, cerebrovascular, or respiratory disease, acute (narrow-angle) glaucoma, and the possibility of pregnancy. Obtain a drug history including allergies, current prescription and OTC drugs, and herbal preparations. Be alert to possible drug interactions. • Evaluate appropriate laboratory findings such as hepatic or renal function studies. • Obtain baseline vital signs, urinary output, bowels sounds, and cardiac rhythm if appropriate. • Assess the patient's ability to receive and understand instruction. Include the family and caregivers as needed.	• *Decreased Cardiac Output* • *Urinary Retention* • *Constipation* • *Deficient Knowledge* (drug therapy) • *Risk for Impaired Body Temperature* • *Risk for Impaired Oral Mucous Membranes* • *Risk for Injury,* related to adverse effects of drug therapy *NANDA I © 2014
Assessment throughout administration: • Assess for desired therapeutic effects dependent on the reason for the drug (e.g., increased ease of breathing, cardiac rhythm stable, BP within normal range). • Continue frequent and careful monitoring of vital signs and urinary output and cardiac monitoring as appropriate. • Assess for and promptly report adverse effects: tachycardia, hypertension, dysrhythmias, tremors, dizziness, headache, or decreased urinary output. Seizures or ventricular tachycardia may signal drug toxicity and should be immediately reported.	

IMPLEMENTATION

Interventions and (Rationales)	Patient-Centered Care
Ensuring therapeutic effects: • Continue frequent assessments as described earlier for therapeutic effects dependent on the reason the drug therapy is given. (Pulse, BP, and respiratory rate should be within normal limits or within parameters set by the health care provider. Gastric motility and cramping have slowed.)	• Teach the patient, family, or caregiver how to monitor the pulse and BP. Ensure the proper use and functioning of any home equipment obtained.
• Provide supportive nursing measures; e.g., proper positioning for dyspnea. (Nursing measures such as raising the head of the bed during dyspnea will supplement therapeutic drug effects and optimize outcomes.)	• Instruct the patient that sips of water, ice chips, or hard candies as allowed, or oral rinses free of alcohol may ease mouth dryness. Avoid alcohol-based rinses because these may dry the mouth further.
Minimizing adverse effects: • Monitor for signs of excessive ANS stimulation such as drowsiness, blurred vision, tachycardia, dry mouth, urinary hesitancy, and decreased sweating. (Side effects are due to the blockade of muscarinic receptors. Anticholinergics are contraindicated in patients with acute/narrow angle glaucoma because mydriasis will increase intraocular pressure. **Lifespan:** Children and older adults may be more sensitive to the effects of anticholinergic drugs and require frequent monitoring.)	• Instruct the patient to immediately report palpitations, shortness of breath, dizziness, dysphagia, or syncope to the health care provider. • Older and debilitated patients should report excessive drowsiness or CNS stimulation occurring, even at usual doses of anticholinergics.
• Notify the health care provider if the BP or pulse exceeds established parameters. Continue frequent cardiac monitoring as appropriate (e.g., ECG) and urine output. (Because anticholinergic drugs stimulate heart rate and increase the chance for dysrhythmias, they must be closely monitored to avoid adverse effects. External monitoring devices will detect early signs of adverse effects as well as monitoring for therapeutic effects.)	• To allay possible anxiety, teach the patient about the rationale for all equipment used and the need for frequent monitoring as applicable.

continued

Nursing Practice Application *continued*

IMPLEMENTATION

Interventions and (Rationales)	Patient-Centered Care
• Monitor the patient for abdominal distention and auscultate for bowel sounds. Palpate for bladder distention and monitor output. (Anticholinergics may decrease tone and motility of intestinal and bladder smooth muscle. **Lifespan:** The older adult is at increased risk of constipation due to slowed peristalsis. Be aware that the male older adult with an enlarged prostate is at higher-risk for mechanical obstruction.)	• Teach the patient about the importance of drinking extra fluids and increasing fiber intake. Instruct the patient to notify the health care provider if difficulty with urination occurs or if constipation is severe.
• Minimize exposure to heat and strenuous exercise. (Anticholinergics can inhibit sweat gland secretions. Sweating is necessary for patients to cool down, so the drug can increase their risk for heat exhaustion and heat stroke. **Lifespan:** "Atropine fever"–hyperpyrexia due to suppression of perspiration and heat loss–increases the risk of heatstroke in young children and older adults.)	• Instruct the patient to avoid prolonged or strenuous activity in warm or hot environments, especially on humid days. Extra-hot showers and hot tubs should also be avoided. Immediately report dizziness, change in mental status, pale skin, muscle cramping, and nausea because these are signs of an impending heat exhaustion or heat stroke. Children and older adults should be monitored frequently.
• Provide for eye comfort such as a darkened room, soft cloth over eyes, and sunglasses. (Anticholinergic drugs cause mydriasis and photosensitivity to light.)	• Instruct the patient that photosensitivity may occur, and sunglasses may be needed in bright light or for outside activities. Caution should be taken with driving until drug effects are known.
Patient understanding of drug therapy: • Use opportunities during administration of medications and during assessments to provide patient education. (Using time during nursing care helps to optimize and reinforce key teaching areas.)	• The patient, family, or caregiver should be able to state the reason for the drug; appropriate dose and scheduling; what adverse effects to observe for and when to report; equipment needed as appropriate and how to use that equipment; and the required length of medication therapy needed with any special instructions regarding renewing or continuing the prescription as appropriate.
Patient self-administration of drug therapy: • When administering the medications, instruct the patient, family, or caregiver in proper self-administration of an inhaler or ophthalmic drops. (Using time during nurse administration of these drugs helps to reinforce teaching.) • **Lifespan:** Child fatalities have occurred from systemic absorption of anticholinergic eye drops. (Accidental ingestion of a parent's, family member's, or caregiver's eye drops may be fatal.)	• Instruct the patient in proper administration techniques, followed by teach-back. • The patient, family, or caregiver is able to discuss appropriate dosing and administration needs. • **Safety:** Instruct parents of young children to keep eye drops and all medications secured and out of the reach of children.

See Table 12.2 for a list of drugs to which these nursing actions apply.

bright light. Symptoms of overdose (cholinergic crisis) include fever, visual changes, difficulty swallowing, psychomotor agitation, and/or hallucinations. (Use this simile to remember the signs of cholinergic crisis: "Hot as hades, blind as a bat, dry as a bone, mad as a hatter.") The development of safer and more effective drugs has greatly decreased the current use of anticholinergics. An example is ipratropium (Atrovent), an anticholinergic used for patients with COPD. Because it is delivered via aerosol spray, this agent produces more localized action with fewer systemic side effects than atropine.

Chapter Review

KEY Concepts

The numbered key concepts provide a succinct summary of the important points from the corresponding numbered section within the chapter. If any of these points are not clear, refer to the numbered section within the chapter for review.

12.1 The central nervous system is comprised of the brain and spinal cord. The peripheral nervous system is divided into sensory and motor divisions. The motor division has a somatic portion, which is under voluntary control, and an autonomic portion, which is involuntary and controls smooth muscle, cardiac muscle, and glandular secretions.

12.2 Stimulation of the parasympathetic division of the autonomic nervous system induces rest-and-digest responses whereas stimulation of the sympathetic branch causes actions of the fight-or-flight response.

12.3 Drugs can affect parasympathetic nervous transmission across a synapse by binding receptors at the effector organs; or by preventing destruction of the neurotransmitter acetylcholine.

12.4 Acetylcholine is the neurotransmitter that binds with nicotinic receptors in the ganglia of both the sympathetic and parasympathetic division of the autonomic nervous system. It is also the neurotransmitter that binds with nicotinic receptors in skeletal muscle and the CNS. Acetylcholine binds with muscarinic receptors in organs targeted by the parasympathetic nervous system.

12.5 Parasympathomimetics stimulate target tissue innervated by parasympathetic nerves whereas anticholinergics inhibit functionality of the parasympathetic branch.

12.6 Cholinergic drugs act directly by stimulating cholinergic receptors (cholinergic agonists) or indirectly by inhibiting acetylcholinesterase enzyme (cholinesterase inhibitors). Cholinergic agonists have few therapeutic uses because of their numerous side effects.

12.7 Anticholinergics act by blocking the effects of acetylcholine at muscarinic receptors, and they are used to dry secretions, treat asthma, and prevent motion sickness.

REVIEW Questions

1. The nurse is preparing a plan of care for a patient with myasthenia gravis. Which of the following outcome statements would be appropriate for a patient receiving a cholinergic agonist such as pyridostigmine (Mestinon) for this condition? The patient will exhibit:
    1. An increase in pulse rate, blood pressure, and respiratory rate.
    2. Enhanced urinary elimination.
    3. A decrease in muscle weakness, ptosis, and diplopia.
    4. Prolonged muscle contractions and proprioception.
2. Anticholinergics may be ordered for which of the following conditions? (Select all that apply.)
    1. Peptic ulcer disease
    2. Bradycardia
    3. Decreased sexual function
    4. Irritable bowel syndrome
    5. Urine retention
3. Which factor in the patient's history would cause the nurse to question a medication order for atropine?
    1. A 32-year-old man with a history of drug abuse
    2. A 65-year-old man with benign prostatic hyperplasia
    3. An 8-year-old boy with chronic tonsillitis
    4. A 22-year-old woman on the second day of her menstrual cycle
4. Older adult patients taking bethanechol (Urecholine) need to be assessed more frequently because of which of the following adverse effects?
    1. Tachycardia
    2. Hypertension
    3. Dizziness
    4. Urinary retention

5. The patient taking benztropine (Cogentin) should be provided education on methods to manage which common adverse effect?
   1. Heartburn
   2. Constipation
   3. Hypothermia
   4. Increased gastric motility

6. The patient or family of a patient taking neostigmine (Prostigmin) should be taught to be observant for which of the following adverse effects that may signal that a possible overdose has occurred?
   1. Excessive sweating, salivation, and drooling
   2. Extreme constipation
   3. Hypertension and tachycardia
   4. Excessively dry eyes and reddened sclera

PATIENT-FOCUSED Case Study

Katisha Moore is a 68-year-old who enjoys working in her large rose garden. This morning, she noticed that insects had infested the plants. To avoid further damage, she powdered the plants with an insecticide. In her rush to finish, she accidentally contaminated herself with the insecticide and kept working for several hours before showering.

Mrs. Moore is brought into the local emergency department (ED) by her husband that afternoon. She has nausea, dizziness, sweating, excessive salivation, weepy eyes, and a runny nose. She reports intermittent twitching of her upper extremities and uncoordinated movement.

Her initial assessment reveals a 64-kg (142-lb) Caucasian female with a past medication history of hypertension diagnosed 5 years ago. She is married and has two adult children. Her vital signs are blood pressure, 158/94 mmHg; heart rate, 58; respiratory rate, 30; and temperature, 37.3°C (99.2°F). Her skin is pale and moist. She exhibits copious lacrimation and rhinorrhea. Both pupils are constricted. Crackles are heard bilaterally in all lung fields on inspiration. Since admission to the ED she has vomited twice and had one large diarrhea stool.

She is diagnosed with acute organophosphate poisoning. Mrs. Moore is started on oxygen therapy, and the nurse will observe her closely for further respiratory distress. Atropine 2 mg is administered IV every 15 minutes over the next hour.

1. What is the mechanism of action associated with atropine.
2. Why is this drug being given to Mrs. Moore?
3. What adverse effects should you expect for the patient from the administration of atropine?

CRITICAL THINKING Questions

1. A 74-year-old female patient required an indwelling bladder (Foley) catheter for 4 days postoperatively and, after removal, she was still unable to void. She was recatheterized, and a bladder rehabilitation program was begun that included bethanechol (Urecholine). What nursing diagnosis should be considered as a part of this patient's plan of care given this new drug regimen?
2. A 42-year-old male was diagnosed with Parkinson's disease 4 years ago. He is being treated with a regimen that includes benztropine (Cogentin). The nurse recognizes Cogentin as an anticholinergic drug. What assessment data should the nurse gather from this patient? Discuss the potential side effects of benztropine for which the nurse should assess in this patient.

Visit www.pearsonhighered.com/nursingresources for answers and rationales for all activities.

REFERENCES

Herdman, T. H., & Kamitsuru, S. (Eds.). (2014). *NANDA International Nursing Diagnoses: Definitions and Classification, 2015–2017*. Oxford, United Kingdom: Wiley-Blackwell.

SELECTED BIBLIOGRAPHY

Brown, J. H., & Laiken, N. (2011). Muscarinic receptor agonists and antagonists. In L. L. Brunton, B. A. Chabner, & B. C. Knollmann (Eds.), *Goodman and Gilman's the pharmacological basis of therapeutics* (12th ed.). New York, NY: McGraw-Hill.

Katzung, B. G. (2015). Introduction to autonomic pharmacology. In B. G. Katzung & A. J. Trevor (Eds.), *Basic and Clinical Pharmacology* (13th ed.). New York, NY: McGraw-Hill.

Nunn, N., Womack, M., Dart, C., & Barrett-Jolley, R. (2011). Function and pharmacology of spinally-projecting sympathetic pre-autonomic neurons in the paraventricular nucleus of the hypothalamus. *Current Neuropharmacology, 9*, 262–277. doi:10.2174/157015911795596531

Pappano A. J. (2015) Cholinoceptor-blocking drugs. In B. G. Katzung & A. J. Trevor (Eds.), *Basic and Clinical Pharmacology* (13th ed.). New York, NY: McGraw-Hill.

Serra, A., Ruff, R., Kaminski, H., & Leigh, R. J. (2011). Factors contributing to failure of neuromuscular transmission in myasthenia gravis and the special case of the extraocular muscles. *Annals of the New York Academy of Sciences, 1233*, 26–33. doi:10.1111/j.1749-6632.2011.06123.x

van Gestel, A. J., & Steier, J. (2010). Autonomic dysfunction in patients with chronic obstructive pulmonary disease (COPD). *Journal of Thoracic Disease*, 2, 215–222.

Westfall, T. C., & Westfall, D. P. (2011). Neurotransmission: The autonomic and somatic motor nervous systems. In L. L. Brunton, B. A. Chabner, & B. C. Knollmann (Eds.), *Goodman and Gilman's the pharmacological basis of therapeutics* (12th ed.). New York, NY: McGraw-Hill.

Pharmacotherapy Illustrated

13.1 | Impulses and Actions Resulting From the Synthesis, Storage, and Release of Catecholamines, and the Reuptake and Destruction of NE.

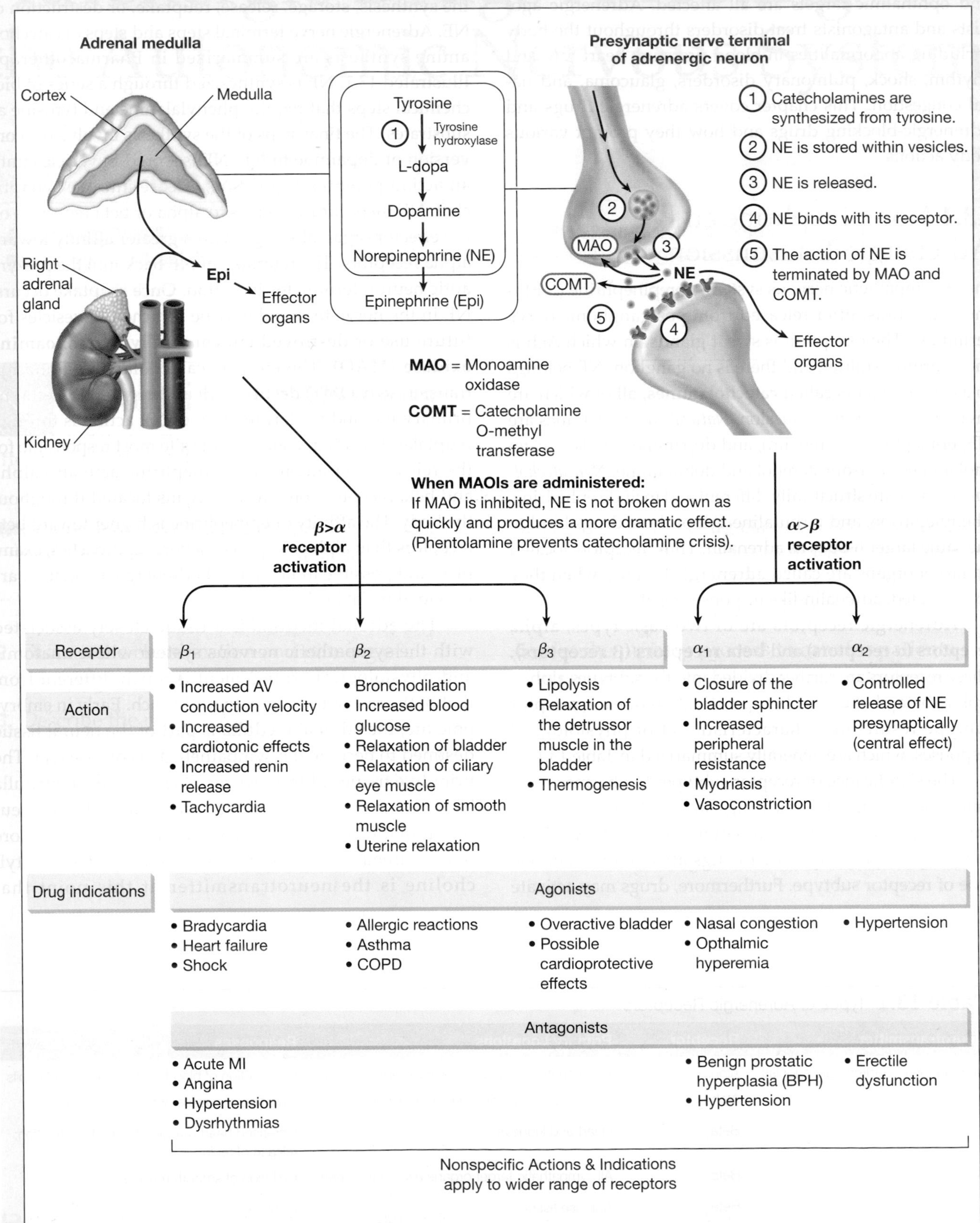
Adrenal medulla
Cortex
Medulla
Right adrenal gland
Kidney
Epi
Effector organs
Tyrosine
1 Tyrosine hydroxylase
L-dopa
Dopamine
Norepinephrine (NE)
Epinephrine (Epi)
Presynaptic nerve terminal of adrenergic neuron
1 Catecholamines are synthesized from tyrosine.
2 NE is stored within vesicles.
3 NE is released.
4 NE binds with its receptor.
5 The action of NE is terminated by MAO and COMT.
MAO
COMT
NE
Effector organs
MAO = Monoamine oxidase
COMT = Catecholamine O-methyl transferase
When MAOIs are administered:
If MAO is inhibited, NE is not broken down as quickly and produces a more dramatic effect. (Phentolamine prevents catecholamine crisis).
β>α receptor activation
α>β receptor activation

	β_1	β_2	β_3	α_1	α_2
Receptor	β_1	β_2	β_3	α_1	α_2
Action	• Increased AV conduction velocity • Increased cardiotonic effects • Increased renin release • Tachycardia	• Bronchodilation • Increased blood glucose • Relaxation of bladder • Relaxation of ciliary eye muscle • Relaxation of smooth muscle • Uterine relaxation	• Lipolysis • Relaxation of the detrussor muscle in the bladder • Thermogenesis	• Closure of the bladder sphincter • Increased peripheral resistance • Mydriasis • Vasoconstriction	• Controlled release of NE presynaptically (central effect)
Drug indications — Agonists	• Bradycardia • Heart failure • Shock	• Allergic reactions • Asthma • COPD	• Overactive bladder • Possible cardioprotective effects	• Nasal congestion • Opthalmic hyperemia	• Hypertension
Antagonists	• Acute MI • Angina • Hypertension • Dysrhythmias			• Benign prostatic hyperplasia (BPH) • Hypertension	• Erectile dysfunction

Nonspecific Actions & Indications apply to wider range of receptors

Table 13.2 General Approaches Affecting Adrenergic Neuronal Transmission

Approach	Example	Indications
Drugs may affect the synthesis of neurotransmitter in the nerve terminal. • Drugs that decrease the amount of neurotransmitter synthesis will inhibit nervous system activity. • Those drugs that increase neurotransmitter synthesis will promote nervous system activity.	*Alpha methyl para tyrosine (αMPT)* This drug temporarily inhibits tyrosine hydroxylase, the rate-limiting step in the synthesis of dopamine.	*Historical interest in the control of hypertension; current possible usefulness for various neuropsychiatric disorders.* Due to weakened release of dopamine, this drug was once thought useful in the treatment of hypertension. Applications more recently include dystonia, dyskinesia, Huntington's chorea, mania, obsessive-compulsive disorder, substance abuse disorders, and schizophrenia.
Drugs can prevent the storage of the neurotransmitter in vesicles within the presynaptic nerve. • Prevention of neurotransmitter storage will inhibit nervous system activity.	*Reserpine* This drug depletes stores of catecholamines in the brain and in the adrenal medulla.	*Antihypertensive symptoms in patients diagnosed with schizophrenia.* Mild essential hypertension or as adjunctive therapy for patients with psychotic symptoms.
Drugs can influence the release of the neurotransmitter from the presynaptic nerve. • Promoting neurotransmitter release will stimulate nervous system activity. Slowing neurotransmitter release will have the opposite effect.	*Amphetamine, dextroamphetamine mixed salts (Adderall)* These drugs increase the release of monoamines and they block the reuptake of norepinephrine and dopamine into the presynaptic neuron.	*Patients diagnosed with ADHD or narcolepsy.* For the treatment of attention deficit/hyperactivity disorder (ADHD) and patients having difficulty staying awake.
Drugs can prevent the normal destruction or reuptake of the neurotransmitter • Drugs that cause the neurotransmitter to remain in the synapse for a longer time will stimulate nervous system activity.	*Monoamine oxidase inhibitors (MAOIs)* These drugs block the degradation of dopamine and norepinephrine within central and peripheral adrenergic nerve terminals.	*For patients diagnosed with clinical depression not controlled by other antidepressants, (i.e., selective serotonin reuptake inhibitors, atypical antidepressants and tricyclic antidepressants (TCAs).*
Drugs can bind to the receptor site on the postsynaptic target tissue. • Drugs that bind to postsynaptic receptors and stimulate target tissue will increase nervous system activity. • Drugs that attach to the postsynaptic targets and prevent the neurotransmitter from reaching its receptors will inhibit nervous system activity.	*Beta blockers* Beta blockers exert their effects by preventing catecholamines from binding to beta receptors in the body.	*Widely used for the control of hypertension.* For high blood pressure, heart failure, and for patients with a history of myocardial infarction (MI). Treatments may help to alleviate signs of heart palpitations and tremulousness.

stimulates the *chromaffin cells* or neuroendocrine cells of the adrenal medulla to release epinephrine directly into the bloodstream. Once released, epinephrine travels to target organs, where it elicits the classic fight-or-flight symptoms (see chapter 12, Figure 12.2). The action of epinephrine is terminated through hepatic metabolism, rather than reuptake.

Other types of adrenergic receptors exist. Although dopamine was once thought to function only as a chemical precursor to NE, research has determined that it serves a larger role as the dedicated neurotransmitter. Five dopaminergic receptors (D_1 through D_5) have been discovered in the central nervous system (CNS). Dopaminergic receptors in the CNS are important to the action of antipsychotic medicines (see chapter 17) and in the treatment of Parkinson's disease (see chapter 20). Dopamine receptors in the peripheral nervous system are located in the arterioles of the kidney and other viscera. Although these receptors likely have a role in autonomic function, their therapeutic importance has yet to be fully discovered.

ADRENERGIC DRUGS (SYMPATHOMIMETICS)

The adrenergic drugs, also known as adrenergic agonists or **sympathomimetics,** stimulate the sympathetic nervous system and induce symptoms characteristic of the fight-or-flight response. These drugs have clinical applications in the treatment of shock and hypotension.

13.2 Clinical Applications of Adrenergic Drugs

Sympathomimetics produce many of the same responses as the anticholinergics. However, because the sympathetic nervous system has alpha and beta subreceptors, the actions of sympathomimetics are more specific and have wider therapeutic application (Table 13.3).

As mentioned, sympathomimetics may be described chemically as *catecholamines* or *noncatecholamines*. The catecholamines share the same biochemical structure as NE and have a short duration of action. They must be

Table 13.3 Selected Adrenergic Drugs

Drug	Primary Receptor Subtype	Primary Uses
albuterol (Proventil, Ventolin, VoSpire) (see page 662 for the Prototype Drug box)	$Beta_2$	Asthma, chronic obstructive pulmonary disease (COPD)
clonidine (Catapres, Kapvay)	$Alpha_2$ in CNS	Hypertension, ADHD, pain
dobutamine (Dobutrex)	$Beta_1$	Cardiac stimulant
dopamine (Dopastat, Intropin) (see page 435 for the Prototype Drug box)	$Alpha_1$ and $beta_1$	Shock
droxidopa (Northera)	$Beta_3$	Neurogenic orthostatic hypotension
epinephrine (Adrenalin, others) (see page 440 for the Prototype Drug box)	Alpha and beta	Cardiac arrest, asthma; anaphylactic and allergic reactions
formoterol (Foradil, Perforomist)	$Beta_2$	Asthma, COPD
isoproterenol (Isuprel)	$Beta_1$ and $beta_2$	Asthma, dysrhythmias, heart failure
metaproterenol (Alupent)	$Beta_2$	Asthma
methyldopa (Aldomet)	$Alpha_2$ in CNS	Hypertension
midodrine (ProAmatine)	Alpha	Hypertension
mirabegron (Myrbetriq)	$Beta_3$	Overactive bladder
norepinephrine (Levophed)	Alpha and $beta_1$	Shock
oxymetazoline (Afrin, others) page 648 for the Prototype Drug box)	Alpha	Nasal congestion
phenylephrine (Neo-Synephrine)	Alpha	Hypertension, nasal congestion
pseudoephedrine (Sudafed and others)	Alpha and beta	Nasal congestion
salmeterol (Serevent)	$Beta_2$	Asthma
terbutaline	$Beta_2$	Asthma

administered parenterally. The noncatecholamines can be taken orally and have longer durations of action because they are not rapidly destroyed by MAO or COMT.

Sympathomimetics act either directly or indirectly. Most sympathomimetics act directly by binding to and activating adrenergic receptors. Examples include the three endogenous catecholamines: epinephrine, norepinephrine, and dopamine. Other medications in this class act indirectly by causing the release of NE from its vesicles within the presynaptic terminal or by inhibiting the reuptake or destruction of NE. Those that act by indirect mechanisms, such as amphetamine or cocaine, are used for their central effects in the brain rather than their autonomic effects. A few drugs, such as ephedrine, act by both direct and indirect mechanisms.

Most effects of sympathomimetics are predictable based on their autonomic actions, dependent on which adrenergic receptor subtypes are stimulated. Because the receptor responses are so different, the student will need to memorize the specific subclass(es) of receptors activated by each sympathomimetic. Specific subclasses of receptors and therapeutic applications are as follows:

- $Alpha_1$ receptor. Treatment of nasal congestion or hypotension; causes dilation of the pupil (mydriasis) during ophthalmic examinations.
- $Alpha_2$ receptor. Treatment of hypertension through a centrally acting mechanism. Autonomic $alpha_2$ receptors are also located on presynaptic membranes of postganglionic neurons; when activated, they reduce the release of NE within the axon terminal.
- $Beta_1$ receptor. Treatment of cardiac arrest, heart failure, and shock.
- $Beta_2$ receptor. Treatment of asthma and premature labor contractions.
- $Beta_3$ receptor. Treatment of overactive bladder

Some sympathomimetics are nonselective, stimulating more than one type of adrenergic receptor. For example, epinephrine stimulates all five types of adrenergic receptors and is used for cardiac arrest and asthma. Pseudoephedrine (Sudafed and others) stimulates both $alpha_1$ and $beta_2$ receptors and is used as a nasal decongestant. Isoproterenol (Isuprel) stimulates both $beta_1$ and $beta_2$ receptors and is used to increase the rate, force, and conduction speed of the heart and, occasionally, for asthma. The nonselective drugs generally cause more autonomic-related side effects than the selective drugs.

The side effects of the sympathomimetics are mostly extensions of their autonomic actions. Cardiovascular effects such as tachycardia, hypertension, and dysrhythmias are

Community-Oriented Practice

USE OF EPINEPHRINE AUTO-INJECTORS

The EpiPen® and the Auvi-Q® are examples of auto-injectors containing epinephrine that are used to prevent and treat anaphylaxis and severe allergic reactions to insect stings, foods, or drugs. As its name suggests, the EpiPen is a cylinder-shaped device approximately the size of a large pen. The Auvi-Q is shaped like a rectangular cell phone. The Auvi-Q has the additional property of providing voice instructions for the use of the device. Increased awareness of the severity of some allergies, and an increased incidence of anaphylaxis to substances and foods such as peanuts, have led to increased prescriptions for epinephrine auto-injectors (Campbell, Manivannan, Hartz, & Sadosty, 2012). These devices are designed to be easy to operate, although the word *auto* sometimes gives people a false sense of security that the injector is foolproof. In a study of children with peanut allergies who had received prescriptions for an auto injector, Chad et al. (2013) found that a majority of parents remained fearful of using the device after instructions were given. Over 32% reported that they were afraid of using the device incorrectly.

The nurse has a key responsibility in teaching parents and older children the correct use of an epinephrine auto-injector. Nurses should be familiar with the common types of auto-injectors used in their clinical agency and read the directions well in advance of teaching patients. In addition to teaching patients or families the proper administration techniques, the following information should also be included:

- Call 911 and seek medical attention any time epinephrine is required.
- Inject the drug into the thigh only, not into the buttock or hip (dorsogluteal) regions.
- Take the used auto-injector to the emergency department or provider's office for proper disposal.
- Keep the auto-injector on hand at all times and an extra one available. Store the additional device in a cool, dark place, but refrigeration is not recommended.

particularly troublesome and may limit therapy. Large doses can induce CNS excitement and seizures. Other sympathomimetic responses that may occur are dry mouth, nausea, and vomiting. Some of these drugs cause anorexia, which has led to their historical use as appetite suppressants. However, because of prominent cardiovascular side effects, sympathomimetics are now rarely used for this purpose.

Drugs in this class are found as prototypes in many other chapters in this textbook. For additional prototypes of drugs in this class, see dopamine (Dopastat, Intropin), epinephrine (Adrenalin), and norepinephrine (Levophed) in chapter 29; oxymetazoline (Afrin) in chapter 39; and albuterol (Proventil, Ventolin, VoSpire) in chapter 40.

ADRENERGIC-BLOCKING DRUGS

Adrenergic-blocking drugs or antagonists inhibit the sympathetic nervous system and produce many of the same rest-and-digest symptoms as the parasympathomimetics. They have wide therapeutic application in the treatment of hypertension.

13.3 Clinical Applications of Adrenergic-Blocking Drugs

Adrenergic antagonists are drugs that act by directly blocking adrenergic receptors. A less used description of these drugs is **sympatholytics.** The actions of these drugs are specific to either alpha or beta blockade. Medications in this class have great therapeutic application and are the most widely prescribed class of autonomic drugs (Table 13.4).

Alpha-adrenergic antagonists, or simply alpha blockers, are used for their effects on vascular smooth muscle. By relaxing vascular smooth muscle in small arteries, $alpha_1$ blockers such as doxazosin (Cardura) cause vasodilation, decreasing blood pressure. They may be used either alone or in combination with other drugs in the treatment of hypertension (see chapter 26). A second use is in the treatment of BPH, due to their ability to increase urine flow by relaxing smooth muscle in the bladder neck, prostate, and urethra (see chapter 47).

The most common adverse effect of alpha blockers is orthostatic hypotension, which occurs when a patient abruptly changes from a recumbent to an upright position. Reflex tachycardia, nasal congestion, and impotence are other important side effects that may occur as a consequence of increased parasympathetic activity.

Phentolamine (Regitine) is used as an aid in the diagnosis of pheochromocytoma. **Pheochromocytoma** is a rare, catecholamine-secreting tumor on the adrenal gland that may precipitate life-threatening hypertension. Sudden and marked reduction in blood pressure following parenteral administration of phentolamine is brought about by the *nonspecific* blockade of alpha receptors. Other indications for phentolamine are hypertensive crises caused by methoxamine and phenylephrine treatment, or excess plasma levels of catecholamines in patients taking MAOIs. Phentolamine is a specific antidote for catecholamine overdose and is injected intradermally for catecholamine extravasation.

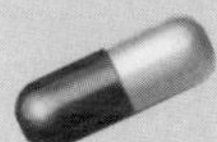

Prototype Drug | Phenylephrine *(Neo-Synephrine)*

Therapeutic Class: Nasal decongestant; mydriatic drug; antihypotensive
Pharmacologic Class: Adrenergic drug (sympathomimetic)

Actions and Uses

Phenylephrine is a selective alpha-adrenergic agonist that is available in different formulations, including intranasal, ophthalmic, intramuscular (IM), subcutaneous, and intravenous (IV). All its actions and indications are extensions of its sympathetic stimulation.

Intranasal Administration: When applied intranasally by spray or drops, phenylephrine reduces nasal congestion by constricting small blood vessels in the nasal mucosa.

Topical Administration*:* Applied topically to the eye during ophthalmic examinations, phenylephrine can dilate the pupil without causing significant cycloplegia.

Parenteral Administration: The parenteral administration of phenylephrine can reverse acute hypotension caused by spinal anesthesia or vascular shock. Because phenylephrine lacks beta-adrenergic agonist activity, it produces relatively few cardiac side effects at therapeutic doses. Its longer duration of activity and lack of significant cardiac effects gives phenylephrine some advantages over epinephrine or norepinephrine in treating acute hypotension.

Administration Alerts

- Parenteral administration can cause tissue injury with extravasation.
- Phenylephrine ophthalmic drops may damage soft contact lenses.
- Pregnancy category C.

PHARMACOKINETICS

Onset	Peak	Duration
Immediate IV; 10–15 min IM/subcutaneous	5–10 min IV; 15–30 min IM/subcutaneous	15–20 min IV; 30–120 min IM/subcutaneous; 3–6 h topical

Adverse Effects

When the drug is used topically or intranasally, side effects are uncommon. Intranasal use can cause burning of the mucosa and rebound congestion if used for prolonged periods (see chapter 39). Ophthalmic preparations can cause narrow-angle glaucoma secondary to their mydriatic effect. High doses can cause reflex bradycardia due to the elevation of blood pressure caused by stimulation of alpha$_1$ receptors.

When used parenterally, the drug should be used with caution in patients with advanced coronary artery disease, hypertension, or hyperthyroidism. Anxiety, restlessness, and tremor may occur due to the drug's stimulation effect on the CNS. Patients with hyperthyroidism may experience a severe increase in basal metabolic rate, resulting in increased blood pressure and ventricular tachycardia.

Black Box Warning: Severe reactions, including death, may occur with IV infusion even when appropriate dilution is used to avoid rapid diffusion. Therefore, restrict IV use for situations in which other routes are not feasible.

Contraindications: This drug should not be used in patients with acute pancreatitis, heart disease, hepatitis, or narrow-angle glaucoma.

Interactions

Drug–Drug: Drug interactions may occur with MAO inhibitors (MAOIs), causing a hypertensive crisis. Increased effects may also occur with tricyclic antidepressants, ergot alkaloids, and oxytocin. Inhibitory effects occur with alpha blockers and beta blockers. Phenylephrine is incompatible with iron preparations (ferric salts). Phenylephrine may cause dysrhythmias when taken in combination with digoxin.

Lab Tests: Unknown.

Herbal/Food: Unknown.

Treatment of Overdose: Overdose may cause tachycardia and hypertension. Treatment with an alpha blocker such as phentolamine (Regitine) may be indicated to decrease blood pressure.

Nursing Practice Application
Pharmacotherapy With Adrenergic Drugs

ASSESSMENT	POTENTIAL NURSING DIAGNOSES*
Baseline assessment prior to administration: • Obtain a complete health history including cardiovascular, cerebrovascular, respiratory disease, or diabetes. Obtain a drug history including allergies, current prescription and over-the-counter (OTC) drugs, and herbal preparations. Be alert to possible drug interactions. • Evaluate appropriate laboratory findings such as hepatic or renal function studies. • Obtain baseline vital signs, weight, and urinary and cardiac output as appropriate. • Assess the nasal mucosa for excoriation or bleeding prior to beginning therapy for nasal congestion. • Assess the patient's ability to receive and understand instruction. Include the family and caregivers as needed.	• *Decreased Cardiac Output* • *Ineffective Tissue Perfusion* • *Impaired Gas Exchange* • *Ineffective Airway Clearance* • *Deficient Knowledge* (drug therapy) • *Risk for Injury,* related to adverse effects of drug therapy or administration • *Risk for Disturbed Sleep Pattern,* related to adverse effects of drug therapy *NANDA I © 2014
Assessment throughout administration: • Assess for desired therapeutic effects dependent on the reason for the drug (e.g., increased ease of breathing, blood pressure (BP) within normal range, nasal congestion improved). • Continue frequent and careful monitoring of vital signs and urinary and cardiac output as appropriate, especially if IV administration is used. • Assess for and promptly report adverse effects: tachycardia, hypertension, dysrhythmias, tremors, dizziness, headache, and decreased urinary output. Immediately report severe hypertension, seizures, and angina which may signal drug toxicity.	

IMPLEMENTATION

Interventions and (Rationales)	Patient-Centered Care
Ensuring therapeutic effects: • Continue frequent assessments for therapeutic effects dependent on the reason the drug therapy is given. (Pulse, BP, and respiratory rate should be within normal limits or within the parameters set by the health care provider. Nasal congestion should be decreased; reddened, irritated sclera should be improved.)	• Teach the patient, family, or caregiver how to monitor the pulse and BP, as appropriate. Ensure the proper use and functioning of any home equipment obtained.
• Provide supportive nursing measures; e.g., proper positioning for dyspnea, shock, etc. (Supportive nursing measures will supplement therapeutic drug effects and optimize the outcome.)	• Teach the patient to report increasing dyspnea despite medication therapy and to not take more than the prescribed dose unless instructed otherwise by the health care provider.
Minimizing adverse effects: • Monitor for signs of excessive autonomic nervous system stimulation and notify the health care provider if the BP or pulse exceeds established parameters. Continue frequent cardiac monitoring (e.g., ECG, cardiac output) and urine output if IV adrenergics are given. (Because adrenergic drugs stimulate the heart rate and raise BP, they must be closely monitored to avoid adverse effects. **Lifespan:** The older adult may be at greater risk due to previously existing cardiovascular disease. **Diverse Patients:** Research suggests African Americans may experience an impaired [diminished] vascular response to isoproterenol, and vital signs should be monitored frequently during administration.)	• Instruct the patient to report palpitations, shortness of breath, chest pain, excessive nervousness or tremors, headache, or urinary retention immediately. • Teach the patient to limit or eliminate the use of foods and beverages that contain caffeine because these may cause excessive nervousness, insomnia, and tremors.
• Closely monitor the IV infusion site when using IV adrenergics. All IV adrenergic drips should be given via infusion pump. (Blanching at the IV site is an indicator of extravasation and the IV infusion should be immediately stopped and the provider contacted for further treatment orders. Infusion pumps allow precise dosing of the medication.)	• To allay possible anxiety, teach the patient about the rationale for all equipment used and the need for frequent monitoring.

continued

Nursing Practice Application *continued*

IMPLEMENTATION	
Interventions and (Rationales)	**Patient-Centered Care**
• Monitor oral and nasal mucosa and breath sounds in patients taking inhaled adrenergic drugs. (Inhaled epinephrine and other adrenergic drugs may reduce bronchial secretions, making removal of mucus more difficult.) • Inspect nasal mucosa for irritation, rhinorrhea, or bleeding after nasal use. Avoid prolonged use of adrenergic nasal sprays. (Vasoconstriction may cause transient stinging, excessive dryness, or bleeding. Rebound congestion with chronic rhinorrhea may result after prolonged treatment.)	• Continue to monitor blood glucose and appropriate laboratory work. (Adrenergic drugs affect a wide range of body systems. A change in antidiabetes medications or dosing may be required if glucose remains elevated.) • Teach the patient with diabetes to monitor his or her blood glucose more frequently and to notify the health care provider if a consistent increase is noted. • Teach the patient to increase fluid intake to moisten airways and assist in the expectoration of mucus, unless contraindicated. • Instruct the patient not to use nasal spray longer than 3–5 days without consulting the provider. OTC saline nasal sprays may provide comfort if mucosa is dry and irritated. Increasing oral fluid intake may also help with hydration. • **Lifespan:** Teach the family or caregiver that adrenergic nasal sprays and other decongestants are not recommended in children and should be used only under a provider's supervision.
• Provide for eye comfort such as darkened room, soft cloth over eyes, and sunglasses. Transient stinging after installation of eyedrops may occur. (Adrenergic drugs can cause mydriasis and photosensitivity to light. Localized vasoconstriction may cause stinging of the eyes.)	• Instruct the patient that photosensitivity may occur, and sunglasses may be needed in bright light or for outside activities. The provider should be notified if irritation or sensitivity occurs beyond 12 hours after the drug has been discontinued. Soft contact lens users should check with the provider before using, as some solutions may stain lenses. **Lifespan & Safety**: Assist the older adult with ambulation if blurred vision or light-sensitivity occurs, to prevent falls.
Patient understanding of drug therapy: • Use opportunities during administration of medications and during assessments to provide patient education. (Using time during nursing care helps to optimize and reinforce key teaching areas.)	• The patient, family, or caregiver should be able to state the reason for the drug; appropriate dose and scheduling; what adverse effects to observe for and when to report; equipment needed as appropriate and how to use that equipment; and the required length of medication therapy needed with any special instructions regarding renewing or continuing the prescription as appropriate.
Patient self-administration of drug therapy: • When administering medications, instruct the patient, family, or caregiver in proper self-administration of an inhaler, epinephrine injection kit, nasal spray, or ophthalmic drops. (Using time during nurse administration of these drugs helps to reinforce teaching.)	• Instruct the patient in proper administration techniques, followed by teach-back. Inhalation forms should only be dispensed when the patient is upright to properly aerosolize the drug and prevent overdosage from excessively large droplets. • Teach the patient, family, or caregiver proper technique for epinephrine auto-injector and to have on hand for emergency use at all times. If epinephrine auto-injector is needed and used, 911 and the health care provider should be called immediately after use. • Teach the patient, family, or caregiver to not share nasal sprays with other people to prevent infection. • The patient, family, or caregiver is able to discuss appropriate dosing and administration needs.

See Table 13.3 for a list of drugs to which these nursing actions apply.

Table 13.1 Selected Adrenergic-Blocking Drugs (Antagonists)

Drug	Primary Receptor Subtype	Primary Uses
acebutolol (Sectral)	$Beta_1$	Hypertension, dysrhythmias, angina
alfuzosin (UroXatral)	$Alpha_1$	Benign prostatic hyperplasia (BPH)
atenolol (Tenormin)	$Beta_1$	Hypertension, angina
bisoprolol (Zebeta)	$Beta_1$	Hypertension, heart failure
carteolol (Cartrol)	$Beta_1$ and $beta_2$	Hypertension, glaucoma
carvedilol (Coreg)	$Alpha_1$, $beta_1$, and $beta_2$	Hypertension, heart failure, acute MI
doxazosin (Cardura)	$ALPHA_1$	Hypertension, BPH
esmolol (Brevibloc)	$Beta_1$	Hypertension, dysrhythmias
metoprolol (Lopressor, Toprol)	$Beta_1$	Hypertension, acute MI, heart failure
nadolol (Corgard)	$Beta_1$ and $beta_2$	Hypertension, angina
phentolamine (Regitine)	Alpha	Severe hypertension
prazosin (Minipress)	$Alpha_1$	Hypertension
propranolol (Inderal, Innopran XL) (see page 453 for the Prototype Drug box)	$Beta_1$ and $beta_2$	Hypertension, dysrhythmias, heart failure
sotalol (Betapace, Sorine)	$Beta_1$ and $beta_2$	Dysrhythmias
tamsulosin (Flomax)	$Alpha_1$	BPH
terazosin (Hytrin)	$Alpha_1$	Hypertension
timolol (Blocadren, Timoptic) (see page 871 for the Prototype Drug box)	$Beta_1$ and $beta_2$	Hypertension, acute MI, glaucoma

Note: This is a partial list of adrenergic-blocking drugs. For additional drugs and doses, refer to the chapter containing the primary use.

Beta-adrenergic antagonists may block either $beta_1$ receptors, or $beta_2$ receptors, or both types of receptors. Regardless of their receptor specificity, all beta blockers are used therapeutically for their effects on the cardiovascular system. Beta blockers decrease the rate and force of contraction of the heart and slow electrical conduction through the atrioventricular node. Drugs that selectively block $beta_1$ receptors, such as atenolol (Tenormin), are called *cardioselective* drugs. Because they have little effect on noncardiac tissue, they exert fewer side effects than nonselective drugs such as propranolol (Inderal, InnoPran XL).

The primary use of beta blockers is in the treatment of hypertension. Although the exact mechanism by which beta blockers reduce blood pressure is not completely understood, it is thought that the reduction may be due to decreased cardiac output or to suppression of renin release by the kidneys. See chapter 26 for a more comprehensive description of the use of beta blockers in hypertension management.

Beta-adrenergic antagonists have several other important therapeutic applications that are discussed in many chapters in this textbook. By decreasing the cardiac workload, beta blockers can ease the pain associated with migraines (see chapter 18) and angina pectoris (see chapter 28). By slowing electrical conduction across the myocardium, beta blockers are useful in treating certain types of dysrhythmias (see chapter 30). Other therapeutic uses include the treatment of heart failure (see chapter 27), MI (see chapter 28), and narrow-angle glaucoma (see chapter 50).

Adverse effects may occur with beta-adrenergic blockade. Beta blockers may exacerbate heart failure in some patients with pre-existing myocardial conditions. Increased risk of hypotension and bradycardia may occur. Adverse non-cardiac effects include significant bronchial constriction, which may be harmful especially in patients with respiratory conditions such as asthma or COPD. Beta blockers may cause hypoglycemia or hyperglycemia and mask the symptoms of hypoglycemia in diabetic patients. Other adverse effects are diarrhea, nausea, vomiting, muscle cramps, rash, blurred vision, fatigue, depression, and problems with erections in men. Beta blockers should be discontinued gradually. Abrupt discontinuation can bring on an acute resurgence of symptoms. Notable reactions in some patients are heart palpitations, a rise in blood pressure, or recurrence of chest pain.

Check Your Understanding 13.1

A 64-year old man is taking atenolol (Tenormin) for treatment of hypertension. His seasonal allergies have been worse this year, and he is considering an OTC decongestant, pseudoephedrine (Sudafed), which a friend recommended. Is this medication safe for him to take? *Visit www.pearsonhighered.com/nursingresources for the answer.*

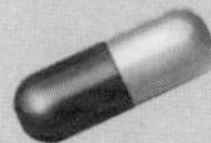

Prototype Drug | Prazosin (*Minipress*)

Therapeutic Class: Antihypertensive **Pharmacologic Class:** Adrenergic-blocking drug

Actions and Uses

Prazosin is a selective alpha$_1$-adrenergic antagonist that competes with norepinephrine at its receptors on vascular smooth muscle in arterioles and veins. Its major action is a rapid decrease in peripheral resistance that reduces blood pressure. It has little effect on cardiac output or heart rate, and it causes less reflex tachycardia than some other drugs in this class. Tolerance to prazosin's antihypertensive effect may occur. Its most common use is in combination with other drugs, such as beta blockers or diuretics, in the pharmacotherapy of hypertension. Prazosin has a short half-life and is often taken two or three times per day.

Administration Alerts

- Give a low first dose to avoid severe hypotension.
- Safety during pregnancy (category C) or lactation is not established.

Onset	Peak	Duration
2 H	2–4 H	LESS THAN 24 H

Adverse Effects

Like other alpha blockers, prazosin tends to cause orthostatic hypotension due to alpha$_1$ inhibition in vascular smooth muscle. In rare cases, this hypotension can cause unconsciousness about 30 minutes after the first dose. To avoid this situation, the first dose should be very low and given at bedtime. Dizziness, drowsiness, or light-headedness may occur. Reflex tachycardia may result from the rapid fall in blood pressure. Alpha blockade may cause nasal congestion or inhibition of ejaculation.

Contraindications: Safety during pregnancy and lactation is not established.

Interactions

Drug–Drug: Concurrent use of antihypertensives and diuretics results in extremely low blood pressure. Alcohol should be avoided.

Lab Tests: Prazosin increases urinary metabolites of vanillylmandelic acid (VMA) and norepinephrine, which are measured to screen for pheochromocytoma (adrenal tumor). Prazosin will cause false-positive results.

Herbal/Food: Do not use saw palmetto or nettle root products. Saw palmetto blocks alpha$_1$ receptors, resulting in the dilation of blood vessels and a hypotensive response.

Treatment of Overdose: Overdose may cause hypotension. Blood pressure may be elevated by the administration of fluid expanders, such as normal saline, or vasopressors, such as dopamine or dobutamine.

Nursing Practice Application

Pharmacotherapy With Adrenergic-Blocker Drugs

ASSESSMENT

Baseline assessment prior to administration:

- Obtain a complete health history including cardiovascular, cerebrovascular, respiratory disease, or diabetes. Obtain a drug history including allergies, current prescription and OTC drugs, herbal preparations, and alcohol use. Be alert to possible drug interactions.
- Evaluate appropriate laboratory findings including electrolytes, glucose, and hepatic and renal function studies.
- Obtain baseline weight, vital signs, and cardiac monitoring (e.g., ECG, cardiac output as appropriate).
- For treatment of BPH, assess urinary output.
- Assess the patient's ability to receive and understand instruction. Include the family and caregivers as needed.

POTENTIAL NURSING DIAGNOSES*

- *Decreased Cardiac Output*
- *Ineffective Tissue Perfusion*
- *Impaired Gas Exchange*
- *Ineffective Airway Clearance*
- *Impaired Urinary Elimination*
- *Activity Intolerance*
- *Deficient Knowledge* (drug therapy)
- *Risk for Falls,* related to adverse effects of drug therapy
- *Risk for Injury,* related to adverse effects of drug therapy
- *Risk for Disturbed Sleep Pattern,* related to adverse effects of drug therapy
- *Risk for Sexual Dysfunction,* related to adverse effects of drug therapy

*NANDA I © 2014

Nursing Practice Application *continued*

ASSESSMENT	POTENTIAL NURSING DIAGNOSES*
Assessment throughout administration: • Assess for desired therapeutic effects dependent on the reason for the drug (e.g., BP within normal range, dysrhythmias/palpitations relieved, greater ease in urination). • Continue frequent and careful monitoring of vital signs, daily weight, and urinary and cardiac output as appropriate, especially if IV administration is used. • Assess for and promptly report adverse effects: bradycardia, hypotension, dysrhythmias, reflex tachycardia (from too-rapid decrease in BP or hypotension), dizziness, headache, and decreased urinary output. Severe hypotension, seizures, and dysrhythmias/palpitations may signal drug toxicity and should be immediately reported.	

IMPLEMENTATION

Interventions and (Rationales)	Patient-Centered Care
Ensuring therapeutic effects: • Continue frequent assessments as described earlier for therapeutic effects dependent on the reason the drug therapy is given. Daily weights should remain at or close to baseline weight. (Pulse, BP, and respiratory rate should be within normal limits or within parameters set by the health care provider. Urinary hesitancy or frequency should be decreased and urine output improved. An increase in weight over 1 kg per day may indicate excessive fluid gain. **Diverse Patients:** Research indicates differing responses to antihypertensive therapy, including with adrenergic blocking drugs, in ethnically diverse populations compared to non-Hispanic whites.)	• Teach the patient, family, or caregiver how to monitor the pulse and BP as appropriate. Ensure the proper use and functioning of any home equipment obtained. • Have the patient weigh self daily along with BP and pulse measurements. The pulse rate should be taken for one full minute at a pulse point most easily felt. Report a weight gain or loss of more than 1 kg (2 lb) in a 24 hour period.
Minimizing adverse effects: • Continue to monitor vital signs. Take BP lying, sitting, and standing to detect orthostatic hypotension. Be particularly cautious with older adults, who are at increased risk for hypotension. Notify the health care provider if the BP or pulse decrease beyond established parameters or if hypotension is accompanied by reflex tachycardia. (Adrenergic drugs decrease heart rate and cause vasodilation, resulting in lowered BP. Orthostatic hypotension may increase the risk of falls or injury. **Lifespan:** Be aware that dizziness may increase the risk of falls in the older adult. Reflex tachycardia may signal that the BP has dropped too quickly or too substantially.)	• **Safety:** Teach the patient to rise from lying to sitting or standing slowly to avoid dizziness or falls. If dizziness occurs, the patient should sit or lie down and not attempt to stand or walk, until the sensation passes. • Instruct the patient to stop taking medication if BP is 90/60 mmHg or below, or parameters set by the health care provider, and immediately notify the provider.
• Continue cardiac monitoring (e.g., ECG) as ordered for dysrhythmias in the hospitalized patient. (External monitoring devices will detect early signs of adverse effects as well as monitoring for therapeutic effects.)	• Instruct the patient to immediately report palpitations, chest pain, or dyspnea.
• Weigh the patient daily and report a weight gain or loss of 1 kg (2 lb) or more in a 24-hour period. (Daily weight is an accurate measure of fluid status and takes into account intake, output, and insensible losses. Weight gain or edema may signal that BP has lowered too quickly, stimulating renin release or is an adverse effect.)	• Have the patient weigh self daily, ideally at the same time of day, and record weight along with BP and pulse measurements. Have the patient report a weight gain or loss of more than 1 kg (2 lb) in a 24-hour period.
• Monitor urine output and symptoms of dysuria such as hesitancy or retention when given for BPH. (Continued or worsening urinary symptoms may indicate need for further evaluation of the condition. **Lifespan:** Be aware that the male older adult with an enlarged prostate is at higher risk for mechanical obstruction.)	• Have the patient promptly report urinary hesitancy, feelings of bladder fullness, or difficulty starting urinary stream.
• **Safety:** Give the first dose of the drug at bedtime. (A first-dose response may result in a greater initial drop in BP than subsequent doses.)	• Instruct the patient to take the first dose of medication at bedtime, immediately before going to bed, and to avoid driving for 12 to 24 hours after the first dose or when the dosage is increased until the effects are known.

continued

Nursing Practice Application *continued*

IMPLEMENTATION	
Interventions and (Rationales)	**Patient-Centered Care**
• Continue to monitor blood glucose and appropriate laboratory work. (Adrenergic-blocking drugs affect a wide range of body systems. They may also interfere with some oral diabetic drugs or change the way a hypoglycemic reaction is perceived.) • Assess the patient's mental status and mood. (Adrenergic blockers may cause depression or dysphoria.)	• Teach the patient with diabetes to monitor blood glucose more frequently and to be aware of subtle signs of possible hypoglycemia (e.g., nervousness, irritability). The patient on oral antidiabetic drugs should promptly report any consistent changes in blood sugar levels to the health care provider. • Teach the patient to report unusual feelings of sadness, despondency, apathy, or depression that may warrant a change in medication.
• Provide for eye comfort such as adequately lighted room. (Adrenergic-blocking drugs can cause miosis and difficulty seeing in low-light levels.)	• **Safety**: Caution the patient about driving or other activities in low-light conditions or at night until the effects of the drug are known.
• Do not abruptly stop the medication. (Rebound hypertension and tachycardia may occur.)	• Teach the patient, family, or caregiver not to stop the medication abruptly and to call the health care provider if the patient is unable to take the medication for more than 1 day due to illness.
Patient understanding of drug therapy:	
• Use opportunities during administration of medications and during assessments to provide patient education. (Using time during nursing care helps to optimize and reinforce key teaching areas.)	• The patient, family, or caregiver should be able to state the reason for the drug; appropriate dose and scheduling; what adverse effects to observe for and when to report; equipment needed as appropriate and how to use that equipment; and the required length of medication therapy needed with any special instructions regarding renewing or continuing the prescription as appropriate.
Patient self-administration of drug therapy:	
• When administering medications, instruct the patient, family, or caregiver in the proper self-administration of drugs and ophthalmic drops. (Using time during nurse administration of these drugs helps to reinforce teaching.)	• Instruct the patient in proper administration techniques, followed by teach-back. • The drug should be taken at the same time each day when possible. • The patient, family, or caregiver is able to discuss appropriate dosing and administration needs.

See Table 13.4 for a list of drugs to which these nursing actions apply.

Chapter Review

KEY Concepts

The numbered key concepts provide a succinct summary of the important points from the corresponding numbered section within the chapter. If any of these points are not clear, refer to the numbered section within the chapter for review.

13.1 Norepinephrine is the primary neurotransmitter released at adrenergic receptors, which are divided into alpha and beta subtypes. Drugs can affect nervous transmission across a synapse by preventing the synthesis, storage, or release of the neurotransmitter; by preventing the destruction of the neurotransmitter; or by influencing the binding of neurotransmitters to the receptors.

13.2 Sympathomimetics act by directly activating adrenergic receptors, or indirectly by increasing the release of norepinephrine from nerve terminals. They are used primarily for their effects on the heart (hypertension, cardiac arrest), bronchial tree (asthma, COPD), and nasal passages (nasal congestion).

13.3 Adrenergic-blocking drugs are used primarily for treatment of hypertension (minor use for BPH) and are the most widely prescribed class of autonomic drugs.

REVIEW Questions

1. Following administration of phenylephrine (Neo-Synephrine), the nurse would assess for which of the following adverse drug effects?
   1. Insomnia, nervousness, and hypertension
   2. Nausea, vomiting, and hypotension
   3. Dry mouth, drowsiness, and dyspnea
   4. Increased bronchial secretions, hypotension, and bradycardia

2. A patient is started on atenolol (Tenormin). Which is the most important action to be included in the plan of care for this patient related to this medication?
   1. Monitor apical pulse and blood pressure
   2. Elevate the head of the bed during meals
   3. Take the medication after meals
   4. Consume foods high in potassium

3. Propranolol (Inderal) has been ordered for a patient with hypertension. Because of adverse effects related to this drug, the nurse would carefully monitor for which adverse effect?
   1. Bronchodilation
   2. Tachycardia
   3. Edema
   4. Bradycardia

4. The health care provider prescribes epinephrine (adrenalin) for a patient who was stung by several wasps 30 minutes ago and is experiencing an allergic reaction. The nurse knows that the primary purpose of this medication for this patient is to:
   1. Stop the systemic release of histamine produced by the mast cells.
   2. Counteract the formation of antibodies in response to an invading antigen.
   3. Increase the number of white blood cells produced to fight the primary invader.
   4. Increase a declining blood pressure and dilate constricting bronchi associated with anaphylaxis.

5. To avoid the first-dose phenomenon, the nurse knows that the initial dose of prazosin (Minipress) should be:
   1. Very low and given at bedtime.
   2. Doubled and given before breakfast.
   3. The usual dose and given before breakfast.
   4. The usual dose and given immediately after breakfast.

6. A patient who is taking an adrenergic-blocker for hypertension reports being dizzy when first getting out of bed in the morning. The nurse should advise the patient to:
   1. Move slowly from the recumbent to the upright position.
   2. Drink a full glass of water before rising to increase vascular circulatory volume.
   3. Avoid sleeping in a prone position.
   4. Stop taking the medication.

PATIENT-FOCUSED Case Study

Tyrone Mathey is a 48-year-old African American man who is an attorney at a large law firm. He has made an appointment with his provider today for increased feelings of anxiety, headaches, and "just not feeling well." His medical and family histories indicate that both of his parents died within the last 10 years. His father died of a stroke and his mother died of a heart attack. Mr. Mathey states that he has been prescribed prazosin (Minipress) in the past but he stopped taking it. When questioned about why he chose not to take the medication, he reluctantly confides in you that he suspected the medication was causing adverse sexual effects. His body temperature is 37°C (98.6°F), heart rate is 88 beats/min, respiratory rate is 18 breaths/min, and blood pressure is 160/90 mmHg. During the examination an ECG and laboratory test results were all within normal limits.

1. Identify the mechanism of action associated with prazosin (Minipress).
2. Could the prazosin (Minipress) be the cause of his sexual adverse effects?
3. As this patient's nurse, how would you approach the topic of medication-induced sexual dysfunction?

CRITICAL THINKING Questions

1. A 24-year-old patient is evaluated for seasonal allergies by his provider. Phenylephrine (Neo-Synephrine) nasal spray is recommended by the provider to treat symptoms related to allergic rhinitis. When teaching this patient about his medication, what therapeutic effects will the phenylephrine (Neo-Synephrine) provide? What adverse effects should the patient be observant for?
2. A 66-year-old man has had increasing trouble with urination, including difficulty starting to urinate and feeling that his bladder has not completely emptied. His provider prescribes doxazocin (Cardura) for treatment of BPH. The patient is alarmed and asks the nurse, "Why was I prescribed this? My brother takes it for high blood pressure and my blood pressure is normal!" As the nurse, how would you respond?

Visit www.pearsonhighered.com/nursingresources for answers and rationales for all activities.

REFERENCES

Campbell, R. L., Manivannan, V., Hartz, M. F., & Sadosty, A. T. (2012). Epinephrine auto-injector pandemic. *Pediatric Emergency Care, 28*, 938–942. doi:10.1097/PEC.0b013e318267f689

Chad, L., Ben-Shoshan, M., Asai, Y., Cherkaoui, S., Alizadehfar, R., St-Pierre, Y., . . . Clarke, A. (2013). A majority of parents of children with peanut allergy fear using the epinephrine auto-injector. *Allergy, 68*, 1605–1609. doi:10.1111/all.12262

Herdman, T. H., & Kamitsuru, S. (Eds.). (2014). *NANDA International nursing diagnoses: Definitions and classification, 2015–2017*. Oxford, United Kingdom: Wiley-Blackwell.

SELECTED BIBLIOGRAPHY

Biaggioni, I., & Robertson, D. (2015). Adrenoceptor agonists & sympathomimetic drugs. In B. G. Katzung, S. B. Masters, & A. J. Trevor (Eds.), *Basic and clinical pharmacology* (13th ed., pp. 152–168). New York, NY: McGraw-Hill.

De Lima, L. G., Saconato, H., Atallah, A. N., & da Silva, E. M. (2014). Beta-blockers for preventing stroke recurrence. *Cochrane Database of Systematic Reviews, 10*, Article No.:CD007890. doi:10.1002/14651858.CD007890.pub3

Larochelle, P., Tobe, S. W., & Lacourcière, Y. (2014). -Blockers in hypertension: Studies and meta-analyses over the years. *Canadian Journal of Cardiology, 30*(5 Suppl), S16–S22. doi:10.1016/j.cjca.2014.02.012.

Lieberman P., Nicklas, R. A., Oppenheimer, J., Kemp, S. F., Lang, D. M., Bernstein, D. I., . . . Wallace, D. (2010). The diagnosis and management of anaphylaxis practice parameter: 2010 update. *Journal of Allergy and Clinical Immunology, 126*, 477–480. doi:10.1016/j.jaci.2010.06.022

Lymperopoulos, A., Garcia, D., Walklett, K. (2014). Pharmacogenetics of cardiac inotropy. *Pharmacogenomics, 15*, 1807–1821. doi:10.2217/pgs.14.120

Sacco, E., Bientinesi, R., Tienforti, D., Racioppi, M., Gulino, G., D'Agostino, D., . . . Bassi, P. (2014). Discovery history and clinical development of mirabegron for the treatment of overactive bladder and urinary incontinence. *Expert Opinion on Drug Discovery, 9*, 433–448. doi:10.1517/17460441.2014.892923

Westfall T. C., & Westfall, D. P. (2011). Adrenergic agonists and antagonists. In: L. L. Brunton, B. A. Chabner, & B. C. Knollmann (Eds.), *Goodman and Gilman's the pharmacological basis of therapeutics* (12th ed.). New York, NY: McGraw-Hill.

Chapter 14

Drugs for Anxiety and Insomnia

Drugs at a Glance

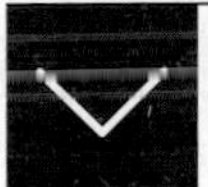

Learning Outcomes

After reading this chapter, the student should be able to:

1. Identify the major types of anxiety disorders.
2. Identify the regions of the brain associated with anxiety, sleep, and wakefulness.
3. Discuss factors contributing to anxiety and explain some nonpharmacologic therapies used to cope with this disorder.
4. Identify the three classes of medications used to treat anxiety and sleep disorders.
5. Explain the pharmacologic management of anxiety and insomnia.
6. Describe the nurse's role in the pharmacologic management of anxiety and insomnia.
7. Identify normal sleep patterns and explain how these might be affected by anxiety and stress.
8. Categorize drugs used for anxiety and insomnia based on their classification and mechanism of action.
9. For each of the drug classes listed in Drugs at a Glance, know representative drugs and explain their mechanisms of action, primary actions, and important adverse effects.
10. Use the nursing process to care for patients receiving pharmacotherapy for anxiety and insomnia.

(pill icon) indicates a prototype drug, each of which is featured in a Prototype Drug box.

Patients experience nervousness and tension more often than any other neurologic symptoms. Seeking relief, they often turn to a variety of pharmacologic and complementary and alternative medicine (CAM) therapies. Although drugs do not cure the underlying problem, most health care providers agree that they can provide temporary help to calm patients who are experiencing acute anxiety or who have simple sleep disorders. This chapter deals with drugs that treat anxiety, cause sedation, or help patients sleep.

ANXIETY DISORDERS

According to the *International Classification of Diseases*, 10th edition (ICD-10), **anxiety** is a state of apprehension, tension, or uneasiness resulting from imminent or perceived danger, the source of which is largely unknown. Anxious individuals can often identify at least some factors that bring on their symptoms. Most people state that their feelings of anxiety are disproportionate to any factual dangers.

14.1 Types of Anxiety Disorders

The anxiety experienced by people faced with a stressful environment is called **situational anxiety.** To a degree, situational anxiety is beneficial because it motivates people to promptly accomplish tasks—if for no other reason than to eliminate the source of nervousness. Situational stress may be intense, though patients often learn coping mechanisms to deal with the stress without seeking conventional medical intervention.

Generalized anxiety disorder (GAD) is a difficult-to-control, excessive anxiety that lasts 6 months or more. It focuses on a variety of life events or activities and interferes with normal day-to-day functions. It is the most common type of stress disorder and the one most frequently encountered by the nurse. Symptoms include restlessness, fatigue, muscle tension, nervousness, inability to focus or concentrate, an overwhelming sense of dread, and sleep disturbances. Autonomic signs of sympathetic nervous system activation that accompany anxiety include blood pressure elevation, heart palpitations, varying degrees of respiratory change, and dry mouth. Parasympathetic responses may consist of abdominal cramping, diarrhea, fatigue, and urinary urgency. Women are slightly more likely to experience GAD than men, and its prevalence is highest in the 20–35 age group.

A second category of intense anxiety, called **panic disorder,** is characterized by intense feelings of immediate apprehension, fearfulness, terror, or impending doom, accompanied by increased autonomic nervous system activity. Although panic attacks usually last less than 10 minutes, patients may describe them as seemingly endless. Up to 5% of the population will experience one or more panic attacks during their lifetime with women being affected about twice as often as men.

Other categories of anxiety disorders include phobias, obsessive–compulsive disorder, and post-traumatic stress disorder. **Phobias** are fearful feelings attached to situations or objects. Common phobias include fear of snakes, spiders, crowds, or heights. A persistent and unreasonable fear of being judged, ridiculed, or embarrassed by others is termed **social anxiety disorder,** or social phobia. Performing and speaking in public may cause feelings of dread, nervousness, or apprehension termed *performance anxiety*. Some anxiety is normal when a person faces or performs for a crowd, but extreme fear to the point of phobia is not normal. Symptoms of phobias include sweating, tachycardia, trembling, and bowel cramping.

Obsessive–compulsive disorder (OCD) involves recurrent, intrusive thoughts or repetitive behaviors that interfere with normal activities or relationships. Common examples include fear of exposure to germs and repetitive hand washing. **Post-traumatic stress disorder (PTSD)** is a type of extreme situational anxiety that develops in response to reexperiencing a previous life event. Traumatic life events such as war, physical or sexual abuse, rape and domestic violence, natural disasters, or homicidal situations may lead to a sense of helplessness and reexperiencing of the traumatic event. The terrorist attacks on September 11, 2001 and hurricane Katrina in 2005 are examples of situations that triggered many cases of PTSD around the turn of the millennium. Years of the war in Vietnam, Afghanistan, and Iraq have brought PTSD to the attention of the American public as military personnel continue to integrate into civilian society. People who experience lingering traumatic life events are at risk for developing signs and symptoms of PTSD. In those experiencing PTSD, the risk of attempted suicide is very high.

14.2 Specific Regions of the Brain Responsible for Anxiety and Wakefulness

Neural systems in the brain associated with anxiety and restlessness include the limbic system and the reticular activating system. These are illustrated in Pharmacotherapy Illustrated 14.1.

The **limbic system** is an area in the middle of the brain responsible for emotional expression, learning, and memory. Signals routed through the limbic system ultimately connect with the hypothalamus. Emotional states associated with this connection include anxiety, fear, anger, aggression, remorse, depression, sexual drive, and euphoria.

Pharmacotherapy Illustrated

14.1 | Regions of the Brain Affected by Antianxiety Medications

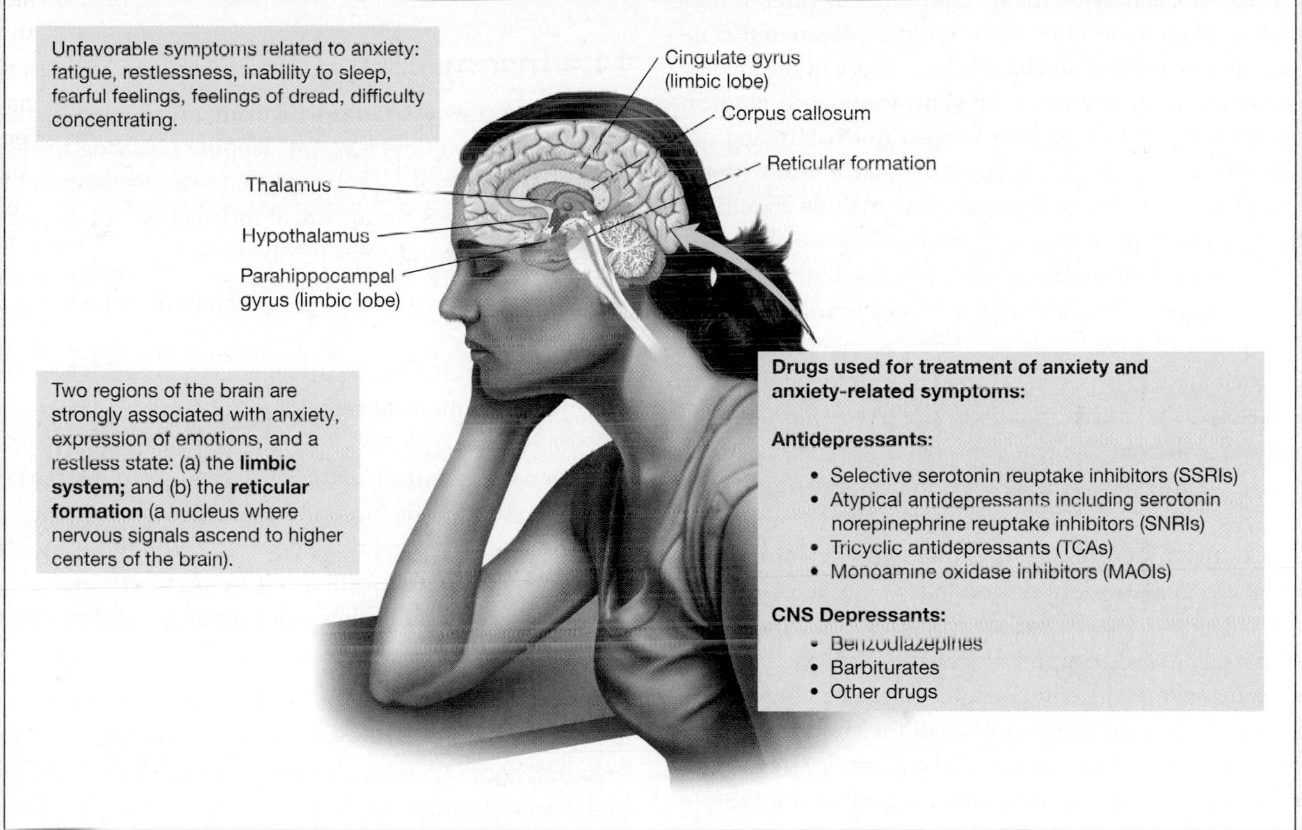
Unfavorable symptoms related to anxiety: fatigue, restlessness, inability to sleep, fearful feelings, feelings of dread, difficulty concentrating.
Cingulate gyrus (limbic lobe)
Corpus callosum
Reticular formation
Thalamus
Hypothalamus
Parahippocampal gyrus (limbic lobe)
Two regions of the brain are strongly associated with anxiety, expression of emotions, and a restless state: (a) the **limbic system;** and (b) the **reticular formation** (a nucleus where nervous signals ascend to higher centers of the brain).
Drugs used for treatment of anxiety and anxiety-related symptoms:
Antidepressants:
• Selective serotonin reuptake inhibitors (SSRIs)
• Atypical antidepressants including serotonin norepinephrine reuptake inhibitors (SNRIs)
• Tricyclic antidepressants (TCAs)
• Monoamine oxidase inhibitors (MAOIs)
CNS Depressants:
• Benzodiazepines
• Barbiturates
• Other drugs

The hypothalamus is an important center responsible for unconscious responses to extreme stress such as high blood pressure, elevated respiratory rate, and dilated pupils. These are responses associated with the fight-or-flight response of the autonomic nervous system, as presented in chapter 13. The many endocrine functions of the hypothalamus are discussed in chapter 44.

PharmFacts

ANXIETY DISORDERS

- Over 19 million Americans are diagnosed with anxiety every year.
- Illnesses that commonly coexist with anxiety include depression, eating disorders, and substance abuse.
- Prevalent anxiety disorders occur between the ages of 18 and 54:
  1. Phobia
  2. Post-traumatic stress disorder
  3. Generalized anxiety disorder
  4. Obsessive–compulsive disorder
  5. Panic disorder

As shown in Pharmacotherapy Illustrated 14.1, the hypothalamus connects with the **reticular formation,** a network of neurons found along the entire length of the brainstem. Stimulation of the reticular formation causes heightened alertness and arousal; inhibition causes general drowsiness and the induction of sleep.

The larger area in which the reticular formation is found is called the **reticular activating system (RAS).** This structure projects from the brainstem to the thalamus. The RAS is responsible for sleeping and wakefulness and performs an alerting function for the entire cerebral cortex. It helps a person focus attention on individual tasks by transmitting information to higher brain centers.

If signals are prevented from passing through the RAS, no emotion-related signals are sent to the brain, resulting in a reduction in general brain activity. If signals coming from the hypothalamus are allowed to proceed, then those signals are further routed through the RAS and on to integrative brain centers. This is the neural mechanism thought to be responsible for feelings such as anxiety and fear. It is also the mechanism associated with restlessness and an interrupted sleeping pattern.

14.3 Anxiety Management Through Pharmacologic and Nonpharmacologic Strategies

Although stress may be incapacitating, it is often only a symptom of an underlying disorder. It is considered more productive to uncover and address the cause of the anxiety rather than to merely treat the symptoms with medications. Patients should be encouraged to explore and develop nonpharmacologic coping strategies to deal with the underlying causes. Such strategies may include cognitive–behavioral therapy, counseling, biofeedback techniques, meditation, herbal products such as valerian, and other CAM therapies. One model for stress management is shown in Figure 14.1.

When anxiety becomes severe enough to significantly interfere with activities of daily living (ADLs), pharmacotherapy is indicated. In most types of stress, **anxiolytics,** or drugs having the ability to relieve anxiety, are quite effective. These include medications found within a number of therapeutic categories: central nervous system (CNS) agents such as antidepressants and CNS depressants; drugs for seizures (see chapter 15); emotional and mood disorder drugs (see chapter 16); antihypertensive agents (see chapter 26); and antidysrhythmics (see chapter 30). Anxiolytics provide treatment for all the conditions mentioned in Section 14.1: phobias, post-traumatic stress disorder, generalized anxiety disorder, obsessive–compulsive disorder, and panic attack.

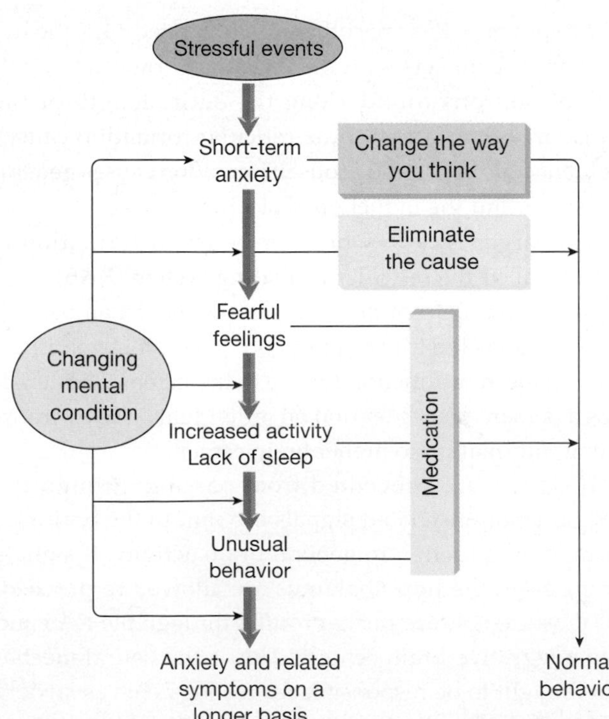

FIGURE 14.1 A model of anxiety in which stressful events or a changing mental condition can produce unfavorable symptoms, some of which may be controlled by medication

INSOMNIA

Insomnia is a condition characterized by a patient's inability to fall asleep or remain asleep. Pharmacotherapy may be indicated if the sleeplessness interferes with ADLs.

14.4 Insomnia and Its Link to Anxiety

Why is it that we need sleep? During an average lifetime, about 33% of the time is spent sleeping or trying to sleep. Although it is well established that sleep is essential for wellness, scientists are unsure of its function or how much is needed. Following are some theories:

- Inactivity during sleep gives the body time to repair itself.
- Sleep is a function that evolved as a protective mechanism. Throughout history, night-time was the safest time of day.
- Sleep deals with "electrical" charging and discharging of the brain. The brain needs time for processing and filing new information collected throughout the day. When this is done without interference from the outside environment, these vast amounts of data can be retrieved through memory.

The acts of sleeping and waking are synchronized to many different bodily functions. Body temperature, blood pressure, hormone levels, and respiration all fluctuate on a cyclic basis throughout the 24-hour day, known as the circadian rhythm. Disruption of the circadian rhythm may occur when traveling through multiple time zones (jet lag) or in those who alternate day and night shifts at work. When this cycle becomes impaired, pharmacologic or other interventions may be needed to readjust it.

PharmFacts

INSOMNIA

- One third of the world's population has trouble sleeping during part of the year.
- Insomnia is more common in women than in men.
- Patients who are older than 65 sleep less than patients in any other age group.
- Only about 70% of people with insomnia ever report this problem to their health care providers.
- People buy over-the-counter (OTC) sleep medications and combination drugs with sleep additives more often than any other drug category. Examples of trade-name products are Anacin PM, Excedrin PM, Nytol, Sleep-Eze, Sominex, Tylenol PM, and Unisom.
- As a natural solution for sleep, some patients consider melatonin or herbal remedies such as valerian (see chapter 10) (Bernert, Turvey, Conwell, and Joiner, 2014).

Insomnia, or sleeplessness, is a disorder sometimes associated with anxiety. There are several major types of insomnia. **Short-term** or **behavioral insomnia** may be attributed to stress caused by a hectic lifestyle or the inability to resolve day-to-day conflicts within the home environment or the workplace. Worries about work, marriage, children, and health are common reasons for short-term loss of sleep. When stress interrupts normal sleeping patterns, patients cannot sleep because their minds are too active.

Some people are consistently tired during the day. A drowsy state during the day could be due to loss of sleep at night, or the patient may have narcolepsy. **Narcolepsy** is characterized by overwhelming daytime drowsiness and sudden attacks of sleep during the day. Additional sleep disorders that cause daytime sleepiness are sleep apnea and restless legs syndrome. Provigil (Modafinil) is a wakefulness-promoting drug approved by the U.S. Food and Drug Administration (FDA) for oral (PO) administration to treat narcolepsy.

Some consumed substances and medications can be linked with a restless sleep pattern. Foods or beverages containing stimulants such as caffeine may interrupt sleep. Patients may also find that the use of tobacco products makes them restless and edgy. Alcohol, although often enabling a person to fall asleep, may produce vivid dreams and frequent awakenings that prevent restful sleep. Ingestion of a large meal, especially one high in protein and fat, consumed close to bedtime can interfere with sleep, due to the increased metabolic rate needed to digest the food. Certain medications cause CNS stimulation, and these should not be taken immediately before bedtime.

Stressful conditions such as too much light, uncomfortable room temperature (especially one that is too warm), snoring, and recurring nightmares also interfere with sleep. **Long-term insomnia,** that which lasts 30 days or longer, is often caused by depression, manic disorders, and or chronic pain. Mental health disorders and certain medical conditions are often linked with an interrupted sleep pattern.

Nonpharmacologic means should be attempted prior to initiating drug therapy for sleep disorders. Long-term use of sleep medications is likely to worsen insomnia and may cause physical or psychological dependence. Some patients experience a phenomenon referred to as **rebound insomnia.** This condition occurs when a sedative drug is discontinued abruptly or after it has been taken for a long time; sleeplessness and symptoms of anxiety then become markedly worse.

Older patients are more likely to experience medication-related sleep problems. Drugs may seem to help the insomnia of an elderly patient for a night or two, only to produce generalized brain dysfunction as the medication accumulates in the system. The agitated patient may then be mistakenly overdosed with further medication. Nurses, especially those who work in geriatric settings, are responsible for making accurate observations and reporting patient responses to drugs so the health care provider can determine the lowest effective maintenance dose. When as needed (prn) medication is required for sleep, the nurse needs to conduct an individualized assessment of the patient as well as follow-up evaluation and documentation of the medication's effect.

14.5 Use of the Electroencephalogram to Diagnose Sleep Disorders

The **electroencephalogram (EEG)** is a tool for diagnosing sleep disorders, seizure activity, depression, and dementia. Four types of brain waves—alpha, beta, delta, and theta—are identified by their shape, frequencies, and height on a graph. Brain waves give the health care provider an idea of how brain activity changes during various stages of sleep and consciousness. For example, alpha waves indicate an awake but drowsy patient. Beta waves indicate an alert patient whose mind is active.

Two distinct types of sleep can be identified with an EEG: nonrapid eye movement (NREM) sleep and rapid eye movement (REM) sleep. There are three progressive stages that advance into REM sleep. The stages of sleep are shown in Table 14.1. After NREM sleep has gone through

Complementary and Alternative Therapies

MELATONIN

Melatonin is a natural hormone produced during the night by the pineal gland. The secretion of melatonin is stimulated by darkness and inhibited by light. As melatonin production rises, alertness decreases and body temperature starts to fall, both of which make sleep more inviting. Melatonin production is related to age. Children manufacture more melatonin than older adults; however, melatonin production begins to drop at puberty.

Melatonin appears to help people, particularly older adults, to fall asleep faster. The National Center for Complementary and Integrative Health (NCCIH, 2014) cites evidence that melatonin also appears to be useful in people with insomnia related to disrupted circadian rhythm cycles. It is believed that melatonin helps to reset the circadian rhythm for these patients, rather than cause drowsiness. Melatonin appears to be safe for short-term use but it is not free of side effects. It may cause nausea, headache, or dizziness, and has been noted to adversely affect mood in patients with dementia (NCCIH, 2014).

PharmFacts

INSOMNIA LINKED TO INSULIN RESISTANCE

- Chronic lack of sleep may make people more prone to developing type 2 diabetes.
- Chronic lack of sleep can provide the impetus for the body to develop a reduced sensitivity to insulin.
- Healthy adults who sleep less during the night tend to secrete more insulin than those who sleep more hours during the same period.
- Exercise and outside activities tend to reverse unfavorable metabolic signs, especially in older patients.
- Sleep deprivation (6.5 hours or less per night) is possibly one of the factors why type 2 diabetes is becoming more prevalent.

the three stages, the sequence may go in reverse. Under normal circumstances, after returning from the depths of stage 3 back to stage 1 of NREM, a person will still not awaken. Sleep quality begins to change; it is not as deep, and hormone levels and body temperature begin to rise. At that point, REM sleep occurs. **Rapid eye movement (REM) sleep** is often called paradoxical sleep, because the brain wave pattern of this stage is similar to that when persons are drowsy but awake. This is the stage during which dreaming occurs. People with normal sleep patterns move from NREM to REM sleep about every 90 minutes.

Patients who are deprived of stage 3 NREM sleep experience depression and a feeling of apathy and fatigue. Stage 3 NREM sleep appears to be linked to repair and restoration of the physical body, whereas REM sleep is associated with learning, memory, and the capacity to adjust to changes in the environment. It appears that the body requires the REM dream state to keep the psyche functioning normally. When test subjects are deprived of REM sleep, they experience a **sleep debt** and become frightened, irritable, paranoid, and even emotionally disturbed. Judgment is impaired, and reaction time is slowed. It is speculated that to make up for their lack of dreaming, these persons experience far more daydreaming and fantasizing throughout the day.

CENTRAL NERVOUS SYSTEM DRUGS

CNS drugs can produce profound activity in the brain and spinal cord. **CNS depressants** are drugs that slow neuronal activity in the brain. Patients experiencing anxiety or sleep disorders benefit from four general classes of medications: antidepressants, benzodiazepines, barbiturates, and nonbenzodiazepine/nonbarbiturate CNS depressants.

Table 14.1 Stages of Sleep

Stage	Description
NREM stage 1	At the onset of sleep, the patient is in a stage of drowsiness for about 5 to 10 minutes. During this time, the patient can be easily awakened.
NREM stage 2	The patient is still in light sleep. The heart rate slows and the body temperature drops.
NREM stage 3	This the deepest stage of sleep. It is harder to wake up the patient in this stage. The patient is disoriented for a brief time.
REM sleep	This stage is characterized by eye movement and loss of muscle tone. Eye movement occurs in bursts of activity. Dreaming takes place in this stage. The mind is very active and resembles a normal waking state.

Additional drug classes have anxiolytic activity and prevent stressful reactions in the body.

14.6 Treating Anxiety and Insomnia With CNS Drugs

Anxiolytic drugs have an ability to reduce anxiety symptoms by altering levels of two important neurotransmitters in the brain, norepinephrine and serotonin. Restoration of normal neurotransmitter balance helps to reduce symptoms associated with depression, panic, obsessive–compulsive behavior, and phobia.

CNS depressants used for anxiety and sleep disorders are categorized into four major classes: the antidepressants, benzodiazepines, nonbenzodiazepine anxiolytics, and barbiturates. Other CNS depressants that have a calming effect in the body include the opioids (see chapter 18) and ethyl alcohol (see chapter 22).

CNS depression should be viewed as a continuum ranging from relaxation, to sedation, to the induction of sleep and anesthesia. Coma and death are the end stages of CNS depression. Some drug classes are capable of producing the full range of CNS depression from calming to anesthesia, whereas others are less efficacious. Medications that depress the CNS are sometimes called **sedatives** because of their ability to sedate or relax a patient. At higher doses, some of these drugs are called **hypnotics** because of their ability to induce sleep. Thus, the term **sedative–hypnotic** is often used to describe a drug with the ability to produce a calming effect at lower doses and the ability to induce sleep at higher doses. **Tranquilizer** is an older term that is sometimes used to describe a drug that produces a calm or tranquil feeling.

Many CNS depressants can cause physical and psychological dependence, as discussed in chapter 22. The withdrawal syndrome for some CNS depressants can cause life-threatening neurologic reactions, including fever, psychosis, and seizures. Other withdrawal symptoms

Community-Oriented Practice

SAFETY OF ANTIHISTAMINES FOR SLEEP

Antihistamines, particularly the older first-generation "sedating" forms such as diphenhydramine (Benadryl, Sominex, others), are commonly found in OTC sleep remedies and are widely used to help promote sleep. While the drowsiness and sedation caused by these drugs may be an annoying side effect when the drugs are used for allergies, it is this property that helps to induce sleep when used for nighttime sedation. Residual daytime sleepiness and effects on cognitive function have been noted (Katayose et al., 2012). Recent studies have also shown that both original and second-generation antihistamines may have an effect on quality of sleep, mood, reaction time, and motor movement (Kavanaugh, Grant, & Anoopkumar-Dukie, 2012; Naicker, Anoopkumar-Dukie, Grant, & Kavanaugh, 2013; Ozdemir et al., 2014).

Patients who use OTC antihistamine sleep aids should be cautioned about the potential for daytime drowsiness. They should also be taught that more subtle effects such as slowed reaction time, impaired cognitive function, and other systemic effects, may occur even when daytime drowsiness is not evident. This is particularly important when used by older adults and by patients with existing movement difficulties. When used to promote sleep, they should be used short-term only (Vande Griend & Anderson, 2012). Because tolerance to these drugs develops over time, continued insomnia should be evaluated by the provider to ensure appropriate treatment.

include increased heart rate and lowered blood pressure; loss of appetite; muscle cramps; impairment of memory, concentration, and orientation; abnormal sounds in the ears and blurred vision; and insomnia, agitation, anxiety, and panic. Obvious withdrawal symptoms typically last from 2 to 4 weeks. Subtle ones can last months.

Antidepressants

Until the 1980s, **antidepressants** or medications that enhance mood were used mainly to treat depression or depression that accompanied anxiety. Today, antidepressants are used not only to treat major depression (see chapter 16), but also anxiety conditions including GAD, OCD, panic, social phobia, and PTSD.

14.7 Antidepressants for Symptoms of Panic and Anxiety

For most patients, panic symptoms come in two stages. The first stage is termed *anticipatory anxiety*, in which the patient begins to think about an upcoming challenge and starts to experience feelings of dread. The second stage is when physical symptoms such as shortness of breath, accelerated heart rate, and muscle tension start to emerge. Many of the stressful symptoms are associated with activation of the autonomic nervous system (see chapter 13). For panic attacks, the most useful therapy is to help the patient become motivated to face his or her fear and to suppress symptoms in one or more of these stages. If drugs can reduce the negative thoughts associated with the anticipatory component of panic, then there is less likelihood that the patient will feel stressed. Drugs also reduce neuronal activity and actually suppress the autonomic nervous system, helping the patient to remain calm. The patient can then use self-help skills to control his or her behavior.

Historically, antidepressant medications used to reduce symptoms of panic and anxiety have been the tricyclic antidepressants (TCAs), monamine oxidase inhibitors (MAOIs), and selective serotonin reuptake inhibitors (SSRIs). The newer first-line SSRIs have treated not only panic symptoms but also symptoms of GAD, OCD, PTSD, and phobias (Table 14.2). Popular SSRIs available for treatment of anxiety symptoms and depression include citalopram (Celexa), escitalopram (Lexapro), fluoxetine (Prozac), paroxetine (Paxil), and sertraline (Zoloft). Escitalopram (Lexapro) is featured as a prototype drug primarily used for treating GAD.

Atypical antidepressants are drugs that do not fall conveniently into the other categories. Mirtazapine may be useful in managing sleep disturbances or agitation. Adverse effects for mirtazapine involve weight gain, constipation, and dry mouth. Trazodone may be used along with an SSRI to help with restlessness and insomnia. Blurred vision, headache, and nausea are among the adverse effects expected with trazadone.

Because of adverse reactions, some patients might find antidepressant treatment unacceptable. In 2004, the FDA issued a black box warning pointing out the potential warning signs of suicide in adults and children at the beginning of antidepressant treatment and when doses are changed. Also, many symptoms that are the focus of anxiety therapy might be expected to occur with the use of antidepressants. These signs include irritability, panic attacks, agitation, insomnia, and hostility. See chapter 16 for important primary actions and adverse effects of antidepressant drugs in general.

Following is a brief summary of additional important considerations for each class of antidepressant:

Table 14.2 Antidepressants for Treatment of Anxiety Symptoms, Restlessness, and Depression

Drug	Route and Adult Dose (max dose where indicated)	Adverse Effects
SELECTIVE SEROTONIN REUPTAKE INHIBITORS (SSRIs)		
citalopram (Celexa)	PO: start at 20 mg/day; may increase to 40 mg/day if needed	*Nausea, vomiting, dry mouth, insomnia, somnolence, headache, nervousness, anxiety, gastrointestinal (GI) disturbances, anorexia, sexual dysfunction, agitation, dizziness, fatigue* Stevens–Johnson syndrome (SJS), extreme mania/hypomania, and suicidality (especially in children), abnormal bleeding, extreme psychomotor disturbances, seizures, autonomic instability with possible rapid fluctuations of vital signs, severe hyperthermia, serotonin syndrome
escitalopram (Lexapro)	PO: 10 mg/day; may increase to 20 mg/day if needed after 1 wk	
fluoxetine (Prozac)	PO: 20 mg/day in a.m.; may increase by 20 mg/day at weekly intervals (max: 80 mg/day); when stable may switch to one 90-mg sustained-release capsule per week (max: 90 mg/wk)	
fluvoxamine (Luvox)	PO: start with 50 mg/day; may increase slowly up to 300 mg/day given at bedtime or divided bid	
paroxetine (Paxil, Pexeva, others)	PO: 20–60 mg/day	
sertraline (Zoloft) (see page 206 for the Prototype Drug box)	PO: begin with 50 mg/day; gradually increase every few weeks according to response (range: 50–200 mg)	
ATYPICAL ANTIDEPRESSANTS		
duloxetine (Cymbalta)	PO: 40–60 mg/day in one or two divided doses	*Erratic heart rate and blood pressure, orthostatic hypotension, dry mouth, dizziness, somnolence, nausea, vomiting, sweating* Severe hostility, impulsivity, mental status changes that include extreme agitation progressing to delirium and coma, suicidality (especially in children)
mirtazapine (Remeron)	PO: 15 mg/day in a single dose at bedtime; may increase every 1–2 wk (max: 45 mg/day)	
trazodone (Desyrel, Oleptro)	PO: 150 mg/day in divided doses; may increase by 50 mg/day over 3–4 days (max: 400–600 mg/day)	
venlafaxine (Effexor)	PO: start with 37.5 mg/day sustained release and increase to 75–225 mg/day sustained release	
TRICYCLIC ANTIDEPRESSANTS (TCAs)		
amitriptyline (Elavil)	PO: 75–100 mg/day, may gradually increase to 150–300 mg/day (use lower doses in nonhospitalized patients)	*Drowsiness, sedation, dizziness, orthostatic hypotension, dry mouth, constipation, urine retention, weight gain, tremor, dysrhythmias, blurred vision, slight mydriasis* Agranulocytosis; bone marrow depression; seizures; heart block; myocardial infarction (MI); angioedema of the face, tongue, or generalized
clomipramine (Anafranil)	PO: 75–300 mg/day in divided doses	
desipramine (Norpramin)	PO: 75–100 mg/day at bedtime or in divided doses; may gradually increase to 150–300 mg/day (use lower doses in older adult patients)	
doxepin (Silenor)	PO: 30–150 mg/day at bedtime or in divided doses; may gradually increase to 300 mg/day (use lower doses in older adult patients)	
imipramine (Tofranil) (see page 208 for the Prototype Drug box)	PO: 75–100 mg/day (max: 300 mg/day) in single or divided doses	
nortriptyline (Aventyl, Pamelor)	PO: 25 mg tid or qid, gradually increased to 100–150 mg/day	
trimipramine (Surmontil)	PO: 75–100 mg/day (max 300 mg/day) in divided doses	
MONOAMINE OXIDASE INHIBITORS (MAOIs)		
phenelzine (Nardil) (see page 209 for the Prototype Drug box)	PO: 15 mg tid, rapidly increasing to at least 60 mg/day; may need up to 90 mg/day	*Orthostatic hypotension, constipation, dry mouth, nausea*
tranylcypromine (Parnate)	PO: 30 mg/day in two divided doses (20 mg in a.m., 10 mg in p.m.); may increase by 10 mg/day at 3-wk intervals (max: 60 mg/day)	Hypertensive crisis, hyperthermia

Note: *Italics* indicate common adverse effects; underlining indicates serious adverse effects.

- *SSRIs.* Safer than other classes of antidepressants; less common sympathomimetic effects (increased heart rate and hypertension) and fewer anticholinergic effects; SSRIs can cause weight gain and sexual dysfunction; an overdose of this medication can cause confusion, anxiety, restlessness, hypertension, tremors, sweating, fever, and lack of muscle coordination. Patients taking these medications must be carefully monitored for changes in behavior or suicidal tendencies.

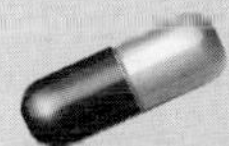

Prototype Drug | Escitalopram *(Lexapro)*

Therapeutic Class: Antidepressant; anxiolytic
Pharmacologic Class: Selective serotonin reuptake inhibitor (SSRI)

Actions and Uses
Escitalopram is an SSRI that increases the availability of serotonin at specific postsynaptic receptor sites located within the CNS. Selective inhibition of serotonin reuptake results in antidepressant activity without production of symptoms of sympathomimetic or anticholinergic activity. This medication is indicated for conditions of generalized anxiety and depression. Off-label uses include the treatment of panic disorders.

Administration Alerts

- This medication should not be started until 14 days have elapsed after discontinuing any MAOI drugs.
- In cases of renal or hepatic impairment or in older adults, reduced doses are advised.
- Dose increments should be separated by at least 1 week.
- Pregnancy category C.

PHARMACOKINETICS

Onset	Peak	Duration
With once-daily dosing, steady-state plasma concentrations can be reached within 1 wk	5 h	Variable

Adverse Effects
Serious reactions include dizziness, nausea, insomnia, somnolence, confusion, and seizures if taken in overdose.

Black Box Warning*:* Antidepressants increase the risk of suicidal thinking and behavior in children, adolescents, and young adults with major depressive disorder and other psychiatric disorders. This drug is not approved for pediatric patients less than 12 years of age.

Contraindications: This drug should not be used in patients who are breast-feeding or within 14 days of MAOI therapy.

Interactions
Drug–Drug: MAOIs should be avoided due to serotonin syndrome, marked by autonomic hyperactivity, hyperthermia, rigidity, diaphoresis, and neuroleptic malignant syndrome. Combination with MAOIs could result in hypertensive crisis, hyperthermia, and autonomic instability.

Escitalopram will increase plasma levels of metoprolol and cimetidine. Concurrent use of alcohol and other CNS depressants may enhance CNS depressant effects; patients should avoid alcohol when taking this drug.

Lab Tests: Unknown.

Herbal/Food: Use caution with herbal supplements such as St. John's wort, which may cause serotonin syndrome and increase the effects of escitalopram.

Treatment of Overdose: There is no specific treatment for overdose. Treat symptoms, as indicated, including dizziness, confusion, nausea, vomiting, tremor, sweating, tachycardia, and seizures.

- *Atypical antidepressants including serotonin–norepinephrine reuptake inhibitors (SNRIs).* Adverse effects include abnormal dreams, sweating, constipation, dry mouth, loss of appetite, weight loss, tremor, abnormal vision, headaches, nausea and vomiting, dizziness, and loss of sexual desire. Patients taking these medications must be carefully monitored for changes in behavior or suicidal tendencies.
- *TCAs.* Not recommended in patients with a history of heart attack, heart block, or arrhythmia; patients often have annoying anticholinergic effects such as dry mouth, blurred vision, urine retention, and hypertension (see chapter 12); most TCAs are pregnancy category C or D; concurrent use with alcohol or other CNS depressants should be avoided; patients with asthma, GI disorders, alcoholism, schizophrenia, or bipolar disorder should take TCAs with extreme caution.
- *MAOIs.* Patients must strictly avoid foods containing tyramine, a form of the amino acid tyrosine, to avoid a hypertensive crisis and should refrain from caffeine intake; MAOIs potentiate the effects of insulin and other diabetic drugs; common adverse effects include orthostatic hypotension, headache, and diarrhea; rarely used because of the potential for serious adverse effects.

Benzodiazepines

The benzodiazepines are one of the most widely prescribed drug classes. The root word *benzo* refers to an aromatic compound. Characteristic of an aromatic is its carbon ring structure, which may be attached to another carbon ring or to a different grouping of atoms. Two nitrogen atoms incorporated into the basic chemical structure of the compound account for the *diazepine* name (*di* = two; *azepine* = nitrogen-containing).

14.8 Treating Anxiety and Insomnia With Benzodiazepines

The benzodiazepines are preferred drugs for various anxiety disorders and for insomnia (Table 14.3). Since the introduction of the first benzodiazepines—chlordiazepoxide (Librium) and diazepam (Valium)—in the 1960s, the class has become one of the most widely prescribed in medicine. Although many benzodiazepines are available, all have the same actions and adverse effects and differ primarily in their onset and duration of action. Although used for other therapies, some, such as midazolam (Versed), have a rapid onset time of 15 to 30 minutes; others, such as halazepam (Paxipam), take 1 to 3 hours to reach peak serum levels. The benzodiazepines are categorized as Schedule IV drugs, although they produce considerably less physical dependence and result in less tolerance than the barbiturates.

Benzodiazepines act by binding to the gamma-aminobutyric acid (GABA) receptor–chloride channel molecule. These drugs intensify the effect of GABA, which is a natural inhibitory neurotransmitter found throughout the brain. Most are metabolized in the liver to active metabolites and are excreted primarily in urine. One major advantage of the benzodiazepines is that they do not produce life-threatening respiratory depression or coma if taken in excessive amounts. Death is unlikely, unless the benzodiazepines are taken in large quantities in combination with other CNS depressants, or if the patient suffers from sleep apnea.

Most benzodiazepines are given orally. Those that can be given parenterally, such as diazepam (Valium) and lorazepam (Ativan), should be monitored carefully due to their rapid onset of CNS effects and due to potential respiratory depression with adjunctive therapies.

The benzodiazepines are preferred drugs for the short-term treatment of insomnia caused by anxiety and have replaced the barbiturates because of their greater margin of safety. Benzodiazepines shorten the length of time it takes to fall asleep and reduce the frequency of interrupted sleep. Although most benzodiazepines increase total sleep time, some reduce stage 3 sleep, and some affect REM sleep. In general, the benzodiazepines used to treat short-term insomnia are different from those used to treat GAD.

Benzodiazepines have a number of other important indications. Diazepam (Valium) is featured as a prototype drug for treating seizure disorders in chapter 15. Other uses include treatment of alcohol withdrawal symptoms (see chapter 22), central muscle relaxation (see chapter 21), and as induction agents in general anesthesia (see chapter 19).

Table 14.3 Benzodiazepines for Anxiety and Insomnia

Drug	Route and Adult Dose (max dose where indicated)	Adverse Effects
ANXIETY THERAPY		
alprazolam (Xanax)	For anxiety: PO: 0.25–0.5 mg tid (max: 4 mg/day) For panic attacks: PO: 1–2 mg tid (max: 8 mg/day)	*Drowsiness, sedation, lethargy, ataxia* Physical dependence, acute hyperexcited states, hallucinations, increased muscle spasticity, renal impairment, congenital defects among women who are pregnant, respiratory impairment due to hypersalivation, respiratory depression, laryngospasm, cardiovascular collapse
chlordiazepoxide (Librium)	Mild anxiety: PO: 5–10 mg tid or qid; IM/IV: 50–100 mg 1 h before a medical procedure Severe anxiety: PO: 20–25 mg tid or qid; IM/IV: 50–100 mg followed by 25–50 mg tid or qid	
clonazepam (Klonopin)	PO: 1–2 mg/day in divided doses (max: 4 mg/day)	
clorazepate (Tranxene)	PO: 15 mg/day at bedtime (max: 60 mg/day in divided doses)	
diazepam (Valium) (see page 190 for the Prototype Drug box)	PO: 2–10 mg bid IM/IV: 2–10 mg: repeat if needed in 3–4 h	
lorazepam (Ativan)	PO: 2–6 mg/day in divided doses (max: 10 mg/day)	
oxazepam (Serax)	PO: 10–30 mg tid or qid	
INSOMNIA THERAPY		
estazolam (Prosom)	PO: 1 mg at bedtime; may increase to 2 mg if necessary	*Drowsiness, somnolence, headache, memory impairment* Agranulocytosis, coma
flurazepam (Dalmane)	PO: 15–30 mg at bedtime	
quazepam (Doral)	PO: 7.5–15 mg at bedtime	
temazepam (Restoril)	PO: 7.5–30 mg at bedtime	
triazolam (Halcion)	PO: 0.125–0.25 mg at bedtime (max: 0.5 mg/day)	

Note: *Italics* indicate common adverse effects; underlining indicates serious adverse effects.

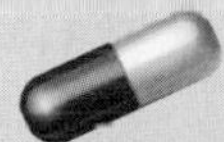

Prototype Drug | Lorazepam *(Ativan)*

Therapeutic Class: Sedative–hypnotic; anxiolytic; anesthetic adjunct
Pharmacologic Class: Benzodiazepine; $GABA_A$-receptor agonist

Actions and Uses
Lorazepam is a benzodiazepine that acts by potentiating the effects of GABA, an inhibitory neurotransmitter, in the thalamic, hypothalamic, and limbic levels of the CNS. It is one of the most potent benzodiazepines. It has an extended half-life of 10 to 20 hours, which allows for once- or twice-a-day oral dosing. In addition to being used as an anxiolytic, lorazepam is used as a preanesthetic medication to provide sedation and for the management of status epilepticus. Unlabeled uses include the treatment of chemotherapy-induced nausea and vomiting.

Administration Alerts

- When administering intravenous (IV), monitor respirations every 5 to 15 minutes. Have airway and resuscitative equipment accessible.
- Pregnancy category D.

PHARMACOKINETICS

Onset	Peak	Duration
1–5 min IV; 15–30 min IM; 30 minutes PO	90 min IM; 2 h PO	Variable

Adverse Effects
The most common adverse effects of lorazepam are drowsiness and sedation, which may decrease with time. When given in higher doses or by the IV route, more severe effects may be observed, such as amnesia, weakness, disorientation, ataxia, sleep disturbance, blood pressure changes, blurred vision, double vision, nausea, and vomiting.

Contraindications: This drug should not be used in patients with acute narrow angle glaucoma, closed-angle glaucoma, misuse or excessive use of drugs, liver disease, impaired brain function, or thoughts of suicide.

Interactions
Drug–Drug: Lorazepam interacts with multiple drugs. For example, concurrent use of CNS depressants, including alcohol, potentiates sedative effects and increases the risk of respiratory depression and death. Symptoms include visual changes, nausea, vomiting, dizziness, and confusion. Lorazepam may decrease the antiparkinsonism effects of levodopa and increase phenytoin levels.

Lab Tests: Unknown.

Herbal/Food: Use cautiously with herbal supplements. For example, sedation-producing herbs such as kava, valerian, chamomile, or hops may have an additive effect with medication. Stimulant herbs such as gotu kola and ma huang may reduce the drug's effectiveness.

Treatment of Overdose: If overdose occurs, flumazenil (Romazicon), a specific benzodiazepine receptor antagonist, can be administered to reverse CNS depressant effects.

Barbiturates

Barbiturates are drugs derived from barbituric acid. They are powerful CNS depressants prescribed for their sedative, hypnotic, and antiseizure effects that have been used in pharmacotherapy since the early 1900s.

14.9 Use of Barbiturates as Sedatives

Until the discovery of the benzodiazepines, barbiturates were the drugs of choice for treating anxiety and insomnia (Table 14.4). Although barbiturates are still indicated for several conditions, they are rarely, if ever, prescribed for treating anxiety or insomnia because of significant adverse effects and the availability of more effective medications. The risk of psychological and physical dependence is high—several are Schedule II drugs. The withdrawal syndrome from barbiturates is extremely severe and can be fatal. Overdose results in profound respiratory depression, hypotension, and shock. Barbiturates have been used to commit suicide, and death due to overdose is not uncommon.

Barbiturates are capable of depressing CNS function at all levels. Like benzodiazepines, barbiturates act by binding to GABA receptor–chloride channel molecules, intensifying the effect of GABA throughout the brain. At low doses they reduce anxiety and cause drowsiness. At moderate doses they inhibit seizure activity (see chapter 15) and promote sleep, presumably by inhibiting brain impulses traveling through the limbic system and the RAS. At higher doses, some barbiturates can induce anesthesia (see chapter 19).

Check Your Understanding 14.1
Benzodiazepines are among the first-line drugs for treating insomnia and anxiety disorders. Why would these drugs pose a safety risk in the older adult? What are the nursing considerations for these drugs when used in the older adult population? *Visit www.pearsonhighered.com/nursingresources for the answers.*

Table 14.4 Barbiturates With Sedative and Hypnotic Properties

Drug	Route and Adult Dose (max dose where indicated)	Adverse Effects
SHORT ACTING		
pentobarbital (Nembutal)	Hypnotic: IM: 150–200 mg	Respiratory depression, laryngospasm, apnea
secobarbital (Seconal)	Hypnotic: PO: 100 mg at bedtime	
INTERMEDIATE ACTING		
butabarbital (Butisol)	Hypnotic: PO: 100 mg at bedtime	*Residual sedation* Agranulocytosis, angioedema, SJS, respiratory depression, circulatory collapse, apnea, laryngospasm
LONG ACTING		
phenobarbital (Luminal) (see page 189 for the Prototype Drug box)	Sedative/Hypnotic: PO: 30–120 mg/day; IV/IM: 100–200 mg/day	*Drowsiness, somnolence* Agranulocytosis, respiratory depression, SJS, exfoliative dermatitis (rare), CNS depression, coma, death

Note: *Italics* indicate common adverse effects; underlining indicates serious adverse effects.

When taken for prolonged periods, barbiturates stimulate the microsomal enzymes in the liver that metabolize medications. Thus, barbiturates can stimulate their own metabolism as well as that of hundreds of other drugs that use these enzymes for their breakdown. With repeated use, tolerance develops to the sedative effects of the drug; this includes cross-tolerance to other CNS depressants such as the opioids. Tolerance does not develop, however, to the respiratory depressant effects. (See chapter 15, for Nursing Practice Application: Pharmacotherapy with Antiseizure Drugs.)

Nonbenzodiazepine, Nonbarbiturate CNS Depressants

These drugs reduce anxiety symptoms but are chemically different from the other anxiolytic drug classes.

14.10 Other CNS Depressants for Anxiety and Sleep Disorders

The final group of CNS depressants used for anxiety and sleep disorders consists of miscellaneous agents that are chemically unrelated to either benzodiazepines or barbiturates (Table 14.5). In addition to nonbenzodiazepine, nonbarbiturate CNS depressants, other drugs used mainly for treatment of social anxiety symptoms include the antiseizure medication valproate (Depakote) and the beta blockers propranolol (Inderal) and atenolol (Tenormin). Drugs used mainly for insomnia therapy include zaleplon (Sonata), eszopiclone (Lunesta), and zolpidem (Ambien, Edluar, Intermezzo). Older CNS depressants such as paraldehyde (Paracetaldehyde), meprobamate (Equanil), and glutethimide (Doriglute) have only historical interest, because they are so rarely prescribed due to their potential for serious adverse effects. Buspirone (BuSpar) and zolpidem (Ambien, Edluar, Intermezzo) are commonly prescribed for their anxiolytic effects. Zolpidem (Ambien, Edluar, Intermezzo), ramelteon (Rozerem) and eszopiclone (Lunesta) have been used primarily for their hypnotic effects.

The mechanism of action for buspirone (BuSpar) is unclear but appears to be related to D_2 dopamine receptors in the brain. The drug has agonist effects on presynaptic dopamine receptors and a high affinity for serotonin receptors. Buspirone is less likely than benzodiazepines to affect cognitive and motor performance and rarely interacts with other CNS depressants. Common adverse effects include dizziness, headache, and drowsiness. Dependence and withdrawal problems are less of a concern with buspirone. Therapy may take several weeks to achieve optimal results.

Zolpidem (Ambien, Edluar, Intermezzo) is a Schedule IV controlled substance limited to the short-term treatment of insomnia. It is highly specific to the GABA receptor (see chapter 15) and produces muscle relaxation and anticonvulsant effects only at doses much higher than the hypnotic doses. As with other CNS depressants, it should be used cautiously in patients with respiratory impairment, in older adults, and when used concurrently with other CNS depressants. Lower dosages may be necessary. Also, because of the rapid onset of this drug (7 to 27 minutes), it should be taken just prior to expected sleep. Because zolpidem is metabolized in the liver and excreted by the kidneys, impaired liver or kidney function can increase serum drug levels. Zolpidem is in pregnancy category B. It should be used with caution in individuals with a high risk of suicide because there is a potential for intentional overdose. Adverse reactions are usually minimal (mild nausea,

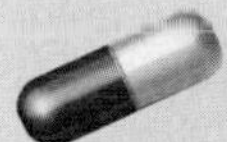

Prototype Drug | Zolpidem *(Ambien, Edluar, Intermezzo)*

Therapeutic Class: Sedative–hypnotic

Pharmacologic Class: Nonbenzodiazepine $GABA_A$ receptor agonist; nonbenzodiazepine, nonbarbiturate CNS depressant

Actions and Uses

Although it is a nonbenzodiazepine, zolpidem acts in a similar fashion to facilitate GABA-mediated CNS depression in the limbic, thalamic, and hypothalamic regions. It preserves stage 3 of sleep and has only minor effects on REM sleep. The only indication for zolpidem is for short-term insomnia management (7 to 10 days). The drug is available in sublingual tablets (Edluar) and oral spray (Zolpimist) formulations. In January 2013, the FDA lowered the recommended dose due to adverse effects observed especially among women.

Administration Alerts

- Because of rapid onset, 7–27 minutes, give immediately before bedtime.
- Pregnancy category B.

Onset	Peak	Duration
7–27 min	0.5–2.3 h	6–8 h

Adverse Effects

Adverse effects include daytime sedation, confusion, amnesia, dizziness, depression with suicidal thoughts, nausea, and vomiting. Zolpidem has been associated with the development of adverse neuropsychiatric reactions, such as hallucinations, sensory distortion, sleepwalking, and nocturnal eating. Women have been found to have a significantly higher serum zolpidem concentration than men. Adverse reactions that develop are dose dependent.

Contraindications: Lactating women should not take this drug.

Interactions

Drug–Drug: Drug interactions with zolpidem include an increase in sedation when used concurrently with other CNS depressants, including alcohol. Phenothiazines augment CNS depression.

Lab Tests: Unknown.

Herbal/Food: When taken with food, absorption is slowed significantly, and the onset of action may be delayed.

Treatment of Overdose: Generalized symptomatic and supportive measures should be applied with immediate gastric lavage where appropriate. IV fluids should be administered as needed. Use of flumazenil (Romazicon) as a benzodiazepine receptor antagonist may be helpful.

dizziness, diarrhea, daytime drowsiness), but rebound insomnia may occur when the drug is discontinued. Other adverse effects are amnesia, somnambulism (sleepwalking), or other activities that may be performed during sleep (e.g., sleepdriving).

Although structurally unrelated to other drugs used to treat insomnia, eszopiclone (Lunesta) has properties similar to those of zolpidem (Ambien, Edluar, Intermezzo). The effectiveness of eszopiclone has been shown in outpatient and sleep laboratory studies, but the drug has not directly been compared with zolpidem or other hypnotics. However, eszopiclone's longer elimination half-life, about twice as long as that of zolpidem, may give it an advantage in maintaining sleep and decreasing early-morning awakening. On the other hand, eszopiclone is more likely to cause daytime sedation.

Zaleplon (Sonata) may be useful for people who fall asleep but awake early in the morning, for example, 2:00 a.m. or 3:00 a.m. It is sometimes used for travel purposes and has been advertised by pharmaceutical companies for this purpose.

In 2005, ramelteon (Rozerem) was approved by the FDA in a single 8-mg dose. Ramelteon is a melatonin receptor agonist that has been shown to mainly improve sleep induction. It has a relatively short onset of action (30 minutes), and its duration is comparable to the non–extended-release form of zolpidem.

In 2014, tasimelteon (Hetlioz) was approved by the FDA as a second melatonin receptor agonist. This drug was indicated for the treatment of non-24-hour sleep-wake disorder. The most common adverse effects of Hetlioz, although minor in occurrence, have been headaches and abnormal dreams. Patients should avoid use of tasimelteon in combination with fluvoxamine (Luvox) or rifampin (Rifadin) due to overlapping cytochrome enzyme mechanisms within the body. Mild toxicity or reduced efficacy could occur if the drugs are taken together. The FDA indications for ramelteon, zolpidem, or tasimelteon are not limited to short-term use, because they do not appear to produce dependence or tolerance to the dose.

Table 14.5 Miscellaneous Drugs for Anxiety and Insomnia

Drug	Route and Adult Dose (max dose where indicated)	Adverse Effects
NONBENZODIAZEPINE, NONBARBITURATE CNS DEPRESSANTS		
buspirone (BuSpar)	Sedative: PO: 7.5–15 mg in divided doses; may increase by 5 mg/day every 2–3 days if needed (max: 60 mg/day)	*Dizziness, headache, drowsiness, nausea, fatigue, ataxia, vomiting, bitter metallic taste, dry mouth, diarrhea, hypotension*
dexmedetomidine (Precedex)	Sedative: IV: loading dose 1 mcg/kg over 10 min; maintenance dose 0.2–0.7 mcg/kg/h	Angioedema, cardiac arrest, exfoliative dermatitis (rare); SJS, anaphylaxis, respiratory failure, coma, sudden death
eszopiclone (Lunesta)	Hypnotic: PO: 2 mg at bedtime; depending on the age, clinical response, and tolerance of the patient, dose may be lowered to 1 mg	
zaleplon (Sonata)	Hypnotic: PO: 10 mg at bedtime (max: 20 mg/day)	
zolpidem (Ambien, Edluar, Intermezzo)	Hypnotic: PO: 5–10 mg at bedtime; Sublingual: 5-10 mg with at least 7-8 h remaining before the planned time of awakening	
ANTISEIZURE MEDICATIONS		
valproic acid (Depakene, Depakote) (see page 192 for the Prototype Drug box)	Social anxiety symptoms: PO: 250 mg tid (max: 60 mg/kg/day)	*Sedation, drowsiness, nausea, vomiting, prolonged bleeding time* Deep coma with overdose, liver failure, pancreatitis, prolonged bleeding time, bone marrow suppression
BETA BLOCKERS		
atenolol (Tenormin) (see page 422 for the Prototype Drug box)	Social anxiety symptoms: PO: 25–100 mg/day	*Bradycardia, hypotension, confusion, fatigue, drowsiness*
propranolol (Inderal) (see page 453 for the Prototype Drug box)	Social anxiety symptoms: PO: 40 mg bid (max: 320 mg/day)	Anaphylactic reactions, SJS, toxic epidermal necrolysis, exfoliative dermatitis, agranulocytosis, laryngospasm, bronchospasm
MELATONIN RECEPTOR DRUGS		
ramelteon (Rozerem)	Hypnotic: PO: 8 mg at bedtime	*Somnolence, dizziness, nausea*
tasimelteon (Hetlioz)	Hypnotic: PO: 20 mg per day taken before bedtime, at the same time every night	Respiratory tract infection
OREXIN RECEPTOR BLOCKER		
suvorexant (Belsomra)	Hypnotic: PO: taken in 5, 10, 15, or 20-mg strengths within 30 min of bed and no more than once per night (max: 20 mg/day)	*Daytime sleepiness* No serious adverse effects

Note: *Italics* indicate common adverse effects; underlining indicates serious adverse effects.

Nursing Practice Application

Pharmacotherapy for Anxiety or Sleep Disorders

ASSESSMENT

Baseline assessment prior to administration:

- Obtain a complete health history including hepatic, renal, respiratory, cardiovascular or neurologic disease, mental status, narrow-angle glaucoma, and pregnancy or breast-feeding. Obtain a drug history including allergies, current prescription and OTC drugs, herbal preparations, and caffeine and alcohol use. Be alert to possible drug interactions.
- Assess stress and coping patterns (e.g., existing or perceived stress, duration, coping mechanisms or remedies).
- Obtain a sleep history (e.g., quality and quantity of sleep, restlessness or frequent wakefulness, snoring or apnea, remedies used for sleep, concerns).
- Evaluate appropriate laboratory findings (e.g., hepatic or renal function studies).
- Obtain baseline vital signs and weight. Assess the patient's risk for falls.
- Assess the patient's ability to receive and understand instruction. Include the family and caregivers as needed.

POTENTIAL NURSING DIAGNOSES*

- *Anxiety*
- *Disturbed Sleep Pattern*
- *Fatigue*
- *Ineffective Coping*
- *Activity Intolerance*
- *Deficient Knowledge* (drug therapy)
- *Risk for Injury, related to adverse effects of drug therapy*
- *Risk for Falls,* related to adverse effects of drug therapy

*NANDA I © 2014

Nursing Practice Application *continued*

ASSESSMENT	POTENTIAL NURSING DIAGNOSES*
Assessment throughout administration: • Assess for desired therapeutic effects (e.g., statements of improvement in anxiety, appetite, ability to carry out ADLs, and sleep patterns normalized). • Continue periodic monitoring of liver and renal function studies. • Assess vital signs and weight periodically or if symptoms warrant. • Assess for and promptly report adverse effects: excessive dizziness, drowsiness, light-headedness, confusion, agitation, palpitations, tachycardia, and musculoskeletal weakness.	

IMPLEMENTATION

Interventions and (Rationales)	Patient-Centered Care
Ensuring therapeutic effects: • Continue assessments as described earlier for therapeutic effects. (If the drug is given for anxiety, the patient reports decreased anxiety, improved sleep and eating habits, improved coping, and ability to carry out ADLs without anxiety. If the drug is given for sleep, the patient reports the ability to fall and remain asleep and improved daytime wakefulness. **Diverse Patients:** Barbiturates induce P450 enzymes and may interact with other drugs. Ethnically diverse populations may also experience effects that are less than, or more than the expected effects of the drug. Nonbenzodiazepine sedative-hypnotic drugs are also metabolized through the P450 pathways. Women may metabolize some sublingual drugs (e.g., zolpidem [Ambien] more slowly, and the dosage may need to be halved by the provider.)	• Encourage the patient to keep a sleep diary of usual bedtime, the time involved trying to fall asleep, the quality and quantity of sleep, and daytime sleepiness. • **Collaboration:** Assist the patient in developing healthy coping strategies and sleep habits with referral to appropriate health care providers as needed. • **Diverse Patients:** Teach ethnically diverse patients to observe for optimal therapeutic effects and to report promptly.
Minimizing adverse effects: • Continue to monitor vital signs, mental status, and coordination and balance periodically. **Lifespan:** Be particularly cautious with older adults who are at increased risk for falls. (Drugs used for anxiety and sleep may cause excessive drowsiness and dizziness, increasing the risk of falls and injury. **Lifespan:** Many benzodiazepines and all barbiturates are included in the Beers List of potentially inappropriate drugs for older adults and warrant careful monitoring.)	• **Safety:** Teach the patient to rise from lying or sitting to standing slowly to avoid dizziness or falls. If dizziness occurs, the patient should sit or lie down and not attempt to stand or walk until the sensation passes.
• Ensure patient safety, especially in older adults. Observe for light-headedness or dizziness. Monitor and assist with ambulation as needed. (Dizziness and drowsiness for a prolonged period may occur, depending on the drug's half-life. Daytime drowsiness may impair walking or the ability to carry out usual ADLs. Subtle changes to mental alertness, cognitive functioning, or motor coordination may occur, even in the absence of sleepiness.)	• **Safety:** Instruct the patient to call for assistance prior to getting out of bed or attempting to walk alone, and to avoid driving or other activities requiring mental alertness or physical coordination until the effects of the drug are known.
• Assess for changes in level of consciousness, disorientation or confusion, or agitation. (Neurologic changes may indicate overmedication or effects of sleep deprivation.)	• Instruct the patient or caregiver to immediately report increasing lethargy, disorientation, confusion, changes in behavior or mood, slurred speech, or ataxia. • Have caregivers observe for nighttime behavioral activities such as sleepwalking, sleep-eating or sleep-driving if nonbenzodiazepine sedative-hypnotic drugs are given, and report immediately. The patient may not remember or be aware of these activities.
• Assess for changes in visual acuity, blurred vision, loss of peripheral vision, seeing rainbow halos around lights, acute eye pain, or any of these symptoms accompanied by nausea and vomiting and report immediately. (Increased intraoptic pressure in patients with narrow-angle glaucoma may occur in patients taking benzodiazepines.)	• Instruct the patient to immediately report any visual changes or eye pain.

continued

Nursing Practice Application *continued*

IMPLEMENTATION	
Interventions and (Rationales)	**Patient-Centered Care**
• Monitor affect and emotional status. (Drugs may increase risk of mental depression, especially in patients with suicidal tendencies. Concurrent use of alcohol and other CNS depressants increase the effects and the risk.)	• Instruct the patient to report significant mood changes, especially depression, and to avoid alcohol and other CNS depressants while taking the drug. • Teach the patient about the need for continued monitoring, especially if pre-existing depression is present.
• Encourage appropriate lifestyle changes: lowered caffeine intake including OTC medications that contain caffeine, increased exercise during the day but not immediately before bedtime, limited or no alcohol intake, and smoking cessation. (Healthy lifestyle changes will support and minimize the need for drug therapy. Caffeine and nicotine may decrease the effectiveness of the drug. Alcohol and other CNS depressants may increase the adverse effects of the drugs.)	• Encourage the patient to adopt a healthy lifestyle of decreased or abstinence from caffeine, nicotine, and alcohol; and increased exercise. Avoiding caffeine, decreasing stimulation (e.g., TV, Internet use) before bedtime, and regular bedtime habits help to promote sleep. • Advise the patient to discuss all OTC medications with the health care provider to ensure that caffeine or alcohol is not included in the formulation.
• Avoid abrupt discontinuation of therapy. (Withdrawal symptoms, including rebound anxiety and sleeplessness, are possible with abrupt discontinuation after long-term use.)	• Instruct the patient to take the drug exactly as prescribed and to not stop it abruptly.
• Assess home storage of medications and identify risks for corrective action. (Overdosage may occur if the patient takes additional doses when drowsy or disoriented from medication effects.)	• **Safety**: Instruct the patient that these drugs should not be kept at the bedside to avoid taking additional doses when drowsy.
• Assess prior methods of stress reduction or sleep hygiene. Reinforce previously used effective methods and teach new coping skills. (Drug therapy is used for the shortest amount of time possible. Developing other coping skills or improved sleep hygiene may lessen the need for drug therapy.)	• **Collaboration:** Teach the patient nonpharmacologic methods for stress relief and for improved sleep hygiene. Refer to appropriate health care providers or support groups as needed.
Patient understanding of drug therapy: • Use opportunities during administration of medications and during assessments to provide patient education. (Using time during nursing care helps to optimize and reinforce key teaching areas.)	• The patient should be able to state the reason for the drug; appropriate dose and scheduling; what adverse effects to observe for and when to report; and the anticipated length of medication therapy.
Patient self-administration of drug therapy: • When administering the medication, instruct the patient, family, or caregiver in proper self-administration of drug, e.g., taking only the amount prescribed. (Using time during nurse administration of these drugs helps to reinforce teaching.)	• The patient is able to discuss appropriate dosing and administration needs. • Teach patients to not open, chew, or crush extended release tablets (e.g., zopidem [Ambien]); swallow them whole with plenty of water. Sublingual forms of the drug (e.g., zolpidem [Edluar]) should be allowed to dissolve under the tongue; water should not be taken.

See Tables 14.2, 14.3, and 14.4 for lists of drugs to which these nursing actions apply.

Also in 2014, the FDA approved a brand new drug in its own class. Suvorexant (Belsomra) tablets are approved for difficulty in falling and staying asleep. Suvorexant is a receptor antagonist that blocks the action of orexin, a chemical involved in the sleep-wake cycle in the brain. The expected action of orexin is uninterrupted sleep lasting for about 7 hours. Although early animal studies proposed questions about impaired cognition in some subjects, human clinical trials have not born out this fact. It is believed that learning and memory are not impaired, although studies are continuing. Suvorexant is taken within 30 minutes of bedtime.

Drugs not listed in Table 14.5 include diphenhydramine (Benadryl) and hydroxyzine (Vistaril). These are antihistamines that produce drowsiness and may be beneficial in calming patients. They offer the advantage of not causing dependence, although their use is often limited by anticholinergic adverse effects. Diphenhydramine (see chapter 39) is a common component of OTC sleep aids, such as Nytol and Sominex. Doxylamine (Unisom) is another antihistamine medication commonly used as a nighttime OTC sleep aid.

Chapter Review

KEY Concepts

The numbered key concepts provide a succinct summary of the important points from the corresponding numbered section within the chapter. If any of these points are not clear, refer to the numbered section within the chapter for review.

14.1 Generalized anxiety disorder is the most common type of anxiety; panic attacks, phobias, obsessive–compulsive disorder, and post-traumatic stress disorder are other important categories.

14.2 The limbic system and the reticular activating system are specific regions of the brain responsible for anxiety and wakefulness.

14.3 Anxiety can be managed through pharmacologic and nonpharmacologic strategies.

14.4 Insomnia is a sleep disorder that may be caused by anxiety. Nonpharmacologic means should be attempted prior to initiating pharmacotherapy.

14.5 The electroencephalogram records brain waves and is used to diagnose sleep and seizure disorders.

14.6 Central nervous system (CNS) agents, including anxiolytics, sedatives, and hypnotics, are used to treat anxiety and insomnia.

14.7 When taken properly, antidepressants can reduce symptoms of panic and anxiety. First-line medications include the selective serotonin reuptake inhibitors (SSRIs) and other antidepressants; tricyclic antidepressants (TCAs) and monoamine oxidase inhibitors (MAOIs) are older drug groups.

14.8 Benzodiazepines are preferred drugs for the management of some anxiety disorders and for insomnia.

14.9 Because of their adverse effects and high potential for dependency, barbiturates are rarely used to treat insomnia.

14.10 Some commonly prescribed drugs and CNS depressants not related to the benzodiazepines or barbiturates are used for the treatment of anxiety and insomnia. Antiseizure medications, beta blockers, melatonin receptor drugs, and a new class of medications called orexin blockers are included in this category.

REVIEW Questions

1. The nurse should assess a patient who is taking lorazepam (Ativan) for the development of which of these adverse effects?
   1. Tachypnea
   2. Astigmatism
   3. Ataxia
   4. Euphoria

2. A patient is receiving temazepam (Restoril). Which of these responses should a nurse expect the patient to have if the medication is achieving the desired effect?
   1. The patient sleeps in 3-hour intervals, awakens for a short time, and then falls back to sleep.
   2. The patient reports feeling less anxiety during activities of daily living.
   3. The patient reports having fewer episodes of panic attacks when stressed.
   4. The patient reports sleeping 7 hours without awakening.

3. A 32-year-old female patient has been taking lorazepam (Ativan) for her anxiety and is brought into the emergency department after taking 30 days' worth at one time. What antagonist for benzodiazepines may be used in this case?
   1. Epinephrine
   2. Atropine
   3. Flumazenil
   4. Naloxone

4. A 17-year-old patient has been prescribed escitalopram (Lexapro) for increasing anxiety uncontrolled by other treatment measures. Because of this patient's age, the nurse will ensure that the patient and parents are taught what important information?
   1. Cigarette smoking will counteract the effects of the drug.
   2. Signs of increasing depression or thoughts of suicide should be reported immediately.

3. The drug causes dizziness and alternative schooling arrangements may be needed for the first two months of use.
4. Anxiety and excitability may increase during the first two weeks of use but then will have significant improvement.

5. Zolpidem (Ambien, Edluar, Intermezzo) has been ordered for a patient for the treatment of insomnia. What information will the nurse provide for this patient? (Select all that apply.)
   1. Be cautious when performing morning activities because it may cause a significant "hangover" effect with drowsiness and dizziness.
   2. Take the drug with food; this enhances the absorption for quicker effects.
   3. Take the drug immediately before going to bed; it has a quick onset of action.
   4. If the insomnia is long-lasting, this drug may safely be used for up to one year.
   5. Alcohol and other drugs that cause CNS depression (e.g., antihistamines) should be avoided while taking this drug.

6. Education given to patients about the use of all drugs to treat insomnia should include an emphasis on what important issue?
   1. They will be required long-term to achieve lasting effects.
   2. They require frequent blood counts to avoid adverse effects.
   3. They are among the safest drugs available and have few adverse effects.
   4. Long-term use may increase the risk of adverse effects, create a "sleep debt," and cause rebound insomnia when stopped.

PATIENT-FOCUSED Case Study

George Orland is a 59-year-old salesman working at a local insurance company in the community. Due to the economy, his income has dropped significantly because it is partially based on commission and he is worried that he is not able to provide for his family. He begins to experience insomnia, difficulty concentrating, and other symptoms related to his anxiety. His health care provider prescribes a short-term course of lorazepam (Ativan) to help him through this difficult period.

1. What adverse effects are associated with this drug therapy?
2. What information should George receive about this medication?
3. What nonpharmacologic measures can the nurse recommend to George to assist him in feeling better about his current situation?

CRITICAL THINKING Questions

1. A 58-year-old male patient underwent an emergency coronary artery bypass graft. He is still experiencing a high degree of pain and also states that he cannot fall asleep. The patient has been ordered estazolam (Prosom) at night for sleep and an opioid (narcotic) analgesic for pain. As the nurse, explain to the student nurse why both medications should be administered.
2. A 42-year-old female patient with ovarian cancer suffered profound nausea and vomiting after her first round of chemotherapy. The oncologist has added lorazepam (Ativan) 2 mg per IV in addition to a previously ordered antinausea medication as part of the prechemotherapy regimen. What is the purpose for adding this benzodiazepine?

Visit www.pearsonhighered.com/nursingresources for answers and rationales for all activities.

REFERENCES

Bernert, R. A., Turvey, C. L., Conwell, Y., and Joiner, T. E. (2014). Association of poor subjective sleep quality with risk for death by suicide during a 10-year period: A longitudinal, population-based study of late life. *JAMA Psychiatry, 71,* 1129–1137. doi:10.1001/jamapsychiatry.2014.1126

Herdman, T. H., & Kamitsuru, S. (Eds.). (2014). *NANDA International nursing diagnoses: Definitions and classification, 2015–2017.* Oxford, United Kingdom: Wiley-Blackwell.

Katayose, Y., Aritake, S., Kitamura, S., Enomoto, M., Hida, A., Takahashi, K., & Mishima, K. (2012). Carryover effect on next-day sleepiness and psychomotor performance of nighttime administered antihistaminic drugs: A randomized controlled trial. *Human Psychopharmacology, 27,* 428–436. doi:10.1002/hup.2244

Kavanaugh, J. J., Grant, G. D., & Anoopkumar-Dukie, S. (2012). Low dosage promethazine and loratidine negatively affect neuromuscular function. *Clinical Neurophysiology, 123,* 780–786. doi:10.1016/j.clinph.2011.07.046

Naicker, P., Anoopkumar-Dukie, S., Grant, G. D., & Kavanaugh, J. J. (2013). The effects of antihistamines with varying anticholinergic properties on voluntary and involuntary movement. *Clinical Neurophysiology, 129,* 1840–1845. doi:10.1016/j.clinph.2013.04.003

National Center for Complementary and Integrative Health. (2014). *Melatonin: What you need to know.* Retrieved from https://nccih.nih.gov/health/melatonin

Ozdemir, P. G., Karadag, A. S., Selvi, Y., Boysan, M., Bilgili, S. G., Aydin, A., & Onder, S. (2014) Assessment of the effects of antihistamine drugs on mood, sleep quality, sleepiness, and dream anxiety. *International Journal of Psychiatry in Clinical Practice, 18,* 161–168. doi:10.3109/13651501.2014.907919

Vande Griend, J. P., & Anderson, S. L. (2012). Histamine-1 receptor antagonism for treatment of insomnia. *Journal of the American Pharmacists Association, 52*(6), e210–e219. doi:10.1331/JAPhA.2012.12051

World Health Organization. (2012). International classification of diseases, tenth edition (ICD-10). Washington, D.C.: Author.

SELECTED BIBLIOGRAPHY

American Sleep Association. (n.d.). *About Insomnia,* Retrieved from https://www.sleepassociation.org/patients-general-public/insomnia/insomnia/

Boelen, P. A., & Carleton, R. N. (2012). Intolerance of uncertainty, hypochondriacal concerns, obsessive-compulsive symptoms, and worry. *The Journal of Nervous and Mental Disease, 200,* 208–213. doi:10.1097/NMD.0b013e318247cb17

Friedman, M. J. (2014). Literature on DSM-5 and ICD-11. *PTSD Research Quarterly, 25*(2), 1–9.

Ghafoori, B., Barragan, B., Tohidian, N., & Palinkas, L. (2012). Racial and ethnic differences in symptom severity of PTSD, GAD, and depression in trauma-exposed, urban, treatment-seeking adults. *Journal of Traumatic Stress, 25,* 106–110. doi:10.1002/jts.21663

Gonçalves, D. C., & Byrne, G. J. (2013). Who worries most? Worry prevalence and patterns across the lifespan. *International Journal of Geriatric Psychiatry, 28,* 41–49. doi:10.1002/gps.3788

Grandner, M. A., Martin, J. L., Patel, N. P., Jackson, N. J., Gehrman, P. R., Pien, G., . . . Gooneratne, N. S. (2012). Age and sleep disturbances among American men and women: Data from the U.S. Behavioral Risk Factor Surveillance System. *Sleep, 35*(3), 395–406. doi:10.5665/sleep.1704

Maercker, A., Brewin, C. R., Bryant, R. A., Cloitre, M., Reed, G. M., van Ommeren, M., . . . Saxena, S. (2013). Proposals for mental disorders specifically associated with stress in the International Classification of Diseases-11. *Lancet, 381,* 1683–1685. doi:10.1016/S0140-6736(12)62191-6

National Institute of Mental Health. (n.d.). *Anxiety disorders,* Retrieved from http://www.nimh.nih.gov/health/publications/anxiety-disorders/index.shtml?rf=53414

Roh, J. H., Jiang, H., Finn, M. B., Stewart, F. R., Mahan, T. E., Cirrito, J. R., . . . Holtzman, D. M. (2014). Potential role of orexin and sleep modulation in the pathogenesis of Alzheimer's disease. *Journal of Experimental Medicine, 211,* 2487–2496. doi:10.1084/jem.20141788

Takayanagi, Y., Spira, A. P., Bienvenu, O. J., Hock, R. S., Carras, M. C., Eaton, W. W., & Mojtabai, R. (2015). Antidepressant use and lifetime history of mental disorders in a community sample: Results from the Baltimore Epidemiologic Catchment Area Study. *Journal of Clinical Psychiatry, 76,* 40-44. doi:10.4088/JCP.13m08824

Torres, R., Kramer, W. G., Baroldi, P. (2015). Pharmacokinetics of the dual melatonin receptor agonist tasimelteon in subjects with hepatic or renal impairment. *Journal of Clinical Pharmacology, 55,* 525–533. doi:10.1002/jcph.440

United States Drug Enforcement Agency. (2011). *Drugs of abuse: Benzodiazepines.* Retrieved from http://www.dea.gov/pr/multimedia-library/publications/drug_of_abuse.pdf#page=53

United States Drug Enforcement Agency. (2011). *Drugs of abuse: Depressants.* Retrieved from http://www.dea.gov/druginfo/drug_data_sheets/Depressants.pdf

Vázquez, G. H., Baldessarini, R. J., Tondo, L. (2014). Co-occurrence of anxiety and bipolar disorders: Clinical and therapeutic overview. *Depression and Anxiety, 31,* 196–206. doi:10.1002/da.22248

Chapter 15

Drugs for Seizures

Drugs at a Glance

Learning Outcomes

After reading this chapter, the student should be able to:

1. Compare and contrast the terms *seizures*, *convulsions*, and *epilepsy*.
2. Recognize possible causes of seizures.
3. Relate signs and symptoms to specific types of seizures.
4. Describe the nurse's role in the pharmacologic management of seizures of an acute nature and epilepsy.
5. Explain the importance of patient drug compliance in the pharmacotherapy of epilepsy and seizures.
6. For each of the drug classes listed in Drugs at a Glance, know representative drug examples and explain their mechanism of drug action, primary actions, and important adverse effects.
7. Categorize drugs used in the treatment of seizures based on their classification and mechanism of action.
8. Use the nursing process to care for patients receiving pharmacotherapy for epilepsy and seizures.

indicates a prototype drug, each of which is featured in a Prototype Drug box.

As the most common neurologic disease, **epilepsy** affects more than 2 million Americans. By definition, epilepsy is any disorder characterized by recurrent seizures. Symptoms of epilepsy depend on the type of seizure and may include blackouts, fainting spells, sensory disturbances, jerking body movements, and temporary loss of memory. This chapter examines the pharmacotherapy used to treat epilepsy and different kinds of seizures.

SEIZURES

A **seizure** or clinically detectable sign of epilepsy is a disturbance of electrical activity in the brain that may affect consciousness, motor activity, and sensation. Seizures are caused by abnormal or uncontrolled neuronal discharges. Uncontrolled charges may remain in one area of the brain or **focus** (plural: *foci*) or propagate to other areas of the brain. As a valuable tool in measuring uncontrolled neuronal activity, the electroencephalogram (EEG) is useful in diagnosing seizure disorders. Figure 15.1 compares normal and abnormal neuronal tracings.

The terms seizure and convulsion are not synonymous. **Convulsions** specifically refer to involuntary, violent spasms of the large skeletal muscles of the face, neck, arms, and legs. Although some types of seizures involve convulsions, other seizures do not. Thus, it may be stated that all convulsions are seizures, but not all seizures are convulsions. Because of this difference, drugs described in this chapter are generally referred to as antiseizure drugs rather than anticonvulsants. Recognizing also that antiseizure drugs are commonly called antiepileptic drugs (AEDs), the term antiseizure in this chapter applies to the treatment of all seizure-related symptoms, including signs of epilepsy.

15.1 Causes of Seizures

A seizure is symptomatic of an underlying disorder, rather than being considered a disease in and of itself. Triggers for seizures include exposure to strobe or flickering lights or the occurrence of small fluid and electrolyte imbalances. Seizure patients appear to have a lower tolerance to environmental triggers. Seizures occur more often when patients are sleep deprived.

There are many different etiologies of seizure activity. In over 50% of cases, no specific cause of seizure activity can be identified. Seizures represent the most common serious neurologic problem affecting children, with an overall incidence approaching 2% for febrile seizures and 1% for idiopathic epilepsy. Medications for mood disorders, psychoses, and local anesthesia when given in high doses may cause seizures, possibly due to toxicity or increased levels of stimulatory neurotransmitters. Seizures may also occur from drug abuse, as with cocaine abuse, or during withdrawal from alcohol or sedative–hypnotic drugs.

Seizures may present as an acute situation, or they may occur on a chronic basis. Seizures that result from an acute complication generally do not recur after the situation has been resolved. On the other hand, if a brain abnormality exists following an acute complication, recurrent seizures are likely. The following are known causes of seizures:

- *Infectious diseases.* Acute infections such as meningitis and encephalitis can cause inflammation in the brain.
- *Trauma.*Physical trauma such as direct blows to the skull may increase intracranial pressure; chemical trauma such as the presence of toxic substances or the ingestion of poisons may cause brain injury.
- *Metabolic disorders.* Changes in fluid and electrolytes such as hypoglycemia, hyponatremia, and water

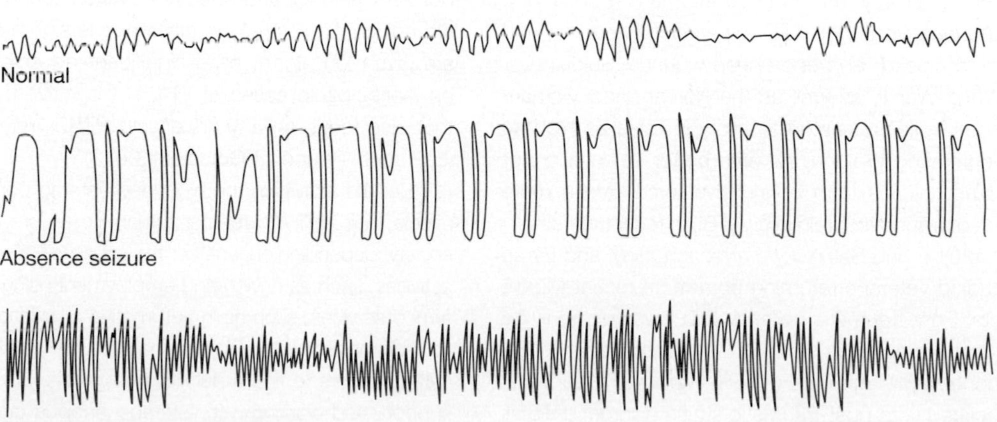

FIGURE 15.1 EEG recordings showing the differences among normal, absence, and generalized tonic–clonic seizure tracings

intoxication may cause seizures by altering electrical impulse transmission at the cellular level.

- *Vascular diseases.* Changes in oxygenation such as those caused by respiratory hypoxia and carbon monoxide poisoning, and changes in perfusion such as those caused by hypotension, stroke, shock, and cardiac dysrhythmias may be causes.
- *Pediatric disorders.* Rapid increase in body temperature may result in a **febrile seizure.**
- *Neoplastic disease.* Tumors, especially rapidly growing ones, may occupy space, increase intracranial pressure, and damage brain tissue by disrupting blood flow.

An important topic when discussing epilepsy and seizure treatment is pregnancy. Because several antiseizure drugs decrease the effectiveness of hormonal contraceptives, additional barrier methods of birth control should be practiced to avoid unintended pregnancy. Prior to pregnancy and considering the serious nature of seizures, patients should consult with their health care provider to determine the most appropriate plan of action for seizure control. When patients become pregnant, extreme caution is necessary. Most antiseizure drugs are pregnancy category D. Some antiseizure drugs may cause folate deficiency, a condition correlated with fetal neural tube defects. Vitamin supplements may be necessary. **Eclampsia** is a severe hypertensive disorder of pregnancy, characterized by seizures, coma, and perinatal mortality. Eclampsia is likely to occur from around the 20th week of gestation until at least 1 week after delivery of the baby. Approximately 25% of women with eclampsia experience seizures within 72 hours postpartum. For years, one of the approaches used to prevent or treat eclamptic seizures was magnesium sulfate. The mechanism for this substance's antiseizure activity is not well understood. A prototype feature for magnesium sulfate is presented in chapter 46.

Seizures can have a significant impact on the quality of life. They may cause serious injury if they occur while a person is driving a vehicle or performing a dangerous activity. Almost all states will not grant, or will take away, a driver's license and require a seizure-free period before granting a driver's license. Without successful pharmaco therapy, epilepsy can severely limit participation in school, employment, and social activities and can definitely affect self-esteem. Chronic depression may accompany poorly controlled seizures. Important considerations in nursing care include identifying patients at risk for seizures, documenting the pattern and type of seizure activity, and implementing needed safety precautions. In collaboration with the patient, the health care provider, pharmacist, and nurse are instrumental in achieving positive therapeutic outcomes. Through a combination of pharmacotherapy, patient–family support, and education, effective seizure control can be achieved in a majority of patients.

15.2 Types of Seizures

The differing presentation of seizures relates to their signs and symptoms. Symptoms may range from sudden, violent shaking and total loss of consciousness to muscle twitching or slight tremor of a limb. Staring into space, altered vision, and difficulty speaking are other behaviors a person may exhibit. Determining the cause of recurrent seizures is important for appropriate drug selection and planning or treatment options. Proper diagnosis, therefore, is essential.

Methods of classifying epilepsy have changed over time. For example, the terms *grand mal* and *petit mal* epilepsy have, for the most part, been replaced by more descriptive and detailed labels. Epilepsies are typically identified using the International Classification of

Treating the Diverse Patient: Epilepsy in Veterans Following Traumatic Brain Injury

Epilepsy occurring after any form of head trauma is a possibility, and soldiers returning from war have experienced seizures and epilepsy related to closed- and open-head wounds. Soldiers returning from World War II, as well as the Korean, and Vietnam wars, experienced epilepsy related to injury in rates as high as 53% after a penetrating brain injury. With better defense armor and helmets, blast injuries from concussive forces are a more common source of traumatic brain injury (TBI) in recent wars.

Chen et al. (2014) and Salinksky, Storzbach, Goy, and Evrad (2014) have studied veterans returning from more recent Middle Eastern conflicts. Post-traumatic epilepsy (PTE) was found to be more likely to occur in cases of severe TBI. In cases of mild TBI, psychogenic nonepileptic seizures (PNES) were more common and often associated with post-traumatic stress disorder (PTSD). Seizure-like activity and other neurological symptoms occurred, but EEG readings and videotapes taken during seizure-like activity did not confirm PTE. The difference is significant because AEDs are given long-term, have significant adverse effects, and may be ineffective in cases of PNES. Cognitive-behavioral therapies that also focus on any underlying PTSD may be more effective (LaFrance, Reuber, & Goldstein, 2013).

Seizure activity in the wounded veteran population significantly affects their ability to reenter civilian life as productive members of society. Depending on whether the cause is PTE or PNES, normal life activities, such as driving and employment using skills learned in the armed services, such as in automotive or aviation jobs, may be difficult or impossible to obtain or maintain. By working with other health care providers to find a definitive diagnosis, providing teaching and support, and working with veterans' support groups, the nurse can help ease the transition for these veterans when they return home.

Table 15.1 Classification of Seizures and Symptoms

Classification	Type	Symptoms
Partial	Simple partial	• Olfactory, auditory, and visual hallucinations • Intense emotions • Twitching of arms, legs, and face
	Complex partial (psychomotor)	• Aura (preceding) • Brief period of confusion or sleepiness afterward with no memory of seizure (*postictal confusion*) • Fumbling with or attempting to remove clothing • No response to verbal commands
Generalized	Absence (petit mal)	• Lasting a few seconds • Seen most often in children (child stares into space, does not respond to verbal stimulation, may have fluttering eyelids or jerking) • Misdiagnosed often (especially in children) as attention deficit/hyperactivity disorder (ADHD) or daydreaming
	Atonic (drop attacks)	• Falling or stumbling for no reason • Lasting a few seconds
	Tonic–clonic (grand mal)	• Aura (preceding) • Intense muscle contraction (tonic phase) followed by alternating contraction and relaxation of muscles (clonic phase) • Crying at the beginning as air leaves lungs; loss of bowel/bladder control; shallow breathing with periods of apnea; usually lasting 1–2 minutes • Disorientation and deep sleep after seizure (*postictal state*)
Special syndromes	Febrile seizure	• Tonic–clonic activity lasting 1–2 minutes • Rapid return to consciousness • Occurs in children usually between 3 months and 5 years of age
	Myoclonic seizure	• Large jerking movements of a major muscle group, such as an arm • Falling from a sitting position or dropping what is held
	Status epilepticus	• Considered a medical emergency • Continuous seizure activity, which can lead to coma and death

Epileptic Seizures nomenclature. These are termed partial (focal), generalized, and special epileptic syndromes (Table 15.1). Types of **partial (focal)** or **generalized seizures** may be recognized based on symptoms observed during a seizure episode. Some symptoms are subtle and reflect the specific nature of neuronal misfiring; others are more complex.

15.3 General Concepts of Antiseizure Pharmacotherapy

The choice of drug for antiseizure pharmacotherapy depends on signs presented by the patient, the patient's previous medical history, and associated pathologies. Once a medication is selected, the patient is placed on a low initial dose. The amount is gradually increased until seizure control is achieved, or until drug side effects prevent additional increases in dose. Serum drug levels may be obtained to assist the health care provider in determining the most effective drug concentration. If seizure activity continues, a different medication is added in small-dose increments while the dose of the first drug is slowly reduced. Because seizures are likely to occur if antiseizure drugs are abruptly withdrawn, the medication is usually discontinued over a period of 6 to 12 weeks.

Traditional and more recently approved antiseizure drugs with indications are shown in Table 15.2. The more recently approved antiseizure drugs offer advantages over the traditional drugs, because they exhibit fewer troublesome side effects. Due to the limited induction of drug-metabolizing enzymes, the pharmacokinetic profiles of the newer drugs have been less complicated. In addition, they have been generally well-tolerated and have posed less of a health risk in pregnancy.

In recent years, the U.S. Food and Drug Administration (FDA) has analyzed reports from clinical studies involving patients taking a variety of antiseizure medications, mostly nontraditional drugs or drugs used to treat conditions outside of seizures. Patients with epilepsy, bipolar disorder, psychoses, migraines, and neuropathic

Table 15.2 Selected Antiseizure Drugs With Indications*

	PARTIAL SEIZURES	GENERALIZED SEIZURES		SPECIAL
		Absence	Tonic–Clonic	Myoclonic
DRUGS THAT POTENTIATE GABA				
diazepam (Valium)		✔	✔	✔
gabapentin (Gralise, Horizant, Neurontin)	✔			
lorazepam (Ativan)			✔	
phenobarbital (Luminal)	✔		✔	
pregabalin (Lyrica)	✔			
primidone (Mysoline)	✔		✔	
tiagabine (Gabitril)	✔			
topiramate (Topamax, Qudexy XR)	✔		✔	✔
HYDANTOIN AND RELATED DRUGS				
carbamazepine (Tegretol)	✔		✔	
lamotrigine (Lamictal)	✔	✔	✔	✔
levetiracetam (Keppra)	✔			
oxcarbazepine (Trileptal, Oxtellar XR)	✔		✔	
phenytoin (Dilantin)	✔		✔	
valproic acid (Depakene)	✔	✔	✔	✔
zonisamide (Zonegran)	✔	✔	✔	✔
SUCCINIMIDES				
ethosuximide (Zarontin)		✔		

*Antiseizure drugs approved for use in adjunctive therapy or monotherapy. Checkmarks include off-label as well as approved indications.

PharmFacts

EPILEPSY

- The word epilepsy is derived from the Greek word *epilepsia*, meaning "to take hold of or to seize."
- About 3 million Americans have epilepsy.
- Each year at least 200,000 people are diagnosed with epilepsy.
- In two-thirds of patients diagnosed with epilepsy, the cause is unknown.
- Most people with seizures are younger than 45 years of age.
- Contrary to popular belief, it is impossible to swallow the tongue during a seizure, and one should never force an object into the mouth of someone who is having a seizure.
- Epilepsy is not a mental illness; children with epilepsy have IQ scores equivalent to those of children without the disorder.
- Famous people who had or may have had epilepsy include Julius Caesar, Alexander the Great, Napoleon, Vincent van Gogh, Charles Dickens, Joan of Arc, Socrates, Agatha Christie, Truman Capote, and Richard Burton.
- Among adult alcoholics receiving treatment for withdrawal, over half will experience seizures within 6 hours upon arriving for treatment.

pain have been among the disorders studied. Compared to placebo trials, many of the popular antiseizure drug have been found to almost double the risk of suicidal behavior and ideation among patients. In a warning issued by the FDA, health care providers were instructed to carefully *balance clinical need for antiseizure drug treatment with risk for suicide*. Patients and caregivers should be encouraged to pay close attention to changes in mood and not to discontinue any antiseizure medication without consulting their health care provider. The reports indicate that both the established antiseizure drugs and the more recently approved medications have had serious clinical drawbacks.

In most cases, effective seizure management can be obtained using only a single drug. However, if seizure activity continues, adjunctive therapy in which two antiseizure medications are prescribed is used, although unwanted side effects may occur. Some antiseizure drug combinations may actually increase the incidence of seizures due to unfavorable drug interactions. Health care providers should consult with current literature regarding drug compatibility before a second antiseizure drug is added to the regimen.

15.4 Mechanisms of Action of Antiseizure Drugs

The goal of antiseizure pharmacotherapy is to suppress neuronal activity just enough to prevent abnormal or repetitive firing. To this end, there are three general mechanisms by which antiseizure drugs act:

- Stimulating an influx of chloride ions, an effect associated with the neurotransmitter gamma-aminobutyric acid (GABA).
- Delaying an influx of sodium.
- Delaying an influx of calcium.

Antiseizure pharmacotherapy is directed at controlling the movement of electrolytes across neuronal membranes or affecting neurotransmitter balance. In a resting state, neurons are normally surrounded by a higher concentration of sodium, calcium, and chloride ions. Potassium levels are higher inside the cell. An influx of sodium or calcium into the neuron *enhances* neuronal activity, whereas an influx of chloride ions or an efflux of potassium ions *suppresses* neuronal activity.

Altered ion fluxes have prompted drug researchers to try to understand more clearly various drug mechanisms and to develop newer drugs. Recently, a fourth mechanism has been recognized and studied—antagonism of the primary excitatory neurotransmitter glutamate. Glutamate works in concert with the cell's Na^+-K^+ ATPase pump, which helps to restore ion balances across neuronal membranes after firing. Any drug that blocks glutamate activity indirectly prevents an influx of positive ions into the cell, so this is consistent with the last two general mechanisms. A related observation has been low levels of the inhibitory amino acid taurine in damaged neuronal tissue. Thus, it has been proposed that taurine stabilizes neuronal cell membranes primarily by reducing glutamate-induced positive ion (sodium and calcium) influxes. Therefore, higher levels of glutamate seem to be associated with neuronal damage. Restoring amino acid–related ion balances has been among the approaches for the general treatment of recurrent and sudden seizure attacks.

DRUGS THAT POTENTIATE GABA ACTION

Several important antiseizure drugs act by changing the action of **gamma-aminobutyric acid (GABA),** the primary inhibitory neurotransmitter in the brain. These drugs mimic the effects of GABA by stimulating an influx of chloride ions through the GABA receptor channel. A model of this receptor is shown in Pharmacotherapy Illustrated 15.1. When the receptor is stimulated and chloride ions move into the cell, the abnormal firing of neurons is suppressed, and seizure activity may be prevented or terminated.

A number of drugs have GABA-related potentiation. Drugs may bind directly to the GABA receptor through specific binding sites. Well-characterized sites have been designated as $GABA_A$ and $GABA_B$. Drugs may enhance GABA release, or drugs may block the reuptake of GABA into nerve cells and glia. Some drugs increase the amount of GABA in the nerve terminal by inhibiting GABA-degrading enzymes. Barbiturates, benzodiazepines, and other GABA-related drugs reduce seizure activity by intensifying GABA action. The predominant effect of GABA potentiation is central nervous system (CNS) depression. These drugs are listed in Table 15.3.

Drugs that potentiate GABA action are used for a variety of other conditions including depression, migraines, and the management of neuropathic pain associated with diabetic peripheral neuropathy, postherpetic neuralgia, fibromyalgia, and spinal cord injury. In addition, some antiseizure drugs have been used for the management of anxiety and bipolar disorder symptoms. Two antiseizure

Complementary and Alternative Therapies

THE KETOGENIC DIET FOR EPILEPSY

The ketogenic diet is used when seizures cannot be controlled through pharmacotherapy or when there are unacceptable adverse effects to the medications. Before antiepileptic drugs were developed, this diet was a primary treatment for epilepsy. Recent studies have examined the possibility that the ketogenic diet could provide symptomatic benefit for patients with Alzheimer's disease (Levy, Cooper, Giri, & Pulman, 2012).

The ketogenic diet is a stringently calculated diet that is high in fat and low in carbohydrates and protein. It limits water intake to avoid ketone dilution and carefully controls caloric intake. Each meal has a ketogenic ratio of 3 or 4 g of fat to 1 g of protein and carbohydrate (Schachter, Kossoff, & Sirven, 2013). Extra fat is usually given in the form of heavy cream, butter, mayonnaise, or vegetable oils such as canola or olive oil.

Research suggests that the diet produces a high success rate for certain patients. Improvement may be noted rapidly after an average of 5 days in some children. The diet appears to be equally effective for every seizure type. The most frequently reported adverse effects include vomiting, fatigue, constipation, diarrhea, and hunger. Kidney stones, acidosis, and slower growth rates are possible risks. Those interested in trying the diet must consult with their health care provider; this is not a do-it-yourself diet and may be harmful if not carefully monitored by skilled professionals.

PHARMACOTHERAPY ILLUSTRATED

15.1 | Model of the GABA Receptor–Chloride Channel Molecules in Relationship to Antiseizure Pharmacotherapy

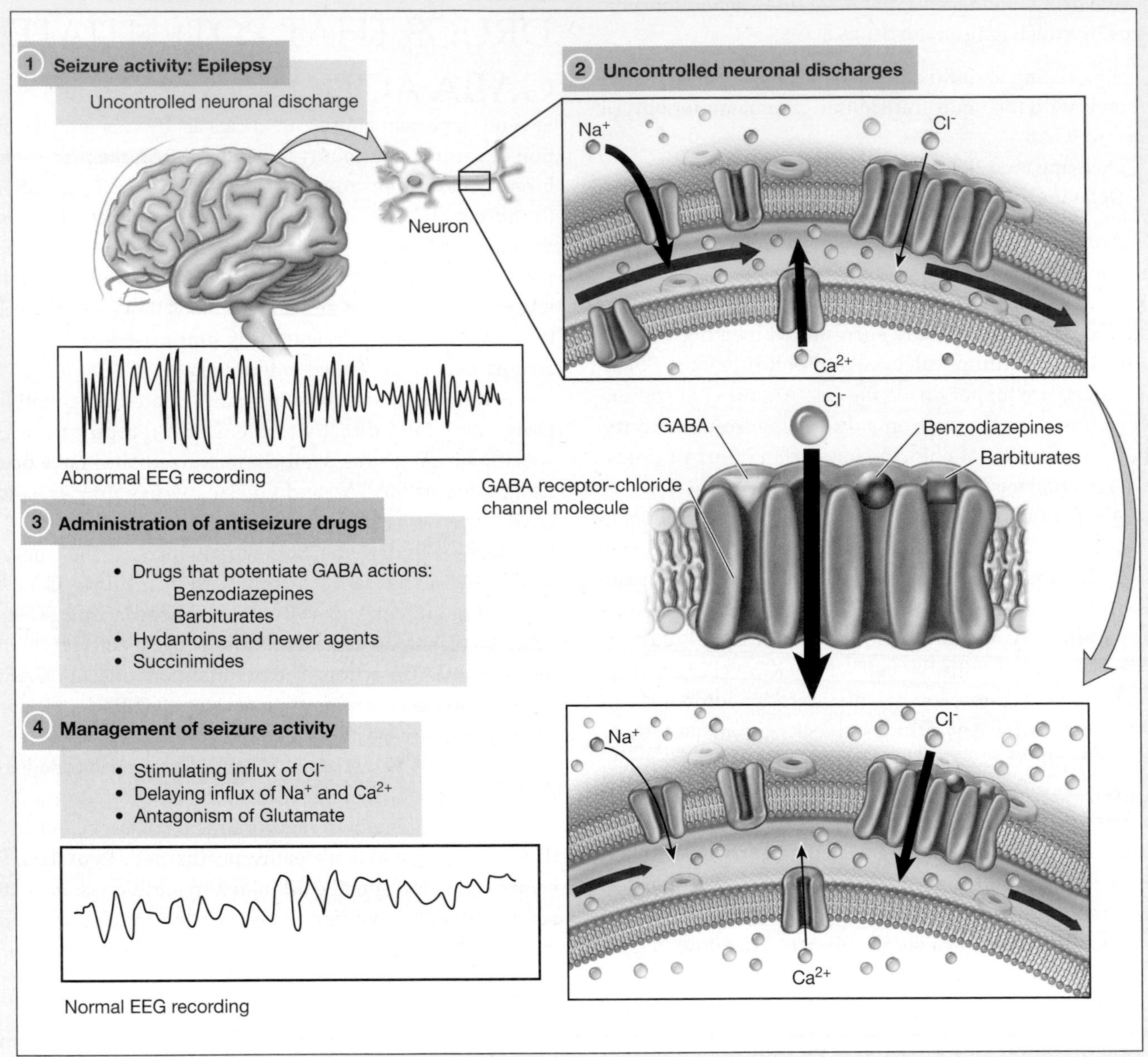

drugs, gabapentin (Gralise, Horizant, Neurontin) and pregabalin (Lyrica) stand out as approaches for the successful management of neuropathic pain and postherpetic neuralgia. Topiramate (Topamax, Qudexy XR) has been used in the treatment of trigeminal neuralgia.

Barbiturates

Barbiturates are organic compounds derived from barbituric acid. These drugs intensify the effect of GABA in the brain and generally depress the firing of CNS neurons.

15.5 Treating Seizures With Barbiturates

The antiseizure properties of phenobarbital were discovered in 1912, and this drug is still occasionally prescribed for seizures. As a class, barbiturates generally have a low margin for safety, a high potential for dependence, and they cause profound CNS depression. Phenobarbital, however, is able to suppress abnormal neuronal discharges without causing sedation. It is inexpensive, long acting, and produces a low incidence of adverse effects. When the drug is given orally

Table 15.3 Antiseizure Drugs That Potentiate GABA Action

Drug	Route and Adult Dose (max dose where indicated)	Adverse Effects
BARBITURATES		
phenobarbital (Luminal)	For partial and generalized seizures: PO: 100–300 mg/day; IV/IM: 200–600 mg up to 20 mg/kg For status epilepticus: IV: 15–18 mg/kg in single or divided doses (max: 20 mg/kg)	*Somnolence* <u>Agranulocytosis, Stevens–Johnson syndrome, angioedema, laryngospasm, respiratory depression, CNS depression, coma, death</u>
primidone (Mysoline)	PO: 250 mg/day, increased by 250 mg/wk up to max of 2 g in two to four divided doses	
BENZODIAZEPINES		
clobazam (Onfi)	Lennox–Gastaut syndrome: PO: 5 mg/day in divided doses, titrated to 10–20 mg daily; dose escalation should not proceed more rapidly than every 7 days (max: 20–40 mg daily based on weight may be started on day 21)	*Drowsiness, sedation, ataxia* <u>Laryngospasm, respiratory depression, cardiovascular collapse, coma</u>
clonazepam (Klonopin)	PO: 1.5 mg/day in three divided doses, increased by 0.5–1 mg every 3 days until seizures are controlled	
clorazepate (Tranxene)	PO: 7.5 mg tid; dose bid–tid; increase dose by 7.5 mg at weekly intervals (max: 90 mg/day)	
diazepam (Valium)	IV push: administer emulsion at 5 mg/min IM/IV: 5–10 mg (repeat as needed at 10–15 min intervals up to 30 mg; repeat again as needed every 2–4 h)	
lorazepam (Ativan) (see page 171 for the Prototype Drug box)	IV: 4 mg injected slowly at 2 mg/min; if inadequate response after 10 min, may repeat once	
OTHER DRUGS THAT POTENTIATE GABA		
ezogabine (Potiga)	PO: 100 mg tid gradually increased to 200 mg–400 mg tid	*Drowsiness, dizziness, fatigue, sedation, somnolence, vertigo, ataxia, confusion, asthenia, headache, tremor, nervousness, memory difficulty, difficulty concentrating, psychomotor slowing, nystagmus, paresthesia, nausea, vomiting, anorexia* <u>Serious disfiguring and debilitating rashes; sudden unexplained death in epilepsy (SUDEP); withdrawal seizures on discontinuation of drug; vision loss</u>
gabapentin (Gralise, Horizant, Neurontin)	PO (Children age 3–12): 10–15 mg/kg/day gradually increased to 40 mg/kg/day PO (Adult and children older than 12): 300 mg tid gradually increased to 1,800–2,400 mg/day	
pregabalin (Lyrica)	PO: 150 mg/day gradually increased up to 600 mg/day	
tiagabine (Gabitril)	PO: 4 mg/day gradually increased up to 56 mg/day in two to four divided doses	
topiramate (Topamax, Qudexy XR)	PO: 50 mg/day gradually increased up to 400 mg/day	
vigabatrin (Sabril)	PO (infantile spasms): 50 mg/kg/day bid, gradually increased up to 150 mg/kg/day PO (adults): 500 mg bid gradually increased up to 1.5 grams bid	

Note: *Italics* indicate common adverse effects; <u>underlining</u> indicates serious adverse effects.

(PO), several weeks may be necessary to achieve optimal effects. Phenobarbital is sometimes a preferred drug for the pharmacotherapy of neonatal seizures.

Overall, barbiturates are effective against all major seizure types except absence seizures. Primidone (Mysoline) has a pharmacologic profile similar to phenobarbital and is among the drugs used effectively to potentiate GABA action. Although used less frequently, barbiturates were once used on a regular basis to terminate the condition of **status epilepticus.** Intravenous (IV) administration of diazepam or lorazepam is now the preferred treatment for this condition.

Benzodiazepines

Like barbiturates, benzodiazepines intensify the effect of GABA in the brain. The benzodiazepines bind directly to the GABA receptor, suppressing abnormal neuronal foci.

15.6 Treating Seizures With Benzodiazepines

Benzodiazepines used in treating epilepsy include clonazepam (Klonopin), clorazepate (Tranxene), lorazepam (Ativan), and diazepam (Valium). Indications include **absence seizures** and **myoclonic seizures**. Parenteral diazepam (Valium) and lorazepam (Ativan) are used to terminate status epilepticus. Because tolerance may begin to develop after only a few months of therapy with benzodiazepines, seizures may recur unless the dose is periodically adjusted. These drugs are generally not used alone in seizure pharmacotherapy, but instead serve as adjuncts to other antiseizure drugs for short-term seizure control.

The benzodiazepines are one of the most widely prescribed classes of drugs, used not only to control seizures but also for anxiety, skeletal muscle spasms, and alcohol withdrawal symptoms.

DRUGS THAT SUPPRESS SODIUM INFLUX

Several drugs dampen CNS activity by delaying an influx of sodium ions across neuronal membranes. Hydantoins and related antiseizure drugs act by this mechanism.

Hydantoins and Related Drugs

Sodium channels guide the movement of sodium ions across neuronal membranes into the intracellular space. Sodium ion movement is the major factor that determines whether a neuron will undergo an action potential. If these channels are temporarily inactivated, neuronal activity will be suppressed. With hydantoin and phenytoin-related drugs, sodium channels are not blocked; they are just desensitized. If channels are blocked, neuronal activity completely stops, as occurs with local anesthetic drugs. Several drugs in this group may not desensitize sodium channels directly, but they may affect the threshold of neuronal firing, or they may interfere with transduction of the excitatory neurotransmitter glutamate. These actions are slightly removed from the direct suppression of sodium influx; however, the result (delayed depolarization of the neuron) is the same. These drugs are listed in Table 15.4.

15.7 Treating Seizures With Hydantoins and Related Drugs

Phenytoin (Dilantin) is a widely used medication. Approved in the 1930s, phenytoin is a broad-spectrum hydantoin drug, useful in treating all types of seizures except absence seizures. It provides effective seizure suppression

Table 15.4 Hydantoins and Related Drugs

Drug	Route and Adult Dose (max dose where indicated)	Adverse Effects
HYDANTOINS		
ethotoin (Peganone)	PO: 1 g/day in four to six divided doses. Usual maintenance dosage is 2–3 g/day	*Somnolence, drowsiness, dizziness, nystagmus, gingival hyperplasia*
fosphenytoin (Cerebyx)	IV: initial dose 15–20 mg PE*/kg at 100–150 mg PE/min followed by 4–6 mg PE/kg/day	Agranulocytosis, aplastic anemias; bullous, exfoliative, or purpuric dermatitis; Stevens–Johnson syndrome; toxic epidermal necrolysis; cardiovascular collapse; cardiac arrest
phenytoin (Dilantin)	PO: 15–18 mg/kg or 1-g initial dose; then 300 mg/day in one to three divided doses; may be gradually increased to 100 mg/wk (max: 600 mg daily) IV: 10–15 mg/kg IV loading dose followed by maintenance dose of 100 mg PO or IV every 6–8 h	
PHENYTOIN-RELATED DRUGS		
carbamazepine (Tegretol)	PO: 200 mg bid, gradually increased to 800–1200 mg/day in three to four divided doses	*Dizziness, ataxia, somnolence, headache, diplopia, blurred vision, transient indigestion, rhinitis, leukopenia, prolonged bleeding time, nausea, vomiting, anorexia*
eslicarbazepine (Aptiom)	PO: 400 mg/day for one wk, then increase to 800 mg/day at weekly intervals (max: 1200 mg/day)	Agranulocytosis; aplastic anemias; bullous, exfoliative dermatitis; Stevens–Johnson syndrome; toxic epidermal necrolysis; bone marrow depression; acute liver failure; pancreatitis; heart block; respiratory depression
felbamate (Felbatol)	PO (Lennox–Gastaut syndrome): 15 mg/kg/day in three to four divided doses gradually increased up to 45 mg/kg/day	
lamotrigine (Lamictal)	PO (adults): 1200 mg/day in three to four divided doses gradually increased up to 3600 mg/day	
levetiracetam (Keppra)	PO: 25–50 mg/day gradually increased up to 700 mg/day	
oxcarbazepine (Oxtellar XR, Trileptal)	PO: 500 mg bid (max: 3000 mg total per day)	
rufinamide (Banzel)	PO: 400 to 800 mg/day gradually increased up to 3,200 mg/day	
valproic acid (Depakene)**	PO/IV: 10–15 mg/kg/day in divided doses, gradually increased up to 60 mg/kg/day	
zonisamide (Zonegran)	PO: 100–400 mg/day gradually increased up to 400 mg/day	

*PE = phenytoin equivalents
** Other formulations of valproic acid include its salts, valproate, and divalproex sodium.
Note: *Italics* indicate common adverse effects; underlining indicates serious adverse effects.

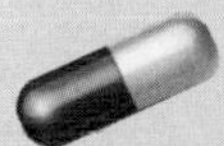

Prototype Drug | Phenobarbital *(Luminal)*

Therapeutic Class: Antiseizure drug; sedative
Pharmacologic Class: Barbiturate; $GABA_A$ receptor agonist

Actions and Uses

Phenobarbital is a long-acting barbiturate used for the management of a variety of seizures. It is also used to promote sleep. Phenobarbital should not be used for pain relief, because it may increase a patient's sensitivity to pain.

Phenobarbital acts biochemically by enhancing the action of the GABA neurotransmitter, which is responsible for suppressing abnormal neuronal discharges that can cause epilepsy.

Administration Alerts

- Parenteral phenobarbital is a soft-tissue irritant. Intramuscular (IM) injections may produce a local inflammatory reaction. IV administration is rarely used, because extravasation may produce tissue necrosis.
- Controlled substance: Schedule IV.
- Pregnancy category D.

PHARMACOKINETICS

Onset	Peak	Duration
20–60 min PO; 5 min IV	4–12 h PO; 30 min IV	10–16 h PO; 4–10 h IV

Adverse Effects

Phenobarbital is a Schedule IV drug that may cause dependence. Common side effects include drowsiness, vitamin deficiencies (vitamin D, folate [B_9]; and B_{12}), and laryngospasms. With overdose, phenobarbital may cause severe respiratory depression, CNS depression, coma, and death.

Contraindications: Administration of phenobarbital is inadvisable in cases of hypersensitivity to barbiturates, severe uncontrolled pain, pre-existing CNS depression, porphyrias, severe respiratory disease with dyspnea or obstruction, and glaucoma or prostatic hypertrophy.

Interactions

Drug–Drug: Phenobarbital interacts with many other drugs. For example, it should not be taken with alcohol or other CNS depressants. These substances potentiate barbiturate action, increasing the risk of life-threatening respiratory depression or cardiac arrest. Phenobarbital increases the metabolism of many other drugs, reducing their effectiveness.

Lab Tests: Barbiturates may affect bromsulphalein tests and increase serum phosphatase.

Herbal/Food: Kava and valerian may potentiate sedation.

Treatment of Overdose: There is no specific treatment for overdose. Drug removal may be accomplished by gastric lavage or use of activated charcoal. Hemodialysis may be effective in facilitating removal of phenobarbital from the body. Treatment is supportive and consists mainly of endotracheal intubation and mechanical ventilation. Treatment of bradycardia and hypotension may be necessary.

without the abuse potential or CNS depression associated with barbiturates. Patients vary significantly in their ability to metabolize phenytoin; therefore, dosages are highly individualized. Because of the very narrow range between a therapeutic dose and a toxic dose, patients must be carefully monitored. Phenytoin and fosphenytoin are first-line drugs in the treatment of status epilepticus.

Phenytoin-related drugs share a mechanism of action similar to that of the hydantoins, including carbamazepine (Tegretol), oxcarbazepine (Oxtellar XR, Trileptal), and valproic acid (Depakene), which is also available as valproate sodium and divalproex sodium. Because carbamazepine produces fewer adverse effects than other phenytoin-related drugs or phenobarbital, it is a preferred drug for tonic–clonic and partial seizures. Carbamazepine is also available in extended release forms (Carbatrol CR, Equetro, Tegretol XR). Oxcarbazepine is a derivative of carbamazepine, so its treatment profile is similar. Oxcarbazepine is slightly better tolerated than carbamazepine although serious skin and organ hypersensitivity reactions have been noted. Valproic acid is a preferred drug for absence and myoclonic seizures and is used in combination with other drugs for partial seizures. Both carbamazepine and valproic acid are used for bipolar disorder (see chapter 16). Divalproex sodium (Depakote) is dispensed as an enteric-coated tablet; other forms are Depakote sprinkle capsules and Depakote ER, an extended-release formulation. Depakene/Depakote are used for generalized tonic–clonic, myoclonic, partial, and absence seizures. These can be taken as monotherapy or in combination with other antiseizure drugs. Other indications are panic disorder (see chapter 14) and prophylaxis of migraine headaches (see chapter 18).

A number of antiseizure drugs show promise in treatment for a range of disorders including absence seizures,

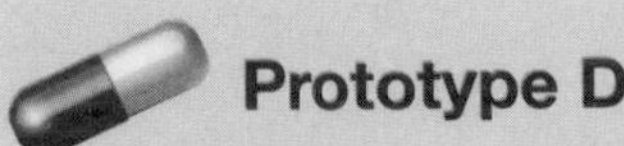

Prototype Drug | Diazepam (*Valium*)

Therapeutic Class: Antiseizure drug **Pharmacologic Class:** Benzodiazepine; $GABA_A$ receptor agonist

Actions and Uses

Diazepam binds to the GABA receptor–chloride channels throughout the CNS. It produces its effects by suppressing neuronal activity in the limbic system and subsequent impulses that might be transmitted to the reticular activating system. Effects of this drug are suppression of abnormal neuronal foci that may cause seizures, calming without strong sedation, and skeletal muscle relaxation. When used orally, maximum therapeutic effects may take from 1 to 2 weeks. Tolerance may develop after about 4 weeks. When given IV, effects occur in minutes, and its anticonvulsant effects last about 20 minutes.

Administration Alerts

- When administering IV, monitor respirations every 5 to 15 minutes. Have airway and resuscitative equipment accessible.
- Pregnancy category D.

PHARMACOKINETICS

Onset	Peak	Duration
30–60 min PO; 15–30 min IV	1–2 h PO; 15 min IM; 1–5 min IV	2–3 h PO; 15–60 min IV

Adverse Effects

Because of tolerance and dependency, use of diazepam is reserved for short-term seizure control or for status epilepticus. When given IV, hypotension, muscular weakness, tachycardia, and respiratory depression are common.

Contraindications: When administered in injectable form, this medication should be avoided under the following conditions: shock, coma, depressed vital signs, obstetrical patients, and infants less than 30 days of age. In tablet form, the medication should not be administered to infants less than 6 months of age, to patients with acute narrow-angle glaucoma or untreated open-angle glaucoma, or within 14 days of monoamine oxidase inhibitor (MAOI) therapy.

Interactions

Drug–Drug: Diazepam should not be taken with alcohol or other CNS depressants because of combined sedation effects. Other drug interactions include cimetidine, oral contraceptives, valproic acid, and metoprolol, which potentiate diazepam's action; and levodopa and barbiturates, which decrease diazepam's action. Diazepam increases the levels of phenytoin in the bloodstream and may cause phenytoin toxicity.

Lab Tests: Unknown.

Herbal/Food: Kava and chamomile may cause an increased drug effect.

Treatment of Overdose: If an overdose occurs, administer flumazenil (Romazicon), a specific benzodiazepine receptor antagonist to reverse CNS depression.

partial seizures, myoclonic seizures, generalized tonic–clonic seizures, and mood disorders. The most common adverse effects of the more recently approved antiseizure drugs are somnolence, drowsiness, dizziness, and blurred vision. Lamotrigine (Lamictal) has become a first-line drug for the management of partial, absence, and tonic-clonic seizures and is also FDA-approved for bipolar disorder. This drug's duration of action is greatly affected by other drugs that inhibit or enhance hepatic metabolizing enzymes. Levetiracetam (Keppra) and zonisamide (Zonegran) are approved for adjunctive therapy of partial seizures in adults. Among the approved antiseizure drugs, levetiracetam is generally less reactive and has less adverse effects than the other antiseizure medications. Conversely, zonisamide is a sulfonamide and can trigger hypersensitivity reactions in some patients. Felbamate (Felbatol) can also cause potentially fatal reactions in patients such as aplastic anemia and liver failure.

In a severe form of epilepsy called Lennox-Gastaut syndrome (LGS), valproic acid derivatives (Depakene, Depakote), lamotrigine (Lamictal), felbamate (Felbatol), topiramate (Topamax, Trokendi XR), and rufinamide (Banzel) are often used for treatment. LGS is characterized by tonic, atonic, atypical absence, and myoclonic symptoms. There is usually no single antiseizure medication that will control symptoms of this particular syndrome.

DRUGS THAT SUPPRESS CALCIUM INFLUX

Neurotransmitters, hormones, and some medications bind to neuronal membranes, stimulating the entry of calcium. Without calcium influx, neuronal transmission would not be possible. Succinimides delay entry of calcium into neurons by blocking low-threshold calcium channels, increasing the electrical threshold of the neuron, and reducing the likelihood that an action potential will be generated. By raising the seizure threshold, succinimides keep neurons from firing too quickly, thus

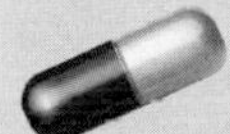

Prototype Drug | Phenytoin *(Dilantin)*

Therapeutic Class: Antiseizure drug; antidysrhythmic **Pharmacologic Class:** Hydantoin; sodium influx–suppressing drug

Actions and Uses

Phenytoin acts by desensitizing sodium channels in the CNS responsible for neuronal responsivity. Desensitization prevents the spread of disruptive electrical charges in the brain that produce seizures. It is effective against most types of seizures except absence seizures. Phenytoin has anti-dysrhythmic activity similar to that of lidocaine (class IB). An unlabeled use is for digitalis-induced dysrhythmias.

Administration Alerts

- When administering IV, mix with saline only, and infuse at the maximum rate of 50 mg/min. Mixing with other medications or dextrose solutions produces precipitate.
- Always prime or flush IV lines with saline before hanging phenytoin as a piggyback, because traces of dextrose solution in an existing main IV or piggyback line can cause microscopic precipitate formation which become emboli if infused. Use an IV line with filter when infusing this drug.
- Phenytoin injectable is a soft-tissue irritant that causes local tissue damage following extravasation. To reduce the risk of soft-tissue damage, do not give IM; inject into a large vein or via a central venous catheter.
- Avoid using hand veins to prevent serious local vaso-constrictive response (purple glove syndrome).
- Pregnancy category D.

PHARMACOKINETICS

Onset	Peak	Duration
Slowly and variably absorbed PO	1.5–3 h prompt release; 4–12 h sustained release	15 days

Adverse Effects

Phenytoin may cause dysrhythmias, such as bradycardia or ventricular fibrillation, severe hypotension, and hyperglycemia. Severe CNS reactions include headache, nystagmus, ataxia, confusion and slurred speech, paradoxical nervousness, twitching, and insomnia. Peripheral neuropathy may occur with long-term use. Phenytoin can cause multiple blood dyscrasias, including agranulocytosis and aplastic anemia.

This medication may cause severe skin reactions, such as rashes, including exfoliative dermatitis and Stevens–Johnson syndrome. Connective tissue reactions include lupus erythematosus, hypertrichosis, hirsutism, and gingival hypertrophy.

Black Box Warning: The rate of IV Dilantin administration should not exceed 50 mg/min in adults and 1–3 mg/kg/min (or 50 mg/min, whichever is slower) in pediatric patients because of the risk of severe hypotension and cardiac arrhythmias. Careful cardiac monitoring is needed during and after administering IV Dilantin.

Contraindications: Patients with hypersensitivity to hydantoin products should be cautious. Rash, seizures due to hypoglycemia, sinus bradycardia, and heart block are contraindications.

Interactions

Drug–Drug: Phenytoin interacts with many other drugs, including oral anticoagulants, glucocorticoids, H_2 antagonists, antituberculin drugs, and food supplements such as folic acid, calcium, and vitamin D. It impairs the efficacy of drugs such as digitoxin, doxycycline, furosemide, estrogens and oral contraceptives, and theophylline. When combined with tricyclic antidepressants, phenytoin can trigger seizures.

Lab Tests: Hydantoins may produce lower-than-normal values for dexamethasone or metyrapone tests. Phenytoin may increase serum levels of glucose, bromsulphalein, and alkaline phosphatase, and may decrease protein-bound iodine and urinary steroid levels.

Herbal/Food: Herbal laxatives (buckthorn, cascara sagrada, and senna) may increase potassium loss. Ginkgo may reduce the therapeutic effectiveness of phenytoin.

Treatment of Overdose: There is no specific treatment for overdose. Drug removal may be accomplished by gastric lavage, use of activated charcoal, or laxative. Treatment is supportive and consists mainly of maintaining the airway and breathing, monitoring phenytoin blood levels, and appropriately treating adverse symptoms.

suppressing abnormal foci. Amino acid compounds are thought to reduce neuronal damage and associated seizure-related symptoms. They tend to reduce intracellular accumulation of calcium while suppressing positive ion fluxes across cell membranes.

Succinimides

Succinimides are medications that suppress seizures by delaying calcium influx into neurons. They are generally only effective against absence seizures. The succinimides are listed in Table 15.5.

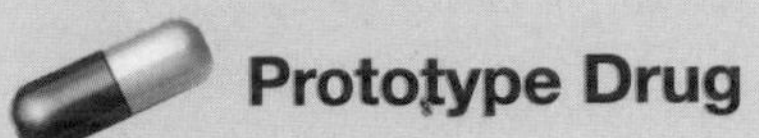

Prototype Drug | Valproic Acid *(Depakene)*

Therapeutic Class: Antiseizure drug **Pharmacologic Class:** Valproate

Actions and Uses

The mechanism of action of valproic acid (valproate) and its derivatives is widespread. Valproic acid (Depakene) and divalproex sodium (Depakote) are closely related drugs used for the treatment of petit mal, grand mal, mixed, and akinetic-myoclonic seizures. Valproate sodium (Depacon) is indicated as an IV alternative in patients for whom oral administration of valproate products is temporarily not feasible. Valproic acid has the same action as that of phenytoin, although effects on GABA and calcium channels also make this drug similar to benzodiazepines and succinimides. It is useful for a wide range of seizure types, including absence seizures and mixed types of seizures. Other uses include prevention of migraine headaches and treatment of bipolar disorder.

Administration Alerts

- Valproic acid is a gastrointestinal (GI) irritant. Advise patients not to chew extended-release tablets because mouth soreness will occur.
- Do not mix valproic acid syrup with carbonated beverages because it will trigger immediate release of the drug, which causes severe mouth and throat irritation.
- Open capsules and sprinkle on soft foods if the patient cannot swallow them.
- Pregnancy category D.

PHARMACOKINETICS

Onset	Peak	Duration
Readily absorbed from the GI tract	1–4 h	Variable

Adverse Effects

Side effects include sedation, drowsiness, GI upset, and prolonged bleeding time. Other effects include visual disturbances, muscle weakness, tremor, psychomotor agitation, bone marrow suppression, weight gain, abdominal cramps, rash, alopecia, pruritus, photosensitivity, erythema multiforme, and fatal hepatotoxicity.

Black Box Warning: May result in fatal hepatic failure, especially in children under the age of 2 years. Nonspecific symptoms often precede hepatic toxicity: weakness, facial edema, anorexia, and vomiting. Liver function tests should be performed prior to treatment and at specific intervals during the first 6 months of treatment. Valproic acid can produce life-threatening pancreatitis and teratogenic effects including spina bifida.

Contraindications: Hypersensitivity may occur. This medication should not be administered to patients with liver disease, bleeding dysfunction, pancreatitis, and congenital metabolic disorders.

Interactions

Drug–Drug: Valproic acid interacts with many drugs. For example, aspirin, cimetidine, chlorpromazine, erythromycin, and felbamate may increase valproic acid toxicity. Concomitant warfarin, aspirin, or alcohol use can cause severe bleeding. Alcohol, benzodiazepines, and other CNS depressants potentiate CNS depressant action. Use of clonazepam concurrently with valproic acid may induce absence seizures. Valproic acid increases serum phenobarbital and phenytoin levels. Lamotrigine, phenytoin, and rifampin lower valproic acid levels.

Lab Tests: Unknown.

Herbal/Food: Unknown.

Table 15.5 Succinimides

Drug	Route and Adult Dose (max dose where indicated)	Adverse Effects
ethosuximide (Zarontin)	PO: 250 mg bid, increased every 4–7 days (max: 1.5 g/day)	*Drowsiness, dizziness, ataxia, epigastric distress, weight loss, anorexia, nausea, vomiting*
methsuximide (Celontin)	PO: 300 mg/day; may increase every 4–7 days (max: 1.2 g/day)	Agranulocytosis, pancytopenia, aplastic anemia, granulocytopenia

Note: *Italics* indicate common adverse effects; underlining indicates serious adverse effects.

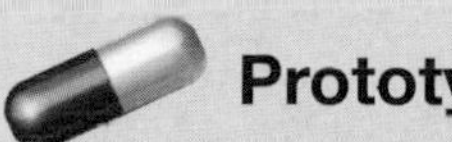

Prototype Drug | Ethosuximide *(Zarontin)*

Therapeutic Class: Antiseizure drug **Pharmacologic Class:** Succinimide

Actions and Uses

Ethosuximide is a preferred drug for managing absence seizures. It depresses the activity of neurons in the motor cortex by elevating the neuronal threshold. It is usually ineffective against psychomotor or tonic–clonic seizures; however, it may be given in combination with other medications that better treat these conditions. It is available in tablet and flavored-syrup formulations.

Administration Alerts

- Do not abruptly withdraw this medication because doing so may induce tonic–clonic seizures.
- Pregnancy category C.

PHARMACOKINETICS

Onset	Peak	Duration
Readily absorbed from the GI tract	4 h	Variable

Adverse Effects

Ethosuximide may impair mental and physical abilities. Psychosis or extreme mood swings, including depression with overt suicidal intent, can occur. Behavioral changes are more prominent in patients with a history of psychiatric illness. CNS effects include dizziness, headache, lethargy, fatigue, ataxia, sleep pattern disturbances, attention difficulty, and hiccups. Bone marrow suppression and blood dyscrasias are possible, as is systemic lupus erythematosus.

Other reactions include gingival hypertrophy and tongue swelling. Common side effects are abdominal distress and weight loss.

Contraindications: Hypersensitivity may occur. Do not use this medication in cases of severe liver or kidney disease. Safety in children younger than 3 years of age has not been established.

Interactions

Drug–Drug: Ethosuximide increases phenytoin serum levels. Valproic acid causes ethosuximide serum levels to fluctuate (increase and decrease).

Lab Tests: Unknown.

Herbal/Food: Ginkgo may reduce the therapeutic effectiveness of ethosuximide.

Treatment of Overdose: There is no specific treatment for overdose. Drug removal may include emesis unless the patient is comatose or convulsing. Treatment may be accomplished by gastric lavage, use of activated charcoal or cathartics, and general supportive measures. Hemodialysis may be effective in facilitating removal of ethosuximide from the body.

15.8 Treating Seizures With Succinimides

Ethosuximide (Zarontin) is the most commonly prescribed drug in this class. It remains a preferred choice for absence seizures, although valproic acid is also effective for these types of seizures. Some of the newer antiseizure drugs, such as lamotrigine (Lamictal) and zonisamide (Zonegran), are being investigated for their roles in treating absence seizures. Lamotrigine has also been found to be effective in patients with partial seizures, usually in combination with other antiseizure medications.

☑ Check Your Understanding 15.1

If an antiseizure drug must be discontinued, how will this be accomplished and why is this method necessary? *Visit www.pearsonhighered.com/nursingresources for the answer.*

Amino Acid Compounds

Some amino acid compounds reduce brain excitability by suppressing positive ion influxes in a manner differently from the other seizure medications. These compounds may suppress ischemia-associated glutamate release. With reduced glutamate release, positive ion influxes and accumulation of intracellular calcium are slowed.

15.9 Treating Seizures With Amino Acid Compounds

Successful administration of amino acids to children with epilepsy has prompted researchers to explore additional approaches in seizure therapy. Administration of amino acid compounds has been particularly effective on the paroxysmal and psychopathologic component of epilepsy. For infants with epilepsy, administration of natural amino acids (e.g., taurine) has supported mental and speech development, which often suffer because of repeated seizures.

Acetazolamide (Diamox) and lacosamide (Vimpat) are two drugs with properties useful in the treatment of a range of conditions and seizures. These drugs restore ionic and thus neurologic imbalances similar to natural amino acids. Acetazolamide is a carbonic hydrase inhibitor approved for the symptomatic relief of glaucoma, for altitude sickness, and for a range of conditions including nausea, dizziness, drowsiness, and fatigue. Its main nervous system application is the treatment of absence and myoclonic seizures. The generic acetazolamide also has diuretic properties. Lacosamide is a prescription medication chemically related to serine. Although this drug does not produce effects through suppression of voltage-gated calcium channels, other membrane protein channels are likely involved. Lacosamide is used in combination with other drugs to treat adult patients with partial-onset seizures. Drawbacks to amino acid therapy are potential allergic reactions, drowsiness, dizziness, irregular heartbeat, and problems with coordination.

Nursing Practice Application

Pharmacotherapy With Antiseizure Drugs

ASSESSMENT	POTENTIAL NURSING DIAGNOSES*
Baseline assessment prior to administration: • Obtain a complete health history including hepatic, renal, cardiovascular, or neurologic disease; mental status; narrow-angle glaucoma; and pregnancy or breast-feeding. Obtain a drug history including allergies, current prescription and over-the-counter (OTC) drugs, and herbal preparations. Be alert to possible drug interactions. • Obtain a seizure history (e.g., frequency, duration, physical symptoms, prodromal warnings, length of postictal period). • Obtain baseline vital signs, weight, and, in pediatric patients, height. • Obtain a developmental history in pediatric patients (e.g., DDST-II level of growth and development, school performance). • Evaluate appropriate laboratory findings (e.g., complete blood count [CBC], electrolytes, hepatic or renal function studies). • Assess the patient's ability to receive and understand instruction. Include the family and caregivers as needed.	• *Situational Low Self-Esteem* • *Social Isolation* • *Deficient Knowledge (drug therapy)* • *Risk for Injury,* related to seizures or adverse drug effects *NANDA I © 2014
Assessment throughout administration: • Assess for desired therapeutic effects (e.g., diminished or absence of seizure activity). • Continue periodic monitoring of CBC and liver and renal function studies. • Assess vital signs and weight periodically or if symptoms warrant. **Lifespan:** Assess height and weight of all pediatric patients. • Assess for and promptly report adverse effects: excessive dizziness, drowsiness, light-headedness, confusion, agitation, palpitations, tachycardia, blurred or double vision, continuous seizure activity, skin rashes, bruising or bleeding, abdominal pain, jaundice, change in color of stool, flank pain, and hematuria.	

IMPLEMENTATION

Interventions and (Rationales)	Patient-Centered Care
Ensuring therapeutic effects: • Continue assessments as described earlier for therapeutic effects. (Antiseizure drugs may not completely resolve symptoms but frequency and severity of seizures should be diminished.)	• Teach the patient, family, or caregiver to keep a seizure diary of frequency, type, length, prodromal symptoms, and postictal period.

Nursing Practice Application *continued*

IMPLEMENTATION	
Interventions and (Rationales)	**Patient-Centered Care**
Minimizing adverse effects: • Continue to monitor vital signs, mental status, coordination, and balance periodically. **Lifespan:** Ensure patient safety, being particularly cautious with older adults who are at increased risk for falls. (Antiseizure drugs may cause drowsiness and dizziness, hypotension, or impaired mental and physical abilities, increasing the risk of falls and injury.) • **Lifespan:** Continue to monitor height, weight, and developmental level in pediatric patients. In the school-age child, assess school performance. (Adverse effects of antiseizure drugs or unresolved seizures may hinder normal growth and development.)	• **Safety:** Teach the patient to rise from lying or sitting to standing slowly to avoid dizziness or falls. If dizziness occurs, the patient should sit or lie down and not attempt to stand or walk, until the sensation passes. **Lifespan:** Teach the patient, family, or caregiver to be especially cautious with the older adult who is at greater risk for falls. • **Safety:** Instruct the patient to call for assistance prior to getting out of bed or attempting to walk alone, and to avoid driving or other activities requiring mental alertness or physical coordination until the effects of the drug are known. • Teach the patient's family or caregiver to keep regularly scheduled appointments with the health care provider and report any developmental lags or concerns.
• Continue to monitor drug levels, CBC, renal and hepatic function, and pancreatic enzymes. (Antiseizure drugs require periodic drug levels to correlate the level with symptoms. Antiseizure drugs may cause hepatotoxicity and valproic acid may cause pancreatitis as an adverse effect. **Diverse Patients:** Some antiseizure drugs induce or inhibit P450 enzymes and may interact with other drugs. Ethnically diverse populations may also experience less than optimal effects of the drug.)	• Instruct the patient on the need to return periodically for laboratory work. • **Diverse Patients:** Teach all patients, but especially ethnically diverse patients, to observe for less than optimal effects and report promptly. • Instruct the patient to carry a wallet identification card or wear medical identification jewelry indicating a seizure disorder and antiseizure medication. • Teach the patient to promptly report any abdominal pain, particularly in the upper quadrants; changes in stool color; yellowing of sclera or skin; or darkened urine.
• Assess for changes in the level of consciousness, disorientation or confusion, or agitation. (Neurologic changes may indicate overmedication or adverse drug effects.)	• Instruct the patient, family, or caregiver to immediately report increasing lethargy, disorientation, confusion, changes in behavior or mood, slurred speech, or ataxia.
• Assess for changes in visual acuity, blurred vision, decrease of peripheral vision, seeing rainbow halos around lights, acute eye pain, or any of these symptoms accompanied by nausea and vomiting, and report immediately. (Increased intraoptic pressure in patients with narrow-angle glaucoma may occur in patients taking benzodiazepines.)	• Instruct the patient to immediately report any visual changes or eye pain.
• Assess for bruising, bleeding, or signs of infection. (Antiseizure drugs may cause blood dyscrasias and increased chances of bleeding or infection.)	• Teach the patient to promptly report any signs of increased bruising, bleeding, or infections (e.g., sore throat and fever, skin rash).
• Monitor affect and emotional status. (Antiseizure drugs may increase the risk of mental depression and suicide. Concurrent use of alcohol or other CNS depressants increase the effects and the risk.)	• Instruct the patient, family, or caregiver to report significant mood changes, especially depression, and to avoid alcohol and other CNS depressants while taking the drug.
• Assess the condition of gums and oral hygiene measures. (Hydantoins and phenytoin-related drugs may cause gingival hyperplasia, increasing the risk of oral infections.)	• Instruct the patient to maintain excellent oral hygiene and keep regularly scheduled dental appointments.
• Encourage appropriate lifestyle and dietary changes. (Caffeine and nicotine may decrease the effectiveness of the benzodiazepines. Barbiturates, drugs with GABA action, and hydantoins and phenytoin-related drugs affect the absorption of vitamins K, D, folic acid, and B vitamins. Alcohol and other CNS depressants may increase the adverse effects of the antiseizure drugs.)	• Encourage the patient to decrease or abstain from caffeine, nicotine, and alcohol; and increase intake of folic acid, and vitamins B-, D-, and K–rich foods. • Advise the patient to discuss all OTC medications with the health care provider to ensure that caffeine or alcohol is not included in the formulation.
• **Lifespan:** Monitor children for paradoxical response to barbiturates. (Hyperactivity may occur.)	• Instruct the patient, family, or caregiver to notify the health care provider if the patient exhibits hyperactive behavior.

continued

Nursing Practice Application *continued*

IMPLEMENTATION	
Interventions and (Rationales)	**Patient-Centered Care**
• **Lifespan:** Assess women of child-bearing age for the possibility of pregnancy, plans for pregnancy, breast-feeding, and contraceptive use. (Antiseizure medications are category D in pregnancy. Barbiturates decrease the effectiveness of oral contraceptives and additional forms of contraception should be used.)	• **Collaboration:** Discuss pregnancy and family planning with women of child-bearing age. Explain the effect of medications on pregnancy and breast-feeding and the need to discuss any pregnancy plans with the health care provider. Discuss the need for additional forms of contraception, including barrier methods, with patients taking barbiturates for seizure control.
• Avoid abrupt discontinuation of therapy. (Status epilepticus may occur with abrupt discontinuation.)	• Instruct the patient to take the drug exactly as prescribed and to not stop it abruptly.
• Assess home storage of medications and identify risks for corrective action. (Overdosage may occur if the patient takes additional doses when drowsy or disoriented from medication effects. Overdosage with barbiturates may prove fatal.)	• **Safety:** Instruct the patient that these drugs should not be kept at the bedside and to avoid taking additional doses when drowsy.
• Provide emotional support and appropriate referrals as needed. (Treatment with antiseizure drugs may require using combinations of drugs, and seizure activity may diminish but may not be resolved. Social isolation and low self-esteem may occur with continued seizure disorder.)	• **Collaboration:** Teach the patient, family, or caregiver about support groups and make appropriate referrals as needed.
• Closely monitor the IV infusion site when using IV antiseizure drugs. All IV drips should be given via infusion pump. (Benzodiazepines, hydantoins, and barbiturates are irritating to the vein. Blanching and pain at the IV site are indicators of extravasation and the IV infusion should be immediately stopped and the provider contacted for further treatment orders. Infusion pumps will allow precise dosing of the medication.)	• Teach the patient to immediately report pain or burning at the IV site or in the extremity with IV.
Patient understanding of drug therapy:	
• Use opportunities during administration of medications and during assessments to provide patient education. (Using time during nursing care helps to optimize and reinforce key teaching areas.)	• The patient should be able to state the reason for the drug; appropriate dose and scheduling; what adverse effects to observe for and when to report; and the anticipated length of medication therapy.
Patient self-administration of drug therapy:	
• When administering the medication, instruct the patient, family, or caregiver in proper self-administration of the drug. (Using time during nurse administration of these drugs helps to reinforce teaching.)	• Teach the patient to take the medication as follows: • Exactly as ordered and the same manufacturer's brand each time the prescription is filled. (Switching brands may result in differing pharmacokinetics and alterations in seizure control.) • Read label directions for how to take the medication. Some forms may not be opened or chewed; others require chewing thoroughly. When it doubt, consult with a pharmacist or other health care provider. • Take a missed dose as soon as it is noticed, but do not take double or extra doses to "catch up." • Take with food to decrease GI upset. • Do not abruptly discontinue the medication.

See Tables 15.3, 15.4, and 15.5 for lists of drugs to which these nursing actions apply. (See also the Nursing Practice Application table in chapter 14, information related to benzodiazepine and nonbenzodiazepine drugs.)

Chapter Review

KEY Concepts

The numbered key concepts provide a succinct summary of the important points from the corresponding numbered section within the chapter. If any of these points are not clear, refer to the numbered section within the chapter for review.

15.1 Seizures are symptomatic of an underlying disorder and are associated with many causes, including brain infection, head trauma, fluid and electrolyte imbalance, hypoxia, stroke, brain tumors, and high fever in children. Pregnancy and quality of life are important issues to consider when discussing epilepsy and seizure management.

15.2 The three broad categories of seizures are partial seizures, generalized seizures, and special epileptic syndromes. Each seizure type has a characteristic set of signs. Control of seizures requires proper diagnosis and drug selection.

15.3 Both traditional and nontraditional antiseizure drugs are indicated for seizures. Both drug classes have serious drawbacks.

15.4 The goal of antiseizure pharmacotherapy is to suppress neuronal activity just enough to prevent abnormal or repetitive fire. There are three general mechanisms by which antiseizure drugs act: stimulating an influx of chloride ions, delaying an influx of sodium, and delaying an influx of calcium.

15.5 GABA-potentiating barbiturates, mainly phenobarbital and primidone, are effective against all kinds of seizures except for absence seizures. GABA-related drugs may be used for a variety of conditions

15.6 Benzodiazepines reduce seizure activity by potentiating GABA action. Their use is limited to short-term therapy for absence seizures and myoclonic seizures and to terminate status epilepticus.

15.7 Hydantoin and related drugs act by delaying sodium influx into neurons. Phenytoin, carbamazepine, and oxcarbazepine are broad-spectrum drugs used for all types of epilepsy except absence seizures. Valproic acid and lamotrigine treat all major types of seizures. Several drugs in this class act by more than one mechanism.

15.8 Succinimides act by delaying calcium influx into neurons. Ethosuximide (Zarontin) is a preferred choice for absence seizures.

15.9 Amino acid compounds reduce the onset of seizures and neuronal damage presumably by keeping positive ion fluxes balanced. Examples are taurine, acetazolamide (Diamox), and lacosamide (Vimpat).

REVIEW Questions

1. An 8-year-old boy is evaluated and diagnosed with absence seizures. He is started on ethosuximide (Zarontin). Which information should the nurse provide the parents?
   1. After-school sports activities will need to be stopped because they will increase the risk of seizures.
   2. Monitor height and weight to assess that growth is progressing normally.
   3. Fractures may occur, so increase the amount of vitamin D and calcium-rich foods in the diet.
   4. Avoid dehydration with activities and increase fluid intake.

2. The nurse is providing education for a 12-year-old patient with partial seizures currently prescribed valproic acid (Depakene). The nurse will teach the patient and the parents to immediately report which symptom?
   1. Increasing or severe abdominal pain
   2. Decreased or foul taste in the mouth
   3. Pruritus and dry skin
   4. Bone and joint pain

3. The nurse is caring for a 72-year-old patient taking gabapentin (Gralise, Horizant, Neurontin) for a seizure disorder. Because of this patient's age, the nurse would establish which nursing diagnosis related to the drug's common adverse effects?
   1. Risk for Deficient Fluid Volume
   2. Risk for Impaired Verbal Communication
   3. Risk for Constipation
   4. Risk for Falls
4. A patient has been taking phenytoin (Dilantin) for control of generalized seizures, tonic–clonic type. The patient is admitted to the medical unit with symptoms of nystagmus, confusion, and ataxia. What change in the phenytoin dosage does the nurse anticipate will be made based on these symptoms?
   1. The dosage will be increased.
   2. The dosage will be decreased.
   3. The dosage will remain unchanged; these are symptoms unrelated to the phenytoin.
   4. The dosage will remain unchanged but an additional antiseizure medication may be added.
5. Teaching for a patient receiving carbamazepine (Tegretol) should include instructions that the patient should immediately report which symptom?
   1. Leg cramping
   2. Blurred vision
   3. Lethargy
   4. Blister-like rash
6. Which of the following medications may be used to treat partial seizures? (Select all that apply.)
   1. Phenytoin (Dilantin)
   2. Valproic acid (Depakene)
   3. Diazepam (Valium)
   4. Carbamazepine (Tegretol)
   5. Ethosuximide (Zarontin)

PATIENT-FOCUSED Case Study

Joelle Birdwell, 16 years old, presents to the clinic with fatigue and pallor. She has a history of a generalized tonic-clonic seizure disorder that has been managed well on carbamazepine (Tegretol). In addition to her pallor and fatigue, Joelle has multiple small petechiae and bruises on her arms and legs. Her hematocrit is 26%.

1. In which drug classification does carbamazepine (Tegretol) belong?
2. What are adverse effects associated with carbamazepine?
3. Can Joelle's symptoms be related to her use of carbamazepine?

CRITICAL THINKING Questions

1. A 24-year-old woman is brought to the emergency department by her husband. He tells the triage nurse that his wife has been treated for seizure disorder secondary to a head injury she received in an automobile accident. She takes phenytoin (Dilantin) 100 mg every 8 hours. He relates a history of increasing drowsiness and lethargy in his wife over the past 24 hours. A phenytoin level is performed, and the nurse notes that the results are 24 mcg/dL. What does this result signify, and what changes does the nurse anticipate will be made to this patient's treatment? (A laboratory guide may need to be consulted.)
2. The nurse is admitting a 17-year-old female patient with a history of seizure disorder. The patient has broken her leg in a car accident in which she was the driver. The patient states that she hates having to take her phenytoin (Dilantin) and that she stopped the drug because she was not allowed to drive and it was making her angry. Explain the possible long-term effects of phenytoin therapy and their impact on patient compliance with the treatment plan. What additional information could the nurse provide for this patient?

Visit www.pearsonhighered.com/nursingresources for answers and rationales for all activities.

REFERENCES

Chen, L. L. K., Baca, C. B., Choe, J., Chen, J. W., Ayad, M. E., & Cheng, E. M. (2014). Posttraumatic epilepsy in Operation Enduring Freedom/Operation Iraqi Freedom veterans. *Military Medicine, 179,* 492–496. doi:10.7205/MILMED-D-13-00413

Herdman, T. H., & Kamitsuru, S. (Eds.). (2014). *NANDA International nursing diagnoses: Definitions and classification, 2015–2017.* Oxford, United Kingdom: Wiley-Blackwell.

LaFrance, W. C., Reuber, M., & Goldstein, L. H. (2013). Management of psychogenic nonepileptic seizures. *Epilepsia, 54*(Suppl. 1), 53–67. doi:10.111/epi.12106

Levy, R. G., Cooper, P. N., Giri, P., & Pulman, J. (2012). Ketogenic diet and other dietary treatments for epilepsy. *Cochrane Database of Systematic Reviews, 3,* Art. No.: CD001903. doi:10.1002/14651858.CD001903.pub2

Salinsky, M., Storzbach, D., Goy, E., & Evrad, C. (2014). Traumatic brain injury and psychogenic seizures in veterans. *The Journal of Head Trauma Rehabilitation, 30*(1), E65–E70. doi:10.1097/HTR.0000000000000057

Schachter, S. C., Kossoff, E., & Sirven, J. (2013.). *Ketogenic diet.* Retrieved from http://www.epilepsy.com/learn/treating-seizures-and-epilepsy/dietary-therapies/ketogenic-diet

SELECTED BIBLIOGRAPHY

Asconapé, J. J. (2014). Use of antiepileptic drugs in hepatic and renal disease. *Handbook of Clinical Neurology, 119,* 417–432. doi:10.1016/B978-0-7020-4086-3.00027-8

Bialer, M. (2012). Why are antiepileptic drugs used for nonepileptic conditions? *Epilepsia. 53*(Suppl. 7), 26–33. doi:10.1111/j.1528-1167.2012.03712.x

Borthen, I., & Gilhus, N. E. (2012). Pregnancy complications in patients with epilepsy. *Current Opinion in Obstetrics and Gynecology 24,* 78–83. doi:10.1097/GCO.0b013e32834feb6a

Cervenka, M. C., Terao, N. N., Bosarge, J. L., Henry, B. J., Klees, A. A., Morrison, P. F., & Kossoff, E. H. (2012). E-mail management of the modified Atkins Diet for adults with epilepsy is feasible and effective. *Epilepsia, 53,* 728–732. doi:10.1111/j.1528–1167.2012.03406.x

Citizens United for Research in Epilepsy (CURE). (n.d.). *Epilepsy facts,* Retrieved from http://www.cureepilepsy.org/aboutepilepsy/facts.asp

Dalkara, S., & Karakurt, A. (2012). Recent progress in anticonvulsant drug research: Strategies for anticonvulsant drug development and applications of antiepileptic drugs for non-epileptic central nervous system disorders. *Current Topics in Medicinal Chemistry, 12*(9), 1033–1071. doi:10.2174/156802612800229215

Di Filippo, T., Parisi, L., & Roccella, M. (2012). Evaluation of creative thinking in children with idiopathic epilepsy (absence epilepsy). *Minerva Pediatrica, 64,* 7–14.

Foreman, B., & Hirsch, L. J. (2012). Epilepsy emergencies: Diagnosis and management. *Neurologic Clinics, 30,* 11–41. doi:10.1016/j.ncl.2011.09.005

Hirsch, L. J. (2012). Intramuscular versus intravenous benzodiazepines for prehospital treatment of status epilepticus. *New England Journal of Medicine, 366,* 659–660.

Oja, S. S., Saransaari, P. (2013). Taurine and epilepsy. *Epilepsy Research, 104,* 187–194. doi:10.1016/j.eplepsyres.2013.01.010

Pizzol, A. D., Martin, K. C., Mattiello, C. M., de Souza, A. C., Torres, C. M., Bragatti, J. A., & Bianchin, M. M. (2012). Impact of the chronic use of benzodiazepines prescribed for seizure control on the anxiety levels of patients with epilepsy. *Epilepsy and Behavior, 23,* 373–376. doi:10.1016/j.yebeh.2011.12.009

Prince, N. J., & Hill, C. (2011). Purple glove syndrome following intravenous phenytoin administration. *Archives of Disease in Childhood, 96,* 734. doi:10.1136/archdischild-2011-300236

Sirikonda, N. S., Patten, W. D., Phillips, J. R., & Mullett, C. J. (2012). Ketogenic diet: Rapid onset of selenium deficiency-induced cardiac decompensation. *Pediatric Cardiology, 33,* 834–838. doi:10.1007/s00246-012-0219-6

Wang, Y., & Khanna, R. (2011). Voltage-gated calcium channels are not affected by the novel anti-epileptic drug lacosamide. *Translational Neuroscience, 2,* 13–22. doi:10.2478/s13380-011-0002-9

Wang, H. R., Woo, Y. S., & Bahk, W. M. (2014). Anticonvulsants to treat post-traumatic stress disorder. *Human Psychopharmacology, 29,* 427–433. doi:10.1002/hup.2425

Chapter 16

Drugs for Emotional, Mood, and Behavioral Disorders

Drugs at a Glance

Learning Outcomes

After reading this chapter, the student should be able to:

1. Identify the two major categories of mood disorders and their symptoms.
2. Identify the symptoms of attention deficit/hyperactivity disorder.
3. Explain the etiology of major depressive disorder.
4. Discuss the nurse's role in the pharmacologic management of patients with depression, bipolar disorder, or attention deficit/hyperactivity disorder.
5. For each of the drug classes listed in Drugs at a Glance, recognize representative drug examples, and explain their mechanism of action, primary actions, and important adverse effects.
6. Categorize drugs used for mood, emotional, and behavioral disorders based on their classification and drug action.
7. Use the nursing process to care for patients receiving pharmacotherapy for mood, emotional, and behavioral disorders.

(pill icon) indicates a prototype drug, each of which is featured in a Prototype Drug box.

Inappropriate or unusually intense emotions are common characteristics of mental health disorders. Although mood changes are a normal part of life, when those changes become severe and impair functionality within the family, work environment, or relationships, an individual may be diagnosed as having a **mood disorder.** The two major categories of mood disorders are depression and bipolar disorder. A third behavioral disorder, attention deficit/hyperactivity disorder, is also included in this chapter.

DEPRESSION

Depression is an emotional disorder characterized by a sad or despondent mood. Many symptoms are associated with depression, including lack of energy, sleep disturbances, abnormal eating patterns, and feelings of despair, guilt, or hopelessness. Depression is the most common mental health disorder of older adults, encompassing a variety of physical, emotional, cognitive, and social considerations.

16.1 Characteristics and Forms of Depression

Among the most common forms of mental illness, **major depressive disorder** or **clinical depression** is estimated to affect 5% to 10% of adults in the United States. The American Psychiatric Association's *Diagnostic and Statistical Manual of Mental Disorders,* 5th edition (DSM-5), describes the following criteria for diagnosis of a major depressive disorder: a depressed affect plus at least five of the following symptoms lasting for a minimum of 2 weeks:

- Difficulty sleeping or sleeping too much
- Extremely tired; without energy
- Abnormal eating patterns (eating too much or not enough)
- Vague physical symptoms (gastrointestinal [GI] pain, joint/muscle pain, or headaches)
- Inability to concentrate or make decisions
- Feelings of despair, guilt, and misery; lack of self-worth
- Obsessed with death (expressing a wish to die or to commit suicide)
- Avoiding psychosocial and interpersonal interactions
- Lack of interest in personal appearance or sex
- Delusions or hallucinations.

The majority of depressed patients are not found in psychiatric hospitals but in mainstream society. For proper diagnosis and treatment to occur, recognition of depression is often a collaborative effort among health care providers. For example, it might be the pharmacist who recognizes that a customer is depressed when the customer buys natural or over-the-counter (OTC) remedies to control anxiety symptoms or to induce sleep.

Situational depression occurs when the depression is the result of a circumstance in a person's life, for example, loss of a job or unfavorable event at home such as death, children leaving home, or divorce. **Dysthymic disorder** is characterized by less severe depressive symptoms that may last several years and prevent a person from feeling well or functioning normally. Because depressed patients may be found in multiple settings, every nurse should be proficient in the assessment of patients afflicted with these conditions.

Some women experience intense mood shifts associated with hormonal changes during the menstrual cycle, pregnancy, childbirth, and menopause. Up to 80% of women who give birth experience **postpartum depression** during the first several weeks after birth of their baby. About 10% of new mothers experience a major depressive episode within 6 months related to the dramatic hormonal shifts that occur during postdelivery. Along with the hormonal changes, additional situational stresses, such as responsibilities at home or work, single parenthood, and caring for children or for aging parents, may contribute to the onset of symptoms. If mood is severely depressed and persists long enough, many women will likely benefit from medical treatment, including women with premenstrual dysphoric disorder, depression during pregnancy, postpartum mood disorders, or menopausal distress.

Because of the possible consequences of perinatal mood disorders, some state agencies mandate that all new mothers receive information about mood shifts prior to their discharge after giving birth. Health care providers in obstetricians' offices, pediatric outpatient settings, and family medicine centers are encouraged to conduct routine screening for symptoms of perinatal mood disorders.

During the dark winter months, some patients experience **seasonal affective disorder (SAD).** This type of depression is associated with enhanced release of the brain neurohormone melatonin due to lower levels of natural light. Exposing patients on a regular basis to specific wavelengths of light may relieve SAD depression and prevent future episodes.

Psychotic depression is characterized by the expression of intense mood shifts and unusual behaviors. Depressive signs and loss of contact with reality, hallucinations, delusions, and disorganized speech patterns are the behaviors observed. For patients with psychosis and for patients with extreme mood swings, severe behaviors are often treatable with antipsychotic therapy. See section 16.8 of this chapter and chapter 17.

16.2 Assessment and Treatment of Depression

The first step in implementing appropriate treatment for depression is a complete health examination. Certain drugs, such as corticosteroids, levodopa, and oral contraceptives, can cause the same symptoms as depression, and the health care provider should rule out this possibility. Depression may be mimicked by a variety of medical and neurologic disorders, ranging from B-vitamin deficiencies to thyroid gland problems to early Alzheimer's disease. If physical

Treating the Diverse Patient: Cultural Influences and the Treatment of Depression

Depression and other mental illnesses are universal to all cultures but the symptoms, willingness to talk about the symptoms, and a person's decision to seek health care and follow a health care provider's recommendations for treatment are not universal. Age, gender, and cultural factors play a role. Because there is a stigma associated with mental illness, assuming there are cultural patterns associated with depression may hinder the nurse and other health care providers from fully understanding the patient's symptoms and providing needed treatment that is acceptable to the patient.

Mood disorders such as depression may not be viewed as a mental health issue but as one that has a foundation in morally or socially accepted norms. In many cultures, it is often considered more appropriate and acceptable to discuss physical symptoms than mental ones. *Somatization*, or experiencing physical symptoms in response to emotional or mental distress, may then become a possible reason for health care–seeking behaviors.

The nurse has the opportunity to help patients gain optimal health by listening to the patient's explanations for an illness as much as by assessing for physical symptoms. Subtle cues and possible symptoms such as fatigue, GI complaints, or lack of concentration may indicate depression. The nurse can ask the patient for help in understanding the cultural meaning of those symptoms to the patient. By avoiding stereotypes related to culture, the nurse can help increase the opportunity for patients with depression to receive appropriate treatment that works within their own culture and beliefs.

causes for the depression are ruled out, a psychological evaluation is often performed to confirm the diagnosis.

During initial health examinations, the nurse should make inquiries about alcohol and drug use and any thoughts about death or suicide. This exam should include questions about any family history of depressive illness. If other family members have been treated for depression, the nurse should document what therapies they may have received and which were effective or helpful.

To determine a course of treatment, the nurse assesses for well-accepted symptoms of depression. In general, severe depressive illness, particularly that which is recurrent, will require both medication and psychotherapy to achieve the best response. Counseling therapies help patients gain insight into and resolve their problems through verbal interaction with the therapist. Behavioral therapies help patients learn how to obtain more satisfaction and rewards through their own actions and how to unlearn the behavioral patterns that contribute to or result from mood shifts.

Helpful short-term psychotherapies for some forms of depression are *interpersonal* and *cognitive–behavioral therapies*. Interpersonal therapies focus on the patient's disturbed personal relationships that both cause and exacerbate the depression. Cognitive–behavioral therapies help patients change the negative styles of thought and behavior often associated with their depression.

Psychodynamic therapies focus on resolving the patient's internal conflicts. These therapies are often postponed until the depressive symptoms are significantly improved.

In patients unresponsive to cognitive-behavioral or psychodynamic therapies, **electroconvulsive therapy (ECT)** continues to be a useful treatment. ECT has the highest rates of response and remission of any form of antidepressant treatment. Although results have been variable, over 70% of patients treated with ECT show improvement. Although ECT is found to be safe, there are still deaths (1 in 10,000 patients). Other serious complications related to seizure activity and anesthesia may be caused by ECT.

Studies suggest that repetitive transcranial magnetic stimulation (rTMS) is an effective somatic treatment for major depressive disorder. This treatment requires surgical implant of the device. In contrast to ECT, rTMS produces minimal effects on memory, does not require general anesthesia, and is helpful without the overt risk of generalized seizures.

Even with the best professional care, the patient with depression may take a long time to recover. Many individuals with major depression have multiple bouts of the illness over the course of a lifetime. This can take its toll on the patient's family, friends, and other caregivers who may sometimes feel burned out, frustrated, or even depressed themselves. They may experience episodes of anger toward the depressed loved one, only to subsequently suffer reactions of guilt over being angry. Although such feelings are common, they can be distressing, and the caregiver may not know where to turn for help. It is often the nurse who is best able to assist the family members of a person suffering from depression. Family members may need counseling themselves.

ANTIDEPRESSANTS

Antidepressants are medications that treat depression by enhancing mood. Over the years, the term *mood* has been defined more broadly to encompass phobias, obsessive–compulsive behavior, panic, and anxiety. Antidepressants are often prescribed for these disorders as well. Research studies have linked depression and anxiety to similar neurotransmitter dysfunction, and both seem to respond to treatment with antidepressant medications (see chapter 14). Antidepressants are also beneficial in treating psychological and physical signs of pain (see chapter 18), especially in patients without major depressive disorder, for example, when mood problems are associated with debilitating conditions such as fibromyalgia or muscle spasticity (see chapter 21).

There is one important warning about antidepressants: The U.S. Food and Drug Administration (FDA) has issued a black box warning to be included in drug package inserts and

PharmFacts

PATIENTS WITH DEPRESSIVE SYMPTOMS

- Major depression, bipolar disorder, and situational depression are common mental health challenges worldwide.
- Clinical depression affects more than 19 million Americans each year. The strongest risk factor for suicide is depression.
- For young people 15–24 years old, suicide is the second leading cause of death in the United States.
- Fewer than half of the people who suffer from depression seek medical treatment. 80% of people who seek treatment for depression are treated successfully.
- Most patients consider depression a weakness rather than an illness.
- There are no common age, sex, or ethnic factors related to depression—it can happen to anyone.

drug information sheets. The advisory is issued to patients, families, and health professionals to closely monitor adults and children who are taking antidepressants for warning signs of suicide, especially at the beginning of treatment. In these cases, doses may be changed. The FDA further advises that signs of anxiety, panic attacks, agitation, irritability, insomnia, impulsivity, hostility, and mania may be expected with some patients. Children, adolescents, and young adults are at a greater risk for suicidal ideation than older adults.

16.3 Mechanism of Action of Antidepressants

Depression is associated with an imbalance of neurotransmitters in regions of the brain associated with focused cognition and emotion. Although medication may not completely restore normal chemical balance, it may help reduce depressive symptoms while the patient develops effective means of coping.

As shown in Pharmacology Illustrated 16.1, antidepressants are theorized to exert effects through actions on specific neurotransmitters in the brain, including norepinephrine, serotonin, and dopamine. The two basic mechanisms of drug action are (1) blocking the enzymatic breakdown of norepinephrine; and (2) slowing the reuptake of serotonin and norepinephrine. In axon terminals, monoamine oxidase (MAO) enzymes normally break down catecholamines and recycle them for further use (see chapter 13). The primary classes of antidepressant drugs, shown in Table 16.1, are as follows:

- Selective serotonin reuptake inhibitors (SSRIs)
- Atypical antidepressants, including serotonin–norepinephrine reuptake inhibitors (SNRIs)
- Tricyclic antidepressants (TCAs)
- Monoamine oxidase inhibitors (MAOIs).

Selective Serotonin Reuptake Inhibitors

Drugs that slow the reuptake of serotonin into presynaptic nerve terminals are called **selective serotonin reuptake inhibitors (SSRIs).** They have become preferred drugs for the treatment of depression.

16.4 Treating Depression With SSRIs

Serotonin is a natural neurotransmitter in the central nervous system (CNS), found in high concentrations within neurons of the hypothalamus, limbic system, medulla, and spinal cord. It is important to several body functions, including cycling between REM and non-REM sleep, pain perception, and emotional states. Lack of adequate serotonin in the CNS can lead to depression. Serotonin is metabolized to a less active substance by the enzyme MAO. Serotonin is also known by its chemical name, 5-hydroxytryptamine (5-HT).

In the 1970s, it became increasingly clear that serotonin had a more substantial role in depression than had previously been thought. Clinicians knew that other drugs altered the sensitivity of serotonin to populations of receptors in the brain, but they did not know how this change was connected to depression. Ongoing efforts to find antidepressants with fewer side effects led to the development of the SSRIs.

SSRIs have approximately the same efficacy at relieving depression as the MAOIs and the TCAs. The major advantage of the SSRIs, and the one that makes them preferred drugs, is their greater safety profile. Sympathomimetic effects (increased heart rate and hypertension) and anticholinergic effects (dry mouth, blurred vision, urinary retention, and constipation) are less common with this drug class. Sedation is also experienced less frequently, and cardiotoxicity is not observed. All drugs in the SSRI class have equal efficacy and similar side effects. In general, SSRIs elicit a therapeutic response more quickly than TCAs.

Whereas the tricyclic class inhibits the reuptake of both norepinephrine and serotonin into presynaptic nerve terminals, the SSRIs selectively target serotonin. Increased levels of serotonin in the synaptic gap induce complex neurotransmitter changes in presynaptic and postsynaptic neurons. Presynaptic receptors become less sensitive, and postsynaptic receptors become more sensitive.

One of the most common side effects of SSRIs relates to sexual dysfunction. Up to 70% of both men and women experience decreased libido and lack of ability to reach orgasm. In men, delayed ejaculation and impotence may occur. For patients who are sexually active, these side effects may result in noncompliance with pharmacotherapy. Other common side effects of SSRIs include nausea, headache, weight gain, anxiety, and insomnia. Weight gain may also lead to noncompliance.

Serotonin syndrome (SES) may occur when the patient is taking another medication that affects the

Pharmacotherapy Illustrated

16.1 | Antidepressants Treat Depressive Symptoms

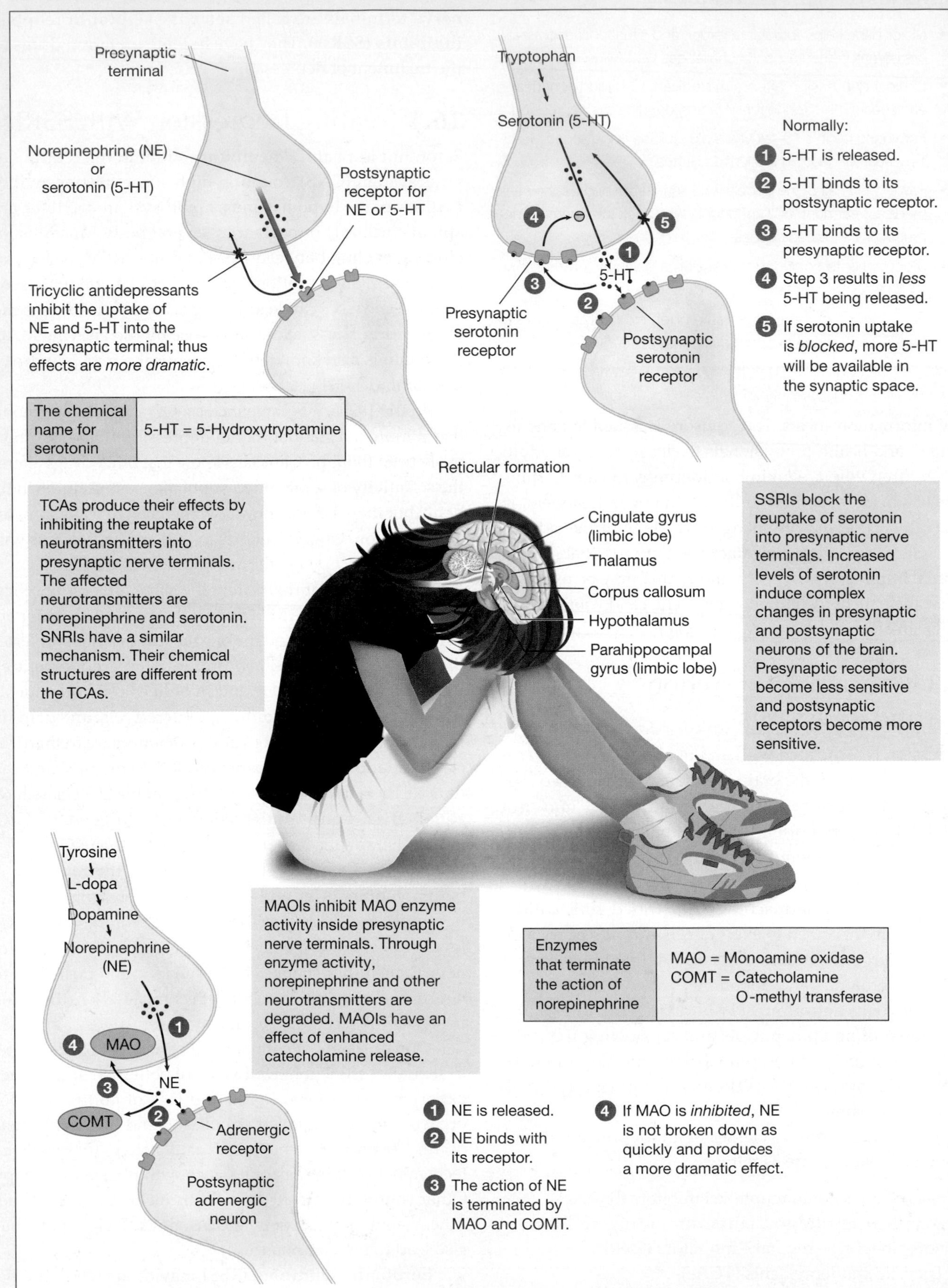

Presynaptic terminal
Norepinephrine (NE) or serotonin (5-HT)
Postsynaptic receptor for NE or 5-HT
Tricyclic antidepressants inhibit the uptake of NE and 5-HT into the presynaptic terminal; thus effects are *more dramatic*.
Tryptophan
Serotonin (5-HT)
5-HT
Presynaptic serotonin receptor
Postsynaptic serotonin receptor
Normally:
1 5-HT is released.
2 5-HT binds to its postsynaptic receptor.
3 5-HT binds to its presynaptic receptor.
4 Step 3 results in *less* 5-HT being released.
5 If serotonin uptake is *blocked*, more 5-HT will be available in the synaptic space.
Reticular formation
Cingulate gyrus (limbic lobe)
Thalamus
Corpus callosum
Hypothalamus
Parahippocampal gyrus (limbic lobe)
Tyrosine
L-dopa
Dopamine
Norepinephrine (NE)
MAO
NE
COMT
Adrenergic receptor
Postsynaptic adrenergic neuron
1 NE is released.
2 NE binds with its receptor.
3 The action of NE is terminated by MAO and COMT.
4 If MAO is *inhibited*, NE is not broken down as quickly and produces a more dramatic effect.

The chemical name for serotonin	5-HT = 5-Hydroxytryptamine

TCAs produce their effects by inhibiting the reuptake of neurotransmitters into presynaptic nerve terminals. The affected neurotransmitters are norepinephrine and serotonin. SNRIs have a similar mechanism. Their chemical structures are different from the TCAs.

SSRIs block the reuptake of serotonin into presynaptic nerve terminals. Increased levels of serotonin induce complex changes in presynaptic and postsynaptic neurons of the brain. Presynaptic receptors become less sensitive and postsynaptic receptors become more sensitive.

MAOIs inhibit MAO enzyme activity inside presynaptic nerve terminals. Through enzyme activity, norepinephrine and other neurotransmitters are degraded. MAOIs have an effect of enhanced catecholamine release.

Enzymes that terminate the action of norepinephrine	MAO = Monoamine oxidase COMT = Catecholamine O-methyl transferase

Table 16.1 Antidepressants

Drug	Route and Adult Dose (max dose where indicated)	Adverse Effects
SELECTIVE SEROTONIN REUPTAKE INHIBITORS (SSRIs)		
citalopram (Celexa)	PO: start at 20 mg/day (max: 40 mg/day)	*Nausea, dry mouth, insomnia, somnolence, headache, nervousness, anxiety, GI disturbances, dizziness, anorexia, fatigue, sexual dysfunction* Suicidal ideation, serotonin syndrome Stevens–Johnson syndrome (SJS)
escitalopram oxalate (Lexapro) (see page 169 for the Prototype Drug box)	PO: 10 mg/day; may increase to 20 mg after 1 wk	
fluoxetine (Prozac)	PO: 20 mg/day in the a.m., may increase by 20 mg/day at weekly intervals (max: 80 mg/day); when stable may switch to a 90-mg sustained-release capsule once weekly (max: 90 mg/wk)	
fluvoxamine (Luvox)	PO: start with 50 mg/day (max: 300 mg/day)	
paroxetine (Paxil, Pexeva)	Depression: PO: 10–50 mg/day (max: 80 mg/day); Obsessive–compulsive disorder: PO: 20–60 mg/day; Panic attacks: PO: 40 mg/day	
sertraline (Zoloft)	Adult: PO: start with 50 mg/day; gradually increase every few weeks to a range of 50–200 mg; Geriatric: start with 25 mg/day	
vilazodone (Viibryd)	Adult: PO: start with 10 mg/day for 7 days; follow with 20 mg once daily for an additional 7 days; increase to 40 mg once daily	
ATYPICAL ANTIDEPRESSANTS (INCLUDING SNRIs)		
bupropion (Wellbutrin, Zyban)	PO: 75–100 mg tid (greater than 450 mg/day increases risk for adverse reactions)	*Insomnia, nausea, dry mouth, constipation, increased blood pressure and heart rate, dizziness, somnolence, sweating, agitation, blurred vision, headache, tremor, vomiting, drowsiness, increased appetite, orthostatic hypotension, sexual dysfunction* suicidal ideation, serotonin syndrome
duloxetine (Cymbalta)	PO: 40–60 mg/day in one or two divided doses	
mirtazapine (Remeron)	PO: 15 mg/day in a single dose at bedtime; may increase every 1–2 wk (max: 45 mg/day)	
nefazodone	PO: 50–100 mg bid; may increase up to 300–600 mg/day	
trazodone (Oleptro)	PO: 150 mg/day; may increase by 50 mg/day every 3–4 days up to 400–600 mg/day	
venlafaxine (Effexor, Effexor XR)	PO: 25–125 mg tid; XR form is taken once daily	
vortioxetine (Brintellix)	PO: 5–20 mg/day once daily	
TRICYCLIC ANTIDEPRESSANTS (TCAs)		
amitriptyline (Elavil)	Adult: PO: 75–100 mg/day (may gradually increase to 150–300 mg/day), Geriatric: PO: 10–25 mg at bedtime (may gradually increase to 25–150 mg/day)	*Drowsiness, sedation, dizziness, orthostatic hypotension, dry mouth, constipation, urinary retention, blurred vision, mydriasis, sexual dysfunction* Suicidal ideation, serotonin syndrome, agranulocytosis; bone marrow depression; seizures; heart block; myocardial infarction (MI); angioedema of the face, tongue, or generalized
amoxapine (Asendin)	Adult: PO: begin with 100 mg/day (may increase on day 3 to 300 mg/day); Geriatric: PO: 25 mg at bedtime; may increase every 3–7 days to 50–150 mg/day (max: 300 mg/day)	
clomipramine (Anafranil)	PO: 75–300 mg/day in divided doses	
desipramine (Norpramin)	PO: 75–100 mg/day; may increase to 150–300 mg/day	
doxepin (Silenor)	PO: 30–150 mg/day at bedtime; may gradually increase to 300 mg/day	
imipramine (Tofranil)	PO: 75–100 mg/day (max: 300 mg/day)	
maprotiline (Ludiomil)	Mild to moderate depression: PO: start at 75 mg/day; gradually increase every 2 wk to 150 mg/day; Severe depression: PO: start at 100–150 mg/day; gradually increase to 300 mg/day	
nortriptyline (Aventyl, Pamelor)	PO: 25 mg tid or qid; may increase to 100–150 mg/day	
protriptyline (Vivactil)	PO: 15–40 mg/day in three to four divided doses (max: 60 mg/day)	
trimipramine (Surmontil)	PO: 75–100 mg/day (max: 300 mg/day)	
MAO INHIBITORS (MAOIs)		
isocarboxazid (Marplan)	PO: 10–30 mg/day (max: 30 mg/day)	*Drowsiness, insomnia, orthostatic hypotension, blurred vision, nausea, constipation, anorexia, dry mouth, urinary retention, sexual dysfunction* Suicidal ideation, serotonin syndrome, respiratory collapse, hypertensive crisis, circulatory collapse
phenelzine (Nardil)	PO: 15 mg tid (max: 90 mg/day)	
selegiline (Emsam)	Transdermal patch: applied to dry, intact skin on the upper torso, upper thigh, or the outer surface of the upper arm once every 24 hours; the recommended starting dose and target dose is 6 mg/24 h	
tranylcypromine (Parnate)	PO: 30 mg/day (give 20 mg in a.m. and 10 mg in p.m.); may increase by 10 mg/day at 3-wk intervals up to 60 mg/day	

Note: *Italics* indicate common adverse effects; underlining indicates serious adverse effects.

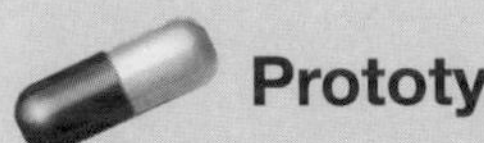

Prototype Drug | Sertraline *(Zoloft)*

Therapeutic Class: Antidepressant **Pharmacologic Class:** Selective serotonin reuptake inhibitor (SSRI)

Actions and Uses

Sertraline is used for the treatment of depression, anxiety, obsessive-compulsive disorder, and panic. The antidepressant and anxiolytic properties of this drug can be attributed to its ability to inhibit the reuptake of serotonin in the brain. Other uses include premenstrual dysphoric disorder, post-traumatic stress disorder, and social anxiety disorder. Therapeutic actions include enhancement of mood and improvement of affect with maximum effects observed after several weeks.

Administration Alerts

- It is recommended that sertraline be given in the morning or evening.
- When administering sertraline as an oral liquid, mix with water, ginger ale, lemon/lime soda, lemonade, or orange juice. Follow the manufacturer's instructions.
- Do not give concurrently with an MAOI or within 5 weeks of discontinuing MAOI medication.
- Pregnancy category C.

PHARMACOKINETICS

Onset	Peak	Duration
2–4 wk	Unknown	Variable (due to extensive binding with serum proteins)

Adverse Effects

Adverse effects include agitation, insomnia, headache, dizziness, somnolence, and fatigue. Take extreme precautions in patients with cardiac disease, hepatic impairment, seizure disorders, suicidal ideation, mania, or hypomania.

Black Box Warning: Antidepressants increase the risk of suicidal thinking and behavior, especially in children, adolescents, and young adults with major depressive disorder and other psychiatric disorders. This drug is not approved for use in pediatric patients for major depressive disorder, but it is approved for obsessive compulsive disorder in children under 6 years of age.

Contraindications: Concomitant use of sertraline and MAOIs or primozide is not advised. Antabuse should be avoided because of the alcohol content of the drug concentrate.

Interactions

Drug–Drug: Highly protein bound medications such as digoxin and warfarin should be avoided due to risk of toxicity and increased blood concentrations leading to increased bleeding. MAOIs may cause neuroleptic malignant syndrome, extreme hypertension, and SES, characterized by confusion, anxiety, restlessness, hypertension, tremors, sweating, hyperpyrexia, or ataxia.

Use cautiously with other centrally acting drugs to avoid adverse CNS effects.

Lab Tests: Sertraline results in asymptomatic elevated liver function tests and a slight decrease in uric acid levels.

Herbal/Food: Patients should use caution if taking St. John's wort or L-tryptophan to avoid serotonin syndrome.

Treatment of Overdose: There is no specific treatment for overdose. Emergency medical attention and general supportive measures may be necessary. Symptoms of overdose include nausea, vomiting, tremor, seizures, agitation, dizziness, hyperactivity, mydriasis, tachycardia, and coma.

metabolism, synthesis, or reuptake of serotonin, causing serotonin to accumulate in the body. Symptoms can begin as early as 2 hours after taking the first dose or as late as several weeks after the initiating pharmacotherapy. SES can be produced by the concurrent administration of an SSRI with an MAOI, a TCA, lithium, or a number of other medications. Symptoms of SES include mental status changes (confusion, anxiety, restlessness), hypertension, tremors, sweating, hyperpyrexia, or ataxia. Conservative treatment is to discontinue the SSRI and provide supportive care. In severe cases, mechanical ventilation and muscle relaxants may be necessary. If left untreated, death may occur.

Atypical Antidepressants

In terms of classification, the atypical antidepressants do not fit conveniently into the other antidepressant drug classes. Thus, "atypical" in this case really refers to the unique chemical structures represented in the group.

16.5 Treating Depression With Atypical Antidepressants

Duloxetine (Cymbalta) and venlafaxine (Effexor), sometimes considered to be in their own class, are the **serotonin–norepinephrine reuptake inhibitors (SNRIs).** They specifically inhibit the reabsorption of serotonin and norepinephrine and elevate mood. In many cases, levels of dopamine are also affected by the SNRIs. In addition to being approved for the treatment of major depression, duloxetine (Cymbalta) is also approved for the treatment of generalized anxiety disorder and for neuropathic pain characteristic of fibromyalgia and diabetic neuropathy. Venlafaxine (Effexor), approved to treat depression and generalized anxiety disorder, is available in an intermediate-release form that requires two or three doses a day and an extended-release (XR) form that allows the patient to take the medication just once a day.

Bupropion (Wellbutrin) not only inhibits the reuptake of serotonin but also affects the activity of norepinephrine and dopamine. It is contraindicated in patients with seizure disorders because it lowers the seizure threshold. Bupropion is marketed as Zyban for use in cessation of smoking. Mirtazapine (Remeron) is used for depression and blocks presynaptic serotonin and norepinephrine receptors, thereby enhancing release of these neurotransmitters. Nefazodone is similar to Remeron. It was originally designed to treat depression, and causes minimal cardiovascular effects, fewer anticholinergic effects, less sedation, and less sexual dysfunction than the other antidepressants. Due to the risk of heptatoxicity, precautions should be noted with this drug. Trazodone (Oleptro) is often used to treat insomnia, rather than as an antidepressant. The high levels of trazodone needed for the improvement of depression causes sedation in many patients.

Tricyclic Antidepressants

Named for their three-ring chemical structure, **tricyclic antidepressants (TCAs)** were the mainstay of depression pharmacotherapy from the early 1960s until the 1980s and are still used today.

Complementary and Alternative Therapies

ST. JOHN'S WORT FOR DEPRESSION

One of the most popular herbs in the United States, St. John's wort (*Hypericum perforatum*), is found growing throughout Asia, Europe, and North America. Its modern use is as an antidepressant. It gets its name from a legend that red spots once appeared on its leaves on the anniversary of the beheading of St. John the Baptist. The word *wort* is a British term for "plant."

The primary active ingredients found in St. John's wort are hypericin and hyperforin, which are believed to selectively inhibit serotonin reuptake in certain brain neurons. A number of clinical studies suggest that St. John's wort is an effective treatment for mild to moderate depression, that it may be just as effective as standard antidepressants, and that it causes fewer adverse effects than traditional drugs. However, the National Center for Complementary and Integrative Health (NCCIH, 2013) has found that study results are mixed with no conclusive evidence that St. John's wort is effective.

St. John's wort may interact with many medications, including hormonal contraceptives, antiseizure medications, warfarin, digoxin, and cyclosporine. It is generally well tolerated, but may produce mild side effects such as GI distress, fatigue, headache, dry mouth, and allergic skin reactions. The herb contains compounds that photosensitize the skin; thus, patients should be advised to apply sunscreen or wear protective clothing when outdoors (NCCIH, 2012).

16.6 Treating Depression With Tricyclic Antidepressants

TCAs act by inhibiting the presynaptic reuptake of both norepinephrine and serotonin. TCAs are used predominately for major depression and occasionally for milder situational depression. Clomipramine (Anafranil) is approved for treatment of obsessive–compulsive disorder, and doxepin (Sinequan) is approved for generalized anxiety disorders, neuropathic pain, and fibromyalgia. Doxepin, available in generic or trade product form (Silenor), is used to treat insomnia or difficulty falling asleep. Common side effects include nausea and drowsiness. Other TCAs are sometimes used off-label for panic disorder and social anxiety disorder. One use for TCAs, not related to psychopharmacology, is the treatment of childhood enuresis (bed-wetting).

Shortly after their approval as antidepressants in the 1950s, it was found that the TCAs produced fewer side effects and were less dangerous than MAOIs. However, TCAs have some unpleasant and serious side effects. The most common side effect is orthostatic hypotension, due to $alpha_1$ blockade on blood vessels. The most serious adverse effect occurs when TCAs accumulate in cardiac tissue. Although rare, cardiac dysrhythmias can occur.

Sedation is a frequently reported complaint at the initiation of therapy, though patients may become tolerant to this effect after several weeks of treatment. Most TCAs used to treat depression have a long half-life, which increases the risk of side effects, especially for patients with delayed excretion. Anticholinergic effects, such as dry mouth, constipation, urinary retention, excessive perspiration, blurred vision, and tachycardia, are common. These effects are less severe if the drug is gradually increased to the therapeutic dose over 2 to 3 weeks. Significant drug interactions can occur with CNS depressants, sympathomimetics, anticholinergics, and MAOIs. Since the advent of newer antidepressants with fewer adverse effects, TCAs are less frequently used as first-line drugs in the treatment of depression and/or anxiety.

Monoamine Oxidase Inhibitors

Monoamine oxidase inhibitors (MAOIs) inhibit MAO, the enzyme that terminates the actions of neurotransmitters such as dopamine, norepinephrine, epinephrine, and serotonin. Because of their low safety margin, these drugs are reserved for patients who have not responded to SSRIs or TCAs.

16.7 Treating Depression With MAOIs

The action of norepinephrine at adrenergic synapses is terminated either by (1) reuptake into the presynaptic nerve

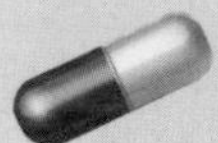

Prototype Drug | Imipramine *(Tofranil)*

Therapeutic Class: Antidepressant; treatment of nocturnal enuresis in children
Pharmacologic Class: Tricyclic antidepressant

Actions and Uses

Imipramine blocks the reuptake of serotonin and norepinephrine into nerve terminals. It is used mainly for major depression, although it is occasionally used for the treatment of nocturnal enuresis (bed wetting) in children. The nurse may find imipramine prescribed for a number of unlabeled uses, including intractable pain, anxiety disorders, and withdrawal syndromes from alcohol and cocaine. Therapeutic effectiveness may not occur for 2 or more weeks.

Administration Alerts

- Paradoxical diaphoresis can be a side effect of TCAs; therefore, diaphoresis may not be a reliable indicator of other disease states such as hypoglycemia.
- Imipramine causes anticholinergic effects and may potentiate effects of anticholinergic drugs administered during surgery.
- Do not discontinue abruptly because rebound dysphoria, irritability, or sleeplessness may occur.
- Pregnancy category C.

PHARMACOKINETICS

Onset	Peak	Duration
Less than 1 h	1–2 h PO; 30 min IM	Variable

Adverse Effects

Side effects include sedation, drowsiness, blurred vision, dry mouth, and cardiovascular symptoms such as dysrhythmias, heart block, and extreme hypertension. Agents that mimic the action of norepinephrine or serotonin should be avoided because imipramine inhibits their metabolism and may produce toxicity. Some patients may experience photosensitivity and hypersensitivity to tricyclic drugs.

Black Box Warning: Antidepressants increase the risk of suicidal thinking and behavior, especially in children, adolescents, and young adults with major depressive disorder and other psychiatric disorders. This drug is not approved for use in pediatric patients.

Contraindications: This drug should not be used in cases of acute recovery after MI, defects in bundle-branch conduction, narrow-angle glaucoma, and severe renal or hepatic impairment. Patients should not use this drug within 14 days of discontinuing MAOIs.

Interactions

Drug–Drug: Concurrent use of other CNS depressants, including alcohol, may cause sedation. Cimetidine (Tagamet) may inhibit the metabolism of imipramine, leading to increased serum levels and possible toxicity. Imipramine may reverse the antihypertensive effects of clonidine and potentiate CNS depression. Use of oral contraceptives may increase or decrease imipramine levels. Disulfiram may lead to delirium and tachycardia. Antithyroid agents may produce agranulocytosis. Phenothiazines cause increased anticholinergic and sedative effects. Sympathomimetics may result in cardiac toxicity. Methylphenidate or cimetidine may increase the effects of imipramine and cause toxicity. Phenytoin is less effective when taken with imipramine. MAOIs may result in neuroleptic malignant syndrome.

Lab Tests: Imipramine produces altered blood glucose tests. Elevation of serum bilirubin and alkaline phosphatase is likely.

Herbal/Food: Herbal supplements such as evening primrose oil or ginkgo may lower the seizure threshold. St. John's wort used concurrently may cause SES.

Treatment of Overdose: There is no specific treatment for overdose. General supportive measures are recommended. Ensure an adequate airway, oxygenation, and ventilation. Monitor cardiac rhythm and vital signs. Gastric lavage may be indicated. Activated charcoal should be administered.

or (2) enzymatic destruction by the enzyme MAO. By decreasing the effectiveness of the enzyme MAO, the MAOIs limit the breakdown of norepinephrine, dopamine, and serotonin in the CNS. This creates higher levels of these neurotransmitters to alleviate symptoms of depression. As shown in Pharmacotherapy Illustrated 16.1, MAO is located within presynaptic nerve terminals.

In the 1950s, the MAOIs were the first drugs approved to treat depression. Because of drug–drug and food–drug interactions, hepatotoxicity, and the development of safer antidepressants, MAOIs are now reserved for patients who are not responsive to other antidepressant classes.

Common side effects of the MAOIs include orthostatic hypotension, headache, insomnia, and diarrhea. A primary concern is that these agents interact with a large number of foods and other medications, sometimes with serious effects. A hypertensive crisis can occur when an MAOI is used concurrently with other antidepressants or sympathomimetic drugs. Combining an MAOI with an SSRI can produce serotonin syndrome. If MAOIs are given with

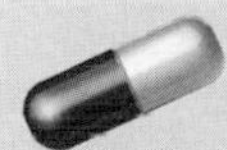

Prototype Drug | Phenelzine *(Nardil)*

Therapeutic Class: Antidepressant **Pharmacologic Class:** Monoamine oxidase inhibitor (MAOI)

Actions and Uses

Phenelzine produces its effects by irreversible inhibition of MAO; therefore, it intensifies the effects of norepinephrine in adrenergic synapses. It is used to manage symptoms of depression that are not responsive to other types of pharmacotherapy and is occasionally used for panic disorder. Drug effects may persist for 2 to 3 weeks after therapy is discontinued.

Administration Alerts

- Washout periods of 2 to 3 weeks are required before introducing other drugs.
- Abrupt discontinuation of this drug may cause rebound hypertension.
- Pregnancy category C.

PHARMACOKINETICS

Onset	Peak	Duration
2 weeks	Variable	48–96 h

Adverse Effects

Common side effects are constipation, dry mouth, orthostatic hypotension, insomnia, nausea, and loss of appetite. It may increase heart rate and neural activity, leading to delirium, mania, anxiety, and convulsions. Severe hypertension may occur when ingesting foods containing tyramine. Seizures, respiratory depression, circulatory collapse, and coma may occur in cases of severe overdose.

Black Box Warning: Antidepressants increase the risk of suicidal thinking and behavior, especially in children, adolescents, and young adults with major depressive disorder and other psychiatric disorders. This drug is not approved for use in pediatric patients.

Contraindications: Patients with cardiovascular or cerebrovascular disease, hepatic or renal impairment, and pheochromocytoma should not use this drug.

Interactions

Drug–Drug: Many drugs affect the action of phenelzine. Concurrent use of TCAs and SSRIs should be avoided because the combinations can cause temperature elevation and seizures. Opiates should be avoided due to increased risk of respiratory failure or hypertensive crisis. Sympathomimetics may precipitate a hypertensive crisis. Caffeine may result in cardiac dysrhythmias and hypertension.

Lab Tests: Phenelzine can produce a slightly false increase in serum bilirubin. Because platelet functioning can be affected, careful attention should be devoted to complete blood count (CBC) results.

Herbal/Food: Concurrent use of ginseng may cause headaches, tremors, mania, insomnia, irritability, and visual hallucinations. Concurrent use of ma huang, ephedra, or St. John's wort may result in a hypertensive crisis.

Treatment of Overdose: Intensive symptomatic and supportive treatment may be required. Induction of emesis or gastric lavage with instillation of charcoal slurry may be helpful. Signs and symptoms of CNS stimulation, including seizures, should be treated with IV diazepam, given very slowly. Hypertension should be treated appropriately with calcium channel blockers. Hypotension and vascular collapse should be treated with IV fluids and, if necessary, blood pressure titration with an IV infusion of a dilute pressor agent. Body temperature should be monitored closely, and respiration should be supported with appropriate measures.

antihypertensives, the patient can experience severe hypotension. MAOIs also potentiate the hypoglycemic effects of insulin and oral antidiabetic drugs. Hyperpyrexia (elevation of body temperature) is known to occur in patients taking MAOIs with meperidine (Demerol), dextromethorphan (Pedia Care and others), and TCAs.

A hypertensive crisis can also result from an interaction between MAOIs and foods containing **tyramine,** a form of the amino acid tyrosine. Tyramine is usually degraded by MAO in the intestines. If a patient takes MAOIs, however, tyramine enters the bloodstream in high concentrations and displaces norepinephrine within presynaptic nerve terminals. The result is a sudden release of norepinephrine, causing acute hypertension. Symptoms usually occur within minutes of ingesting the food and include occipital headache, stiff neck, flushing, palpitations, diaphoresis, and nausea. Myocardial infarctions and cerebral vascular accidents, though rare, are possible consequences. Calcium channel blockers may be given as an antidote. Because of their serious side effects when taken with food and drugs, MAOIs are rarely used and are limited to patients with symptoms that are resistant to more traditional therapies and to patients who are more likely to comply with food restrictions. Examples of foods containing tyramine are listed in Table 16.2.

☑ Check Your Understanding 16.1

Is there a "drug of choice" for depression? With so many drug groups available, why would one be preferred over another? *Visit www.pearsonhighered.com/nursingresources for the answers.*

Table 16.2 Foods Containing Tyramine

Fruits	Dairy Products	Alcohol	Meats
Avocados	Cheese (cottage cheese is okay)	Beer	Beef or chicken liver
Bananas	Sour cream	Wines (especially red wines)	Paté
Raisins	Yogurt		Meat extracts
Papaya products, including meat tenderizers			Pickled or kippered herring
Canned figs			Pepperoni
			Salami
			Sausage
			Bologna/hot dogs
Vegetables	**Sauces**	**Yeast**	**Other Foods to Avoid**
Pods of broad beans (fava beans)	Soy sauce	All yeast or yeast extracts	Chocolate

BIPOLAR DISORDER

Once known as *manic depression*, **bipolar disorder** is characterized by episodes of depression alternating with episodes of mania. Bipolar disorder likely results from abnormal functioning of neurotransmitters or receptors in the brain. It is important to distinguish mania from the effects of drug use or abuse and also from schizophrenia (see chapter 17).

16.8 Characteristics of Bipolar Disorder

During the depressive stages of bipolar disorder, patients exhibit the symptoms of major depression described earlier in this chapter (see section 16.1). Patients with bipolar disorder also display signs of **mania,** an emotional state characterized by high psychomotor activity and irritability. Symptoms of mania, as described in the following list, are generally the opposite of depressive symptoms:

- Inflated self-esteem or grandiosity
- Decreased need for sleep (e.g., feels rested after only 3 hours of sleep)
- Increased talkativeness or pressure to keep talking
- Flight of ideas or subjective feeling that thoughts are racing
- Distractibility (i.e., attention too easily drawn to unimportant or irrelevant external stimuli)
- Increased goal-directed activity (either socially, at work or school, or sexually) or psychomotor agitation
- Excessive involvement in pleasurable activities that have a high potential for painful consequences (e.g., unrestrained buying sprees, sexual indiscretions, or foolish business investments).

For a person to be diagnosed with bipolar disorder, manic symptoms must be present for at least 1 week. Hypomania is characterized by the same symptoms, but they are less severe. Hypomania may involve an excess of excitatory neurotransmitters (such as norepinephrine or glutamate) or a deficiency of inhibitory neurotransmitters such as gamma-aminobutyric acid (GABA) (see chapter 15).

DRUGS FOR BIPOLAR DISORDER

Drugs for bipolar disorder are sometimes called **mood stabilizers,** because they have the ability to moderate extreme shifts in emotions between mania and depression. Lithium, antiseizure drugs, and atypical antipsychotic drugs are also used for mood stabilization in bipolar patients.

16.9 Pharmacotherapy of Bipolar Disorder

For years, the traditional treatment of bipolar disorder was lithium (Eskalith) as monotherapy or in combination with other drugs. Lithium was approved in the United States in 1970. It remains effective for purely manic or purely depressive episodes. Lithium has a narrow therapeutic index and is monitored via serum levels every 4–5 days due to needing to wait 5 days to reach steady state (5 half-lives). Levels are monitored 5 days after any dose change again to reach a steady state. To ensure therapeutic action, concentrations of lithium in the blood must remain within the range of 0.6 to 1.5 mEq/L. Close monitoring encourages compliance and helps prevent toxicity. Lithium acts like sodium in the body so conditions in which sodium is lost (e.g., excessive sweating or dehydration) can cause lithium toxicity. Therefore, it is necessary to also monitor sodium levels. Lithium overdose may be treated with hemodialysis and supportive care. Baseline studies of renal, cardiac, electrolyte, and thyroid status are indicated.

For the most complete control of bipolar disorder, it is not unusual for other drugs to be used in combination with lithium. If the patient is currently taking a mood stabilizer, a TCA or an atypical antidepressant such as bupropion (Wellbutrin) may be necessary during depressed stages. During

Table 16.3 Drugs for Bipolar Disorder

Drug	Route and Adult Dose (max dose where indicated)	Adverse Effects
MOOD STABILIZERS		
lithium (Eskalith)	PO: initial: 600 mg tid; maintenance: 300 mg tid (max: 2.4 g/day)	*Headache, lethargy, fatigue, recent memory loss, nausea, vomiting, anorexia, abdominal pain, diarrhea, dry mouth, muscle weakness, hand tremors, reversible leukocytosis, nephrogenic diabetes insipidus* Peripheral circulatory collapse
ANTISEIZURE DRUGS		
carbamazepine (Tegretol)	PO: 200 mg bid, gradually increased to 800–1,200 mg/day in three to four divided doses	*Dizziness, ataxia, somnolence, headache, nausea, diplopia, blurred vision, sedation, drowsiness, nausea, vomiting, prolonged bleeding time* Heart block, aplastic anemia, respiratory depression, exfoliative dermatitis, SJS, toxic epidermal necrolysis, deep coma, death (with overdose), liver failure, pancreatitis
lamotrigine (Lamictal)	PO: 50 mg/day for 2 weeks, then 50 mg bid for 2 weeks; may increase gradually up to 300–500 mg/day in two divided doses (max: 700 mg/day)	
valproic acid (Depakene, Depakote) (see page 192 for the Prototype Drug box)	PO: 250 mg tid (max: 60 mg/kg/day)	
ATYPICAL ANTIPSYCHOTIC DRUGS		
aripiprazole (Abilify)	PO: 10–15 mg/day (max: 30 mg/day)	*Tachycardia, transient fever, sedation, dizziness, headache, light-headedness, somnolence, anxiety, nervousness, hostility, insomnia, nausea, vomiting, constipation, parkinsonism, akathisia* Agranulocytosis, neuroleptic malignant syndrome (rare), increased risk of death in older adults with dementia-related psychosis
asenapine (Saphris)	Adult: 10 mg sublingually twice daily (monotherapy); 5 mg sublingually twice daily (adjunct to lithium or valproic acid therapy)	
olanzapine (Zyprexa)	Adult: PO: start with 5–10 mg/day; may increase by 2.5–5 mg every week (range 10–15 mg/day; max: 20 mg/day). Geriatric: PO: start with 5 mg/day	
quetiapine (Seroquel)	PO: start with 25 mg bid; may increase to a target dose of 300–400 mg/day in divided doses	
risperidone (Risperdal) (see page 235 for the Prototype Drug box)	PO: 1–6 mg bid; increase by 2 mg daily to an initial target dose of 6 mg/day	
ziprasidone (Geodon)	PO: 20 mg bid (max: 80 mg bid)	

Note: Italics indicate common adverse effects; underlining indicates serious adverse effects.

manic phases, a benzodiazepine will moderate manic symptoms (see chapter 14). In cases of extreme agitation, delusions, or hallucinations, antipsychotic drugs may be indicated (see chapter 17). Continued patient compliance is essential to achieving successful pharmacotherapy because some patients do not perceive their condition as abnormal.

Today, antiseizure drugs (see chapter 15) and atypical antipsychotic drugs (see chapter 17) have emerged as probably the most effective agents for mood stabilization. For example, valproic acid (Depakene, Depakote), carbamazepine (Tegretol), and lamotrigine (Lamictal) are the antiseizure drugs most often used in the treatment of rapidly cycling and mixed states of bipolar disorder. In addition, gabapentin (Neurontin, Gralise, Horizant), oxcarbazepine (Trileptal, Oxtellar), topiramate (Topamax, Qudexy XR), and zonisamide (Zonegran) all have beneficial effects. Several atypical antipsychotics are very effective for the treatment of extreme mania and bipolar disorder. These include aripiprazole (Abilify), asenapine (Saphris), olanzapine (Zyprexa), quetiapine (Seroquel), risperidone (Risperdal), and ziprasidone (Geodon). The atypical antipsychotics carry a black box warning that they are not to be used for patients with dementia-related psychosis due to an increased risk of death in this population. Longer term stabilization of extreme and unusual behaviors with atypical antipsychotics is covered in chapter 17. Table 16.3 lists selected drugs used to treat bipolar disorder.

ATTENTION DEFICIT/ HYPERACTIVITY DISORDER

A condition characterized by poor attention span, behavior control issues, and/or hyperactivity is called **attention deficit/hyperactivity disorder (ADHD).** Although the condition has normally most often been diagnosed in childhood, symptoms of ADHD may extend into adulthood, and an increasing number of adults are being evaluated for ADHD.

16.10 Characteristics of Attention Deficit/Hyperactivity Disorder

ADHD is neither an emotional disorder nor a mood disorder. It is a behavioral disorder that affects as many as 5% of all children. Most children diagnosed with this condition are between the ages of 3 and 7 years, and boys are four to eight times more likely to be diagnosed than girls.

ADHD is characterized by developmentally inappropriate behaviors involving difficulty in paying attention or

Nursing Practice Application

Pharmacotherapy for Mood Disorders

ASSESSMENT	POTENTIAL NURSING DIAGNOSES*
Baseline assessment prior to administration: • Obtain a complete health history including hepatic, renal, urologic, cardiovascular, or neurologic disease; current mental status; narrow-angle glaucoma; pregnancy; or breast-feeding. Obtain a drug history including allergies, current prescription and OTC drugs, and herbal preparations. Be alert to possible drug interactions. • Obtain a history of depression or mood disorder, including a family history of same and severity. Use objective screening tools when possible (e.g., Patient Health Questionnaire [PHQ-9]). If symptoms warrant, also consider use of the Mini Mental State Exam for dementia screening. • Obtain baseline vital signs and weight. • Evaluate appropriate laboratory findings (e.g., CBC, electrolytes, glucose, hepatic and renal function studies). • Assess the patient's ability to receive and understand instruction. Include the family and caregivers as needed.	• *Impaired Mood Regulation* • *Ineffective Coping* • *Powerlessness* • *Anxiety* • *Disturbed Sleep Pattern* • *Self-Care Deficit* (Bathing, Feeding, Dressing) • *Overweight or Obesity* • *Imbalanced Nutrition: Less Than Body Requirements* • *Complicated Grieving* • *Social Isolation* • *Impaired Social Interaction* • *Interrupted Family Processes* • *Urinary Retention,* related to adverse drug effects • *Noncompliance,* related to adverse drug effects • *Deficient Knowledge* (drug therapy) • *Risk for Self-Directed Violence* • *Risk for Self-Mutilation* • *Risk for Suicide* • *Risk for Injury* *NANDA I © 2014
Assessment throughout administration: • Assess for desired therapeutic effects (e.g., increased or stabilized mood, lessening depression, increased activity level, return to normal activities of daily living [ADLs], appetite and sleep patterns; if used for other uses, e.g., neuropathic pain, assess for appropriate therapeutic effects). • Continue periodic monitoring of CBC, electrolytes, glucose, hepatic and renal function studies, and therapeutic drug levels as needed. Frequent sodium levels may be required for patients taking lithium. • Assess vital signs and weight periodically or as symptoms warrant. • Assess for and promptly report adverse effects: dizziness or light-headedness, drowsiness, confusion, agitation, suicidal ideations, palpitations, tachycardia, blurred or double vision, muscle weakness, slight tremors, thirst, nausea, vomiting, diarrhea, dry mouth, increased urinary output, short-term memory loss, skin rashes, bruising or bleeding, abdominal pain, jaundice, change in color of stool, flank pain, and hematuria.	

IMPLEMENTATION

Interventions and (Rationales)	Patient-Centered Care
Ensuring therapeutic effects: • Continue assessments as described earlier for therapeutic effects. (Drugs used for depression may take 2 to 8 weeks before full effects are realized. Lithium may take 2 to 3 weeks before full effects are realized. Use objective measures, e.g., PHQ-9, when possible to help quantify therapeutic results. For outpatient therapy, prescriptions may be limited to 7 days' worth of medication. Have the patient sign a "No Harm/No Suicide" contract as appropriate. When used for anxiety or insomnia, nonpharmacologic measures may be needed until the drug reaches full effects.)	• Teach the patient that full effects may not occur for several weeks or longer but that some improvement should be noticeable after beginning therapy. • Encourage the patient to keep all appointments with the therapist and to discuss ongoing symptoms of depression or mania, reporting any suicidal ideations immediately. • Teach the patient to wear or carry medical identification stating the type of drug therapy used, especially if MAOIs are taken.

Nursing Practice Application *continued*

IMPLEMENTATION	
Interventions and (Rationales)	**Patient-Centered Care**
Minimizing adverse effects: • Continue to monitor vital signs, mental status, and coordination and balance periodically. Ensure patient safety: monitor ambulation until the effects of the drug are known. **Lifespan:** Be particularly cautious with older adults who are at increased risk for falls. (Antidepressant drugs may cause drowsiness and dizziness, hypotension, or impaired mental and physical abilities, increasing the risk of falls and injury.)	• **Safety:** Teach the patient to rise from lying or sitting to standing slowly to avoid dizziness or falls. If dizziness occurs, the patient should sit or lie down and not attempt to stand or walk, until the sensation passes. **Lifespan:** Teach the patient, family, or caregiver to be especially cautious with the older adult who is at greater risk for falls. • Instruct the patient to call for assistance prior to getting out of bed or attempting to walk alone and to avoid driving or other activities requiring mental alertness or physical coordination until the effects of the drug are known.
• Continue to monitor CBC, electrolytes, renal and hepatic function, and drug levels. (Antidepressant drugs may cause hepatotoxicity as an adverse effect. **Diverse Patients:** SSRIs are metabolized through the P450 system and may result in less than optimal therapeutic results based on differences in enzymes. Monitor ethnically diverse patients more frequently in the early stages of drug therapy.)	• Instruct the patient on the need to return periodically for laboratory work. • Teach the patient to promptly report any abdominal pain, particularly in the upper quadrants, changes in stool color, yellowing of sclera or skin, or darkened urine. • **Diverse Patients:** Teach ethnically diverse patients to observe for under- or over-therapeutic effects and report promptly.
• Weigh the patient taking lithium daily and report a weight gain or loss of 1 kg (2 lb) or more in a 24-hour period. Measure intake and output in the hospitalized patient. (Daily weight is an accurate measure of fluid status and takes into account intake, output, and insensible losses. Diuresis is indicated by output significantly greater than intake.) • Maintain a normal fluid balance. (Lithium is an elemental salt, and the body will conserve or lose lithium related to the sodium level. Serum sodium should be drawn with each drug level. Dehydration or overhydration will also result in loss or gain of lithium.)	• Have the patient weigh self daily, ideally at the same time of day, and record weight. Have the patient report a weight loss or gain of more than 1 kg (2 lb) in a 24-hour period. • Advise the patient to continue to consume enough liquids to remain adequately, but not overly, hydrated. Drinking when thirsty, avoiding alcoholic beverages and caffeine, and ensuring adequate but not excessive salt intake will assist in maintaining a normal fluid and drug balance. • Instruct the patient to maintain a normal salt and fluid intake, without unusual or dramatic increases or decreases in normal diet. • Teach the patient that conditions such as dehydration may result in abnormal drug levels and to immediately report any symptoms such as thirst, dizziness, confusion, or muscle weakness and to be cautious with exercising on hot days, as excessive sweating may lead to fluid and sodium loss. Promptly report excessive thirst or urination.
• Assess for changes in level of consciousness, disorientation or confusion, or agitation. (Neurologic changes may indicate under- or overmedication, exacerbation of other psychiatric illness, or adverse drug effects.)	• Instruct the patient, family, or caregiver to immediately report increasing lethargy, disorientation, confusion, changes in behavior or mood, agitation or aggression, slurred speech, or ataxia.
• Assess for changes in visual acuity, blurred vision, loss of peripheral vision, seeing rainbow halos around lights, acute eye pain, or these symptoms accompanied by nausea and vomiting, and report immediately. (Increased intraoptic pressure in patients with narrow-angle glaucoma may occur in patients taking TCAs.)	• Instruct the patient to immediately report any visual changes or eye pain.
• Monitor cardiovascular status. (Early signs of SES include rapid increases in blood pressure and pulse. Headache, palpitations, fever, and neck stiffness may signal a life-threatening hypertensive crisis in a patient taking MAOIs. Lithium toxicity may result in cardiac dysrhythmias or angina.)	• Instruct the patient to immediately report severe headache, dizziness, paresthesias, palpitations, tachycardia, chest pain, nausea or vomiting, diaphoresis, or fever.
• Monitor renal status, blood urea nitrogen [BUN], creatinine, uric acid, and urinalysis periodically in patients taking lithium. (Lithium may cause degenerative changes in the kidney, which increases drug toxicity.)	• Instruct the patient to promptly report decreased urine output, hematuria, or urine sediment; lower abdominal tenderness or flank pain; nausea; or diarrhea to the health care provider.

continued

Nursing Practice Application *continued*

IMPLEMENTATION

Interventions and (Rationales)	Patient-Centered Care
• Assess for bruising, bleeding, or signs of infection. (TCAs may cause blood dyscrasias and increased chances of bleeding or infection.)	• Teach the patient to promptly report any signs of increased bruising, bleeding, or infections (e.g., sore throat and fever, skin rash).
• Assess for dry mouth, blurred vision, urinary retention, and sexual dysfunction. (Anticholinergic-like effects and sexual dysfunction, including loss of libido and impotence, are common antidepressant adverse effects. **Lifespan:** Be aware that the male older adult with an enlarged prostate is at higher-risk for mechanical obstruction. Tolerance to anticholinergic effects usually develops in 2 to 4 weeks.)	• Teach the patient to use ice chips, frequent sips of water, chewing gum, or hard candy to alleviate dry mouth and to avoid alcohol-based mouthwashes, which may increase dryness. • Use of "dry eye" drops and resting eyes periodically may help to decrease dry eye feeling. Teach the patient to report any feelings of scratchiness or eye pain immediately. • Instruct the patient to promptly report difficulty with urination, hesitancy, or dysuria. • Encourage the patient to discuss concerns about sexual functioning and refer to the health care provider if concerns affect medication compliance.
• For patients taking MAOIs, assess usual dietary intake and provide instruction on foods, beverages, and medications to exclude. (Foods and beverages containing tyramine, alcohol, CNS stimulants and adrenergic-like drugs, narcotics, and other CNS depressants may cause significant adverse effects including hypertensive crisis or profound hypotension.)	• Instruct the patient, family, or caregiver in dietary and medication restrictions. Provide written and verbal instruction. • Instruct the patient to immediately report severe headache, dizziness, paresthesias, palpitations, tachycardia, chest pain, nausea or vomiting, diaphoresis, or fever.
• Avoid abrupt discontinuation of therapy. (Profound depression, seizures, or withdrawal symptoms may occur with abrupt discontinuation.)	• Instruct the patient to take the drug exactly as prescribed and to not stop it abruptly.
Patient understanding of drug therapy: • Use opportunities during administration of medications and during assessments to provide patient education. (Using time during nursing care helps to optimize and reinforce key teaching areas.)	• The patient should be able to state the reason for the drug; appropriate dose and scheduling; and what adverse effects to observe for and when to report them.
Patient self-administration of drug therapy: • When administering the medication, instruct the patient, family, or caregiver in proper self-administration of the drug, e.g., take the drug as prescribed and do not substitute brands. (Using time during nurse administration of these drugs helps to reinforce teaching.)	• Teach the patient to take the medication as follows: • Take exactly as ordered and use the same manufacturer's brand each time the prescription is filled. Switching brands may result in differing pharmacokinetics and alterations in therapeutic effect. • Take a missed dose as soon as it is noticed but do not take double or extra doses to "catch up." • Take with food to decrease GI upset. • If medication causes drowsiness, take at bedtime. • Do not abruptly discontinue medication. • Immediately report any increase in dilute urine, diarrhea, fever, or changes in mobility. • Drink adequate fluids to avoid dehydration. • Practice reliable contraception and notify the health care provider if pregnancy is planned or suspected. • Patients taking MAOIs should be given explicit instructions, written as well as verbal, on foods and beverages that must be avoided while taking the medication.

See Table 16.1 for a list of drugs to which these nursing actions apply.

focusing on tasks. ADHD may be diagnosed when the child's hyperactive behaviors significantly interfere with normal play, sleep, or learning activities. Hyperactive children usually have increased motor activity that is manifested by a tendency to be fidgety and impulsive, and to interrupt and talk excessively during their developmental years; therefore, they may not be able to interact with others appropriately at home, school, or on the playground. In boys, the activity levels are usually more overt. Girls show less aggression and impulsiveness but more anxiety, mood swings, social withdrawal, and cognitive and language delays. Girls also tend to be older at the time of diagnosis, so problems and setbacks related to the disorder exist for a longer time before treatment interventions are undertaken. Symptoms of ADHD are described in the following list:

- Easy distractibility
- Failure to receive or follow instructions properly
- Inability to focus on one task at a time and jumping from one activity to another
- Difficulty remembering
- Frequent loss or misplacement of personal items
- Excessive talking and interrupting other children in a group
- Inability to sit still when asked to do so repeatedly
- Impulsiveness
- Sleep disturbance.

Most children with ADHD have associated challenges. Many find it difficult to concentrate on tasks assigned in school. Even if children are gifted, their grades may suffer because they have difficulty following a conventional routine; discipline may also be a problem. Teachers are often the first to suggest that a child be examined for ADHD and receive medication when behaviors in the classroom escalate to the point of interfering with learning. A diagnosis is based on psychological and medical evaluations.

The etiology of ADHD is not clear. For many years, scientists described this disorder as mental brain dysfunction and hyperkinetic syndrome, focusing on abnormal brain function and overactivity. A variety of physical and neurologic disorders have been implicated; only a small percentage of those affected have a known cause. Purported causes have included contact with high levels of lead in childhood and prenatal exposure to alcohol and drugs. Genetic factors may also play a role, although a single gene has not been isolated and a specific mechanism of genetic transmission is not known. The interplay of genetics and environment may be a contributing dynamic. Recent evidence suggests that hyperactivity may be related to a deficit or dysfunction of dopamine, norepinephrine, or serotonin in the reticular activating system of the brain. Although once thought to be the culprits, sugars, chocolate, high-carbohydrate foods and beverages, and certain food additives have been refuted as causative or aggravating factors for ADHD.

The nurse is often involved in the screening and the mental health assessment of children with suspected ADHD. When a child is referred for testing, it is important to remember that both the child and family must be assessed. The family is screened with, or prior to, the child's evaluation. It is the nurse's responsibility to collect comprehensive data about the character and extent of the child's physical, psychological, and developmental health situation, to formulate the nursing diagnoses, and to create an individualized plan of care. A relevant nursing care plan can be created only if it is based on appropriate communication that fosters rapport and trust.

Once ADHD is diagnosed, the nurse is instrumental in educating the family regarding behavioral strategies that might be used to manage the demands of a child who is hyperactive. For the school-age child, the nurse often serves as the liaison to parents, teachers, and school administrators. The parents and child need to understand the importance of appropriate expectations and behavioral consequences. The child, from an early age and based on his or her developmental level, must be educated about the disorder and understand that there are consequences to inappropriate behavior. Self-esteem must be fostered in the child so that strengths in self-worth can develop. It is important for the child to develop a trusting relationship with health care providers and learn the importance of medication management and compliance.

One-third to one-half of children diagnosed with ADHD also experience symptoms of attention dysfunction in their adult years. Symptoms of ADHD in adults appear similar to mood disorders. Symptoms include anxiety, mania, restlessness, and depression, which can cause difficulties in interpersonal relationships. Some patients have difficulty holding jobs and may have an increased risk for alcohol and drug abuse. Untreated ADHD has been linked to low self-esteem, diminished social success, and criminal or violent behaviors.

PharmFacts

ATTENTION DEFICIT/HYPERACTIVITY DISORDER IN CHILDREN

- ADHD is the major reason children are referred for mental health treatment.
- About half are also diagnosed with oppositional defiant or conduct disorder.
- About one fourth are also diagnosed with anxiety disorder.
- About one third are also diagnosed with depression.
- About one fifth also have a learning disability.

DRUGS FOR ATTENTION DEFICIT/HYPERACTIVITY DISORDER

The traditional drugs used to treat ADHD in children have been the CNS stimulants. These drugs stimulate specific areas of the CNS that heighten alertness and increase focus. In 2006, the FDA's Drug Safety and Risk Management Advisory Committee voted to issue black box warnings for CNS stimulants used to treat ADHD, due to the possible adverse cardiovascular and psychiatric effects observed with these drugs. By 2010, several non-CNS stimulants were approved to treat ADHD. Agents for treating ADHD are listed in Table 16.4.

16.11 Pharmacotherapy of ADHD

The main treatment for ADHD is CNS stimulants. Stimulants reverse many of the symptoms, helping patients to focus on tasks. Drugs prescribed for ADHD include D- and L-amphetamine racemic mixture (Adderall), dexmethylphenidate (Focalin), dextroamphetamine (Dexedrine), lisdexamfetamine (Vyvanse), methamphetamine (Desoxyn) and methylphenidate (Ritalin). Intermediate- and

Table 16.4 Drugs for Attention Deficit/Hyperactivity Disorder

Drug	Route and Adult Dose (max dose where indicated)	Adverse Effects
CNS STIMULANTS		
D- and L-amphetamine racemic mixture (Adderall, Adderall-XR)	3–5 years old: PO: 2.5 mg one to two times/day; may increase by 2.5 mg at weekly intervals 6 years old: PO: 5 mg one or two times/day; may increase by 5 mg at weekly intervals (max: 40 mg/day).	*Irritability, nervousness, restlessness, insomnia, euphoria, palpitations* Sudden death (reported in children with structural cardiac abnormalities), circulatory collapse, exfoliative dermatitis, anorexia, liver failure, psychological dependence
dexmethylphenidate (Focalin)	Older than 6 years: PO: 2.5 mg bid may increase by 2.5–5 mg/wk (max: 20 mg/day); 5 mg/day extended release may increase by 5 mg/wk Adult: PO: 2.5 mg bid; may increase by 2.5–5 mg/day at weekly intervals (max: 20 mg/day)	
dextroamphetamine (Dexedrine)	3–5 years old: PO: 2.5 mg one or two times/day; may increase by 2.5 mg at weekly intervals 6 years old: PO: 5 mg one or two times/day; increase by 5 mg at weekly intervals (max: 40 mg/day)	
lisdexamfetamine (Vyvanse)	PO: 30 mg once daily in the a.m. (max: 70 mg/day)	
methamphetamine (Desoxyn)	6 years old: PO: 2.5–5 mg one or two times/day; may increase by 5 mg at weekly intervals (max: 20–25 mg/day)	
methylphenidate (Ritalin, Concerta, Daytrana, Metadate, Methylin)	Children older than age 6: PO: 5–10 mg before breakfast and lunch, with gradual increase of 5–10 mg/wk as needed (max: 60 mg/day) Adult: PO: 5 to 20 mg (prompt-release tablets) bid to tid. Once maintenance dosage is determined, may switch to extended release. Doses will vary depending on the drug formulation and product	
NONSTIMULANTS FOR ADHD		
atomoxetine (Strattera)	Adolescents and children less than 70 kg: PO: 0.5 mg/kg/day initially, may be increased every 3 days to a target dose of 1.2 mg/kg (max of 1.4 mg/kg or 100 mg/day, whichever is less) Adult: PO: 40 mg once daily or 20 mg bid	*Headache, insomnia, upper abdominal pain, vomiting, decreased appetite, dry mouth* Severe liver injury (rare), suicidal ideation (atomoxetine)
clonidine (Kapvay)	PO: dosing should be initiated with one 0.1 mg tablet at bedtime, and the daily dosage should be adjusted in increments of 0.1 mg/day at weekly intervals until the desired response is achieved	
guanfacine (Intuniv)	PO: start with 1 mg once daily; adjust up to 4 mg once daily until the desired response is achieved	

Note: *Italics* indicate common adverse effects, underlining indicates serious adverse effects.

Lifespan Considerations Cardiovascular Effects of ADHD Medications in Children

With the FDA mandate to place black box warnings for increased risk of adverse cardiovascular events on the packaging of the traditional drugs used for ADHD, health care providers may reconsider the use of these drugs and parents may be concerned about their use. Although the events are rare, the FDA found cause to issue the warnings. Research conducted since that time has started to clarify whether the risk is global, that is, affecting all aspects of cardiovascular health, or if there are some specific risks.

Hailpern et al. (2014) used data obtained from the large National Health and Nutrition Examination Survey (NHANES), an ongoing study into the health and nutritional status of children and adults in the United States. They found evidence that ADHD medication use increases heart rate, but did not find conclusive evidence that it had the same effect on blood pressure. While tachycardia is a risk factor for hypertension in adults, it is not known whether it is also a risk factor in children. The study also found that in boys taking ADHD medication, body mass index was lower and there were increased levels of C-reactive protein, a marker of inflammation that is associated with cardiovascular disease. Because this was not true for all study participants, further study is needed into the connection.

The nurse should take the patient's personal and family history of cardiac disease prior to a prescription for stimulant ADHD medications. When patients are taking these drugs, any symptoms of palpitations, shortness of breath, or other cardiac related symptoms should be immediately reported to the health care provider. Blood pressure and pulse should be assessed prior to medication therapy and at each office visit thereafter. Tachycardia should be reported to the provider.

longer-release forms of methylphenidate, marketed as Concerta, Metadate, and Methylin, are available. For greater flexibility in dosing, a methylphenidate patch marketed as Daytrana was approved by the FDA in 2006. In 2013, a daily liquid form of methylphenidate called Qillivant was approved for treatment of ADHD.

Patients taking CNS stimulants must be carefully monitored. CNS stimulants used to treat ADHD may

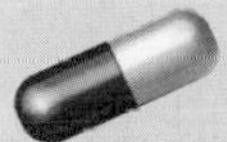

Prototype Drug | Methylphenidate *(Ritalin, Concerta, Daytrana, Metadate, Methylin)*

Therapeutic Class: Attention deficit–hyperactivity disorder drug **Pharmacologic Class:** CNS stimulant

Actions and Uses

Methylphenidate activates the reticular activating system, causing heightened alertness in various regions of the brain, particularly those centers associated with focus and attention. Activation is partially achieved by the release of neurotransmitters such as norepinephrine and dopamine. Impulsiveness, hyperactivity, and disruptive behavior are usually reduced within a few weeks. These changes promote improved psychosocial interactions and academic performance. A transdermal, extended-release form of methyphenidate was approved in 2006 (Daytrana).

Administration Alerts

- Sustained-release tablets must be swallowed whole. Breaking or crushing SR tablets causes immediate release of the entire dose.
- Controlled substance: Schedule II drug.
- Pregnancy category C.

PHARMACOKINETICS

Onset	Peak	Duration
Less than 60 min	2 h; 3–8 sustained release	3–6 h; 8 h sustained release; 8–12 h extended release

Adverse Effects

In a non-ADHD patient, methylphenidate causes nervousness and insomnia. All patients are at risk for irregular heartbeat, high blood pressure, and liver toxicity. Because methylphenidate is a Schedule II drug, it has the potential for causing dependence when used for extended periods. Periodic drug-free "holidays" are recommended to reduce drug dependence and to assess the patient's condition.

Black Box Warning: Methylphenidate is a Schedule II drug with high abuse potential. Give cautiously to patients with a history of drug dependence or alcoholism. Misuse may cause sudden death or a serious cardiovascular adverse event.

Contraindications: Patients with a history of marked anxiety, agitation, psychosis, suicidal ideation, glaucoma, motor tics, or Tourette's disease should not use this drug.

Interactions

Drug–Drug: Methylphenidate interacts with many drugs. For example, it may decrease the effectiveness of anticonvulsants, anticoagulants, and guanethidine. Concurrent therapy with clonidine may increase adverse effects. Antihypertensives or other CNS stimulants could potentiate the vasoconstrictive action of methylphenidate. MAOIs may produce hypertensive crisis.

Lab Tests: Unknown.

Herbal/Food: Administration times relative to meals and meal composition may need individual titration.

Treatment of Overdose: There is no specific treatment for overdose. Signs and symptoms of acute overdose result principally from overstimulation of the CNS and from excessive sympathomimetic effects. Emergency medical attention and general supportive measures may be necessary.

create paradoxical hyperactivity. Adverse reactions include insomnia, nervousness, anorexia, and weight loss. Occasionally, a patient may suffer from dizziness, depression, irritability, nausea, or abdominal pain. CNS stimulants are Schedule II controlled substances and labeled as pregnancy category C. Methylphenidate abuse has been increasing, especially among teens who take the drug to stay awake or as an appetite suppressant to lose weight.

Non-CNS stimulants when taken alone for ADHD exhibit less efficacy, but generally these drugs are more effective as adjunctive therapy. Atomoxetine (Strattera) selectively inhibits the presynpatic release of norepinephrine in the brain, thereby producing a calming effect in patients with ADHD. Other non-CNS stimulants are continuously effective for 24-month treatment periods with few and tolerable adverse effects. Patients taking atomoxetine show improved ability to focus on tasks and reduced hyperactivity. Efficacy appears to be equivalent to methylphenidate (Ritalin). Common side effects include headache, insomnia, upper abdominal pain, decreased appetite, and cough. Unlike methylphenidate, it is not a scheduled drug; thus, parents who are hesitant to place their child on stimulants now have a reasonable alternative. All children treated with atomexetine should be monitored closely for increased risk of suicide ideation.

Clonidine (Kapvay) is indicated for the treatment of ADHD as monotherapy and as adjunctive therapy to stimulant medications. Guanfacine is specifically indicated for children and adolescents diagnosed with ADHD between the ages of 6 to 17 years. Intuniv is a once-daily extended-release formulation of guanfacine for longer-term efficacy. Atomoxetine, clonidine, and guanfacine are all drugs selective for alpha$_2$-adrenergic receptors. Atypical antidepressants such as bupropion (Wellbutrin) and tricyclics such as desipramine (Norpramine) and imipramine (Tofranil) are considered second-choice drugs when CNS stimulants and nonstimulants fail to work or are contraindicated.

Nursing Practice Application

Pharmacotherapy for Attention Deficit/Hyperactivity Disorder

ASSESSMENT	POTENTIAL NURSING DIAGNOSES*
Baseline assessment prior to administration: • Obtain a complete health history including hepatic, renal, cardiovascular, or neurologic disease, including epilepsy. Obtain a drug history including allergies, current prescription and OTC drugs, and herbal preparations. Be alert to possible drug interactions. • Obtain a social and behavioral history. Use objective screening tools when possible. • Obtain a nutritional history and assess normal sleep patterns. • Obtain baseline vital signs and height and weight. • Evaluate appropriate laboratory findings (e.g., electrolytes, CBC, hepatic and renal function studies). • Assess the patient's ability to receive and understand instruction. Include the family and caregivers as needed.	• *Imbalanced Nutrition, Less Than Body Requirements* • *Disturbed Sleep Pattern* • *Dysfunctional Family Processes* • *Deficient Knowledge* (drug therapy) • *Risk for Disproportionate Growth,* related to adverse drug effects • *Risk for Social Isolation* • *Risk for Impaired Social Interaction* *NANDA I © 2014
Assessment throughout administration: • Assess for desired therapeutic effects (e.g., increased ability to focus, normalized activity levels with lessened impulsivity, maintenance of normal appetite and sleep patterns). • Continue periodic monitoring of electrolytes, CBC, and hepatic and renal function studies. • Continue to monitor vital signs and height and weight weekly. **Lifespan:** Be aware that the child, adolescent, or older adult is at greater risk for cardiovascular effects and may be more likely to experience anorexia from the drug. • Assess for and promptly report adverse effects: dizziness, lightheadedness, anxiety, agitation, excessive physical activity, tachycardia, increased blood pressure, hypertension, and palpitations.	

IMPLEMENTATION

Interventions and (Rationales)	Patient-Centered Care
Ensuring therapeutic effects: • Continue assessments as described earlier for therapeutic effects. (Therapeutic effects include the ability to focus and stay-on-task, lessened impulsivity, and improved social interactions.)	• Teach the patient, family, or caregiver to keep a social/behavioral diary. Involve school faculty and other caregivers (e.g., after-school care).
• Continue to monitor the pulse and blood pressure on health care visits. (Tachycardia, increased blood pressure, or hypertension may occur if the dose is excessive.)	• Teach the patient, family, or caregiver to take the pulse along with weekly height and weight or any time symptoms warrant (e.g., child complains of chest discomfort or palpitations). Assist the patient, family, or caregiver to find pulse location most easily felt and have the patient, family, or caregiver teach-back pulse taking before going home.
• Weigh the patient weekly and obtain the patient's height. Report any weight loss or failure to gain weight during the expected growth periods. Assess nutrition and use of other stimulating products (e.g., energy drinks, caffeinated beverages). (Diminished appetite or anorexia from stimulating effects of the drug, or use of other stimulants, may impair the normal nutrition needed for growth and development. **Lifespan:** Children, adolescents, and older adults are more likely to experience anorexia from the drug.)	• Teach the patient, family, or caregiver to obtain height and weight weekly and to report any loss of weight or lack of expected growth. • Encourage the patient, family, or caregiver to administer the drug after the morning meal to avoid impact on appetite, especially if shorter-acting formulations are used. • Discuss the need to avoid or eliminate all foods, beverages, or OTC drugs that contain caffeine or other stimulants.
• Continue to monitor sleep patterns. (Stimulatory effects of drug may affect normal sleeping patterns and may indicate excessive dosage.)	• Instruct the patient, family, or caregiver to inform the provider of disruption to sleep, increased agitation or excessive sleepiness during the day (possible effect from lack of sleep at night). • Have the patient take the dose early in the day and before 4:00 p.m. to help alleviate insomnia unless extended-release formulation is used. Take extended-release formulations in the morning.

Nursing Practice Application *continued*

IMPLEMENTATION	
Interventions and (Rationales)	**Patient-Centered Care**
• Assess for excessive stimulatory effects: agitation, aggression, tremors, or seizures and report immediately. (Excessive CNS stimulation may cause seizures as an adverse effect.)	• Instruct the patient, family, or caregiver to immediately report tremors or seizures to the health care provider.
• Assess for urinary retention periodically. (Atomoxetine [Strattera] and other norepinephrine reuptake inhibitors may cause urinary retention as an adverse effect. **Lifespan:** Be aware that the male older adult with an enlarged prostate is at higher-risk for mechanical obstruction.)	• Instruct the patient to immediately report an inability to void, increasing bladder pressure, or pain.
• Continue to monitor for dermatologic effects including red or purplish skin rash, blisters, or sunburn. (Armodafinil and methylphenidate have been associated with severe skin effects including SJS and exfoliative dermatitis. Sunscreen and protective clothing should be used.)	• Teach the patient to wear sunscreen and protective clothing for sun exposure and to avoid tanning beds. Immediately report any severe sunburn or rashes.
• Assess the need for continuous medication or drug holidays with the patient, family, caregiver, and health care provider based on the social/behavioral diary findings. (Dependent on the degree of behavior, drug holidays over non–school days or vacation periods may be recommended to avoid dependence on the drug and to assess current symptoms of ADHD. If symptoms suggest improvement, a lower dose or medication-free period may be recommended.)	• Teach the patient, family, or caregiver about the use of drug holidays and explore options. If the drug dose is at the upper range, consider tapering the dose prior to beginning the drug holiday to avoid rebound hyperactivity or agitation.
• Assess the home environment for medication safety and the need for appropriate interventions. Advise the family on restrictions about prescription renewal. (Methylphenidate is a Schedule II drug and may not be used by any other person than the patient. Safeguard medication in the home to prevent overdosage.)	• Instruct the patient, family, or caregiver in proper medication storage and the need for the drug to be used by the patient only. • Teach the family or caregiver about prescription renewal restrictions (i.e., new prescription each time, no refills, prescription may not be called in) and explore school policies regarding in-school use (e.g., single-dose sent each day, secured blister-pack used if multidoses are sent).
Patient understanding of drug therapy: • Use opportunities during administration of medications and during assessments to provide patient education. (Using time during nursing care helps to optimize and reinforce key teaching areas.)	• The patient, family, or caregiver should be able to state the reason for the drug; appropriate dose and scheduling; and what adverse effects to observe for and when to report them.
Patient self-administration of drug therapy: • When administering the medication, instruct the patient, family, or caregiver in the proper self-administration of drug, e.g., take the drug as prescribed and do not substitute brands. |(Using time during nurse administration of these drugs helps to reinforce teaching.)	• Teach the patient to take the medication as follows: • Take exactly as ordered and in the morning to prevent insomnia. • Do not take double or extra doses to increase mental focus or to prevent sleepiness. The drug will not achieve these effects but will increase the adverse effects. • Do not open, chew, or crush extended release tablets; swallow them whole with plenty of water. • Do not abruptly discontinue the medication without consulting the health care provider.

See Table 16.4 for lists of drugs to which these nursing actions apply.

Chapter Review

KEY Concepts

The numbered key concepts provide a succinct summary of the important points from the corresponding numbered section within the chapter. If any of these points are not clear, refer to the numbered section within the chapter for review.

16.1 Clinical depression is a common emotional disorder characterized by a despondent mood lasting for a minimum of two weeks. It may be manifested in different ways, such as situational depression, dysthymic disorder, postpartum depression, seasonal affective disorder, and psychotic depression.

16.2 Approaches to treatment of major depression involve a proper health examination, medications, psychotherapeutic techniques, and possibly electroconvulsive or rTMS therapy. There is an important warning from the FDA about antidepressants.

16.3 Antidepressants act by correcting neurotransmitter imbalances in the brain. The two basic mechanisms of action are blocking the enzymatic breakdown of norepinephrine and slowing the reuptake of serotonin. The primary classes of antidepressants are the SSRIs, atypical antidepressants, TCAs, and MAOIs.

16.4 SSRIs act by selectively blocking the reuptake of serotonin in nerve terminals. Because of fewer side effects, SSRIs are drugs of choice in the pharmacotherapy of depression. Serotonin syndrome is a serious concern for SSRIs.

16.5 Atypical antidepressants to do not fit conveniently into the other antidepressant classes. One subgroup is the serotonin-norepinephrine reuptake inhibitors (SNRIs), such as duloxetine and venlafaxine. Another group, which includes bupropion, not only inhibits reuptake of serotonin and norepinephrine, but also inhibits reuptake of dopamine.

16.6 TCAs are older medications used mainly for the treatment of major depression, obsessive–compulsive disorders, and panic attacks. They have unpleasant and serious side effects.

16.7 MAOIs are usually prescribed when other antidepressants have not been successful. They have more serious side effects than other antidepressants.

16.8 Patients with bipolar disorder display not only signs of depression but also signs of mania, a state characterized by high psychomotor activity and irritability.

16.9 Lithium (Eskalith), antiseizure drugs, and atypical antipsychotic drugs are used to treat bipolar disorder. Lithium is effective for purely manic or purely depressive stages. Antiseizure drugs are more effective in the treatment of mania or for cycling and mixed states of bipolar disorder. Atypical antipsychotics are more effective for the treatment of acute mania and for the longer-term treatment of psychotic depression.

16.10 ADHD is a behavioral condition diagnosed primarily in children and characterized by difficulty paying attention, hyperactivity, and impulsiveness.

16.11 The most efficacious drugs for symptoms of ADHD are the CNS stimulants such as methylphenidate (Ritalin). The nonstimulant drug, atomoxetine (Strattera) is an alternative for patients with ADHD.

REVIEW Questions

1. The nurse is monitoring the patient for early signs of lithium (Eskalith) toxicity. Which symptoms, if present, may indicate that toxicity is developing? (Select all that apply.)
   1. Persistent gastrointestinal upset (e.g., nausea, vomiting)
   2. Confusion
   3. Increased urination
   4. Convulsions
   5. Ataxia
2. The parents of a young patient receiving methylphenidate (Ritalin) express concern that the health care provider has suggested the child have a "holiday" from the drug. What is the purpose of a drug-free period?
   1. To reduce or eliminate the risk of drug toxicity
   2. To allow the child's "normal" behavior to return
   3. To decrease drug dependence and assess the patient's status
   4. To prevent the occurrence of a hypertensive crisis
3. A 16-year-old patient has taken an overdosage of citalopram (Celexa) and is brought to the emergency department. What symptoms would the nurse expect to be present?
   1. Seizures, hypertension, tachycardia, extreme anxiety
   2. Hypotension, bradycardia, hypothermia, sedation
   3. Miosis, respiratory depression, absent bowel sounds, hypoactive reflexes
   4. Manic behavior, paranoia, delusions, tremors
4. A 77-year-old female patient is diagnosed with depression and anxiety and is started on imipramine. Because of this patient's age, which adverse effects would take priority when planning care?
   1. Dry mouth and photosensitivity
   2. Anxiety, headaches, insomnia
   3. Drowsiness and sedation
   4. Urinary frequency
5. Which of the following would be a priority component of the teaching plan for a patient prescribed phenelzine (Nardil) for treatment of depression?
   1. Headaches may occur. Over-the-counter medications will usually be effective.
   2. Hyperglycemia may occur and any unusual thirst, hunger, or urination should be reported.
   3. Read labels of food and over-the-counter drugs to avoid those with substances that should be avoided as directed.
   4. Monitor blood pressure for hypotension and report any blood pressure below 90/60.
6. The nurse determines that the teaching plan for a patient prescribed sertraline (Zoloft) has been effective when the patient makes which statement?
   1. "I should not decrease my sodium or water intake."
   2. "The drug can be taken concurrently with the phenelzine (Nardil) that I'm taking."
   3. "It may take up to a month for the drug to reach full therapeutic effects and I'm feeling better."
   4. "There are no other drugs I need to worry about; Zoloft doesn't react with them."

PATIENT-FOCUSED Case Study

Margot Cinotti is a 26-year-old mother of three young children who has been followed since her last pregnancy when she experienced post-partum depression. She was placed on sertraline (Zoloft) and experienced improvement, but not complete resolution of her depression. Lately, her husband reports that she seems increasingly depressed and disinterested in the usual activities around the house or with the children that she used to enjoy. He is concerned that the drug is not working.

1. Which drug classification does sertraline (Zoloft) belong to? What are some of the adverse effects associated with this class?
2. What assessment data should be gathered at this time to help determine the cause of Mrs. Cinotti's increased depression?
3. What changes might be made to her treatment plan?

CRITICAL THINKING Questions

1. A 12-year-old girl has been diagnosed with ADHD. Her parents have been reluctant to agree with the pediatrician's recommendation for pharmacologic management; however, the child's performance in school has deteriorated. A school nurse notes that the child has been placed on amphetamine and dextroamphetamine (Adderall). What information do her parents need about this medication?
2. A 56-year-old female patient has been diagnosed with clinical depression following the death of her husband. She says that she has not been able to sleep for weeks and that she is drinking a lot of coffee. She is also smoking more than she usually has. The health care provider prescribes fluoxetine (Prozac). The patient seeks reassurance from the nurse regarding when she should begin feeling "more like myself." How should the nurse respond?

Visit www.pearsonhighered.com/nursingresources for answers and rationales for all activities.

REFERENCES

Hailpern, S. M., Egan, B. M., Lewis, K. D., Wagner, C., Shattat, G. F., Al Qaoud, D. I., & Shatat, I. F. (2014). Blood pressure, heart rate, and CNS stimulant medication use in children with and without ADHD: Analysis of NHANES data. *Frontiers in Pediatrics, 2*, 100. doi:10.3389/ped.2014.00100

Herdman, T. H., & Kamitsuru, S. (Eds.). (2014). *NANDA International nursing diagnoses: Definitions and classification, 2015–2017*. Oxford, United Kingdom: Wiley-Blackwell.

National Center for Complementary and Integrative Health. (2012). *St. John's wort*. Retrieved from http://www.nccam.nih.gov/health/stjohnswort/ataglance.htm

National Center for Complementary and Integrative Health. (2013). *St. John's wort and depression*. Retrieved from http://www.nccam.nih.gov/health/stjohnswort/sjw-and-depression.htm

SELECTED BIBLIOGRAPHY

American Psychiatric Association. (2013). Diagnostic and statistical manual of mental disorders (5th Ed.: DSM-5). Arlington, VA: Author. doi:10.1176/appi.books.9780890425596.dsm04

Antshel, K. M. (2015). Psychosocial interventions in attention-deficit/hyperactivity disorder: Update. *Child and Adolescent Psychiatric Clinics of North America, 24*, 79–97. doi:10.1016/j.chc.2014.08.002

Berlim M. T., Van den Eynde, F., & Daskalakis, Z. J. (2013). High frequency repetitive transcranial magnetic stimulation accelerates and enhances the clinical response to antidepressants in major depression: A meta-analysis of randomized, double-blind, and sham-controlled trials. *Journal of Clinical Psychiatry, 74*(2), e122–e129. doi:10.4088/JCP.12r07996

Cheung K., Aarts, N., Noordam, R., van Blijderveen, J. C., Sturkenboom, M. C., Ruiter, R., . . . Stricker, B. H. (2014). Antidepressant use and the risk of suicide: A population-based cohort study. *Journal of Affective Disorders, 174*, 479–484. doi:10.1016/j.jad.2014.12.032

DeJesus, S. A., Diaz, V. A., Gonsalves, W. C., & Carek, P. J. (2011). Identification and treatment of depression in minority populations. *International Journal of Psychiatry in Medicine, 42*, 69–83. doi:10.2190/PM.42.1.e

Huang, Y. S., & Tsai, M. H. (2011). Long-term outcomes with medications for attention-deficit hyperactivity disorder: Current status of knowledge. *CNS Drugs, 25*, 539–554. doi:10.2165/11589380-000000000-00000

Jerrell, J. M., McIntyre, R. S., & Park, Y. M. (2014). Correlates of incident bipolar disorder in children and adolescents diagnosed with attention-deficit/hyperactivity disorder. *Journal of Clinical Psychiatry, 75*(11), e1278–1283. doi:10.4088/JCP.14m09046

Karaosmanoğlu, A. D., Butros, S. R., Arellano, R. (2013). Imaging findings of renal toxicity in patients on chronic lithium therapy. *Diagnostic and Interventional Radiology, 19*, 299–303. doi:10.5152.dir.2013.097

Morrissette, D. A., & Stahl, S. M. (2014). Modulating the serotonin system in the treatment of major depressive disorder. *CNS Spectrums, 19* (Suppl. 1), 54–68. doi:10.1017/S1092852914000613

Schatzberg, A. F., Blier, P., Culpepper, L., Jain, R., Papakostas, G. I., & Thase, M. E. (2014). An overview of vortioxetine. *Journal of Clinical Psychiatry, 75*, 1411–1418. doi:10.4088/JCP.14027ah1

UK ECT Review Group. (2003). Efficacy and safety of electroconvulsive therapy in depressive disorders: A systematic review and meta-analysis. *Lancet, 361*(9360), 799–808.

Wang, S., Han, C., & Pae, C. (2015). Criticisms of drugs in early development for the treatment of depression: What can be improved? *Expert Opinion on Investigational Drugs, 24*, 445–453. doi:10.1517/13543784.2014.985784

Chapter 17

Drugs for Psychoses

Drugs at a Glance

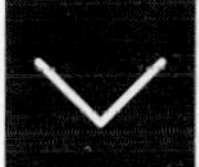

Learning Outcomes

After reading this chapter, the student should be able to:

1. Explain theories for the etiology of schizophrenia.
2. Compare and contrast the positive and negative symptoms of schizophrenia.
3. Discuss the rationale for selecting a specific antipsychotic drug for the treatment of schizophrenia.
4. Explain the importance of patient drug compliance in the pharmacotherapy of schizophrenia.
5. Describe the nurse's role in the pharmacologic management of schizophrenia.
6. Explain the symptoms associated with extrapyramidal symptoms of antipsychotic drugs.
7. For each of the drug classes listed in Drugs at a Glance, know representative drug examples and explain their mechanism of action, primary actions, and important adverse effects.
8. Categorize drugs used for psychoses based on their classification and drug action.
9. Use the nursing process to care for patients receiving pharmacotherapy for psychoses.

(pill icon) indicates a prototype drug, each of which is featured in a Prototype Drug box.

Psychosis is a broad term that refers to a serious mental disorder in which there is a loss of contact with reality. Severe mental illness can be incapacitating for the patient and intensely frustrating for family members and those interacting with the patient on a regular basis. Before the 1950s, patients with psychoses were institutionalized, often for their entire lives. With the introduction of chlorpromazine in the 1950s and the subsequent development of newer drugs, antipsychotic drugs have revolutionized the treatment of mental illness. With proper medical management, patients with serious mental disorders can now lead normal or near normal lives as functioning members of society.

PSYCHOSES

17.1 The Nature of Psychoses

Patients with psychoses often are unable to distinguish what is real from what is illusion. Because of this, patients may be viewed as medically and legally incompetent. The following signs are characteristic of psychosis:

- *Delusions* (strong belief in something that is false or not based on reality); for example, the patient may believe that someone is planting thoughts in his or her head.
- *Hallucinations* (seeing, hearing, or feeling something that is not there); for example, the patient may hear voices or see spiders crawling on walls that others around the patient do not hear or see.
- *Illusions* (distorted or misleading perceptions of something that is actually real); for example, the patient may see a shadow and believe it is really a person.
- *Disorganized behavior;* for example, the patient may wear clothes in an entirely inappropriate manner and for no apparent reason, such as dressing up with layers of clothes including a hat, sunglasses, and several pairs of socks over the hands and feet.
- *Difficulty relating to others*; for example, the patient may become withdrawn from other people in the room, showing signs of distress, maybe even turning combative if confronted or questioned. Signs may range from total inactivity to extreme agitation.
- *Paranoia* or tendency on the part of an individual toward irrational distrust; for example, the patient may have an extreme suspicion that he or she is being followed, or that someone is trying to kill him or her.

Psychoses may be classified as *acute* or *chronic*. Acute psychotic episodes occur over hours or days, whereas chronic psychoses develop over months or years. Sometimes a cause may be attributed to the psychosis, such as traumatic brain injury, overdoses of certain medications, chronic alcoholism, or drug addiction. Additional causes may be extreme depression, bipolar disorder, Alzheimer's disease or schizophrenia. Genetic factors are known to play a role in some psychoses. Unfortunately, the vast majority of psychoses have no identifiable cause.

People with psychosis are usually unable to function in society without long-term drug therapy. Patients must see their health care provider periodically, and medication must be taken for life. Family members and social support groups are important sources of help for patients who cannot function without continuous drug therapy.

17.2 Schizophrenia

Schizophrenia is a type of psychosis characterized by abnormal thoughts and thought processes, disordered communication, and withdrawal from other people and the outside environment. This disorder has a high risk for suicide. Several subtypes of schizophrenic disorders are based on clinical presentation.

Schizophrenia is the most common psychotic disorder, affecting 1% to 2% of the population. Symptoms generally begin to appear in early adulthood with a peak incidence in men 15 to 24 years of age and in women 25 to 34 years of age. Patients potentially experience a variety of symptoms that may change over time. The following symptoms may appear quickly or take longer to develop.

- Hallucinations, delusions, or paranoia
- Strange behavior, such as communicating in rambling statements or made-up words
- Rapid alternation between extreme hyperactivity and stupor
- Attitude of indifference or detachment toward life activities
- Strange or irrational actions and movements
- Deterioration of personal hygiene and job or academic performance
- Marked withdrawal from social interactions and interpersonal relationships.

When observing a patient with schizophrenia, the nurse should look for both positive and negative symptoms. **Positive symptoms** are those that *add* on to normal behavior. These include hallucinations, delusions, and a disorganized thought or speech pattern. **Negative symptoms** are those that *subtract* from normal behavior. These symptoms include a lack of interest, motivation, responsiveness, or pleasure in daily activities. Negative symptoms are characteristic of the indifferent personality exhibited by many people with schizophrenia. They are harder to associate with schizophrenia because they are sometimes mistaken for depression or even laziness. Proper identification of positive and negative symptoms is important for the selection of the appropriate antipsychotic drug.

The cause of schizophrenia has not been determined, although several theories have been proposed. There appears to be a genetic component, because many schizophrenic patients have family members who have been afflicted with the same disorder. Another theory suggests that the disorder is caused by imbalances of neurotransmitters in specific brain regions. This theory suggests the possibility of overactive dopaminergic pathways in the basal nuclei, an area of the brain responsible for motor activity. Neurons in the substantia nigra project to the caudate nucleus and putamen, which are regions of the corpus striatum. The corpus striatum is responsible for synchronized motor activity, actions such as the starting and stopping of leg and arm motions during walking. Also, ventral tegmental neurons project to the hippocampus, nucleus accumbens, and areas of the frontal cortex. Tegmental neurons are thought to precipitate an interest in sights, sounds, ideas, and thoughts. Collectively, neuronal pathways seem to be associated with reinforcement learning and motivational behavior. Important dopaminergic pathways are depicted in Figure 17.1.

Symptoms of schizophrenia seem to be connected with **dopamine type 2 (D_2) receptors.** The basal nuclei are particularly rich in D_2 receptors, whereas areas of the frontal cortex are filled with reverberating subcortical circuits contingent on dopamine levels. Neural circuitries project back to the origin of dopamine synthesis and stimulate the release of more dopamine. All antipsychotic drugs act by entering dopaminergic synapses and compete with the binding of dopamine to receptors. By blocking a majority of the D_2 receptors, antipsychotic drugs reduce positive feedback-type impulses and mitigate symptoms of schizophrenia.

PharmFacts

PSYCHOSES

- Symptoms of psychosis are often associated with other mental health problems including substance abuse, depression, and dementia.
- Psychotic disorders are among the most misunderstood mental health disorders in North America.
- Approximately 3 million Americans have schizophrenia.
- Patients with psychosis often develop symptoms between the ages of 13 and the early 20s.
- As many as 50% of homeless people in America have schizophrenia.
- The probability of developing schizophrenia is 1 in 100 for the general population, 1 in 10 if one parent has the disorder, and 1 in 4 if both parents have schizophrenia.

Schizoaffective disorder is a condition in which the patient exhibits symptoms of both schizophrenia and mood disorder. For example, an acute schizoaffective reaction may include distorted perceptions, hallucinations, and delusions, followed by extreme depression. Over time, both positive and negative psychotic symptoms will appear.

Many conditions can cause bizarre behavior, and these should be distinguished from schizophrenia. Chronic use of amphetamines or cocaine can create a paranoid syndrome. Complex partial seizures (see chapter 15) can cause unusual symptoms that may be mistaken for psychoses. Brain neoplasms, infections, or hemorrhage can also cause bizarre, psychotic-like symptoms.

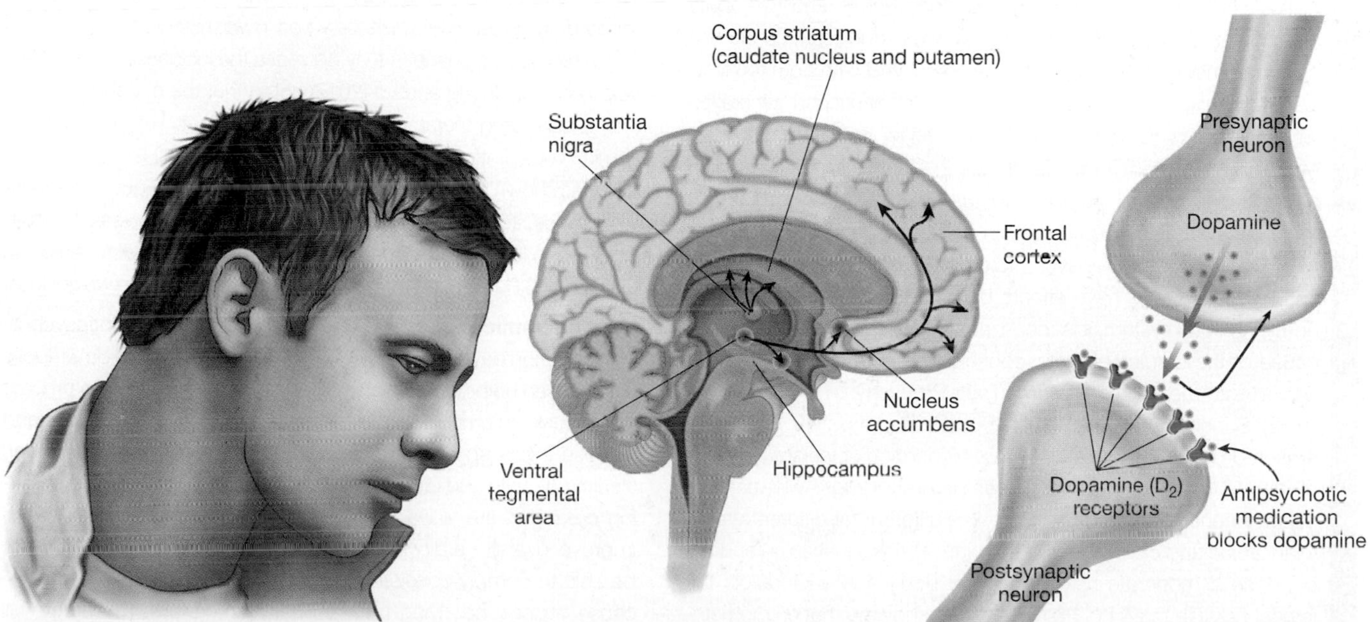

FIGURE 17.1 Overactive dopaminergic pathways in the substantia nigra and ventral tegmental area may be responsible for schizophrenia symptoms; antipsychotic drugs occupy D_2 receptors, preventing dopamine from stimulating postsynaptic neurons

Source: *Core Concepts in Pharmacology* (4th Ed.), by N. Holland, M. Adams, & C. Urban, 2015. Reprinted and electronically reproduced by permission of Pearson Education, Inc., Upper Saddle River, New Jersey.

17.3 Pharmacologic Management of Psychoses

Management of severe mental illness is always challenging for health care providers. Many patients do not see their behavior as abnormal and have difficulty understanding the need for medication. When that medication produces undesirable side effects, such as severe twitching or loss of sexual function, adherence diminishes and patients exhibit symptoms of their pretreatment illness. Agitation, distrust, and extreme frustration are common, because patients cannot comprehend why others are unable to think and see the same way as they do. It should be remembered that unless deemed overtly dangerous to themselves or other people, patients cannot be held for long periods of hospitalization against their wishes. Once released into the community, patients may choose not to take their antipsychotic medication, against the advice of their health care provider. Patients with schizophrenia have a very high noncompliance rate.

The primary therapeutic goal for patients with schizophrenia is to reduce psychotic symptoms to a level that allows the patient to maintain normal social relationships and perform normal activities of daily living (ADLs) independently or with minimal assistance. From a pharmacologic perspective, therapy has both a positive and a negative side. Although many symptoms of psychosis can be controlled with current drugs, adverse effects are common and sometimes severe. The antipsychotic drugs do not cure mental illness, and symptoms remain in remission only as long as the patient chooses to take the drug. The relapse rate for patients who discontinue their medication is 60% to 80%.

In terms of efficacy, there is little difference among the various antipsychotic drugs. There is no single drug of choice for schizophrenia. Clearly, the newer antipsychotic drugs have a lower incidence of adverse effects. With the exception of clozapine, guidelines allow for the use of first and second generation antipsychotics as first line treatments for schizophrenia. However, the selection of a specific drug is highly individualized and based on clinician experience, the occurrence of specific adverse effects, and needs of the patient. For example, patients with psychoses as well as Parkinson's symptoms need an antipsychotic with minimal extrapyramidal symptoms. **Extrapyramidal symptoms (EPS)** are a particularly serious set of adverse reactions to antipsychotic drugs. Those who operate machinery need a drug that does not cause sedation. Men and

Evidence-Based Practice: Cardiometabolic Effects of Antipsychotic Drugs

Clinical Question: Do antipsychotic drugs increase the risk of developing cardiometabolic disease?

Evidence: Landmark research into the effectiveness of antipsychotic drugs such as the CATIE (Clinical Antipsychotic Trials of Intervention Effectiveness) and the SATIETY (Second-Generation Antipsychotic Treatment Indications, Effectiveness, and Tolerability in Youth) studies determined that there were significant cardiovascular and metabolic adverse effects associated with both the first-generation (typical) antipsychotics and the newer second-generation (atypical) drugs (Correll et al., 2009; DeLisi & Nasrallah, 2005; McEvoy et al., 2005). In those studies, cardiovascular effects such as hypertension, and metabolic disturbances such as weight gain and obesity, hyperlipidemia, insulin resistance, and diabetes were found to occur with antipsychotic drugs of both classes. Because antipsychotic drugs have effects on neurochemicals in the autonomic nervous system, it is theorized that these effects may be the cause of the cardiometabolic consequences that have been observed with these drugs (Leung, Barr, Procyshyn, Honer, & Pang, 2012). Subsequent research has found that low-potency first-generation drugs are associated with a higher risk of weight gain and metabolic dysfunction than higher potency drugs, whereas the second-generation drugs' impact was different for different drugs. Olanzapine and clozapine had the highest risk, quetiapine and risperidone a moderate risk, and ziprasidone and aripiprazole the lowest risk (Chang & Lu, 2012). Despite knowing that cardiometabolic adverse effects occur commonly with antipsychotic drugs, one study found that there was a fairly low treatment rate for these complications. Diabetes was the most common condition treated (52% of study patients), with approximately 26% receiving treatment for hypertension, and only 19% for hyperlipidemia (Steylen et al., 2013). The potential cost savings of treatment with lower-risk drugs is also significant. Ward et al. (2013) estimated a cost savings in diabetes treatment by over $450,000, and over $80,000 for cardiovascular heart disease when lower-risk drugs were used.

While lifestyle changes may decrease the incidence of these adverse effects, Chang and Lu (2012) noted that the metabolic effects may require drug therapy for adequate treatment. The oral hypoglycemic drug, metformin, may be given to improve insulin sensitivity and was shown to be most effective with lifestyle changes to promote weight loss. Topiramate, an anticonvulsant, may be given as an off-label use to lessen weight gain and other metabolic effects. Amantadine, an anti-Parkinson's drug, may also slow or promote weight loss.

Nursing Implications: Knowing that patients taking antipsychotic medication have a significantly increased risk of cardiometabolic disease can help nurses plan strategies with the patient to prevent these from occurring. Weight, pulse, blood pressure, and lipid and glucose levels should be checked on each visit to the provider. Healthy lifestyle and dietary habits, increasing exercise, and smoking cessation are ways to counteract the metabolic effects and improve overall cardiovascular functioning. The patient may not be able to comply consistently with these nondrug strategies because of the underlying mental illness. Therefore, the nurse will require patience and creativity to work with the patient to achieve desired outcomes.

women who are sexually active may want a drug without negative effects on sexual interaction. The experience and skills of the health care provider and mental health nurse are particularly valuable in achieving successful psychiatric pharmacotherapy.

The pharmacotherapy of psychosis has undergone three major "generations" of drugs. The first generation drugs are often called the "typical" or "conventional" antipsychotics. Drugs such as chlorpromazine appeared in the early 1950s. The "second-generation" or "atypical" antipsychotic drugs were discovered in the 1970s and 1980s. Atypical antipsychotics are more frequently prescribed because they produce significantly fewer adverse effects, which increases patient compliance. The latest drugs, some still in development, are called "third generation." Classified as dopamine-serotonin system stabilizers, these are still considered "atypical" antipsychotics. Aripiprazole (Abilify) is an example thought to reduce the risk of hyperglycemia and diabetes with longer-term use. These drugs stabilize both dopamine and serotonin levels in the brain.

CONVENTIONAL ANTIPSYCHOTIC DRUGS

Because of neurologic side effects, antipsychotic drugs are sometimes referred to as **neuroleptics.** The two basic categories of antipsychotic drugs are conventional antipsychotics and atypical antipsychotics. The conventional drugs for psychoses include the phenothiazines and nonphenothiazine drugs.

Phenothiazines

The phenothiazines are most effective at treating the positive signs of schizophrenia, such as hallucinations and delusions, and have been the treatment of choice for psychoses for over 60 years.

17.4 Treating Psychoses With Phenothiazines

The phenothiazines are listed in Table 17.1. Within each category, drugs are generally named by their chemical structure.

The first effective drug used to treat schizophrenia was the low-potency phenothiazine chlorpromazine, approved by the U.S. Food and Drug Administration (FDA) for this use in 1954. A number of phenothiazines are now available to treat mental illness. All block the excitement associated with the positive symptoms of schizophrenia, although they differ in potency and side-effect profiles. Hallucinations and delusions often begin to diminish within days. Other symptoms, however, may require as long as 7 to 8 weeks of pharmacotherapy to improve. Because of the high rate of recurrence of psychotic episodes, pharmacotherapy should be considered long term, often for the life of the patient. Phenothiazines are thought to act by preventing dopamine and serotonin from occupying critical neurologic receptor sites. For the conventional antipsychotics, dopamine has higher affinity for the receptor.

Although phenothiazines revolutionized the treatment of severe mental illness, they exhibit numerous adverse effects that can limit pharmacotherapy. These are listed in Table 17.2. Anticholinergic effects such as dry mouth, postural hypotension, and urinary retention are common. Ejaculation disorders occur in a high percentage of patients taking phenothiazines; delay in achieving orgasm (in both men and women) is a common cause for noncompliance, and menstrual disorders are common. High fever, tachycardia, incontinence, confusion, and other signs of **neuroleptic malignant syndrome (NMS)** may occur. Each phenothiazine has a slightly different side-effect spectrum. For example, perphenazine has a low incidence of anticholinergic effects, whereas chlorpromazine has a high incidence of anticholinergic effects. Thioridazine (Mellaril) frequently causes sedation, whereas this side effect is less common with trifluoperazine. Although prochlorperazine tablets have

Table 17.1 Conventional Antipsychotic Drugs: Phenothiazines

Drug	Route and Adult Dose (max dose where indicated)	Adverse Effects
chlorpromazine	PO: 25–100 mg tid or qid (max: 1000 mg/day) IM/IV: 25–50 mg (max: 600 mg q4-6h)	*Sedation, drowsiness, dizziness, extrapyramidal symptoms, constipation, photosensitivity, orthostatic hypotension, urinary retention* Increased risk for suicide, agranulocytosis, pancytopenia, anaphylactoid reaction, tardive dyskinesia, neuroleptic malignant syndrome, hypothermia, adynamic ileus, sudden unexplained death
fluphenazine (Prolixin decanoate injection)	PO: 0.5–10 mg/day (max: 20 mg/day) IM/subcutaneous; long-acting injections range from 12.5 mg to 37.5 mg every 2–3 weeks	
perphenazine	PO: 4–16 mg bid to qid (max: 64 mg/day)	
prochlorperazine (Compazine) (see page 706 for the Prototype Drug box)	PO: 0.5–10 mg/day (max: 20 mg/day)	
thioridazine (Mellaril)	PO: 50–100 mg tid (max: 800 mg/day)	
Trifluoperazine	PO: 1–2 mg bid (max: 20 mg/day)	

Note: *Italics* indicate common adverse effects; underlining indicates serious adverse effects.

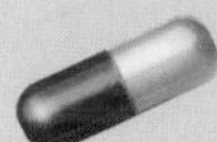

Prototype Drug | Chlorpromazine

Therapeutic Class: Conventional antipsychotic; schizophrenia drug
Pharmacologic Class: D_2 dopamine receptor antagonist; phenothiazine

Actions and Uses

Chlorpromazine provides symptomatic relief of positive symptoms of schizophrenia and controls manic symptoms in patients with schizoaffective disorder. Many patients must take chlorpromazine for 7 or 8 weeks before they experience improvement. Extreme agitation may be treated with intramuscular (IM) or intravenous (IV) injections, which begin to act within minutes. Chlorpromazine can also control severe nausea and vomiting.

Administration Alerts

- Do not crush or open sustained-release forms.
- When administered IM, give deep IM, only in the upper outer quadrant of the buttocks; the patient should remain supine for 30 to 60 minutes after injection and then rise slowly.
- The drug must be gradually withdrawn over 2 to 3 weeks, and nausea, vomiting, dizziness, tremors, or dyskinesia may occur.
- IV forms should be used only during surgery or for severe hiccups.
- Pregnancy category C.

PHARMACOKINETICS

Onset	Peak	Duration
30–60 min	2–4 h PO; 15–20 min IM/IV	30 h

Adverse Effects

Strong blockade of alpha-adrenergic receptors and weak blockade of cholinergic receptors explain some of chlorpromazine's adverse effects. Common adverse effects are dizziness, drowsiness, and orthostatic hypotension.

EPS occur more commonly in elderly, female, and pediatric patients who are dehydrated. Neuroleptic malignant syndrome (NMS) may also occur. Patients taking chlorpromazine who are exposed to warmer temperatures should be monitored more closely for symptoms of NMS.

Black Box Warning: Elderly patients with dementia-related psychosis are at increased risk for death when taking conventional antipsychotics.

Contraindications: Use is not advised during alcohol withdrawal or when the patient is in a comatose state. Caution should be used with other conditions, including subcortical brain damage, bone marrow depression, and Reye's syndrome.

Interactions

Drug–Drug: Chlorpromazine interacts with several drugs. For example, concurrent use with sedative medications such as phenobarbital should be avoided. Taking chlorpromazine with tricyclic antidepressants can elevate blood pressure. Concurrent use of chlorpromazine with antiseizure medication can lower the seizure threshold.

Lab Tests: Chlorpromazine may increase cephalin flocculation and possibly other liver function tests. False-positive results may occur for amylase, 5-hydroxyindole acetic acid, porphobilinogens, urobilinogen, and urine bilirubin. False-positive or false-negative pregnancy tests may result.

Herbal/Food: Kava and St. John's wort may increase the risk and severity of dystonia.

Treatment of Overdose: There is no specific treatment for overdose; patients are treated symptomatically. EPS may be treated with antiparkinsonism drugs, barbiturates, anticholinergics (benztropine [Cogentin]), or diphenhydramine (Benadryl). Avoid producing respiratory depression with these treatments.

been used to treat symptoms of schizophrenia, prochlorperazine suppositories and tablets are most often used in the control of severe nausea and vomiting. Promethazine (Phenergan) for example, is chemically described as a phenothiazine; it is found in the same drug class as prochlorperazine. Promethazine is most often used as a sedating antihistamine for short-term insomnia, allergic reactions, travel sickness, and adjunctive medication during anesthesia (see chapter 19). It is worth emphasizing that some phenothiazines have a broader spectrum of application than just psychoses; for example, many have a calming effect and ease restlessness.

Unlike many other drugs whose primary action is on the central nervous system ([CNS] e.g., amphetamines, barbiturates, anxiolytics, alcohol), antipsychotic drugs do not cause physical or psychological dependence. They also have a wide safety margin between a therapeutic and a lethal dose; deaths due to overdoses of antipsychotic drugs are uncommon.

Extrapyramidal symptoms include acute dystonia, akathisia, secondary parkinsonism, and tardive dyskinesia. Acute **dystonias** occur early in the course of pharmacotherapy and involve severe muscle spasms, particularly of the back, neck, tongue, and face. **Akathisia,** the most common EPS, is an

Table 17.2 Adverse Effects of Phenothiazine Drugs

Effect	Description
Acute dystonia	Severe spasms, particularly the back muscles, tongue, and facial muscles; twitching movements
Akathisia	Constant pacing with repetitive, compulsive movements
Anticholinergic effects	Dry mouth, tachycardia, blurred vision
Disparity	High risk of suicide among patients receiving antipsychotic therapy
Hypotension	Particularly severe when the patient moves quickly from a recumbent to an upright position
Neuroleptic malignant syndrome	High fever, confusion, muscle rigidity, and high serum creatine kinase; can be fatal
Secondary parkinsonism	Tremor, muscle rigidity, stooped posture, and shuffling gait
Sedation	Usually diminishes with continued therapy
Sexual dysfunction	Impotence and diminished libido
Tardive dyskinesia	Bizarre tongue and face movements such as lip smacking and wormlike motions of the tongue; puffing of cheeks, uncontrolled chewing movements

inability to rest or relax. The patient paces, has trouble sitting or remaining still, and has difficulty sleeping. Symptoms of phenothiazine-induced **secondary parkinsonism** include tremor, muscle rigidity, stooped posture, and a shuffling gait. Long-term use of phenothiazines may lead to **tardive dyskinesia**, which is characterized by unusual tongue and face movements such as lip smacking and wormlike motions of the tongue. If EPS are reported early and the drug is withdrawn or the dosage reduced, the side effects can be reversible. With higher doses given for prolonged periods, the EPS may become permanent. The nurse must be vigilant in observing and reporting EPS, because prevention is the best treatment.

With the conventional antipsychotics, it is not always possible to control the disabling symptoms of schizophrenia without producing some degree of EPS. In these patients, drug therapy may be warranted to treat EPS symptoms. Concurrent pharmacotherapy with an anticholinergic drug may prevent some of the EPS (see chapter 12). For acute dystonia, benztropine (Cogentin) may be given parenterally. Medications containing levodopa are usually avoided, because dopamine antagonizes the action of the phenothiazines. Beta-adrenergic blockers and benzodiazepines are sometimes given to reduce signs of akathisia.

Nonphenothiazines

Nonphenothiazines have efficacy equal to that of the phenothiazines. Although the incidence of sedation and anticholinergic adverse effects is less, EPS may be common, particularly in older adults. The nonphenothiazine antipsychotic class (Table 17.3) consists of drugs whose chemical structures are dissimilar to the phenothiazines.

17.5 Treating Psychoses With Nonphenothiazines

Introduced shortly after the phenothiazines, the nonphenothiazines were initially expected to produce fewer side effects. Unfortunately, this has not been the case. The spectrum of adverse effects for the nonphenothiazines is identical to that for the phenothiazines, although the degree to which a particular effect occurs depends on the specific drug. In general, the nonphenothiazine drugs cause less sedation and fewer anticholinergic adverse effects than chlorpromazine but may still produce EPS. Concurrent therapy with other CNS depressants must be carefully monitored because of the potential additive effects.

Drugs in the nonphenothiazine class have the same therapeutic effects and efficacy as the phenothiazines. They are also believed to act by the same mechanism as the phenothiazines, that is, by blocking postsynaptic D_2 dopamine receptors. As a class, they offer no significant advantages over the phenothiazines in the treatment of schizophrenia.

Table 17.3 Conventional Antipsychotic Drugs: Nonphenothiazines

Drug	Route and Adult Dose (max dose where indicated)	Adverse Effects
haloperidol (Haldol)	PO: 0.2–5 mg bid or tid IV/IM lactate injections: 2–5 mg q4h. Doses up to 8 to 10 mg may be given IM. Acutely agitated patients may require hourly injections. Long-acting IM decanoate injections: initial dose 10 to 15 times the previous PO daily dose every 3 to 4 weeks. The initial dose should not exceed 100 mg. The balance should be given in 3 to 7 days. There is limited experience with doses greater than 450 mg/month. Do not give IV.	*Sedation, transient drowsiness, EPS, tremor, orthostatic hypotension* Tardive dyskinesia, neuroleptic malignant syndrome, laryngospasm, respiratory depression, hepatotoxicity, acute renal failure, sudden unexplained death, agranulocytosis
loxapine (Loxitane)	PO: start with 20 mg/day and rapidly increase to 60–100 mg/day in divided doses (max: 250 mg/day)	
pimozide (Orap)	PO: 1–2 mg/day in divided doses; gradually increase every other day to 7–16 mg/day (max: 10 mg/day)	
thiothixene (Navane)	PO: 2 mg tid; may increase up to 15 mg/day (max: 60 mg/day)	

Note: *Italics* indicate common adverse effects; underlining indicates serious adverse effects.

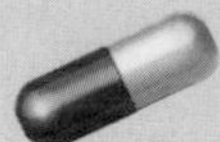

Prototype Drug | Haloperidol *(Haldol)*

Therapeutic Class: Conventional antipsychotic; schizophrenia drug
Pharmacologic Class: D_2 dopamine receptor antagonist; nonphenothiazine

Actions and Uses

Haloperidol is classified chemically as a butyrophenone. Its primary use is for the management of acute and chronic psychotic disorders. It may be used to treat patients with Tourette's syndrome and children with severe behavior problems such as unprovoked aggressiveness and explosive hyperexcitability. It is approximately 50 times more potent than chlorpromazine but has equal efficacy in relieving symptoms of schizophrenia. Haldol LA is a long-acting preparation that lasts for approximately 3 weeks following IM or subcutaneous administration. This is particularly beneficial for patients who are uncooperative or unable to take oral medications.

Administration Alerts

- Do not abruptly discontinue, or severe adverse reactions may occur.
- The patient must take the medication as ordered for therapeutic results to occur.
- If the patient does not comply with oral (PO) therapy, injectable long-acting haloperidol should be considered.
- Pregnancy category C.

PHARMACOKINETICS

Onset	Peak	Duration
30–35 min	2–6 h PO; 10–20 min IM	Variable

Adverse Effects

Haloperidol produces less sedation and hypotension than chlorpromazine, but the incidence of EPS is high. Older adults are more likely to experience adverse effects and often are prescribed half the adult dose until the adverse effects of therapy can be determined. Although the incidence of NMS is rare, it can occur.

Black Box Warning: Elderly patients with dementia-related psychosis are at increased risk for death when taking conventional antipsychotics.

Contraindications: Pharmacotherapy with nonphenothiazines is not advised if the patient is receiving medication for any of the following conditions: Parkinson's disease, seizure disorders, alcoholism, and severe mental depression.

Interactions

Drug–Drug: Haloperidol interacts with many drugs. For example, the following drugs decrease the effects/absorption of haloperidol: aluminum- and magnesium-containing antacids, levodopa (also increases chances of levodopa toxicity), lithium (increases chance of a severe neurologic toxicity), phenobarbital, phenytoin (also increases chances of phenytoin toxicity), rifampin, and beta blockers (may increase blood levels of haloperidol, thus leading to possible toxicity). Haloperidol inhibits the action of centrally acting antihypertensives.

Lab Tests: Unknown.

Herbal/Food: Kava may increase the effect of haloperidol.

Treatment of Overdose: In general, the symptoms of overdose are an exaggeration of known pharmacologic effects and adverse reactions, the most prominent of which would be severe EPS, hypotension, or sedation. With EPS, antiparkinsonism medication should be administered. Hypotension should be counteracted with IV fluids, plasma, or concentrated albumin, or vasopressor drugs.

☑ Check Your Understanding 17.1

A patient is experiencing significant adverse effects from his antipsychotic drug, and because there are few symptoms of his original disease (schizophrenia) decides that he is cured and stops taking his medication. As the nurse, how would you respond? *Visit www.pearsonhighered.com/nursingresources for the answer.*

ATYPICAL ANTIPSYCHOTIC DRUGS

Atypical antipsychotics treat both positive and negative symptoms of schizophrenia. They have become first-line drugs for treating psychoses.

17.6 Treating Psychoses With Atypical Antipsychotics

The approval of clozapine (Clozaril), the first atypical antipsychotic, marked the first major advance in the pharmacotherapy of psychoses since the discovery of chlorpromazine decades earlier. Clozapine, and the other drugs in this class, are called second generation, or atypical, because they have a broader spectrum of action than the conventional antipsychotics, controlling both the positive and negative symptoms of schizophrenia (Table 17.4). Furthermore, at therapeutic doses they exhibit their antipsychotic actions without producing the EPS effects of the

Table 17.4 Atypical Antipsychotic Drugs

Drug	Route and Adult Dose (max dose where indicated)	Adverse Effects
aripiprazole (Abilify, extended-release injectable)	PO: 10–15 mg/day (max: 30 mg/day) IM extended-release injection: 400 mg IM once a month; 200 to 300 mg IM if drug-drug interactions, poor cytochrome P450 metabolism, or adverse effects	*Tachycardia, transient fever, sedation, dizziness, headache, light-headedness, somnolence, anxiety, nervousness, hostility, insomnia, nausea, dry mouth, vomiting, constipation, secondary parkinsonism, akathisia, EPS* Agranulocytosis, orthostatic hypotension, neuroleptic malignant syndrome (rare), sudden unexplained death
asenapine (Saphris)	Adult: sublingually 5 mg bid (max: 10 mg bid)	
brexpiprazole (Rexulti)	PO: 2–4 mg daily (max 4 mg/day)	
clozapine (Clozaril)	PO: start at 25–50 mg/day and titrate to a target dose of 350–450 mg/day in 3 days; may increase further (max: 900 mg/day)	
iloperidone (Fanapt)	Adult: PO: 12 to 24 mg/day bid	
lurasidone (Latuda)	Adult: PO: 40 mg once daily (max: 80 mg/day)	
olanzapine (Zyprexa, Zypadhera injection)	Adult: PO: start with 5–10 mg/day; may increase by 2.5–5 mg every week (range 10–15 mg/day; max: 20 mg/day). Geriatric: PO: start with 5 mg/day IM long-acting embonate injection: Starting dose: 210–300 mg/2 weeks; Maintenance dose: 150–300 mg/2 weeks	
paliperidone (Invega, Invega Sustenna)	PO: 6 mg/day (max: 12 mg/day) IM long acting injection; initial dose of 234 mg on treatment day 1 and 156 mg one week later, both administered in the deltoid muscle. The recommended monthly maintenance dose is 117 mg	
quetiapine (Seroquel, Seroquel XR)	PO: start with 25 mg bid; may increase to a target dose of 300–400 mg/day in divided doses (max: 800 mg/day) Extended-release: available in 50-mg, 150-mg, 200-mg, 300-mg, and 400-mg tablet strengths. Meds should be taken in the evening, within 3–4 h before bedtime, without food or with a light meal. Titrate to the recommended dose of 300 mg/day by day 4.	
risperidone (Risperdal, Risperdal Consta)	PO: 1–6 mg bid; increase by 2 mg daily to an initial target dose of 6 mg/day IM long acting injection: 25 mg every 2 weeks. Some patients not responding to 25 mg may benefit from a higher dose of 37.5 mg or 50 mg. The maximum dose should not exceed 50 mg.	
ziprasidone (Geodon)	PO: 20 mg bid (max: 80 mg bid) IM: 10 mg q2h (max: 40 mg/day)	

Note: *Italics* indicate common adverse effects; underlining indicates serious adverse effects.

conventional drugs. Some drugs, such as clozapine, are especially useful for patients in whom other drugs have proved unsuccessful.

The mechanism of action of the atypical drugs is largely unknown, but they are thought to act by blocking different receptor types in the brain. Like the phenothiazines, the atypical drugs block dopamine D_2 receptors. However, the atypical antipsychotics also block serotonin (5-HT) and alpha-adrenergic receptors, which is thought to account for some of their properties. Because the atypical drugs are only loosely bound to D_2 receptors, they produce fewer EPS than the conventional antipsychotics.

Although there are fewer side effects with atypical antipsychotics, adverse effects are still significant, and patients must be carefully monitored. The use of atypical antipsychotics has been differentially associated with an increased risk of weight gain, diabetes, and hypertriglyceridemia. In addition, they have been associated with a possible increased risk of cerebrovascular events and higher mortality rates. Although most antipsychotics cause weight gain, the atypical drugs are specifically associated with obesity and its risk factors. There is an increased risk for death if they are used to treat dementia-related psychosis in older adults. Risperidone (Risperdal) and some of the other antipsychotic drugs increase prolactin levels, which can lead to menstrual disorders, decreased libido, and osteoporosis in women. In men, high prolactin levels can cause lack of libido, impotence, or gynecomastia. There is also concern that some atypical drugs alter glucose metabolism, attributing to the onset of type 2 diabetes.

Nursing Practice Application

Pharmacotherapy With Antipsychotic Drugs

ASSESSMENT	POTENTIAL NURSING DIAGNOSES*
Baseline assessment prior to administration: • Obtain a complete health history including hepatic, renal, urologic, cardiovascular, respiratory, or neurologic disease (especially Parkinson's disease or seizures), current mental status, pregnancy, or breast-feeding. Obtain a drug history including allergies, current prescription and over-the-counter (OTC) drugs, alcohol use, smoking, and herbal preparations. Be alert to possible drug interactions. • Obtain a history of depression or mental disorders, including a family history of same and severity. • Assess for disturbances in thought processes, perception, verbal communication, affect, behavior, interpersonal relationships, and self-care. Use objective screening tools per the health care agency. • Obtain baseline vital signs and weight. • Evaluate appropriate laboratory findings (e.g., complete blood count [CBC], electrolytes, glucose, hepatic and renal function studies, drug screening). • Assess the patient's ability to receive and understand instruction. Include the family and caregivers as needed.	• *Disturbed Personal Identity* • *Anxiety* • *Impaired Verbal Communication* • *Impaired Social Interaction* • *Ineffective Health Maintenance* • *Ineffective Health Management* • *Noncompliance* • *Deficient Knowledge* (drug therapy) • *Risk for Self-Directed Violence* • *Risk for Other-Directed Violence* • *Risk for Self-Mutilation* *NANDA I © 2014
Assessment throughout administration: • Assess for desired therapeutic effects (e.g., normalizing thought processes, lessening delusions, hallucinations, improvement in positive or negative symptoms, ability to return to normal ADLs, improvement in appetite and sleep patterns; if used for other uses, e.g., severe nausea and vomiting, assess for appropriate therapeutic effects). • Continue periodic monitoring of CBC, electrolytes, glucose, hepatic and renal function studies, and therapeutic drug levels. • Assess vital signs, especially orthostatic blood pressure, and weigh periodically. • Assess for and promptly report adverse effects: dizziness or light-headedness, confusion, agitation, suicidal ideations, hypotension, tachycardia, increase in temperature, blurred or double vision, skin rashes, bruising or bleeding, abdominal pain, jaundice, change in color of stool, flank pain, and hematuria. • Assess for and promptly report EPS including secondary parkinsonism, acute dystonias, akathisia, and tardive dyskinesias (see "Minimizing adverse effects" in the following section). • Immediately report signs and symptoms of NMS: unstable blood pressure, elevated temperature, diaphoresis, dyspnea, muscle rigidity, and incontinence.	

IMPLEMENTATION

Interventions and (Rationales)	Patient-Centered Care
Ensuring therapeutic effects: • Continue assessments, as described earlier, for therapeutic effects. (Drugs used for psychoses and schizophrenia do not cure the underlying disorder; rather, they improve positive and negative symptoms of the disorder. Gradual improvement over several weeks to months may be noted.)	• Teach the patient, family, or caregiver that full effects may not occur immediately but that some improvement should be noticeable after beginning therapy. • Supportive, inpatient care may be required during the acute, early period of therapy.
• Monitor patient compliance to the drug regimen. (The presence of severe mental disorders may result in noncompliance to medications. Regular, consistent dosing is essential to correcting the underlying disorder. Because the drugs do not cure the underlying disorder, if regular administration is disrupted, symptoms may return abruptly. Alternative drug forms such as PO disintegrating tablets or IM depot injections may need to be considered if noncompliance continues.)	• Involve the family and caregiver to the extent possible in ensuring that the patient remains on regular medication routines. • Ensure that the patient takes the medication as prescribed. *Never* leave medications at the bedside. • Question the possibility of noncompliance if original symptoms or adverse effects suddenly increase in frequency or severity.

Nursing Practice Application *continued*

IMPLEMENTATION	
Interventions and (Rationales)	**Patient-Centered Care**
Minimizing adverse effects: • Continue to monitor vital signs periodically, especially blood pressure. Keep the patient supine for 30 minutes to 1 hour after giving parenteral medications, and recheck blood pressure measurements every 15 to 30 minutes. Ensure patient safety; monitor ambulation until the effects of the drug are known. **Lifespan:** Be particularly cautious with older adults who are at an increased risk for falls. (Antipsychotic drugs may cause hypotension, increasing the risk of falls and injury.)	• Have the patient rise from lying or sitting to standing slowly to avoid dizziness or falls. If dizziness occurs, the patient should sit or lie down and not attempt to stand or walk, until the sensation passes. • **Safety:** Instruct the patient to call for assistance prior to getting out of bed or attempting to walk alone. For patients on at-home/outpatient medication, avoid driving or other activities requiring mental alertness or physical coordination until effects of the drug are known.
• Continue to monitor motor activity, coordination and balance, and for EPS. (EPS may be an unavoidable adverse effect of drug therapy but the drug dose will be reduced or stopped or the medication will be changed when possible.) • Ensure adequate nutrition and fluid intake if tardive dyskinesias are present. (Severe choreiform tongue movement may significantly hinder or prevent adequate nutrition.) • Ensure patient safety if secondary parkinsonism affects gait or if akathisia is present. Acute dystonias may require treatment with other medications to halt spasms. (Bradykinesias, slow-to-start ambulation, and a slow, shuffling gait may predispose the patient to falls. Akathisia with pacing may significantly impair the patient's ability to rest and sleep. Additional medications may be required for treatment. Anticholinergics or other drugs may be required to stop spasms.)	• Instruct the patient, family, or caregiver to immediately report EPS for additional treatment. • Encourage the patient, family, or caregiver to obtain and record a weight weekly to ensure that dietary needs are being met if tardive dyskinesias are present.
• Monitor for and immediately report signs and symptoms of NMS. (NMS is a rare but potentially fatal syndrome that must be recognized and treated immediately.)	• Instruct the patient, family, or caregiver to immediately report any changes in level of consciousness, elevated temperature, excessive sweating, severe muscle rigidity, increased respirations or shortness of breath, or incontinence.
• **Lifespan:** Monitor cardiovascular and respiratory function more frequently, particularly in the older adult with existing disease or dementia. (An increased risk of death from cardiovascular events [e.g., heart failure, sudden cardiac death], or from respiratory infection has been noted in some patients, particularly those taking atypical antipsychotic drugs.)	• Instruct the patient, family, or caregiver to immediately report dizziness, palpitations, tachycardia, chest pain, cough, chest congestion, fever, or breathing difficulties.
• Continue to monitor CBC, electrolytes, renal and hepatic function, and therapeutic drug levels. (Antipsychotic drugs may cause bone marrow depression and hepatotoxicity as adverse effects. Atypical antipsychotic drugs such as risperidone may cause an increase in glucose levels, and clozapine may cause bone marrow depression. Some of the atypical antipsychotics may cause an increase in lipid levels [hyperlipidemia]. **Diverse Patients:** Most antipsychotic drugs are metabolized through the P450 system and may result in different effects based on differences in enzymes. Monitor ethnically diverse patients more frequently to ensure optimal therapeutic effects and minimal adverse effects especially in early stages of drug therapy.)	• Instruct the patient on the need to return periodically for laboratory work. • Teach the patient to promptly report any abdominal pain, particularly in the upper quadrants; changes in stool color, yellowing of sclera or skin; darkened urine, skin rashes; low-grade fevers, general malaise or changes in behavior or activity level; or redness or swelling around sites of injury. • Teach the patient with diabetes, the family, or the caregiver to monitor blood glucose more frequently and to report consistent elevations to the health care provider. • **Diverse Patients:** Teach ethnically diverse patients to observe for appropriate effects, especially in early drug therapy, and promptly report suboptimal or adverse effects.
• Monitor for anticholinergic effects, including dry mouth, drowsiness, blurred vision, constipation, and urinary retention. Provide symptomatic treatment to ease effects. (Anticholinergic symptoms are common adverse effects of antipsychotic drugs. Tolerance to anticholinergic effects usually develops over time. **Lifespan:** Be aware that the male older adult with an enlarged prostate is at higher risk for mechanical obstruction.)	• Encourage sips of water, ice chips, hard candy, or chewing gum to ease mouth dryness. Avoid alcohol-based mouthwashes, which are drying to the mucosa and which the patient may drink. • Increase dietary fiber intake and adequate fluid intake. • Promptly report urinary frequency, hesitancy, or retention to the health care provider.

continued

Nursing Practice Application *continued*

IMPLEMENTATION	
Interventions and (Rationales)	**Patient-Centered Care**
• Monitor for sunburning or rashes. (Antipsychotic drugs cause photosensitivity.)	• Teach the patient, family, or caregiver to apply sunscreen (SPF 15 or above) prior to sun exposure or to ensure that protective clothing is worn. Promptly report sunburn to the health care provider.
• Monitor for weight gain, gynecomastia, and changes in secondary sexual characteristics (e.g., amenorrhea, impotence). (Some antipsychotic drugs may cause weight gain and have pituitary effects. Impotence and weight gain may be significant reasons for nonadherence.)	• Teach the patient, family, or caregiver to weigh the patient weekly and to report a significant weight gain of 2 kg (5 lb) or more per week to the health care provider. • Encourage a healthy diet and increased exercise. • Address sexual concerns and refer as appropriate to the health care provider.
• **Lifespan:** Monitor for the possibility of pregnancy in women of childbearing age. (Most antipsychotic drugs are Category C and the benefits of the use of any particular drug must be weighed against possible fetal effects.)	• Encourage the patient, family, or caregiver to discuss family planning with the health care provider. • Teach the patient, family, or caregiver to promptly report a positive pregnancy test or suspicion of pregnancy to the provider.
• **Lifespan:** Monitor adolescents under 24 and older adults for unusual symptoms or expressed thoughts of suicide. (Children and adolescents younger than 24, and the older adult, particularly with dementia, are at greater risk for suicide and risk of death than other patients.)	• Encourage the patient, family, or caregiver to keep all appointments with the health care provider and to promptly report overt symptoms of depression, suicidal ideations, or other unusual behaviors.
• Monitor for alcohol and illegal drug use. (Used concurrently, these cause an increased CNS depressant effect or an exacerbation in psychotic symptoms.)	• Instruct the patient to avoid alcohol and illegal drug use. **Collaboration:** Refer the patient to community support groups such as AA or NA as appropriate.
• Monitor caffeine use. (Use of caffeine-containing substances may negate the effects of antipsychotics.)	• Teach the patient, family, or caregiver to avoid caffeine-containing beverages, foods, and OTC medications, and to read food labels when in doubt of whether the product contains caffeine.
• Monitor for smoking. (Heavy smoking may decrease the metabolism of some antipsychotics such as haloperidol, leading to decreased efficacy.)	• Instruct the patient to stop or decrease smoking. Refer the patient to smoking cessation programs, if indicated.
Patient understanding of drug therapy: • Use opportunities during administration of medications and during assessments to provide patient education. Use brief explanations during times of delusions or hallucinations. (Using time during nursing care helps to optimize and reinforce key teaching areas. Brief, consistent explanations assist to interrupt delusional periods.)	• The patient, family, or caregiver should be able to state the reason for the drug; appropriate dose and scheduling; and what adverse effects to observe for and when to report them.
Patient self-administration of drug therapy: • When administering the medication, instruct the patient, family, or caregiver in proper self-administration of the drug, e.g., take the drug as prescribed and do not substitute brands. (Using time during nurse administration of these drugs helps to reinforce teaching.)	• Teach the patient, family, or caregiver to take the medication as follows: • Take exactly as ordered and use the same manufacturer's brand each time the prescription is filled. Switching brands may result in differing pharmacokinetics and alterations in therapeutic effect. • Ensure that all medication is taken exactly when and as ordered. Use of a calendar to track doses may be helpful. • Unless otherwise directed, mix liquid drug solutions with water, milk, or non-grapefruit juices. Do not mix with cola, tea, or caffeine-containing beverages. • Administer IM injections by deep gluteal injection using enclosed diluent and safety needle if provided by the manufacturer. Check the enclosed directions about refrigerating dosages. • If the medication causes drowsiness, take at bedtime. Tolerance to anticholinergic effects such as drowsiness usually develops over time. • Do not abruptly discontinue the medication.

See Tables 17.1 and 17.3 for lists of drugs to which these nursing actions apply.

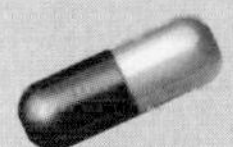

Prototype Drug | Risperidone *(Risperdal)*

Therapeutic Class: Atypical antipsychotic; schizophrenia drug
Pharmacologic Class: D_2 dopamine receptor antagonist (weaker affinity for D_1 receptors); serotonin (5-HT) receptor antagonist

Actions and Uses
Therapeutic effects of risperidone include treatment and prevention of schizophrenia relapse and expression of bipolar mania symptoms. Risperidone also treats symptoms of irritability in children with autism. Expected results are a reduction of excitement, paranoia, or negative behaviors associated with psychosis. Effects occur primarily from blockade of dopamine type 2, serotonin type 2, and alpha$_2$-adrenergic receptors located within the CNS. For a full range of effectiveness, the drug is sometimes combined with lithium (Eskalith) or valproate (Depakene, Depacon). Risperidone is a long-acting preparation, which, following IM administration, releases only a small amount. After a 3-week lag, the rest of the drug releases and lasts for approximately 4–6 weeks. PO preparations release sooner and have a 1–2 week onset of action.

Administration Alerts
- Several weeks are required for therapeutic effectiveness.
- When switching from other antipsychotics, discontinue medications to avoid overlap.
- Pregnancy category C.

PHARMACOKINETICS

Onset	Peak	Duration
1–2 wk PO; 3 wk IM	4–6 wk	6 wk

Adverse Effects
Common adverse effects are EPS (involuntary shaking of the head, neck, and arms), hyperactivity, fatigue, nausea, dizziness, visual disturbances, fever, and orthostatic hypotension. Risperidone may cause weight gain and hyperglycemia, thus worsening glucose control in diabetic patients.

Black Box Warning: Elderly patients with dementia-related psychosis are at increased risk for death when taking atypical antipsychotics.

Contraindications: If older adults with dementia-related psychoses are given risperidone, they are at an increased risk for heart failure, pneumonia, or sudden death. Patients with underlying cardiovascular disease may be especially prone to dysrhythmias and hypotension. Risperidone should be avoided in patients with a history of seizures, suicidal ideations, or kidney/liver disease.

Interactions
Drug–Drug: Patients taking risperidone should avoid CNS depressants such as alcohol, antihistamines, sedative–hypnotics, or opioid analgesics. These can increase some of the adverse effects of risperidone. Due to inhibition of liver enzymes, other drugs that increase adverse effects of risperidone include selective serotonin reuptake inhibitors (SSRIs) such as paroxetine (Paxil), sertraline (Zoloft), and fluoxetine (Prozac) and antifungal drugs such as fluconazole (Diflucan), itraconazole (Sporanox), and ketoconazole (Nizoral). Risperidone may interfere with elimination by the kidneys of clozapine (Clozaril), which also increases the risk of adverse reactions.

Lab Tests: Risperidone may cause increased serum prolactin levels and increased ALT (alanine aminotransferase) and AST (aspartate aminotransferase) liver enzyme levels. Other potential lab changes are anemia, thrombocytopenia, leukocytosis, and leukopenia.

Herbal/Food: Use with caution with herbal supplements, such as kava, valerian, or chamomile, which may increase risperidone's CNS depressive effects.

Treatment of Overdose: Activated charcoal, which may be used with sorbitol, may be as or more effective than emesis or gastric lavage, and should be considered in treating overdosage. Establish and maintain the airway; ensure adequate oxygenation and ventilation. Maintain cardiovascular function.

DOPAMINE-SEROTONIN SYSTEM STABILIZERS

17.7 Treating Psychoses With Dopamine-Serotonin System Stabilizers

In 2002, due to side effects caused by conventional and atypical antipsychotic medications, a new drug class was developed to better meet the needs of patients with psychoses. This class, sometimes considered a third generation class of antipsychotics, is the *dopamine-serotonin system stabilizers (DSSs)* or dopamine partial agonists. Aripiprazole (Abilify) was the first drug in this class, and brexpiprazole was approved in 2015. Because these medications control both the positive and negative symptoms of schizophrenia, they are grouped in Table 17.4 with the atypical antipsychotic drugs.

The dopamine partial agonists are generally well tolerated in patients with schizophrenia. In particular, their use seems to be associated with a lower incidence of EPS than haloperidol and fewer weight-gain issues than other atypical antipsychotics, for example, olanzapine. Anticholinergic adverse effects are virtually nonexistent. In fact, the incidence of adverse effects compared to the other atypical antipsychotic drugs is generally very low. Aripiprazole is also used to treat bipolar disorder and mixed episodes of mania and depression, as monotherapy or adjunctive (add-on) therapy. For major depressive disorder, aripiprazole and brexpiprazole are used as adjunctive therapy. Notable side effects, however, include headache, nausea and vomiting, fever, constipation, and anxiety.

Chapter Review

KEY Concepts

The numbered key concepts provide a succinct summary of the important points from the corresponding numbered section within the chapter. If any of these points are not clear, refer to the numbered section within the chapter for review.

17.1 Psychoses are severe mental and behavioral disorders characterized by disorganized mental capacity and an inability to recognize reality.

17.2 Schizophrenia is a type of psychosis characterized by abnormal thoughts and thought processes, disordered communication, withdrawal from other people and the environment, and a high risk for suicide.

17.3 Pharmacologic management of psychoses is difficult because the adverse effects of the drugs may be severe, and patients often do not understand the need for medication.

17.4 The phenothiazines have been effectively used for the treatment of psychoses for more than 60 years; however, they have a high incidence of adverse effects. Extrapyramidal symptoms (EPS) and neuroleptic malignant syndrome (NMS) are two particularly serious conditions.

17.5 The conventional nonphenothiazine antipsychotics have the same therapeutic applications and adverse effects as the phenothiazines.

17.6 Atypical antipsychotics are often preferred because they address both positive and negative symptoms of schizophrenia and produce less dramatic side effects.

17.7 Dopamine-serotonin system stabilizers are the newest antipsychotic class. The incidence of adverse effects compared to the other atypical antipsychotic drugs is very low.

REVIEW Questions

1. The patient states that he has not taken his antipsychotic drug for the past 2 weeks because it was causing sexual dysfunction. What is the nurse's primary concern at this time?
    1. A hypertensive crisis may occur with such abrupt withdrawal of the drug.
    2. Significant muscle twitching may occur, increasing fall risk.
    3. Extrapyramidal symptoms such as secondary parkinsonism are likely to occur.
    4. Symptoms of psychosis are likely to return.

2. Prior to discharge, the nurse plans for patient teaching related to side effects of phenothiazines to the patient, family, or caregiver. Which of the following should be included?
    1. The patient may experience withdrawal and slowed activity.
    2. Severe muscle spasms may occur early in therapy.
    3. Tardive dyskinesia is likely early in therapy.
    4. Medications should be taken as prescribed to prevent adverse effects.

3. A 20-year-old man is admitted to the psychiatric unit for treatment of acute schizophrenia and is started on risperidone (Risperdal). Which patient effects should the nurse assess for to determine whether the drug is having therapeutic effects?
   1. Restful sleep, elevated mood, and coping abilities
   2. Decreased delusional thinking and lessened auditory/visual hallucinations
   3. Orthostatic hypotension, reflex tachycardia, and sedation
   4. Relief of anxiety and improved sleep and dietary habits

4. Nursing implications of the administration of haloperidol (Haldol) to a patient exhibiting psychotic behavior include which of the following? (Select all that apply.)
   1. Take 1 hour before or 2 hours after antacids.
   2. The incidence of extrapyramidal symptoms is high.
   3. It is therapeutic if ordered on an as-needed (prn) basis.
   4. Haldol is contraindicated in Parkinson's disease, seizure disorders, alcoholism, and severe mental depression.
   5. Crush the sustained-release form for easier swallowing.

5. A patient is treated for psychosis with fluphenazine. What drug will the nurse anticipate may be given to prevent the development of acute dystonia?
   1. Benztropine (Cogentin)
   2. Diazepam (Valium)
   3. Haloperidol (Haldol)
   4. Lorazepam (Ativan)

6. The nurse should immediately report the development of which of the following symptoms in a patient taking antipsychotic medication?
   1. Fever, tachycardia, confusion, incontinence
   2. Pacing, squirming, or difficulty with gait such as bradykinesia
   3. Severe spasms of the muscles of the tongue, face, neck, or back
   4. Sexual dysfunction or gynecomastia

PATIENT-FOCUSED Case Study

John Delarcy, a 68-year-old patient has been started on olanzapine (Zyprexa) for treatment of acute psychoses. He has both positive symptoms (e.g., hallucinations and disorganized thought patterns) and negative symptoms (e.g., lack of responsiveness).

1. What is a priority of care for this patient?
2. What teaching is important for this patient?

CRITICAL THINKING Questions

1. A 22-year-old male patient has been on haloperidol (Haldol LA) for 2 weeks for the treatment of schizophrenia. During a follow-up assessment, the nurse notices that the patient keeps rubbing his neck and is complaining of neck spasms. What is the nurse's initial action? What is the potential cause of the sore neck and what would be the potential treatment? What teaching is appropriate for this patient?
2. A 20-year-old newly diagnosed patient with schizophrenia has been on chlorpromazine and is doing well. Today the nurse notices that the patient appears more anxious and is demonstrating increased paranoia. What is the nurse's initial action? What is the potential problem? What patient teaching is important?

Visit www.pearsonhighered.com/nursingresources for answers and rationales for all activities.

REFERENCES

Chang, S. C., & Lu, M. L. (2012). Metabolic and cardiovascular adverse effects associated with treatment with antipsychotic drugs. *Journal of Experimental and Clinical Medicine*, 4(2), 103–107. doi:10.1016/j.jecm.2012.01.007

Correll, C. U., Manu, P., Olshanskiy, V., Napolitano, B., Kane, J. M., & Malhotra, A. K. (2009). Cardiometabolic risk of second-generation antipsychotic medications during first-time use in children and adolescents. *JAMA*: The *Journal of the American Medical Association, 302*, 1765–1773. doi:10.1001/jama.2009.1549

DeLisi, L. E., & Nasrallah, H. A. (2005). The CATIE schizophrenia effectiveness trial. *Schizophrenia Research, 80*, v–vi. doi:10.1016/j.schres.2005.10.004

Herdman, T. H., & Kamitsuru, S. (Eds.). (2014). *NANDA International nursing diagnoses: Definitions and classification, 2015–2017*. Oxford, United Kingdom: Wiley-Blackwell.

Leung, J. Y. T., Barr, A. M., Procyshyn, R. M., Honer, W. G., & Pang, C. C. Y. (2012). Cardiovascular side-effects of antipsychotic drugs: The role of the autonomic nervous system. *Pharmacology & Therapeutics, 135*, 113–122. doi:10.1016/j.pharmthera.2012.04.003

McEvoy, J. P., Meyer, J. M., Goff, D. C., Nasrallah, H. A., Davis, S. M., Sullivan, L., . . . Lieberman, J. A. (2005). Prevalence of the metabolic syndrome in patients with schizophrenia: Baseline results from the Clinical Antipsychotic Trials of Intervention Effectiveness (CATIE) schizophrenia trial and comparison with national estimates from NHANES III. *Schizophrenia Research, 80*, 19–32. doi:10.1016/j.schres.2005.07.014

Steylen, P. M., van der Heijden, F. M., Kok, H. D., Sijben, N. A., & Verhoeven, W. M. (2013). Cardiometabolic comorbidity in antipsychotic treated patients: Need for systematic evaluation and treatment. *International Journal of Psychiatry in Clinical Practice, 17*, 125–130. doi:10.3109/13651501.2013.779000

Ward, A., Quon, P., Abouzaid, S., Haber, N., Ahmed, S., & Kim, E. (2013). Cardiometabolic consequences of therapy for chronic schizophrenia using second-generation antipsychotic agents in a Medicaid population: Clinical and economic evaluation. *P & T: A Peer-Reviewed Journal for Managed Care and Hospital Formulary Management, 38*, 109–115.

SELECTED BIBLIOGRAPHY

Abou-Setta, A. M., Mousavi, S. S., Spooner, C., Schouten, J. R., Pasichnyk, D., Armijo-Olivo, S., . . . Hartling, L. (2012). First-generation versus second-generation antipsychotics in adults: Comparative effectiveness. *Comparative Effectiveness Reviews, No. 63*. Rockville, MD: Agency for Healthcare Research and Quality. Retrieved from http://www.ncbi.nlm.nih.gov/books/NBK107254/

Murri, M. B., Guaglianone, A., Bugliani, M., Calcagno, P., Respino, M., Serafini, G., . . . Amore, M. (2015). Second-generation antipsychotics and neuroleptic malignant syndrome: Systematic review and case report analysis. *Drugs in R&D, 15*, 45–62. doi:10.1007/s40268-014-0078-0

Dunlop, J., & Brandon, N. J. (2015). Schizophrenia drug discovery and development in an evolving era: Are new drug targets fulfilling expectations? *Journal of Psychopharmacology, 29*, 230–238. Advance online publication. doi:10.1177/0269881114565806

Gierisch, J. M., Nieuwsma, J. A., Bradford, D. W., Wilder, C. M., Mann-Wrobel, M. C., McBroom, A. J., . . . Williams, J. W. (2013). Interventions to improve cardiovascular risk factors in people with serious mental illness. *Comparative Effectiveness Reviews, No. 105*. Rockville, MD: Agency for Healthcare Research and Quality. Retrieved from http://www.ncbi.nlm.nih.gov/books/NBK138237/

Leucht, S., Cipriani, A., Spineli, L., Mavridis, D., Orey, D., Richter, F., . . . Davis, J. M. (2013). Comparative efficacy and tolerability of 15 antipsychotic drugs in schizophrenia: A multiple-treatments meta-analysis. *Lancet, 382*, 951–962. doi:10.1016/S0140-6736(13)60733-3

Maglione, M., Maher, A. R., Hu, J., Wang, Z., Shanman, R., Shekelle, P. G., . . . Perry, T. (2011). Off-label use of atypical antipsychotics: An update. *Comparative Effectiveness Reviews, No. 43*. Rockville, MD: Agency for Healthcare Research and Quality. Retrieved from http://www.ncbi.nlm.nih.gov/books/NBK66081/

McDonagh, M., Peterson, K., Carson, S., Fu, R., Thakurta, S. (2010). *Drug class review: Atypical antipsychotic drugs: Final update 3 report*. Portland, OR: Oregon Health & Science University. Retrieved from http://www.ncbi.nlm.nih.gov/books/NBK50583/

National Institutes of Health, National Institute of Mental Health. (n.d.). *Any anxiety disorder among adults*. Retrieved from http://www.nimh.nih.gov/statistics/1ANYDIS_ADULT.shtml

Seida, J. C., Schouten, J. R., Mousavi, S. S., Hamm, M., Beaith, A., Dryden, D. M., . . . Carrey, N. (2012). *First- and second-generation antipsychotics for children and young adults* [Internet]. Rockville, MD: Agency for Healthcare Research and Quality (Comparative Effectiveness Reviews, No. 39.). Retrieved from http://www.ncbi.nlm.nih.gov/books/?term=abilify

Chapter 18

Drugs for the Control of Pain

Drugs at a Glance

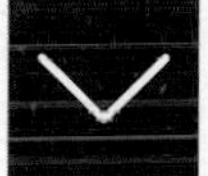

Learning Outcomes

After reading this chapter, the student should be able to:

1. Relate the importance of pain assessment to effective pharmacotherapy.
2. Explain the neural mechanisms at the level of the spinal cord responsible for pain.
3. Explain how pain can be controlled by inhibiting the release of spinal neurotransmitters.
4. Describe the role of complementary and alternative therapies in pain management.
5. Compare and contrast the types of opioid receptors and their importance in effective management of pain.
6. Explain the role of opioid antagonists in the diagnosis and treatment of acute opioid toxicity.
7. Describe the long-term treatment of opioid dependence.
8. Compare the pharmacotherapeutic approaches of preventing migraines with those of aborting migraines.
9. For each of the drug classes listed in Drugs at a Glance, know representative drug examples, and explain the mechanisms of drug action, primary actions, and important adverse effects.
10. Categorize drugs used in the treatment of pain based on their classification and mechanism of action.
11. Use the nursing process to care for patients receiving pharmacotherapy for pain and for migraines.

(pill icon) indicates a prototype drug, each of which is featured in a Prototype Drug box.

Pain is a physiological and psychological experience characterized by unpleasant feelings, usually associated with trauma or disease. On a basic level, pain may be viewed as a defense mechanism that helps us to avoid potentially damaging situations and encourages us to seek medical help. Although the neural and chemical mechanisms for pain are fairly straightforward, many emotional processes are a part of this experience. Anxiety, fatigue, and depression can increase the perception of pain; positive attitudes and support from health care providers may reduce the perception of pain. For example, some patients tolerate their pain better if they know the source of trauma and the medical courses available to treat their discomfort. There are many options for pain assessment and the treatment of pain-associated disorders.

ACUTE OR CHRONIC PAIN

The purpose of pain assessment is to guide the appropriate course of medical treatment. Pain can be characterized as acute or chronic. *Acute pain* is an intense pain occurring over a brief time, usually from time of injury until tissue repair. *Chronic pain* is longer lasting pain that may persist for weeks, months, or years. Pain lasting longer than six months can interfere with activities of daily living (ADLs) and can contribute to feelings of helplessness or hopelessness.

18.1 Assessment and Classification of Pain

The psychological reaction to pain is subjective. During physical assessment, the same degree and type of pain that would be described as excruciating or unbearable by one patient may not even be mentioned by another patient. Several numeric scales and survey instruments are available to help health care providers standardize the patient's conveyance of pain and subsequently measure the progress of drug therapies. Successful pain management depends not only on an accurate assessment of how the patient feels but an understanding of the underlying disorder causing the suffering. Selection of appropriate therapy is dependent on both the nature and characteristic of pain.

Besides being termed acute or chronic, pain can also be described by its source. Injury to tissues produces *nociceptor pain*. This type of pain may be further subdivided into *somatic pain*, which produces sharp, localized sensations in the body, or *visceral pain*, which produces generalized dull and internal throbbing or aching pain. The term **nociceptor** refers to activation of receptor nerve endings that receive and transmit pain signals to the central nervous system (CNS). **Neuropathic pain** is caused by direct injury to the nerves. Whereas nociceptor pain responds well to conventional pain relief medications, neuropathic pain responds less successfully. Common types of neuropathic pain are shown in Table 18.1.

Table 18.1 Common Types of Neuropathic Pain

EXAMPLES	DESCRIPTION
Carpal tunnel syndrome	Pain due to nerve compression in the wrist, thumb, and fingers
Central pain syndrome	General pain caused by damage of nerves in the CNS, i.e., due to stroke or multiple sclerosis
Degenerative disk disease	Back pain due to damage of nerves entering or exiting the spinal cord
Diabetic neuropathy	Burning or stabbing pain in the hands and feet of patients suffering from diabetes
Intractable cancer pain	Pain due to progressive or metastatic spread of cancer
Phantom limb pain	Pain occurring in some patients after a limb is amputated
Postherpetic neuralgia	Pain brought on by herpes and herpes–related viruses or the outbreak of shingles
Postsurgical pain	Pain after a surgical procedure
Sciatica	Leg pain due to compression or irritation of the sciatic nerve
Trigeminal neuralgia	Shooting pain in the upper neck and jaw

18.2 Complementary and Alternative Approaches for Pain Management

Although drugs are effective at relieving pain for most patients, many drugs have significant side effects. For example, at high doses, aspirin may cause gastrointestinal (GI) bleeding. Some opioids have the potential for dependency and most cause significant drowsiness. To assist patients in obtaining adequate pain relief, nonpharmacologic techniques may be used alone or as adjunctive therapy. When used concurrently with traditional medications, nonpharmacologic techniques may result in fewer drug-related adverse effects and allow for lower doses of medications. Techniques used for reducing pain are as follows:

- Acupuncture
- Biofeedback therapy
- Massage
- Heat or cold packs
- Meditation or prayer
- Relaxation therapy
- Art or music therapy
- Guided imagery
- Chiropractic manipulation
- Hypnosis
- Physical therapy
- Therapeutic or physical touch
- Transcutaneous electrical nerve stimulation (TENS)
- Natural agents applied to the skin to produce a warming sensation.

All of the these techniques have an advantage in that they can help improve the patient's mood, reduce anxiety, and provide the patient with a sense of control. Depending on the technique, nonpharmacologic strategies often relax muscles, strengthen coping abilities, and generally improve the patient's quality of life. There are many determinants of successful therapy depending on the type, duration, and severity of pain. The success of therapy will also vary from patient to patient and will depend on many factors including the patient's age, attitude, tolerance, and level of compliance. The patient's coping skills, capabilities, and commitment will play a role in both pain management and recovery. Costs of health care, availability of support from family members, and support from members of the community are extremely important.

Patients with *intractable* or not easy to relieve pain, may require additional therapy. In this case, adjuvant analgesics or *co-analgesics* may be used. **Adjuvant analgesics** are drugs not typically classified as analgesics, but which can provide relief for specific types of pain. For example, certain antiseizure drugs and local anesthetics are examples of drug categories approved by the U.S. Food and Drug Administration (FDA) for successful management of pain. Carbamazepine (Tegretol) is approved for treatment of pain due to trigeminal neuralgia. Valproic acid (Depakene) is approved for the treatment of pain due to migraines. Gabapentin (Neurontin) is prescribed for the management of postherpetic neuralgia. Pregabalin (Lyrica) is approved for treatment of fibromyalgia, postherpetic neuralgia, and pain due to peripheral diabetic neuropathy. All of these drugs were originally developed to treat conditions other than pain, and were found useful for difficult to manage pain.

Anesthetic nerve blocking drugs are another type of adjuvant analgesic used for the management of acute and chronic pain, and are administered in a variety of ways for different purposes. Lidoderm, for example, is a local anesthetic patch with 5% lidocaine used to reduce pain or discomfort caused by skin irritations such as sunburn, insect bites, plant resins, minor cuts, scratches, and burns, and for post-shingles and post-surgical pain. Corticosteroids reduce inflammation and can also control certain types of inflammatory pain.

Some well-established medications are occasionally used off-label for pain management. Examples include the tricyclic antidepressants (TCAs) amitriptyline (Elavil), nortriptyline (Aventyl, Pamelor) and imipramine (Tofranil), which have been used to supress a variety of pain impulses characterized as chronic and neuropathic. Neuropathic pain impulses may also be slowed by certain antidysrhythmic drugs when TCAs are not effective. Thus, cardiovascular drugs have even found a place in pain management. Examples are mexiletine (Mexitil) and flecainide (Tambocor).

PharmFacts

PAIN

Pain is a common symptom, reflected by the following statistics:

- Every year in America, approximately 16 million people experience chronic arthritic pain.
- More than 31 million adults have reported low back pain, whereas 19 million people have experienced this pain on a more chronic basis.
- At least 50 million people are fully or partially disabled due to pain.
- More than 50% of adults experience muscle pain each year.
- Up to 40% of people with cancer report moderate to severe pain with treatment.
- More than two thirds of older Americans suffer from multiple, chronic conditions, and treatment for these conditions makes up 66% of the U.S. health care budget.

18.3 The Neural Mechanisms of Pain

The process of pain transmission begins when nociceptors are stimulated. **Nociceptors** are free nerve endings located throughout the entire body. The nerve impulse signaling the pain is sent to the spinal cord along two types of sensory neurons, called Aδ and C fibers. **Aδ fibers** are thinly wrapped in myelin, a fatty substance that speeds up nerve transmission. They signal sharp, well-defined pain. **C fibers** are unmyelinated, thus, they carry nerve impulses more slowly and conduct dull, poorly localized pain.

Once pain impulses reach the spinal cord, neurotransmitters pass the message along to the next neuron. Here, a neurotransmitter called **substance P** is thought to be responsible for continuing the pain message, although other neurotransmitter candidates have been proposed. Spinal substance P is critical because it controls whether pain signals will continue to the brain. The activity of substance P may be affected by other neurotransmitters released from neurons in the CNS. One group of these neurotransmitters, called **endogenous opioids,** includes endorphins, dynorphins, and enkephalins. Figure 18.1 shows one point of contact where endogenous opioids modify sensory information at the level of the spinal cord. If pain impulses reach the brain, many possible actions may occur, ranging from immediate reaction to the stimulus, persistent aching and suffering, or thoughts of mental depression if the pain signal is repetitive and long-lasting.

Because pain signals begin at nociceptors located within peripheral body tissues and then proceed throughout the CNS, there are several targets where medications can work to stop pain transmission. In general, two major classes of drugs are employed to manage pain: opioid analgesics and nonopioid analgesics such as the nonsteroidal

Community-Oriented Practice

APPROPRIATE RESOURCES FOR A PATIENT IN PAIN

Experiencing pain, particularly chronic pain, may lead patients to increase their efforts to seek health information from sources other than their health care providers. Providers should not assume that patients find the most reputable sources with current information. This is especially true for patients with low health literacy. Ellis, Mullan, Worsley, & Pai (2012) found that patients with low health literacy most often turned to newspaper, television, or their own social networks, whereas patients with high health literacy found sought information from the Internet or specialist health information sources. For low-income or disabled patients, the Internet may be a luxury they can't afford. Choi and Dinitto (2013) found that among homebound older adults, African American and Hispanic patients were more likely to have never used the Internet than other patient groups. The older adult may be more likely to have difficulty remembering verbal instructions given (McCarthy et al., 2012). Pain intensity itself may decrease the knowledge about pain medication use (Devraj, Herndon, & Griffin, 2013). Since pain may be an overwhelming experience, patients may not have the physical, mental, or emotional reserves for knowledge recall.

Improving a patient's medication knowledge, especially about pain treatment, is a primary role of the nurse. An assessment of whether the patient has sought additional resources and information, and the quality of those sources, should be included in a patient's pain assessment. Reputable sites such as the NIH Pain Consortium's "Pain Information Brochure" (2014) can provide valuable information tailored to the type of pain the patient is experiencing. The nurse should also teach and reinforce the use of nonpharmacologic strategies for pain control, how to read labels on over-the-counter (OTC) medications to avoid excessive doses of drugs such as acetaminophen, and the ideal administration timing of pain medications for optimal relief.

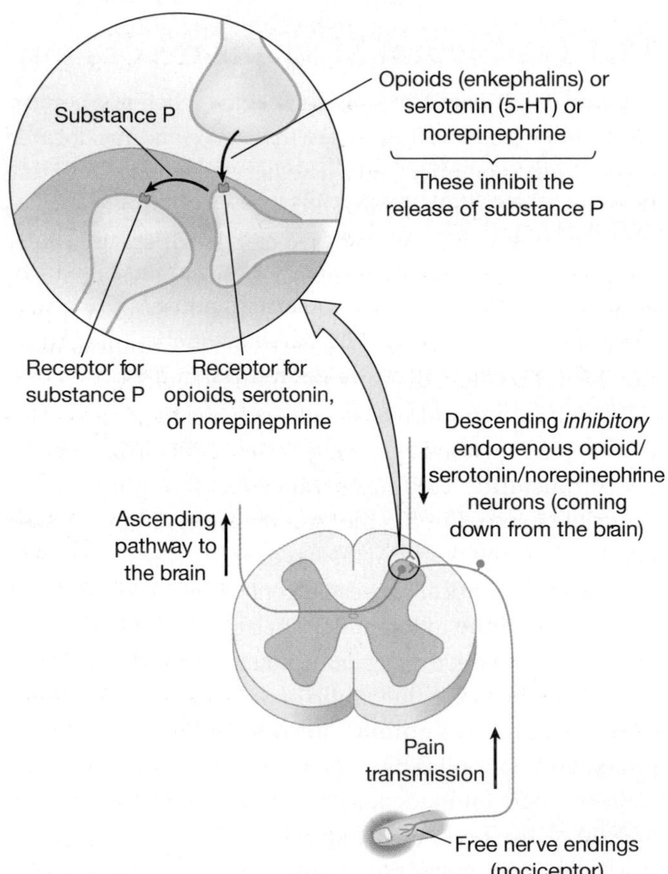

FIGURE 18.1 Neural pathways for pain

anti-inflammatory drugs (NSAIDs). Opioids act within the CNS, whereas NSAIDs act at the nociceptor level. There are multiple sites throughout the CNS where centrally acting drugs can produce their effects, and there are many peripheral targets as well, depending on the approach of drug therapy.

OPIOID ANALGESICS FOR SEVERE PAIN

An opioid analgesic is a natural or synthetic morphine-like substance responsible for reducing moderate to severe pain. Opioids are **narcotic** substances, meaning that they can produce numbness or stupor-like symptoms.

18.4 Classification of Opioids

By definition, **analgesics** are medications used to relieve pain. Terminology of the narcotic analgesic medications may be confusing. Several of these drugs are obtained from opium, a milky extract from the unripe seeds of the poppy plant, which contains more than 20 different chemicals having pharmacologic activity. Opium consists of 9% to 14% morphine and 0.8% to 2.5% codeine. These natural substances are called **opiates.** In a search for safer analgesics, chemists have created several dozen synthetic drugs with activity similar to that of the opiates. For example, morphine is a natural narcotic; meperidine is a synthetic narcotic. **Opioid** is a general term referring to any of these substances, natural or synthetic, having opiate-like activity.

Narcotic often describes opioid drugs that produce analgesia and CNS depression. In the context of drug enforcement, however, the term *narcotic* describes a much broader range of abused illegal drugs such as hallucinogens, heroin, amphetamines, and marijuana. This is an important fact to remember when relating use of opioids to members of law enforcement.

Opioids exert their actions by interacting with at least four major types of receptors: mu, kappa, delta, and an opioid-like receptor called nociceptin or orphanin FQ peptide. From the perspective of pain management, the **mu receptors**

Table 18.2 Responses Produced by Activation of Specific Opioid Receptors

Response	Mu Receptor	Kappa Receptor
Analgesia	✓	✓
Decreased GI motility	✓	✓
Euphoria	✓	
Miosis		✓
Physical dependence	✓	
Respiratory depression	✓	
Sedation	✓	✓

and **kappa receptors** have been the ones traditionally targeted. Although delta receptors have a role in analgesia, they are connected with the emotional and affective components of the pain experience. Thus, delta receptors have been studied as targets for modulation of the emotional pain experience. Responses produced by activation of mu and kappa receptors are listed in Table 18.2.

Because there are multiple opioid receptors, three general types of drug–receptor interactions are possible.

Opioid agonist. Drugs that activate both mu and kappa receptors; for example, morphine and codeine (see Section 18.5)

Opioid antagonist. Drugs that block both mu and kappa receptors; for example, naloxone (Evzio, Narcan) (see Section 18.6)

Mixed opioid agonist-antagonist. Drugs that occupy one receptor and block (or have no effect) on the other; for example, pentazocine (Talwin), butorphanol (Stadol), and buprenorphine (Buprenex)

Figure 18.2 illustrates actions resulting from stimulation of mu and kappa receptors.

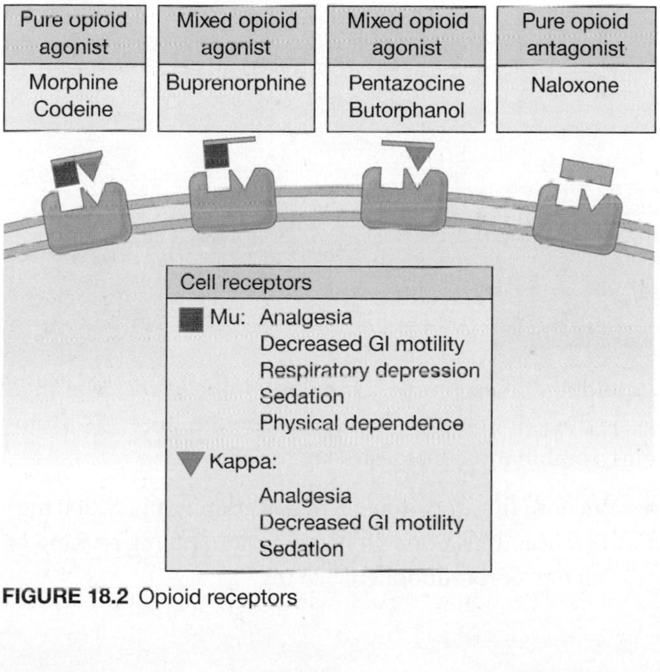

FIGURE 18.2 Opioid receptors

Opioid Agonists

Narcotic opioid agonists bind to opioid receptors and produce multiple responses throughout the body. Morphine is the prototype drug used to treat severe pain. It is considered the standard by which the effectiveness of other opioids is compared.

18.5 Pharmacotherapy With Opioid Agonists

Opioids are the first-line drugs for severe to extreme pain that cannot be controlled with other classes of analgesics. More than 20 different opioids are available as medications. They may be classified by similarities in their chemical structures, by their mechanisms of action, or by their effectiveness (Table 18.3). Experience has borne out that single to multiple doses of orally (PO) and intravenously (IV) administered opioids can alleviate severe pain without producing respiratory depression. For details of all of the various methods of opioid administration, nursing students should refer to a comprehensive drug guide.

Opioids produce many important effects other than analgesia. They are effective at suppressing the cough reflex and at slowing the motility of the GI tract for cases of severe diarrhea. As powerful CNS depressants, opioids can cause sedation, which may be either therapeutic or determined a side effect, depending on the patient's disease state. Some patients experience euphoria and intense relaxation, which are reasons why opiates are sometimes abused. There are many adverse effects, including nausea, vomiting, constipation, sedation, and respiratory depression. In 2014, the FDA approved naloxegol (Movantik), a drug that provides treatment for adult patients with chronic non-cancer pain who have opioid-induced constipation.

All opioids have the potential to cause physical and psychological dependence, as discussed in chapter 22. The better known Schedule II opioids are fentanyl, hydromorphone, methadone, morphine, oxycodone, and oxymorphone. Over the years, health care providers and nurses have hesitated to administer the proper amount of opioid analgesics for fear of causing patient dependence or of producing serious adverse effects such as sedation or respiratory depression. Because of this tendency, some patients have not received complete pain relief.

When used according to accepted medical practice, patients can, and indeed should, receive the pain relief they need without fear of addiction or adverse effects. One method available is **patient-controlled analgesia (PCA).** With a PCA Pump, patients are able to self-medicate with opioid medication by pressing a limited rate-controlled button. Safe levels of scheduled pain medication are delivered with an infusion pump.

In the pharmacologic management of pain, it is common practice to combine opioids and nonnarcotic analgesics into a single tablet or capsule. The two classes of

Table 18.3 Opioids for Pain Management

Drug	Route and Adult Dose (max dose where indicated)	Adverse Effects
OPIOID AGONISTS WITH HIGH EFFECTIVENESS		
fentanyl (Actiq, Abstral, Duragesic, Fentora, Lazanda, Onsolis, Oralet)	Transdermal patch: 25 mcg/h PO: 100 mcg initial dose (max: 100 mcg units provided at a time) Nasal spray: 100 mcg initial dose (max 800 mcg) Buccal transmucosal: 200 mcg initial dose (max: no more than six 200-mcg units should be in the patient's possession for titration)	*Pruritus, constipation, nausea, sedation, drowsiness, dizziness* Anaphylactoid reaction, cardiac arrest, severe respiratory depression or arrest, convulsions, abuse potential
hydromorphone (Dilaudid, Exalgo)	PO/Subcutaneous/IM/IV: 1–4 mg every 4–6 h prn	
levorphanol (Levo-Dromoran)	PO: 2–3 mg tid—qid prn Subcutaneous/IV: 1–2 mg q6-8h	
meperidine (Demerol)	PO: 50–150 mg q3–4h IM: 50–100 mg q3–4h IV: 1–1.5 mg/kg q3–4h	
methadone (Dolophine)	PO: 2.5–10 mg q3–4h prn	
morphine (Astramorph PF, Duramorph, others)	PO: 10–30 mg q4h prn Sustained release: 15–30 mg q8–12h IM: 10 mg q4h IV: 2–10 mg q2–4h	
oxymorphone (Opana)	Subcutaneous: 1–1.5 mg q4–6h Rectal: 1 suppository (5 mg) q4–6h PO (extended release): 5–20 mg bid	
OPIOID AGONISTS WITH MODERATE EFFECTIVENESS		
codeine	PO: 15–60 mg qid IM: 15–30 mg q4–6h	*Sedation, nausea, constipation, dizziness* Hepatotoxicity, respiratory depression, circulatory collapse, coma, abuse potential
hydrocodone (Hycodan)	PO: 5–10 mg q4–6h prn (max: 15 mg/dose)	
oxycodone (OxyContin, Oxecta)	PO: 5–10 mg qid prn Controlled release: 10–20 mg q12h	
OPIOID ANTAGONISTS		
naloxone (Evzio, Narcan)	IV: 0.4–2 mg; may be repeated q2–3min up to 10 mg if necessary	*Muscle and joint pain, sleep anxiety, headache, nervousness, withdrawal symptoms, vomiting, diarrhea, insomnia* Hepatotoxicity
naltrexone (ReVia, Trexan, Vivitrol)	PO: 25 mg followed by another 25 mg in 1 h if no withdrawal response (max: 800 mg/day)	
OPIOIDS WITH MIXED AGONIST–ANTAGONIST EFFECTS		
buprenorphine (Buprenex, Butrans, Suboxone)	IM/IV: 0.3 mg q6h (max: 0.6 mg q4h) Topical: one patch every 7 days Sublingual: 12–16 mg/day	*Drowsiness, dizziness, light-headedness, euphoria, nausea, clammy skin, sweating, insomnia, abdominal pain, constipation* Respiratory depression, shock
butorphanol (Stadol)	IM: 1–4 mg q3–4h prn (max: 4 mg/dose) IV: 2.5–10 mg (usually 5 mg) q2–4h	
dezocine (Dalgan)	IM: 5–10 mg (usually 10 mg) q3–4h	
nalbuphine (Nubain)	Subcutaneous/IM/IV: 10–20 mg q3–6h prn (max: 160 mg/day)	
pentazocine (Talwin)	PO: 50–100 mg q3–4h (max: 600 mg/day) Subcutaneous/IM/IV: 30 mg q3–4h (max: 360 mg/day)	

Note: *Italics* indicate common adverse effects; underlining indicates serious adverse effects.

analgesics work synergistically to relieve pain, and the dose of the opioid can be kept small to avoid narcotic-related side effects. With growing concern over the risk of hepatic toxicity related to combining large doses of opioid and nonopioid products (e.g., acetaminophen, NSAIDs), it should be noted that additional doses of *combination* products may raise the dose of both drug products to unacceptable levels. Additional doses of a combination product should not be used unless the dose of the *nonnarcotic* analgesic does not exceed the recommended dose. As examples, combination analgesics are as follows:

- Vicodin (hydrocodone, 5 mg; acetaminophen, 300 mg)
- Percocet (oxycodone hydrochloride, 2.5 mg or 5 mg or 7.5 mg; acetaminophen, 325 mg)

- Percodan (oxycodone hydrochloride, 4.5 mg; oxycodone terephthalate, 0.38 mg; aspirin, 325 mg)
- Empirin with Codeine No. 2 (codeine phosphate, 15 mg; aspirin, 325 mg)
- Ascomp with Codeine or Fiorinal (codeine phosphate, 30 mg; aspirin, 325 mg; caffeine, 40 mg; butalbital, 50 mg)
- Fioricet with Codeine (codeine phosphate, 30 mg; acetaminophen, 325 mg; caffeine, 40 mg; butalbital, 50 mg)
- Tylenol with Codeine (single dose may contain from 15 to 60 mg of codeine phosphate and from 300 to 325 mg of acetaminophen).

Some opioids are used primarily for conditions other than general complaints of pain. For example, alfentanil (Alfenta), remifentanil (Ultiva), and sufentanil (Sufenta) are used to provide continuous pain relief during and after surgery or for use during the induction and maintenance of general anesthesia. These are discussed further in chapter 19. Codeine is most often prescribed as a cough suppressant and is covered in chapter 39. Opioids used in treating diarrhea are presented in chapter 42.

Fentanyl is available for several different routes of administration. The fentanyl transdermal system (Duragesic patch) is a strong prescription medication used for the control of moderate to severe chronic pain. The patch enables longer lasting relief from persistent pain. Fentanyl (Lazanda) nasal spray is available for quick delivery across nasal mucous membranes. Fentanyl is also administered

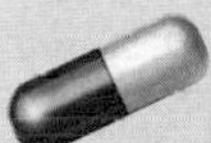

Prototype Drug | Morphine *(Astramorph PF, Duramorph, others)*

Therapeutic Class: Opioid analgesic **Pharmacologic Class:** Opioid receptor agonist

Actions and Uses

Morphine binds with both mu and kappa receptor sites to produce profound analgesia. It causes euphoria, constriction of the pupils, and stimulation of cardiac muscle. It is used for symptomatic relief of serious acute and chronic pain after nonnarcotic analgesics have failed, as preanesthetic medication, to relieve shortness of breath associated with heart failure and pulmonary edema, and for acute chest pain connected with MI.

Administration Alerts

- The oral solution may be given sublingually.
- The oral solution comes in multiple strengths; carefully observe drug orders and labels before administering.
- Morphine causes peripheral vasodilation, which results in orthostatic hypotension.
- Patients should never open capsules or crush extended release forms of opioids unless directed to do so by the health care provider.
- Pregnancy category B (D in long-term use or with high doses).

PHARMACOKINETICS

Onset	Peak	Duration
Less than 60 min	60 min PO; 20–60 min rectally; 50–90 min subcutaneously; 30–60 min IM; 20 min IV	Up to 7 h

Adverse Effects

Morphine may cause dysphoria (restlessness, depression, and anxiety), hallucinations, nausea, constipation, dizziness, and an itching sensation. Overdose may result in severe respiratory depression or cardiac arrest. Tolerance develops to the sedative, nausea-producing, and euphoric effects of the drug. Cross-tolerance also develops between morphine and other opioids such as heroin, methadone, and meperidine. Physical and psychological dependence develops when high doses are taken for prolonged periods.

Black Box Warning: When morphine is administered as an epidural drug, due to the risk of adverse effects, patients must be observed in a fully equipped and staffed environment for at least 24 hours. Morphine administered as extended-release tablets has an abuse liability similar to other opioid analgesics. Morphine is a Schedule II controlled substance and should be taken properly according to dispensing instructions (i.e., tablets/capsules should be taken whole and not broken, chewed, dissolved, or crushed). Alcohol should be avoided with morphine products (e.g., Avinza). Failure to follow these warnings could result in fatal respiratory depression.

Contraindications: Morphine may intensify or mask the pain of gallbladder disease, due to biliary tract spasms. Morphine should also be avoided in cases of acute or severe asthma, GI obstruction, and severe hepatic or renal impairment.

Interactions

Drug–Drug: Morphine interacts with several drugs. For example, concurrent use of CNS depressants, such as alcohol, other opioids, general anesthetics, sedatives, and antidepressants such as monoamine oxidase inhibitors (MAOIs) and TCAs, potentiate the action of opiates, increasing the risk of severe respiratory depression and death.

Lab Tests: Unknown.

Herbal/Food: Yohimbe, kava kava, valerian, and St. John's wort may potentiate the effect of morphine.

Treatment of Overdose: IV administration of naloxone is the specific treatment. Other treatments include activated charcoal, a laxative, and a counteracting narcotic antagonist. Multiple doses may be needed.

as a lozenge (Actiq, Oralet), tablet (Fentora, Onsolis), or via sublingual (Abstral) administration. These slowly dissolve in the mouth, and drugs are absorbed via the mouth's mucous membranes. Buccal fentanyl is indicated for the management of breakthrough cancer pain in adult patients who are already receiving and who might already be tolerant to opioid therapy. These medications should not be used to treat pain other than chronic cancer pain or in the management of acute or postoperative pain, including headaches and migraines. Fentanyl may cause serious harm or death if used accidentally by a child or by an adult who does not have a higher level of tolerance to opioids. Respiratory depression and fatal overdose are risks.

Opioid Antagonists

Opioid antagonists are substances that prevent the effects of opioid agonists. Many drugs are considered competitive antagonists because they compete with opioids for access to the opioid receptor.

Check Your Understanding 18.1

Combination products containing an opioid analgesic with an adjuvant drug such as acetaminophen, may be used so that the dose of the opioid can be lower as it works synergistically with the adjuvant drug to control pain. Refer to Table 18.3, Opioids for Pain Management, and using Vicodin (hydrocodone and acetaminophen) as an example, explain why a combination product may not always be the best practice for pain control. *Visit www.pearsonhighered.com/nursingresources for the answer.*

18.6 Pharmacotherapy With Opioid Antagonists

Opioid overdose can occur as a result of overly aggressive pain therapy, attempted suicide, or substance abuse. Any opioid may be abused for its psychoactive effects;

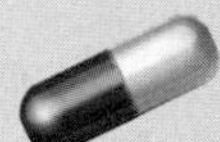

Prototype Drug | Naloxone *(Evzio, Narcan)*

Therapeutic Class: Drug for treatment of acute opioid overdose and misuse
Pharmacologic Class: Opioid receptor antagonist

Actions and Uses

Naloxone is a pure opioid antagonist, blocking both mu and kappa receptors. It is used for complete or partial reversal of opioid effects in emergency situations when acute opioid overdose is suspected. Given IV, it begins to reverse opioid-initiated CNS and respiratory depression within minutes. It will immediately cause opioid withdrawal symptoms in patients physically dependent on opioids. It is also used to treat postoperative opioid depression. It is occasionally given as adjunctive therapy to reverse hypotension caused by septic shock.

In 2014, the FDA approved a prescription treatment that can be used by family members or caregivers to treat a person known or suspected to have had an opioid overdose. Evzio (naloxone subcutaneous injection) rapidly delivers a single dose of the drug naloxone via a hand-held auto-injector that can be carried in a pocket or stored in a medicine cabinet. Narcan may be administered intravenously, intramuscularly, or subcutaneously.

Administration Alerts

- Administer for a respiratory rate of fewer than 10 breaths/minute. Keep resuscitative equipment accessible.
- Pregnancy category B.

PHARMACOKINETICS

Onset	Peak	Duration
1–2 min IV; 2–5 min IM; 2–5 min subcutaneously	5–15 min	45 min

Adverse Effects

Naloxone itself has minimal toxicity. However, reversal of the effects of opioids may result in rapid loss of analgesia, increased blood pressure, tremors, hyperventilation, nausea and vomiting, and drowsiness.

Black Box Warning: None; however, naltrexone, a similar opioid receptor antagonist, has the capacity to produce hepatic injury when taken in excessive doses or if taken by patients with hepatic injury or acute liver disease.

Contraindications: Naloxone should not be used for respiratory depression caused by nonopioid medications.

Interactions

Drug–Drug: Drug interactions include a reversal of the analgesic effects of opioid agonists and mixed agonist drugs.

Lab Tests: Unknown.

Herbal/Food: Echinacea may increase the risk of hepatotoxicity.

Treatment of Overdose: Naloxone overdose requires the use of oxygen, IV fluids, vasopressors, and other supportive measures as indicated. These treatments may be useful in combination drug overdoses (for example, pentazocine with naloxone [Talwin NX]).

Nursing Practice Application

Pharmacotherapy for Pain

ASSESSMENT	POTENTIAL NURSING DIAGNOSES*
Baseline assessment prior to administration: • Obtain a complete health history including cardiovascular, neurologic, respiratory, hepatic, renal, cancer, gallbladder, or urologic disease; pregnancy; or breast-feeding. Note recent surgeries or injuries. Obtain a drug history including allergies, current prescription and OTC drugs, and herbal preparations. Be alert to possible drug interactions. • Assess the level of pain. Use objective screening tools when possible (e.g., FLACC [face, limbs, arms, cry, consolability] for infants or very young children, Wong-Baker FACES scale for children or older adults, numerical rating scale for adults). Assess history of pain and what has worked successfully or not for the patient in the past. • Obtain baseline vital signs and weight. • Evaluate appropriate laboratory findings (e.g., complete blood count [CBC], hepatic and renal function studies). • Assess the patient's ability to receive and understand instruction. Include the family and caregivers as needed.	• *Acute Pain* • *Chronic Pain* • *Ineffective Breathing Pattern* • *Constipation,* related to adverse drug effects • *Deficient Knowledge* (drug therapy) • *Risk for Injury,* related to adverse drug effects • *Risk for Falls,* related to adverse drug effects *NANDA I © 2014
Assessment throughout administration: • Assess for desired therapeutic effects (e.g., absent or greatly diminished pain, ability to move more easily without pain, carry out postoperative treatment care). Continue to use a pain-rating scale to quantify the level of improvement. • Continue periodic monitoring of CBC and hepatic and renal function studies. • Assess vital signs, especially blood pressure, pulse, and respiratory rate. • Assess for and report adverse effects: excessive dizziness, drowsiness, confusion, agitation, hypotension, tachycardia, bradypnea, and pinpoint pupils.	

IMPLEMENTATION

Interventions and (Rationales)	Patient-Centered Care
Ensuring therapeutic effects: • Continue assessments as described earlier for therapeutic effects. Give the drug *before* the start of acute pain and encourage regularly scheduled doses for the first 24 to 48 hours postoperatively. Provide additional comfort measures to supplement drug therapy. (Consistent use of a pain rating scale by all providers will help quantify the level of pain relief and lead to better pain control. Watch for subtle signs of pain: hesitancy to move, shallow breaths to avoid increasing pain, grimacing on movement.)	• Teach the patient that pain relief, rather than merely control, is the goal of therapy. • Encourage the patient to take the drug consistently during the acute postoperative or procedure period rather than requesting only when pain is severe. • Explain the rationale behind the pain rating scale (i.e., it allows consistency among all providers). • Encourage the patient, family, or caregiver to use additional, nonpharmacologic pain relief techniques (e.g., distraction with television or music, backrubs, guided imagery).
Minimizing adverse effects: • Continue to monitor vital signs, especially respirations and pulse oximetry as ordered, postoperatively and in patients with acute pain. For terminal cancer pain, obtain instructions from the oncologist or hospice provider on any dose restrictions. (Respiratory depression is most common with the first dose of an opioid and when given in the presence of other CNS depressants (e.g., postoperatively when the patient may still be experiencing effects of general anesthesia). Count respirations *before* giving the opioid drug and contact the provider before giving if the respirations are below 12 breaths per minute in the adult patient, or per health care provider's parameters and as ordered in the child. Continue to assess the respiratory rate every 15 to 30 minutes for the first 4 hours. For terminal cancer pain, the drug may not be withheld regardless of the respiratory rate, and depending on the provider.)	• Encourage the patient to take deep breaths in the postoperative period. • Encourage consistent pain medication usage to increase activity tolerance. • Encourage the patient with terminal cancer to take the dose consistently around the clock with as-needed (prn) doses as required. Advise the family or caregiver on the provider's instructions for adequate pain relief and to contact the provider if any pain remains.

continued

Nursing Practice Application *continued*

IMPLEMENTATION	
Interventions and (Rationales)	**Patient-Centered Care**
• Monitor the blood pressure and pulse periodically or if symptoms warrant. Ensure patient safety. **Lifespan:** Be particularly cautious with older adults who are at an increased risk for falls. (Opioids may cause hypotension as an adverse effect and increase the risk of falls or injuries.)	• Teach the patient to rise from lying or sitting to standing slowly to avoid dizziness or falls. If dizziness occurs, the patient should sit or lie down and not attempt to stand or walk, until the sensation passes. • **Safety:** Instruct the patient to call for assistance prior to getting out of bed or attempting to walk alone, and to avoid driving or other activities requiring mental alertness or physical coordination until the effects of the drug are known.
• Continue to assess bowel sounds. Increase fluid intake and dietary fiber intake. (Decreased peristalsis is an adverse effect of opioid drugs. **Lifespan:** The older adult is at increased risk of constipation due to slowed peristalsis as a result of the aging process. Significantly diminished or absent bowel sounds are reported to the health care provider immediately. Additional medications such as Miralax or Colace may be required.)	• Teach the patient to increase fluids to 2 L per day and to increase the intake of dietary fiber such as fruits, vegetables, and whole grains. • Instruct the patient to report severe constipation to the health care provider for additional advice on laxatives or stool softeners.
• Monitor for itching or complaints of itching. (Opioids may cause histamine release and itching or a sensation of itching. In severe cases, antihistamines may be required. Assess for signs and symptoms of true allergy/anaphylaxis: changes in vital signs, especially hypotension and tachycardia, dyspnea, or urticaria.)	• Teach the patient to report itching to the health care provider, especially if itching is severe or increasing. • Instruct the patient to immediately report any itching associated with dizziness or light-headedness, difficulty breathing, palpitations, or significant hives.
• Assess for changes in level of consciousness and neurologic changes. (Neurologic changes may indicate overmedication, increased intracranial pressure, or adverse drug effects. **Lifespan:** Older adults may be at risk for confusion and falls.)	• Instruct the patient, family, or caregiver to immediately report increasing lethargy, disorientation, confusion, changes in behavior or mood, agitation or aggression, slurred speech, ataxia, or seizures. Ensure patient safety if disorientation is present.
• Assess for urinary retention, especially in the postoperative period. (Opioids may cause urinary retention as an adverse effect. **Lifespan:** Be aware that the male older adult with an enlarged prostate is at higher-risk for mechanical obstruction.)	• Encourage the patient to move about in bed and to start early ambulation as soon as allowed postoperatively. Assist to a normal voiding position if unable to use the bathroom or commode. • Instruct the patient to immediately report an inability to void, increasing bladder pressure, or pain.
• Monitor pain relief in patients on PCA pumps. If a basal dose is not given continuously, assess that pain relief is adequate and contact the provider if pain remains present. (PCA-administered pain control has greatly improved pain relief for patients with regular dosing but is only effective when taken as needed. Review dosage history and patient symptoms to ensure adequate pain relief. Contact the provider if dose, frequency, or basal dose seems inadequate for relief.)	• Instruct the patient, family, or caregiver on the use of the PCA pump. Encourage use on a prn basis whenever pain is present or increasing, and before activities. Emphasize the limitations present to protect the patient (i.e., overdose is not possible).
• Administer antiemetics 30 to 60 minutes before opioid dose if nausea and vomiting occur. (Nausea and vomiting are common adverse effects.)	• Encourage the patient to report nausea if it occurs. Small amounts of food intake (e.g., dry crackers) and sips of carbonated beverages (e.g., ginger ale) may help if the patient is not NPO (nothing by mouth).
• For IV push administration, dilute the drug with 4 to 5 mL of sterile normal saline and administer over 4 to 5 minutes unless otherwise ordered. The patient should remain supine to prevent dizziness or hypotension. Monitor blood pressure, pulse rate, and respiratory rate before and after the dose. (Opioids may cause hypotension and significant dizziness. Keeping the patient supine will limit these effects.)	• **Safety:** Explain the rationale to the patient for the need to remain flat during the drug administration and for 15 to 30 minutes after the dose, and to call for assistance before getting out of bed.
• Assess the home environment for medication safety and need for appropriate interventions. Advise the family on restrictions of prescription renewal. (Opioids are scheduled drugs and may not be used by any person other than the patient. Safeguard medication in the home to prevent overdose.)	• Instruct the patient, family, or caregiver in proper medication storage and need for the drug to be used by the patient only. • Teach the family or caregiver about prescription renewal restrictions (i.e., new prescription each time, no refills, prescription may not be called in) as appropriate for the Schedule of the drug.

Nursing Practice Application *continued*

IMPLEMENTATION	
Interventions and (Rationales)	**Patient-Centered Care**
Patient understanding of drug therapy: • Use opportunities during administration of medications and during assessments to provide patient education. (Using time during nursing care helps to optimize and reinforce key teaching areas.)	• The patient should be able to state the reason for the drug, appropriate dose and scheduling, and what adverse effects to observe for and when to report them.
Patient self-administration of drug therapy: • When administering the medication, instruct the patient, family, or caregiver in proper self-administration of drug (e.g., take the drug as prescribed when needed). (Using time during nurse administration of these drugs helps to reinforce teaching.)	• Teach the patient to take the medication as follows: • Before the pain becomes severe and for cancer pain, as consistently as possible. • If using a PCA pump: use the self-dosage button whenever pain begins to increase or before activities such as sitting at the bedside. • Take with food to decrease GI upset. • Do not open, chew, or crush extended release tablets (e.g., oxycodone [OxyContin]); swallow them whole with plenty of water. • Because opioids are Scheduled drugs (most often C-II through IV), federal law restricts the sale and use of the drug to the person receiving the prescription only. Additional prescriptions may be necessary if the drug is continued beyond the first prescription (e.g., phone-in refills are not allowed for C-II drugs). Do not share with any other person and do not discard any unused drug down drains, flush down the toilet (dependent on state law), or place in the garbage. Return any unused drug to the pharmacy or health care provider for proper disposal.

See Table 18.3 for a list of drugs to which these nursing actions apply.

however, morphine, meperidine, oxycodone, and heroin are preferred because of their potency. Although heroin is currently available as a legal analgesic in many countries, it is deemed too dangerous for therapeutic use by the FDA and is a major drug of abuse. Once injected or inhaled, heroin rapidly crosses the blood–brain barrier to enter the brain, where it is metabolized to morphine. Thus, the effects and symptoms of heroin administration are actually caused by the activation of mu and kappa receptors by morphine. The initial effect is an intense euphoria, called a *rush,* followed by several hours of deep relaxation.

Opioid antagonists are blockers of opioid activity. They are often used to reverse the severe symptoms of opioid intoxication such as sedation or respiratory distress. Infusion with the opioid antagonist naloxone (Evzio, Narcan) may be used to reverse respiratory depression and other acute symptoms. In cases where the patient is unconscious or unclear as to which drug has been taken, opioid antagonists may be given to diagnose the overdose. If the opioid antagonist fails to quickly reverse the acute symptoms, the overdose may be attributed to a nonopioid substance.

Opioid antagonists are often provided in combination with opioids for patients with respiratory ailments. Antagonists provide protection against respiratory depressant properties of opioids while providing optimal pain relief. Naltrexone mixed with morphine (Embeda) is used for moderate to severe pain control when a continuous, around-the-clock opioid analgesic is needed for an extended period. Targiniq ER, a combination of oxycodone plus naloxone, may also be indicated for the management of pain severe enough to require daily, long-term opioid treatment.

Opioids With Mixed Agonist–Antagonist Activity

Narcotic opioids that have mixed agonist–antagonist activity stimulate the opioid receptor; thus, they cause analgesia. However, the withdrawal symptoms or adverse effects are not as intense due to partial activity of receptor subtypes.

18.7 Treatment for Opioid Dependence

Although effective at relieving pain, the opioids have a greater risk for dependence than almost any other class of medications. Tolerance to the euphoric effects of opioids develops relatively quickly, causing abusers to escalate their doses and take the drugs more frequently. The higher and more frequent doses rapidly cause physical dependence in opioid users.

When physically dependent patients attempt to discontinue drug use, they experience extremely uncomfortable symptoms that convince many to continue their drug-taking behavior. As long as the drug is continued, they feel "normal," and many can continue work or social activities. In cases when the drug is abruptly discontinued, the patient experiences about 7 days of withdrawal symptoms before overcoming the physical dependence.

The intense craving characteristic of psychological dependence may occur for many months, and even years, following discontinuation of opioids. This often results in a return to drug-seeking behavior unless significant support groups are established.

One method of treating opioid dependence has been to switch the patient from IV and inhalation forms of illegal drugs to methadone (Dolophine). Although oral methadone is an opioid, it does not cause the same degree of euphoria as the injectable opioids. Methadone also does not cure the dependence, and the patient must continue taking the drug to avoid withdrawal symptoms. This therapy, called **methadone maintenance,** may continue for many months or years, until the patient decides to enter a total withdrawal treatment program. Methadone maintenance allows patients to return to productive work and social relationships without the physical, emotional, and criminal risks of illegal drug use.

A newer treatment option is to administer buprenorphine (Buprenex, Butrans, Suboxone), a mixed opioid agonist–antagonist, by the sublingual or transdermal route. Buprenorphine is used early in opioid abuse therapy to prevent opioid withdrawal symptoms. Bunavail, Suboxone and Zubsolv, which contain both buprenorphine and naloxone, have become popular alternatives to methadone maintenance. It is unlikely that a person would abuse these drugs because the naloxone component would induce unpleasant withdrawal-like symptoms. Furthermore, treatment with Bunavail, Suboxone and Zubsolve can be managed in an office environment, rather than a person reporting daily to a methadone clinic for their dose.

It is important to note that use of the naloxone injector product (Evzio) along with buprenorphine or pentazocine, may result in incomplete reversal of respiratory depression in patients with respiratory conditions. This is because large doses of naloxone may be required to antagonize these opioid agonists. Evzio is a take-home naloxone auto-injector that patients, family members, and other caregivers can have close by in case of an opioid overdose (see naloxone Prototype drug box).

Health care providers should always be aware that the pain-blocking properties of opioids with mixed agonist–antagonist activity are reduced when administered in combination with opioid agonists. Thus, there may be a tendency to overprescribe mixed opioids, promoting drug misuse. This is true even though in most cases the potential for causing opioid addiction is lower with mixed agonist–antagonists compared with pure opioid agonists.

NONOPIOID ANALGESICS FOR MODERATE PAIN

The nonopioid analgesics include NSAIDs and a few centrally acting drugs, for example acetaminophen. The role of the NSAIDs in the treatment of inflammation and fever is discussed more thoroughly in chapter 33. Therefore, there is only brief mention here. Table 18.4 highlights the more common nonopioid analgesics.

Nonsteroidal Anti-Inflammatory Drugs

The NSAIDs act by inhibiting pain mediators at the nociceptor level. When tissue is damaged, chemical mediators are released locally, including histamine, potassium ion, hydrogen ion, bradykinin, and prostaglandins. Bradykinin is associated with the initial sensory impulse of pain. Prostaglandins can induce pain through the formation of free radicals.

18.8 Pharmacotherapy With NSAIDS

NSAIDs inhibit **cyclooxygenase (COX),** an enzyme responsible for the formation of prostaglandins. When cyclooxygenase is inhibited, inflammation and pain are reduced. NSAIDs are drugs of choice for mild to moderate pain, especially for pain associated with inflammation. These drugs have many advantages over the opioids because they have antipyretic and anti-inflammatory activity as well as analgesic properties.

Aspirin, Ibuprofen, and COX-2 Inhibitors

Aspirin and ibuprofen are available OTC and are inexpensive NSAIDs. Ibuprofen and related medications are available in many different formulations, including those designed for children. They are safe and well tolerated by most patients when used at low to moderate doses.

After tissue damage, prostaglandins are formed with the help of two enzymes called cyclooxygenase type 1 (COX-1) and cyclooxygenase type 2 (COX-2). Aspirin and ibuprofen-related drugs inhibit both COX-1 and COX-2. Thus, COX inhibition is the basis of NSAID therapy. Because the COX-2 enzyme is more specific for the synthesis of inflammatory prostaglandins, the selective COX-2 inhibitors provide more specific and peripheral pain relief. Celecoxib (Celebrex) is the representative COX-2 inhibitor. Other COX-2 inhibitors are available outside of the United States. Figure 18.3 illustrates the mechanism of pain transmission at the nociceptor level.

Table 18.4 Nonopioid Analgesics

Drug	Route and Adult Dose (max dose where indicated)	Adverse Effects
NSAIDs: ASPIRIN AND OTHER SALICYLATES		
aspirin (acetylsalicylic acid, ASA)	PO: 350–650 mg q4h (max: 4 g/day)	*Heartburn, stomach pains, ulceration*
salsalate (Disalcid)	PO: 325–3,000 mg/day in divided doses (max: 4 g/day)	Bronchospasm, anaphylactic shock, hemolytic anemia
NSAIDs: IBUPROFEN AND SIMILAR DRUGS		
diclofenac (Cambia, Cataflam, Voltaren, Zipsor)	PO: 50 mg bid–qid (max: 200 mg/day)	*Indigestion, nausea, occult blood loss, anorexia, headache, drowsiness, dizziness*
diflunisal	PO: 1,000 mg followed by 500 mg bid–tid	
etodolac	PO: 200–400 mg tid–qid	Aplastic anemia, drug-induced peptic ulcer, GI bleeding, agranulocytosis, laryngospasm, laryngeal edema; peripheral edema, anaphylaxis, acute renal failure; vomiting, constipation, diarrhea
fenoprofen (Nalfon)	PO: 200 mg tid–qid	
flurbiprofen (Ansaid, Ocuten)	PO: 50–100 mg tid–qid (max: 300 mg/day)	
ibuprofen (Advil, Motrin, others) (see page 506 for the Prototype Drug box)	PO: 400 mg tid–qid (max: 1,200 mg/day)	
indomethacin (Indocin, Tivorbex)	PO: 25–50 mg bid–tid (max: 200 mg/day), or 75 mg sustained release one to two times/day	
ketoprofen (Actron, Orudis)	PO: 12.5–50 mg tid–qid	
ketorolac (Toradol)	PO: 10 mg qid prn (max: 40 mg/day)	
mefenamic acid (Ponstel)	PO: Loading dose: 500 mg; Maintenance dose: 250 mg q6h prn	
meloxicam (Mobic)	PO: 7.5 mg/day (max: 15 mg/day) 7.5–15 mg daily	
nabumetone (Relafen)	PO: 1,000 mg/day (max: 2,000 mg/day)	
naproxen (Naprelan, Naprosyn)	PO: 500 mg followed by 200–250 mg tid–qid (max: 1,250 mg/day)	
naproxen sodium (Aleve, Anaprox, others)	PO: 250–500 mg bid (max: 1,000 mg/day naproxen)	
oxaprozin (Daypro)	PO: 600–1,200 mg/day (max: 1,800 mg/day)	
piroxicam (Feldene)	PO: 10–20 mg one to two times/day (max: 20 mg/day)	
sulindac (Clinoril)	PO: 150–200 mg bid (max: 400 mg/day)	
tolmetin (Tolectin)	PO: 400 mg tid (max: 2 g/day)	
NSAIDs: COX-2 INHIBITORS		
celecoxib (Celebrex)	PO: 100–200 mg q6-8h or 200 mg qid	*Abdominal pain, dizziness, headache, sinusitis, hypersensitivity* Cautious use due to FDA review
CENTRALLY ACTING DRUGS		
acetaminophen (Tylenol, others) (see page 509 for the Prototype Drug box)	PO: 325–650 mg q4-6h (max 3g/day)	*Hypotension, dry mouth, constipation, drowsiness, sedation, dizziness, vertigo, fatigue, headache*
tramadol (Ultram)	PO: 50–100 mg q4-6h prn (max: 400 mg/day); may start with 25 mg/day, and increase by 25 mg every 3 days up to 200 mg/day	Anaphylactic reaction, hepatotoxicity, hepatic coma, acute renal failure
ziconotide (Prialt)	Intrathecal 0.1 mcg/h via infusion, may increase by 0.1 mcg/h every 2–3 days (max: 0.8 mcg/h)	

Note: *Italics* indicate common adverse effects; underlining indicates serious adverse effects.

Although aspirin and ibuprofen have similar efficacy at relieving pain and inflammation and share certain side effects, there are important differences. Aspirin has a greater effect on blood coagulation than ibuprofen; thus, aspirin is used for the prophylaxis of cardiovascular events but ibuprofen is not. Aspirin poses a greater risk for GI bleeding, especially at high doses. The ibuprofen-like drugs are available in a wider variety of formulations, including parenteral and extended-release forms.

Centrally Acting Drugs

Centrally acting drugs are drugs that exert effects directly within the brain and spinal cord. Any analgesic drug that has a *central effect* bypasses the nociceptor level. Acetaminophen is a centrally acting nonopioid analgesic. Acetaminophen reduces fever by direct action at the level of the hypothalamus and causes dilation of peripheral blood vessels, enabling sweating and dissipation of heat. It is the primary alternative to NSAIDs

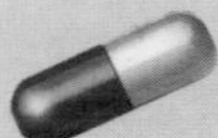

Prototype Drug | Aspirin *(Acetylsalicylic Acid, ASA)*

Therapeutic Class: Nonopioid analgesic; nonsteroidal anti-inflammatory drug (NSAID); antipyretic
Pharmacologic Class: Salicylate; cyclooxygenase (COX) inhibitor

Actions and Uses

Aspirin inhibits prostaglandin synthesis involved in the processes of pain and inflammation and produces mild to moderate relief of fever. It has limited effects on peripheral blood vessels, causing vasodilation and sweating. Aspirin has significant anticoagulant activity, and this property is responsible for its ability to reduce the risk of mortality following MI, and to reduce the incidence of strokes. Aspirin has also been found to reduce the risk of colorectal cancer, although the mechanism by which it affords this protective effect is unknown.

Administration Alerts

- Platelet aggregation inhibition caused by aspirin is irreversible. Aspirin should be discontinued 1 week prior to surgery.
- Aspirin is excreted in the urine and affects urine testing for glucose and other metabolites, such as vanillylmandelic acid (VMA).
- Pregnancy category D.

PHARMACOKINETICS

Onset	Peak	Duration
1 h	2–4 h	24 h

Adverse Effects

At high doses, such as those used to treat severe inflammatory disorders, aspirin may cause gastric discomfort and bleeding because of its antiplatelet effects. Enteric-coated tablets and buffered preparations are available for patients who experience GI side effects.

Contraindications: Because aspirin increases bleeding time, it should not be given to patients receiving anticoagulant therapy such as warfarin and heparin.

Interactions

Drug–Drug: Concurrent use of phenobarbital, antacids, and glucocorticoids may decrease aspirin's effects. Aspirin may potentiate the action of oral hypoglycemic drugs. Effects of NSAIDs, uricosuric drugs such as probenecid, beta blockers, spironolactone, and sulfa drugs may be decreased when combined with aspirin. Insulin, methotrexate, phenytoin, sulfonamides, and penicillin may increase effects. When aspirin is taken with alcohol, pyrazolone derivatives, steroids, or other NSAIDs, there is an increased risk for gastric ulcers.

Lab Tests: Aspirin may cause prolonged prothrombin time by decreasing prothrombin production. Aspirin may also interfere with pregnancy tests and decrease serum levels of cholesterol, potassium, PBI, T_3, and T_4. High salicylate levels may cause abnormalities in liver function tests.

Herbal/Food: Feverfew, garlic, ginger, and ginkgo may increase the risk of bleeding.

Treatment of Overdose: Treatment may include any of the following: activated charcoal, gastric lavage, laxative, or drug therapy for overdose symptoms such as dizziness, drowsiness, abdominal pain, or seizures.

when patients cannot take aspirin or ibuprofen. Acetaminophen does not produce GI bleeding or ulcers and it does not exhibit cardiotoxicity. The safety profile of acetaminophen is excellent when administered in proper therapeutic doses, although hepatotoxicity can occur with misuse and overdose. Aspirin and acetaminophen have similar efficacies in relieving pain and reducing fever. Acetaminophen is featured as a prototype drug for the treatment of fever in chapter 33.

Tramadol (Ultram) and ziconotide (Prialt) are also centrally acting analgesics. Of the two drugs, tramadol is the most widely prescribed. Tramadol has weak opioid activity, although it is not thought to relieve pain by this mechanism. Its main action is to inhibit reuptake of norepinephrine and serotonin in spinal neurons. Tramadol is well tolerated, but common adverse effects are vertigo, dizziness, headache, nausea, vomiting, constipation, and lethargy.

TENSION HEADACHES AND MIGRAINES

Headaches are some of the most common complaints of patients. Living with headaches can interfere with ADLs, thus causing great distress. The pain and inability to focus and concentrate result in work-related absences and in difficulties caring for home and family. When the headaches are persistent, or occur as migraines, drug therapy is warranted.

18.9 Classification of Headaches

Of the several varieties of headaches, the most common type is the **tension headache.** This condition occurs when muscles of the head and neck become very tight because of stress, causing a steady and lingering pain. Although quite painful, tension headaches are self-limiting and generally considered an annoyance rather than a medical emergency.

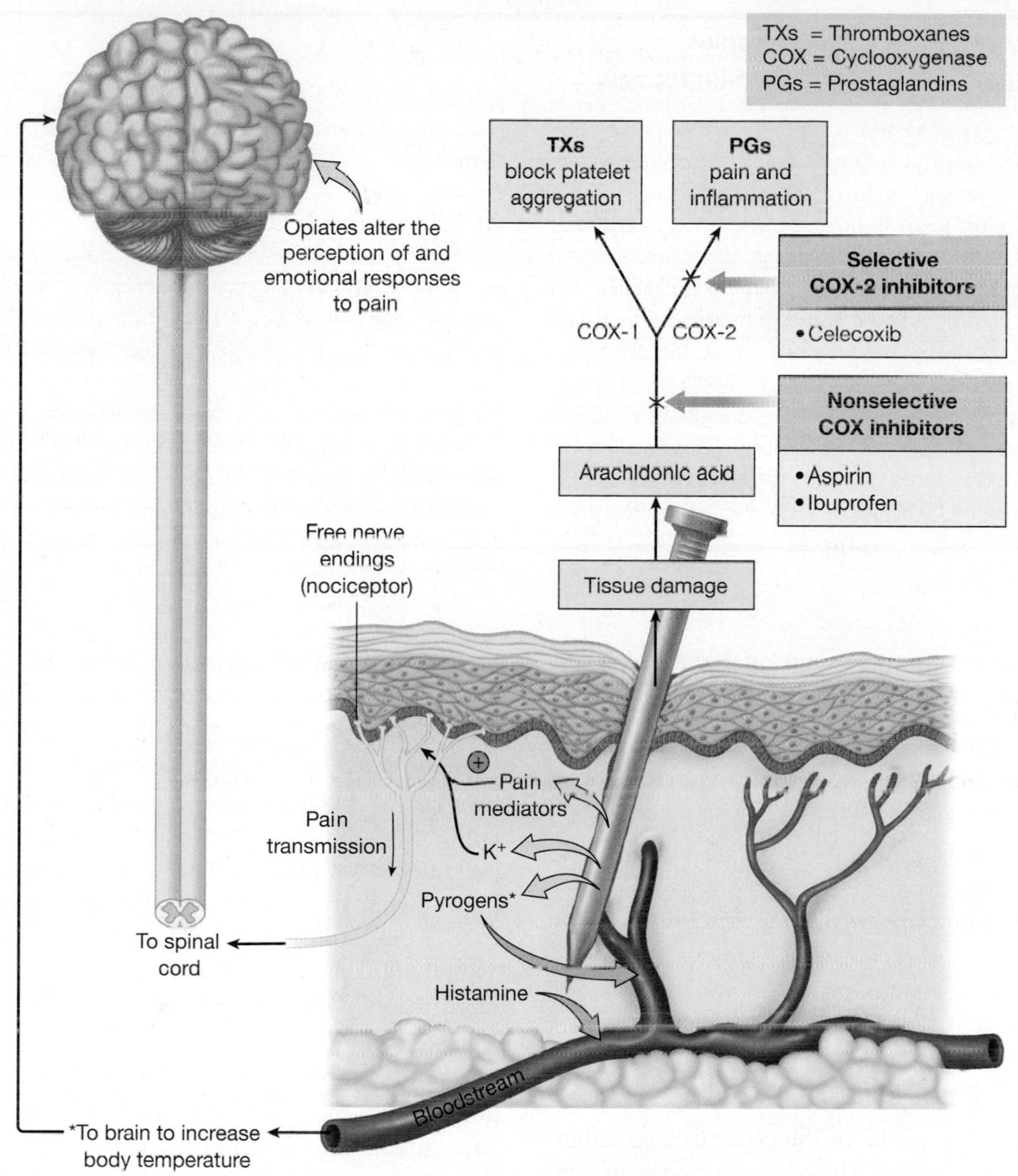

FIGURE 18.3 Mechanisms of pain transmission at the nociceptor level

PharmFacts

HEADACHES AND MIGRAINES

- Migraine is the most common cause of recurrent moderate to severe headache.
- Over 28 million Americans suffer from migraines.
- Of all migraines, 95% are controlled by drug therapy and other measures.
- Before puberty, boys generally have more migraines than girls.
- After puberty, the occurrence of migraines among women is four to eight times higher than men.
- Headaches and migraines appear mostly among people in their 20s and 30s. An alternate diagnosis is usually considered with onset after the age of 50.
- Persons with a family history of headache or migraine have a higher chance of developing these disorders.

The most painful type of headache is the **migraine,** which is characterized by throbbing or pulsating pain, sometimes preceded by an aura. **Auras** are sensory cues that let the patient know that a migraine attack is coming soon. Examples of sensory cues are jagged lines or flashing lights or special smells, tastes, or sounds. Most migraines are accompanied by nausea and vomiting. Triggers for migraines include nitrates, monosodium glutamate (MSG)—found in many Asian foods—red wine, perfumes, food additives, caffeine, chocolate, and aspartame. By avoiding foods containing these substances, some patients can prevent the onset of a migraine attack.

Drug Therapy for Tension Headaches

Tension headaches can usually be effectively treated with OTC analgesics such as aspirin, ibuprofen, or acetaminophen. As tension headaches escalate, prescription combination

Complementary and Alternative Therapies

NONPHARMACOLOGIC APPROACHES FOR CHRONIC PAIN

Chronic pain is difficult for a patient to experience and difficult for a provider to manage. The National Center for Complementary and Integrative Health (NCCIH, 2014) provides recommendations for nonpharmacologic approaches to chronic pain. Among the strategies recommended are massage therapy, yoga, acupuncture, spinal manipulation, and glucosamine and chondroitin. Acupuncture is discussed in chapter 38. Glucosamine and chondroitin are discussed in chapter 48.

The role of a patient's perceptions of benefit from nonpharmacologic therapies plays an important role. Schafer et al. (2012) and Sherman et al. (2014) found that patients' expectations of nonpharmacologic therapy included pain relief, improved function and fitness, and improved well-being. They also found that these expectations changed over time. For these reasons providers need to manage expectations as to what is or is not an appropriate outcome of complementary and alternative medicine (CAM) (Hsu et al., 2014; Sherman et al., 2012).

Further research with randomized clinical trials is needed to determine what CAM is most effective, and at what "dose." For example, Sherman et al. (2012) studied whether massage therapy for 30 minutes or 60 minutes was most effective for chronic neck pain when given between one and three times per week. In their study, 60 minute massages were more effective.

Until more research is conducted into CAM therapies for chronic pain, the nurse should help to manage the patient's expectations appropriately and stay up-to-date with current research (NCCIH, 2014).

drugs may offer more effective pain relief. For example, the following are stronger nonopioid alternatives for treatment of tension headaches:

- Ascomp (aspirin, 325 mg; caffeine, 40 mg; butalbital, 50 mg)
- Fioricet (acetaminophen, 325 mg; caffeine, 40 mg; butalbital, 50 mg)
- Phrenilin (acetaminophen, 325 mg; butalbital, 50 mg tablet)
- Phrenilin Forte (acetaminophen, 650 mg; butalbital, 50 mg capsule).

Antimigraine Drugs

There are two primary goals for the pharmacologic therapy of migraines (Table 18.5). The first is to stop migraines in progress, and the second is to prevent migraines from occurring. Mostly, the drugs used to abort migraines are different from those used for prophylaxis. Drug therapy is most effective if begun before a migraine has reached a severe pain level.

18.10 Drug Therapy for Migraines

The two major drug classes used as antimigraine drugs, the triptans and the ergot alkaloids, are both serotonin (5-HT) agonists. Serotonergic receptors are found throughout the CNS and in the cardiovascular and GI systems. At least five receptor subtypes have been identified. In addition to the triptans, other drugs acting at serotonergic receptors include the popular antianxiety drugs fluoxetine (Prozac) and buspirone (BuSpar).

Pharmacotherapy of migraine termination generally begins with acetaminophen or NSAIDs. If OTC or milder prescription analgesics are unable to abort the migraine, the drugs of choice are often the triptans. These drugs are selective for the 5-HT_1-receptor subtype, and they are thought to act by constricting intracranial vessels. They are effective in aborting migraines with or without auras. Although oral forms of the triptans are most convenient, patients who experience nausea and vomiting during the migraine may require an alternative dosage form. Intranasal formulations and prefilled syringes of triptans are available for patients who are able to self-administer the medication. All triptans have similar effectiveness and side effects.

For patients who are unresponsive to triptans, the ergot alkaloids may be used to abort migraines. The first purified alkaloid, ergotamine (Ergostat), was isolated from the ergot fungus in 1920, although the actions of the ergot alkaloids had been known for thousands of years. Ergotamine is an inexpensive drug that is available in oral, sublingual, and suppository forms. Modifications of the original molecule have produced a number of other pharmacologically useful drugs, such as dihydroergotamine mesylate (D.H.E. 45, Migranal). Dihydroergotamine is given parenterally and as a nasal spray. Because the ergot alkaloids interact with adrenergic and dopaminergic receptors as well as serotonergic receptors, they produce multiple actions and side effects. Many ergot alkaloids are pregnancy category X drugs.

Drugs for migraine prophylaxis include various classes of drugs that are discussed in other chapters of this textbook. These include antiseizure drugs, beta-adrenergic blockers, calcium channel blockers, antidepressants, and neuromuscular blockers. Because all these drugs have the potential to produce side effects, prophylaxis is initiated only if the incidence of migraines is high and the patient is

Table 18.5 Antimigraine Drugs

Drug	Route and Adult Dose (max dose where indicated)	Adverse Effects
TRIPTANS		
almotriptan (Axert)	PO: 6.25–12.5 mg; may repeat in 2 h if necessary (max: 2 tabs/day)	*Asthenia, tingling, warming sensation, dizziness, vertigo*
eletriptan (Relpax)	PO: 20–40 mg; may repeat in 2 h if necessary (max: 80 mg/day)	Coronary artery vasospasm, MI, cardiac arrest
frovatriptan (Frova)	PO: 2.5 mg; may repeat in 2 h if necessary (max: 7.5 mg/day)	
naratriptan (Amerge)	PO: 1–2.5 mg; may repeat in 4 h if necessary (max: 5 mg/day)	
rizatriptan (Maxalt)	PO: 5–10 mg; may repeat in 2 h if necessary (max: 30 mg/day); 5 mg with concurrent propranolol (max: 15 mg/day)	
sumatriptan (Imitrex)	PO: 25 mg for 1 dose (max: 100 mg)	
zolmitriptan (Zomig)	PO: 2.5–5 mg; may repeat in 2 h if necessary (max: 10 mg/day)	
ERGOT ALKALOIDS		
dihydroergotamine (D.H.E. 45, Migranal)	IM/subcutaneous: 1 mg; may be repeated at 1-h intervals to a total of 3 mg (max: 6 mg/wk) Nasal: 1 spray (0.5 mg) each nostril, may repeat once in 15 min	*Weakness, nausea, vomiting, abnormal pulse, pruritus* Delirium, convulsive seizures, intermittent claudication
ergotamine (Ergostat), ergotamine with caffeine (Cafergot, Ercaf, others)	PO: 1–2 mg followed by 1–2 mg every 30 min until headache stops (max: 6 mg/day or 10 mg/wk) Sublingual: 2 mg, may repeat in 30 min for total three doses/24 h or five doses/wk	
ANTISEIZURE DRUGS		
topiramate (Topamax)	PO: start with 50 mg/day, increase by 50 mg/wk to effectiveness (max: 1600 mg/day)	*Nausea, vomiting, sedation, drowsiness, weakness*
valproic acid (Depakene) (see page 192 for the Prototype Drug box)	PO: 250 mg bid (max: 100 mg/day)	Liver failure, bone marrow depression
BETA-ADRENERGIC BLOCKERS		
atenolol (Tenormin) (see page 422 for the Prototype Drug box)	PO: 25–50 mg/day (max: 100 mg/day)	*Bradycardia, hypotension, heart failure (HF), confusion, drowsiness, insomnia*
metoprolol (Lopressor) (see page 404 for the Prototype Drug box)	PO: 50–100 mg one to two times/day (max: 450 mg/day)	Bronchospasm, exfoliative dermatitis, agranulocytosis, membrane irritation, rash, heart block, cardiac arrest, anaphylaxis, Stevens–Johnson syndrome
propranolol (Inderal) (see page 453 for the Prototype Drug box)	PO: 80–240 mg/day in divided doses; may need 160–240 mg/day	
timolol (Blocadren) (see page 871 for the Prototype Drug box)	PO: 10 mg bid; may increase to 60 mg/day in two divided doses	
CALCIUM CHANNEL BLOCKERS		
nifedipine (Procardia) (see page 385 for the Prototype Drug box)	PO: 10–20 mg tid (max: 180 mg/day)	*Dizziness, light-headedness, facial flushing, heat sensitivity, diarrhea, peripheral edema, headache, hypotension, constipation*
nimodipine (Nimotop)	PO: 60 mg q4h for 21 days; start therapy within 96 hours of subarachnoid hemorrhage	Myocardial infarction (MI), atrioventricular (AV) block, hepatotoxicity
verapamil (Isoptin SR) (see page 456 for the Prototype Drug Box)	PO: 40–80 mg tid (max: 360 mg/day)	
TRICYCLIC ANTIDEPRESSANTS		
amitriptyline (Elavil)	PO: 75–100 mg/day	*Sedation, drowsiness, orthostatic hypotension, blurred vision, slight mydriasis, dry mouth, urinary retention, constipation*
imipramine (Tofranil) (see page 208 for the Prototype Drug box)	PO: 75–100 mg/day (max: 300 mg/day)	
protriptyline (Vivactil)	PO: 15–40 mg/day in three to four divided doses (max: 60 mg/day)	MI, dysrhythmias, heart block, agranulocytosis, angioedema, bone marrow depression
MISCELLANEOUS DRUGS		
onabotulinumtoxin A (Botox)	IM: 155 units administered intramuscularly (IM) to muscles of the head and neck area	*Nausea, vomiting, sedation, drowsiness, weakness,*
methysergide (Sansert)	PO: 4–8 mg/day in divided doses	*discoloration of urine (for vitamin B_2), painful urination*
riboflavin (vitamin B_2)	As a supplement: PO: 5–10 mg/day For deficiency: PO: 5–30 mg/day in divided doses	Shortness of breath

Note: *Italics* indicate common adverse effects; underlining indicates serious adverse effects.

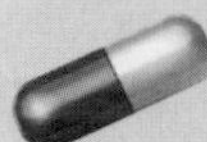

Prototype Drug | Sumatriptan *(Imitrex)*

Therapeutic Class: Antimigraine drug
Pharmacologic Class: Triptan; 5-HT (serotonin) receptor drug; vasoconstrictor of intracranial arteries

Actions and Uses

Sumatriptan belongs to a relatively newer group of antimigraine drugs known as the triptans. The triptans act by causing vasoconstriction of cranial arteries. This vasoconstriction is moderately selective and does not usually affect overall blood pressure. Sumatriptan is available in oral, intranasal, and subcutaneous forms. Subcutaneous administration terminates migraine attacks in 10 to 20 minutes; the dose may be repeated 60 minutes after the first injection to a maximum of two doses per day. If taken orally, sumatriptan should be administered as soon as possible after the migraine is suspected or has begun.

Administration Alerts

- Sumatriptan may produce cardiac ischemia in susceptible persons with no previous cardiac events. Health care providers may opt to administer the initial dose of sumatriptan in the health care setting.
- Sumatriptan's systemic vasoconstrictor activity may cause hypertension and may result in dysrhythmias or MI. Keep resuscitative equipment accessible.
- Sumatriptan selectively reduces carotid arterial blood flow. Monitor changes in level of consciousness and observe for seizures.
- Pregnancy category C.

PHARMACOKINETICS

Onset	Peak	Duration
15 min nasal; 30 min PO; 10 min subcutaneous	2 h PO; 12 min subcutaneous, 60–90 min nasal	24–48 h

Adverse Effects

Some dizziness, drowsiness, or a warming sensation may be experienced after taking sumatriptan; however, these effects are not normally severe enough to warrant discontinuation of therapy.

Contraindications: Because of its vasoconstricting action, the drug should be used cautiously, if at all, in patients with recent MI, or with a history of angina pectoris, hypertension, or diabetes. Sumatriptan is contraindicated in patients with serious renal or hepatic impairment.

Interactions

Drug–Drug: Sumatriptan interacts with several drugs. For example, an increased effect may occur when taken with MAOIs and selective serotonin reuptake inhibitors (SSRIs). Further vasoconstriction can occur when taken with ergot alkaloids and other triptans.

Lab Tests: Unknown.

Herbal/Food: Ginkgo, ginseng, echinacea, and St. John's wort may increase triptan toxicity.

Treatment of Overdose: Treatment may include drug therapy for the following symptoms: weakness, lack of coordination, watery eyes and mouth, tremors, seizures, or breathing problems.

unresponsive to the drugs used to abort migraines. Of the various drugs, the beta blocker propranolol (Inderal) is one of the most commonly prescribed. Amitriptyline (Elavil), an antidepressant, is preferred for patients who may have a mood disorder or suffer from insomnia in addition to their migraines. In 2010, onabotulinumtoxinA (Botox) was approved for the treatment of chronic migraines in cases where other medications were not successful. Botox inhibits neuromuscular transmission by blocking the release of acetylcholine from axon terminals innervating skeletal muscle. With this approach, IM injections are divided across specific muscles of the head and neck. When muscles are blocked, migraines subside for a period of up to 3 months. More indications for Botox therapy are discussed in chapter 21.

Nursing Practice Application
Pharmacotherapy for Migraines

ASSESSMENT	POTENTIAL NURSING DIAGNOSES*
Baseline assessment prior to administration: • Obtain a complete health history including cardiovascular, neurologic, hepatic, or renal disease; pregnancy; or breast-feeding. Obtain a drug history including allergies, current prescription and OTC drugs, herbal preparations, caffeine, nicotine, and alcohol use. Be alert to possible drug interactions. • Obtain baseline vital signs, apical pulse, level of consciousness, and weight. • Assess the level of pain. Use objective screening tools when possible (e.g., Wong-Baker FACES scale for children, numerical rating scale for adults). Assess the history of the pain and what has worked successfully or not for the patient in the past. • Evaluate appropriate laboratory findings (e.g., CBC, hepatic or renal function studies). • Assess the patient's ability to receive and understand instruction. Include the family and caregivers as needed.	• *Acute Pain* • *Ineffective Health Management* • *Ineffective Coping* • *Deficient Knowledge* (drug therapy) *NANDA I © 2014
Assessment throughout administration: • Assess for desired therapeutic effects (e.g., headache pain is decreased or absent). • Continue monitoring level of consciousness and neurologic symptoms (e.g., numbness or tingling). • Assess vital signs, especially blood pressure and pulse, periodically. • Continue periodic monitoring of hepatic and renal function studies. • Assess stress and coping patterns for possible symptom correlation (e.g., existing or perceived stress, duration, coping mechanisms or remedies). • Assess for and promptly report adverse effects: chest pain or tightness, palpitations, tachycardia, hypertension, dizziness, light headedness, confusion, and numbness or tingling in the extremities.	

IMPLEMENTATION

Interventions and (Rationales)	Patient-Centered Care
Ensuring therapeutic effects: • Continue assessments as described earlier for therapeutic effects. Give the drug *before* the start of acute pain when possible. (Consistent use of a pain rating scale by all providers will help quantify the level of pain relief and leads to better pain control. Pain relief begins within the first several minutes after administration.)	• Teach the patient that pain relief, rather than merely control, is the goal of therapy. • Encourage the patient to take the drug before a headache becomes severe and consistently as ordered. • Explain the rationale behind the pain rating scale (i.e., it allows consistency among all providers). • Encourage the patient to use additional, nonpharmacologic pain relief techniques (e.g., quiet, darkened, cool room).
Minimizing adverse effects: • Monitor the blood pressure and pulse periodically, especially in patients at risk for undiagnosed cardiovascular disease. Cardiovascular status should be monitored frequently following the first dose given. (Triptans cause vasoconstriction. **Lifespan:** Postmenopausal women, men over 40, smokers, and people with other known coronary artery disease risk factors may be at the greatest risk. Older adults may have undetected cardiovascular disease, placing them at greater risk for adverse effects.)	• Instruct the patient to report any chest pain, tightness, or pulsating activity that is severe or continues following drug dosage.
• Observe for changes in severity, character, or duration of headache. (Sudden severe headaches of "thunderclap" quality can signal subarachnoid hemorrhage. Headaches that differ in quality and are accompanied by such signs as fever, rash, or stiff neck may herald meningitis.)	• Instruct the patient to immediately report changes in character or duration of headache or if accompanied by additional symptoms such as fever, rash, or stiff neck.

continued

Nursing Practice Application *continued*

IMPLEMENTATION	
Interventions and (Rationales)	**Patient-Centered Care**
• Continue to monitor neurologic status periodically. (Neurologic changes may indicate adverse drug effects or may signal cerebral ischemia.)	• Instruct the patient to immediately report increasing dizziness, light-headedness, or blurred vision.
• Monitor dietary intake of foods that contain tyramine, caffeine, alcohol, or other food triggers. (Some foods or beverages may trigger an acute migraine. Correlating symptoms with food or beverages assists in relieving the cause of the headache.)	• Encourage the patient to keep a food diary and correlate symptoms with specific foods or beverages. Teach the patient to avoid or limit foods containing tyramine, such as pickled foods, beer, wine, and aged cheeses, because they are common triggers for migraines.
• Encourage the patient to discuss other methods of migraine control if ergot alkaloids are required for more than short-term use. (Ergot alkaloids cause significant vasoconstriction and cause dependence. Other, safer drugs may be needed for long-term relief of migraines.)	• Instruct the patient to discuss treatment options for long-term migraine relief with the health care provider.
• **Lifespan:** Women who are planning pregnancy, pregnant, or breast-feeding, should discuss the use of drug therapy and alternative treatment before using antimigraine drugs. (Triptans are known to cause birth defects in animals. Ergotamine and other ergot alkaloids are category X drugs.)	• Teach women of childbearing age to discuss the use of antimigraine drugs before planning pregnancy and to discontinue use if pregnant or breast-feeding unless directed otherwise by the provider.
Patient understanding of drug therapy: • Use opportunities during administration of medications and during assessments to provide patient education. (Using time during nursing care helps to optimize and reinforce key teaching areas.)	• The patient should be able to state the reason for the drug; appropriate dose and scheduling; and what adverse effects to observe for and when to report them.
Patient self-administration of drug therapy: • When administering the medication, instruct the patient, family, or caregiver in the proper self-administration of the drug (e.g., take the drug as prescribed when needed). (Using time during nurse administration of these drugs helps to reinforce teaching.)	• Teach the patient to take the medication before the pain becomes severe or at the first symptoms of a migraine, if possible. • Use the drug exactly as prescribed; overuse can lead to rebound headaches. • Teach the patient the proper administration of subcutaneous medication. Have the patient or caregiver teach-back the technique. (Pain or redness at the injection site is common but usually disappears within an hour after the dose is taken.) • Instruct the patient that an appropriate intranasal dose is one spray into ONE nostril unless otherwise ordered by the health care provider.

See under "Triptans" in Table 18.5 for a list of drugs to which these nursing actions apply.

Chapter Review

KEY Concepts

The numbered key concepts provide a succinct summary of the important points from the corresponding numbered section within the chapter. If any of these points are not clear, refer to the numbered section within the chapter for review.

18.1 Pain is assessed and classified as acute or chronic, nociceptor or neuropathic.

18.2 Nonpharmacologic techniques such as massage, biofeedback therapy, and meditation may be used alone or with adjunctive pharmacotherapy in effective pain management.

18.3 Two main classes of pain medications are employed to manage pain. Centrally acting drugs suppress pain impulses by activating opioid receptors; peripherally acting drugs reduce inflammation.

18.4 Opioids are natural or synthetic substances extracted from the poppy plant that exert their effects through interaction with mu and kappa receptors.

18.5 Opioids are the drugs of choice for extreme to severe pain. They also have other important therapeutic effects including dampening of the cough reflex and slowing of the motility of the GI tract.

18.6 Opioid antagonists may be used to reverse the symptoms of opioid toxicity or overdose, such as sedation and respiratory depression.

18.7 Opioid withdrawal can result in severe symptoms, and opioid dependence is often treated with methadone maintenance and newer drug combination therapies.

18.8 Nonopioid analgesics, such as aspirin, acetaminophen, and the selective COX-2 inhibitors, are effective in treating mild to moderate pain and fever.

18.9 Headaches are classified as tension headaches or migraines. Migraines may be preceded by auras, and symptoms include nausea and vomiting.

18.10 The goals of pharmacotherapy for migraines are to stop them in progress and to prevent them from occurring. Triptans, ergot alkaloids, and other drug classes are used to treat migraines.

REVIEW Questions

1. The nurse teaches the patient relaxation techniques and guided imagery as an adjunct to medication for treatment of pain. What is the main rationale for the use of these techniques as adjuncts to analgesic medication?
   1. They are less costly techniques.
   2. They may allow lower doses of drugs with fewer adverse effects.
   3. They can be used at home.
   4. They do not require self-injection.

2. The emergency department nurse is caring for a patient with a migraine. Which drug would the nurse anticipate administering to abort the patient's migraine attack?
   1. Morphine
   2. Propranolol (Inderal)
   3. Ibuprofen (Motrin)
   4. Sumatriptan (Imitrex)

3. A patient admitted with hepatitis B is prescribed hydrocodone with acetaminophen (Vicodin) 2 tablets for pain. What is the most appropriate action for the nurse to take?
   1. Administer the drug as ordered.
   2. Administer 1 tablet only.
   3. Recheck the order with the health care provider.
   4. Hold the drug until the health care provider arrives.

4. The nurse administers morphine 4 mg IV to a patient for treatment of severe pain. Which of the following assessments require immediate nursing interventions? (Select all that apply.)
   1. The patient's blood pressure is 110/70 mmHg.
   2. The patient is drowsy.
   3. The patient's pain is unrelieved in 15 minutes.
   4. The patient's respiratory rate is 10 breaths per minute.
   5. The patient becomes unresponsive.

5. Planning teaching needs for a patient who is to be discharged postoperatively with a prescription for oxycodone with acetaminophen (Percocet) should include which of the following?
   1. Refer the patient to a drug treatment center if addiction occurs.
   2. Encourage increased fluids and fiber in the diet.
   3. Monitor for GI bleeding.
   4. Teach the patient to self-assess blood pressure.

6. What is the most appropriate method to ensure adequate pain relief in the immediate postoperative period from an opioid drug?
   1. Give the drug only when the family members report that the patient is complaining of pain.
   2. Give the drug every time the patient complains of acute pain.
   3. Give the drug as consistently as possible for the first 24 to 48 hours.
   4. Give the drug only when the nurse observes signs and symptoms of pain.

PATIENT-FOCUSED Case Study

Lee Sutter, 45 years old, is on a PCA pump to manage postoperative pain related to recent cancer surgery. The PCA is set to deliver a basal rate of morphine of 6 mg/h. As his nurse, you discover Lee to be unresponsive with a respiratory rate of 8 breaths per minute and oxygen saturation of 84%.

1. What should be your first response?
2. What do you anticipate will be needed after that initial response?
3. What follow-up is needed after this time?

CRITICAL THINKING Questions

1. A 64-year-old patient has had a long-standing history of migraines as well as coronary artery disease, type 2 diabetes, and hypertension. On review of the medical history, the nurse notes that this patient has recently started on sumatriptan (Imitrex), prescribed by the patient's new neurologist. What intervention and teaching is appropriate for this patient?
2. A 58-year-old woman with a history of a recent MI is on beta-blocker and anticoagulant therapy. The patient also has a history of arthritis and during a recent flare-up began taking aspirin because it helped control pain in the past. What teaching or recommendation would the nurse have for this patient?

Visit www.pearsonhighered.com/nursingresources for answers and rationales for all activities.

REFERENCES

Choi, N. G., & Dinitto, D. M. (2013). The digital divide among low-income homebound older adults: Internet use patterns, eHealth literacy, and attitudes toward computer/Internet use. *Journal of Medical Internet Research, 15*(5), e93. doi:10.2196/jmir.2645

Devraj, R., Herndon, C. M., & Griffin, J. (2013). Pain awareness and medication knowledge: A health literacy evaluation. *Journal of Pain & Palliative Care Pharmacotherapy, 27*, 19–27. doi:10.3109/15360288.2012.751955

Ellis, J., Mullan, J., Worsley, A., & Pai, N. (2012). The role of health literacy and social networks in arthritis patients' health information-seeking behavior: A qualitative study. *International Journal of Internal Medicine, 2012*, Article ID 397039. doi:10.1155/2012/397039

Herdman, T. H., & Kamitsuru, S. (Eds.). (2014). *NANDA International nursing diagnoses: Definitions and classification, 2015–2017*. Oxford, United Kingdom: Wiley-Blackwell.

Hsu, C., Sherman, K. J., Eaves, E. R., Turner, J. A., Cherkin, D. C., Cromp, D., Schaefer, L., & Ritenbaugh, C. (2014). New perspectives on patient expectations of treatment outcomes: Results from qualitative interviews with patients seeking complementary and alternative medicine treatments for chronic low back pain. *BMC Complementary and Alternative Medicine, 14*, 276. doi:10.1186/1472-6882-14-276

McCarthy, D. M., Waite, K. R., Curtis, L. M., Engel, K. G., Baker, D. W., & Wolf, M. S. (2012). What did the doctor say? Health literacy and recall of medical instructions. *Medical Care, 50*, 277–282. doi:10.1097/MLR.0b013e318241e8e1

National Center for Complementary and Integrative Health. (2014). *Chronic pain and complementary health approaches: What you need to know*. Retrieved from https://nccih.nih.gov/health/pain/chronic.htm

NIH Pain Consortium. (2014). *Pain information brochure*. Retrieved from http://painconsortium.nih.gov/News_Other_Resources/pain_index.html#Anchor-Bac-14817

Schafer, L. M., Hsu, C., Eaves, E. R., Ritenbaugh, C., Turner, J., Cherkin, D. C., . . . Sherman, K. J. (2012). Complementary and alternative medicine (CAM) providers' views of chronic low back pain patients' expectation of CAM therapies: A qualitative study. *BMC Complementary and Alternative Medicine, 12*, 234. doi:10.1186/1472-6882-12-234

Sherman, K. J., Cook, A. J., Wellman, R. D., Hawkes, R. J., Kahn, J. R., Deyo, R. A., & Cherkin, D. C. (2014). Five-week outcomes from a dosing trial of therapeutic massage for chronic neck pain. *Annals of Family Medicine, 12*, 112–120. doi:10.1370/afm.1602

SELECTED BIBLIOGRAPHY

Agius, A. M., Jones, N. S., & Muscat, R. (2013). A randomized controlled trial comparing the efficacy of low-dose amitriptyline, amitriptyline with pindolol and surrogate placebo in the treatment of chronic tension-type facial pain. *Rhinology, 51*, 143–153.

Centers for Disease Control and Prevention. (2013). *The state of aging and health in America 2013*. Atlanta, GA: Author.

Crespin, D. J., Griffin, K. H., Johnson, J. R., Miller, C., Finch, M. D., Rivard, R. L.,. . . Dusek, J. A. (2015). Acupuncture provides short-term pain relief for patients in a total joint replacement program. *Pain Medicine, 16*, 1195–1203. doi:10.1111/pme.12685

Finnerup, N. B., Attal, N., Haroutounian, S., McNicol, E., Baron, R., Dworkin, R. H.,. . . Wallace, M. (2015). Pharmacotherapy for neuropathic pain in adults: A systematic review and meta-analysis. *Lancet Neurology, 14*, 162–173. doi:10.1016/S1474-4422(14)70251-0

Fornasari, D. (2012). Pain mechanisms in patients with chronic pain. *Clinical Drug Investigation, 32*(Suppl. 1), 45–52.

Govenden, D., & Serpell, M. (2014). Improving outcomes for chronic pain in primary care. The *Practitioner, 258*(1774), 13–17.

Howard-Anderson, J., Ganz, P. A., Bower, J. E., & Stanton, A. L. (2012). Quality of life, fertility concerns, and behavioral health outcomes in younger breast cancer survivors: A systematic review. *Journal of the National Cancer Institute, 104*, 386–405. doi:10.1093/jnci/djr541

Institute of Medicine of the National Academies. (2011). *Relieving pain in America: A blueprint for transforming prevention, care, education and research*. Washington, D. C.: The National Academies Press. Retrieved from http://books.nap.edu/openbook.php?record_id=13172&page=1

Molton, I. R., & Terrill, A. L. (2014). Overview of persistent pain in older adults. *American Psychologist, 69*(2), 197–207. doi:10.1037/a0035794

National Headache Foundation. (n.d.). *Learn about headaches*. Retrieved from http://www.headaches.org/headache-fact-sheets/

Penprase, B., Brunetto, E., Dahmani, E., Forthoffer, J. J., & Kapoor, S. (2015). The efficacy of preemptive analgesia for postoperative pain control: A systematic review of the literature. *AORN Journal, 101*, 94–105.e8. doi:10.1016/j.aorn.2014.01.030

Reddy, D. S. (2013). The pathophysiological and pharmacological basis of current drug treatment of migraine headache. *Expert Review of Clinical Pharmacology, 6*, 271–288. doi:10.1586/ecp.13.14

Silberstein, S. D. (2011). *Migraine*. Retrieved from http://www.merckmanuals.com/professional/neurologic_disorders/headache/migraine

Torpy, J. M., & Livingston, E. H. (2013). JAMA patient page. Aspirin therapy. *JAMA, The Journal of the American Medical Association, 309*, 1645. doi:10.1001/jama.2013.3866

Chapter 19

Drugs for Local and General Anesthesia

Drugs at a Glance

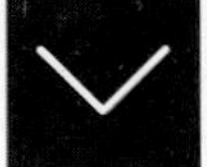

Learning Outcomes

After reading this chapter, the student should be able to:

1. Compare and contrast the five major clinical techniques for administering local anesthetics.
2. Describe differences between the two major chemical classes of local anesthetics.
3. Explain why epinephrine and sodium bicarbonate are sometimes included in local anesthetic cartridges.
4. Identify the actions of general anesthetics on the central nervous system.
5. Compare and contrast the two primary ways that general anesthesia may be induced.
6. Identify the four stages of general anesthesia.
7. For each of the drug classes listed in Drugs at a Glance, know representative drug examples, and explain their mechanisms of action, primary actions, and important adverse effects.
8. Categorize drugs used before, during, and after anesthesia based on their classification and drug action.
9. Use the nursing process to care for patients who are receiving pharmacotherapy with anesthetic agents.

indicates a prototype drug, each of which is featured in a Prototype Drug box.

Anesthesia is a medical procedure performed by administering drugs that cause loss of sensation. **Local anesthesia** occurs when sensation is lost to a limited part of the body without loss of consciousness. **General anesthesia** requires different classes of drugs that cause loss of sensation to the entire body, usually resulting in loss of consciousness. This chapter examines drugs used for both local and general anesthesia, including select drugs used before, during, and after surgical procedures.

LOCAL ANESTHESIA

Local anesthesia is loss of sensation to a relatively small part of the body without loss of consciousness to the patient. This procedure may be necessary for a brief medical or dental procedure.

19.1 Regional Loss of Sensation Using Local Anesthesia

Although local anesthesia often results in loss of sensation to a small, limited area, it sometimes affects larger portions of the body, such as an entire limb. Thus, some local anesthetic treatments are more accurately called *surface* anesthesia or *regional* anesthesia, depending on how the drugs are administered and their resulting effects.

The five major routes for applying local anesthetics are shown in Figure 19.1. The method used is dependent on the location and the amount of anesthesia that is needed. For example, some local anesthetics are applied topically before a needlestick or for minor skin surgery. Others are used to block sensations to larger areas such as the limbs or lower abdomen. The different methods of local and regional anesthetic administration are summarized in Table 19.1.

LOCAL ANESTHETICS

Local anesthetics are drugs that produce a rapid loss of sensation to a limited part of the body. They produce their therapeutic effect by blocking the entry of sodium ions into neurons.

19.2 Mechanism of Action of Local Anesthetics

The mechanism of action of local anesthetics is well-known. The concentration of sodium ions is normally higher on the outside of neurons than on the inside. A rapid influx of sodium ions into cells is necessary for neurons to fire.

As illustrated in Pharmacotherapy Illustrated 19.1, local anesthetics act by blocking sodium channels. Because

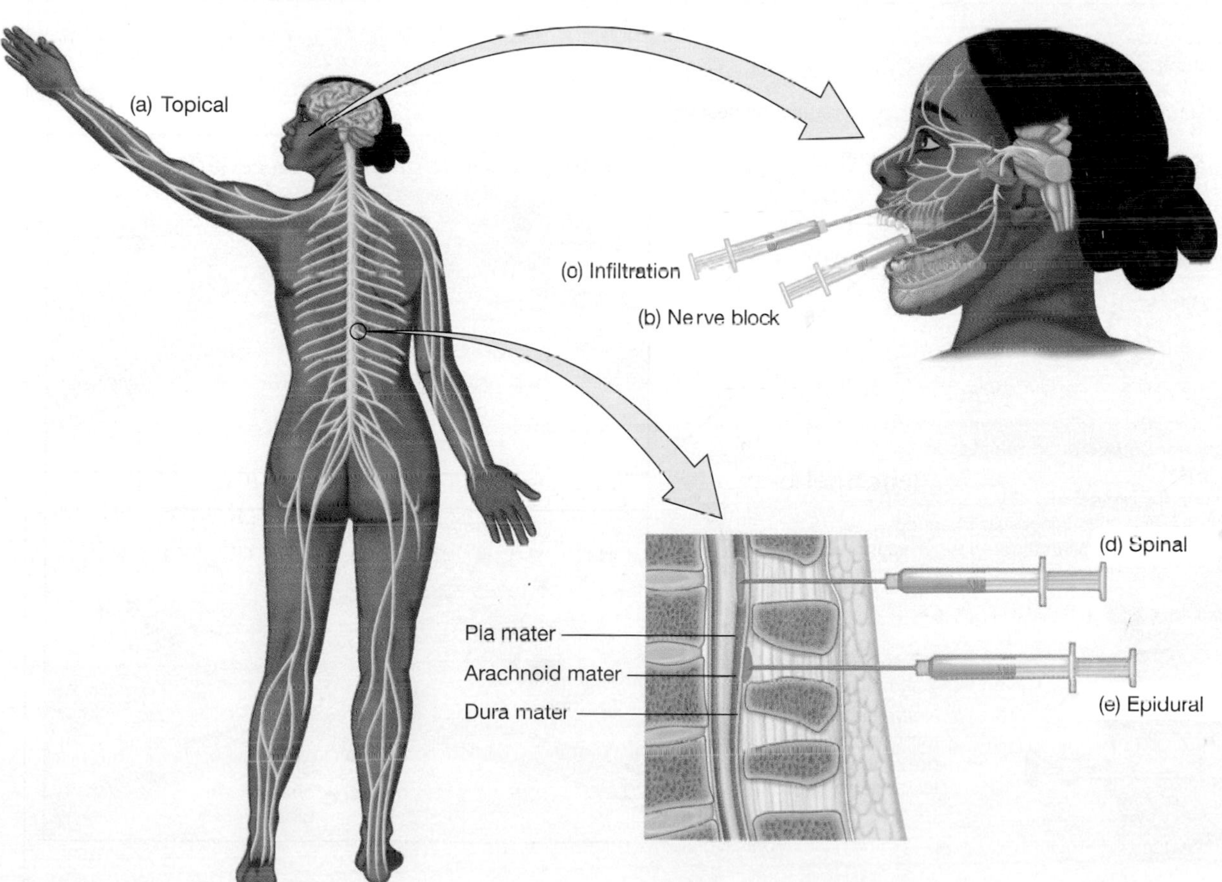

FIGURE 19.1 Techniques for applying local anesthesia: (a) topical; (b) infiltration; (c) nerve block; (d) spinal; and (e) epidural

Table 19.1 Methods of Local Anesthetic Administration

Route	Formulation/Method	Description
Topical (surface) anesthesia	Creams, sprays, suppositories, drops, and lozenges	Applied to mucous membranes including the eyes, lips, gums, nasal membranes, and throat
Infiltration (field block) anesthesia	Direct injection into tissue immediate to the surgical site	Drug diffuses into tissue to block a specific group of nerves in a small area close to the surgical site
Nerve block anesthesia	Direct injection into tissue that may be distant from the operation site	Drug affects nerve bundles serving the surgical area; used to block sensation in a limb or large area of the face
Spinal anesthesia	Injection into the cerebral spinal fluid (CSF)	Drug affects a large, regional area such as the lower abdomen and legs
Epidural anesthesia	Injection into the epidural space of the spinal cord	Most commonly used in obstetrics during labor and delivery

this action is a nonselective process, both sensory and motor impulses are affected. Thus, both sensation and muscle activity will temporarily diminish in the area treated with local anesthetics. Because of their mechanism of action, local anesthetics are called *sodium channel blockers*.

During a medical or surgical procedure, it is essential that an anesthetic lasts long enough to complete the procedure. Small amounts of epinephrine are sometimes added to the anesthetic solution in order to constrict blood vessels in the immediate area. This keeps the anesthetic localized, thus extending its duration of action. Epinephrine added to lidocaine (Xylocaine) for example, may increase the local anesthetic action from about 20 minutes to as long as 60 minutes. This is important for short surgical or dental

Pharmacotherapy Illustrated

19.1 | Mechanism of Action of Local Anesthetics

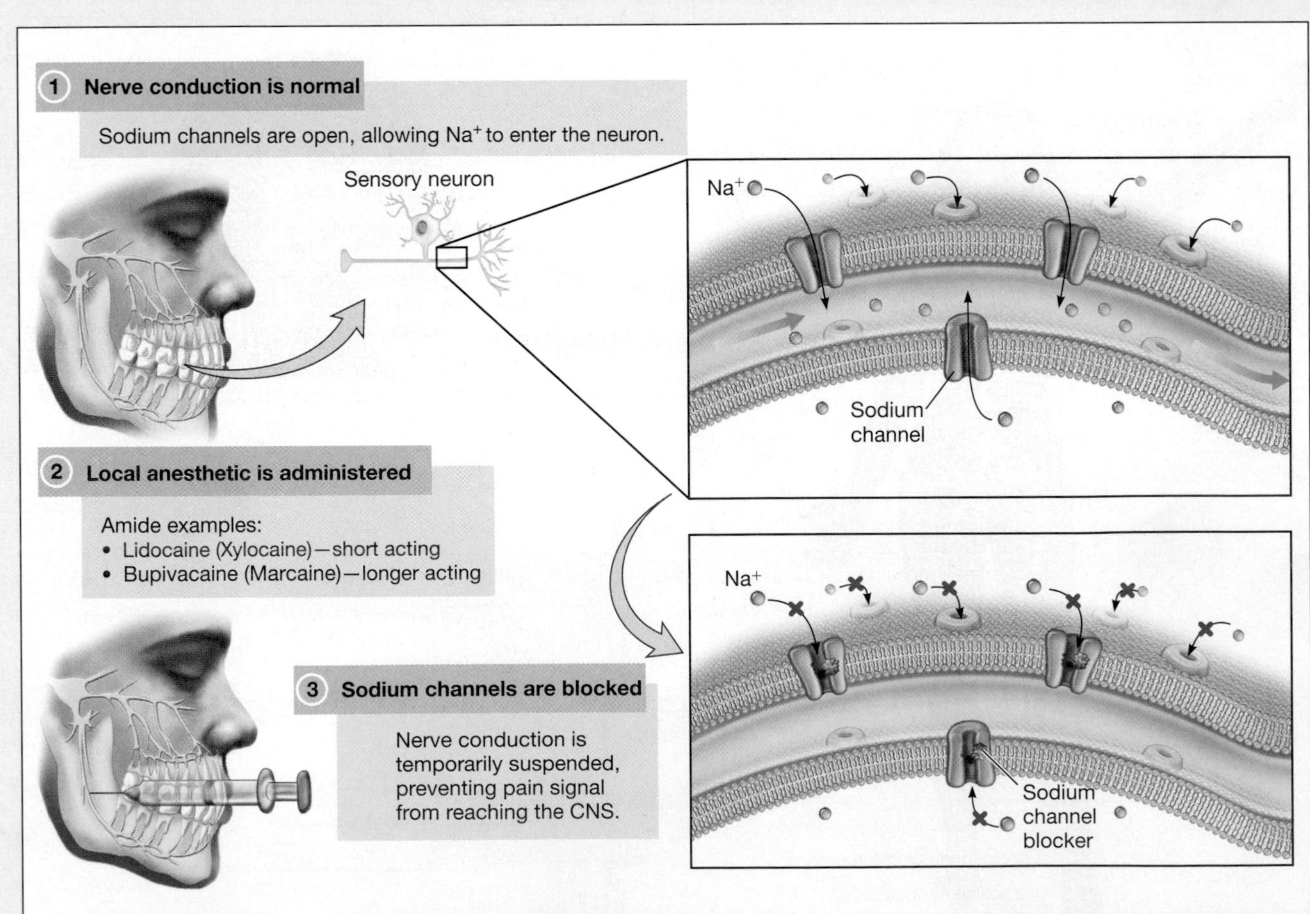

PharmFacts

ANESTHESIA AND ANESTHETICS

- More than 20 million people receive general anesthetics each year in the United States.
- About half of all general anesthetics are administered by a nurse anesthetist.
- Some of the first medical applications of anesthetics in the United States were in 1842, using ether, and in 1846, using nitrous oxide.
- Herbal products may interact with anesthetics. For example, St. John's wort may intensify or prolong the effects of some opioids and anesthetics.

procedures that take less than one hour; otherwise, a second injection might be necessary.

Alkaline additives are also included in some anesthetic solutions in order to increase local anesthesia in regions that have local infections or abscesses. Bacteria tend to acidify an infected site, and local anesthetics are less effective in this type of environment. Adding an alkaline solution such as sodium bicarbonate neutralizes the infected area and allows the anesthetic to work better. Methylparaben is another additive that may be added to the anesthetic solution to retard bacterial growth.

19.3 Classification of Local Anesthetics

Local anesthetics are classified by their chemical structures; the two major classes are **amides** and **esters** (Table 19.2). A small number of miscellaneous anesthetics are neither amides nor esters. As illustrated in Figure 19.2, the terms *ester* and *amide* refer to types of chemical linkages found within the anesthetic molecules.

Esters

Esters are mentioned first because they were the first anesthetics to be used in medical procedures. As early as the 1880s, cocaine was routinely used for eye surgery, nerve blocks, and spinal anesthesia. Cocaine is found in the leaves of the plant *Erythroxylon coca*, native to the Andes Mountains of Peru. Even today, cocaine is sometimes applied to the lining of the mouth, nose, and throat (mucous membranes) before biopsy, stitches, and wound cleaning. Its onset is within seconds after application. Cocaine temporarily numbs the area for about 1–2 minutes. It constricts blood vessels, an effect that decreases bleeding and swelling during the procedure. The abuse potential of cocaine is discussed in chapter 22.

Another ester, procaine (Novocain), was the drug of choice for dental procedures from the mid-1900s until the 1960s, when the development of the amide anesthetics led to a significant decline in the use of the ester drug class. One ester, benzocaine (Solarcaine, others), is used as a topical over-the-counter (OTC) agent for treating a large number of painful conditions, including sunburn, insect bites, hemorrhoids, sore throat, and minor wounds. Tetracaine is often sprayed on the skin or mucous membranes to produce loss of feeling before and during surgery or endoscopic procedures. A topical preparation comprised of benzocaine, butamben, and tetracaine (Cetacaine) is used for examination of the esophagus or colon. Proparacaine (Alcaine, Ophthetic) is used for short-term anesthesia during ocular procedures.

Amides

Amides have largely replaced the esters, because they produce fewer side effects and generally have a longer duration of action. Lidocaine (Xylocaine) is the most widely

Table 19.2 Selected Local Anesthetics

Chemical Classification	Drug	General Adverse Effects
Esters	benzocaine (Americaine, Anbesol, Solarcaine, others) chloroprocaine (Nesacaine) procaine (Novocain) proparacaine (Alcaine, Ophthetic) tetracaine (Pontocaine)	*CNS depression and burning, stinging and redness at topical application sites* Respiratory arrest, circulatory failure, anaphylactoid reaction
Amides	articaine (Septocaine, Zorcaine) bupivacaine (Exparel, Marcaine, Sensorcaine) dibucaine (Nupercainal) lidocaine (Anestacon, Dilocaine, Xylocaine, others) mepivacaine (Carbocaine, Isocaine, Polocaine) prilocaine ropivacaine (Naropin)	*Burning, stinging and redness at topical application sites* Difficulty breathing or swallowing, respiratory depression and arrest, convulsions, anaphylactoid reaction, burning, contact dermatitis
Miscellaneous drugs	dyclonine (Dyclone) ethyl chloride or chloroethane pramoxine (Tronothane)	*Burning, stinging, sensation at application site* Respiratory or cardiac arrest

Note: *Italics* indicate common adverse effects; underlining indicates serious adverse effects.

Type	General formula	Example
Ester	$R-\overset{O}{\overset{\|\|}{C}}-O-R$	$H_2N-C_6H_4-\overset{O}{\overset{\|\|}{C}}-O-C_2H_2-N(C_2H_5)_2$ **Procaine**
Amide	$R-NH-\overset{O}{\overset{\|\|}{C}}-R$	$(CH_3)_2C_6H_3-NH-\overset{O}{\overset{\|\|}{C}}-CH_2-N(C_2H_5)_2$ **Lidocaine**

FIGURE 19.2 Chemical structures of ester and amide local anesthetics

used amide for short surgical procedures. Ethyl chloride or chloroethane is a mild topical drug supplied as liquid in a spray bottle. It is used for basic procedures such as removing splinters or small debris from the skin's surface.

Adverse effects to amide anesthesics are uncommon. Allergy is rare. When it does occur, it is often due to sulfites, which are added as preservatives to prolong the shelf life of the anesthetic. Early signs of adverse effects include symptoms of central nervous system (CNS) stimulation such as restlessness or anxiety. Later, drowsiness and unresponsiveness may occur due to CNS depression. Cardiovascular effects, including hypotension and dysrhythmias, are possible. Patients with a history of cardiovascular disease are often given forms of local anesthetics that contain no epinephrine to reduce the possible effects of this sympathomimetic on the heart and blood pressure. CNS and cardiovascular adverse effects are rare unless the local anesthetic is absorbed rapidly or is accidentally injected directly into a blood vessel.

Lifespan Considerations: Geriatric
Cognitive Dysfunction After Surgery

Postoperative cognitive dysfunction (POCD) has been noted after cardiac as well as other surgeries. Periods of confusion and declines in cognitive skills such as word recall and memory impairment may occur, although they are not always long lasting. The older adult, age 60 years or older, has significantly higher rates of POCD than middle-age (40–59 years) or younger (18–39 years) adults experience. Monitoring brain function during surgery may help to prevent POCD by allowing for lower doses of anesthetic. Chan, Cheng, Lee, and Gin (2013) found that intra-operative monitoring and analyzing of brain function by EEG allowed for titration of anesthetic agents to maintain a constant level of brain function, and lower rates of POCD were noted postoperatively. The amount of anesthetic agent used was able to be reduced by up to 27%. Current research is also investigating whether inflammation of the endothelial cells may be a cause of POCD (Riedel, Browne, & Silbert, 2014). The same mechanism that has been implicated in the development of other diseases such as atherosclerotic heart disease may also be the underlying cause of POCD. If so, the discovery could lead to methods of identifying patients at-risk for POCD or new treatments aimed at preventing or reversing the condition. Nurses should observe for any cognitive dysfunction such as delirium, confusion, or memory impairment, even if transitory, in postoperative patients and refer them to their health care provider for appropriate monitoring beyond the immediate postoperative period.

GENERAL ANESTHESIA

General anesthesia is loss of sensation throughout the entire body, accompanied by loss of consciousness. General anesthetics are used when it is necessary for the patient to remain still and without pain for a longer time than could be achieved with local anesthetics.

19.4 Characteristics of General Anesthesia

The goal of general anesthesia is to provide a rapid and complete loss of sensation. Signs of general anesthesia include total analgesia (no feeling of pain) and loss of consciousness, memory, and body movement. Although these signs are similar to those of sleeping, general anesthesia and sleep are not exactly the same. General anesthetics depress most nervous activity in the brain, whereas sleeping stops activity in only very specific areas. In fact, some brain activity actually increases during sleep, as described in chapter 14.

General anesthesia is rarely achieved with a single drug. Instead, multiple medications are used to rapidly induce unconsciousness, cause muscle relaxation, and maintain deep anesthesia. This approach, called **balanced**

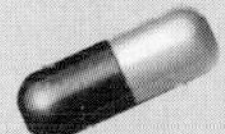

Prototype Drug | Lidocaine *(Xylocaine)*

Therapeutic Class: Anesthetic (local/topical); antidysrhythmic (class IB) **Pharmacologic Class:** Sodium channel blocker; amide

Actions and Uses

Lidocaine, the most frequently used injectable local anesthetic, acts by blocking neuronal pain impulses. It may be injected as a nerve block for spinal and epidural anesthesia. Lidocaine patches may be administered to relieve pain related to postherpetic neuralgia (Lidoderm) or dental procedures (DentiPatch). Zingo (lidocaine hydrochloride monohydrate) is a needle-free intradermal injection system that is indicated for rapid local anesthesia. It works by providing 0.5 mg lidocaine topically. This method is useful for pretreatment in instances such as IV insertions or blood draws. Like other amides, lidocaine acts by blocking sodium channels located within neuronal membranes.

Lidocaine may be given intravenously (IV), intramuscularly (IM), or subcutaneously to treat dysrhythmias, as discussed in chapter 30. Topical forms are also available. Mouthwashes and rinses can be compounded to help ease pain associated with mouth and throat ulcerations. Lidocaine is commonly compounded with antacids, antibiotics, antifungals, antihistamines, and coating agents.

Administration Alerts

- Solutions of lidocaine containing preservatives or epinephrine are intended for local anesthesia only and must never be given parenterally for dysrhythmias.
- Do not apply topical lidocaine to large skin areas or to broken or abraded areas, because significant absorption may occur. Do not allow it to come into contact with the eyes.
- For spinal or epidural block, use only preparations specifically labeled for IV use.
- Pregnancy category B.

PHARMACOKINETICS

Onset	Peak	Duration
45–90 sec IV; 5–15 min IM; 2–5 min topical	Less than 30 min	10–20 min IV; 60–90 min IM; 30–60 min topical; more than 100 min injected for anesthesia

Adverse Effects

When lidocaine is used for anesthesia, side effects are uncommon. An early symptom of toxicity is CNS excitement, leading to irritability and confusion. Serious adverse effects include convulsions, respiratory depression, and cardiac arrest. Until the effect of the anesthetic diminishes, patients may injure themselves by biting or chewing areas of the mouth that have no sensation following a dental procedure.

Black Box Warning: Use of 2% oral viscous lidocaine products especially among infants, may lead to ingestion that cannot be predicted or controlled. When excessive amounts of lidocaine are administered to infants and young children, or they accidentally swallow too much, it can induce seizures, brain injury, cardiac abnormalities, and/or death.

Contraindications: Lidocaine should be avoided in cases of sensitivity to amide-type local anesthetics. Application or injection of lidocaine anesthetic is also contraindicated in the presence of severe trauma or sepsis, blood dyscrasias, dysrhythmias, sinus bradycardia, and severe degrees of heart block.

Interactions

Drug–Drug: Barbiturates may decrease the activity of lidocaine. Increased effects of lidocaine occur if taken concurrently with cimetidine, quinidine, and beta blockers. If lidocaine is used on a regular basis, its effectiveness may diminish when used with other medications.

Lab Tests: Increased creatine phosphokinase (CPK).

Herbal/Food: Unknown.

Treatment of Overdose: Emergency medical attention is needed because of the many associated substantive symptoms such as breathing difficulty, swelling of the lips, chest pain, irregular heartbeat, nausea, vomiting, tremors, and seizure activity. **Lipid infusion therapy (LipidRescue)** is the use of an intravascular infusion of a lipid emulsion to treat severe, systemic drug toxicity or poisoning. This method was originally developed to treat local anesthetic toxicity, a potentially fatal complication of regional anesthesia that can also occur in other situations where patients receive local anesthetic injections. Lipid infusion therapy can also effectively treat a wide variety of nonlocal anesthetic overdoses. These include reversing CNS and cardiovascular signs and symptoms of drug toxicity.

anesthesia, allows the dose of inhalation anesthetic to be lower so that the procedure is safer for the patient.

General anesthesia is a progressive process that occurs in distinct steps, or stages: 1) loss of pain; 2) excitement and hyperactivity; 3) surgical anesthesia; and 4) respiratory and cardiovascular paralysis. The most effective medications can quickly move the patient through the stages, whereas others are only able to affect the lighter stage 1 (mild sedation). Most major surgery occurs in stage 3, where the patient is completely relaxed and

Nursing Practice Application

Pharmacotherapy With Local Anesthetics

ASSESSMENT	POTENTIAL NURSING DIAGNOSES*
Baseline assessment prior to administration: • Obtain a complete health history including cardiovascular, hepatic, renal, respiratory, or neurologic disease; pregnancy; or breast-feeding. Obtain a drug history including allergies, current prescription and OTC drugs, herbal preparations, caffeine, nicotine, and alcohol use. If the patient reports an allergy to "caine" drugs, note the specific reactions the patient experienced. Be alert to possible drug interactions. • Obtain baseline vital signs and weight. • Assess for areas of broken skin, abrasions, burns, or other wounds in the area to be treated with a local anesthetic. • Evaluate laboratory findings appropriate to the procedure (e.g., complete blood count [CBC], electrolytes, hepatic or renal function studies). • Assess the patient's ability to receive and understand instruction. Include the family and caregivers as needed.	• *Acute Pain* • *Deficient Knowledge* (drug therapy) • *Risk for Aspiration* • *Risk for Infection* • *Risk for Injury* *NANDA I © 2014
Assessment throughout administration: • Assess for desired therapeutic effects (e.g., local or regional area numbness). • Assess vital signs, especially blood pressure (BP) and pulse, if regional block is used. Report a BP less than 90/60, pulse above 100, or per parameters as ordered by the health care provider. • Assess the local or regional area blocked. Expect blanching in a localized area if the local anesthetic contained epinephrine. If a regional area was blocked, periodically assess the ability to move limbs distal to the block. • Assess the level of consciousness if a large regional block was given. Report any increasing drowsiness, dizziness, light-headedness, confusion, or agitation immediately. • Assess for and promptly report adverse effects: bradycardia or tachycardia, hypotension or hypertension, and dyspnea.	

IMPLEMENTATION

Interventions and (Rationales)	Patient-Centered Care
Ensuring therapeutic effects: • Continue assessments as described earlier for therapeutic effects. Assess the localized area for numbness and blanching if the local anesthetic included epinephrine. Assess the ability to move limbs distal to the regional anesthetic. (The duration of anesthetic action will depend on the solution used and whether epinephrine is included in the solution. Epinephrine in the anesthetic solution will constrict localized blood vessels and result in blanching of the area.)	• **Safety:** Teach the patient that the area may be numb for several hours after the procedure is completed. • Teach the patient that it is normal that a slight pressure sensation may remain during anesthesia (e.g., sensation of "tugging" during suturing) but that no pain should be felt. Have the patient alert the health care provider if more than a slight pressure sensation or any pain is noticed during anesthesia. • Teach the patient that it is normal to regain some ability to move limbs (e.g., after epidural anesthetic) before the ability to feel the movement.

Nursing Practice Application *continued*

IMPLEMENTATION	
Interventions and (Rationales)	**Patient-Centered Care**
Minimizing adverse effects:	
• Continue to monitor vital signs, especially BP and pulse, for patients given regional anesthesia. Immediately report a BP below 90/60 or per parameters as ordered by the health care provider, tachycardia or bradycardia, changes in level of consciousness, dyspnea, or decrease in respiratory rate. (Adverse effects of local anesthesia are rare. Regional blocks may cause hypotension with the possibility of reflex tachycardia. **Lifespan:** Be particularly cautious with older adults who are at increased risk for hypotension due to physiologic changes related to aging or concurrent vasoactive drug use. Bradycardia, hypotension, decreased level of consciousness, decreased respiratory rate, and dyspnea may signal that the anesthesia has entered the systemic circulation and is acting as a general anesthetic.)	• Instruct the patient to report any increasing nausea, drowsiness, dizziness, light-headedness, confusion, or anxiety immediately.
• **Diverse Patients:** Continue to monitor hepatic function and drug effects. (Because amide anesthetics such as lidocaine are metabolized through the P450 system, they may result in less than optimal results based on differences in enzymes.)	• Teach ethnically diverse patients to observe and report effects of local anesthetic use to ensure therapeutic results.
• Caution the patient not to eat, chew gum, or drink until the mouth sensation has returned if local (dental) or oral/throat anesthesia has been used. If throat anesthesia was used, assess the gag reflex before eating. (Local anesthetics are effective for up to 3 hours or more. Biting injuries to oral mucous membranes may occur while tissue is numb. Aspiration of food or liquids is possible until the swallowing sensation and gag reflex return.)	• **Safety:** Instruct the patient to refrain from eating or drinking for 1 hour or more postanesthesia or until sensation has completely returned to the oral cavity or throat.
• Monitor motor coordination and/or ambulation post–regional block until certain motor movement is unaffected. **Lifespan:** Be particularly cautious with older adults who are at an increased risk for falls. (Numbness or effects on motor ability post–regional anesthetic may impair movement and increase the risk of falls or injuries.)	• **Safety:** Instruct the patient to call for assistance prior to getting out of bed or attempting to walk alone post–epidural block, and to avoid driving or other activities requiring physical coordination (e.g., regional upper limb block) until the residual effects of the drug are known.
• Assess areas of abrasion, burns, or open wounds if a local anesthetic was applied to the area. (Large, open, or denuded areas may increase the amount of drug absorption into the general circulation. Use sterile technique to apply the drug to open areas.)	• Instruct the patient to report increased redness, swelling, or drainage from open areas under treatment.
• Read all labels carefully before using parenteral solutions. (Solutions containing epinephrine must *never* be used IV or for local anesthesia in areas of decreased circulation [e.g., fingertips, toes, earlobes] due to vasoconstrictive effects.)	• Provide an explanation of desired effects of the local anesthetic and the need for postprocedure monitoring.
• Monitor pain relief in patients post–regional block (e.g., epidural). (Pain sensation will increase as the regional block wears off. Additional pain relief may be required.)	• Teach the patient to report any discomfort or pain as the anesthesia wears off.
Patient understanding of drug therapy:	
• Use opportunities during administration of medications and during assessments to provide patient education. (Using time during nursing care helps to optimize and reinforce key teaching areas.)	• The patient should be able to state the reason for the drug, anticipated sensations, and adverse effects to observe for and when to report them.
Patient self-administration of drug therapy:	
• When administering the medication, instruct the patient, family, or caregiver in proper self-administration of the drug (e.g., take the drug as prescribed when needed). (Using time during nurse administration of these drugs helps to reinforce teaching.)	• Teach the patient to take oral medication (e.g., lidocaine viscous) by swishing and spitting if used for oral cavity or by gargling, and do not swallow unless directed by the health care provider. Apply topical medication in a thin layer to the skin area as directed.

See Table 19.2 for a list of drugs to which these nursing actions apply.

Table 19.3 Stages of General Anesthesia

Stage	Characteristics
1	Loss of pain: The patient loses general sensation but may be awake. This stage proceeds until the patient loses consciousness.
2	Excitement and hyperactivity: The patient may be delirious and try to resist treatment. Heart rate and breathing may become irregular and blood pressure can increase. IV agents are administered here to calm the patient.
3	Surgical anesthesia: Skeletal muscles become paralyzed. Cardiovascular and breathing activities stabilize. Eye movements slow and the patient becomes still.
4	Paralysis of the medulla region in the brain (responsible for controlling respiratory and cardiovascular activity): If breathing or the heart stops, death could result. This stage is usually avoided during general anesthesia.

sedated. Thus, stage 3 anesthesia is called **surgical anesthesia.** When seeking surgical anesthesia, the anesthesiologist will try to move quickly through stage 2 because this stage produces distressing symptoms. Often an IV drug will be given to calm the patient. The stages of general anesthesia are described in Table 19.3.

There are two primary methods of producing general anesthesia. *Intravenous (IV) drugs* are usually administered first because they act within a few seconds. After the patient loses consciousness, *inhaled drugs* are used to maintain the anesthesia. During short surgical procedures or those requiring lower stages of anesthesia, the IV drugs may be used alone.

GENERAL ANESTHETICS

General anesthetics are drugs that rapidly produce unconsciousness and total analgesia. To supplement the effects of a general anesthetic, adjunct drugs are given before, during, and after surgery.

Intravenous Drugs

19.5 Pharmacotherapy With Intravenous General Anesthetics

IV general anesthetics, listed in Table 19.4, are important components of balanced anesthesia. Although occasionally used alone, IV anesthetics are most often

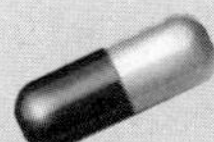

Prototype Drug | Propofol *(Diprivan)*

Therapeutic Class: General anesthetic **Pharmacologic Class:** N-methyl-D-aspartate (NMDA) receptor agonist

Actions and Uses

Propofol has become the most widely used IV anesthetic due to its effectiveness and relative safety profile. Propofol is indicated for the induction and maintenance of general anesthesia. It has almost an immediate onset of action and is used effectively for conscious sedation. Emergence from anesthesia is rapid and few adverse effects occur during recovery. Propofol has an antiemetic effect that can prevent nausea and vomiting.

Administration Alerts

- Compared to standard doses of benzodiazepines and other drugs, propofol may provide faster onset and deeper sedation.
- The drug should be administered only by those who are trained in the administration of general anesthesia.
- Pregnancy category B.

PHARMACOKINETICS

Onset	Peak	Duration
40–60 sec	3–5 min	10–15 min

Adverse Effects

Common adverse effects are pain at the injection site, apnea, respiratory depression, and hypotension. Propofol has been associated with a collection of metabolic abnormalities and organ system failures, referred to as propofol infusion syndrome (PIF). The syndrome is characterized by severe metabolic acidosis, hyperkalemia, lipidemia, rhabdomyolysis, hepatomegaly, and cardiac failure.

Contraindications: Propofol is contraindicated in patients who have a known hypersensitivity reaction to the medication or its emulsion, which contains soybean and egg products. Diprivan injectable emulsion is not recommended for obstetrics, including cesarean section deliveries, or for use in nursing mothers. The drug should be used with caution in patients with cardiac or respiratory impairment.

Interactions

Drug–Drug: The dose of propofol should be reduced in patients receiving preanesthetic medications such as benzodiazepines or opioids. Use with other CNS depressants can cause additive CNS and respiratory depression.

Lab Tests: Unknown.

Herbal/Food: Unknown.

Treatment of Overdose: Overdose will produce cardiac and respiratory depression. Treatment includes mechanical ventilation, increasing the flow rate of IV fluids, and administering vasopressor agents as needed to maintain blood pressure.

Table 19.4 Examples of Intravenous General Anesthetics

Chemical Classification	Drug	General Adverse Effects
Benzodiazepines	diazepam (Valium) lorazepam (Ativan) midazolam (Versed)	*Dizziness, decreased alertness, diminished concentration* Cardiovascular collapse, laryngospasm
Opioids	alfentanil (Alfenta) fentanyl (Sublimaze, others) remifentanil (Ultiva) sufentanil (Sufenta)	*Nausea, gastrointestinal (GI) disturbances* Marked CNS depression
Miscellaneous IV drugs	etomidate (Amidate) ketamine (Ketalar) propofol (Diprivan)	*Dizziness, unsteadiness, dissociation, increased blood pressure and pulse rate, confusion, excitement* Circulatory or respiratory depression with apnea, laryngospasm, anaphylaxis

Note: *Italics* indicate common adverse effects; underlining indicates serious adverse effects.

administered along with inhaled general anesthetics. Concurrent administration of IV and inhaled anesthetics allows the dose of the inhaled agent to be reduced, thus lowering the potential for serious side effects. Also, when IV and inhaled anesthetics are combined, they provide greater analgesia and greater muscle relaxation than could be provided by the inhaled anesthetic alone. If IV anesthetics are administered alone, they are generally reserved for medical procedures that take less than about 15 minutes.

Drugs employed as IV anesthetics include opioids, benzodiazepines, and miscellaneous drugs. Opioids offer the advantage of superior analgesia. Combining the opioid fentanyl (Sublimaze) with the antipsychotic agent droperidol (Inapsine) for example, produces a state known as **neuroleptanalgesia.** In this state, patients are conscious, though insensitive to pain and unconnected with surroundings. The premixed combination of these two agents is marketed as Innovar. A similar conscious, dissociated state is produced with the amnestic drug ketamine (Ketalar).

Inhaled Drugs

19.6 Pharmacotherapy With Inhaled General Anesthetics

Inhaled general anesthetics, listed in Table 19.5, are gases and volatile liquids. These drugs produce their effects by preventing the flow of sodium into neurons in the CNS, thus delaying nerve impulses and producing a dramatic reduction in neural activity. The exact mechanism is not known, although it is likely that gamma-aminobutyric acid (GABA) receptors in the brain are activated. It is not the same mechanism as local anesthetics. There is some inconclusive evidence suggesting that the mechanism may be related to antiseizure drugs. There is no specific receptor that binds to general anesthetics, and they do not appear to affect neurotransmitter release.

Gases

The only gas used routinely for anesthesia is nitrous oxide, commonly called *laughing gas*. Nitrous oxide is used for brief obstetric and surgical procedures and for dental

Table 19.5 Inhaled General Anesthetics

Type	Drug	General Adverse Effects
Gas	nitrous oxide	*Dizziness, drowsiness, nausea, euphoria, vomiting* Apnea, cyanosis
Volatile liquid	desflurane (Suprane) enflurane (Ethrane) isoflurane (Forane) sevoflurane (Sevo, Ultane)	*Drowsiness, nausea, vomiting* Myocardial depression, marked hypotension, pulmonary vasoconstriction, hepatotoxicity, malignant hyperthermia

Note: *Italics* indicate common adverse effects; underlining indicates serious adverse effects.

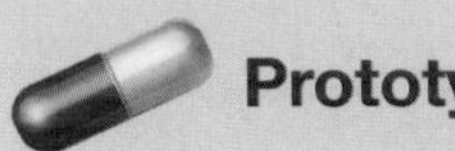

Prototype Drug | Nitrous Oxide

Therapeutic Class: General anesthetic **Pharmacologic Class:** Inhalation gaseous drug

Actions and Uses

The main action of nitrous oxide is analgesia caused by suppression of pain mechanisms in the CNS. This agent has a low potency and does not produce complete loss of consciousness or profound relaxation of skeletal muscle. Because nitrous oxide does not induce surgical anesthesia (stage 3), it is commonly combined with other surgical anesthetic agents. Nitrous oxide is ideal for short surgical or dental procedures because the patient remains conscious and can follow instructions while experiencing full analgesia.

Nitrous oxide is always combined with oxygen (25% to 30%) and is administered in a semiclosed method through a tube or by mask. Nitrous oxide is also used for dental procedures in which the mask is placed over the nose.

Administration Alerts

Establish an IV if one is not already in place in case emergency medications are needed.

PHARMACOKINETICS

Onset	Peak	Duration
–5 min	Less than 10 min	Patients recover from anesthesia rapidly after nitrous oxide is discontinued.

Adverse Effects

When used in low to moderate doses, nitrous oxide produces few adverse effects. At higher doses, patients exhibit some adverse signs of stage 2 anesthesia (see Table 19.3) such as anxiety, excitement, and combativeness. Lowering the inhaled dose will quickly reverse these adverse effects. As nitrous oxide is exhaled, the patient may temporarily have some difficulty breathing at the end of a procedure. Nausea and vomiting following the procedure are more common with nitrous oxide than with other inhalation anesthetics.

Some general anesthetics infrequently produce liver damage. Nitrous oxide has the potential to be abused by users (sometimes medical personnel) who enjoy the relaxed, sedated state that the drug produces.

Contraindications: This drug is contraindicated in patients with an impaired level of consciousness, head injury, inability to comply with instructions, decompression sickness (nitrogen narcosis, air embolism, undiagnosed abdominal pain or marked distention, bowel obstruction, hypotension, shock, chronic obstructive pulmonary disease, cyanosis, chest trauma with pneumothorax, or who are being air transported.

Interactions

Drug–Drug: Sympathomimetics and phosphodiesterase inhibitors may exacerbate dysrhythmias.

Lab Tests: Unknown.

Herbal/Food: Milk thistle taken before and after anesthesia may lower the potential risk of liver damage. Herbal products such as ginger may also provide therapeutic benefit.

Treatment of Overdose: Metoclopramide may help reduce the symptoms of nausea and vomiting associated with inhalation of nitrous oxide.

procedures. It may also be used in conjunction with other general anesthetics, making it possible to decrease other dosages with high effectiveness.

Nitrous oxide should be used cautiously in patients with myasthenia gravis, because it may cause respiratory depression and prolonged hypnotic effects. Patients with cardiovascular disease, especially those with increased intracranial pressure, should be monitored carefully, because hypnotic drug effects may be prolonged or potentiated.

Volatile Liquids

Volatile anesthetics are liquid at room temperature but are converted into a vapor and inhaled to produce their anesthetic effects. Commonly administered volatile agents are desflurane (Suprane) and sevoflurane (Ultane). Some general anesthetics enhance the sensitivity of the heart to drugs such as epinephrine, norepinephrine, dopamine, and serotonin. Volatile liquids have been associated with arrhythmias, some of which may be fatal. Isoflurane (Forane) is featured as the prototype drug in this category. Adverse reactions encountered in the administration of general anesthetics have been respiratory depression, hypotension, and dysrhythmias. Shivering, nausea, vomiting, and obstructive gastrointestinal signs have been observed in the postoperative period. Transient elevations in white blood count have been observed even in the absence of surgical stress. Malignant hyperthermia and elevated carboxyhemoglobin levels are common adverse reactions. The volatile liquids are excreted almost entirely by the lungs through exhalation.

☑ Check Your Understanding 19.1

To improve oxygenation and to prevent secretions from being retained, patients are encouraged to deep breathe following surgery with general anesthetics. Following surgery where inhaled volatile anesthetics were used, why is deep breathing especially essential? *Visit www.pearsonhighered.com/nursingresources for the answer.*

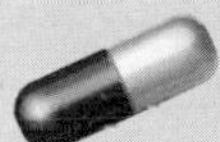

Prototype Drug | Isoflurane *(Forane)*

Therapeutic Class: Inhaled general anesthetic **Pharmacologic Class:** GABA and glutamate receptor agonist

Actions and Uses

Isoflurane produces a potent level of surgical anesthesia that is rapid in onset. It provides the patient with smooth induction with a low degree of metabolism by the body. This drug provides excellent muscle relaxation and may be used off-label as adjuvant therapy in the treatment of status asthmaticus. Isoflurane with oxygen or with an oxygen/nitrous oxide mixture may be used. Compared to other inhaled general anesthetics, cardiac output is well maintained.

Administration Alerts

- Premedication should be selected according to the needs of the patient. Since secretions are weakly stimulated by the use of anticholinergic drugs, premedication is a matter of choice.
- Pregnancy category C.

PHARMACOKINETICS

Onset	Peak	Duration
7–10 min	Rapidly absorbed by the lungs; minimum alveolar concentration values vary with age.	Patients recover from anesthesia in less than 1 hour after the drug is discontinued.

Adverse Effects

Mild nausea, vomiting, and tremor are common adverse effects. The drug produces a dose-dependent respiratory depression and a reduction in blood pressure. Malignant hyperthermia with elevated temperature has been reported.

Contraindications: Patients with a known history of genetic predisposition to malignant hyperthermia should not use isoflurane. Caution should be used when treating patients with head trauma or brain neoplasms due to possible increases in intracranial pressure. Elderly patients are more susceptible to hypotension caused by the drug.

Interactions

Drug–Drug: When isoflurane is used concurrently with nitrous oxide, coughing, breath holding, and laryngospasms may occur. If isoflurane is administered with systemic polymyxin and aminoglycosides, skeletal muscle weakness, respiratory depression, or apnea may occur. Additive effects may occur with isoflurane if administered with other skeletal muscle relaxants. Additive hypotension may result if used concurrently with antihypertensive medications such as beta blockers. Epinephrine, norepinephrine, dopamine, and other adrenergic agonists should be administered with caution due to the possibility of dysrhythmias. Other drugs may cause dysrhythmias including amiodarone, ibutilide, droperidol, and phenothiazines. Levodopa should be discontinued 6 to 8 hours before isoflurane administration.

Lab Tests: Unknown.

Herbal/Food: St. John's wort should be discontinued 2 to 3 weeks prior to administration due to the possible risk of hypotension.

Treatment of Overdose: Since isoflurane causes profound respiratory depression, patients are treated symptomatically until effects of the drug diminish.

Nursing Practice Application

Pharmacotherapy With General Anesthetics

ASSESSMENT	POTENTIAL NURSING DIAGNOSES*
Baseline assessment prior to administration: • Obtain a complete health history including cardiovascular, respiratory, hepatic, renal, or neurologic disease; pregnancy; or breast-feeding. Obtain a drug history including allergies, current prescription and OTC drugs, herbal preparations, caffeine, nicotine, and alcohol use. Be alert to possible drug interactions. • Assess for a previous history of anesthesia and note any significant reactions. Obtain a family history of anesthesia problems, particularly related to the use of neuromuscular blockers (e.g., succinylcholine), or any unusual temperature effects related to surgery.	• *Anxiety* • *Impaired Gas Exchange* • *Ineffective Breathing Pattern* • *Decreased Cardiac Output* • *Nausea,* related to adverse drug effects • *Deficient Knowledge* (drug therapy) • *Risk for Injury* • *Risk for Infection* *NANDA I © 2014

continued

Nursing Practice Application *continued*

ASSESSMENT	POTENTIAL NURSING DIAGNOSES*
• Obtain baseline vital signs, height, and weight. Note the day/hour the patient last ate or drank. • Evaluate laboratory findings appropriate to the procedure (e.g., CBC, electrolytes, hepatic or renal function studies, MRI or CT scan results). • Obtain required preoperative paperwork (e.g., informed consent, completed history and physical). • Administer any preoperative adjunctive drugs (e.g., sedative, analgesic) as ordered. • Assess the level of anxiety and any concerns or questions the patient, family, or caregiver may have. Reinforce preoperative teaching, including deep breathing exercises. Provide the family or caregiver with information on the anticipated length of the procedure, waiting room area, and availability of telephone and eating facilities. • **Lifespan:** When working with pediatric patients, allow parents or the caregiver to stay with the child as long as agency policy permits to decrease patient anxiety. Provide simple explanations of the procedure appropriate for the age of the child. • **Lifespan:** When working with older adults, note assistive devices (e.g., glasses, hearing aids) and remove only when necessary. Give to the family or caregiver, or provide for safekeeping. Ensure that devices are available in the postoperative period. • Initiate an IV access site if required for the procedure. • Assess the patient's ability to receive and understand instruction. Include the family and caregivers as needed.	
Assessment throughout administration: • Assess for desired therapeutic effects (e.g., diminished or loss of consciousness). • Assess vital signs, especially BP and pulse, frequently. Report a BP less than 90/60, pulse above 100, or per parameters as ordered by the health care provider. • Maintain operative sterility throughout the procedure. • Assess the level of consciousness in the postoperative period. Continue frequent monitoring of vital signs and pulse oximetry. • Assess for and promptly report adverse effects: bradycardia or tachycardia, hypotension or hypertension, dyspnea, and rapidly increasing temperature.	

IMPLEMENTATION

Interventions and (Rationales)	Patient-Centered Care
Ensuring therapeutic effects: • Continue assessments as described earlier for therapeutic effects. Provide for patient safety during the preoperative and operative periods and assess the level of consciousness, vital signs, and return of motor and sensory sensation postoperatively. (The duration of anesthetic action will depend on the drugs used and adjunctive or reversal agents used.)	• Provide a quiet environment postoperatively and frequently orient the patient to the postoperative recovery unit.
• Assess for shivering in the postoperative period and provide additional blankets or warmth as needed. (General anesthetics depress the CNS and some autonomic activity. As autonomic activity returns, shivering is common. Warm blankets provide comfort during this period.)	• Continue to orient the patient in the postoperative period and allay anxiety about shivering.

Nursing Practice Application *continued*

IMPLEMENTATION	
Interventions and (Rationales)	**Patient-Centered Care**
Minimizing adverse effects: • Continue to monitor vital signs frequently, including temperature. Report a BP below 90/60 or per parameters as ordered by the health care provider, tachycardia or significant bradycardia, or dyspnea. Report any increase in temperature immediately. (CNS depression will cause decreases in all vital signs but significant bradycardia, hypotension, decreased respiratory rate, or dyspnea should be reported promptly. **Lifespan:** The older adult is more sensitive to the effects of anesthesia and may be more likely to experience adverse effects such as hypotension and delirium. Malignant hyperthermia associated with anesthetics is a rare but potentially fatal adverse effect, and any increase in temperature above the preoperative baseline should be reported immediately.)	• Provide an explanation for all procedures and monitoring to the patient.
• Provide adequate pain relief in the immediate postoperative period. (General anesthetics do not necessarily provide analgesia, depending on the agent. Adequate pain relief begins ideally in the preoperative period. Assess for nonverbal signs of pain such as restlessness or grimacing as the patient regains consciousness.)	• Encourage the patient to request pain medication as able. Assure the patient, family, or caregiver that pain needs will be frequently monitored.
• Encourage the patient to take deep breaths and move the lower extremities frequently in the postoperative period. (General anesthetics given by inhalation are excreted via the lungs. Deep breathing assists in removing the remaining anesthetic. Early range-of-motion exercises may help prevent venous thrombosis and complications.)	• Teach the patient deep breathing exercises in the preoperative period and that early movement of the legs will be encouraged in the early postoperative period, unless otherwise ordered by the provider.
• Frequently orient the patient to the surroundings, day, and time, and maintain a safe environment. (During the period of anesthesia, consciousness is lost along with the ability to orient to day, time, and person. Confusion related to these effects in the postoperative period is common. Use of safety measures such as side rails and soft restraints may be necessary until the patient regains consciousness.)	• Continue to orient the patient frequently and explain all procedures.
• For patients receiving ketamine and other drugs causing neuroleptanalgesia, provide a quiet, calm environment postprocedure. Avoid overstimulating the patient during vital signs, using a soft touch and explanations of all procedures done. (During recovery from neuroleptanalgesia drugs, confusion and misinterpretation of sensory stimulation may cause extreme anxiety, fear, or paranoia. Keep all stimuli to a minimum until the patient regains full consciousness.)	• Explain the full procedure and required postprocedural care to the patient, family, or caregiver. Alert the family or caregiver that visiting may be restricted during the immediate recovery period in order to minimize sensory stimulation.
• Continue to monitor hepatic function. (**Lifespan:** Normal physiologic changes related to aging may increase the risk of toxicity in the older adult requiring drugs with hepatic metabolism).	• Provide an explanation for all procedures and for monitoring to the patient.
• **Diverse Patients**: Monitor for therapeutic and adverse effects frequently in ethnically diverse patients. (Because drugs such as fentanyl and midazolam are metabolized through the P450 system, they may result in less than optimal results based on differences in enzymes.)	• Teach ethnically diverse patients to continue to observe and report unusual effects of the general anesthetic after discharge, such as prolonged drowsiness, restlessness, or confusion.
Patient understanding of drug therapy: • Use opportunities during the preoperative period to provide patient education when the patient is alert, or to the family or caregiver. (Using time during nursing care helps to optimize and reinforce key teaching areas.)	• The patient, family, or caregiver should be able to state the reason for the drug(s), anticipated sensations, and adverse effects to observe for and when to report them.

See Tables 19.4 and 19.5 for lists of drugs to which these nursing actions apply.

ADJUNCTS TO ANESTHESIA

Many drugs are used either to complement the effects of general anesthetics or to treat anticipated side effects of the anesthesia. Some of these agents, listed in Table 19.6, are called *adjuncts* to anesthesia. They may be given prior to, during, or after surgery.

19.7 Drugs as Adjuncts to Surgery

Preoperative drugs are given to relieve anxiety and to provide mild sedation. Anticholinergics such as atropine may be administered to dry secretions and to suppress the bradycardia caused by some anesthetics. Sedative–hypnotic drugs (benzodiazepines) help reduce fear, anxiety, or pain associated with the surgery. Opioids such as morphine may be given to counteract pain that the patient will experience post-surgery.

Neuromuscular Blockers

During surgery, the primary adjunctive agents are the **neuromuscular blockers** (see chapter 21). Neuromuscular blockades cause paralysis without loss of consciousness, which means that without a general anesthetic, patients would be awake and without the ability to move. Remember, breathing muscles are skeletal muscle. This is why patients require intubation and mechanical ventilation. Administration of these drugs also allows a reduced amount of general anesthetic. The following important patient monitoring steps are necessary:

- Baseline neurologic assessment should be performed before neuromuscular blocking drugs are administered.
- Dosage of the neuromuscular blocking drugs should be maintained by using *peripheral nerve stimulation* during the surgical procedure.
- To ensure adequate sedation and continued need for neuromuscular blockade, the nurse and health care staff should monitor the patient during the entire surgery.
- Neuromuscular blockade should be discontinued after surgery and as soon as it is clinically possible.
- Monitor for malignant hyperthermia signs; if triggered, progressive hypermetabolic reactions with sustained muscle contractions could develop with devastating consequences.
- Postneurologic evaluation and continued patient monitoring are necessary steps after surgery is completed.

Table 19.6 Selected Adjuncts to General Anesthesia

Chemical Classification	Drug	Indications
PREOPERATIVE		
Anticholinergic	atropine	General anesthesia as a premedication, in emergency situations or during surgery to increase heart rate and to reverse the effects of some cholinergic drugs
Benzodiazepine	midazolam (Versed)	Generally used before other IV agents for induction of anesthesia
Dopamine blocker	droperidol (Inapsine)	Nausea and vomiting caused by opioids; reduces anxiety and relaxes muscles
Opioids	alfentanil (Alfenta)	Short duration; for induction of anesthesia when endotracheal or mechanical ventilation is needed; provides analgesia
	fentanyl (Actiq, Duragesic, Sublimaze, others); fentanyl/droperidol (Innovar)	Analgesia during or after anesthesia
	morphine	Analgesia during or after anesthesia
	remifentanil (Ultiva)	Analgesia during or after anesthesia; shorter duration of action than fentanyl
	sufentanil (Sufenta)	Primary anesthesia or to provide analgesia during or after anesthesia
DURING SURGERY		
Neuromuscular blockers	mivacurium (Mivacron)	Short duration muscle paralysis; nondepolarizing-type muscle relaxation
	rocuronium (Zemuron)	Intermediate duration muscle paralysis; nondepolarizing-type muscle relaxation
	succinylcholine (Anectine, Quelicin)	Short duration muscle paralysis; depolarizing-type muscle relaxation
	tubocurarine	Long duration muscle paralysis; nondepolarizing-type muscle relaxation
POSTOPERATIVE		
Cholinergic	bethanechol (Urecholine)	Relief of constipation and urinary retention caused by opioids; stimulates GI motility
Phenothiazine	promethazine (Phenazine, Phenergan, others)	Nausea and vomiting caused by obstetric sedation and anesthesia
Serotonin blocker	ondansetron (Zofran, Zuplenz)	Nausea and vomiting caused by cancer chemotherapy, radiation therapy, and surgery

Note: *Italics* indicate common adverse effects; underlining indicates serious adverse effects.

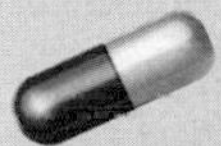

Prototype Drug | Succinylcholine *(Anectine, Quelicin)*

Therapeutic Class: Skeletal muscle paralytic drug; neuromuscular blocker
Pharmacologic Class: Depolarizing blocker; acetylcholine receptor blocking drug

Actions and Uses

Like the natural neurotransmitter acetylcholine, succinylcholine acts on cholinergic receptor sites at neuromuscular junctions. At first, depolarization occurs, and skeletal muscles contract. After repeated contractions, however, the membrane is unable to repolarize as long as the drug stays attached to the receptor. Effects are first noted as muscle weakness and muscle spasms. Eventually, paralysis occurs. Succinylcholine is rapidly broken down by the enzyme cholinesterase; when the IV infusion is stopped, the duration of action is only a few minutes. Use of succinylcholine reduces the amount of general anesthetic needed for procedures. Dantrolene (Dantrium) is a drug used preoperatively or postoperatively to reduce the signs of malignant hyperthermia in susceptible patients.

Administration Alerts

- Pregnancy category C.

PHARMACOKINETICS

Onset	Peak	Duration
0.5–1 min IV; 2–3 min IM	Variable within minutes	2–3 min IV; 10–30 min IM

Adverse Effects

Succinylcholine can cause complete paralysis of the diaphragm and intercostal muscles; thus, mechanical ventilation is necessary during surgery. Bradycardia and respiratory depression are expected adverse effects. If doses are high, the ganglia are affected, causing tachycardia, hypotension, and urinary retention.

Patients with certain genetic defects may experience a rapid onset of extremely high fever with muscle rigidity—a serious condition known as malignant hyperthermia. Succinylcholine should be employed with caution in patients with fractures or muscle spasms, because the initial muscle fasciculations may cause additional trauma. Neuromuscular blockade may be prolonged in patients with hypokalemia, hypocalcemia, or low plasma pseudocholinesterase levels.

Black Box Warning: Succinylcholine should be administered in a facility with trained personnel to monitor, assist, and control respiration. Cardiac arrest has been reported resulting from hyperkalemic rhabdomyolysis most frequently in infants or children with undiagnosed skeletal muscle myopathy or Duchenne's muscular dystrophy. This drug is reserved for use in children in cases of emergency intubation or in instances when immediate securing of airway is necessary.

Contraindications: Succinylcholine should be used with extreme caution in patients with severe burns or trauma, neuromuscular diseases, or glaucoma. Succinylcholine is contraindicated in patients with a family history of malignant hyperthermia or conditions of pulmonary, renal, cardiovascular, metabolic, or hepatic dysfunction.

Interactions

Drug–Drug: Additive skeletal muscle blockade will occur if succinylcholine is given concurrently with clindamycin, aminoglycosides, furosemide, lithium, quinidine, or lidocaine. The effect of succinylcholine may be increased if given concurrently with phenothiazines, oxytocin, promazine, tacrine, or thiazide diuretics. The effect of succinylcholine is decreased if given with diazepam.

If this drug is given concurrently with nitrous oxide, an increased risk of bradycardia, dysrhythmias, sinus arrest, apnea, and malignant hyperthermia exists. If succinylcholine is given concurrently with cardiac glycosides, there is increased risk of cardiac dysrhythmias. If narcotics are given concurrently with succinylcholine, there is increased risk of bradycardia and sinus arrest.

Lab Tests: Unknown.

Herbal/Food: Unknown.

Treatment of Overdose: Treatment may involve drug therapy for the following symptoms: weakness, lack of coordination, watery eyes and mouth, tremors, and seizures. Problems with breathing require emergency medical measures.

Neuromuscular blocking agents are classified as *depolarizing* blockers or *nondepolarizing* blockers. The only depolarizing blocker is succinylcholine (Anectine, Quelicin), which works by binding to acetylcholine receptors at neuromuscular junctions to cause total skeletal muscle paralysis. Malignant hyperthermia may be produced when succinylcholine is used during surgery; therefore, precautions should be taken. As with general anesthetics, Dantrolene (Dantrium) is used to reduce the signs of malignant hyperthermia in susceptible patients. One indication for succinylcholine is for ease of tracheal intubation. Mivacurium (Mivacron), a short acting nondepolarizing blocker is rarely used but is mentioned here due to historical interest. Tubocurarine, also rarely used, is a longer-acting neuromuscular blocker. Rocuronium (Zemuron) is routinely indicated for outpatients as an adjunct to general anesthesia for skeletal muscle relaxation during surgery or for mechanical ventilation. Rocuronium may be used to facilitate tracheal intubation. The nondepolarizing blockers compete with acetylcholine for cholinergic receptors at the neuromuscular junction. Once attached to cholinergic receptors, the nonpolarizing blockers have the same general action as the depolarizing blockers—muscle paralysis.

Postoperative drugs include analgesics for pain and antiemetics such as promethazine (Phenergan, others) for the nausea and vomiting that sometimes occurs during recovery from anesthesia. Occasionally following surgery a parasympathomimetic such as bethanechol (Urecholine) is administered to stimulate the urinary tract and smooth muscle of the bowel to begin peristalsis. Bethanechol is featured as a prototype drug in chapter 12.

Chapter Review

KEY Concepts

The numbered key concepts provide a succinct summary of the important points from the corresponding numbered section within the chapter. If any of these points are not clear, refer to the numbered section within the chapter for review.

19.1 Regional loss of sensation is achieved by administering local anesthetics topically or through the infiltration, nerve block, spinal, or epidural routes.

19.2 Local anesthetics act by blocking sodium channels in neurons. Epinephrine is sometimes added to prolong the duration of anesthetic action.

19.3 Local anesthetics are classified as amides or esters. The amides, such as lidocaine (Xylocaine), have largely replaced the esters because they have fewer averse effects and a longer duration of action.

19.4 General anesthesia produces a complete loss of sensation accompanied by loss of consciousness, memory, and body movement. Four stages of general anesthesia are (1) loss of pain; (2) excitement and hyperactivity; (3) surgical anesthesia; and (4) respiratory and cardiovascular paralysis.

19.5 IV anesthetics are used alone, for short procedures, or in combination with inhalation anesthetics.

19.6 Inhaled general anesthetics are used to maintain surgical anesthesia. Some, such as nitrous oxide, have low efficacy, whereas others, such as isoflurane (Forane), can induce deep anesthesia.

19.7 Numerous nonanesthetic medications, including antianxiety drugs, opioids, and neuromuscular blockers are administered as adjuncts to surgery. Important patient monitoring steps are necessary.

REVIEW Questions

1. The patient received lidocaine viscous before a gastroscopy was performed. Which of the following would be a priority for the nurse to assess during the postprocedural period?

1. Return of gag reflex
2. Ability to urinate
3. Leg pain
4. Ability to stand

2. A young patient requires suturing of a laceration to the right forearm and the provider will use lidocaine (Xylocaine) with epinephrine as the local anesthetic prior to the procedure. Why is epinephrine included in the lidocaine for this patient?

1. It will increase vasodilation at the site of the laceration.
2. It will prevent hypotension.
3. It will ensure that infection risk is minimized postsuturing.
4. It will prolong anesthetic action at the site.

3. The patient who is scheduled to have a minor in-office surgical procedure will receive nitrous oxide and expresses concern to the nurse that the procedure will hurt. Which of the following would be the nurse's best response?
   1. "You may feel pain during the procedure but you won't remember any of it."
   2. "You will be unconscious the entire time and won't feel any pain."
   3. "You will not feel any pain during the procedure because the drug blocks the pain signals."
   4. "You will feel pain but you won't perceive it the same way; that's why it's called 'laughing gas.'"
4. The patient returns to the postanesthesia recovery unit (PACU) for observation and recovery following surgery with a general anesthetic. Which of the following assessment findings may the nurse expect to find during this recovery period? (Select all that apply.)
   1. Bradycardia
   2. Severe headache
   3. Hypertension
   4. Respiratory depression
   5. Urinary frequency
5. A patient is admitted to the postanesthesia recovery unit (PACU) after receiving ketamine (Ketalar) after his minor orthopedic surgery. What is the most appropriate nursing action in the recovery period for this patient?
   1. Frequently orient the patient to time, place, and person.
   2. Keep the patient in a bright environment so there is less drowsiness.
   3. Frequently assess the patient for sensory deprivation.
   4. Place the patient in a quiet area of the unit with low lights and away from excessive noise.
6. A patient has received succinylcholine (Anectine, Quelicin) along with the general anesthetic in surgery. Which of the following abnormal findings in the recovery period should be reported immediately to the provider?
   1. Temperature 38.9°C (102°F)
   2. Heart rate 56
   3. Blood pressure 92/58
   4. Respiratory rate 15

PATIENT-FOCUSED Case Study

Rob Valetti is a 28-year-old steelworker for a heating and cooling company. While on the job he cut his right hand with a piece of steel for an air-conditioning vent. He is admitted to the emergency department for sutures to the right middle and ring fingers, and palm. The laceration will be anesthetized with lidocaine prior to suturing.

1. What is the action of lidocaine?
2. Why do some solutions of lidocaine contain epinephrine?
3. As the nurse, what post-procedure instructions will you give Rob?

CRITICAL THINKING Questions

1. An older adult patient, age 77, is scheduled for an open reduction with internal fixation of the right hip for a fracture. When preparing the postoperative care plan, what should be included for this patient in the immediate postoperative recovery period?
2. A patient who has a history of cardiac dysrhythmias returns from surgery during which the patient received isoflurane (Forane) as a general anesthetic. What adverse effect of isoflurane might occur related to this patient's past medical history? What priority assessment data will the nurse gather in the recovery period related to this?

Visit www.pearsonhighered.com/nursingresources for answers and rationales for all activities.

REFERENCES

Chan, M. T. V., Cheng. B. C. P., Lee. T. M. C., & Gin, T. (2013). BIS-guided anesthesia decreases postoperative delirium and cognitive decline. *Journal of Neurosurgical Anesthesiology, 25,* 33–42. doi:10:1097/ANA.0b013e3182712fba

Herdman, T. H., & Kamitsuru, S. (Eds.). (2014). *NANDA International nursing diagnoses: Definitions and classification, 2015–2017.* Oxford, United Kingdom: Wiley-Blackwell.

Riedel, B., Browne, K., & Silbert, B. (2014). Cerebral protection: Inflammation, endothelial dysfunction, and postoperative cognitive dysfunction. *Current Opinion in Anaesthesiology, 27,* 89–97. doi:10.1097/ACO.0000000000000032

SELECTED BIBLIOGRAPHY

Brown, E. N., Purdon, P. L., & Van Dort, C. J. (2011). General anesthesia and altered states of arousal: A systems neuroscience analysis. *Annual Review of Neuroscience, 34,* 601–628. doi:10.1146/annurev-neuro-060909-153200

Derry, S., Wiffen, P. J., Moore, R. A., & Quinlan, J. (2014). Topical lidocaine for neuropathic pain in adults. *Cochrane Database of Systematic Reviews, 7,* Art. No.: CD010958. doi:10.1002/14651858.CD010958.pub2

History of Anesthaesia Society. (n.d.). *Timeline of important dates and events in the development of anaesthesia.* Retrieved from http://www.histansoc.org.uk/timeline.html

Humble, S. R., Dalton, A. J., & Li, L. (2014). A systematic review of therapeutic interventions to reduce acute and chronic post-surgical pain after amputation, thoracotomy or mastectomy. *European Journal of Pain, 19, 451–465.* doi:10.1002/ejp.567

Kye, Y. C., Rhee, J. E., Kim, K., Kim, T., Jo, Y. H., Jeong, J. H., & Lee, J. H. (2012). Clinical effects of adjunctive atropine during ketamine sedation in pediatric emergency patients. *The American Journal of Emergency Medicine, 30,* 1981–1985. doi:10.1016/j. ajem.2012.04.030

Persson, J. (2013). Ketamine in pain management. *CNS Neuroscience & Therapeutics, 19,* 396–402. doi:10.1111/cns.12111

Reed, K. L., Malamed, S. F., & Fonner, A. M. (2012). Local anesthesia part 2: Technical considerations. *Anesthesia Progress, 59* (3), 127–137. doi:10.2344/0003-3006-59.3.127

Theanesthesiaconsultant Blog. (2015). *The obese patient and anesthesia.* Retrieved from http://theanesthesiaconsultant.com/2013/03/07/anesthesia-facts-for-non-medical-people-obesity-and-anesthesia/

To, D., Kossintseva, I., & de Gannes, G. (2014). Lidocaine contact allergy is becoming more prevalent. *Dermatologic Surgery, 40,* 1367–1372. doi:10.1097/DSS.0000000000000190

Weinberg, G. (n.d.). *LipidRescue™ resuscitation for drug toxicity,* . Retrieved from http://lipidrescue.org/

Chapter 20

Drugs for Degenerative Diseases of the Nervous System

Drugs at a Glance

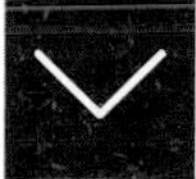

Learning Outcomes

After reading this chapter, the student should be able to:

1. Identify the most common degenerative diseases of the central nervous system.
2. Describe symptoms of Parkinson's disease.
3. Explain the neurochemical basis for Parkinson's disease, focusing on the roles of dopamine and acetylcholine in the brain.
4. Describe the nurse's role in the pharmacologic management of Parkinson's disease and Alzheimer's disease.
5. Describe symptoms of Alzheimer's disease and explain theories about why these symptoms develop.
6. Explain the goals of pharmacotherapy for Alzheimer's disease and the efficacy of existing medications.
7. Describe the signs and basis for development of multiple sclerosis symptoms.
8. Categorize drugs used in the treatment of Alzheimer's disease, Parkinson's disease, and multiple sclerosis based on their classification and mechanism of action.
9. For each of the drug classes listed in Drugs at a Glance, know representative drug examples, and explain their mechanisms of action, primary action, and important adverse effects.
10. Use the nursing process to care for patients receiving pharmacotherapy for degenerative diseases of the central nervous system.

indicates a prototype drug, each of which is featured in a Prototype Drug box.

Table 20.2 Drugs for Parkinson's Disease

Drug	Route and Adult Dose (max dose where indicated)	Adverse Effects
DOPAMINE AGONISTS AND RELATED DRUGS		
amantadine (Symmetrel)	PO: 100 mg one to two times/day	*Skin irritation, dizziness, light-headedness, difficulty concentrating, confusion, anxiety, headache, sleep dysfunction, weight loss, fatigue, nausea, vomiting, constipation, orthostatic hypotension, choreiform and involuntary movements, dystonia, dyskinesia* Acute myocardial infarction (MI), shock, neuroleptic malignant syndrome, hallucinations, agranulocytosis, depression with suicidal tendencies, EPS, fulminant liver failure, severe hepatocellular injury, hallucinations with higher doses of levodopa
apomorphine	Subcutaneous: 2 mg for the first dose (max: 6 mg)	
bromocriptine (Parlodel)	PO: 1.25–2.5 mg/day up to 100 mg/day in divided doses	
levodopa-carbidopa (Parcopa, Sinemet)	PO: 1 tablet containing 10 mg carbidopa/100 mg levodopa or 25 mg carbidopa/100 mg levodopa tid (max: 6 tabs/day)	
levodopa-carbidopa-entacapone (Stalevo)	PO: 500 mg–1 g/day; may be increased by 100–750 mg every 3–7 days	
pramipexole (Mirapex)	PO: Start with 0.125 mg tid for 1 wk and gradually increase to a target dose of 1.5 mg tid	
ropinirole (Requip)	PO: Start with 0.25 mg tid and gradually increase to a target dose of 1 mg tid	
rotigotine transdermal system (Neupro)	Transdermal patch: Applied once per day to clean, dry, intact healthy skin on the front of the abdomen, thigh, hip, flank, shoulder, or upper arm.	
MAO-B INHIBITORS AND OTHER ENZYME-INHIBITING DRUGS		
entacapone (Comtan)	PO: 200 mg given with levodopa-carbidopa up to eight times/day	*Nausea, vomiting, cramps, heartburn, headache, joint pain, muscle pain, dry mouth, insomnia, mental confusion, constipation, gastric upset, mouth sores* Hallucinations, hepatotoxicity, seizures, convulsions, sudden numbness
rasagiline (Azilect)	PO: 0.5–1 mg once daily	
selegiline (Eldepryl, Zelapar)	PO: 5 mg/dose bid (max: 10 mg/day)	
tolcapone (Tasmar)	PO: 100 mg tid (max: 600 mg/day)	

Note: *Italics* indicate common adverse effects; underlining indicates serious adverse effects.

disorder, symptoms may be dramatically reduced in some patients.

Antiparkinson's drugs are given to restore the balance of dopamine and acetylcholine in specific regions of the brain. This balance may be achieved by either increasing the levels of dopamine (dopamine agonists and monoamine oxidase-B inhibitors [MAO-B inhibitors]) or by inhibiting the excitatory actions of acetylcholine (cholinergic blockers). Drugs for PD are listed in Table 20.2.

Dopamine Agonists and MAO-B Inhibitors

Dopamine agonists stimulate dopamine receptors. MAO-B inhibitors help to block the enzymatic breakdown of dopamine within nerve terminals. Both drug classes are core treatments in PD and slow the progression of debilitating symptoms.

20.3 Treating Parkinson's Disease With Dopamine-Enhancing Drugs

Drug therapy for PD attempts to restore the functional balance of dopamine and acetylcholine in the corpus striatum of the brain. Dopamine-enhancing drugs are used to increase dopamine levels in this region. As shown in Pharmacotherapy Illustrated 20.1, levodopa is a precursor of dopamine synthesis. Supplying it directly leads to increased biosynthesis of dopamine within the nerve terminals. Whereas levodopa can cross the blood–brain barrier, dopamine cannot; thus, dopamine itself is not useful for therapy. The effectiveness of levodopa is "boosted" by combining it with carbidopa. Without carbidopa, only 1% of a dose of levodopa reaches the CNS. This combination, marketed as Parcopa or Sinemet, makes more levodopa available to enter the CNS. If the fixed dose combination of levodopa-carbidopa does not give satisfactory therapeutic results, "extra" carbidopa (Lodosyn) can be administered. In 2015 the FDA approved two other formulations of levodopa-carbidopa. Rytary is an extended-release capsule that allows for once daily dosing, and Duopa is an enteral suspension administered through a gastrostomy tube.

Other approaches to enhancing dopamine are used in treating PD. Apomorphine (Apokyn), bromocriptine (Parlodel), pramipexole (Mirapex), and ropinirole (Requip) directly activate the dopamine receptor and are called *dopamine agonists. Rotigotine (Neupro)* is a dopamine agonist that is used to treat the signs and symptoms of idiopathic PD and moderate-to-severe restless leg syndrome. *Neupro* is a transdermal delivery system that provides *rotigotine* continuously over a 24-hour period. This patch can be used alone or with other medications. Amantadine (Symmetrel), an antiviral agent with limited efficacy, causes the release of dopamine from nerve terminals.

Complementary and Alternative Therapies

GINKGO BILOBA FOR DEMENTIA

The seeds and leaves of ginkgo biloba have been used in traditional Chinese medicine for thousands of years. The seeds of the plant contain a toxic substance and a standardized extract of the leaves are used. The tree is planted throughout the world, including the United States. In Western medicine, the focus has been on treating depression and memory loss.

Ginkgo has been claimed to improve mental functioning and slow the dementia characteristic of Alzheimer's disease. The mechanism of action seems to be related to increasing the blood supply to the brain by dilating blood vessels, decreasing the viscosity of the blood, and modifying the neurotransmitter system. As with research with other herbals, most research into the usefulness of ginkgo suffers from lack of consistent control groups and small numbers of participants. Recent studies have suggested that ginkgo may stabilize or slow the decline in mental functioning in patients with cognitive impairment or dementia, and there appears to be a protective effect that gingko provides against the cellular apoptosis (Jahanshahi, Nickmahzar, & Babakordi, 2013; Solfrizzi & Panza, 2015). Ginkgo exhibits a relatively low incidence of side effects, with nausea, gastrointestinal (GI) upset, diarrhea, headache, and dizziness being the most common (National Center for Complementary and Integrative Health, 2013). Gingko may increase the risk of bleeding and patients taking anticoagulants or planning surgical or dental procedures should alert their provider if they use gingko.

Pharmacotherapy Illustrated

20.1 | Antiparkinson Drugs Restore Dopamine Function and Block Cholinergic Activity in the Nigrostriatal Pathway

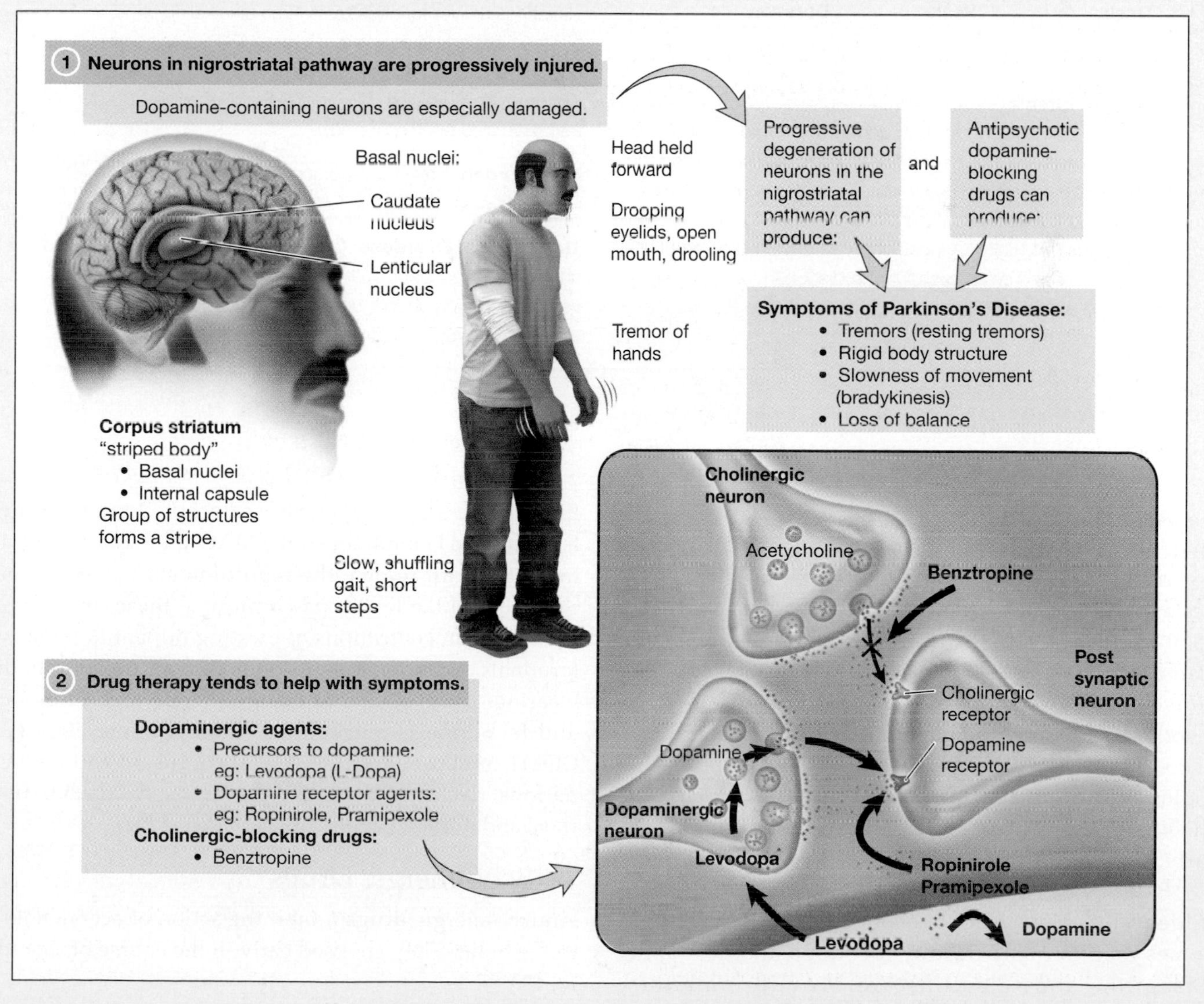

1 Neurons in nigrostriatal pathway are progressively injured.
Dopamine-containing neurons are especially damaged.
Basal nuclei:
Caudate nucleus
Lenticular nucleus
Corpus striatum
"striped body"
• Basal nuclei
• Internal capsule
Group of structures forms a stripe.
Head held forward
Drooping eyelids, open mouth, drooling
Tremor of hands
Slow, shuffling gait, short steps
Progressive degeneration of neurons in the nigrostriatal pathway can produce:
and
Antipsychotic dopamine-blocking drugs can produce:
Symptoms of Parkinson's Disease:
• Tremors (resting tremors)
• Rigid body structure
• Slowness of movement (bradykinesis)
• Loss of balance
2 Drug therapy tends to help with symptoms.
Dopaminergic agents:
• Precursors to dopamine: eg: Levodopa (L-Dopa)
• Dopamine receptor agents: eg: Ropinirole, Pramipexole
Cholinergic-blocking drugs:
• Benztropine
Cholinergic neuron
Acetycholine
Benztropine
Post synaptic neuron
Cholinergic receptor
Dopamine receptor
Dopamine
Dopaminergic neuron
Levodopa
Ropinirole
Pramipexole
Levodopa
Dopamine

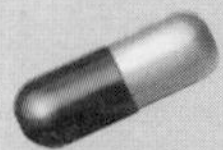

Prototype Drug | Levodopa, Carbidopa, and Entacapone *(Stalevo)*

Therapeutic Class: Antiparkinson drug

Pharmacologic Class: Dopamine precursor; dopamine-enhancing drug combination

Actions and Uses

Stalevo restores the neurotransmitter dopamine in extrapyramidal areas of the brain, thus relieving some Parkinson's symptoms, especially tremor, bradykinesia, gait, and muscle rigidity. To increase its effect, levodopa is combined with two other drugs, carbidopa and entacapone, which prevent its enzymatic breakdown. Several months may be needed to achieve maximum therapeutic effects.

Administration Alerts

- The patient may be unable to self-administer medication and may need assistance.
- Administer exactly as ordered.
- Abrupt withdrawal of the drug can result in Parkinson's-like symptoms or neuroleptic malignant syndrome (NMS).
- Pregnancy category C.

PHARMACOKINETICS

Onset	Peak	Duration
Less than 30 min	1–2 h	Variable

Adverse Effects

Side effects of Stalevo include uncontrolled and purposeless movements such as extending the fingers and shrugging the shoulders, involuntary movements, loss of appetite, nausea, and vomiting. Muscle twitching and spasmodic winking are early signs of toxicity. Orthostatic hypotension is common in some patients. The drug should be discontinued gradually, because abrupt withdrawal can produce acute Parkinson's-like symptoms.

Contraindications: Stalevo is contraindicated in the treatment of narrow-angle glaucoma. This drug is contraindicated in patients with suspicious pigmented lesions or a history of melanoma. This medication should be avoided in cases of acute psychoses and severe psychoneurosis within 2 weeks of therapy with monoamine oxidase inhibitors (MAOIs).

Interactions

Drug–Drug: Stalevo interacts with many drugs. Haloperidol taken concurrently may antagonize the therapeutic effects of Stalevo. Methyldopa may increase toxicity. Antihypertensives may cause increased hypotensive effects. Anticonvulsants may decrease the therapeutic effects of Stalevo. Antacids containing magnesium, calcium, or sodium bicarbonate may increase Stalevo absorption, which could lead to toxicity. Pyridoxine reverses the antiparkinson effects of Stalevo.

Lab Tests: Abnormalities in laboratory tests may include elevations of liver function tests such as alkaline phosphatase, aspartate aminotransferase (AST), alanine aminotransferase (ALT), lactic dehydrogenase, and bilirubin. Abnormalities in blood urea nitrogen and positive Coombs' test have also been reported.

Herbal/Food: Kava may worsen the symptoms of Parkinson's.

Treatment of Overdose: General supportive measures should be taken along with immediate gastric lavage. Intravenous (IV) fluids should be administered judiciously, and an adequate airway should be maintained.

A few studies have focused on dopamine agonists as an adjunctive line of treatment for PD. Studies have purported that ropinirole (Requip) delays the onset of dyskinesia better than additional doses of levodopa carbidopa combination drugs. Patients taking ropinirole alone may also experience less progressive dyskinesia symptoms. However, in terms of ADLs, most have reported that levodopa-carbidopa combination drugs may control motor symptoms better. Pramipexole (Mirapex) and ropinirole (Requip) have proven to be safe and effective for the initial sole therapy and when combined with carbidopa-levodopa.

Entacapone (Comtan), rasagiline (Azilect), selegiline (Eldepryl, Zelapar), and tolcapone (Tasmar) inhibit enzymes that normally destroy levodopa and dopamine. Rasagiline and selegiline are MAO-B inhibitors. Entacapone and tolcapone are catechol-O-methyl transferase (COMT) inhibitors. Like MAO-B inhibitors, COMT inhibitors can reduce the requirements for levodopa-carbidopa. Like levodopa-carbidopa, these drugs have increased concentrations of existing dopamine in nerve terminals and improve motor fluctuations relating to the wearing-off effect. Entacapone combined with carbidopa and levodopa is marketed as Stalevo. Side effects of COMT inhibitors include mental confusion and hallucinations, nausea and vomiting, cramps, headache, diarrhea, and possible liver damage.

Anticholinergic Drugs

Anticholinergic drugs inhibit the action of acetylcholine in the brain. They are used early in the course of therapy for PD.

Table 20.3 Anticholinergic Drugs and Drugs With Anticholinergic Activity Used for Parkinson's Disease

Drug	Route and Adult Dose (max dose where indicated)	Adverse Effects
benztropine (Cogentin)	PO: 0.5–1 mg/day; gradually increase as needed (max: 6 mg/day)	*Sedation, nausea, constipation, dry mouth, blurred vision, drowsiness, dizziness, tachycardia, hypotension, confusion, nervousness*
biperiden (Akineton)	PO: 2 mg one to four times/day	<u>Paralytic ileus, cardiovascular collapse, loss of balance, hallucinations</u>
diphenhydramine (Benadryl) (see page 645 for the Prototype Drug box)	PO: 25–50 mg tid–qid (max: 300 mg/day)	
trihexyphenidyl (Artane)	PO: 1 mg on day 1; 2 mg on day 2; then increase by 2 mg every 3–5 days up to 6–10 mg/day (max: 15 mg/day)	

Note: *Italics* indicate common adverse effects; <u>underlining</u> indicates serious adverse effects.
For the complete nursing process applied to anticholinergic therapy, see Nursing Practice Application: Pharmacotherapy With Anticholinergic Drugs, in chapter 12.

20.4 Treating Parkinson's Disease With Anticholinergic Drugs

Another approach to changing the balance between dopamine and acetylcholine in the brain is to give cholinergic blockers, or anticholinergic drugs. By blocking the effect of acetylcholine, anticholinergics inhibit the overactivity of this neurotransmitter in the corpus striatum, thus allowing dopamine to exert more influence in this region. These drugs, which help to control tremors and restlessness are listed in Table 20.3. The student should review chapter 12 for a complete discussion of the actions and side effects of anticholinergics.

Anticholinergics such as atropine were the first drugs used to treat tremors and uncontrolled muscle movements caused by PD. The large number of peripheral adverse effects has limited the uses of this drug class. The anticholinergics now used for treatment of Parkinson's-like symptoms are centrally acting, and they produce fewer side effects. Autonomic effects such as dry mouth, blurred vision, tachycardia, urinary retention, and constipation are still troublesome. In older adults, these drugs sometimes produce confusion, delusions, and even hallucinations.

ALZHEIMER'S DISEASE

Alzheimer's disease (AD) affects memory, thinking, and behavior. It is one of the forms of dementia that gradually gets worse over time. By age 85, as many as 50% of the population may be affected by AD. Drugs may help slow the rate at which symptoms become worse, but there is no cure for the disorder.

20.5 Characteristics of Alzheimer's Disease

Alzheimer's disease (AD) is responsible for 70% of all dementia. **Dementia** is a degenerative disorder characterized by progressive memory loss, confusion, and an inability to think or communicate effectively. Consciousness and perception are usually unaffected. Known causes of dementia include multiple cerebral infarcts, severe infections, and toxins. Although the cause of most dementia is unknown, it is usually associated with cerebral atrophy or other structural changes within the brain. The patient generally lives 5 to 10 years following diagnosis; AD is the fourth leading cause of death in the United States.

Despite extensive, ongoing research, the etiology of AD remains unknown. The early-onset familial form of this disorder, accounting for about 10% of cases, is associated with gene defects on chromosome 1, 14, or 21. Chronic inflammation and excess free radicals may cause neuronal damage. Environmental, immunologic, and nutritional factors, as well as viruses, are considered possible sources of brain damage.

Although the cause may be unknown, structural damage in the brain of patients with AD has been well documented. **Amyloid plaques** and **neurofibrillary tangles,** found within the brain at autopsy, are present in nearly all patients with AD. It is suspected that these structural changes are caused by chronic inflammatory or oxidative cellular damage to the surrounding neurons. There is a loss in both the number and function of neurons.

Patients with AD experience a dramatic loss of ability to perform tasks that require acetylcholine as the neurotransmitter. Because acetylcholine is a major neurotransmitter within the **hippocampus,** an area of the brain responsible for learning and memory, and other parts of the cerebral cortex, neuronal functioning within these brain areas is especially affected. Thus, an inability to remember and to recall information is among the early symptoms of AD. Symptoms of this disease are as follows:

- Impaired memory and judgment
- Confusion or disorientation
- Inability to recognize family or friends
- Aggressive behavior
- Depression
- Psychoses, including paranoia and delusions
- Anxiety.

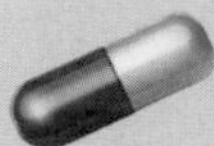

Prototype Drug | Benztropine *(Cogentin)*

Therapeutic Class: Antiparkinson drug **Pharmacologic Class:** Centrally acting cholinergic receptor blocker

Actions and Uses

Benztropine acts by blocking excess cholinergic stimulation of neurons in the corpus striatum. It is used for relief of Parkinson's-like symptoms and for the treatment of EPS brought on by antipsychotic pharmacotherapy. This medication suppresses tremors but is not effective at relieving tardive dyskinesia.

Administration Alerts

- The patient may be unable to self-administer medication and may need assistance.
- Benztropine may be taken in divided doses, two to four times a day, or the entire day's dose may be taken at bedtime.
- If muscle weakness occurs, the dose should be reduced.
- Pregnancy category C.

PHARMACOKINETICS

Onset	Peak	Duration
15 min IM/IV; 1 h PO	1–2 h	6–10 h

Adverse Effects

As expected from its autonomic action, benztropine can cause typical anticholinergic side effects such as dry mouth, constipation, and tachycardia. Adverse general effects include sedation, drowsiness, dizziness, restlessness, irritability, nervousness, and insomnia.

Contraindications: Contraindications include narrow-angle glaucoma, myasthenia gravis, blockage of the urinary tract, severe dry mouth, hiatal hernia, severe constipation, enlarged prostate, and liver disease.

Interactions

Drug–Drug: Benztropine interacts with many drugs. Common medications that should not be used in combination with benztropine are aripiprazole (Abilify), lorazepam (Ativan), docusate (Colace), divalproex sodium (Depakote), gabapentin, ziprasidone (Geodon), haloperidol (Haldol), clonazepam (Klonopin), lamotrigine (Lamictal), lisinopril, lithium, metformin, fluoxetine (Prozac), risperidone (Risperdal), quetiapine (Seroquel), levothyroxine (Synthroid), topiramate (Topamax), trazodone, bupropion (Wellbutrin), sertraline (Zoloft), and olanzapine (Zyprexa). Over-the-counter (OTC) cold medicines should be avoided. Drugs that enhance dopamine release or activate dopamine receptors may produce additive effects. Haloperidol decreases the effectiveness of benzotropine. Benztropine should not be taken with alcohol because of combined sedative effects. Antihistamines, phenothiazines, tricyclic antidepressants, disopyramide, and quinidine may increase anticholinergic effects, and antidiarrheals may decrease absorption.

Lab Tests: Unknown.

Herbal/Food: Unknown.

Treatment of Overdose: Physostigmine 1 to 2 mg subcutaneously or IV, will reverse symptoms of anticholinergic intoxication. A second injection may be given after 2 hours, if required. Otherwise, treatment is symptomatic and supportive.

DRUGS FOR ALZHEIMER'S DISEASE

Drugs are used to slow memory loss and other progressive symptoms of dementia. Some drugs are given to treat associated symptoms such as depression, anxiety, or psychoses. The **cholinesterase inhibitors** are the most widely used class of drugs for treating AD. Representative drugs are listed in Table 20.4. Memantine (Namenda) was the first in a newer class of drugs called *glutamatergic inhibitors*, approved for treatment of AD. Other drugs purported to prevent or help slow the onset of AD progression have included NSAIDs, vitamin E, and selegiline (MAO-B inhibitor).

Cholinesterase Inhibitors

The U.S. Food and Drug Administration (FDA) has approved only a few drugs for AD. The most effective of these medications act by intensifying the effect of acetylcholine at the cholinergic receptor, as shown in Pharmacotherapy Illustrated 20.2.

20.6 Treating Alzheimer's Disease With Cholinesterase Inhibitors

Acetylcholine is naturally degraded in the synapse by the enzyme **acetylcholinesterase (AchE).** When AchE is inhibited, acetylcholine levels become elevated and produce a more profound effect on the receptor. As described in chapter 12, the AchE inhibitors are indirect-acting cholinergic drugs.

The goal of pharmacotherapy in the treatment of AD is to improve function in three domains: ADLs, behavior, and cognition. Although the AchE inhibitors improve all three domains, their efficacy is modest at best. Therapy is begun as soon as the diagnosis of AD is established. These agents are ineffective in treating the severe stages of this disorder, probably because so many neurons have died.

Table 20.4 Cholinesterase Inhibitors Used for Alzheimer's Disease

Drug	Route and Adult Dose (max dose where indicated)	Adverse Effects
donepezil (Aricept)	PO: 5–10 mg at bedtime	*Headache, dizziness, insomnia, nausea, diarrhea, vomiting, muscle cramps, anorexia, abdominal pain* Hepatotoxicity, renal toxicity, bradycardia, heart block, extreme weight loss
galantamine (Razadyne, Reminyl)	PO; Initiate with 4 mg bid for at least 4 wk; if tolerated, may increase by 4 mg bid every 4 wk to a target dose of 12 mg bid (max: 8–16 mg bid)	
rivastigmine (Exelon)	PO: Start with 1.5 mg bid with food; may increase by 1.5 mg bid every 2 wk if tolerated; target dose 3–6 mg bid (max: 12 mg bid) Exelon Patch: initial dose one patch 4.6 mg/24 h once daily; maintenance dose one patch 9.5 mg/24 h once daily	

Note: *Italics* indicate common adverse effects; underlining indicates serious adverse effects.
For the complete nursing process applied to anticholinesterase therapy, see Nursing Practice Application: Pharmacotherapy With Cholinergic Drugs, in chapter 12.

Increasing the level of acetylcholine is effective only if there are functioning neurons present. Often, as the disease progresses, the AchE inhibitors are discontinued; their therapeutic benefit does not outweigh their expense or the risks of side effects.

All AchE inhibitors used to treat AD have equal efficacy. Side effects are those expected of drugs that enhance actions of the parasympathetic nervous system (see chapter 12). The GI system is most affected, with nausea, vomiting, and diarrhea being reported. Weight loss, a potentially serious side effect of AchE inhibitors is observed in some older adults. When therapy is discontinued, doses of the AchE inhibitors should be lowered gradually.

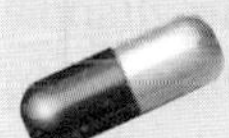

Prototype Drug | Donepezil *(Aricept)*

Therapeutic Class: Alzheimer's disease drug **Pharmacologic Class:** Cholinesterase inhibitor

Actions and Uses

Donepezil is an AchE inhibitor that improves memory in cases of mild to moderate Alzheimer's dementia by enhancing the effects of acetylcholine in neurons in the cerebral cortex that have not been damaged. Patients should receive pharmacotherapy for at least 6 months prior to assessing maximum benefits of drug therapy. Improvement in memory may be observed as early as 1 to 4 weeks following medication. The therapeutic effects of donepezil are often short lived, and the degree of improvement is modest, at best. An advantage of donepezil over other drugs in its class is that its long half-life permits it to be given once daily.

Administration Alerts

- Give medication prior to bedtime.
- Medication is most effective when given on a regular schedule.
- Pregnancy category C.

PHARMACOKINETICS

Onset	Peak	Duration
Less than 20 min	3–4 h	Variable

Adverse Effects

Common side effects of donepezil are vomiting and diarrhea. Less common effects are abnormal dreams, fainting, and darkened urine. CNS side effects include insomnia, syncope, depression, headache, and irritability. Musculoskeletal side effects include muscle cramps, arthritis, and bone fractures. Generalized side effects include headache, fatigue, chest pain, increased libido, hot flashes, urinary incontinence, dehydration, and blurred vision. Hepatotoxicity has not been observed. Patients with bradycardia, hypotension, asthma, hyperthyroidism, or active peptic ulcer disease should be monitored carefully.

Contraindications: Donepezil is contraindicated in patients with GI bleeding and jaundice.

Interactions

Drug–Drug: Donepezil will cause anticholinergics to be less effective. Donepezil interacts with several other drugs. For example, bethanechol causes a synergistic effect. Phenobarbital, phenytoin, dexamethasone, and rifampin may speed the elimination of donepezil. Quinidine or ketoconazole may inhibit the metabolism of donepezil. Because donepezil acts by increasing cholinergic activity, two cholinergic drugs should not be administered concurrently.

Lab Tests: Unknown.

Herbal/Food: Unknown.

Treatment of Overdose: Anticholinergics such as atropine may be used as an antidote for donepezil overdosage. IV atropine sulfate titrated to effect is recommended: an initial dose of 1 to 2 mg IV with subsequent doses based on clinical response.

REFERENCES

Aviles-Olmos, I., Dickson, J., Kefalopoulou, Z, Djamshidian, A., Ell, P., Soderlund, T., . . . Foltynie, T. (2013). Exenatide and the treatment of patients with Parkinson's disease. *Journal of Clinical Investigation, 123,* 2730–2736. doi:10.1172/JCI68295

Aviles-Olmos, I., Limousin, P., Lees, A., & Foltynie, T. (2013). Parkinson's disease, insulin resistance and novel agents of neuroprotection. *Brain, 136,* 374–384. doi:10.1093/brain/aws009

Aviles-Olmos, I., Dickson, J., Kefalopoulou, Z., Djamshidian, A., Kahan, J., Ell, P., . . . Foltynie, T. (2014). Motor and cognitive advantages persist 12 months after exenatide exposure in Parkinson's disease. *Journal of Parkinson's Disease, 4,* 337–344. doi:10.3233/JPD-14036

Herdman, T. H., & Kamitsuru, S. (Eds.). (2014). *NANDA International nursing diagnoses: Definitions and classification, 2015–2017.* Oxford, United Kingdom: Wiley-Blackwell.

Jahanshahi, M., Nickmahzar, E. G., & Babakordi, F. (2013). Effect of gingko biloba extract on scopolamine-induced apoptosis in the hippocampus of rats. *Anatomical Science International, 88,* 217–222. doi:10.1007/s12565-013-0188-8

National Center for Complementary and Integrative Health. (2013). *Gingko.* Retrieved from https://nccih.nih.gov/health/ginkgo/ataglance.htm

Salcedo, I., Tweedie, D., Li, Y., & Greig, N. H. (2012). Neuroprotective and neurotrophic actions of glucagon-like peptide-1: An emerging opportunity to treat neurodegenerative and cerebrovascular disorders. *British Journal of Pharmacology, 166,* 1586–1599. doi:10.1111/j.1476-5381.2012.01971.x

Sofrizzi, V., & Panza, F. (2015). Plant-based nutraceutical interventions against cognitive impairment and dementia: Meta-analytic evidence of efficacy of a standardized gingko biloba extract. *Journal of Alzheimer's Disease, 43,* 605–611. doi:10.3233/JAD-141887

SELECTED BIBLIOGRAPHY

Alzheimer's Association. (2014). 2014 Alzheimer's disease: Facts and figures. *Alzheimer's & Dementia, 10*(2). Retrieved from http://www.alz.org/downloads/Facts_Figures_2014.pdf

Arnold, D. L., Calabresi, P. A., Kieseier, B. C., Sheikh, S. I., Deykin, A., Zhu, Y., . . . Hung, S. (2014). Effect of peginterferon beta-1a on MRI measures and achieving no evidence of disease activity: Results from a randomized controlled trial in relapsing-remitting multiple sclerosis. *BMC Neurology, 14,* 240. doi:10.1186/s12883-014-0240-x

Breitner, J. C., Baker, L. D., Montine, T. J., Meinert, C. L., Lyketsos, C. G., Ashe, K. H., . . . Tariot, P. N. (2011). Extended results of the Alzheimer's disease anti-inflammatory prevention trial. *Alzheimer's & Dementia, 7,* 402–411.

Bruno, D., Grothe, M. J., Nierenberg, J., Zetterberg, H., Blennow, K., Teipel, S., & Pomara, N. (2015). A study on the specificity of the association between hippocampal volume and delayed primacy performance in cognitively intact elderly individuals. *Neuropsychologia, 69,* 1–8. doi:10.1016/j.neuropsychologia.2015.01.025

Drugs.com. (n.d.). *Carbidopa and levodopa.* Retrieved from http://www.drugs.com/pro/carbidopa-and-levodopa.html

Féger, J., & Hirsch, E. C. (2015). In search of innovative therapeutics for neuropsychiatric disorders: The case of neurodegenerative diseases. *Annales Pharmaceutiques Francaises, 73,* 3–12. doi:10.1016/j.pharma.2014.10.001

Genetics Home Reference. (2013). *Multiple sclerosis.* Retrieved from http://ghr.nlm.nih.gov/condition/multiple-sclerosis

Hagmeyer, S., Haderspeck, J. C., Grabrucker, A. M. (2015). Behavioral impairments in animal models for zinc deficiency. *Frontiers in Behavioral Neuroscience, 8,* 443. doi:10.3389/fnbeh.2014.00443

Havrdova, E., Horakova, D., Kovarova, I. (2015). Alemtuzumab in the treatment of multiple sclerosis: Key clinical trial results and considerations for use. *Therapeutic Advances in Neurological Disorders, 8,* 31–45. doi:10.1177/1756285614563522

Hoozemans, J. J., Veerhusi, R., Rozemuller, J. M., & Eikelenboom, P. (2011). Soothing the inflamed brain: Effect of non-steroidal anti-inflammatory drugs on Alzheimer's disease. *CNS & Neurological Disorders Drug Targets, 10* (1), 57–67.

Hu, X., Seddighzadeh, A., Stecher, S., Zhu, Y., Goyal, J., Matson, M., . . . Hung, S. (2015). Pharmacokinetics, pharmacodynamics, and safety of peginterferon beta-1a in subjects with normal or impaired renal function. *Journal of Clinical Pharmacology, 55,* 179–188. doi:10.1002/jcph.390

Jaturapatpom, D., Isaac, M. G., McCleery, J., & Tabet, N. (2012). Aspirin, steroidal and non-steroidal anti-inflammatory drugs for the treatment of Alzheimer's disease. *Cochrane Database of Systematic Reviews, 2,* Art. No.: CD006378. doi:10.1002/14651858.CD006378.pub2

Milo, R. (2015). Effectiveness of multiple sclerosis treatment with current immunomodulatory drugs. *Expert Opinion on Pharmacotherapy, 16,* 659–673. doi:10.1517/14656566.2015.1002769

National Multiple Sclerosis Society. (n.d.). *Multiple sclerosis FAQs.* Retrieved from http://www.nationalmssociety.org/What-is-MS/MS-FAQ-s

National Parkinson Foundation. (n.d.). *Carbidopa/levodopa.* Retrieved from http://www.parkinson.org/Parkinson-s-Disease/Treatment/Medications-for-Motor-Symptoms-of-PD/Carbidopa-levodopa

Parkinson's Disease Foundation. (n.d.). *Statistics on Parkinson's.* Retrieved from http://www.pdf.org/en/parkinson_statistics

Pietrangelo, A., & Higuera, V. (2015). *Multiple sclerosis by the numbers: Facts, statistics, and you.* Retrieved from http://www.healthline.com/health/multiple-sclerosis/facts-statistics-infographic

Samuel, M., Rodriguez-Oroz, M., Antonini, A., Brotchie, J. M., Chaudhuri K. R., Brown, R. G., . . . Lang A. E. (2015). Management of impulse control disorders in Parkinson's disease: Controversies and future approaches. *Movement Disorders, 30,* 150–159. doi:10.1002/mds.26099

Chapter 21

Drugs for Neuromuscular Disorders

Drugs at a Glance

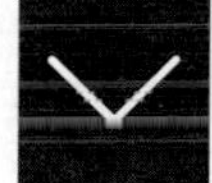

Learning Outcomes

After reading this chapter, the student should be able to:

1. Identify the different body systems contributing to muscle movement.
2. Discuss pharmacologic and nonpharmacologic therapies used to treat muscle spasms and spasticity.
3. Explain the goals of pharmacotherapy with skeletal muscle relaxants.
4. Describe the nurse's role in the pharmacologic management of muscle spasms.
5. Compare and contrast the roles of the following drug categories in treating muscle spasms and spasticity: centrally acting skeletal muscle relaxants, direct-acting antispasmodics, and skeletal muscle relaxants for short medical procedures.
6. For each of the drug classes listed in Drugs at a Glance, know representative drugs, and explain their mechanisms of action, primary actions, and important adverse effects.
7. Use the nursing process to care for patients who are receiving pharmacotherapy for muscle spasms.

indicates a prototype drug, each of which is featured in a Prototype Drug box.

Disorders associated with movement are some of the most difficult conditions to treat because their underlying mechanisms span other important systems in the body: the nervous, muscular, endocrine, and skeletal systems. Proper body movement depends not only on intact neural pathways but also on proper functioning of muscles, bones, and joints (see chapter 48), which in turn depend on the levels of minerals such as sodium, potassium, and calcium in the bloodstream (see chapters 25 and 48). The pharmacotherapy of muscular disorders including muscle spasms, spasticity, and treatments involving the neuromuscular junction are the focus of this chapter.

MUSCLE SPASMS

Muscle spasms are involuntary contractions of a muscle or groups of muscles. The muscles become tightened and fixed, causing intense pain which usually diminishes after a few minutes. Chronic muscle spasms can impair joint function.

21.1 Causes of Muscle Spasms

Muscle spasms are a common condition usually associated with excessive use of and local injury to the skeletal muscle. Another possible cause of muscle spasms is overmedication with antipsychotic drugs (see chapter 17). Disorders and conditions such as epilepsy, hypocalcemia, dehydration, and neurologic disorders are linked with muscle spasms. Poor blood circulation to the legs, known as *intermittent claudication*, is a common cause of muscle cramping in the lower kegs. Patients with muscle spasms may experience inflammation, edema, and pain at the affected muscle, loss of coordination, and reduced mobility. When a muscle spasms, it locks in a contracted state. A single, prolonged contraction is a **tonic spasm,** whereas multiple, rapidly repeated contractions are **clonic spasms.** Both nonpharmacologic and pharmacologic strategies are approaches to treat muscle spasms.

21.2 Pharmacologic and Nonpharmacologic Strategies to Treat Muscle Spasms

To determine the etiology of muscle spasms, patients require a careful history assessment and physical exam. After diagnosis, nonpharmacologic therapies are applied in conjunction with medications. Examples of nonpharmacologic therapies include immobilization of the affected muscle, application of heat or cold, hydrotherapy, therapeutic ultrasound, supervised exercises, massage, physical therapy, and manipulation. Patients may prefer to treat minor muscle aches and spasms with herbal remedies. Examples are topical formulations of black cohosh, castor oil packs, or capsaicin, a substance derived from cayenne peppers (see the Complementary and Alternative Therapies feature on page 303). Oral therapy with vitamin B_6 (pyridoxine) has been found to reduce the intensity and duration of leg muscle cramping in some patients.

Pharmacotherapy for muscle spasm may include combinations of analgesics, anti-inflammatory drugs, and centrally acting skeletal muscle relaxants. Most skeletal muscle relaxants relieve symptoms of muscular stiffness and rigidity due to muscular injury or degenerative diseases (e.g., multiple sclerosis [MS]). Drugs help improve mobility in cases where patients have restricted movements. The therapeutic goals are to minimize pain and discomfort, increase range of motion, and improve the patient's ability to function independently.

PharmFacts

MUSCLE SPASMS

- More than 12 million people worldwide have muscle spasms.
- Muscle spasms that are severe enough for drug therapy are often found in patients who have other debilitating disorders such as stroke, injury, neurodegenerative diseases, or cerebral palsy.
- Cerebral palsy is usually associated with events that occur before or during birth but may be acquired during the first few months or years of life as the result of head trauma or infection.
- Dystonia affects over 250,000 people in the United States; it is the third most common movement disorder following essential tremor and Parkinson's disease.
- Researchers have recognized multiple forms of inheritable dystonia and identified at least five genes responsible for the various manifestations.

CENTRALLY ACTING SKELETAL MUSCLE RELAXANTS

Many muscle relaxants generate their effects by inhibiting upper motor neuron activity within the brain and/or spinal cord. Thus, the origin of drug action is within the central nervous system (CNS).

21.3 Treating Muscle Spasms at the Brain and Spinal Cord Levels

Skeletal muscle relaxants act at various levels of the CNS. Although their exact mechanisms are not fully understood, it is believed that they generate their effects within the brain and/or spinal cord. Ultimately, upper motor neuron activity is inhibited in the brain, and simple reflexes are altered in the spinal cord.

Table 21.1 Centrally Acting Drugs That Relax Skeletal Muscles

Drug	Route and Adult Dose (max dose where indicated)	Adverse Effects
SKELETAL MUSCLE RELAXANTS		
baclofen (Lioresal)	PO: 5 mg tid (max: 80 mg/day)	*Drowsiness, dizziness, dry mouth, sedation, ataxia, light-headedness, urinary hesitancy or retention, hypotension, bradycardia* Angioedema, anaphylactic reaction, respiratory depression, coma, laryngospasm, cardiovascular collapse
carisoprodol (Soma)	PO: 350 mg tid	
chlorzoxazone (Paraflex, Parafon Forte)	PO: 250–500 mg tid–qid (max: 3 g/day)	
cyclobenzaprine (Amrix, Flexeril)	PO: 10–20 mg bid–qid (max: 60 mg/day); 15 mg once daily for extended-release capsules (max: 30 mg/day)	
metaxalone (Skelaxin)	PO: 800 mg tid–qid (max: 10 mg/day)	
methocarbamol (Robaxin)	PO: 1.5 g qid for 2–3 days; then reduce to 1 g qid IV/IM: 1–3 g once daily for 3 days; repeat after a drug-free interval of 48 h if necessary; do not exceed 3 mL/min	
orphenadrine (Norflex)	PO: 100 mg bid	
IMIDAZOLINES		
clonidine (Catapres, transdermal patch)	PO: 0.1 mg bid, with titration to 0.2 to 0.6 mg bid; transdermal patch changed every 7 days	
tizanidine (Zanaflex)	PO: 4–8 mg tid–qid (max: 36 mg/day)	
BENZODIAZEPINES		
clonazepam (Klonopin)	PO: 1.5 mg tid, may be increased in increments of 0.5–1 mg every 3 days	*Drowsiness, dizziness, sedation, ataxia, light-headedness* Respiratory depression
diazepam (Valium) (see page 190 for the Prototype Drug box)	PO: 4–10 mg bid–qid	
lorazepam (Ativan) (see page 171 for the Prototype Drug box)	PO: 1–2 mg bid–tid (max: 10 mg/day) IM/IV: 2–10 mg, repeat if needed in 3–4 h IV pump: administer emulsion at 5 mg/min	

Note: *Italics* indicate common adverse effects; underlining indicates serious adverse effects.

After injury, antispasmodic drugs are used to treat localized spasms. Drugs may be prescribed alone or in combination with other medications to reduce pain and increase range of motion. Commonly used skeletal muscle relaxants are baclofen (Lioresal) and cyclobenzaprine (Amrix, Flexeril) among other medications. Tizanidine (Zanaflex) and clonidine (Catapres) are imidazolines, a chemical classification commonly associated with agents that treat nasal congestion or irritated eyes. Although not classified as antispasmodics and generally indicated for treatment of anxiety-related symptoms, benzodiazepines such as diazepam (Valium), clonazepam (Klonopin), and lorazepam (Ativan), have skeletal muscle relaxant properties. Centrally acting drugs that relax skeletal muscles are summarized in Table 21.1.

Baclofen (Lioresal) is structurally similar to the inhibitory neurotransmitter gamma-aminobutyric acid (GABA). Baclofen has been employed to reduce muscle spasms in patients with MS, cerebral palsy (CP), and spinal cord injury. Baclofen is popular due to its wide safety margin. Common side effects of baclofen are drowsiness, dizziness,

Lifespan Considerations: Pediatric Intrathecal Baclofen for Children With Spastic Cerebral Palsy

Over 70% of patients with CP have spasticity associated with other motor disorders. Spasticity can be painful, increases metabolic needs, and may severely limit activities of daily living (ADLs). Prior drug therapy for patients with CP has included diazepam (Valium), dantrolene (Dantrium), and oral baclofen (Lioresal). Because these drugs are given PO, they cause systemic adverse effects that also affect ADLs. These effects include drowsiness, dizziness, confusion, and hypotension. Intrathecal baclofen, delivered directly into the spinal fluid circulation by an implanted pump, has demonstrated significant improvements in the treatment of spastic CP with reduced systemic effects. It has also been noted to have overall patient and caregiver satisfaction with the outcomes (Baker, Tann, Mutlu, & Gaebler-Spira, 2014). It appears effective in managing the pain and startle response common in CP and improves the ease of care. Complications related to the baclofen pump have been reported, but the majority were related to the delivery device (e.g., infections, scarring) and not the baclofen (Borrini et al., 2014). In a study of patients who had used intrathecal baclofen for 10 years or longer, decreased pain and spasms and improved sleep were noted (Mathur, Chu, McCormick, Chang Chien, & Marciniak, 2014). Because nurses work closely with patients who have chronic conditions such as CP, they are often the primary providers of education for families and for school nurses on the use of the baclofen pump, care needs such as site care, and how to monitor drug effects. Intrathecal baclofen is also used in other spastic disorders such as MS, spinal cord injury, brain injury, and stroke.

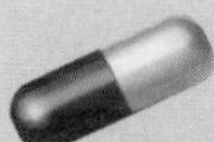

Prototype Drug | Cyclobenzaprine *(Amrix, Flexeril)*

Therapeutic Class: Centrally acting skeletal muscle relaxant **Pharmacologic Class:** Catecholamine reuptake inhibitor

Actions and Uses

Cyclobenzaprine relieves muscle spasms of local origin without interfering with general muscle function. This drug acts by depressing motor activity primarily in the brainstem; limited effects also occur in the spinal cord. Cyclobenzaprine increases circulating levels of norepinephrine, blocking presynaptic uptake. Its mechanism of action is similar to that of tricyclic antidepressants (see chapter 16). The drug causes muscle relaxation in cases of acute muscle spasticity, but it is not effective in cases of CP or diseases of the brain and spinal cord. This medication is structurally similar to amitriptyline, thus the same adverse drug reactions should be expected and precautions taken. Cyclobenzaprine is meant to provide therapy for only 2 to 3 weeks.

Administration Alerts

- The drug is not recommended for pediatric use.
- Use with great caution in patients older than age 65 because this population is more likely to experience confusion, hallucinations, and adverse cardiac events from the drug.
- Maximum effects may take 1 to 2 weeks.
- Pregnancy category B.

PHARMACOKINETICS

Onset	Peak	Duration
1 h	3–8 h	12–14 h

Adverse Effects

Adverse reactions to cyclobenzaprine include drowsiness, blurred vision, dizziness, dry mouth, rash, and tachycardia. One reaction, although rare, is angioedema (swelling of the tongue).

Contraindications: Cyclobenzaprine should be used with caution in patients with myocardial infarction (MI), dysrhythmias, hypothyroidism or severe cardiovascular disease.

Interactions

Drug–Drug: Alcohol, phenothiazines, and other CNS depressants may cause additive sedation. Cyclobenzaprine should not be used within 2 weeks of a monoamine oxidase inhibitor (MAOI) therapy because hyperpyretic crisis and convulsions may occur.

Lab Tests: Unknown.

Herbal/Food: Unknown.

Treatment of Overdose: The intravenous (IV) administration of 1 to 3 mg of physostigmine is reported to reverse symptoms of poisoning by drugs with anticholinergic activity. Physostigmine may be helpful in the treatment of cyclobenzaprine overdose.

weakness, and fatigue. Intrathecal use of baclofen in children is discussed in the Lifespan Considerations feature.

Clonidine (Catapres) and tizanidine (Zanaflex) are centrally acting alpha$_2$-adrenergic agonists that inhibit motor neurons mainly at the spinal cord level. Patients receiving high doses report drowsiness; thus, these drugs also have depressant effects within the brain. Though uncommon, one adverse effect of tizanidine is hallucinations. The most frequent side effects are dry mouth, fatigue, dizziness, and sleepiness. Tizanidine is as efficacious as baclofen and preferred by many health care providers.

As discussed in chapter 14, benzodiazepines inhibit both sensory and motor neuron activity by enhancing the effects of GABA. Common adverse side effects include drowsiness and ataxia (loss of coordination). Benzodiazepines are usually prescribed for sedation and relief of muscle tension when baclofen and tizanidine fail to produce adequate therapeutic effects.

SPASTICITY

Spasticity is a condition in which muscle groups remain in a continuous state of contraction, usually resulting from neuronal motor damage or neurologic disorders. Contracted muscles become stiff with increased muscle tone. Other signs and symptoms include mild to severe pain, exaggerated deep tendon reflexes, localized muscle spasms, scissoring (involuntary crossing of the legs), and fixed joints.

21.4 Causes and Treatment of Spasticity

Muscle spasticity has a different etiology than muscle spasm. Spasticity usually results from damage to the motor areas of the cerebral cortex that control muscle movement. Etiologies most commonly associated with this condition include CP, severe head injury, spinal cord injury or lesions, and stroke. **Dystonia,** a chronic neurologic disorder, is characterized by continuous, involuntary muscle contractions that force body parts into abnormal, occasionally painful movements or postures. It affects the muscle tone of the arms, legs, trunk, neck, eyelids, face, or vocal cords. Spasticity can be distressing and greatly affects an individual's quality of life, whether the condition is short- or long-lived. In addition to causing pain, impaired physical mobility influences the ability to perform ADLs and diminishes the patient's sense of independence.

Effective treatments for spasticity are both physical therapy and medications. Medications alone are not adequate in reducing the complications of spasticity. Regular and consistent physical therapy exercises have been shown to decrease the severity of symptoms. Types of exercise treatments include muscle stretching to help prevent contractures, muscle-group strengthening activities, and repetitive-motion exercises for improvement of mobility. In extreme cases, surgery to release tendons or to sever the nerve–muscle pathway has been performed. Centrally acting antispasmodics and drugs that focus on the neuromuscular junction and muscle tissue are effective in the treatment of spasticity.

☑ Check Your Understanding 21.1

What is a major drawback to all of the centrally-acting muscle relaxant drugs used to treat muscle spasms or spasticity? *Visit www.pearsonhighered.com/nursingresources for the answer.*

DIRECT-ACTING ANTISPASMODICS

Whereas the centrally acting drugs inhibit neurons at the level of the CNS, direct-acting drugs work at the level of the neuromuscular junction and skeletal muscles. As shown in Pharmacotherapy Illustrated 21.1, dantrolene (Dantrium) and botulinum toxins are direct-acting drugs. The direct-acting medications produce antispasmodic effects directly at the muscle tissue level.

Complementary and Alternative Therapies

CAPSAICIN FOR NEUROPATHIC AND OTHER PAIN

Capsaicin (*Capsicum annum*), also known as cayenne, chili pepper, paprika, or red pepper, has been used as a remedy for minor muscle pain or tension. Capsaicin, the active ingredient in cayenne and other peppers, diminishes the chemical messengers that travel through the sensory nerves, thereby decreasing the sensation of pain. Capsaicin cream (0.025% to 0.075%) is available over the counter and may be applied directly to the affected area up to four times a day. The highest dose (8%) is available as a patch by prescription and its use must be carefully monitored by a health care provider. The Qutenza (capsaicin) patch has been shown to be effective for neuropathic pain in several studies (Mou et al., 2014; Wagner, Poole, & Roth-Daniek, 2013). Applying cool compresses prior to application of the patch was found to be effective in relieving localized pain at the patch site (Knolle et al., 2013). The topical creams are well tolerated, with reddening of the skin and local stinging being the most common side effects. It should be kept away from the eyes and mucous membranes to avoid burning, and the hands must be washed thoroughly after use.

21.5 Treating Muscle Spasms Directly at the Muscle Tissue

Dantrolene relieves spasticity by interfering with the release of calcium ions in skeletal muscle. Calcium released from the sarcoplasmic reticulum is necessary for skeletal muscle contraction. If the release of calcium is blocked, muscle tension will be reduced.

Botulinum toxin is an unusual drug because, in higher quantities, it acts as a poison. *Clostridium botulinum* is the bacterium responsible for botulism food poisoning. At lower doses however, this agent can be safely and effectively used as a muscle relaxant. Botulinum toxin produces its effect by blocking the release of acetylcholine from cholinergic nerve terminals (see chapter 12). Acetylcholine is the natural neurotransmitter necessary for the voluntary contraction of skeletal muscles.

Two antigenically distinct serotypes, botulinum toxin type A and botulinum toxin type B, are currently available for relaxing muscle. Botulinum type A drugs acting directly at the neuromuscular junction include abobotulinumtoxinA (Dysport), incobotulinumtoxinA (Xeomin), and onabotulinumtoxinA (Botox). The only botulinum toxin type B drug is rimabotulinumtoxinB (Myobloc). Direct-acting drugs are summarized in Table 21.2.

Because of the potential for extreme muscle weakness associated with botulinum, precautions are often needed when applying it. To circumvent major problems with mobility or posture, botulinum toxin is often applied to small muscle groups. Sometimes this drug is administered with centrally acting oral medications to increase functional use of a range of muscle groups. Indications for botulinum toxin are provided in Table 21.3.

Importantly, these medications can spread to other parts of the body, causing serious and potentially fatal adverse effects. Effects can occur hours or even weeks after the injection. Serious adverse effects are angina, difficulty breathing, extreme muscle weakness, dysrhythmias, difficulty swallowing, and loss of bladder control. Children being treated for muscle spasms have the greatest risk of adverse effects, as well as patients with debilitating conditions such as muscular dystrophy or musculoskeletal disorders. The chances of serious adverse effects occurring are unlikely when botulinum toxin is used to treat migraines, skin conditions such as wrinkles or eye spasm, or for excessive sweating in adults.

Pharmacotherapy Illustrated

21.1 | Mechanism of Action of Direct-Acting Antispasmodics

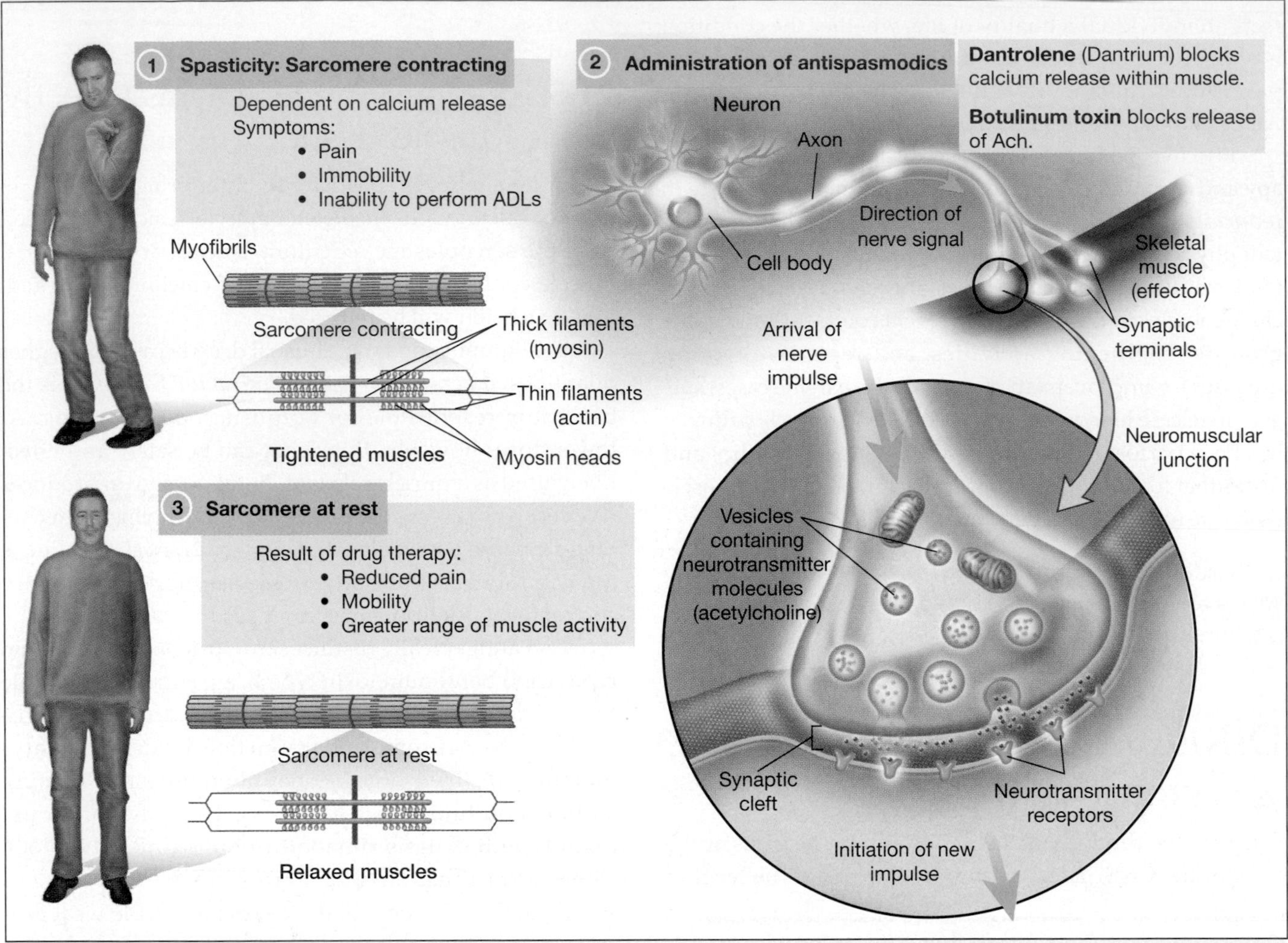

Table 21.2 Direct-Acting Antispasmodic Drugs

Drug	Route and Adult Dose (max dose where indicated)	Adverse Effects
NEUROMUSCULAR JUNCTION		
abobotulinumtoxinA (Dysport)	50 units in five equal aliquots injected directly into target muscle	*Headache, dysphagia, ptosis, local muscle weakness, pain, muscle tenderness* Anaphylaxis, dysphagia, death
incobotulinumtoxinA (Xeomin)	120 units injected per treatment session directly into target muscle	
onabotulinumtoxinA (Botox)	25 units injected directly into target muscle (max: 30-day dose should not exceed 200 units)	
rimabotulinumtoxinB (Myobloc)	2500–5000 units/dose injected directly into target muscle; doses should be divided among muscle groups	
SKELETAL MUSCLE		
dantrolene (Dantrium)	PO: 25 mg/day; increase to 25 mg bid–qid; may increase every 4–7 days up to 100 mg bid–tid	*Muscle weakness, dizziness, diarrhea* Hepatic necrosis

Note: *Italics* indicate common adverse effects; underlining indicates serious adverse effects.

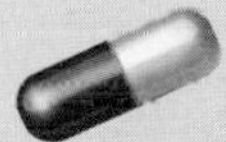

Prototype Drug | Dantrolene Sodium *(Dantrium)*

Therapeutic Class: Skeletal muscle relaxant **Pharmacologic Class:** Direct-acting antispasmodic; calcium release blocker

Actions and Uses

Dantrolene is often used for spasticity, especially for spasms of the head and neck. It directly relaxes muscle spasms by interfering with the release of calcium ions from storage areas inside skeletal muscle cells. It does not affect cardiac or smooth muscle. Dantrolene is especially useful for muscle spasms when they occur after spinal cord injury or stroke and in cases of CP or MS. Occasionally, it is useful for the treatment of muscle pain after heavy exercise. An IV form (Revonto) is a preferred drug for the treatment of malignant hyperthermia.

Administration Alerts

- Use oral suspension within several days because it does not contain a preservative.
- IV solution has a high pH and therefore is extremely irritating to tissue.
- Pregnancy category C.

PHARMACOKINETICS

Onset	Peak	Duration
1–2 h	5 h	Variable

Adverse Effects

Adverse effects include muscle weakness, drowsiness, dry mouth, dizziness, nausea, diarrhea, tachycardia, erratic blood pressure, photosensitivity, and urinary retention.

Black Box Warning: This drug has the potential for hepatoxicity. Liver dysfunction may be evidenced by abnormal chemical blood enzyme levels. The risk of hepatic injury is increased in females over 35 years of age and after 3 months of therapy. There is also a higher proportion of hepatic events with fatal outcome in older patients receiving dantrolene. This is due to the greater likelihood of drug-induced, potentially fatal, hepatocellular diseases observed in these groups. Therapy should be discontinued after 45 days with no observable benefit.

Contraindications: Patients with impaired cardiac or pulmonary function or hepatic disease should not take this drug.

Interactions

Drug–Drug: Dantrolene interacts with many other drugs. For example, it should not be taken with over-the-counter (OTC) cough preparations and antihistamines, alcohol, or other CNS depressants. Verapamil, diltiazem, and other calcium channel blockers that are taken with dantrolene increase the risk of ventricular fibrillation and cardiovascular collapse.

Lab Tests: Unknown.

Herbal/Food: Unknown.

Treatment of Overdose: For acute overdosage, general supportive measures should be used.

Table 21.3 Indications for Botulinum Toxin

	Axillary Hyperhidrosis	Blepharospasm	Cervical Dystonia	Glabellar Lines	Overactive bladder	Chronic Migraine	Strabismus	Upper Limb Spasticity
abobotulinumtoxinA (Dysport)			X	X				
incobotulinumtoxinA (Xeomin)		X	X	X				
onabotulinumtoxinA (Botox)	X	X	X	X	X	X	X	X
onabotulinumtoxinA (Botox Cosmetic)				X				
rimabotulinumtoxinB (Myobloc)			X					

21.6 Blocking the Effect of Acetylcholine at the Receptor

Neuromuscular blockers bind to nicotinic receptors located on the surface of skeletal muscle. For pharmacotherapy, *nicotinic blocking agents* interfere with the binding of acetylcholine, thereby preventing voluntary muscle contraction. Remember that nicotinic blocking drugs are cholinergic in nature (see chapter 12).

Neuromuscular blocking drugs (see chapter 19) are separated into two major classes: nondepolarizing blockers and depolarizing blockers. *Nondepolarizing blockers* compete with acetylcholine for the receptor. As long as agents interfere with the binding of acetylcholine, muscles remain relaxed. By a related mechanism, *depolarizing blockers* bind to the acetylcholine receptor and produce a state of continuous depolarization. This action first results in small fasciculations or brief repeated muscle movements, followed by relaxation of muscle tissue. Relaxation is short-lived until charges across the muscle membrane are restored (in other words after repolarization of muscle tissue). Importantly, patients treated with neuromuscular blockers are able to feel pain. Thus, for surgical procedures, concomitant use of anesthetic drugs is essential.

An important fact to mention is that nicotinic blocking drugs, although acting at the neuromuscular junction are different from *ganglionic blocking drugs* that target the autonomic nervous system. In this instance, acetylcholine does indeed bind to nicotinic receptors, but the resulting actions are involuntary and do not involve skeletal muscle contraction (see chapter 12). Ganglionic blockers dampen parasympathetic tone and produce effects like increased heart rate, dry mouth, urinary retention, and reduced GI activity. They also dampen sympathetic tone, resulting in reduced sweating and less norepinephrine being released from postsynaptic nerve terminals (see chapter 13). As an example, mecamylamine (Inversine) is a ganglionic blocker primarily used to treat patients with essential hypertension (see chapter 26).

The classic example of a nondepolarizing blocker is tubocurarine. It is of important historical interest, having been replaced by newer, safer medications. Tubocurarine and related blocking drugs used to relax the muscles of patients being prepared for longer surgical procedures are summarized in Table 21.4. Although not preferred for mechanical ventilation or endotracheal intubation, small doses of these drugs may be used for intermediate surgical procedures (see chapter 19). A concern of tubocurarine-like treatment is over-relaxation of muscles. As examples, normal breathing activity (involving the diaphragm, glottis, and intercostal muscles) and swallowing activity (involving neck and esophageal muscles) require contraction of skeletal muscle and those actions may be impaired by these drugs.

Depolarizing drugs are used primarily to relax the muscles of patients receiving electroconvulsive therapy (ECT) (see chapter 16) and for shorter surgical procedures, for example, mechanical ventilation and endotracheal intubation. Succinylcholine (Anectine, Quelicin) is the prototype example of a depolarizing blocker (see chapter 19). Adverse effects include persistent paralysis in some patients, elevated blood levels of potassium, malignant hyperthermia, and postoperative muscle pain.

Table 21.4 Neuromuscular Blocking Drugs

Drug	Duration and Administration Route
NONDEPOLARIZING BLOCKERS	
atracurium (Tracrium)	Long duration; IV
cisatracurium (Nimbex)	Long duration; IV
mivacurium (Mivacron)	Shorter duration; IV
pipecuronium (Arduan)	Longest duration; IV
rocuronium (Zemuron)	Long duration; IV
tubocurarine	Longest duration; oldest of the nondepolarizing drugs IV and IM
vecuronium (Norcuron)	Long duration; IV
DEPOLARIZING BLOCKERS	
succinylcholine (Anectine, Quelicin) (see page 277 for the Prototype Drug box)	Shortest duration; IV and IM

Note: See chapter 19 for a Nursing Practice Application specific to neuromuscular blocking drugs.

Malignant hyperthermia is a rare, life-threatening, anesthetic-related disorder that occurs in susceptible patients following the administration of a triggering agent, such as inhaled halogenated volatile anesthetics or succinylcholine. Once triggered, a rapidly progressive hypermetabolic reaction involving sustained muscle contraction occurs with potentially devastating consequences. Treatment of malignant hyperthermia requires rapid identification of signs and symptoms, discontinuation of the triggering agent, institution of dantrolene therapy, and control of associated symptoms. The signs of malignant hyperthermia include muscle rigidity, rapid heart rate, high body temperature, muscle breakdown, and increased acid content.

After the acute crisis has been controlled, dantrolene (Revonta) 1 mg/kg every 4 to 6 hours or alternatively 0.25 mg/kg/hr continuous infusion for 24 hours is recommended. Adverse effects associated with dantrolene include loss of grip strength, muscle weakness, drowsiness, dizziness, and injection site reactions, including pain, erythema, and swelling.

Nursing Practice Application

Pharmacotherapy for Muscle Spasms or Spasticity

ASSESSMENT	POTENTIAL NURSING DIAGNOSES*
Baseline assessment prior to administration: • Obtain a complete health history including cardiovascular, respiratory, hepatic, renal, or musculoskeletal diseases. Obtain a drug history including allergies, current prescription and OTC drugs, and herbal preparations. Be alert to possible drug interactions. • Obtain a history of the current condition and symptoms, exacerbating conditions, and ability to carry out ADLs, particularly related to mobility. • If present, assess the level of pain. Use objective screening tools when possible (e.g., FLACC [face, limbs, arms, cry, consolability] for infants or very young children, Wong-Baker FACES scale for children, numerical rating scale for adults). Assess the history of pain associated with muscle spasms and what has worked or not worked for the patient in the past. • Evaluate appropriate laboratory findings such as hepatic or renal function studies. • Obtain baseline vital signs, muscle strength, and the presence and type of muscle spasms (tonic, clonic, mixed). • Assess the patient's ability to receive and understand instruction. Include the family or caregivers as needed. **Assessment throughout administration:** • Assess for desired therapeutic effects dependent on the reason for the drug (e.g., decreased muscle spasm, rigidity, decreased pain). • Continue periodic monitoring of vital signs and motor function. • Assess for and promptly report adverse effects: fatigue, drowsiness, dizziness, dry mouth, orthostatic hypotension, tachycardia, palpitations, swelling of tongue or face, diplopia, urinary retention, diarrhea, or constipation.	• *Acute Pain* • *Chronic Pain* • *Impaired Physical Mobility* • *Self-Care Deficit* (feeding, bathing, hygiene, toileting) • *Disturbed Body Image* • *Fatigue* • *Deficient Knowledge* (drug therapy) • *Risk for Injury,* related to disease condition, adverse drug effects *NANDA I © 2014

IMPLEMENTATION

Interventions and (Rationales)	Patient-Centered Care
Ensuring therapeutic effects: • Continue assessments as described earlier for therapeutic effects. Drug therapy may take several days to have the full effect with lessening pain and tenderness, increased range of motion, and before an increased ability to complete ADLs is noted. Support the patient in self-care activities as necessary until improvement is observed. (An ability to carry out ADLs gradually improves with consistent usage.)	• Teach the patient that improvement may gradually be noted over several days' time and full therapeutic effects may take one week or longer. Nonpharmacologic measures may be needed until the full medication effect is noted.
Minimizing adverse effects: • Monitor motor coordination and/or ambulation and other essential motor activities. **Lifespan:** Be particularly cautious with older adults who are at an increased risk for falls. (Gradual improvement in symptoms may be noticed over several weeks but pain or spasms may affect motor skills. Particular care with ambulation is required because pain, spasms, or rigidity may increase the risk of falls. **Lifespan:** Cyclobenzaprine is included in the Beers List of potentially inappropriate drugs for older adults and warrants careful monitoring.)	• **Safety:** Instruct the patient to call for assistance prior to getting out of bed or attempting to walk alone if pain, spasms, or rigidity are particularly severe. • **Collaboration:** Assess the ability of the patient, family, or caregiver to carry out ADLs at home, and explore the need for additional health care referrals if the disability will require long-term physical therapy (e.g., CP). • **Safety:** Instruct the patient to avoid driving or other activities requiring mental alertness or physical coordination until the effects of the drug are known.

continued

Nursing Practice Application *continued*

IMPLEMENTATION	
Interventions and (Rationales)	**Patient-Centered Care**
• Continue to monitor vital signs, particularly blood pressure. Take the blood pressure lying, sitting, and standing to detect orthostatic hypotension. **Lifespan:** Be particularly cautious with older adults who are at an increased risk for hypotension. Notify the health care provider if the blood pressure decreases beyond established parameters or if hypotension is accompanied by reflex tachycardia. (Orthostatic hypotension is a possible adverse effect and, in addition to muscles spasms, pain, or rigidity, may increase the risk of falls or injury. Cyclobenzaprine (Amrix, Flexeril) may cause tachycardia and palpitations.)	• **Safety:** Teach the patient to rise from lying to sitting or standing slowly to avoid dizziness or falls. If dizziness occurs, the patient should sit or lie down and not attempt to stand or walk, until the sensation passes. • Have the patient immediately report dizziness, lightheadedness, rapid heart rate, palpitations, or syncope.
• Monitor muscle tone, range of motion, and degree of muscle spasm. (Improvement should be observed over the first week or two of therapy. Increasing ability of range of motion and decreased muscle tenderness and rigidity helps to determine effectiveness of drug therapy.)	• Teach the patient how to perform gentle range-of-motion exercises, exercising only to the point of mild physical discomfort but never pain, throughout the day.
• Provide additional pain relief measures such as positional support, gentle massage, and moist heat or ice packs. (Supportive nursing measures may increase pain relief and supplement drug therapy.)	• Teach the patient complementary pain interventions such as positioning, gentle massage, application of heat or cold to the painful area, distraction with television or music, or guided imagery.
• Continue to monitor renal and hepatic function periodically if the patient is on long-term use of the drug. (Muscle relaxants and antispasmodic drugs may cause hepatotoxicity as an adverse effect. **Lifespan:** Women over the age of 35 taking dantrolene (Dantrium) are at greater risk for hepatotoxicity and should be monitored frequently.)	• Instruct the patient on the need to return periodically for laboratory work.
• Assess bowel sounds periodically if constipation or diarrhea is problematic. Increase fluid intake and dietary fiber intake to prevent gastrointestinal (GI) effects and to ease dry mouth effects. (Muscle relaxant drugs may decrease peristalsis as an adverse effect. Significantly diminished or absent bowels sounds are immediately reported to the health care provider. **Lifespan:** The older adult is at increased risk of constipation due to slowed peristalsis. Additional fluids and fiber may ease constipation and prevent diarrhea but additional medications such as Miralax or Colace may be required if the constipation is severe.)	• Teach the patient to increase fluids to 2 L per day and increase the intake of dietary fiber such as fruits, vegetables, and whole grains. • Instruct the patient to report severe constipation to the health care provider for additional advice on laxatives or stool softeners.
• Assess for tongue or facial swelling. (Although rare, cyclobenzaprine may cause swelling of the tongue or face and should be reported immediately.)	• Instruct the patient to immediately report any swelling of the tongue, face, or throat.
• Avoid the use of other CNS depressants, including alcohol, and use with caution concurrently with antihypertensive medications. (CNS depressants and alcohol may increase the sedative properties of the drug. Antihypertensive medications may increase risk of hypotension.)	• Teach the patient to avoid or eliminate alcohol while on the drug. If other sedatives or antihypertensives are ordered, have the patient consult with the health care provider about dose and sequencing. Immediately report any dizziness, palpitations, or syncope.
• Assess for urinary retention periodically. (Muscle relaxants and antispasmodics may cause urinary retention as an adverse effect. **Lifespan:** Be aware that the male older adult with an enlarged prostate is at higher-risk for mechanical obstruction.)	• Instruct the patient to immediately report an inability to void and increasing bladder pressure or pain.
Patient understanding of drug therapy: • Use opportunities during administration of medications and during assessments to provide patient education. (Using time during nursing care helps to optimize and reinforce key teaching areas.)	• The patient should be able to state the reason for the drug, appropriate dose and scheduling, and what adverse effects to observe for and when to report them.

Nursing Practice Application *continued*

IMPLEMENTATION	
Interventions and (Rationales)	**Patient-Centered Care**
Patient self-administration of drug therapy: • When administering the medication, instruct the patient, family, or caregiver in the proper self-administration of the drug (e.g., take the drug as prescribed when needed). (Using time during nurse administration of these drugs helps to reinforce teaching.)	• Instruct the patient in proper administration guidelines. The dose should be taken consistently and not prn for best results unless otherwise ordered. Encourage the patient to maintain a medication log, noting symptoms along with dose and timing of medications, and to bring the log to each health care visit. • Teach patients to not open, chew, or crush extended release tablets (e.g., cylcobenzaprine [Amrix, Flexeril]); swallow them whole with plenty of water. • Take the drug with food or milk if stomach upset occurs.

See Tables 21.1 and 21.2 for lists of drugs to which these nursing actions apply.

Chapter Review

KEY Concepts

The numbered key concepts provide a succinct summary of the important points from the corresponding numbered section within the chapter. If any of these points are not clear, refer to the numbered section within the chapter for review.

21.1 Muscle spasms, which are involuntary contractions of a muscle or group of muscles, most commonly occur because of localized trauma to the skeletal muscle.

21.2 Muscle spasms can be treated through nonpharmacologic and pharmacologic strategies.

21.3 Many muscle relaxants treat muscle spasms at the level of the CNS by generating their effect within the brain and/or spinal cord, usually by inhibiting upper motor neuron activity, causing sedation, or altering simple reflexes.

21.4 Spasticity, a condition in which selected muscles are continuously contracted, results from damage to the CNS. Effective treatment for spasticity includes both physical therapy and medications.

21.5 Some antispasmodic drugs used for spasticity act directly on muscle tissue, relieving spasticity by interfering with the release of calcium ions.

21.6 Neuromuscular blocking drugs are classified as nondepolarizing blockers and depolarizing blockers. Both classes of drugs bind to the acetylcholine nicotinic receptor, relaxing muscles by slightly different mechanisms and duration of action.

REVIEW Questions

1. Cyclobenzaprine (Amrix, Flexeril) is prescribed for a patient with muscle spasms of the lower back. Appropriate nursing interventions would include which of the following? (Select all that apply.)
   1. Assessing the heart rate for tachycardia
   2. Assessing the home environment for patient safety concerns
   3. Encouraging frequent ambulation
   4. Providing oral suction for excessive oral secretions
   5. Providing assistance with activities of daily living such as reading
2. The patient is scheduled to receive rimabotulinumtoxinB (Myobloc) for treatment of muscle spasticity. Which of the following will the nurse teach the patient to report immediately?
   1. Fever, aches, or chills
   2. Difficulty swallowing, ptosis, blurred vision
   3. Continuous spasms and pain on the affected side
   4. Moderate levels of muscle weakness on the affected side
3. A patient has purchased capsaicin over-the-counter cream to use for muscle aches and pains. What education is most important to give this patient?
   1. Apply with a gloved hand only to the site of pain.
   2. Apply the medication liberally above and below the site of pain.
   3. Apply to areas of redness and irritation only.
   4. Apply liberally with a bare hand to the affected limb.
4. A patient has been prescribed clonazepam (Klonopin) for muscle spasms and stiffness secondary to an automobile accident. While the patient is taking this drug, what is the nurse's primary concern?
   1. Monitoring hepatic laboratory work
   2. Encouraging fluid intake to prevent dehydration
   3. Assessing for drowsiness and implementing safety measures
   4. Providing social services referral for patient concerns about the cost of the drug
5. A female patient is prescribed dantrolene (Dantrium) for painful muscle spasms associated with multiple sclerosis. The nurse is writing the discharge plan for the patient and will include which of the following teaching points? (Select all that apply.)
   1. If muscle spasms are severe, supplement the medication with hot baths or showers three times per day.
   2. Inform the health care provider if she is taking estrogen products.
   3. Sip water, ice, or hard candy to relieve dry mouth.
   4. Return periodically for required laboratory work.
   5. Obtain at least 20 minutes of sun exposure per day to boost vitamin D levels.
6. A patient who has been prescribed baclofen (Lioresal) returns to the health care provider after a week of drug therapy, complaining of continued muscle spasms of the lower back. What further assessment data will the nurse gather?
   1. Whether the patient has been taking the medication consistently or only when the pain is severe
   2. Whether the patient has been consuming alcohol during this time
   3. Whether the patient has increased the dosage without consulting the health care provider
   4. Whether the patient's log of symptoms indicates that the patient is telling the truth

PATIENT-FOCUSED Case Study

Nathan Ebbens, a 32-year-old farmer, injured his lower back while unloading a truck at a farm cooperative. His health care provider started him on cyclobenzaprine (Amrix, Flexeril) 10 mg tid for 7 days and referred him to outpatient physical therapy. After 4 days, the patient reports back to the office nurse that he is constipated and having trouble emptying his bladder.

1. What might be the cause of these effects?
2. As the nurse, what orders do you anticipate from the provider?
3. Nathan is switched to baclofen (Lioresal) orally. What additional teaching will he need?

CRITICAL THINKING Questions

1. A 46-year-old male quadriplegic patient has been experiencing severe spasticity in the lower extremities, making it difficult for him to maintain his position in his electric wheelchair. Prior to the episodes of spasticity, the patient was able to maintain a sitting posture. The risks and benefits of therapy with dantrolene (Dantrium) have been explained to him, and he has decided that the benefits outweigh the risks. What assessments should the nurse make to determine whether the treatment is beneficial?

2. A 52-year-old executive has started treatment with onabotulinumtoxinA (Botox) and is preparing to return home after her first injections. What should the nurse teach her?

Visit www.pearsonhighered.com/nursingresources for answers and rationales for all activities.

REFERENCES

Baker, K. W., Tann, B., Mutlu, A., & Gaebler-Spira, D. (2014). Improvements in children with cerebral palsy following intrathecal baclofen: Use of the Rehabilitation Institute of Chicago Care and Comfort Caregiver Questionnaire (RIC CareQ). *Journal of Child Neurology, 29,* 312–317. doi:10.1177/0883073812475156

Borrini, L., Bensmail, D., Thiebaut, J. B., Hugeron, C., Rech, C., & Jourdan, C. (2014). Occurrence of adverse events in long-term intrathecal baclofen infusion: A 1-year follow-up study of 158 adults. *Archives of Physical Medicine and Rehabilitation, 95,* 1032–1038. doi:10.1016/j.apmr.2013.12.019

Herdman, T. H., & Kamitsuru, S. (Eds.). (2014). *NANDA International nursing diagnoses: Definitions and classification, 2015–2017.* Oxford, United Kingdom: Wiley-Blackwell.

Knolle, E., Zadrazil, M., Kovacs, G. G., Medwed, S., Sharbert, G., & Schemper, M. (2013). Comparison of cooling and EMLA to reduce the burning pain during capsaicin 8% patch application: A randomized, double-blind, placebo-controlled study. *Pain, 154,* 2729–2736. doi:10.1016/j.pain.2013.08.001

Mathur, S. N., Chu, S. K., McCormick, Z., Chang Chien, G., & Marciniak, C. M. (2014). Long-term intrathecal baclofen: Outcomes after more than 10 years of treatment. *PM & R: The Journal of Injury, Function, and Rehabilitation, 6,* 506–513. doi:10.1016/j.pmrj.2013.12.005

Mou, J., Paillard, F., Turnbull, B., Trudeau, J., Stoker, M., & Katz, N. P. (2014). Qutenza (capsaicin) 8% patch onset and duration of response and effects of multiple treatments in neuropathic pain patients. *The Clinical Journal of Pain, 30,* 286–294. doi:10.1097/AJP.0b013e31829a4ced

Wagner, T., Poole, C., & Roth-Daniek, A. (2013). The capsaicin 8% patch for neuropathic pain in clinical practice: A retrospective analysis. *Pain Medicine, 14,* 1202–1211. doi:10.1111/pme.12143

SELECTED BIBLIOGRAPHY

American Association of Neurological Surgeons. (2005). *Dystonia,* Retrieved from http://www.aans.org/patient%20information/conditions%20and%20treatments/dystonia.aspx

American Association of Neurological Surgeons. (2006). *Spasticity,* Retrieved from http://www.aans.org/Patient%20Information/Conditions%20and%20Treatments/Spasticity.aspx

Bowman, W. C. (2006). Neuromuscular block. *British Journal of Pharmacology, 147*(Suppl. 1), S277–S286. doi:10.1038/sj.bjp.0706404

Fortuna, R., Horisberger, M., Vaz, M. A., Herzog, W. (2013). Do skeletal muscle properties recover following repeat onabotulinum toxin A injections? *Journal of Biomechanics, 46,* 2426–2433. doi:10.1016/j.jbiomech.2013.07.028

Kheder, A., Padmakumari, K., & Nair, S. (2012). Spasticity: Pathophysiology, evaluation and management. *Practical Neurology, 12*(5), 289–298. doi:10.1136/practneurol-2011-000155

Lam, T. I., Bingham, D., Chang, T. J., Lee, C. C., Shi, J., Wang, D., . . . Liu, J. (2013). Beneficial effects of minocycline and botulinum toxin-induced constraint physical therapy following experimental traumatic brain injury. *Neurorehabilitation Neural Repair, 27,* 889–899. doi:10.1177/1545968313491003

Lecouflet, M., Leux, C., Fenot, M., Célerier, P., & Maillard, H. (2014). Duration of efficacy increases with the repetition of botulinum toxin A injections in primary palmar hyperhidrosis: A study of 28 patients. *Journal of American Academy of Dermatology, 70,* 1083–1087. doi:10.1016/j.jaad.2013.12.035

Lim, E. C., Quek, A. M., & Seet, R. C. (2011). Accurate targeting of botulinum toxin injections: How to and why. *Parkinsonism Related Disorders, 17*(Suppl. 1), S34–S39. doi:10.1016/j.parkreldis.2011.06.016

Matthews, E., & Hanna, M. G. (2014). Repurposing of sodium channel antagonists as potential new anti-myotonic drugs. *Experimental Neurology, 261,* 812–815. doi:10.1016/j.expneurol.2014.09.003

Schneiderbanger, D., Johannsen, S., Roewer, N., & Schuster, F. (2014). Management of malignant hyperthermia: Diagnosis and treatment. *Journal of Therapeutics and Clinical Risk Management, 10,* 355–362. doi:10.2147/TCRM.S47632

Vitale, D. C., Piazza, C., Sinagra, T., Urso, V., Cardì, F., Drago, F., & Salomone, S. (2013). Pharmacokinetic characterization of tizanidine nasal spray, a novel intranasal delivery method for the treatment of skeletal muscle spasm. *Clinical Drug Investigation, 33,* 885–891. doi:10.1007/s40261-013-0137-2

Chapter 22

Substance Abuse

Drugs at a Glance

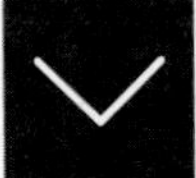

Learning Outcomes

After reading this chapter, the student should be able to:

1. Explain underlying causes of substance abuse.
2. Compare and contrast psychological and physical dependence.
3. Compare withdrawal syndromes for the various substance abuse classes.
4. Discuss how the nurse can recognize drug tolerance in patients.
5. Explain the major characteristics of abuse, dependence, tolerance, and approaches for treatment in the following drug classes: alcohol, nicotine, marijuana, hallucinogens, CNS stimulants, sedatives, and opioids.
6. Describe the role of the nurse in delivering care to individuals who have substance use disorder.

Throughout history, individuals have consumed both natural substances and prescription drugs to improve performance, assist with relaxation, alter psychological state, and enhance social interaction. Substance abuse has a tremendous societal, economic, and health impact. Although the terms *drug abuse* and *substance abuse* have often been used interchangeably, substance abuse is considered more inclusive because of the involved legal and illegal agents, musused household items, and drugs available for medication purposes. By definition, *substance abuse* is considered the self-administration of a drug in a manner that does not conform to the norms within the patient's own culture and society. A newer term recently introduced in the medical literature to describe this condition is **substance use disorder.** This eliminates the word "abuse," which has a negative stigma attached to it.

22.1 Overview of Substance Use Disorder

Abused substances belong to many diverse chemical classes. Drugs have few structural similarities, but they all have in common the ability to affect the brain and central nervous system (CNS). Some substances—such as opium, marijuana, cocaine, nicotine, caffeine, and alcohol—are obtained from natural sources. Others are synthetic or **designer drugs,** created in illegal laboratories for the purpose of profiting from illicit drug trafficking.

Although the public associates substance abuse with illegal drugs, this is not necessarily the case. Alcohol and nicotine, two of the most commonly abused drugs, are both legal for adults. Abused legal CNS-influencing drugs include prescription medications such as methylphenidate (Ritalin) and oxycodone (OxyContin). Legal substances without prescription involve agents such as volatile inhalants. Ketamine and nitrous oxide are examples of misused legal anesthetics. Huffing of organic, household, or industrial chemical products is not uncommon. Aerosols and paint thinners are inhalants that can be obtained without prescription. Athletes often abuse legal anabolic steroids.

Frequently abused illegal substances include heroin (opioids) and hallucinogens such as lysergic acid diethylamide (LSD) and crystalized methamphetamine produced in a chemical laboratory. Phencyclidine hydrochloride (PCP) is a hallucinogen with a history of abuse but not so much at present. Marijuana is now illegal in many states but legal for medical purposes and for recreational use at some locations.

Several drugs once used therapeutically are now illegal due to their high potential for abuse. Cocaine was once widely used as a local anesthetic, but today nearly all the cocaine acquired by users is obtained illegally. Although LSD is now illegal, in the 1940s and 1950s it was used in psychotherapy. Phencyclidine was popular in the early 1960s as an anesthetic but was withdrawn from the market in 1965 because patients reported hallucinations, delusions, and anxiety after recovering from anesthesia. Many amphetamines once used for weight loss and bronchodilation were discontinued in the 1980s after unpleasant psychotic episodes were reported. The sum of this information relates to the diversity of substances and circumstances within our culture, in which patients can either misuse or abuse drugs.

22.2 Neurobiologic and Psychosocial Components of Substance Use Disorder

Addiction is an overwhelming compulsion that drives someone to take drugs repetitively, despite serious health and social consequences. It is impossible to accurately predict whether a person will develop substance use disorder. Attempts to predict a person's addictive tendency using psychological profiles or genetic markers have largely been unsuccessful. Substance use depends on multiple, complex, interacting variables such as described in the following categories:

- *User-related factors.* Genetic factors (e.g., metabolic enzymes, innate tolerance), personality for risk-taking behavior, prior experiences with drugs, disorders that may require a scheduled drug
- *Environmental factors.* Societal and community norms, role models, peer influences, educational level
- *Factors related to the agent or drug.* Cost, availability, dose, mode of administration (e.g., oral [PO], intravenous [IV], inhalation), speed of onset/termination, and length of drug use

In the case of legal prescription drugs, addiction may begin with a legitimate need for pharmacotherapy. For example, narcotic analgesics may be prescribed for pain relief, or sedatives may be taken for a sleep disorder. The drug experience brings some degree of satisfaction or pleasure to the user. Whether it be pain relief, euphoria, sedation, or feelings of well-being or excitement, the substance user finds the drug experience reinforcing and worth repeating.

There is often the concern that the therapeutic use of scheduled drugs creates large numbers of addicted patients. Because of this, medications having a potential for abuse have been prescribed at the lowest effective dose and for the shortest time necessary to treat the medical problem. Prescription drugs in fact rarely cause addiction when used as prescribed and according to accepted medical protocols. As mentioned in chapter 2, numerous laws have been passed in an attempt to limit substance abuse and addiction. The risk of addiction caused by prescription medications is primarily a function of dose and duration of drug therapy. The nurse should be able to administer medications for the relief of patient symptoms without unnecessary fear of producing dependency.

22.3 Physical and Psychological Dependence

Whether a substance is addictive is related to how easily an individual can stop taking the agent on a repetitive basis. When a person has an overwhelming desire to take a drug and cannot stop, this condition is referred to as *substance dependence*. Substance dependence is classified into two categories, physical dependence and psychological dependence.

Physical dependence refers to an altered physical condition caused by the adaptation of the nervous system to repeated substance use. Over time, the body's cells become accustomed to the presence of the abused substance. With physical dependence, uncomfortable symptoms known as *withdrawal* result when the agent is discontinued. Alcohol, sedatives, nicotine, and CNS stimulants are examples of substances that with extended use may easily cause physical dependence. Repeated doses of opioids, such as morphine and heroin, may produce physical dependence rather quickly, particularly when the drugs are taken IV.

In contrast, **psychological dependence** refers to a condition in which no obvious physical signs of discomfort are observed after the agent is discontinued. The user, however, will have an overwhelming desire to continue drug-seeking behavior despite obvious negative economic, physical, or social consequences. Associated intense craving may be connected with the patient's home or social environment. For psychological dependence to occur, relatively high doses of drugs are usually taken for a prolonged period. Examples are antianxiety drugs and drugs for insomnia (e.g., benzodiazepines and sleep aid medication). On the other hand, psychological dependence may develop quickly after only one use, as with crack cocaine, a potent, rather inexpensive, form of cocaine. Whereas physical dependence is often overcome within a few days or weeks after discontinuing the drug, psychological dependence may persist for months or years and be responsible for relapses back to drug-seeking behavior.

22.4 Withdrawal Syndrome

Once a person becomes physically dependent and the substance is abruptly discontinued, **withdrawal syndrome** may occur. Prescription drugs are often used to reduce the severity of withdrawal symptoms. For example, alcohol withdrawal might be treated with the short-acting

PharmFacts

SUBSTANCE USE IN THE UNITED STATES

- Over 28 million Americans have used illicit drugs at least once.
- Nurses and other health care providers are at increased risk for substance use problems especially with benzodiazepines, opioids, and alcohol. It is estimated that 6% to 8% of health professionals have a substance use problem.
- Twenty-five percent of high school students use an illegal drug monthly. Of the most commonly abused substances, marijuana remains at the top of the list. Over 36% of 10th-grade students and over 46% of 12th-grade students have reported using marijuana and hashish.
- An estimated 2.4 million Americans have used heroin during their lifetime.
- About one in five Americans has lived with an alcoholic while growing up. Children of alcoholic parents are four times more likely to become alcoholics than children of nonalcoholic parents.
- Alcohol is an important factor in 68% of manslaughters, 54% of murders, 48% of robberies, and 44% of burglaries.
- Among youth between the ages of 12 and 17, 7.2 million have drunk alcohol at least once. Girls are as likely as boys to drink alcohol.
- Barbiturate overdose is a factor in almost one third of all drug-related deaths.
- Two million Americans have used cocaine on a monthly basis; about 567,000 have used crack cocaine.
- Approximately 70% of the cocaine entering the United States comes from Colombia and passes through south Florida.
- There has been a considerable decline in recent years among 8th and 10th graders in perceived risk associated with inhalant use. Sixteen percent of 8th graders and 11% of 12th graders have reported using volatile inhalants.
- Thirty percent of all Americans are cigarette smokers, including 25% who are between the ages of 12 and 25.
- Forty-three percent of 10th-grade students and 54% of 12th-grade students have reported smoking cigarettes.
- The trend for Ecstasy (MDMA) use has increased slightly since 2013. Over 8% of 12th-grade students have reported using Ecstasy.
- LSD is one of the most potent drugs known, with only 25–150 mcg constituting a dose. Almost 9% of 12th-grade students have reported using LSD.
- The misuse of over-the-counter cough and cold medicines to get high involves medicines that contain the cough-suppressant dextromethorphan. Youngsters sometimes take large doses of these medicines in order to get high, which is a dangerous practice.

Community-Oriented Practice

SUBSTANCE USE DISORDER AND CO-OCCURRING MENTAL DISORDERS

Substance use and transitioning from use to abuse, have been noted in patients with mental disorders at higher rates than patients without mental illness. In patients with mental disorders, diagnoses of personality and psychotic disorders had the highest association with the transition from use to abuse, and this was especially true for nicotine (Lev-Ran, Imtiaz, Rehm, & Le Foll, 2013). Depression as well as suicide attempt are also linked to substance abuse. Ortiz-Gómez, López-Canul, and Arankowsky-Sandoval (2014) conducted a study with patients in drug rehabilitation and found that over 68% of the patients had experienced depression prior to the onset of substance abuse. The rate of suicide attempt was also greater during the rehabilitation process if the patient had had previous attempts before the substance abuse began. For patients seeking help for substance use disorder, improvement of their depression has also been noted. The longer the patient waited before treatment began, there was less chance of improvement in their depression (Chan, Huang, Bradley, & Unützer, 2014). When treating the patient with a substance use disorder, the nurse should be alert to the possibility of other underlying mental disorders, including anxiety and depressive disorders, or the more severe illnesses such as psychosis and schizophrenia. Treating the whole patient, including concurrent disorders, may improve the overall outcome of treatment.

benzodiazepine oxazepam (Serax); opioid withdrawal might be treated with methadone. Symptoms of nicotine withdrawal might be relieved with replacement therapy in the form of nicotine patches or chewing gum. For withdrawal from CNS stimulants, hallucinogens, or inhalants, specific pharmacologic intervention is generally not indicated.

Symptoms of withdrawal may be particularly severe for those who are dependent on alcohol or sedatives. Because of the severity of the symptoms, the process of withdrawal from these agents is generally best accomplished in a treatment facility. Examples of drugs and associated withdrawal symptoms and characteristics are shown in Table 22.1.

With chronic substance use, people will often associate use of the substance with their conditions and surroundings, including social contacts with other users who are also taking the drug. Users tend to revert to drug-seeking behavior when they return to the company of other substance users. Counselors often encourage users to refrain from associating with past social contacts or having relationships with other substance users to lessen the possibility for relapse. The formation of new social contacts within self-help organizations such as Alcoholics Anonymous helps some people transition to a drug-free lifestyle. Residential secondary treatment or "step-down" care from primary treatment may be required for some patients who are not ready to return to the community after detoxification.

22.5 Tolerance

Tolerance is a biologic condition that occurs when the body adapts to a substance after repeated administration. Over time, higher doses of the agent are required to produce the same initial effect. For example, at the start of pharmacotherapy, a patient may find that 2 mg of a sedative is effective for inducing sleep. After taking the medication for several months, the patient notices that it takes 4 mg or perhaps 6 mg to fall asleep. Tolerance should be thought of as a natural consequence of continued drug use

Table 22.1 Selected Drugs, Withdrawal Symptoms, and Characteristics

Drug	Physiological and Psychological Effects	Signs of Toxicity
Alcohol	Tremors, fatigue, anxiety, abdominal cramping, hallucinations, confusion, seizures, delirium	Extreme somnolence, severe CNS depression, diminished reflexes, respiratory depression
Barbiturates	Insomnia, anxiety, weakness, abdominal cramps, tremor, anorexia, seizures, skin hypersensitivity reactions, hallucinations, delirium	Severe CNS depression, tremor, diaphoresis, vomiting, cyanosis, tachycardia, Cheyne–Stokes respirations
Benzodiazepines	Insomnia, restlessness, abdominal pain, nausea, sensitivity to light and sound, headache, fatigue, muscle twitches	Somnolence, confusion, diminished reflexes, coma
Cocaine and amphetamines	Mental depression, anxiety, extreme fatigue, hunger	Dysrhythmias, lethargy, skin pallor, psychosis
Hallucinogens	Rarely observed; dependent on specific drug	Panic reactions, confusion, blurred vision, increase in blood pressure, psychotic-like state
Marijuana	Irritability, restlessness, insomnia, tremor, chills, weight loss	Euphoria, paranoia, panic reactions, hallucinations, psychotic-like state
Nicotine	Irritability, anxiety, restlessness, headaches, increased appetite, insomnia, inability to concentrate, increase in heart rate and blood pressure	Heart palpitations, tachyarrhythmias, confusion, depression, seizures
Opioids	Excessive sweating, restlessness, pinpointed pupils, agitation, goose bumps, tremor, violent yawning, increased heart rate, orthostatic hypotension, nausea/vomiting, abdominal cramps and pain, muscle spasms with kicking movements, weight loss	Respiratory depression, cyanosis, extreme somnolence, coma

and not considered evidence of addiction or substance use disorder. Development of drug tolerance is common for substances that affect the nervous system.

Tolerance does not develop at the same rate for all actions of a drug. The following are a few examples:

- Patients usually develop tolerance to the nausea and vomiting produced by narcotic analgesics after only a few doses.
- Patients will often endure annoying side effects of drugs, such as the sedation caused by antihistamines, if they know that tolerance to these effects will develop quickly.
- Tolerance to mood-altering drugs and their ability to reduce pain develops more slowly.
- Tolerance to the drug's ability to constrict the pupils never develops.

Once tolerance to a substance develops, it often extends to closely related drugs. This phenomenon is known as **cross-tolerance.** For example, a heroin addict will become tolerant to the analgesic effects of other opioids such as morphine or meperidine. Patients who have developed tolerance to alcohol will show tolerance to other CNS depressants such as barbiturates, benzodiazepines, and some general anesthetics. This has important clinical implications for the nurse, because doses of these related medications will need adjustment in order to obtain maximum therapeutic benefit.

The terms *immunity* and *resistance* are often confused with tolerance. These terms more correctly refer to the immune system and infections, respectively. They should not be used interchangeably with tolerance. For example, patients become tolerant to the effects of pain relievers: They do not become immune or resistant. Microorganisms become resistant to the effects of an antibiotic: They do not become tolerant.

22.6 Central Nervous System Depressants

CNS depressants are a group of drugs that cause patients to feel relaxed or sedated. Drugs in this group include barbiturates, nonbarbiturate sedative–hypnotics, benzodiazepines, alcohol, and opioids. Although the majority of these are legal substances, they are controlled due to their abuse potential.

Sedatives and Sedative–Hypnotics

Sedatives, also known as *tranquilizers,* are prescribed for sleep disorders and certain forms of epilepsy. The two primary classes of sedatives are the barbiturates and the nonbarbiturate sedative–hypnotics. Their actions, indications, safety profiles, and addictive potential are roughly equivalent. Physical dependence, psychological dependence, and tolerance develop when these agents are taken for extended periods at high doses (see chapter 2). Patients sometimes abuse these drugs by faking prescriptions or by sharing their medication with friends. Sedatives are commonly combined with other drugs of abuse, such as CNS stimulants or alcohol. Addicts often alternate between amphetamines, which keep them awake for several days, and barbiturates, which are needed to help them relax and fall asleep.

Many sedatives have a long duration of action: Effects may last an entire day, depending on the specific drug. Users may appear dull or apathetic. Higher doses resemble alcohol intoxication, with slurred speech and motor incoordination. Death may result from barbiturate overdose. Four commonly abused barbiturates are pentobarbital (Nembutal), amobarbital (Amytal), secobarbital (Seconal), and a combination of secobarbital and amobarbital (Tuinal). The historic use of barbiturates in treating sleep disorders is discussed in chapter 14, and their use for epilepsy treatment is presented in chapter 15.

The medical use of barbiturates and nonbarbiturate sedative–hypnotics has declined markedly over the past 20 years. Overdoses of these drugs are extremely dangerous. They suppress the respiratory centers in the brain, and the user may stop breathing or lapse into a coma. Withdrawal symptoms resemble those of alcohol withdrawal and may be life threatening.

Benzodiazepines are another group of CNS depressants that have a potential for abuse. They are one of the most widely prescribed classes of drugs and have largely replaced the barbiturates. Their primary indication is anxiety (see chapter 14), although they are also used to prevent seizures (see chapter 15) and for muscle relaxation (see chapter 21). Popular benzodiazepines include alprazolam (Xanax), diazepam (Valium), temazepam (Restoril), triazolam (Halcion), and midazolam (Versed).

As a frequently prescribed drug class, benzodiazepine abuse is fairly common. Patients abusing benzodiazepines may appear carefree, detached, sleepy, or disoriented. Death due to overdose is rare, even with high doses. Users may combine these agents with alcohol, cocaine, or heroin to augment their drug experience. If combined with other agents, overdose may be lethal. The benzodiazepine withdrawal syndrome is less severe than that of barbiturates or alcohol. Due to the longer half-life of benzodiazepines, however, drug levels remain high for several weeks. This makes abuse of benzodiazepines very dangerous.

Opioids

Opioids, also known as *opioid narcotics,* are prescribed for severe pain, persistent cough, and diarrhea. The opioid class includes natural substances obtained from the unripe seeds of the poppy plant such as opium, morphine, and codeine. Synthetic drug examples are meperidine (Demerol), oxycodone (OxyContin), fentanyl (Duragesic, Sublimaze), methadone (Dolophine), and heroin. Vicodin (hydrocodone and acetaminophen combination) is one of the most widely abused of the narcotic drugs, most of which are analgesics. The therapeutic applications of the opioid analgesics are discussed in more detail in chapter 18.

The effects of oral opioids begin within 30 minutes and may last more than a day. *Parenteral* forms produce immediate effects, including the brief, intense rush of euphoria sought by heroin addicts. Individuals experience a range of CNS effects from extreme pleasure to slowed body activities and profound sedation. Signs include constricted pupils, an increase in the pain threshold, and, ultimately, respiratory depression. Overdose of opioids is extremely dangerous and fatal. The pharmacotherapy of opioid blocking drugs is covered in chapter 18.

Addiction to opioids can occur rapidly, and withdrawal can produce intense symptoms. Although extremely unpleasant, withdrawal from opioids is not life threatening, compared to barbiturate withdrawal. Methadone is a narcotic sometimes used to treat opioid addiction. Although methadone has addictive properties of its own, it does not produce the same degree of euphoria as with other opioids, and its effects are longer lasting. Heroin addicts are switched to methadone to prevent unpleasant withdrawal symptoms. Because methadone is taken orally, patients are no longer exposed to serious risks associated with IV drug use, such as hepatitis and AIDS. Withdrawal from methadone is more prolonged than with heroin or morphine, but the symptoms are less intense. Patients sometimes remain on methadone maintenance for a lifetime. A widely used alternative to methadone maintenance is the combination drug buprenorphine with naloxone, marketed as Suboxone or Zubsolv, which is discussed in chapter 18.

Ethyl Alcohol

Ethyl alcohol, commonly referred to as *drinking alcohol*, is one of the most commonly abused drugs. Alcohol is a legal substance for adults, and it is readily available as beer, wine, and liquor. The economic, social, and health consequences of alcohol abuse are staggering. Despite the enormous negative consequences associated with long-term use, small quantities of alcohol consumed on a daily basis may have medical benefits such as the reduced risks of stroke and heart attack.

Alcohol is classified as a CNS depressant because it slows the region of the brain responsible for alertness and wakefulness. Alcohol easily crosses the blood–brain barrier, so its effects are observed within 5 to 30 minutes after consumption. Effects of alcohol are directly proportional to the amount consumed and include relaxation, sedation, memory impairment, loss of motor coordination, reduced judgment, and decreased inhibition. Alcohol also imparts a characteristic odor to the breath and increases blood flow in certain areas of the skin, causing a flushed face, pink cheeks, or red nose. Although these symptoms are easily recognized, the nurse must be aware that other substances and disorders may cause similar effects. For example, many antianxiety agents, sedatives, and antidepressants can cause drowsiness, memory difficulties, and loss of motor coordination. Certain mouthwashes contain alcohol and may cause the breath to smell like alcohol. Other disorders may produce breath smells that can be confused with alcohol. During assessment, the skilled nurse must consider these factors before confirming alcohol use.

The presence of food in the stomach slows the absorption of alcohol, thus delaying the onset of drug action. Detoxification of alcohol by the liver occurs at a slow, constant rate, which is not affected by the presence of food. The average rate is about 15 mL per hour—the practical equivalent of one alcoholic beverage per hour. If consumed at a higher rate, alcohol will accumulate in the blood and produce greater depressant effects on the brain. Acute overdoses of alcohol produce vomiting, severe hypotension, respiratory failure, and coma. Death due to alcohol poisoning is not uncommon. The nurse should teach patients to never combine alcohol consumption with other CNS depressants because their effects are cumulative, and profound sedation or coma may result.

With acute alcohol withdrawal, benzodiazepines are the preferred drug class for treatment (Valium or Librium therapy). Although the use of benzodiazepines is more guarded for longer-term therapy of alcoholism, the reality is that many alcoholics continue to receive benzodiazepines for anxiety disorders and insomnia secondary to alcohol dependence. Seizures are also a risk to the patient, even after weeks of cessation from alcohol consumption; hence, benzodiazepine step-down therapy is often beneficial.

Naltrexone appears to be effective for reducing the craving experienced by people who are alcohol-dependent. Pleasurable effects and craving seem to be opioid–dependent processes physiologically. By blocking craving, and due to its pleasure-blocking properties, naltrexone may enhance the ability of patients to quit drinking.

Chronic alcohol consumption produces both psychological and physiological dependence and results in a large number of adverse health effects. The organ most affected by chronic alcohol abuse is the liver. Alcoholism is a common cause of *cirrhosis*, a debilitating and often fatal failure of the liver to perform its vital functions. Liver impairment causes abnormalities in blood-clotting and nutritional deficiencies. It also sensitizes the patient to the effects of all medications metabolized by the liver. For alcoholic patients, the nurse should begin therapy with reduced medication doses until the adverse effects of pharmacotherapy can be assessed.

Delirium tremens (DT) may occur in individuals who have constantly consumed alcohol for a longer period.

Symptoms are hallucinations, confusion, disorientation, and agitation. Many patients experience anxiety, panic, paranoia, and sensations of something crawling on the skin.

Alcohol withdrawal syndrome is severe and may be life threatening. Antiseizure medications may be used in the treatment of alcohol withdrawal (see chapter 15). Long-term treatment for alcohol abuse includes behavioral counseling and self-help groups such as Alcoholics Anonymous. Disulfiram (Antabuse) is another approach to discourage relapses. Disulfiram inhibits acetaldehyde dehydrogenase, the enzyme that metabolizes alcohol. If a patient consumes alcohol while taking disulfiram, he or she becomes violently ill within 5 to 10 minutes, with headache, shortness of breath, nausea/vomiting, and other unpleasant symptoms. Disulfiram is effective only in highly motivated patients, because the success of pharmacotherapy is entirely dependent on patient adherence. Alcohol sensitivity continues for up to 2 weeks after disulfiram has been discontinued. As a category X drug, disulfiram should never be taken during pregnancy.

In addition to disulfiram, acamprosate calcium (Campral) is an FDA-approved drug for maintaining alcohol abstinence in patients with alcohol dependence. Acamprosate's mechanism of action involves the restoration of neuronal excitation—the alteration of gamma-aminobutyrate and glutamate activity in the CNS—and does not appear to have other CNS actions. Adverse reactions to acamprosate include diarrhea, flatulence, and nausea. The drug is contraindicated in patients with severe renal impairment but may be used in patients at increased risk for hepatotoxicity.

Check Your Understanding 22.1

Opioid drugs such as the narcotics may cause tolerance, dependence, and addiction. What is the difference between these three terms? *Visit www.pearsonhighered.com/nursingresources for the answer.*

Complementary and Alternative Therapies

MILK THISTLE FOR ALCOHOL LIVER DAMAGE

Milk thistle (*Silybum marianum*) is a plant found growing in North America that has been used as an herbal medicine for centuries. The active ingredient in the milk thistle plant has been used to protect the liver in disorders such as hepatitis, cirrhosis, and gallbladder disease. Some studies have suggested that silymarin, which comes from the seeds of the milk thistle is able to neutralize the effects of alcohol and actually stimulate liver regeneration. It may act as an antioxidant and free-radical scavenger. Larger, controlled clinical trials have found no evidence of these protective properties, however (National Center for Complementary and Integrative Health, 2012). For most people, the herb has few side effects, other than mild diarrhea, bloating, and upset stomach. It may lower blood glucose levels, and patients with hypoglycemia or diabetes should discuss the use of milk thistle with their provider before taking it. It may also trigger allergies in patients allergic to the chrysanthemum family of plants (e.g., ragweed, marigolds, daisies).

22.7 Cannabinoids

Cannabinoids are substances obtained from the hemp plant *Cannabis sativa*, which thrives in tropical climates. Cannabinoid agents are usually smoked and include marijuana, hashish, and hash oil. Although more than 61 cannabinoid chemicals have been identified, the ingredient responsible for most of the psychoactive properties is **delta-9-tetrahydrocannabinol (THC).**

Marijuana

Marijuana, also known as *grass, pot, weed, reefer,* and many other names, is a natural product obtained from *C. sativa.* Marijuana is one of the most commonly used federally illicit drugs in the United States, although several states have legalized it. Alcohol outranks marijuana in terms of general use. Use of marijuana slows motor activity, decreases coordination, and causes disconnected thoughts, feelings of paranoia, and euphoria. It increases thirst and craving for food, particularly chocolate and other sweets. One hallmark symptom of marijuana use is red or bloodshot eyes, caused by dilation of blood vessels.

When inhaled, marijuana produces effects that occur within minutes and last up to 24 hours. Because marijuana smoke is inhaled more deeply and held within the lungs for a longer time than cigarette smoke, it introduces four times more particulates (tar) into the lungs than tobacco smoke. Smoking marijuana on a daily basis may increase the risk of lung cancer and other respiratory disorders. Chronic use is associated with a lack of motivation in achieving or pursuing life goals. THC accumulates in the reproductive organs and may cause infertility and birth defects.

Unlike many abused substances, marijuana produces little physical dependence or tolerance. Withdrawal symptoms are mild, if they are experienced at all. Metabolites of THC, however, remain in the body for months to years, allowing laboratory specialists to easily determine whether someone has taken marijuana. For several days after use, THC can also be detected in the urine. Despite numerous attempts to demonstrate therapeutic applications for marijuana, results have been controversial and the full medical value of the drug remains to be proven. Various diseases and conditions have been cited as being improved by marijuana: glaucoma, epilepsy, improved lung capacity in smokers of tobacco, benefit in cancer patients, anxiety, Alzheimer's disease, multiple sclerosis, muscle spasms, lessened side-effects of Hepatitis C treatment, inflammatory bowel disease, arthritis, metabolic benefits in emaciated patients, lupus, Crohn's disease, Parkinson's disease, post-traumatic stress disorder (PTSD), benefit to stroke victims, alcohol cessation treatment, to stimulate the appetite in chemotherapy patients, and to prevent nightmares.

In the United States, over 23 states have legalized medical marijuana. One major concern is the deleterious effects of marijuana among young users. Marijuana use among the youth has been a major debate in areas where there have been drives to legalize cannabis. Debates over marijuana legalization will no doubt continue for years.

"K2" or *"Spice"* refers to a wide variety of herbal mixtures with chemical additives that produce experiences similar to marijuana. Of the illicit drugs most used by high school students, Spice is second only to marijuana.

22.8 Hallucinogens

Hallucinogens consist of a diverse class of chemicals that have in common the ability to produce an altered, dreamlike state of consciousness. The prototype substance for this class, sometimes called **psychedelics,** is LSD. All hallucinogens are Schedule I drugs: They have no medical use.

LSD

For nearly all drugs of abuse, predictable symptoms occur in every user. Effects from hallucinogens, however, are highly variable and dependent on the mood and expectations of the user and the surrounding environment in which the substance is used. Two people taking the same agent will report completely different symptoms, and the same person may report different symptoms with each use. Users who take LSD and psilocybin (magic mushrooms, or "shrooms") (Figure 22.1) may experience symptoms such as laughter, visions, religious revelations, or deep personal insights. Common occurrences are hallucinations and afterimages projected onto people as they move. Users also report seeing unusually bright lights and vivid colors. Some users hear voices; others report smells. Many experience a profound sense of truth and deep-directed thoughts. Unpleasant experiences can be terrifying and may include anxiety, panic attacks, confusion, severe depression, and paranoia.

LSD, also called *acid, the beast, blotter acid, California sunshine,* and other names is derived from a fungus that grows on rye and other grains. LSD is nearly always administered orally and can be manufactured in capsule, tablet, or liquid form. A common and inexpensive method for distributing LSD is to place drops of the drug on paper, often containing the images of cartoon characters or graphics related to drug culture. The paper is dried; users then ingest the paper containing the LSD to produce the drug's effects.

LSD is distributed throughout the body immediately after use. Effects are experienced within an hour and may last from 6 to 12 hours. LSD affects the central and autonomic nervous systems, increasing blood pressure, elevating body temperature, dilating pupils, and increasing the heart rate. Repeated use may cause impaired memory and inability to reason. In extreme cases, patients may develop psychoses. One unusual adverse effect is flashbacks, in which the user experiences the effects of the drug again, sometimes weeks, months, or years after the drug was initially taken. Although tolerance is observed, little or no dependence occurs with the hallucinogens.

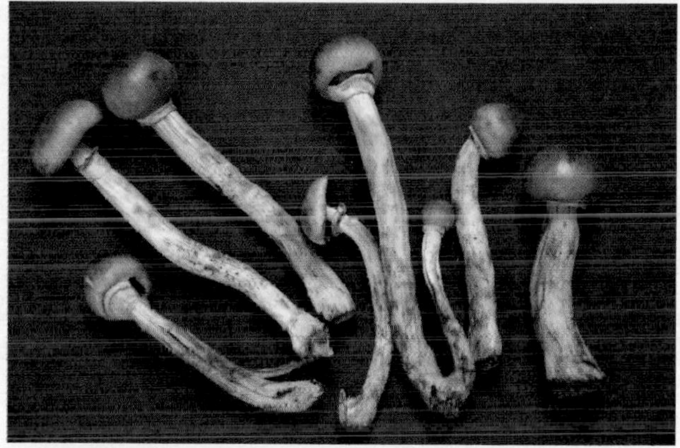

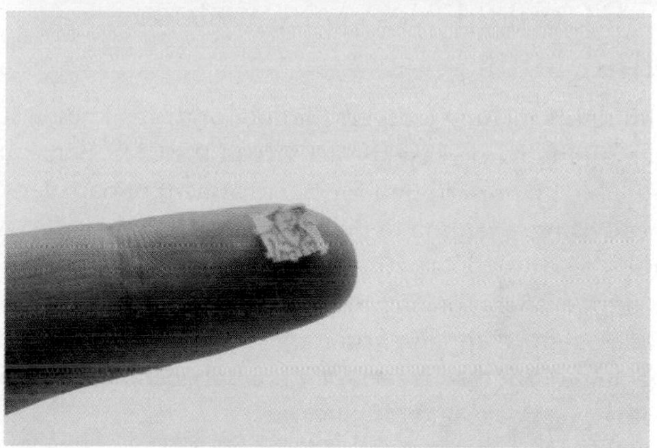

FIGURE 22.1 The hallucinogen psilocyban, derived from mushrooms (top) produces effects in the human body similar to LSD (bottom)
(top) Janine Wiedel Photolibrary/Alamy, (bottom) Joe Bird/Alamy.

Recreational and Club Drugs

In addition to LSD, other abused hallucinogens include the following:

- *Mescaline.* Found in the peyote cactus of Mexico and Central America (Figure 22.2)
- *MDMA (3,4-methylenedioxymethamphetamine; XTC, Ecstasy, or Molly).* An amphetamine originally synthesized for research purposes that has since become popular among teens and young adults

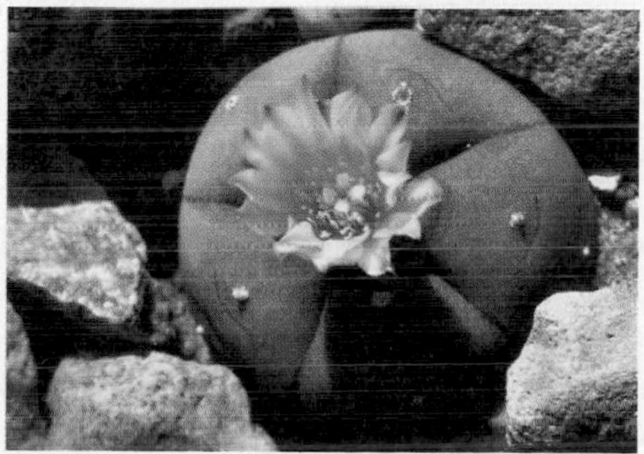

FIGURE 22.2 Mescaline, derived from the peyote cactus
R. Konig/Jacana/Science Source.

- *DOM (2,5 dimethoxy-4-methylamphetamine).* A recreational drug often linked with rave parties as a drug of choice having the name STP
- *MDA (3,4-methylenedioxyamphetamine).* Called the love drug because it is believed to enhance sexual desire
- *Phencyclidine (PCP; angel dust or phenylcyclohexylpiperidine).* Produces a trancelike state that may last for days and results in severe brain damage
- *Ketamine (date rape drug or special coke).* Produces unconsciousness and amnesia; primary legal use is as an anesthetic.

22.9 Central Nervous System Stimulants

Stimulants include a diverse family of drugs known for their ability to increase the activity of the CNS. Some are available by prescription for the treatment of narcolepsy, obesity, and attention deficit/hyperactivity disorder. As drugs of abuse, CNS stimulants are taken to produce a sense of exhilaration, improve mental and physical performance, reduce appetite, prolong wakefulness, or simply "get high." Stimulants include the amphetamines, cocaine, methylphenidate, and caffeine.

Amphetamines and Methylphenidate

CNS stimulants have effects similar to those of the neurotransmitter norepinephrine (see chapter 13). Norepinephrine affects awareness and wakefulness by activating neurons in a part of the brain called the **reticular formation.** High doses of amphetamines give the user a feeling of self-confidence, euphoria, alertness, and empowerment; but just as short-term use induces favorable feelings, long-term use often results in feelings of restlessness, anxiety, and fits of rage, especially when the user is coming down from a "high" induced by the drug.

Most CNS stimulants affect cardiovascular and respiratory activity, resulting in increased blood pressure and increased respiration rate. Other symptoms include dilated pupils, sweating, and tremors. Overdoses of some stimulants lead to seizures and cardiac arrest.

Amphetamines and dextroamphetamines were once widely prescribed for depression, obesity, drowsiness, and congestion. In the 1960s, it was recognized that the medical uses of amphetamines did not outweigh their risk for misuse. Due to the development of safer medications, the current therapeutic uses of these drugs are extremely limited. Most substance users obtain these agents from illegal laboratories which can easily produce amphetamines and make huge profits.

Dextroamphetamine (Dexedrine) may be prescribed for **attention deficit/hyperactivity disorder (ADHD)** and narcolepsy. Methamphetamine, commonly called *ice,* is often used as a recreational drug by users who like the rush that it gives them. It usually is administered in powder or crystal form, but it may also be smoked. Methamphetamine is a Schedule II drug marketed under the trade name Desoxyn, although most users obtain it from illegal methamphetamine (*meth*) laboratories. A structural analogue of methamphetamine, methcathinone (street name, *Cat*), is made illegally and snorted, taken orally, or injected IV. Methcathinone is a Schedule I agent.

Methylphenidate (Ritalin) is a CNS stimulant widely prescribed for children diagnosed with ADHD (see chapter 16). Adderall (dextroamphetamine and amphetamine combination) is another widely abused CNS stimulant used for the same therapeutic purpose. These drugs have a calming effect in children who are inattentive or hyperactive. By stimulating the alertness center in the brain, the child is able to focus on tasks for longer periods. Paradoxically, the calming effects these stimulants have on children are usually the opposite of the effects on adults. The therapeutic applications of methylphenidate and amphetamine combination drugs are discussed in chapter 16.

Ritalin is a Schedule II drug that has many of the same effects as cocaine and amphetamines. It is sometimes abused by adolescents and adults seeking euphoria. Tablets are crushed and used intranasally or dissolved in liquid and injected IV. Ritalin is sometimes mixed with heroin, a combination called *speedball*. Adderall is the most widely abused amphetamine prescription drug.

Cocaine

Cocaine is a natural substance obtained from leaves of the coca plant, which grows in the Andes Mountains region of South America. Documentation suggests that the plant has been used by Andean cultures since 2500 B.C. Natives in this region chew the coca leaves, or make teas of the dried leaves. Because coca is taken orally, absorption is slow, and the leaves contain only 1% cocaine, so users do not suffer the ill effects caused by chemically pure extracts from the plant. In the Andean culture, use of coca leaves is not considered substance abuse because it is part of the social norms of that society.

Cocaine is a Schedule II drug that produces actions similar to those of the amphetamines, although its effects are usually more rapid and intense. Trailing marijuana, it is the one of the most commonly abused federally illicit drugs in the United States. Routes of administration include snorting, smoking, and injecting. In small doses, cocaine produces feelings of intense euphoria, a decrease in hunger, analgesia, illusions of physical strength, and increased sensory perception. Larger doses will magnify these effects and also cause rapid heartbeat, sweating, dilation of the pupils, and an elevated body temperature. After the feelings of euphoria diminish, the user is left with a sense of irritability, insomnia, depression, and extreme distrust. Some users report the sensation that insects are crawling under the skin. Users who snort cocaine develop a chronic runny nose, a crusty redness around the nostrils, and deterioration of the nasal cartilage. Overdose can result in dysrhythmias, convulsions, stroke, or death due to respiratory arrest. The withdrawal syndrome for amphetamines and cocaine is much less intense than from alcohol or barbiturate abuse.

Caffeine

Caffeine is a natural substance found in the seeds, leaves, or fruits of more than 63 plant species throughout the world. Significant amounts of caffeine are consumed in chocolate, coffee, tea, soft drinks, and ice cream. Caffeine is sometimes added to over-the-counter (OTC) pain relievers because it has been shown to increase the effectiveness of these medications. Caffeine travels to almost all parts of the body after ingestion, and several hours are needed for the body to metabolize and eliminate the drug. Caffeine has a pronounced diuretic effect.

Caffeine is considered a CNS stimulant because it produces increased mental alertness, restlessness, nervousness, irritability, and insomnia. The physical effects of caffeine include bronchodilation, increased blood pressure, increased production of stomach acid, and changes in blood glucose levels. Repeated use of caffeine may result in physical dependence and tolerance. Withdrawal symptoms include headaches, fatigue, depression, and impaired performance of daily activities.

22.10 Nicotine

Nicotine is sometimes considered a CNS stimulant, and although it does increase alertness, its actions and long-term consequences place it in a class by itself. Nicotine is unique among abused substances in that it is legal, strongly addictive, and associated with highly carcinogenic products. Furthermore, use of tobacco can cause harmful effects to those in the immediate area who breathe secondhand smoke. Patients often do not consider tobacco use as substance abuse.

Tobacco Use and Nicotine Products

Tobacco is among the top abused legal substances in the United States. The most common method by which nicotine enters the body is through the inhalation of cigarette, pipe, or cigar smoke. Tobacco smoke contains more than 1,000 chemicals, a significant number of which are carcinogens. The primary addictive substance present in cigarette smoke is nicotine. Effects of inhaled nicotine may last from 30 minutes to several hours.

Nicotine affects many body systems including the nervous, cardiovascular, and endocrine systems. Nicotine stimulates the CNS directly, causing increased alertness and ability to focus, feelings of relaxation, and lightheadedness. The cardiovascular effects of nicotine include an accelerated heart rate and increased blood pressure, caused by activation of nicotinic receptors located throughout the autonomic nervous system (see chapter 12). These cardiovascular effects can be particularly serious in patients taking oral contraceptives: The risk of a fatal heart attack is five times greater in smokers than in nonsmokers. Muscular tremors may occur with moderate doses of nicotine, and convulsions may result from very high doses. Nicotine affects the endocrine system by increasing the basal metabolic rate, leading to weight loss. Nicotine also reduces appetite. Chronic smoking leads to bronchitis, emphysema, and lung cancer.

Both psychological and physical dependence occur relatively quickly with nicotine. Once started on tobacco, patients tend to continue their drug use for many years, despite overwhelming medical evidence that the quality of life will be adversely affected and their life span shortened. Discontinuation results in agitation, weight gain, anxiety, headache, and an extreme craving for the drug. Although nicotine replacement patches and gum assist patients in dealing with the unpleasant withdrawal symptoms, only 25% of patients who attempt to stop smoking remain tobacco-free one year later. Bupropion (Zyban) and varenicline (Chantix) are the two main prescription medications prescribed to help people quit smoking.

22.11 The Nurse's Role in Substance Use

The nurse plays a key role in the prevention, diagnosis, and treatment of substance use. A thorough medical history must include questions about substance use. In the case of IV drug users, the nurse must consider the possibility of HIV infection, hepatitis, tuberculosis, and associated diagnoses. Patients are often reluctant to report their drug use, for fear of embarrassment or being arrested. The nurse must be knowledgeable about the signs of substance abuse and withdrawal symptoms, and develop a keen sense of perception during the assessment stage. A trusting nurse–patient relationship is essential to helping patients deal with their dependence. By using therapeutic communication skills and by demonstrating a nonjudgmental, empathetic attitude, the nurse can build a trusting relationship with patients.

It is often difficult for a health care provider not to condemn or stigmatize a patient for his or her substance use. Most nurses are all too familiar with the devastating medical, economic, and social consequences of substance use and misuse. The nurse must be firm in disapproving of these activities, yet compassionate in trying to help patients receive treatment. A list of social agencies dealing with dependency should be readily available for patients needing assistance. When possible, the nurse should attempt to involve family members and other close contacts in the treatment regimen. Educating the patient and family members about the long-term consequences of substance use is essential. Substance use also affects members of the health care community. The nurse should be aware of the ramifications of drug abuse and the impact this would have on personal goals and their career.

Chapter Review

KEY Concepts

The numbered key concepts provide a succinct summary of the important points from the corresponding numbered section within the chapter. If any of these points are not clear, refer to the numbered section within the chapter for review.

22.1 Abused substances belong to many diverse chemical classes. Drugs have few structural similarities, but they all have in common the ability to affect the brain and central nervous system.

22.2 Addiction is an overwhelming compulsion to continue repeated drug use that has both neurobiologic and psychosocial components.

22.3 Certain substances can cause both physical and psychological dependence, which results in continued drug-seeking behavior despite negative health and social consequences.

22.4 The withdrawal syndrome is a set of uncomfortable symptoms that occur when an abused substance is discontinued. The severity of the withdrawal syndrome varies among the different drug classes.

22.5 Tolerance is a biologic condition that occurs with repeated use of certain substances and results in the necessity for higher doses to achieve the same initial response. Cross-tolerance occurs between closely related drugs.

22.6 CNS depressants, which include sedatives, opioids, and ethyl alcohol, decrease the activity of the brain, causing drowsiness, slowed speech, and diminished motor coordination.

22.7 Cannabinoids, which include marijuana, are the most frequently abused class of illegal substances. They cause less physical dependence and tolerance than the CNS depressants.

22.8 Hallucinogens, including LSD, cause an altered state of thought and perception similar to dreams. Their effects are extremely variable and unpredictable.

22.9 CNS stimulants—including amphetamines, methylphenidate, cocaine, and caffeine—increase the activity of the CNS and produce increased wakefulness.

22.10 Nicotine is a powerful and highly addictive cardiovascular and CNS stimulant that has serious adverse effects with chronic use.

22.11 The nurse serves an important role in educating patients about the consequences of drug abuse and in recommending appropriate treatment.

REVIEW Questions

1. Following a surgical procedure, the patient states that he does not want to take narcotic analgesics for pain because he is afraid he will become addicted to the drug. What is the best response by the nurse to the patient's concerns?
   1. Dependence on narcotics is common among postoperative patients but can be managed successfully.
   2. Addiction to prescription drugs is rare when used as prescribed and according to medical protocol such as for pain control.
   3. Older patients are more likely to become addicted.
   4. Addiction is rare if the patient has a high pain threshold.

2. The patient states that she has been increasing the amount and frequency of the antianxiety drug she is using because "it just isn't working like it did before." What effect does this indicate?
   1. Immunity
   2. Resistance
   3. Tolerance
   4. Addiction

3. A 17-year-old confides to the nurse that he smokes marijuana but that "it isn't as bad as tobacco cigarettes; it's not addicting like nicotine!" Which statement would be an appropriate response by the nurse?
   1. Although marijuana may not be addicting in the same way that nicotine is, it damages lung tissue and may cause breathing problems and cancer.
   2. Marijuana is not approved for any use except under highly regulated conditions.
   3. Marijuana is four times as addicting as nicotine.
   4. The effects of marijuana are much more prolonged than nicotine because it stays in the body longer.
4. The patient with a history of alcohol abuse is admitted to the hospital. The nursing care plan includes assessment for symptoms of alcohol withdrawal. What symptoms will the nurse observe for? (Select all that apply.)
   1. Confusion
   2. Violent yawning
   3. Tremors
   4. Constricted pupils
   5. Hallucinations
5. The patient states that she is going to quit smoking "cold turkey." The nurse teaches the patient to expect which of the following symptoms during withdrawal from nicotine? (Select all that apply.)
   1. Headaches
   2. Increased appetite
   3. Tremors
   4. Insomnia
   5. Increased heart rate and blood pressure
6. What is the difference between physical and psychological dependence?
   1. Physical dependence is the adaptation of the body to a substance over time such that when the substance is withdrawn, withdrawal symptoms will result. Psychological dependence is the overwhelming desire to continue using a substance after it is stopped or withdrawn but without physical withdrawal symptoms occurring.
   2. Physical and psychological dependence are terms that are used interchangeably. In both cases, physical withdrawal symptoms will result if the substance is withdrawn from use.
   3. They occur together: psychological dependence is the first type of dependence to occur with a substance, followed by physical dependence.
   4. Psychological dependence develops when the brain adapts over time to the use of the substance. Physical dependence is the active seeking of a substance associated with a desire to continue using the substance.

PATIENT-FOCUSED Case Study

Sulinda Morgan, 16-years-old, is hospitalized in the intensive care unit (ICU) following the ingestion of a high dose of MDMA (Ecstasy) at a street dance. Her mother cannot understand why her daughter could have such serious complications after "just one dose." As the nurse, you are concerned that the mother lacks sufficient knowledge about the drug to be helpful.

1. What is the drug classification of MDMA?
2. What are the adverse effects associated with MDMA?
3. What teaching will you provide for the mother?

CRITICAL THINKING Questions

1. A student nurse has noticed that one of her student colleagues seems to have changed her behavior lately. The student, always anxious about grades and learning the material, is now detached, sleepy during class, and sometimes appears disoriented to what day it is. When questioned, the student admits that she has been taking alprazolam (Xanax) for anxiety and has recently had to keep increasing the amount she takes to control her anxiety. What do the symptoms indicate? If the student stops taking the drug abruptly, what symptoms might result?
2. A 44-year-old businessman travels weekly for his company and has had difficulty sleeping in "one hotel after another." He consulted his health care provider and has been taking secobarbital (Seconal) nightly to help him sleep. The patient has called the nurse at the health care provider's office and has said, "I have to have something stronger. This drug isn't working." What does the nurse consider as part of the assessment?

Visit www.pearsonhighered.com/nursingresources for answers and rationales for all activities.

REFERENCES

Chan, Y. F., Huang, H., Bradley, K., & Unützer, J. (2014). Referral for substance abuse treatment and depression improvement among patients with co-occurring disorders seeking behavioral health services in primary care. *Journal of Substance Abuse Treatment, 46,* 106–112. doi:10.1016/j.sat.2013.08.016

Herdman, T. H., & Kamitsuru, S. (Eds.). (2014). *NANDA International nursing diagnoses: Definitions and classification, 2015–2017.* Oxford, United Kingdom: Wiley-Blackwell.

Lev-Ran, S., Imtiaz, S., Rehm, J., & Le Foll, B. (2013). Exploring the association between lifetime prevalence of mental illness and transition from substance use to substance use disorders: Results from the National Epidemiologic Survey of Alcohol and Related Conditions (NESARC). *The American Journal on Addictions, 22,* 93–98. doi:10.1111/j.1521-0391.2013.00304.x

National Center for Complementary and Integrative Health. (2012). *Milk thistle.* Retrieved from https://nccih.nih.gov/health/milkthistle/ataglance.htm

Ortiz-Gómez, L. D., López-Canul, B., & Arankowsky-Sandoval, G. (2014). Factors associated with depression and suicide attempts in patients undergoing rehabilitation for substance abuse. *Journal of Affective Disorders, 169,* 10–14. doi:10.1016/j.jad.2014.07.033

SELECTED BIBLIOGRAPHY

Brecht, M. L., & Urada, D. (2011). Treatment outcomes for methamphetamine users: California Proposition 36 and comparison clients. *Journal of Psychoactive Drugs, 43*(Suppl. 7), 68–76. doi:10.1080/02791072.2011.602279

Campbell, G., Nielsen, S., Bruno, R., Lintzeris, N., Cohen, M., Hall, W., . . . Degenhardt, L. (2015). The Pain and Opioids IN Treatment study: Characteristics of a cohort using opioids to manage chronic non-cancer pain. *Pain, 156,* 231–242. doi:10.1097/01.j.pain.0000460303.63948.8e

Centers for Disease Control and Prevention. (2011). Quitting smoking among adults—United States, 2001–2010. *Morbidity and Mortality Weekly Report, 60,* 1513–1519.

D'Apolito, K. (2013). Breastfeeding and substance abuse. *Clinical Obstetric Gynecology, 56,* 202–211. doi:10.1097/GRF.0b013e31827e6b71

Davison, S., & Janca, A. (2012). Personality disorder and criminal behaviour: What is the nature of the relationship? *Current Opinion in Psychiatry, 25,* 39–45. doi:10.1097/YCO.0b013e32834d18f0

Fernandez-Calderón, F., Lozano, O. M., Vidal, C., Ortega, J. G., Vergara, E., González-Sáiz, F., . . . Pérez, M. I. (2011). Polysubstance use patterns in underground rave attenders: A cluster analysis. *Journal of Drug Education, 41,* 183–202. doi:10.2190/DE.41.2.d

Fiellin, L. E., Tetrault, J. M., Becker, W. C., Fiellin, D. A., & Hoff, R. A. (2013). Previous use of alcohol, cigarettes, and marijuana and subsequent abuse of prescription opioids in young adults. *Journal of Adolescent Health, 52,* 158–163. doi:10.1016/j.jadohealth.2012.06.010

Fogger, S. A. (2011). Update on ecstasy. *Journal of Psychosocial Nursing and Mental Health Services, 49*(4), 16–18. doi:10.3928/02793695-20110302-03

Gérardin, M., Victorri-Vigneau, C., Louvigné, C., Rivoal, M., & Jolliet, P. (2011). Management of cannabis use during pregnancy: An assessment of healthcare professionals' practices. *Pharmacoepidemiology and Drug Safety, 20,* 464–473. doi:10.1002/pds.2095

Giuliano, M. R., Fikru, B., Schondelmeyer, S. W., & Dann, J. (2015). Medical marijuana: Policy topic for 2015 APhA House of Delegates. *Journal of the American Pharmacists Association, 55,* 10–16. doi:10.1331/JAPhA.2015.15500

Harrington, M., Robinson, J., Bolton, S. L., Sareen, J., & Bolton, J. (2011). A longitudinal study of risk factors for incident drug use in adults: Findings from a representative sample of the US population. *Canadian Journal of Psychiatry, 56,* 686–695.

Heinzerling, K. G., Gadzhyan, J., van Oudheusden, H., Rodriguez, F., McCracken, J., & Shoptaw, S. (2013). Pilot randomized trial of bupropion for adolescent methamphetamine abuse/dependence. *Journal of Adolescent Health, 52,* 502–505. doi:10.1016/j.jadohealth.2012.10.275

Jamison, R. N., Serraillier, J., & Michna, E. (2011). Assessment and treatment of abuse risk in opioid prescribing for chronic pain. *Pain Research and Treatment,* Article ID 941808, 12 pages. doi:10.1155/2011/941808

Johnston, L. D., O'Malley, P. M., Bachman, J. G., & Schulenberg, J. E. (2012). *Monitoring the future national results on adolescent drug use: Overview of key findings, 2011.* Ann Arbor, MI: Institute for Social Research, The University of Michigan.

Kandel, D. B. (2003). Does marijuana use cause the use of other drugs? *JAMA: The Journal of the American Medical Association, 289,* 482–483.

Leece, P., Rajaram, N., Woolhouse, S., & Millson, M. (2013). Acute and chronic respiratory symptoms among primary care patients who smoke crack cocaine. *Journal of Urban Health, 90,* 542–551. doi:10.1007/s11524-012-9780-9

McClure, E. A., Campbell, A. N., Pavlicova, M., Hu, M., Winhusen, T., Vandrey, R. G., . . . Nunes, E. V. (2014). Cigarette smoking during substance use disorder treatment: Secondary outcomes from a national drug abuse treatment clinical trials network study. *Journal of Substance Abuse Treatment, 53,* 39-46. doi:10.1016/j.jsat.2014.12.007

O'Brien, C. P. (2012). Drug addiction and drug abuse. In L. L. Brunton, B. Chabner, and B. Knollman (Eds.), *Goodman & Gilman's the pharmacological basis of therapeutics* (12th ed., pp. 649–668). New York, NY: McGraw-Hill.

Prendergast, M. L. (2011). Issues in defining and applying evidence-based practices criteria for treatment of criminal-justice involved clients. *Journal of Psychoactive Drugs, Suppl. 1,* 10–18.

Thornton, L. K., Baker, A. L., Lewin, T. J., Kay-Lambkin, F. J., Kavanagh, D., Richmond, R., . . . Johnson, M. P. (2012). Reasons for substance use among people with mental disorders. *Addictive Behaviors, 37,* 427–434. doi:10.1016/j.addbeh.2011.11.039

U.S. Department of Health and Human Services, Substance Abuse and Mental Health Services Administration, Center for Behavioral Health Statistics and Quality. (2013). *Results from the 2013 National Survey on Drug Use and Health: Summary of national findings.* Retrieved from http://www.samhsa.gov/data/sites/default/files/NSDUHresultsPDFWHTML2013/Web/NSDUHresults2013.htm

Vilarim, M. M., Rocha Araujo, D. M., & Nardi, A. E. (2011). Caffeine challenge test and panic disorder: A systematic literature review. *Expert Review of Neurotherapeutics, 11,* 1185–1195. doi:10.1586/ern.11.83

Volkow, N. D., & Skolnick, P. (2012). New medications for substance use disorders: Challenges and opportunities. *Neuropsychopharmacology, 37,* 290–292. doi:10.1038/npp.2011.84

Wong, S., Ordean, A., Kahan, M., Maternal Fetal Medicine Committee, Family Physicians Advisory Committee, Medico-Legal Committee, & Society of Obstetricians and Gynaecologists of Canada. (2011). Substance use in pregnancy. *Journal of Obstetrics and Gynaecology Canada, 33*(4), 367–384.

Unit 4

The Cardiovascular and Urinary Systems

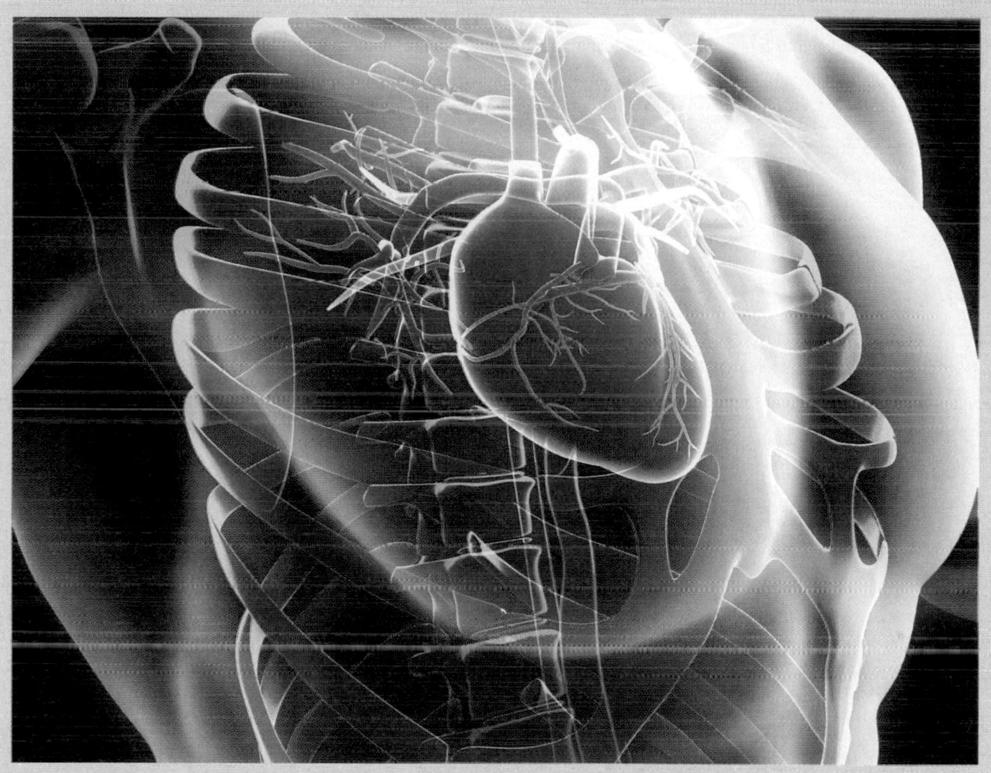

The Cardiovascular and Urinary Systems

Chapter 23

Drugs for Lipid Disorders

Drugs at a Glance

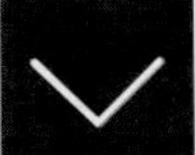

Learning Outcomes

After reading this chapter, the student should be able to:

1. Summarize the link between high blood cholesterol, LDL levels, and cardiovascular disease.
2. Compare and contrast the different types of lipids.
3. Illustrate how lipids are transported through the blood.
4. Compare and contrast the different types of lipoproteins.
5. Give examples of how cholesterol and LDL levels can be controlled through nonpharmacologic means.
6. For each of the drug classes listed in Drugs at a Glance, know representative drug examples, and explain their mechanisms of action, primary actions, and important adverse effects.
7. Explain the nurse's role in the pharmacologic management of lipid disorders.
8. Use the nursing process to care for patients receiving pharmacotherapy for lipid disorders.

indicates a prototype drug, each of which is featured in a Prototype Drug box.

Research over the past 30 years has brought about a nutritional revolution as new knowledge about lipids and their relationship to obesity and cardiovascular disease has encouraged people to make more responsible lifestyle choices. Advances in the diagnosis of lipid disorders have helped identify those patients at greatest risk for cardiovascular disease and those most likely to benefit from pharmacologic intervention. Research in pharmacology has led to safe, effective drugs for lowering lipid levels, thus decreasing the risk of cardiovascular-related diseases. As a result of this knowledge and through advancements in pharmacology, the incidence of death due to most cardiovascular diseases has been declining, although they remain the leading cause of death in the United States.

PharmFacts

HIGH BLOOD CHOLESTEROL

- Approximately 31 million American adults have high total cholesterol values (above 240 mg/dL).
- The percentage of Americans with hypercholesterolemia has been declining since 1960.
- High blood cholesterol peaks at ages 45–54 in men and 55–64 in women.
- The ethnic group with the highest rate of hypercholesterolemia is Mexican Americans in men and Caucasians in women.
- People with high total cholesterol levels have twice the risk of heart disease compared to people with optimal levels.

23.1 Types of Lipids

There are three primary types of lipids important to human nutrition. The most common are the **triglycerides,** or neutral fats, which account for 90% of total lipids in the body. A triglyceride molecule contains glycerol and three fatty acids. The fatty acids may be saturated (all the carbon atoms have hydrogen atoms attached) or unsaturated (one or more carbons are connected by double bonds and fewer hydrogen atoms). If the unsaturated fatty acid has a double bond at its third carbon, it is called an omega-3 fatty acid. High dietary intake of saturated fatty acids is associated with an increased risk for cardiovascular disease. In contrast, unsaturated and omega-3 fatty acids are sometimes called "good" fats because they may provide cardiovascular health benefits. Triglycerides are the major storage form of fat in the body and the only type of lipid that serves as an important energy source.

A second class, the **phospholipids,** is essential to building plasma membranes. The best known phospholipids are **lecithins,** which are found in high concentration in egg yolks and soybeans. Although lecithin was once promoted as a natural treatment for high-cholesterol levels, controlled studies have not shown it to be of any benefit for this disorder.

The third class of lipids is the **steroids,** a diverse group of substances having a common chemical structure called the **sterol nucleus,** or ring structure. Cholesterol is the most widely known of the steroids, and its role in promoting **atherosclerosis** has been clearly demonstrated. Cholesterol is a natural and vital component of plasma membranes. Unlike the triglycerides that provide fuel for the body during times of energy need, cholesterol serves as the building block for a number of essential biochemicals, including vitamin D, bile acids, cortisol, estrogen, progesterone, and testosterone. Although clearly essential for life, the body makes approximately 75% of blood cholesterol from other chemicals; the other 25% comes from cholesterol in the diet. Dietary cholesterol is obtained solely from animal products; humans do not metabolize the sterols produced by plants. The American Heart Association (AHA) recommends that the intake of dietary cholesterol be limited to less than 300 mg per day.

23.2 Lipoproteins

Because lipid molecules are not soluble in plasma, they must be specially packaged for transport through the blood. To accomplish this transport, the body forms complexes called **lipoproteins,** which consist of various amounts of cholesterol, triglycerides, and phospholipids, along with a protein carrier. The protein component is called an **apoprotein** (*apo-* means "separated from" or "derived from").

The three most common lipoproteins are classified according to their composition, size, and weight or density, which is due primarily to the amount of apoprotein present in the complex. Each type varies in lipid and apoprotein makeup and serves a different function in transporting lipids. For example, **high-density lipoprotein (HDL)** contains the most apoprotein, up to 50% by weight. The highest amount of cholesterol is carried by **low-density lipoprotein (LDL).** Figure 23.1 illustrates the three basic lipoproteins and their compositions.

To understand the pharmacotherapy of lipid disorders, it is important to learn the functions of the major lipoproteins and their roles in transporting cholesterol. LDL transports cholesterol from the liver to the tissues and organs, where it is used to build plasma membranes or to synthesize other steroids. Once in the tissues, cholesterol can also be stored for later use. Storage of cholesterol in the lining of blood vessels, however, is not desirable because it contributes to plaque buildup and atherosclerosis. LDL is often called "bad" cholesterol, because this lipoprotein contributes significantly to plaque deposits and coronary artery disease. **Very low-density lipoprotein (VLDL)** is the primary carrier of triglycerides in the blood. Through a series of steps, VLDL is reduced in size to become LDL.

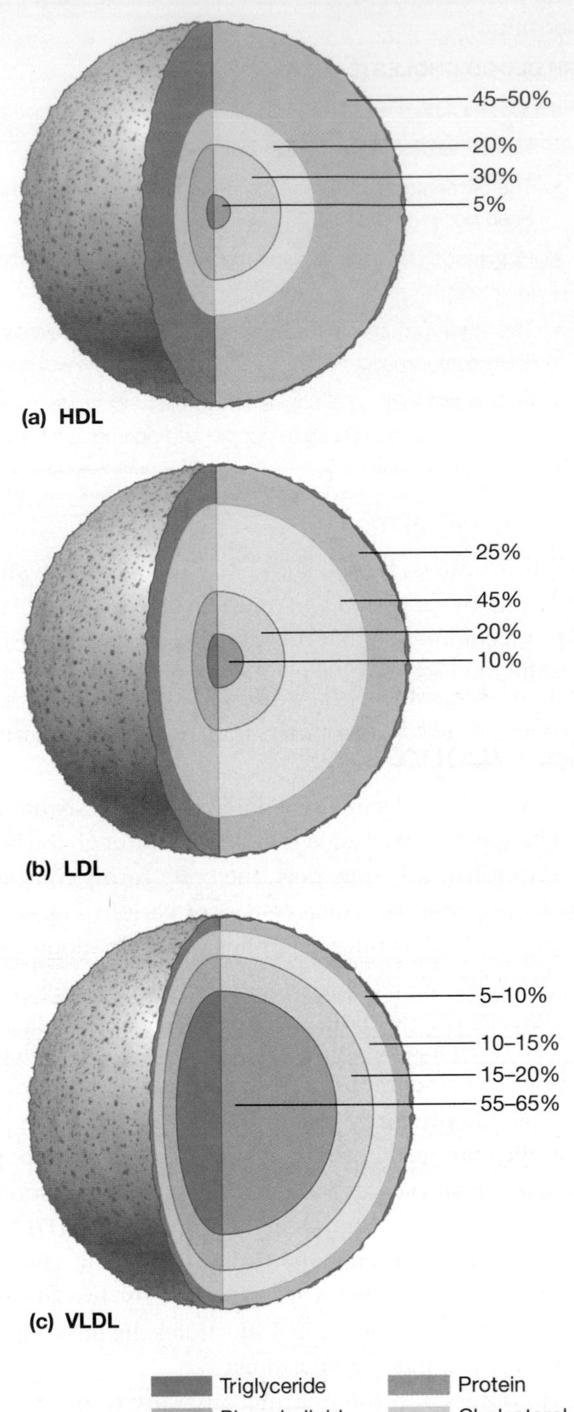

FIGURE 23.1 Composition of lipoproteins: (a) HDL; (b) LDL; (c) VLDL

Reducing LDL levels in the blood has been shown to decrease the incidence of coronary artery disease.

HDL is manufactured in the liver and small intestine and assists in the transport of cholesterol away from the body tissues and back to the liver in a process called **reverse cholesterol transport.** The cholesterol component of the HDL is then broken down to unite with bile that is subsequently excreted in the feces. Excretion via bile is the only route the body uses to remove cholesterol. Because HDL transports cholesterol for destruction and removes it from the body, it is considered "good" cholesterol.

Several terms are used to describe lipid disorders. **Hyperlipidemia,** the general term meaning high levels of lipids in the blood, is a major risk factor for cardiovascular disease. Elevated blood cholesterol, or **hypercholesterolemia,** is the type of hyperlipidemia that is most familiar to the general public. **Dyslipidemia** is the term that refers to abnormal (excess or deficient) levels of lipoproteins. Most patients with these disorders are asymptomatic and do not seek medical intervention until cardiovascular disease produces symptoms such as chest pain or signs of hypertension.

The etiology of hyperlipidemia may be inherited or acquired. Certainly, diets high in saturated fats, trans fats, and refined carbohydrates, and lack of exercise contribute greatly to hyperlipidemia and resulting cardiovascular diseases. However, genetics determines one's ability to metabolize lipids and contributes to high lipid levels in substantial numbers of patients. Dyslipidemias are clearly the result of a combination of genetic and environmental (lifestyle) factors.

23.3 LDL and Cardiovascular Disease

Although high serum cholesterol is associated with cardiovascular disease, it is not adequate to simply measure total cholesterol in the blood. Because some cholesterol is being transported for destruction, a more accurate profile is obtained by measuring LDL and HDL. The goal in maintaining normal cholesterol levels is to maximize the HDL and minimize the LDL. This goal is sometimes stated as a ratio of LDL to HDL. If the ratio is greater than 5.0 (five times more LDL than HDL), the male patient is considered at risk for cardiovascular disease. Because women generally have a higher HDL level, their ratio is different than men. Ratios above 4.4 in women increase their risk of cardiovascular disease.

Scientists have further divided LDL into subclasses of lipoproteins. For example, one variety found in LDL, called lipoprotein (a), has been strongly associated with plaque formation and heart disease. It is likely that further research will discover other varieties, with the expectation that drugs will be designed to be more selective toward the "bad" lipoproteins. Table 23.1 gives the optimal, borderline, and high laboratory values for each of the major lipids and lipoproteins.

Establishing treatment guidelines for dyslipidemia has been difficult because the condition has no symptoms, and the progression to cardiovascular disease may take decades. In 2013, major revisions were made to treatment guidelines by the American College of Cardiology (ACC) and the AHA. The 2013 ACC/AHA guidelines no longer stress specific target goals for LDL levels. Four treatment categories were established, with three of the categories for prevention

Table 23.1 Standard Laboratory Lipid Profiles

Type of Lipid	Laboratory Value (mg/dL)	Standard
Total cholesterol	Less than 200	Desirable
	200–240	Borderline high risk
	Greater than 240	High risk
LDL cholesterol	Less than 100	Optimal
	100–129	Near or above optimal
	130–159	Borderline high risk
	160–189	High risk
	Greater than 190	Very high risk
HDL cholesterol	Less than 40 (men) or 50 (women)	Low risk
	Greater than 60	Desirable
Serum triglycerides	Less than 150	Normal
	150–199	Borderline high risk
	200–499	High risk
	Greater than 500	Very high risk

Source: "Executive Summary of the Third Report of the National Cholesterol Education Program (NCEP) Expert Panel on Detection, Evaluation, and Treatment of High Blood Cholesterol in Adults (Adult Treatment Panel III), by Expert Panel on Detection," 2001, *JAMA, 285*(19), pp. 2486–2497.

Lifespan Considerations: Pediatric
Pediatric Dyslipidemias

Most people consider dyslipidemia a condition that occurs with advancing age. Dyslipidemias, however, are also a concern for some pediatric patients and multiple research studies have demonstrated that the early stage of atherosclerosis begins in childhood. Children who are most at risk include those with a family history of premature coronary artery disease or dyslipidemia and those who have hypertension, diabetes, or are obese. Lipid levels fluctuate in children and tend to be higher in girls. In 2012, the National Heart, Lung, and Blood Institute published guidelines for reducing the risk of cardiovascular disease in children and adolescents (U.S. Department of Health and Human Services, 2012). Nutritional intervention, regular physical activity, and risk factor management are warranted when the LDL level reaches 110 to 129 mg/dL. More aggressive dietary therapy and pharmacotherapy may be warranted in pediatric patients with LDL levels above 130 mg/dL. The long-term effects of lipid-lowering drugs in children have not been clearly established; therefore, drug therapy is not usually recommended below 10 years of age. Most drugs in the statin class are approved by the U.S. Food and Drug Administration (FDA) for lowering lipid levels in adolescents; however, the concern over muscle and cartilage toxicity has led to a reluctance to prescribe them in all but extreme cases. Cholestyramine (Questran) and colestipol (Colestid) also have FDA approval for hypercholesterolemia in children, but side effects sometimes result in poor adherence. Until more research into standardized recommendations for pediatric dyslipidemia treatment is completed, dietary changes along with increased exercise levels remain a recommended option to help pediatric patients decrease lipid levels.

of atherosclerotic cardiovascular disease (ASCVD), which includes coronary heart disease, stroke, and peripheral arterial disease. The new recommendation calls for a discussion of risks, benefits, and patient preferences before starting drug therapy for those groups. The treatment categories are as follow:

1. Adults with ASCVD
2. Adults with diabetes, aged 40 to 75 years with LDL levels between 70 and 189 mg/dL
3. Adults with LDL cholesterol levels of 190 mg/dL or higher
4. Adults aged 40 through 75 years who have LDL levels between 70 and 189 mg/dL and 7.5% or greater 10-year risk of ASCVD.

Based on the results of hundreds of clinical trials over many years, the ACC/AHA guidelines also recommended specific medication classes for treating patients in these categories. The statins are the recommended first-line therapy for all treatment categories. The goal is no longer to use drugs to achieve a target LDL goal. Follow-up measures of LDL, however, will still be used to determine compliance with the drug regimen.

23.4 Controlling Lipid Levels Through Lifestyle Changes

Lifestyle changes should always be included in any treatment plan for managing serum cholesterol levels. Many patients with borderline laboratory values can control their dyslipidemia entirely through nonpharmacologic means. It is important to note that all the lifestyle factors for managing serum cholesterol levels also apply to cardiovascular disease in general. Because many patients taking lipid-lowering drugs also have underlying cardiovascular disease, these lifestyle changes are particularly important.

Patients should be taught that all drugs used for hyperlipidemia have potential adverse effects and that preventing the development of ASCVD *without* pharma cotherapy should be a therapeutic goal. In most cases, pharmacotherapy should be initiated after attempts to lower lipid levels with lifestyle changes fail. Following are the most important lipid-reduction lifestyle modifications:

- Monitor blood lipid levels regularly, as recommended by the health care provider.
- Maintain weight at an optimal level.
- Implement a medically supervised exercise plan.
- Reduce dietary saturated fats, trans fats, and cholesterol.
- Increase soluble fiber in the diet, such as that found in oat bran, apples, beans, and broccoli.
- Eliminate tobacco use.

Nutritionists recommend that the consumption of total dietary fat be less than 35% of the caloric intake (a maximum of 10% from saturated fats). For many years, it was recommended that dietary cholesterol intake be reduced as much as possible and not exceed 300 mg/day. Reviews of recent research, however, suggest that the amount of cholesterol *consumed* is only slightly related to the amount of cholesterol appearing in the *blood*. Why is this the case? The liver reacts to a low-cholesterol diet by making more cholesterol and by inhibiting its excretion when saturated fats are present. Thus when the patient consumes more cholesterol, the body makes less of it, keeping the overall amount in the blood relatively constant. To reduce serum cholesterol, the patient must reduce saturated fat and refined carbohydrates in the diet. The 2013 ACC/AHA guidelines call for a reduction of saturated fat in the diet to 5% to 6% of total calories. In addition, levels of trans fatty acids from meat and dairy fat should be reduced.

Nutritionists also recommend increasing the dietary intake of plant sterols and stanols as a means to reduce blood cholesterol levels. Plant sterols and stanols are essential components of plant membranes. These plant lipids have a structure similar to that of cholesterol and therefore compete with that substance for absorption in the digestive tract. When the body absorbs the plant sterols, cholesterol is excreted from the body. When less cholesterol is delivered to the liver, LDL uptake increases, thereby decreasing serum LDL (the "bad" cholesterol) level. Plant sterols and stanols may be obtained from a variety of sources including wheat, corn, rye, oats, and rice, as well as nuts and olive oil. Commercially, stanols and sterols have been added to products such as certain margarines, salad dressings, cereals, and fruit juices. It is estimated that a daily intake of 2 to 3 g of plant sterols or stanols may reduce cholesterol levels by about 10%.

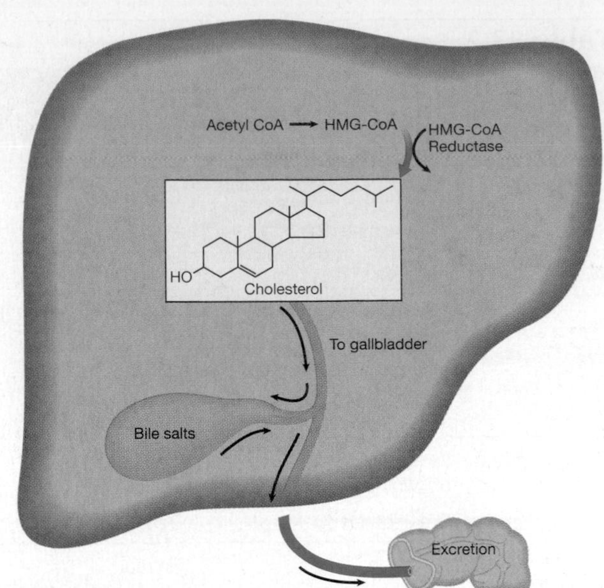

FIGURE 23.2 Cholesterol biosynthesis and excretion

HMG-CoA REDUCTASE INHIBITORS (STATINS)

The statin class of antihyperlipidemics interferes with a critical enzyme in the synthesis of cholesterol. These medications, listed in Table 23.2, are first-line drugs in the treatment of lipid disorders.

23.5 Pharmacotherapy With Statins

In the late 1970s, compounds isolated from various species of fungi were found to inhibit cholesterol synthesis in human cells in the laboratory. This class of drugs, known as the *statins,* has since revolutionized the treatment of lipid disorders. Statins can produce a dramatic reduction in LDL-cholesterol levels, lower triglyceride and VLDL levels, and raise the level of "good" HDL cholesterol. High intensity statin therapy is able to lower LDL levels by more than 50%. About one in every three or four heart attacks, strokes, or blood clots can be prevented with appropriate statin therapy.

Cholesterol is manufactured in the liver by a series of more than 25 metabolic steps, beginning with acetyl CoA, a two-carbon unit that is produced in the breakdown of fatty acids. Of the many enzymes involved in this complex pathway, **HMG-CoA reductase** (3-hydroxy-3-methylglutaryl coenzyme A reductase) serves as the primary regulatory site for cholesterol biosynthesis. Under normal conditions, this enzyme is controlled through negative feedback: High levels of LDL cholesterol in the blood will shut down production of HMG-CoA reductase, thus turning off the cholesterol pathway. Figure 23.2 illustrates selected steps in cholesterol biosynthesis and the importance of HMG-CoA reductase.

The statins act by inhibiting HMG-CoA reductase, which results in less cholesterol biosynthesis. As the liver makes less cholesterol, it responds by making more LDL receptors on the surface of liver cells. The greater number of hepatic LDL receptors increases the removal of LDL from the blood. Blood levels of both LDL and cholesterol are reduced. The drop in lipid levels is not permanent, however, so patients need to remain on these drugs during the remainder of their lives or until their hyperlipidemia can be controlled through dietary or lifestyle changes. Statins have been shown to clearly slow the progression of coronary artery disease and to reduce mortality from cardiovascular disease. This reduction in adverse cardiovascular events is especially high in those patients who have diabetes as a comorbid condition with hyperlipidemia. The mechanisms of action of the statins and other drugs for dyslipdidemia are illustrated in Pharmacotherapy Illustrated 23.1.

All the statins are given orally (PO) and are well tolerated by most patients. Minor side effects include headache,

Table 23.2 Drugs for Dyslipidemias

Drug	Route and Adult Dose (max dose where indicated)	Adverse Effects
HMG COA REDUCTASE INHIBITORS		
atorvastatin (Lipitor)	PO: 10–80 mg daily	*Headache, dyspepsia, abdominal cramping, myalgia, rash or pruritus* Rhabdomyolysis, severe myositis, elevated hepatic enzymes
fluvastatin (Lescol)	PO: 20–80 mg daily	
lovastatin (Altoprev, Mevacor)	PO:10–80 mg daily (immediate release); 20-60 mg daily (extended release)	
pitavastatin (Livalo)	PO: 1–4 mg daily	
pravastatin (Pravachol)	PO: 10–80 mg daily	
rosuvastatin (Crestor)	PO: 5–40 mg daily	
simvastatin (Zocor)	PO: 5–40 mg daily	
BILE ACID SEQUESTRANTS		
cholestyramine (Questran)	PO: 4–8 g bid–qid (max: 24 g/day)	*Constipation, nausea, vomiting, abdominal pain, bloating, dyspepsia* Gastrointestinal (GI) tract obstruction, vitamin deficiencies due to poor absorption
colesevelam (Welchol)	PO: 1.875 g bid (max: 3.75 g/day)	
colestipol (Colestid)	PO: 5–20 g daily in divided doses	
FIBRIC ACID DRUGS		
fenofibrate (Lofibra, Tricor, others)	PO: 54 mg daily (max: 200 mg/day)	*Myalgia, flulike syndrome, nausea, vomiting, increased serum transaminase and creatinine levels* Rhabdomyolysis, cholelithiasis, pancreatitis
fenofibric acid (Fibricor, Trilipix)	PO: (Fibricor: regular release): 35–105 mg once daily PO: (Trilipix: delayed release): 45–135 mg once daily	
gemfibrozil (Lopid)	PO: 600 mg bid (max: 1,500 mg/day)	
OTHER DRUGS FOR DYSLIPIDEMIAS		
alirocumab (Praluent)	Subcutaneous: 75–150 mg every 2 wk	*Itching, swelling, pain, or bruising at injection site, nasopharyngitis, flu* Hypersensitivity reactions
evolocumab (Repatha)	Subcutaneous: 140 mg every 2 wk	*Nasopharyngitis, influenza, back pain,* Hypersensitivity reactions
ezetimibe (Zetia)	PO: 10 mg daily	*Arthralgia, fatigue, upper respiratory tract infection, diarrhea, elevation of hepatic enzymes* Rhabdomyolysis
icosapent (Vascepa)	PO: 4 g daily with food	*Arthralgia* Hypersensitivity
lomitapide (Juxtapid)	PO: 5–60 mg once daily	*Abdominal pain, diarrhea, nausea, vomiting, dyspepsia, reduced absorption of fat soluble vitamins and fatty acids* Fetal toxicity, hepatotoxicity
mipomersen (Kynamro)	Subcutaneous: 200 mg once weekly	*Injection site reactions, flu-like symptoms, nausea and headache* Hepatotoxicity and elevations in serum transaminases
niacin (Niaspan)	Hyperlipidemia: PO: 1.5–3 g daily in divided doses (max: 6 g/day) Niacin deficiency: PO: 10–20 mg daily	*Flushing, nausea, pruritus, headache, bloating, diarrhea* Dysrhythmias
omega-3-acid ethyl esters (Lovaza)	PO: 4 g daily with food	*Eructation, dyspepsia, fishy taste* Hypersensitivity

Note: *Italics* indicate common adverse effects; underlining indicates serious adverse effects.

fatigue, muscle or joint pain, and heartburn. Severe myopathy and rhabdomyolysis are rare but serious adverse effects of the statins. **Rhabdomyolysis** is a breakdown of muscle fibers usually due to muscle trauma or ischemia. During rhabdomyolysis, contents of muscle cells spill into the systemic circulation, causing potentially fatal acute renal failure. The mechanism by which statins cause this disorder is unknown. Macrolide antibiotics such as erythromycin, azole antifungals, fibric acid agents, and certain immunosuppressants should be avoided during statin therapy because these can interfere with statin metabolism and increase the risk of severe myopathy.

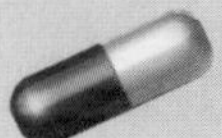

Prototype Drug | Cholestyramine *(Questran)*

Therapeutic Class: Antihyperlipidemic **Pharmacologic Class:** Bile acid sequestrant

Actions and Uses

Cholestyramine is a powder that is mixed with fluid before being taken once or twice daily. It is not absorbed or metabolized once it enters the intestine; thus, it does not produce any systemic effects. It may take 30 days or longer to produce its maximum effect. Questran binds with bile acids (containing cholesterol) in an insoluble complex that is excreted in the feces. Cholesterol levels decline due to fecal loss.

Administration Alerts

- Mix thoroughly with 60 to 180 mL of water, noncarbonated beverages, highly liquid soups, or pulpy fruits (applesauce, crushed pineapple). Have the patient drink it immediately to avoid potential irritation or obstruction in the GI tract.
- Give other drugs more than 2 hours before or 4 hours after the patient takes cholestyramine.
- Pregnancy category C.

PHARMACOKINETICS

Onset	Peak	Duration
24–48 h	1–3 wk	2–4 wk

Adverse Effects

Although cholestyramine rarely produces serious side effects, patients may experience constipation, bloating, gas, and nausea that sometimes limit its use.

Contraindications: This drug is contraindicated in patients with total biliary obstruction and in those with prior hypersensitivity to the drug.

Interactions

Drug–Drug: Because cholestyramine can bind to other drugs, such as digoxin, penicillins, thyroid hormone, and thiazide diuretics, and interfere with their absorption, it should not be taken at the same time as these other medications. Cholestyramine may increase the effects of anticoagulants by decreasing the levels of vitamin K in the body.

Lab Tests: Aspartate aminotransferase (AST), phosphorus, chloride, and alkaline phosphatase (ALP) levels may increase. Serum calcium, sodium, and potassium levels may decrease.

Herbal/Food: Taking cholestyramine with food may interfere with the absorption of the following essential nutrients: beta-carotene, calcium, folic acid, iron, magnesium, vitamin B_{12}, vitamin D, vitamin E, vitamin K, and zinc. Manifestations of nutrient depletion may include weakened immune system, cardiovascular problems, and osteoporosis.

Treatment of Overdose: There is no specific treatment for overdose.

Complementary and Alternative Therapies

COENZYME Q10 FOR HEART DISEASE

CoQ10 is a vitamin-like substance found in most animal cells. It is an essential component in the cell's mitochondria for producing energy or ATP. Because the heart requires high levels of ATP, a sufficient level of CoQ10 is essential to that organ. Foods richest in this substance are pork, sardines, beef heart, salmon, broccoli, spinach, and nuts. Older adults appear to have an increased need for CoQ10.

Reports of the benefits of CoQ10 for treating heart disease began to emerge in the mid-1960s. Subsequent reports have claimed that CoQ10 may possibly be effective for mitochondrial disorders; decreasing the risk of subsequent heart attacks following an MI, hypertension, migraines, or Parkinson's disease; enhancing the immune system; and preventing blood vessel damage following cardiac bypass surgery (National Institutes of Health, 2014). Considerable research has been conducted on this antioxidant.

Statins block an enzyme involved in the production of CoQ10, creating a deficiency of the antioxidant in patients taking statin medications. The myopathy and rhabdomyolysis caused by statins may be due to this decrease in CoQ10 levels. Supplementation with CoQ10 may improve myopathy symptoms. Like most dietary supplements, controlled research studies are often lacking and give conflicting results. At this time, evidence to support the use of CoQ10 in treating patients with heart disease, neurologic disorders, or cancer is weak.

NIACIN

Niacin is a vitamin that is occasionally used to lower lipid levels. It has a number of side effects that limit its use. The dose for niacin is given in Table 23.2.

23.7 Pharmacotherapy With Niacin

Niacin, or nicotinic acid, is a B-complex vitamin. Its ability to lower lipid levels, however, is unrelated to its role as a vitamin because much higher doses are needed to

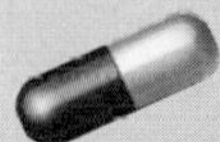

Prototype Drug | Gemfibrozil *(Lopid)*

Therapeutic Class: Antihyperlipidemic **Pharmacologic Class:** Fibric acid drug (fibrate)

Actions and Uses

Gemfibrozil is indicated for the treatment of hypertriglyceridemia and hypercholesterolemia. Effects of gemfibrozil include up to a 50% reduction in VLDL with an increase in HDL. The mechanism of achieving this action is unknown. It is less effective than the statins at lowering LDL; thus, it is not a drug of first choice for reducing LDL levels. Gemfibrozil is taken orally at 600 to 1,200 mg/day.

Administration Alerts

- Administer with meals to decrease GI distress.
- Pregnancy category B.

PHARMACOKINETICS

Onset	Peak	Duration
1–2 h	1–2 h	2–4 months

Adverse Effects

Gemfibrozil produces few serious adverse effects, but it may increase the likelihood of gallstones and may occasionally affect liver function. The most common adverse effects are GI related: dyspepsia, diarrhea, nausea, and cramping.

Contraindications: Gemfibrozil is contraindicated in patients with hepatic impairment, severe renal dysfunction, or pre-existing gallbladder disease, or those with prior hypersensitivity to the drug.

Interactions

Drug–Drug: Concurrent use of gemfibrozil with oral anticoagulants may potentiate anticoagulant effects. Concurrent use with statins should be avoided because this increases the risk of myopathy and rhabdomyolysis. Gemfibrozil may increase the effects of certain antidiabetic agents, statins, sulfonylureas, and vitamin K antagonists.

Lab Tests: May increase liver enzyme values, and CPK and serum glucose levels. May decrease hemoglobin (Hgb), hematocrit (Hct), and white blood cell (WBC) counts.

Herbal/Food: Fatty foods may decrease the efficacy of gemfibrozil.

Treatment of Overdose: There is no specific treatment for overdose.

reduce serum lipid levels. For lowering cholesterol, the usual dose of niacin is 2 to 3 grams per day. When taken as a vitamin, the dose is only 25 mg/day. The primary effect of niacin is to decrease VLDL levels, and because LDL is synthesized from VLDL, the patient experiences a reduction in LDL levels. It also has the desirable effects of reducing triglycerides and increasing HDL levels. As with other lipid-lowering drugs, maximum therapeutic effects may take a month or longer to achieve.

Although effective at reducing LDL levels by as much as 20%, niacin produces a higher incidence of adverse effects than the statins. Flushing and hot flashes occur in almost every patient. In addition, a variety of uncomfortable intestinal effects such as nausea, excess gas, and diarrhea are commonly reported. More serious adverse effects such as hepatotoxicity and gout are possible. Niacin is not usually prescribed for patients with diabetes mellitus, because the drug can raise fasting blood glucose levels. Because of the high frequency of side effects, niacin is most often used in lower doses in combination with a statin or bile acid–binding agent. Taking one aspirin tablet 30 minutes prior to niacin administration can reduce uncomfortable flushing in many patients.

Niacin is rarely used as monotherapy for dyslipidemias. In low doses, however, niacin can boost the effectiveness of the statins in lowering LDL-cholesterol levels. Fixed-dose combinations include niacin with lovastatin (Advicor) and niacin with simvastatin (Simcor).

Although niacin is available as a vitamin supplement without a prescription, patients should be instructed not to attempt self-medication with this drug. One form of niacin available over-the-counter (OTC) as a vitamin supplement called nicotinamide has no lipid-lowering effects. Patients should be informed that if niacin is to be used to lower cholesterol, it should be done under medical supervision.

FIBRIC ACID AGENTS

Once widely used to lower lipid levels, the fibric acid drugs have been largely replaced by the statins. They are sometimes used in combination with the statins. In addition they remain drugs of choice for treating extremely high triglyceride levels. The fibric acid drugs are listed in Table 23.2.

23.8 Pharmacotherapy with Fibric Acid Drugs

The first fibric acid drug, clofibrate (Atromid-S), was widely prescribed until a 1978 study determined that it did not reduce mortality from cardiovascular disease. Although clofibrate is no longer available, other fibric acid medications such as fenofibrate (Lofibra, Tricor), fenofibric acid (Fibricor, Trilipix), and gemfibrozil (Lopid), are sometimes indicated for patients with excessive triglyceride and VLDL levels. They are preferred drugs for treating severe hypertriglyceridemia. Combining a fibric acid with a statin results in greater decreases in serum triglyceride levels than using either drug alone. Fibric acid drugs activate the enzyme lipoprotein lipase, which increases the breakdown and elimination of triglyceride-rich particles from the plasma.

The most common adverse effects of the fibrates relate to the GI system: dyspepsia, diarrhea, abdominal pain, nausea, and vomiting. Taking these medications with meals usually diminishes GI distress. Drugs in this class are generally not used in patients with hepatic impairment or gallbladder disease.

MISCELLANEOUS DRUGS FOR DYSLIPIDEMIA

In recent years, several new approaches have been discovered that are useful in controlling dyslipidemias. These medications are indicated as miscellaneous drugs in Table 23.2.

23.9 Pharmacotherapy With Miscellaneous Drugs for Dyslipidemias

Ezetimibe (Zetia) is the only drug in a class called cholesterol absorption inhibitors. Cholesterol is absorbed from the intestinal lumen by cells in the jejunum of the small intestine. Ezetimibe blocks this absorption by as much as 50%, causing less cholesterol to enter the blood. Unfortunately, the body responds by synthesizing more cholesterol; thus, a statin is usually administered concurrently.

When given as monotherapy, ezetimibe produces a small reduction in serum LDL. Adding a statin to the therapeutic regimen reduces LDL by an *additional* 15% to 20%. Vytorin is a combination tablet containing fixed-dose combinations of ezetimibe and simvastatin and Liptruzet combines ezetimibe with atorvastatin. Because bile acid sequestrants inhibit the absorption of ezetimibe, these drugs should not be taken together.

Serious adverse effects from ezetimibe are uncommon. Nasopharyngitis, myalgia, upper respiratory tract infection, arthralgia, and diarrhea are the most common adverse effects, although these rarely require discontinuation of therapy. Ezetimibe is pregnancy category C.

Omega-3 fatty acid esters (Epanova, Lovaza) and icosapent (Vascepa) are prescription forms of omega-3 fatty acids found in fish oil. Fish oil has long been a natural therapy for lowering blood lipid levels. These drugs are approved as adjuncts to diet in the treatment of severe hypertriglyceridemia. Adverse effects are minor and include eructation, fishy taste, and diarrhea. The drugs should be used with caution in patients who are allergic to seafood, especially shellfish.

Two drugs were approved in 2013 for a very narrow indication: lowering LDL in patients with homozygous familial hypercholesterolemia (HoFH). HoFH is a genetic disorder in which the body has such high levels of cholesterol and LDL that cardiovascular disease begins in childhood and results in death by the mid-thirties. Many of these patients have a diminished response to therapy with statins and other antihyperlipidemics. The two new drugs, lomitapide (Juxtapid) and mipomersen (Kynamro), act by very different and unique mechanisms. Therapy is very costly and will likely limit the widespread use of the two drugs.

Lomitapide is classified as a microsomal triglyceride transfer protein (MTP) inhibitor. Inhibition of MTP lowers plasma levels of LDL. The drug is given orally and is indicated only for HoFH. GI adverse effects such as diarrhea, nausea, vomiting, dyspepsia, and abdominal pain occur in almost all patients. Drug interactions may be serious with medications that inhibit hepatic CYP3A4, such as ketoconazole and lopinavir/ritonavir or telithromycin. These drugs will markedly increase levels of lomitapide. Lomitamide is contraindicated during pregnancy (Category X).

Mipomersan is classified as an inhibitor of apo B synthesis, the primary protein that makes up LDL particles. By preventing the synthesis of apo B, mipomersen is able to lower LDL values in patients with HoFA. Mipomersen is given as a once weekly subcutaneous injection.

Mipomersen and lomitapide carry identical black box warnings that the drugs can cause elevations in serum transaminases and may increase hepatic fat (hepatic steatosis). The drugs are contraindicated in patients with active hepatic disease or elevated transaminases. Mipomersen and lomitapide are only available in restricted use programs that require prescribing physicians and pharmacists to be certified through special training.

Representing a new approach to the pharmacotherapy of hypercholesterolemia, alirocumab (Praluent) and evolocumab (Repatha) were approved in 2015. These drugs are monoclonal antibodies that inhibits a specific protein called PCSK9 (proprotein convertase subtilisin kexin type 9). When the PCSK9 protein is inhibited, the number of LDL receptors in the liver is reduced and more LDL is excreted from the body, thus reducing serum cholesterol. These drugs are indicated for patients with heterozygous

Patient Safety: Concurrent Medication Administration

The nurse administers the following oral medications ordered for a 64-year-old man: tetracycline 500 mg bid, digoxin (Lanoxin) 0.25 mg/day, and cholestyramine (Questran) 4 g bid before meals (a.c.) and at bedtime. At 8:00 a.m., before breakfast, the nurse administers tetracycline 500 mg, digoxin 0.25 mg, and cholestyramine 4 mg. What should the nurse have done differently? *Visit www.pearsonhighered.com/nursingresources for the suggested answer.*

familial hypercholesterolemia (HeFH) who have not responded adequately to statin therapy. They are given by the subcutaneous route once every 2 weeks. The most common side effects of alirocumab and evolocumab include itching, swelling, pain, or bruising at the injection site; nasopharyngitis, and flu.

Nursing Practice Application

Lipid-Lowering Pharmacotherapy

ASSESSMENT	POTENTIAL NURSING DIAGNOSES*
Baseline assessment prior to administration: • Obtain a complete health history including cardiovascular, musculoskeletal (pre-existing conditions that might result in muscle or joint pain), GI (peptic ulcer disease, hemorrhoids, inflammatory bowel disease, chronic constipation, dysphagia or esophageal strictures), and the possibility of pregnancy. Obtain a drug history including allergies, current prescription and OTC drugs, herbal preparations, and alcohol use. Be alert to possible drug interactions. • Evaluate appropriate laboratory findings, especially liver function studies and lipid profiles. • Assess the patient's ability to receive and understand instruction. Include family and caregivers as needed.	• *Imbalanced Nutrition: More Than Body Requirements* • *Ineffective Health Management* • *Chronic Pain*, related to adverse drug effects • *Deficient Knowledge* (drug therapy) *NANDA I © 2014
Assessment throughout administration: • Assess for desired therapeutic effects (e.g., lowered total cholesterol, LDL levels, increased HDL levels). • Continue periodic monitoring of lipid profiles, liver function studies, creatine kinase (CK), and uric acid levels. • Assess for adverse effects: musculoskeletal discomfort, nausea, vomiting, abdominal cramping, and diarrhea. Immediately report severe musculoskeletal pain, unexplained muscle tenderness accompanied by fever, inability to maintain activities of daily living (ADLs) due to musculoskeletal weakness or pain, unexplained numbness or tingling of extremities, yellowing of sclera or skin, severe constipation, or straining with passing of stools or tarry stools.	

IMPLEMENTATION

Interventions and (Rationales)	Patient-Centered Care
Ensuring therapeutic effects: • Follow appropriate administration guidelines. (Many of the lipid-lowering drugs have specific administration requirements. For best results, some should be taken at night when cholesterol biosynthesis is at its highest. Always check administration guidelines.)	• Teach the patient to take the drug following appropriate guidelines (see Patient Self-Administration of Drug Therapy).
• Encourage appropriate lifestyle changes. Provide for dietitian consultation as needed. (Healthy lifestyle changes will support and minimize the need for drug therapy.)	• Encourage the patient and family to adopt a healthy lifestyle of low-fat food choices, increased exercise, decreased alcohol consumption, and smoking cessation. • Encourage increased intake of omega-3 and CoQ10–rich foods (e.g., fish such as salmon and sardines, nuts, extra virgin olive and canola oils, beef and chicken). Supplementation may be needed; instruct the patient to seek the advice of a health care provider before supplements are taken.
Minimizing adverse effects: • Continue to monitor periodic liver function tests and CK levels. (Abnormal liver function tests or increased CK levels may indicate drug-induced adverse hepatic effects or myopathy and should be reported. **Lifespan:** Monitor the older adult more frequently because age-related physiological changes may affect the drug's metabolism or excretion. **Diverse Patients:** Because statins metabolize through the P450 system pathways, monitor ethnically diverse patients to ensure optimal therapeutic effects and to minimize adverse effects.)	• Instruct the patient on the need to return periodically for laboratory work.

continued

Nursing Practice Application *continued*

IMPLEMENTATION	
Interventions and (Rationales)	**Patient-Centered Care**
• Continue to assess for drug-related symptoms, which may indicate adverse effects are occurring. (Lipid-lowering drugs often adversely affect the liver but may also cause drug-specific adverse effects.) • Assess for the possibility of increased adverse effects when a combination of lipid-lowering agents are used. (Lipid-lowering agents may be combined for better effects but this increases the risk of adverse effects.)	• Teach the patient the importance of reporting signs or symptoms related to adverse drug effects as follows: • *Statins.* Report unusual or unexplained muscle tenderness, increasing muscle pain, numbness or tingling of extremities, or effects that hinder normal ADL activities. **Lifespan:** The drug should not be taken during pregnancy, if pregnancy is suspected, or while breast-feeding. • *Bile acid sequestrants.* Report severe nausea, heartburn, constipation, or straining with passing stools. Any tarry stools or yellowing of sclera or skin should also be reported. **Lifespan:** The older adult may have an increased risk of bleeding due to drug-related changes with vitamin K synthesis. • *Niacin.* Report flank, joint, or stomach pain, or yellowing of sclera or skin. • *Fibric acid drugs.* Report unusual bleeding or bruising, right upper quadrant pain, muscle cramping, or changes in the color of the stool. Patients with diabetes on PO medications may need a change in their dosage and should monitor their glucose more frequently in early therapy. **Lifepan & Safety:** Monitor the older adult for dizziness and assist with ambulation to prevent falls. **Diverse Patients:** Research has indicated that Hispanics and Native Americans may have a greater risk for development of gallbladder disease than other ethnic groups. • Instruct the patient who is taking a combination of lipid-lowering drugs to be alert to symptoms related to adverse effects of both drugs, as above.
• If long-term therapy is used, ensure adequate intake of fat-soluble vitamins (A, D, E, K) and folic acid in the diet or consider supplementation. (Lipid-lowering drugs may cause depletion or diminished absorption of these nutrients.)	• Instruct the patient and family about foods high in folic acid and fat-soluble vitamins and about the need to consult with the health care provider about the possible need for vitamin and folic acid supplementation while on long-term therapy.
Patient understanding of drug therapy: • Use opportunities during administration of medications and during assessments to provide patient education. (Using time during nursing care helps to optimize and reinforce key teaching areas.)	• The patient and/or family should be able to state the reason for the drug; appropriate dose and scheduling; what adverse effects to observe for and when to report; and the anticipated length of medication therapy.
Patient self-administration of drug therapy: • When administering the medication, instruct the patient and/or family in proper self-administration of the drug (e.g., during the evening meal). (Using time during nurse administration of these drugs helps to reinforce teaching.)	• The patient and family are able to discuss appropriate dosing and administration needs. • The patient takes the drug following appropriate guidelines: • *Statins.* Take with evening meal; avoid grapefruit and grapefruit juice, which could inhibit the drug's metabolism, leading to toxic levels. • *Bile acid sequestrants.* Take before meals with plenty of fluids, mixing powders or granules thoroughly with liquid. Take other medications 2 hours before, or 4 hours after the bile acid sequestrant is taken. • *Niacin.* Take with cold water to decrease flushing. Take one aspirin tablet (81–325 mg) 30 minutes before the niacin dose. • *Fibric acid agents.* Take with a meal.

Chapter Review

KEY Concepts

The numbered key concepts provide a succinct summary of the important points from the corresponding numbered section within the chapter. If any of these points are not clear, refer to the numbered section within the chapter for review.

23.1 Lipids can be classified into three types, based on their chemical structures: triglycerides, phospholipids, and steroids. Triglycerides and cholesterol are blood lipids that can lead to atherosclerotic plaque.

23.2 Lipids are carried through the blood as lipoproteins; VLDL and LDL are associated with an increased incidence of cardiovascular disease, whereas HDL exerts a protective effect.

23.3 Blood lipid profiles are important diagnostic tools in guiding the therapy of dyslipidemias. The optimal levels of the different lipids are reviewed periodically and adjusted based on the results of current research.

23.4 Before starting pharmacotherapy for hyperlipidemia, patients should seek to control the condition through lifestyle changes such as restriction of dietary saturated fats and cholesterol, increased exercise, and smoking cessation.

23.5 Statins inhibit HMG-CoA reductase, a critical enzyme in the biosynthesis of cholesterol. These agents are safe and effective for most patients and are drugs of choice in reducing blood lipid levels.

23.6 The bile acid sequestrants bind bile and cholesterol and accelerate their excretion. These agents can reduce cholesterol and LDL levels but are not drugs of choice due to their frequent adverse effects.

23.7 Niacin can be effective at lowering LDL cholesterol when given in large amounts. It is not a drug of first choice, but it is sometimes combined in smaller doses with other lipid-lowering agents such as the statins.

23.8 Fibric acid agents lower triglyceride and VLDL levels but have little effect on LDL. They are not preferred drugs because of their potential side effects.

23.9 Several miscellaneous drugs are used to treat dyslipidemias. Ezetimibe lowers cholesterol by inhibiting the absorption of cholesterol. The omega-3 fatty acids Epinova, Lovaza, and Vascepa are used to lower serum triglyceride levels. Lomitapide and mipomerson are newer drugs, approved to treat dyslipidmias in patients with HoFH. Alirocumab is a monoclonal antibody used in patients with HeFH.

REVIEW Questions

1. The patient is to begin taking atorvastatin (Lipitor) and the nurse is providing education about the drug. Which symptom related to this drug should be reported to the health care provider?
   1. Constipation
   2. Increasing muscle or joint pain
   3. Hemorrhoids
   4. Flushing or "hot flash"

2. A patient is receiving cholestyramine (Questran) for elevated low-density lipoprotein (LDL) levels. As the nurse completes the nursing care plan, which of the following adverse effects will be included for continued monitoring?
   1. Abdominal pain
   2. Orange-red urine and saliva
   3. Decreased capillary refill time
   4. Sore throat and fever

3. The nurse is instructing a patient on home use of niacin and will include important instructions on how to take the drug and about its possible adverse effects. Which of the following may be expected adverse effects of this drug? (Select all that apply.)
   1. Fever and chills
   2. Intense flushing and hot flashes
   3. Tingling of the fingers and toes
   4. Hypoglycemia
   5. Dry mucous membranes
4. The community health nurse is working with a patient taking simvastatin (Zocor). Which patient statement may indicate the need for further teaching about this drug?
   1. "I'm trying to reach my ideal body weight by increasing my exercise."
   2. "I didn't have any symptoms even though I had high lipid levels. I hear that's common."
   3. "I've been taking my pill before my dinner."
   4. "I take my pill with grapefruit juice. I've always taken my medications that way."
5. A patient has been on long-term therapy with colestipol (Colestid). To prevent adverse effects related to the length of therapy and lack of nutrients, which of the following supplements may be required? (Select all that apply.)
   1. Folic acid
   2. Vitamins A, D, E, and K
   3. Potassium, iodine, and chloride
   4. Protein
   5. B vitamins
6. A patient has been ordered gemfibrozil (Lopid) for hyperlipidemia. The nurse will first validate the order with the health care provider if the patient reports a history of which disorder?
   1. Hypertension
   2. Angina
   3. Gallbladder disease
   4. Tuberculosis

PATIENT-FOCUSED Case Study

Evelyn Williams is a 49-year-old black female who feels fine. However, she recently had her cholesterol level checked at her church's health fair where she was told that it exceeded the normal value. As directed, she made an appointment and saw her health care provider.

During the office visit, the nurse collects Evelyn's social and health history. Evelyn's vital signs, except for blood pressure, are within normal limits. Her blood pressure is elevated (142/90 mmHg). She is slightly overweight and has been on a diet for 1 week. Her favorite foods are potato chips and all dairy products, especially cheese. She admits to smoking less than a pack of cigarettes per day and occasionally drinks a glass of wine with dinner. Evelyn is divorced and has one teenage son.

A series of laboratory and diagnostic tests is completed during the visit. Evelyn's physical exam is normal, and there are no ECG abnormalities. The blood tests are unremarkable with the exception of the lipid profile.

	Patient Value	Normal Range
Total Cholesterol	240 mg/dL	Less than 200
Triglycerides	199 mg/dL	Less than 150
HDL Cholesterol	30 mg/dL	Greater than 60
LDL Cholesterol	184	Less than 100
Cholesterol-to-HDL Ratio	6.6	Less than 4.5

Evelyn's provider places her on a standard cholesterol-lowering diet and prescribes atorvastatin (Lipitor) 10 mg daily. Evelyn is instructed to return to the office in 1 month for a follow-up visit.

1. How would you respond to Evelyn when she asks you, "Is high cholesterol due to heredity or from what I eat?"
2. What health teaching should you provide the patient about ways to reduce high blood lipid levels?
3. What potential adverse effects of the statin drugs should Evelyn be taught to watch for?

CRITICAL THINKING Questions

1. A patient has been prescribed cholestyramine (Questran) for elevated lipids. What teaching is important for this patient?

2. A male patient with diabetes presents to the emergency department with complaints of being flushed and having "hot flashes." The patient admits to self-medicating with niacin for elevated lipid levels. What is the nurse's best response?

Visit www.pearsonhighered.com/nursingresources for answers and rationales for all activities.

REFERENCES

Expert Panel on Detection. (2001). Executive Summary of the Third Report of the National Cholesterol Education Program (NCEP) Expert Panel on Detection, Evaluation, and Treatment of High Blood Cholesterol in Adults (Adult Treatment Panel III). *JAMA: The Journal of the American Medical Association, 285*, 2486–2497. doi:10.1001/jama.285.19.2486

Herdman, T. H., & Kamitsuru, S. (Eds.). (2014). *NANDA International nursing diagnoses: Definitions and classification, 2015–2017*. Oxford, United Kingdom: Wiley-Blackwell.

Psaty, B. M., & Weiss, N. S. (2014). 2013 ACC/AHA guideline on the treatment of blood cholesterol: A fresh interpretation of old evidence. *JAMA: The Journal of the American Medical Association, 311*, 461–462. doi:10.1001/jama.2013.284203

U.S. Department of Health and Human Services, National Institutes of Health, National Heart, Lung, and Blood Institute. (2012). *Expert panel on integrated guidelines and risk reduction in children and adolescents* (NIH publication No. 12-7486A). Retrieved from http://www.nhlbi.nih.gov/files/docs/peds_guidelines_sum.pdf

SELECTED BIBLIOGRAPHY

Anderson, T. J., Grégoire, J., Hegele, R. A., Couture, P., Mancini, G. B., McPherson, R., . . . Ur, E. (2013). 2012 update of the Canadian Cardiovascular Society guidelines for the diagnosis and treatment of dyslipidemia for the prevention of cardiovascular disease in the adult. *Canadian Journal of Cardiology, 29*, 151–167. doi:10.1016/j.cjca.2012.11.032

Bamba, V. (2014). Update on screening, etiology, and treatment of dyslipidemia in children. *The Journal of Clinical Endocrinology & Metabolism, 99*, 3093–3102. doi:10.1210/jc.2013-3860

Berglund, L., Brunzell, J. D., Goldberg, A. C., Goldberg, I. J., Sacks, F., Murad, M. H., & Stalenhoef, A. F. (2012). Evaluation and treatment of hypertriglyceridemia: An Endocrine Society clinical practice guideline. *The Journal of Clinical Endocrinology & Metabolism, 97*, 2969–2989. doi:10.1210/jc.2011-3213

Bersot, T. P. (2012). Drug therapy for hypercholesterolemia and dyslipidemia. In L. L. Brunton, B. A. Chabner, & B. C. Knollman (Eds.), *Goodman and Gilman's the pharmacological basis of therapeutics* (12th ed., pp. 877–908). New York, NY: McGraw-Hill.

Centers for Disease Control and Prevention. (2015). *Cholesterol: Facts*. Retrieved from http://www.cdc.gov/cholesterol/facts.htm

Citkowitz, E. (2014). *Familial hypercholesterolemia*. Retrieved from http://emedicine.medscape.com/article/121298-overview

Eiland, L. S., & Luttrell, P. K. (2010). Use of statins for dyslipidemia in the pediatric population. *Journal of Pediatric Pharmacology and Therapeutics, 15*, 160–172.

Jellinger, P. S., Smith, D. A., Mehta, A. E., Ganda, O., Handelsman, Y., Rodbard, H. W., . . . Seibel, J. A. (2012). American Association of Clinical Endocrinologists' guidelines for management of dyslipidemia and prevention of atherosclerosis. *Endocrine Practice, 18*, 269–293. doi:10.4158/EP.18.2.269

Keaney, J. F., Jr., Curfman, G. D., & Jarcho, J. A. (2014). A pragmatic view of the new cholesterol treatment guidelines. *New England Journal of Medicine, 370*, 275–278. doi:10.1056/NEJMms1314569

National Institutes of Health. (2014). *Coenzyme Q10*. Retrieved from http://www.nlm.nih.gov/medlineplus/druginfo/natural/938.html

Oldways. (n.d.). *Heritage pyramids and total diet*. Retrieved from http://www.oldwayspt.org/eating-well/introduction-traditional-diet-pyramids

Smith, R. J., & Hiatt, W. R. (2013). Two new drugs for homozygous familial hypercholesterolemia: Managing benefits and risks in a rare disorder. *JAMA Internal Medicine, 173*, 1491–1492. doi:10.1001/jamainternmed.2013.6624

Steinberger, J., & Kelly, A. S. (2008). Challenges of existing pediatric dyslipidemia guidelines: Call for reappraisal. *Circulation, 117*, 9–10. doi:10.1161/circulationaha.107.743104

Stone, N. J., Robinson, J., Lichtenstein, A. H., Merz, C. N. B., Lloyd-Jones, D. M., Blum, C. B., . . . Wilson, P. W. F. (2013). 2013 ACC/AHA guideline on the treatment of blood cholesterol to reduce atherosclerotic cardiovascular risk in adults: A report of the American College of Cardiology/American Heart Association Task Force on Practice Guidelines. *Journal of the American College of Cardiology, 63* (25_PA), 2889–2934. doi:10.1016/j.jacc.2013.11.002

Taylor, F., Ward, K., Moore, T. H. M., Burke, M., Davey-Smith, G., Casas J-P., & Ebrahim, S. (2011). Statins for the primary prevention of cardiovascular disease. *Cochrane Database of Systematic Reviews*, 1, Art. No.: CD004816. doi:10.1002/14651858.CD004816.pub4

Vogel, R. A. (2014). The new cholesterol guidelines: Finally more light than heat. *Journal of the American College of Cardiology, 64*, 920–921. doi:10.1016/j.jacc.2014.06.1175

Weintraub, H. (2013). Update on marine omega-3 fatty acids: Management of dyslipidemia and current omega-3 treatment options. *Atherosclerosis, 230*, 381–389. doi:10.1016/j.atherosclerosis.2013.07.041

Chapter 24

Diuretic Therapy and Drugs for Renal Failure

Drugs at a Glance

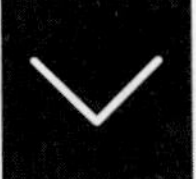

Learning Outcomes

After reading this chapter, the student should be able to:

1. Explain the primary functions of the kidneys.
2. Explain the processes that change the composition of filtrate as it travels through the nephron.
3. Describe the adjustments in pharmacotherapy that must be considered in patients with renal failure.
4. Identify indications for diuretics.
5. Describe the general adverse effects of diuretic pharmacotherapy.
6. Compare and contrast the loop, thiazide, and potassium-sparing diuretics.
7. Describe the nurse's role in the pharmacologic management of renal failure and in diuretic therapy.
8. For each of the classes shown in Drugs at a Glance, know representative drugs, and explain the mechanism of drug action, primary actions, and important adverse effects.
9. Use the nursing process to care for patients who are receiving pharmacotherapy with diuretics.

(pill icon) indicates a prototype drug, each of which is featured in a Prototype Drug box.

The kidneys serve an amazing role in maintaining homeostasis. By filtering a volume equivalent to all the body's extracellular fluid every 100 minutes, the kidneys are able to make immediate adjustments to fluid volume, electrolyte composition, and acid–base balance. This chapter examines diuretics, agents that increase urine output, and other drugs used to treat kidney failure. Chapter 25 presents additional medications for treating fluid, electrolyte, and acid–base imbalances.

PharmFacts

RENAL DISORDERS

- Although more than 16,000 kidney transplants are performed annually, more than 80,500 people are on the waiting list to receive a kidney transplant.
- One of every 750 people is born with a single kidney. A single kidney is larger and more vulnerable to injury from heavy contact sports.
- About 400,000 Americans are treated for kidney failure each year, and 90,000 die annually from causes related to the disease.
- Type 2 diabetes and hypertension account for over two thirds of new cases of chronic kidney failure each year.

THE KIDNEYS

24.1 Functions of the Kidneys

When most people think of the kidneys, they think of excretion. Although this is certainly true, the kidneys have many other homeostatic functions. The kidneys are the primary organs for regulating fluid balance, electrolyte composition, and acid–base balance of body fluids. They also secrete the enzyme renin, which helps regulate blood pressure (see chapter 25), and erythropoietin, a hormone that stimulates red blood cell production. In addition, the kidneys are responsible for the production of calcitriol, the active form of vitamin D, which helps maintain bone homeostasis (see chapter 48). It is not surprising that our overall health is strongly dependent on proper functioning of the kidneys.

The urinary system consists of two kidneys, two ureters, one urinary bladder, and a urethra. Each kidney contains more than 1 million **nephrons,** the functional units of the kidney. Blood enters the nephron through the large renal arteries and is filtered through the glomerulus, a specialized capillary containing pores. Water and other small molecules readily pass through the pores of the glomerulus and enter Bowman's capsule, the first section of the nephron, and then the proximal tubule. Once in the nephron, the fluid is called **filtrate.** After leaving the proximal tubule, the filtrate travels through the loop of Henle and, subsequently, the distal tubule. Nephrons empty their filtrate into common collecting ducts and then into larger and larger collecting structures inside the kidney. Fluid leaving the collecting ducts and entering subsequent portions of the kidney is called urine. Parts of the nephron are illustrated in Figure 24.1.

Many drugs are small enough to pass through the pores of the glomerulus and enter the filtrate. If the drug is bound to plasma proteins, however, it will be too large and will continue circulating in the blood.

24.2 Renal Reabsorption and Secretion

When filtrate enters Bowman's capsule, its composition is very similar to that of plasma. Plasma proteins such as albumin, however, are too large to pass through the filter and will not be present in the filtrate or in the urine of healthy patients. If these proteins *do* appear in urine, it means they were able to pass through the filter due to kidney pathology.

As filtrate travels through the nephron, its composition changes dramatically. Some substances in the filtrate cross the walls of the nephron to reenter the blood, a process known **as tubular reabsorption.** Water is the most important molecule reabsorbed in the tubule. For every 180 L of water entering the filtrate each day, approximately 178.5 L is reabsorbed, leaving only 1.5 L to be excreted in the urine. Glucose, amino acids, and essential ions such as sodium, chloride, calcium, and bicarbonate are also reabsorbed.

Certain ions and molecules that are too large to pass through Bowman's capsule may still enter the urine by crossing from the blood to the filtrate in a process called **tubular secretion.** Potassium, phosphate, hydrogen, and ammonium ions enter the filtrate through active secretion. Acidic drugs secreted in the proximal tubule include penicillin G, ampicillin, sulfisoxazole, nonsteroidal anti-inflammatory drugs (NSAIDs), and furosemide. Basic drugs include procainamide, epinephrine, dopamine, neostigmine, and trimethoprim.

Reabsorption and secretion are critical to the pharmacokinetics of drugs. Some drugs are reabsorbed, whereas others are secreted into the filtrate. For example, approximately 90% of a dose of penicillin G enters the urine through secretion. When the kidney is damaged, reabsorption and secretion mechanisms are impaired and serum drug levels may be dramatically affected. The processes of reabsorption and secretion are illustrated in Figure 24.1.

RENAL FAILURE

Renal failure is a decrease in the kidneys' ability to maintain electrolyte and fluid balance and to excrete waste

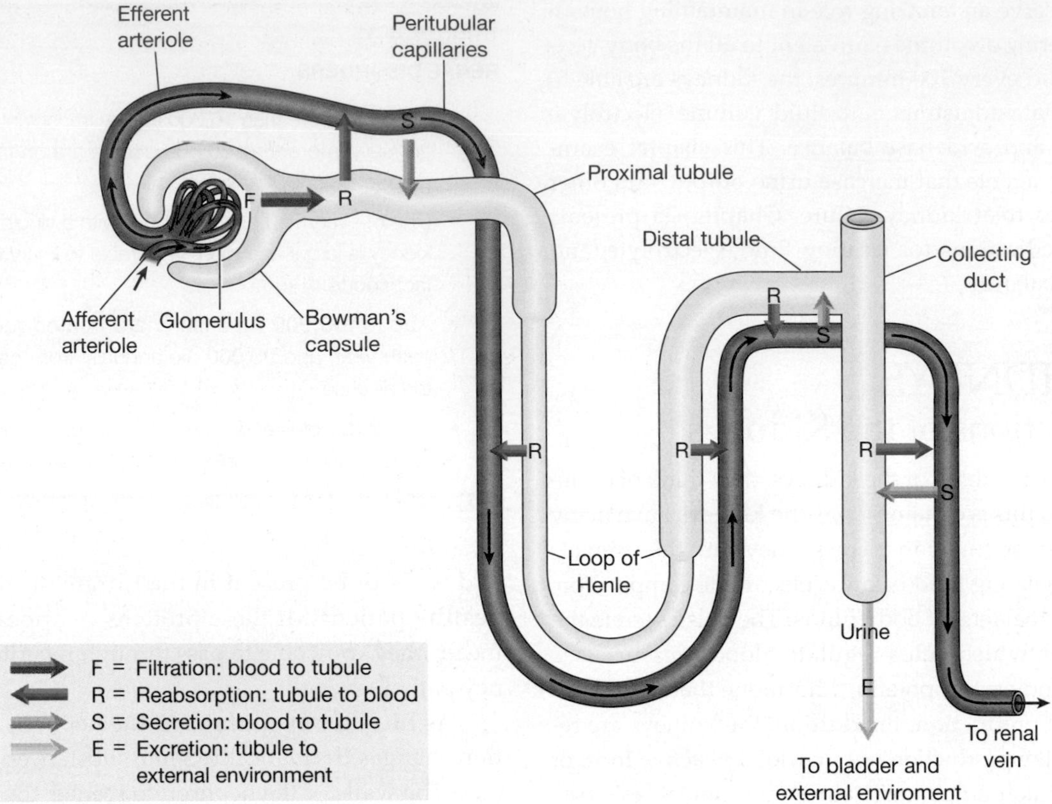

FIGURE 24.1 The nephron

products. The cause of renal failure may be due to pathology within the kidney itself or the result of disorders in other body systems. The primary treatment goals for a patient with renal failure are to maintain blood flow through the kidneys and adequate urine output.

24.3 Diagnosis and Pharmacotherapy of Renal Failure

Before pharmacotherapy is initiated in a patient with renal failure, an assessment of the degree of kidney impairment is necessary. The basic diagnostic test is a **urinalysis,** which examines urine for the presence of blood cells, proteins, pH, specific gravity, ketones, glucose, and microorganisms. The urinalysis can detect proteinuria and albuminuria, which are the primary measures of structural kidney damage. Although it is easy to perform, the urinalysis is nonspecific: Many diseases can cause abnormal urinalysis values. Serum creatinine is an additional measure for detecting kidney disease. To provide a more definitive diagnosis, diagnostic imaging such as computed tomography, sonography, or magnetic resonance imaging may be necessary. Renal biopsy may be performed to obtain a more specific diagnosis.

The best marker for estimating kidney function is the glomerular filtration rate (GFR), which is the volume of filtrate passing through Bowman capsules per minute. The GFR can be used to predict the onset and progression of kidney failure and provides an indication of the ability of the kidneys to excrete drugs from the body. A progressive decline in GFR indicates a decline in the number of functioning nephrons. As nephrons die, however, the remaining healthy nephrons have the ability to compensate by increasing their filtration capacity. Thus, patients with significant kidney damage may exhibit no symptoms until 50% or more of the nephrons have become nonfunctional and the GFR falls to less than half its normal value.

Renal failure is classified as acute or chronic, depending on its onset. Acute renal failure requires immediate treatment because retention of nitrogenous waste products in the body such as urea and creatinine can result in death if untreated. The most frequent cause of acute renal failure is renal hypoperfusion, the lack of sufficient blood flow through the kidneys. Hypoperfusion can lead to permanent destruction of kidney cells and nephrons. To correct this type of renal failure, the cause of the hypoperfusion must be quickly identified and corrected. Potential causes include heart failure, dysrhythmias, hemorrhage, toxins, and dehydration. Because pharmacotherapy with nephrotoxic drugs can also lead to either acute or chronic renal failure, it is good practice for nurses to remember common nephrotoxic drugs, which are listed in Table 24.1. Patients receiving these medications must receive frequent kidney function tests.

Chronic renal failure occurs over a period of months or years. Over half of the patients with chronic renal

Table 24.1 Nephrotoxic Drugs

Drug or Class	Indication/Classification
Aminoglycosides	Antibiotic
Amphotericin B (Amphotec, AmBisome)	Systemic antifungal
Angiotensin-converting enzyme (ACE) inhibitors	Hypertension, heart failure
Cisplatin (Platinol), carboplatin (Paraplatin)	Cancer
Cyclosporine (Neoral, Sandimmune), tacrolimus (Prograf)	Immunosuppressant
Foscarnet (Foscavir)	Antiviral
Nonsteroidal anti-inflammatory drugs (NSAIDs)	Inflammation or pain
Pentamidine (Pentam)	Anti-infective (Pneumocystis)
Radiographic intravenous (IV) contrast agents	Diagnosis of kidney and vascular disorders

failure have a medical history of longstanding hypertension (HTN) or diabetes mellitus. Because of the long, gradual development period and nonspecific symptoms, chronic renal failure may go undiagnosed for many years. By the time the disease is diagnosed, impairment may be irreversible. In end-stage renal disease (ESRD), dialysis and kidney transplantation become treatment alternatives.

Treatment of renal failure attempts to manage the cause of the dysfunction. Diuretics are given to increase urine output, and cardiovascular drugs are administered to treat underlying HTN or heart failure. Dietary management is often necessary to prevent worsening of renal impairment. Depending on the stage of the disease, dietary management may include protein restriction and reduction of sodium, potassium, phosphorus, and magnesium intake. For patients with diabetes, control of blood glucose through intensive insulin therapy may reduce the risk of renal damage. Selected pharmacologic drugs used to prevent and treat kidney failure are summarized in Table 24.2.

Nurses play a key role in recognizing and responding to renal failure. Once a diagnosis is established, all nephrotoxic medications should be either discontinued or used with extreme caution. Because the kidneys excrete most drugs or their metabolites, medications will require a significant dosage reduction in patients with moderate to severe renal failure. The importance of this cannot be overemphasized: *Administering the "average" dose to a patient in severe renal failure can have fatal consequences.*

DIURETICS

Diuretics are drugs that are frequently used in the pharmacotherapy of renal and cardiovascular disorders. They are indicated for the treatment of hypertension, heart failure, and disorders characterized by accumulation of edema fluid.

24.4 Mechanisms of Action of Diuretics

A **diuretic** is a drug that increases the rate of urine flow. The goal of most diuretic therapy is to reverse abnormal fluid retention by the body. Excretion of excess fluid from the body is particularly desirable in the following conditions:

- HTN
- Heart failure
- Kidney failure
- Liver failure or cirrhosis
- Pulmonary edema

The most common mechanism by which diuretics act is by blocking sodium ion (Na^+) reabsorption in the

Table 24.2 Pharmacologic Management of Renal Failure

Complication	Pathogenesis	Treatment
Anemia	Kidneys are unable to synthesize enough erythropoietin for red blood cell production.	Epoetin alfa (Procrit, Epogen) or darbepoietin alfa (Aranesp)
Hyperkalemia	Kidneys are unable to adequately excrete potassium.	Dietary restriction of potassium; polystyrene sulfate (Kayexalate) with sorbitol
Hyperphosphatemia	Kidneys are unable to adequately excrete phosphate.	Dietary restriction of phosphate; phosphate binders such as calcium carbonate (Os-Cal 500, others), calcium acetate (Calphron, PhosLo), lanthanum carbonate (Fosrenol), sucroferric oxyhydroxide (Velphoro) or sevelamer (Renagel)
Hypervolemia	Kidneys are unable to excrete sufficient sodium and water, leading to water retention.	Dietary restriction of sodium; loop diuretics in acute conditions, thiazide diuretics in mild conditions
Hypocalcemia	Hyperphosphatemia leads to loss of calcium.	Usually corrected by reversing the hyperphosphatemia, but additional calcium supplements may be necessary
Metabolic acidosis	Kidneys are unable to adequately excrete metabolic acids.	Sodium bicarbonate or sodium citrate

Pharmacotherapy Illustrated

24.1 | Sites of Action of the Diuretics

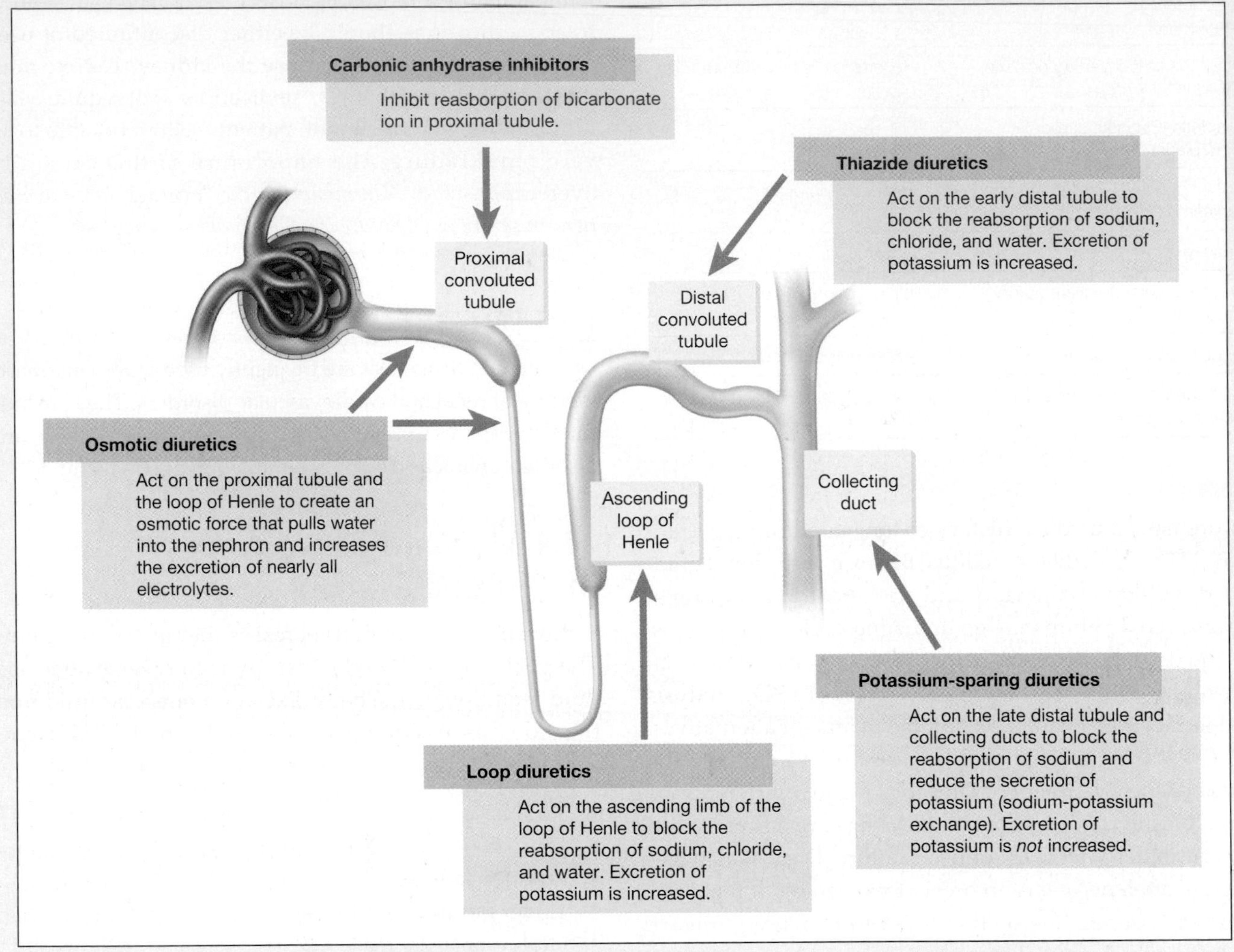

Carbonic anhydrase inhibitors
Inhibit reasborption of bicarbonate ion in proximal tubule.
Thiazide diuretics
Act on the early distal tubule to block the reabsorption of sodium, chloride, and water. Excretion of potassium is increased.
Proximal convoluted tubule
Distal convoluted tubule
Osmotic diuretics
Act on the proximal tubule and the loop of Henle to create an osmotic force that pulls water into the nephron and increases the excretion of nearly all electrolytes.
Ascending loop of Henle
Collecting duct
Potassium-sparing diuretics
Act on the late distal tubule and collecting ducts to block the reabsorption of sodium and reduce the secretion of potassium (sodium-potassium exchange). Excretion of potassium is *not* increased.
Loop diuretics
Act on the ascending limb of the loop of Henle to block the reabsorption of sodium, chloride, and water. Excretion of potassium is increased.

Based on *Pharmacology: Connections to Nursing Practice* (3rd Ed.), by M. Adams and C. Urban, 2016. Reprinted and electronically reproduced by permission of Pearson Education, Inc., Upper Saddle River, New Jersey.

nephron, thus sending more Na^+ to the urine. Chloride ions (Cl^-) follow sodium. Because water molecules also travel with Na^+, blocking the reabsorption of Na^+ will increase the volume of urination, or diuresis. Diuretics may affect the renal excretion of other ions, including magnesium, potassium, phosphate, calcium, and bicarbonate ions.

Diuretics are classified into three major groups and one miscellaneous group based on differences in their chemical structures and mechanism of action. Some drugs, such as furosemide (Lasix), act by preventing the reabsorption of Na^+ in the loop of Henle; thus, they are called *loop* diuretics. Because of the abundance of Na^+ in the filtrate within the loop of Henle, drugs in this class are capable of producing large increases in urine output. Other drugs, such as the *thiazides,* act by blocking Na^+ in the distal tubule. Because most Na^+ has already been reabsorbed from the filtrate by the time it reaches the distal tubule, the thiazides produce less diuresis than furosemide and other loop diuretics. The third major class is named *potassium sparing,* because these diuretics have minimal effect on potassium (K^+) excretion. Miscellaneous drugs include the osmotic diuretics and carbonic anhydrase inhibitors. The sites in the nephron where the various diuretics act are shown in Pharmacotherapy Illustrated 24.1.

It is common practice to combine two or more drugs in the pharmacotherapy of HTN and fluid retention disorders. The diuretics are frequently a component of fixed-dose combinations with drugs from other classes. The primary rationales for combination therapy are that the

Evidence-Based Practice: Diuretics and Risk for Falls

Clinical Question: Does the use of diuretics increase the risk for falls?

Evidence: Falls are a known health problem, particularly for older adults. Falls result in increased hospitalizations and adverse outcomes. Because diuretics may decrease intravascular volume resulting in hypotension, they have been implicated as a potential cause for increased fall risk. Research has been inconclusive or contradictory, however. Several studies have noted that the use of diuretics played a role in falls. Berry et al., 2012, noted that a risk for falls increased substantially the day after there was a change in a loop diuretic prescription. Butt et al., 2013 found that an increased fall risk continued for 45 days following antihypertensive treatment with diuretics. Williams, Szekendi, & Thomas, 2014 noted that the risk of falls almost doubled when patients were taking diuretics, although it was not conclusive that the diuretic, or the need for more frequent toileting, was the causative factor. Other studies, including systematic reviews and meta-analyses have not found a statistical association between diuretic use and falls (de Groot et al., 2013; Zang, 2013).

Nursing Implications: Patients who are receiving diuretic therapy need to be closely monitored for the development of orthostatic hypotension that may cause syncope, and more frequent orthostatic blood pressure monitoring should be implemented. This is especially important when a diuretic has been started or a change in dose has been implemented. Assisting the patient with ambulation after ensuring that blood pressure is stable; teaching the patient, family members, or caregivers to monitor the blood pressure before activities; and ensuring that the patient remains adequately hydrated are safety measures that may prevent falls related to syncope caused by a drop in blood pressure. If significant changes in postural blood pressure readings are noted, the nurse should consult with the health care provider and a change in medication strategies may be warranted.

incidence of adverse effects is decreased and the pharmacologic effects (such as diuresis or reduction in blood pressure) may be enhanced. For patient convenience, some of these drugs are combined in single-tablet formulations. More than 25 different fixed-dose combinations are available to treat HTN (see chapter 26). Examples of single-tablet combinations that include diuretics include the following:

- Accuretic: hydrochlorothiazide and quinapril.
- Aldactazide: hydrochlorothiazide and spironolactone.
- Apresazide: hydrochlorothiazide and hydralazine.
- Tribenzor: hydrochlorothiazide, olmesartan, and amlodipine.
- Zestoretic: hydrochlorothiazide and lisinopril.

Loop Diuretics

24.5 Pharmacotherapy With Loop Diuretics

The most effective diuretics are the *loop* or *high-ceiling* diuretics. Drugs in this class act by blocking the reabsorption of Na^+ and Cl^- in the loop of Henle. When given IV, they have the ability to cause large amounts of fluid to be excreted by the kidney in a very short time. Loop diuretics are used to reduce the edema associated with heart failure, hepatic cirrhosis, or chronic renal failure. Furosemide and torsemide are also approved for HTN. Doses for the loop diuretics are listed in Table 24.3.

Furosemide is the most frequently prescribed loop diuretic. Unlike the thiazide diuretics, furosemide is able to

Table 24.3 Loop Diuretics

Drug	Route and Adult Dose (max dose where indicated)	Adverse Effects
bumetanide (Bumex)	PO: 0.5–2 mg, may repeat at 4- to 5-h intervals if needed (max: 10 mg/day) IV/IM: 0.5–1 mg over 1–2 min, repeated every 2–3 h prn (max: 10 mg/day)	*Minor hypokalemia, postural hypotension, tinnitus, nausea, diarrhea, dizziness, fatigue* Significant hypokalemia, blood dyscrasias, dehydration, ototoxicity, electrolyte imbalances, circulatory collapse
ethacrynic acid (Edecrin)	PO: 50–100 mg one to two times/day, may increase by 25–50 mg PRN (max: 400 mg/day). IV; 0.5–1 mg/kg or 50 mg (max: 100 mg/dose	
furosemide (Lasix)	PO: 20–80 mg in single or divided doses (max: 600 mg/day) IV/IM: 20–40 mg in single or divided doses (max 200 mg/dose) up to 600 mg/day	
torsemide (Demadex)	PO/IV: 10–20 mg/day (max: 200 mg/day), IV may be repeated in 2 h if needed	

Note: *Italics* indicate common adverse effects; underlining indicates serious adverse effects.

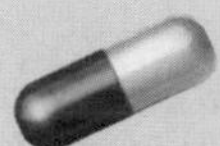

Prototype Drug | Furosemide *(Lasix)*

Therapeutic Class: Drug for heart failure and HTN **Pharmacologic Class:** Diuretic (loop type)

Actions and Uses

Furosemide is often used in the treatment of acute heart failure because it has the ability to remove large amounts of excess fluid from the patient in a short period. When given IV, diuresis begins within 5 minutes, giving patients quick relief from their distressing symptoms. Furosemide acts by preventing the reabsorption of sodium and chloride in the loop of Henle region of the nephron. Compared with other diuretics, furosemide is particularly beneficial when cardiac output and renal flow are severely diminished.

Administration Alerts

- Check the patient's serum potassium levels before administering the drug. If potassium levels are below normal, notify the health care provider before administering.
- Due to the prolonged half-life in premature infants and neonates, the drug must be used with caution.
- Older adults may require lower doses.
- Pregnancy category C.

PHARMACOKINETICS

Onset	Peak	Duration
30–60 min PO; 5 min IV	60–70 min PO; 15-20 min IV	6–8 h PO; 2 h IV

Adverse Effects

Adverse effects of furosemide, like those of most diuretics, involve potential electrolyte imbalances, the most important of which is hypokalemia. Because furosemide is so effective, fluid loss must be carefully monitored to prevent possible dehydration and hypotension. Hypovolemia may cause orthostatic hypotension and syncope. Ototoxicity is rare but may result in permanent hearing deficit.

Black Box Warning: Furosemide is a potent diuretic that, if given in excessive amounts, may lead to profound diuresis with water and electrolyte depletion. Careful medical supervision is required.

Contraindications: Contraindications include hypersensitivity to furosemide or sulfonamides, anuria, hepatic coma, and severe fluid or electrolyte depletion.

Interactions

Drug–Drug: Because hypokalemia may cause dysrhythmias in patients taking cardiac glycosides, combination therapy with digoxin must be carefully monitored. Furosemide should not be used concurrently with aminoglycoside antibiotics due to the possibility of additive nephrotoxicity and ototoxicity. Concurrent use with corticosteroids, amphotericin B, or other potassium-depleting drugs can result in hypokalemia. When given with lithium, elimination of lithium is decreased, causing a higher risk of toxicity. Furosemide may diminish the hypoglycemic effects of sulfonylureas and insulin.

Lab Tests: Furosemide may increase values for the following: blood glucose, blood urea nitrogen (BUN), serum amylase, cholesterol, triglycerides, and serum electrolytes.

Herbal/Food: Use with hawthorn could result in additive hypotensive effects. Ginseng may decrease the effectiveness of loop diuretics. High sodium intake can reduce the effectiveness of diuretics.

Treatment of Overdose: Overdose will result in hypotension and severe fluid and electrolyte loss. Treatment is supportive, with replacement of fluids and electrolytes, and the possible administration of a vasopressor.

increase urine output even when blood flow to the kidneys is diminished, which makes it of particular value in patients with renal failure. Torsemide has a longer half-life than furosemide, which offers the advantage of once-a-day dosing. Bumetanide (Bumex) is 40 times more potent than furosemide but has a shorter duration of action.

The rapid excretion of large amounts of fluid has the potential to produce serious adverse effects, including dehydration and electrolyte imbalances. Signs of dehydration include thirst, dry mouth, weight loss, and headache. Hypotension, dizziness, and fainting can result from the rapid fluid loss. Potassium depletion can be serious and cause dysrhythmias; potassium supplements may be prescribed to prevent hypokalemia. Potassium loss is of particular concern to patients who are also taking digoxin (Lanoxin) because these patients may experience dysrhythmias. Although rare, ototoxicity is possible, and other ototoxic drugs such as the aminoglycoside antibiotics should be avoided during loop diuretic therapy. Because of the potential for serious adverse effects, the loop diuretics are normally reserved for patients with moderate to severe fluid retention, or when other diuretics have failed to achieve therapeutic goals.

Table 24.4 Thiazide and Thiazide-Like Diuretics

Drug	Route and Adult Dose (max dose where indicated)	Adverse Effects
SHORT ACTING		
chlorothiazide (Diuril)	PO: 250 mg–1 g/day IV: 250 mg–1 g/day in single or two divided doses	*Minor hypokalemia, fatigue* Significant hypokalemia, electrolyte depletion, dehydration, hypotension, hyponatremia, hyperglycemia, coma, blood dyscrasias
hydrochlorothiazide (Microzide)	PO: 25–100 mg/day as single or divided dose (max: 50 mg/day for HTN; 100 mg/day for edema)	
INTERMEDIATE ACTING		
bendroflumethiazide and nadolol (Corzide)	PO: 1 tablet/day (40–80 mg nadolol/5 mg bendroflumethiazide)	
metolazone (Zaroxolyn)	PO: 2.5–10 mg once daily (max: 5 mg/day for HTN; 20 mg/day for edema)	
LONG ACTING		
chlorthalidone (Hygroton)	PO: 50–100 mg/day (max: 100 mg/day for HTN; 200 mg/day for edema)	
indapamide (Lozol)	PO: 2.5 mg once daily (max: 5 mg/day	
methyclothiazide (Enduron)	PO: 2.5–10 mg/day (max: 5 mg/day for HTN; 10 mg/day for edema)	

Note: *Italics* indicate common adverse effects; underlining indicates serious adverse effects.

Thiazide Diuretics

24.6 Pharmacotherapy With Thiazide Diuretics

The thiazides constitute the largest, most frequently prescribed class of diuretics. These drugs act on the distal tubule to block Na^+ reabsorption and increase K^+ and water excretion. Their primary use is for the treatment of mild to moderate HTN; however, they are also indicated for edema due to mild to moderate heart failure, liver failure, and renal failure. They are less effective at producing diuresis than the loop diuretics and they are ineffective in patients with severe renal failure. The thiazide diuretics are listed in Table 24.4.

All the thiazide diuretics are available by the oral (PO) route and have equivalent efficacy and safety profiles. They differ, however, in their potency and duration of action. Three drugs—chlorthalidone (Hygroton), indapamide (Lozol), and metolazone (Zaroxolyn)—are not true thiazides, although they are included with this drug class because they have similar mechanisms of action and adverse effects.

The adverse effects of thiazides are similar to those of the loop diuretics, although their frequency is less, and they do not cause ototoxicity. Dehydration and excessive loss of Na^+, K^+, or Cl^- may occur with overtreatment. Concurrent therapy with digoxin requires careful monitoring to prevent dysrhythmias due to potassium loss. Potassium supplements may be indicated during thiazide therapy to prevent hypokalemia. Patients with diabetes should be aware that thiazide diuretics sometimes raise blood glucose levels.

Potassium-Sparing Diuretics

24.7 Pharmacotherapy With Potassium-Sparing Diuretics

Hypokalemia is one of the most serious adverse effects of the thiazide and loop diuretics. The therapeutic advantage of the potassium-sparing diuretics is that increased diuresis can be obtained without affecting blood K^+ levels. Doses for the potassium-sparing diuretics are listed in Table 24.5. There are two distinct mechanisms by which these drugs act.

Table 24.5 Potassium-Sparing Diuretics

Drug	Route and Adult Dose (max dose where indicated)	Adverse Effects
amiloride (Midamor)	PO: 5 mg/day (max: 20 mg/day)	*Minor hyperkalemia, headache, fatigue, gynecomastia (spironolactone)* Dysrhythmias (from hyperkalemia), dehydration, hyponatremia, agranulocytosis, and other blood dyscrasias
eplerenone (Inspra)	PO: 25–50 mg once daily (max: 100 mg/day for HTN; 50 mg/day for heart failure)	
spironolactone (Aldactone)	PO: 25–100 mg one to two times/day (max: 400 mg/day)	
triamterene (Dyrenium)	PO: 50–100 mg bid (max: 300 mg/day)	

Note: *Italics* indicate common adverse effects; underlining indicates serious adverse effects.

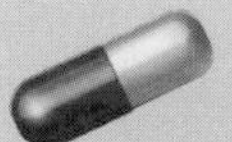

Prototype Drug | Hydrochlorothiazide *(Microzide)*

Therapeutic Class: Drug for hypertension and edema **Pharmacologic Class:** Thiazide diuretic

Actions and Uses

Hydrochlorothiazide is the most widely prescribed diuretic for HTN. Like many diuretics, it produces few serious adverse effects and is effective at producing a 10 to 20 mmHg reduction in blood pressure. Patients with severe HTN or a compelling condition may require the addition of a second drug from a different class to control the disease. Hydrochlorothiazide is the most common medication found in fixed-dose combination drugs for HTN. Hydrochlorothiazide is approved to treat ascites, edema, heart failure, HTN, and nephrotic syndrome. Nurses sometimes use HCTZ as an abbreviation for this drug; however, this should be avoided because it causes confusion between hydrochlorothiazide and hydrocortisone.

Hydrochlorothiazide acts on the kidney tubule to decrease the reabsorption of Na^+. Normally, more than 99% of the sodium entering the kidney is reabsorbed by the body. When hydrochlorothiazide blocks this reabsorption, more Na^+ is sent into the urine. When sodium moves across the tubule, water flows with it; thus, blood volume decreases and blood pressure falls. The volume of urine produced is directly proportional to the amount of sodium reabsorption blocked by the diuretic.

Administration Alert

- Administer the drug early in the day to prevent nocturia.
- Pregnancy category B.

PHARMACOKINETICS

Onset	Peak	Duration
2 h	4 h	6–12 h

Adverse Effects

Hydrochlorothiazide is well tolerated and exhibits few serious adverse effects. The most common adverse effects are potential electrolyte imbalances due to loss of excessive K^+ and Na^1. Because hypokalemia may cause cardiac conduction abnormalities, patients are usually instructed to increase their potassium intake as a precaution. Hydrochlorothiazide may precipitate gout attacks due to its tendency to cause hyperuricemia.

Contraindications: Contraindications include anuria and prior hypersensitivity to thiazides or sulfonamides. Thiazides are contraindicated in pre-eclampsia or other pregnancy-induced HTN.

Interactions

Drug–Drug: When given concurrently, other antihypertensives have additive or synergistic effects with hydrochlorothiazide on blood pressure. Thiazides may reduce the effectiveness of anticoagulants, sulfonylureas, and antidiabetic drugs including insulin. Cholestyramine and colestipol decrease the absorption of hydrochlorothiazide and reduce its effectiveness. Hydrochlorothiazide increases the risk of renal toxicity from NSAIDs. Corticosteroids and amphotericin B increase potassium loss when given with hydrochlorothiazide. Hypokalemia caused by hydrochlorothiazide may increase digoxin toxicity. Hydrochlorothiazide decreases the excretion of lithium and can lead to lithium toxicity.

Lab Tests: Hydrochlorothiazide may increase serum glucose, cholesterol, bilirubin, triglyceride, and calcium levels. The drug may decrease serum magnesium, potassium, and sodium levels.

Herbal/Food: Ginkgo biloba may produce a paradoxical increase in blood pressure. Use with hawthorn could result in additive hypotensive effects.

Treatment of Overdose: Overdose is manifested as electrolyte depletion, which is treated with infusions of fluids containing electrolytes. Infusion of fluids will also prevent dehydration and hypotension.

Normally, sodium and potassium are exchanged in the distal tubule; Na^+ is reabsorbed back into the blood, and K^+ is secreted into the distal tubule. Triamterene and amiloride block this exchange, causing Na^+ to stay in the tubule and ultimately leave through the urine. When Na^+ is blocked, the body retains more K^+. Because most of the Na^+ has already been removed before the filtrate reaches the distal tubule, these potassium-sparing diuretics produce only a mild diuresis. Their primary use is in combination with thiazide or loop diuretics to minimize potassium loss.

The third potassium-sparing diuretic, spironolactone, acts by blocking the actions of the hormone aldosterone. It is sometimes called an aldosterone antagonist and may be used to treat hyperaldosteronism. Blocking aldosterone enhances the *excretion* of Na^+ and the *retention* of K^+. Like the other two drugs in this diuretic class, spironolactone produces only a weak diuresis. Unlike the other two, spironolactone has been found to significantly reduce mortality in patients with heart failure (see chapter 27). Eplerenone (Inspra) is a newer aldosterone antagonist that is claimed to exhibit fewer adverse effects than spironolactone.

Patients taking potassium-sparing diuretics should *not* take potassium supplements or be advised to add

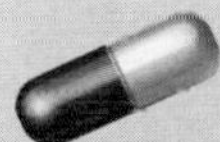

Prototype Drug | Spironolactone *(Aldactone)*

Therapeutic Class: Antihypertensive, drug for reducing edema
Pharmacologic Class: Potassium-sparing diuretic, aldosterone antagonist

Actions and Uses

Spironolactone, the most frequently prescribed potassium-sparing diuretic, is primarily used to treat mild hypertension, often in combination with other antihypertensives. It may be used to reduce edema associated with kidney or liver disease and it is effective in slowing the progression of heart failure.

Spironolactone acts by inhibiting aldosterone, the hormone secreted by the adrenal cortex responsible for increasing the renal reabsorption of Na^+ in exchange for K^+, thus causing water retention. When aldosterone is blocked by spironolactone, Na^+ and water excretion is increased and the body retains more potassium. Because of its anti-aldosterone effect, spironolactone may be used to treat primary hyperaldosteronism. It is available in tablet form and as a fixed-dose combination with hydrochlorothiazide.

Administration Alerts

- Give with food to increase the absorption of the drug.
- Do not give K^+ supplements.
- Pregnancy category C

PHARMACOKINETICS

Onset	Peak	Duration
2–4 hours	6–8 hours	2–3 days or longer

Adverse Effects

Spironolactone does such an efficient job of retaining K^+ that hyperkalemia may develop. The risk of hyperkalemia is increased if the patient takes potassium supplements or is concurrently taking ACE inhibitors. Signs and symptoms of hyperkalemia include muscle weakness, fatigue, and bradycardia. In men, spironolactone can cause gynecomastia, impotence, and diminished libido. Women may experience menstrual irregularities, hirsutism, and breast tenderness. When serum potassium levels are monitored carefully and maintained within normal values, adverse effects from spironolactone are uncommon.

Black Box Warning: Because spironolactone has been found to cause tumors in animals in clinical studies, it should be used only for specified indications.

Contraindications: Spironolactone is contraindicated in patients with anuria, significant impairment of renal function, or hyperkalemia. Spironolactone is contraindicated during pregnancy and lactation.

Interactions

Drug–Drug: When spironolactone is combined with ammonium chloride, acidosis may occur. Aspirin and other salicylates cause increased half-life which can lead to digoxin toxicity. Concurrent use with digoxin may decrease the effects of digoxin. When taken with potassium supplements, ACE inhibitors, and angiotensin-receptor blockers (ARBs), hyperkalemia may result. Concurrent use with antihypertensives will result in an additive hypotensive effect.

Lab Tests: Spironolactone may increase plasma cortisol values and may interfere with serum glucose determination.

Herbal/Food: Use with hawthorn may result in additive hypotensive effects.

Treatment of Overdose: Treatment is supportive and may include agents to replace fluid and electrolytes lost through diuresis and drugs to raise blood pressure.

potassium-rich foods to their diet. Intake of excess potassium when taking these medications may lead to hyperkalemia.

Miscellaneous Diuretics

24.8 Miscellaneous Diuretics for Specific Indications

A few miscellaneous diuretics, listed in Table 24.6, have limited and specific indications. Two of these drugs inhibit **carbonic anhydrase,** an enzyme that affects acid–base balance by its ability to form carbonic acid from water and carbon dioxide. Acetazolamide (Diamox) is a carbonic anhydrase inhibitor used to decrease intraocular fluid pressure in patients with open-angle glaucoma (see chapter 50). In addition to its diuretic effect, acetazolamide has applications as an anticonvulsant and in treating glaucoma. It has also been used to treat acute mountain sickness in patients at very high altitudes. The carbonic anhydrase inhibitors are not commonly used as diuretics, because they produce only a weak diuresis and can contribute to metabolic acidosis.

The osmotic diuretics also have very specific applications. For example, mannitol is used to maintain urine flow in patients with acute renal failure or during prolonged surgery. Since this drug is not reabsorbed in the tubule, it is able to maintain the flow of filtrate even in cases with severe renal hypoperfusion. Mannitol can also be used to lower intraocular pressure in certain types of glaucoma, although it is used for this purpose only when safer

Table 24.6 Miscellaneous Diuretics

Drug	Route and Adult Dose (max dose where indicated)	Adverse Effects
CARBONIC ANHYDRASE INHIBITORS		
acetazolamide (Diamox)	PO: 250–375 mg/day	*Electrolyte imbalances, fatigue, nausea, vomiting, dizziness*
methazolamide (Neptazane)	PO: 50–100 mg bid–tid	<u>Dehydration, blood dyscrasias, pancytopenia, flaccid paralysis, hemolytic anemia, aplastic anemia</u>
OSMOTIC DIURETICS		
glycerin	PO: 1–1.5 g/kg, 1–2 h before ocular surgery	*Electrolyte imbalances, fatigue, nausea, vomiting, dizziness*
mannitol (Osmitrol)	IV: 100 g infused over 2–6 h	<u>Hyponatremia, edema, convulsions, tachycardia</u>

Note: *Italics* indicate common adverse effects, <u>underlining</u> indicates serious adverse effects.

drugs have failed to produce an effect. It is a highly potent diuretic that is given only by the IV route. Unlike other diuretics that draw excess fluid away from tissue spaces, mannitol can worsen edema and thus must be used with caution in patients with pre-existing heart failure or pulmonary edema. The exception is the brain: Mannitol can reduce intracranial pressure due to cerebral edema. Osmotic diuretics are rarely drugs of first choice due to their potential toxicity.

☑ Check Your Understanding 24.1

Why does the location of a diuretic's effect on the renal tubules cause a loop diuretic to be more potent than a thiazide or potassium-sparing diuretic? *Visit www.pearsonhighered.com/nursingresources for the answer.*

Complementary and Alternative Therapies

CRANBERRY FOR URINARY SYSTEM HEALTH

Nearly everyone is familiar with the bright red cranberries that are eaten during holiday times. Native Americans used the colorful, ripe berries to treat wounds, to cure anorexia, and for other digestive complaints. In the 1900s, it was noted that the acidity of the urine increases after eating cranberries; thus began the belief that cranberry juice is a natural cure for urinary tract infections. The herb is taken as juice or dried berries. Some individuals may prefer to take cranberry capsules, which are available at retail pharmacies.

Cranberry contains a significant amount of vitamin C and other antioxidants that can promote health. They contain a substance that can prevent bacteria from sticking to the walls of the bladder. A meta-analysis of research studies that included 1,600 patients concluded that cranberries can indeed prevent symptomatic urinary tract infections (Wang et al., 2012). It is important to note that cranberry should be taken to prevent, not treat, urinary tract infections.

Cranberry is a safe supplement, although large amounts may cause gastrointestinal upset and diarrhea. The juice should be 100% cranberry and not "cocktail" juice because that contains sugar, which enhances bacteria growth and may be contraindicated in patients with diabetes.

Nursing Practice Application

Pharmacotherapy With Diuretics

ASSESSMENT	POTENTIAL NURSING DIAGNOSES*
Baseline assessment prior to administration: • Obtain a complete health history including cardiovascular disease, diabetes, and pregnancy or breast-feeding. Obtain a drug history including allergies; current prescription and over-the-counter (OTC) drugs; herbal preparations; use of digoxin, lithium, or antihypertensive drugs; and alcohol use. Be alert to possible drug interactions. • Evaluate appropriate laboratory findings such as electrolytes, glucose, complete blood count (CBC), hepatic or renal function studies, uric acid levels, and lipid profiles. • Obtain baseline weight, vital signs (especially blood pressure [BP] and pulse), breath sounds, and cardiac monitoring (e.g., ECG, cardiac output) if appropriate. Assess for location and character/amount of edema, if present. Assess baseline hearing and balance.	• *Deficient Fluid Volume* • *Fatigue* • *Decreased Cardiac Output* • *Noncompliance,* related to adverse drug effects • *Deficient Knowledge* (drug therapy) • *Risk for Falls,* related to adverse drug effects • *Risk for Injury,* related to adverse drug effects • *Risk for Urge Incontinence,* related to drug effects *NANDA I © 2014

Nursing Practice Application *continued*

ASSESSMENT	POTENTIAL NURSING DIAGNOSES*
Assessment throughout administration: • Assess for desired therapeutic effects (e.g., adequate urine output, lowered BP if given for HTN). • Continue periodic monitoring of electrolytes, glucose, CBC, lipid profiles, liver function studies, creatinine, and uric acid levels. • Assess for and promptly report adverse effects: hypotension, palpitations, dizziness, musculoskeletal weakness or cramping, nausea, vomiting, abdominal cramping, diarrhea, or headache. Immediately report tinnitus or hearing loss, loss of balance or incoordination, severe hypotension accompanied by reflex tachycardiac dysrhythmias, decreased urine output, and weight gain or loss over 1 kg (2 lb) in a 24-hour period.	

IMPLEMENTATION

Interventions and (Rationales)	Patient-Centered Care
Ensuring therapeutic effects: • Continue frequent assessments as described earlier for therapeutic effects: urine output is increased, and BP and pulse are within normal limits or within parameters set by the health care provider. (Diuresis may be moderate to extreme depending on the type of diuretic given. BP should be within normal limits without the presence of reflex tachycardia.) • Daily weights should remain at or close to baseline weight. (An increase in weight over 1 kg (2 lb) per day may indicate excessive fluid gain. A decrease of over 1 kg (2 lb) per day may indicate excessive diuresis and dehydration.)	• Teach the patient, family, or caregiver how to monitor pulse and BP. Ensure the proper use and functioning of any home equipment obtained. • Have the patient weigh self daily and record weight along with BP and pulse measurements.
Minimizing adverse effects: • Continue to monitor vital signs. Take BP lying, sitting, and standing to detect orthostatic hypotension, especially when a diuretic has been started or dosage has been changed. **Lifespan:** Be cautious with the older adult who is at increased risk for hypotension. (Diuretics reduce circulating blood volume, resulting in lowered BP. Orthostatic hypotension may increase the risk of falls.)	• **Safety:** Teach the patient to rise from lying or sitting to standing slowly to avoid dizziness or falls. If dizziness occurs, the patient should sit or lie down and not attempt to stand or walk until the sensation passes. • Instruct the patient to call for assistance prior to getting out of bed or attempting to walk alone, and to avoid driving or other activities requiring mental alertness or physical coordination until the effects of the drug are known. • Instruct the patient to stop taking the medication if BP is 90/60 mmHg or is below the parameters set by the health care provider, and promptly notify the provider.
• Continue to monitor electrolytes, glucose, CBC, lipid profiles, liver function studies, creatinine, and uric acid levels. (Most diuretics cause loss of Na^+ and K^+ and may increase lipid, glucose, and uric acid levels.)	• Instruct the patient on the need to return periodically for laboratory work and to inform laboratory personnel of diuretic therapy when providing blood or urine samples. • Advise the patient to carry a wallet identification card or wear medical identification jewelry indicating diuretic therapy.
• Continue to monitor hearing and balance, reporting persistent tinnitus or vertigo promptly. (Ototoxicity may occur, especially with loop diuretics. **Lifespan:** Because of pharmacokinetic differences, exercise additional caution when administering diuretics to infants and very young children. Audiology and additional monitoring may be ordered.)	• Have the patient report persistent tinnitus and balance or coordination problems immediately.
• Weigh the patient daily and report significant weight gains or losses. Measure intake and output in the hospitalized patient. (Daily weight is an accurate measure of fluid status and takes into account intake, output, and insensible losses. Diuresis is indicated by output significantly greater than intake.)	• Have the patient weigh self daily, ideally at the same time of day. Have the patient report a weight loss or gain of more than 1 kg (2 lb) in a 24-hour period. • Advise the patient to continue to consume enough liquids to remain adequately, but not overly, hydrated. Drinking when thirsty, avoiding alcoholic beverages, and ensuring adequate but not excessive salt intake will assist in maintaining normal fluid balance. • Teach the patient that excessive heat conditions contribute to excessive sweating and fluid and electrolyte loss, and extra caution is warranted in these conditions.

continued

Nursing Practice Application *continued*

IMPLEMENTATION	
Interventions and (Rationales)	**Patient-Centered Care**
• Monitor nutritional status and encourage appropriate intake to prevent electrolyte imbalances. (Electrolyte imbalances may occur with diuretics. Most diuretics cause Na^+ and K^+ loss. Potassium-sparing diuretics may result in Na^+ loss but K^+ increase. **Lifespan:** Monitor electrolyte levels frequently in older adults because they are at greater risk for imbalances due to age-related physiologic changes.)	• Instruct the patient who is taking potassium-*wasting* diuretics (e.g., thiazides, thiazide-like, and loop diuretics) to consume foods high in potassium: fresh fruits such as strawberries and bananas; dried fruits such as apricots and prunes; vegetables and legumes such as tomatoes, beets, and dried beans; juices such as orange, grapefruit, or prune; and fresh meats. • Instruct the patient who is taking potassium-*sparing* diuretics to avoid foods high in K^+ such as described earlier, not to use salt substitutes (which often contain K^+ salts), and to consult with a health care provider before taking vitamin and mineral supplements or specialized sports beverages. (Typical OTC sports beverages, e.g., Gatorade and Powerade, may have lesser amounts of potassium but have high carbohydrate amounts, which may lead to increased diuresis, diarrhea, and the potential for dehydration from the hyperosmolarity.)
• Observe for signs of hypokalemia or hyperkalemia. Use with caution in patients taking corticosteroids, ACE inhibitors, ARBs, digoxin, or lithium. Promptly report symptoms to the health care provider. (Thiazide, thiazide-like, and loop diuretics can cause hypokalemia; potassium-sparing diuretics may cause hyperkalemia. Concurrent use with corticosteroids may increase the risk of hypokalemia. Concurrent use with ACE inhibitors or ARBs may increase the risk of hyperkalemia. Concurrent use with digoxin increases the risk of potentially fatal dysrhythmias, and concurrent use with lithium may cause toxic levels of the drug.)	• Teach the patient the signs and symptoms of hypokalemia or hyperkalemia, which should be reported immediately to the health care provider. • Teach the patient to follow recommended dietary intake of high- or low-potassium foods as appropriate to the type of diuretic taken to avoid hypokalemia or hyperkalemia.
• Observe for signs of hyperglycemia, especially in patients with diabetes. (Thiazide, thiazide-like, and loop diuretics may cause hyperglycemia, especially in patients with diabetes.)	• Instruct the patient with diabetes to report a consistent elevation in blood glucose to the health care provider. • Teach the patient with diabetes to monitor his or her blood glucose levels more frequently until the effects of the diuretic are known.
• Observe for symptoms of gout. (Diuretics may cause hyperuricemia, which may result in goutlike conditions including warmth, pain, tenderness, swelling, and redness around joints; arthritis-like symptoms; and limited movement in affected joints.)	• Instruct the patient to promptly report signs and symptoms of gout to the health care provider. • Teach the patient who is prone to gout to increase fluid intake and to avoid shellfish, organ meats (e.g., liver, kidneys), alcohol, and high-fructose beverages.
• Observe for sunburning if prolonged sun exposure has occurred. (Many diuretics cause photosensitivity and an increased risk of sunburning.)	• Instruct the patient to wear sunscreen and protective clothing if prolonged sun exposure is anticipated.
• Observe for signs of infection. (Some diuretics may decrease white blood cell counts. Agranulocytosis is a possible adverse effect of diuretic therapy.)	• Instruct the patient to report any flulike symptoms: shortness of breath, fever, sore throat, malaise, joint pain, or profound fatigue.
• **Lifespan:** Assess for the possibility of pregnancy or breast-feeding before beginning the drug. (Some diuretics are pregnancy category D drugs and should not be used during pregnancy.)	• Instruct female patients who may be considering pregnancy, or are pregnant or breast-feeding to notify their provider before starting the drug.
Patient understanding of drug therapy: • Use opportunities during administration of medications and during assessments to provide patient education. (Using time during nursing care helps to optimize and reinforce key teaching areas.)	• The patient, family, or caregiver should be able to state the reason for the drug; appropriate dose and scheduling; what adverse effects to observe for and when to report; and the anticipated length of medication therapy.
Patient self-administration of drug therapy: • When administering the medication, instruct the patient, family, or caregiver in the proper self-administration of the drug (e.g., early in the day to prevent disruption of sleep from nocturia). (Proper administration increases the effectiveness of the drug.)	• The patient, family, or caregiver is able to discuss appropriate dosing and administration needs.

Chapter Review

KEY Concepts

The numbered key concepts provide a succinct summary of the important points from the corresponding numbered section within the chapter. If any of these points are not clear, refer to the numbered section within the chapter for review.

24.1 The kidneys regulate fluid volume, electrolytes, and acid–base balance.

24.2 The three major processes of urine formation are filtration, reabsorption, and secretion. As filtrate travels through the nephron, its composition changes dramatically as a result of the processes of reabsorption and secretion.

24.3 The dosage levels for most medications must be reduced in patients with renal failure. Diuretics may be used to maintain urine output while the cause of the renal impairment is treated.

24.4 Diuretics are drugs that increase urine output, usually by blocking sodium reabsorption. The three primary classes are loop, thiazide, and potassium-sparing diuretics.

24.5 The most efficacious diuretics are the loop or high-ceiling drugs, which block the reabsorption of sodium in the loop of Henle.

24.6 The thiazides act by blocking sodium reabsorption in the distal tubule of the nephron, and are the most widely prescribed class of diuretics.

24.7 Though less effective than the loop diuretics, potassium-sparing diuretics are used in combination with other drugs and help prevent hypokalemia.

24.8 Several less commonly prescribed classes such as the carbonic anhydrase inhibitors and the osmotic diuretics have specific indications in reducing intraocular fluid pressure (acetazolamide) or reversing severe renal hypoperfusion (mannitol).

REVIEW Questions

1. Which of the following actions by the nurse is most important when caring for a patient with renal disease who has an order for furosemide (Lasix)?
   1. Assess urine output and renal laboratory values for signs of nephrotoxicity.
   2. Check the specific gravity of the urine daily.
   3. Eliminate potassium-rich foods from the diet.
   4. Encourage the patient to void every 4 hours.
2. The patient admitted for heart failure has been receiving hydrochlorothiazide (Microzide). Which of the following laboratory levels should the nurse carefully monitor? (Select all that apply.)
   1. Platelet count
   2. White blood cell count
   3. Potassium
   4. Sodium
   5. Uric acid
3. Which of the following clinical manifestations may indicate that the patient taking metolazone (Zaroxolyn) is experiencing hypokalemia?
   1. Hypertension
   2. Polydipsia
   3. Cardiac dysrhythmias
   4. Skin rash
4. The nurse is providing teaching to a patient who has been prescribed furosemide (Lasix). Which of the following should the nurse teach the patient?
   1. Avoid consuming large amounts of kale, cauliflower, or cabbage.
   2. Rise slowly from a lying or sitting position to standing.
   3. Count the pulse for one full minute before taking this medication.
   4. Restrict fluid intake to no more than 1 L per 24-hour period.

5. While planning for a patient's discharge from the hospital, which of the following teaching points would be included for a patient going home with a prescription for chlorothiazide (Diuril)?
   1. Increase fluid and salt intake to make up for the losses caused by the drug.
   2. Increase intake of vitamin-C rich foods such as grapefruit and oranges.
   3. Report muscle cramping or weakness to the health care provider.
   4. Take the drug at night because it may cause drowsiness.

6. A patient with a history of heart failure will be started on spironolactone (Aldactone). Which of the following drug groups should *not* be used, or used with extreme caution in patients taking potassium-sparing diuretics?
   1. Nonsteroidal anti-inflammatory drugs
   2. Corticosteroids
   3. Loop diuretics
   4. Angiotensin-converting enzyme inhibitors or angiotensin-receptor blockers

PATIENT-FOCUSED Case Study

Naomi Saltzman is an 82-year-old with a history of hypertension, and a myocardial infarction resulting in heart failure three years ago, managed by furosemide (Lasix) 20 mg/daily, digoxin (Lanoxin) 0.125 mg/daily, and potassium supplements (KDur) 20 mEq/daily. She has remained active, but relies on a neighbor for transportation to the pharmacy and market. Recently, the neighbor has been out of town for two weeks, and Naomi discovered that she had not calculated the need for medication refills before her neighbor left. She ran out of her KDur, but figured that since it was just a "supplement," it could wait until the neighbor returned.

After taking medical transport services to her provider for her recheck, she is noted to have generalized weakness and fatigue. She has lost 3.6 kg (8 lb) since her last clinic visit 6 weeks ago. Her blood pressure is 104/62 mmHg, her heart rate is 98 beats/min and slightly irregular, her respiratory rate is 20 breaths/min, and her body temperature is 36.2°C (97.2°F). The blood specimen collected showed a serum sodium level of 130 mEq/L and a potassium level of 3.2 mEq/L. Naomi is diagnosed with dehydration and hypokalemia.

1. Discuss fluid and electrolyte imbalances related to the following diuretic therapies:
   a. Loop diuretics.
   b. Thiazide diuretics.
   c. Potassium-sparing diuretics.
   d. Osmotic diuretics.
2. What relationship exists between Naomi's diuretic therapy and hypokalemia?
3. What patient education should the nurse provide Naomi about her medications?

CRITICAL THINKING Questions

1. A 43-year-old man is diagnosed with hypertension following an annual physical examination. The patient is thin and states that he engages in fairly regular exercise, but he describes his job as highly stressful. He also has a positive family history for hypertension and stroke. The health care provider initiates therapy with hydrochlorothiazide (Microzide). The patient asks the nurse, "I have high blood pressure. Why do I need a 'water pill' to help my blood pressure?" How does hydrochlorothiazide reduce blood pressure?
2. A 54-year-old female patient has been treated with chlorothiazide (Diuril) for hypertension. Due to increasing blood pressure, edema, and signs of early heart failure, the provider switches her to a low dose of furosemide (Lasix) and spironolactone (Aldactone). The patient wants to know why she now needs two diuretics and questions the nurse about whether this is a safe thing to do. How should the nurse respond?

Visit www.pearsonhighered.com/nursingresources for answers and rationales for all activities.

REFERENCES

Berry, S. D., Mittleman, M. A., Zhang, Y., Solomon, D. H., Lipsitz, L. A., Mostofsky, E., . . . Kiel, D. P. (2012). New loop diuretic prescriptions may be an acute risk factor for falls in nursing homes. *Pharmacoepidemiology and Drug Safety, 21*, 560–563. doi:10.1002/pds.3256

Butt, D. A., Mamdani, M., Austin, P. C., Tu, K., Gomes, T., & Glazier, R. H. (2013). The risk of falls on initiation of antihypertensive drugs in the elderly. *Osteoporosis International, 24*, 2649–2657. doi:10.1007/s00198-013-2369-7

de Groot, M. H., van Campen, J. P., Moek, M. A., Tulner, L. R., Beijnen, J. H., & Lamoth, C. J. (2013). The effects of fall-risk-increasing drugs on postural control: A literature review. *Drugs & Aging, 30*, 901–920. doi:10.1007/s40266-013-0113-9

Herdman, T. H., and Kamitsuru, S. (2014). *NANDA International nursing diagnoses: Definitions and classification, 2015–2017*. Oxford, United Kingdom: Wiley-Blackwell.

Wang, C. H., Fang, C. C., Chen, N. C., Liu, S. S., Yu, P. H., Wu, T. Y., . . . Chen, S. C. (2012). Cranberry-containing products for prevention of urinary tract infections in susceptible populations: A systematic review and meta-analysis of randomized controlled trials. *Archives of Internal Medicine, 172*, 988–996. doi:10.1001/archinternmed.2012.3004

Williams, T., Szekendi, M., & Thomas, S. (2014). An analysis of patient falls and fall prevention programs across academic medical centers. *Journal of Nursing Care Quality, 29*, 19–29. doi:10.1097/NCQ.0b013e3182a0cd19

Zang, G. (2013). Antihypertensive drugs and the risk of fall injuries: A systematic review and meta-analysis. *The Journal of International Medical Research, 41*, 1408–1417. doi:10.1177/0300060513497562

SELECTED BIBLIOGRAPHY

Armstrong, A. (2013). Practical tips for prescribing in renal impairment. *Nurse Prescribing, 11*, 222–227. doi:10.12968/npre.2013.11.5.222

Cox, Z. L., & Lenihan, D. J. (2014). Loop diuretic resistance in heart failure: Resistance etiology-based strategies to restoring diuretic efficacy. *Journal of Cardiac Failure 20*, 611–622. doi:10.1016/j.cardfail.2014.05.007

National Center for Complementary and Integrative Health. (2012). *Cranberry*. Retrieved from http://nccam.nih.gov/health/cranberry

National Institute of Diabetes and Digestive and Kidney Diseases. (n.d.). *Kidney disease statistics for the United States*. Retrieved from http://www.niddk.nih.gov/health-information/health-statistics/Pages/kidney-disease-statistics-united-states.aspx

National Kidney Foundation (n.d.). *Herbal supplements and kidney disease*. Retrieved from http://www.kidney.org/atoz/content/herbalsupp.cfm

Piepoli, M., Binno, S., Villani, G. Q., & Cabassi, A. (2014). Management of oral chronic pharmacotherapy in patients hospitalized for acute decompensated heart failure. *International Journal of Cardiology, 176*(2), 321–326. doi:10.1016/j.ijcard.2014.07.085

Reilly, R. F., & Jackson, E. K. (2012). Diuretics. In L. L. Brunton, B. A. Chabner, & B. C. Knollman (Eds.), *Goodman and Gilman's the pharmacological basis of therapeutics* (12th ed., pp. 671–720). New York, NY: McGraw-Hill.

Rich, M. W. (2012). Pharmacotherapy of heart failure in the elderly: Adverse events. *Heart Failure Reviews, 17*(4–5), 589–595. doi:10.1007/s10741-011-9263-1

Tamargo, J., Segura, J., & Ruilope, L. M. (2014). Diuretics in the treatment of hypertension. Part 1: Thiazide and thiazide-like diuretics. *Expert Opinion on Pharmacotherapy, 15*, 527–547. doi:10.1517/14656566.2014.879118

Tamargo, J., Segura, J., & Ruilope, L. M. (2014). Diuretics in the treatment of hypertension. Part 2: Loop diuretics and potassium-sparing agents. *Expert Opinion on Pharmacotherapy, 15*, 605–621. doi:10.1517/14656566.2014.879117

von Lueder, T. G., Atar, D., & Krum, H. (2013). Diuretic use in heart failure and outcomes. *Clinical Pharmacology & Therapeutics, 94*, 490–498. doi:10.1038/clpt.2013.140

Chapter 25

Drugs for Fluid Balance, Electrolyte, and Acid–Base Disorders

Drugs at a Glance

- **FLUID REPLACEMENT AGENTS** page 360
  - **Crystalloids and Colloids** page 360
    - *dextran 40 (Gentran 40, LMD, others)* page 362
- **ELECTROLYTES** page 362
  - *sodium chloride (NaCl)* page 365
  - *potassium chloride (KCL)* page 366
- **ACID–BASE AGENTS** page 366
  - *sodium bicarbonate* page 370

Learning Outcomes

After reading this chapter, the student should be able to:

1. Describe conditions for which intravenous fluid therapy may be indicated.
2. Explain how changes in the osmolality or tonicity of a fluid can cause water to move between fluid compartments.
3. Compare and contrast the use of crystalloids and colloids in intravenous therapy.
4. Explain the importance of electrolyte balance in the body.
5. Explain the pharmacotherapy of sodium and potassium imbalances.
6. Discuss common causes of alkalosis and acidosis and the medications used to treat these conditions.
7. Describe the nurse's role in the pharmacologic management of fluid balance, electrolyte, and acid–base disorders.
8. For each of the classes listed in Drugs at a Glance, know representative drugs, and explain the mechanism of drug action, primary actions, and important adverse effects.
9. Use the nursing process to care for patients who are receiving pharmacotherapy for fluid balance, electrolyte, and acid–base disorders.

(pill icon) indicates a prototype drug, each of which is featured in a Prototype Drug box.

The volume and composition of fluids in the body must be maintained within narrow limits. Excess fluid volume can lead to hypertension (HTN), congestive heart failure (CHF), or peripheral edema, whereas depletion results in dehydration and perhaps shock. Body fluids must also contain specific amounts of essential ions or electrolytes and be maintained at particular pH values. Accumulation of excess acids or bases can change the pH of body fluids and rapidly result in death if left untreated. This chapter examines drugs used to reverse fluid balance, electrolyte, or acid–base disorders.

FLUID BALANCE

Body fluids travel between compartments, which are separated by semipermeable membranes. Control of water balance in the various compartments is essential to homeostasis. Fluid imbalances are frequent indications for pharmacotherapy.

25.1 Body Fluid Compartments

The greatest bulk of body fluid consists of water, which serves as the universal solvent in which most nutrients, electrolytes, and minerals are dissolved. Water alone is responsible for about 60% of the total body weight in a middle-age adult. A newborn may contain 80% water, whereas an older adult may contain only 40%.

In a simple model, water in the body can be located in one of two places, or compartments. The **intracellular fluid (ICF) compartment,** which contains water that is *inside* cells, accounts for about two thirds of the total body water. The remaining one third of body fluid resides *outside* cells in the **extracellular fluid (ECF) compartment.** The ECF compartment is further divided into two parts: fluid in the plasma, or intravascular space, and fluid in the interstitial spaces between cells. The relationship between these fluid compartments is illustrated in Figure 25.1.

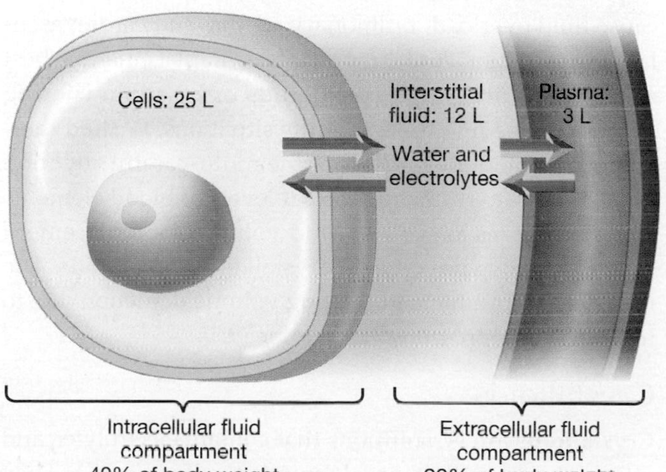

FIGURE 25.1 Major fluid compartments in the body

There is a continuous exchange and mixing of fluids between the various compartments, which are separated by membranes. For example, the plasma membranes of cells separate the ICF from the ECF. The capillary membranes separate plasma from the interstitial fluid. Although water travels freely among the compartments, the movement of large molecules and those with electrical charges is governed by processes of diffusion and active transport. Movement of ions and drugs across membranes is a primary concept of pharmacokinetics (see chapter 4).

25.2 Osmolality, Tonicity, and the Movement of Body Fluids

Osmolality and tonicity are two related terms central to understanding fluid balance in the body. Large changes in the osmolality or tonicity of a body fluid can cause significant shifts in water balance between compartments. Nurses often administer intravenous (IV) fluids to compensate for these changes.

The **osmolality** of a fluid is a measure of the number of dissolved particles, or solutes, in 1 kg (1 L) of water. In most body fluids, three solutes determine the osmolality: sodium, glucose, and urea. Sodium is the greatest contributor to osmolality due to its abundance in most body fluids. The normal osmolality of body fluids ranges from 275 to 295 milliosmols per kilogram (mOsm/kg).

The term **tonicity** is sometimes used interchangeably with osmolality, although they are somewhat different. Tonicity is the ability of a solution to cause a change in water movement across a membrane due to osmotic forces. Whereas osmolality is a laboratory value that can be precisely measured, tonicity is a general term used to describe the *relative* concentration of IV fluids. The tonicity of the plasma is used as the reference point when administering IV solutions: Normal plasma is considered isotonic. Solutions that have the same concentration of solutes as plasma are called *isotonic*. *Hypertonic* solutions contain a greater concentration of solutes than plasma, whereas *hypotonic* solutions have a lesser concentration of solutes than plasma.

Through **osmosis,** water moves from areas of low solute concentration (low osmolality) to areas of high solute concentration (high osmolality). If a *hypertonic* (hyperosmolar) IV solution is administered, the plasma gains more solutes than the interstitial fluid. Water will move, by osmosis, from the interstitial fluid compartment to the plasma compartment. This type of fluid shift removes water from cells and can result in dehydration. Water will move in the opposite direction, from plasma to interstitial fluid, if a *hypotonic* solution is administered. This type of fluid shift could result in hypotension due to movement of water out of the vascular system. Isotonic solutions produce no net fluid shift when infused. These movements are illustrated in Figure 25.2.

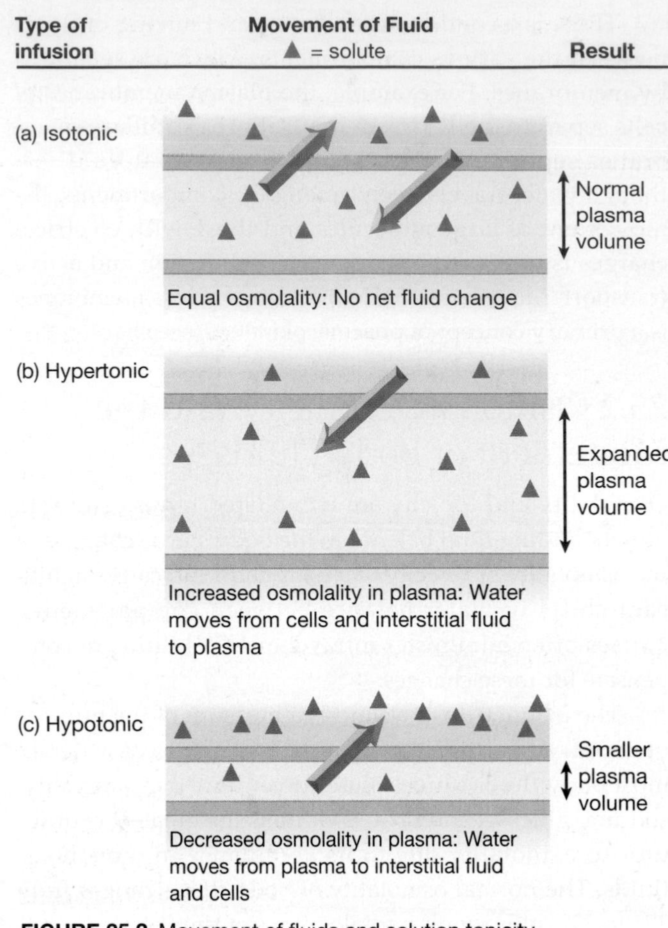

FIGURE 25.2 Movement of fluids and solution tonicity

25.3 Regulation of Fluid Intake and Output

The average adult has a water *intake* of approximately 2,500 mL/day, most of which comes from ingested food and beverages. Water *output* is achieved through the kidneys, lungs, skin, feces, and sweat. To maintain water balance, water intake must equal water output. Net gains or losses of water can be estimated by changes in total body weight.

The most important physiological regulator of fluid intake is the thirst mechanism. The sensation of thirst occurs when osmoreceptors in the hypothalamus sense that the ECF has become hypertonic. Saliva secretion diminishes and the mouth dries, driving the individual to drink liquids. As the ingested water is absorbed, the osmolality of the ECF falls and the thirst center in the hypothalamus is no longer stimulated.

The kidneys are the primary regulators of fluid output. Through activation of the renin–angiotensin–aldosterone system, the hormone aldosterone is secreted by the adrenal cortex. Aldosterone causes the kidneys to retain additional sodium and water in the body, thus increasing the osmolality of the ECF. A second hormone, antidiuretic hormone (ADH), is released by the pituitary gland during periods of high plasma osmolality. ADH acts directly on the distal tubules of the kidney to increase water reabsorption. This increased water in the intravascular space dilutes the plasma, thus lowering its osmolality.

Failure to maintain proper balance between intake and output can result in fluid balance disorders that are indications for pharmacologic intervention. Fluid *deficit* disorders can cause dehydration or shock, which are treated by administering oral or IV fluids. Fluid *excess* disorders are treated with diuretics (see chapter 24). In the treatment of fluid imbalances, the ultimate goal is to diagnose and correct the *cause* of the disorder while administering supporting fluids and medications to stabilize the patient.

FLUID REPLACEMENT AGENTS

Net loss of fluids from the body can result in dehydration and shock. IV fluid therapy is used to maintain blood volume and support blood pressure.

25.4 Intravenous Therapy With Crystalloids and Colloids

When fluid output exceeds fluid intake, volume deficits may result. Shock, dehydration, or electrolyte loss may occur; large deficits are fatal, unless treated. The following are some common reasons for fluid depletion:

- Loss of gastrointestinal (GI) fluids due to vomiting, diarrhea, chronic laxative use, or GI suctioning
- Excessive sweating during hot weather, athletic activity, or prolonged fever
- Severe burns
- Hemorrhage
- Excessive diuresis due to diuretic therapy or uncontrolled diabetic ketoacidosis.

The immediate goal in treating a volume deficit disorder is to replace the depleted fluid. Replacement of depleted fluids should always be conducted in a controlled, stepwise manner because infusing fluids too rapidly can cause fluid overload, pulmonary edema, and cardiovascular stress. In nonacute circumstances, replacement is best achieved by drinking more liquids or by administering fluids via a feeding tube. In acute situations, IV fluid therapy is indicated. Regardless of the route, careful attention must be paid to restoring normal levels of blood elements and electrolytes as well as fluid volume. IV replacement fluids are of two basic types: crystalloids and colloids. The use of blood products in treating volume depletion due to hemorrhage is presented in chapter 29.

Crystalloids

Crystalloids are IV solutions that contain electrolytes and other substances that closely mimic the body's ECF. They are used to replace depleted fluids and to promote urine output. Crystalloid solutions are capable of quickly diffusing

Table 25.1 Selected Crystalloid IV Solutions

Drug	Tonicity
Normal saline (0.9% NaCl)	Isotonic
Hypertonic saline (3% NaCl)	Hypertonic
Hypotonic saline (0.45% NaCl)	Hypotonic
Lactated Ringer's	Isotonic
Plasma-Lyte 148	Isotonic
Plasma-Lyte 56	Hypotonic
DEXTROSE SOLUTIONS	
5% dextrose in water (D_5W)	Isotonic*
5% dextrose in normal saline	Hypertonic
5% dextrose in 0.2% normal saline	Isotonic
5% dextrose in lactated Ringer's	Hypertonic
5% dextrose in Plasma-Lyte 56	Hypertonic

Note: *Because dextrose is metabolized quickly, the solution is sometimes considered hypotonic.

across membranes, thus leaving the plasma and entering the interstitial fluid and ICF. An estimated two thirds of infused crystalloids will distribute in the interstitial space. Isotonic, hypotonic, and hypertonic solutions are available. Sodium is the most common crystalloid added to solutions. Some crystalloids contain dextrose, a form of glucose, commonly in concentrations of 2.5%, 5%, or 10%. Dextrose is added to provide nutritional value: 1 L of 5% dextrose supplies 170 calories. In addition, water is formed during the metabolism of dextrose, enhancing the rehydration of the patient. When dextrose is infused, it is metabolized, and the solution becomes hypotonic. Selected crystalloids are listed in Table 25.1.

Infusion of crystalloids will increase total fluid volume in the body, but the compartment that is most expanded depends on the solute (sodium) concentration of the fluid administered. *Isotonic* crystalloids can expand the circulating intravascular (plasma) fluid volume without causing major fluid shifts between compartments. They are primarily used for hydration and to expand ECF volume. Isotonic crystalloids such as normal saline (NS) are often used to treat fluid loss due to vomiting, diarrhea, or surgical procedures, especially when the blood pressure is low. Because isotonic crystalloids can rapidly expand circulating blood volume, care must be taken not to cause fluid overload in the patient.

Infusion of *hypertonic* crystalloids expands plasma volume by drawing water away from the cells and tissues. These agents are used to relieve cellular edema, especially cerebral edema. When patients are dehydrated and have hypertonic plasma, a solution that is initially hypertonic may be infused, such as D_5 0.45% NS, that matches the tonicity of the plasma. This allows the fluid to enter the vascular compartment without causing a net fluid loss or gain in the cells. As the dextrose is subsequently metabolized, the solution becomes hypotonic. This hypotonic solution then causes water to shift into the intracellular space, relieving the dehydration within the cells. A solution of 3% NS is hypertonic and usually reserved for treating severe hyponatremia. Overtreatment with hypertonic crystalloids such as 3% NS can lead to excessive expansion of the intravascular (plasma) compartment, fluid overload, and hypertension.

Hypotonic crystalloids will cause water to move out of the plasma to the tissues and cells in the *intracellular* compartment; thus, these solutions are not considered efficient plasma volume expanders. Hypotonic crystalloids are indicated for patients with hypernatremia and cellular dehydration. Care must be taken not to cause depletion of the intravascular compartment (hypotension) or too much expansion of the intracellular compartment (peripheral edema). Patients who are dehydrated with *low* blood pressure should be given NS; patients who are dehydrated with *normal* blood pressure should be given a hypotonic solution.

Colloids

Colloids are proteins, starches, or other large molecules that remain in the blood for a long time because they are too large to easily cross the capillary membranes. While circulating, they have the same effect as hypertonic solutions, drawing water molecules from the cells and tissues into the plasma through their ability to increase plasma osmolality and osmotic pressure. Sometimes called *plasma volume expanders*, these solutions are particularly important in treating hypovolemic shock due to burns, hemorrhage, or surgery.

The most commonly used colloid is normal serum albumin, which is featured as a prototype drug for shock in chapter 29. Several colloid products contain dextran, a synthetic polysaccharide. Dextran infusions can double the plasma volume within a few minutes, although its effects last only about 12 hours. Plasma protein fraction is a natural volume expander that contains 83% albumin and 17% plasma globulins. Plasma protein fraction and albumin are also indicated in patients with hypoproteinemia. Hetastarch is a synthetic colloid with properties similar to those of 5% albumin, but with an extended duration of action. Selected colloid solutions are listed in Table 25.2.

Table 25.2 Selected Colloid Solutions (Plasma Volume Expanders)

Drug	Tonicity
5% albumin	Isotonic
Dextran 40 in normal saline	Isotonic
Dextran 40 in D_5W	Isotonic
Dextran 70 in normal saline	Isotonic
Hetastarch 6% in normal saline	Isotonic
Plasma protein fraction	Isotonic

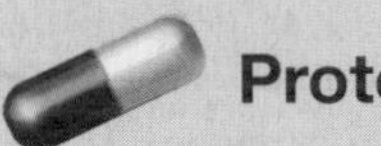

Prototype Drug | Dextran 40 *(Gentran 40, LMD others)*

Therapeutic Class: Plasma volume expander **Pharmacologic Class:** Colloid

Actions and Uses

Dextran 40 is a polysaccharide that is too large to pass through capillary walls. It is similar to dextran 70, except dextran 40 has a lower molecular weight. Dextran 40 acts by raising the osmotic pressure of the blood, thereby causing fluid to move from the interstitial spaces of the tissues to the intravascular space (blood). Given as an IV infusion, it has the capability of expanding plasma volume within minutes after administration. Cardiovascular responses include increased blood pressure, increased cardiac output, and improved venous return to the heart. Dextran 40 is excreted rapidly by the kidneys. Indications include fluid replacement for patients experiencing hypovolemic shock due to hemorrhage, surgery, or severe burns. When given for acute shock, it is infused as rapidly as possible until blood volume is restored.

Dextran 40 also reduces platelet adhesiveness and improves blood flow through its ability to reduce blood viscosity. These properties have led to its use in preventing deep vein thromboses and postoperative pulmonary emboli.

Administration Alerts

- Emergency administration may be given 1.2 to 2.4 g/min.
- Nonemergency administration should be infused no faster than 240 mg/min.
- Discard unused portions once opened because dextran contains no preservatives.
- Pregnancy category C.

PHARMACOKINETICS

Onset	Peak	Duration
Several minutes	Unknown	12–24 h

Adverse Effects

Vital signs should be monitored continuously during dextran 40 infusions to prevent hypertension caused by plasma volume expansion. Signs of fluid overload include tachycardia, peripheral edema, distended neck veins, dyspnea, or cough. A small percentage of patients are allergic to dextran 40, including the possibility of anaphylaxis. The drug should be discontinued immediately if signs of hypersensitivity are suspected.

Contraindications: Dextran 40 is contraindicated in patients with renal failure or severe dehydration. Other contraindications include severe CHF and hypervolemic disorders.

Interactions

Drug–Drug: There are no clinically significant interactions.

Lab Tests: Dextran 40 may prolong bleeding time.

Herbal/Food: Unknown.

Treatment of Overdose: For patients with normal renal function, discontinuation of the infusion will result in reduction of adverse effects. Patients with renal impairment may benefit from the administration of an osmotic diuretic.

ELECTROLYTES

Electrolytes are small charged molecules essential to homeostasis. Too little or too much of an electrolyte can result in serious complications and must be quickly corrected. Table 25.3 describes electrolytes that are important to human physiology.

Table 25.3 Electrolytes Important to Human Physiology

Compound	Formula	Cation	Anion
Calcium chloride	$CaCl_2$	Ca^{2+}	$2Cl^-$
Disodium phosphate	Na_2HPO_4	$2Na^+$	HPO_4^{2-}
Potassium chloride	KCl	K^+	Cl^-
Sodium bicarbonate	$NaHCO_3$	Na^+	HPO_3^-
Sodium chloride	$NaCl$	Na^+	Cl^-
Sodium sulfate	Na_2SO_4	$2Na^+$	SO_4^{2-}

25.5 Physiological Role of Electrolytes

Minerals are inorganic substances needed in very small amounts to maintain homeostasis. Minerals are held together by ionic bonds and dissociate, or ionize, when placed in water. The resulting ions have positive or negative charges and are able to conduct electricity, hence the name **electrolyte.** Positively charged electrolytes are called **cations;** those with a negative charge are **anions.** Electrolyte levels are measured in units of milliequivalents per liter (mEq/L).

Electrolytes are essential to many body functions, including nerve conduction, membrane permeability, muscle contraction, water balance, and bone growth and remodeling. Levels of electrolytes in body fluids are maintained within very narrow ranges, primarily by the kidneys and GI tract. As electrolytes are lost due to normal excretory functions, they must be replaced by adequate intake;

Table 25.4 Electrolyte Imbalances

Ion	Condition	Abnormal Serum Value (mEq/L)	Supportive Treatment*
Calcium	Hypercalcemia	Greater than 11	Hypotonic fluids or calcitonin
	Hypocalcemia	Less than 4	Calcium supplements or vitamin D
Chloride	Hyperchloremia	Greater than 112	Hypotonic fluid
	Hypochloremia	Less than 95	Hypertonic salt solution
Magnesium	Hypermagnesemia	Greater than 4	Hypotonic fluid
	Hypomagnesemia	Less than 0.8	Magnesium supplements
Phosphate	Hyperphosphatemia	Greater than 6	Dietary phosphate restriction
	Hypophosphatemia	Less than 1	Phosphate supplements
Potassium	Hyperkalemia	Greater than 5	Hypotonic fluid, buffers, or dietary potassium restriction
	Hypokalemia	Less than 3.5	Potassium supplements
Sodium	Hypernatremia	Greater than 145	Hypotonic fluid or dietary sodium restriction
	Hyponatremia	Less than 135	Hypertonic salt solution or sodium supplement

Note: *For all electrolyte imbalances, the primary therapeutic goal is to identify and correct the *cause* of the imbalance.

otherwise, electrolyte imbalances will result. Although imbalances can occur with any ion, Na^+, K^+, and Ca^{2+} are of greatest importance. The major body electrolyte imbalance states and their treatments are listed in Table 25.4. Calcium, phosphorous, and magnesium imbalances are discussed in chapter 43; the role of calcium in bone homeostasis is presented in chapter 48.

An electrolyte imbalance is a sign of an underlying medical condition that needs attention. Imbalances are associated with a large number of disorders, with renal impairment being the most common cause. In some cases, drug therapy itself can cause the electrolyte imbalance. For example, aggressive therapy with loop diuretics such as furosemide (Lasix) can rapidly deplete the body of sodium and potassium. The therapeutic goal is to quickly correct the electrolyte imbalance while the underlying condition is being diagnosed and treated. Treatments for electrolyte imbalances depend on the severity of the condition and range from simple adjustments in dietary intake to rapid electrolyte infusions. Serum electrolyte levels must be carefully monitored during therapy to prevent imbalances in the *opposite* direction; levels can change rapidly from hypoconcentrations to hyper-concentrations.

25.6 Pharmacotherapy of Sodium Imbalances

Sodium ion (Na^+) is the most abundant cation in extracellular fluid. Because of sodium's central roles in neuromuscular physiology, acid–base balance, and overall fluid distribution, sodium imbalances can have serious consequences. Although definite sodium monitors or sensors have yet to be discovered in the body, the regulation of sodium balance is well understood.

Sodium balance and water balance are intimately connected. As Na^+ levels increase in a body fluid, solute particles accumulate, and the osmolality increases. Water will move toward this area of relatively high osmolality. In simplest terms, water travels toward or with Na^+. The physiological consequences of this relationship cannot be overstated: As the Na^+ and water content of plasma increases, so does blood volume and blood pressure. Thus, Na^+ movement provides an important link between water retention, blood volume, and blood pressure.

In healthy individuals, the kidney regulates sodium intake to be equal to sodium output. High levels of aldosterone secreted by the adrenal cortex promote Na^+ and water retention by the kidneys as well as K^+ excretion in the urine. Inhibition of aldosterone promotes sodium and water excretion. When a patient ingests high amounts of sodium, aldosterone secretion decreases, thus allowing excess Na^+ to enter the urine. This relationship is illustrated in Figure 25.3.

Hypernatremia

Sodium excess, or **hypernatremia,** occurs when the serum sodium level rises above 145 mEq/L. The most common cause of hypernatremia is decreased Na^+ excretion due to kidney disease. Hypernatremia may also be caused by excessive intake of sodium, either through dietary consumption or by overtreatment with IV fluids containing sodium chloride or sodium bicarbonate. Another cause of hypernatremia is high net water losses, such as occur from inadequate water intake, watery diarrhea, fever, or burns. High doses of corticosteroids or estrogens also promote Na^+ retention.

A high serum sodium level increases the osmolality of the plasma, drawing fluid from interstitial spaces and cells, thus causing cellular dehydration. Manifestations of hypernatremia include thirst, fatigue, weakness, muscle twitching, convulsions, altered mental status, and a decreased level of consciousness. For minor hypernatremia, a low-salt diet may be effective in returning serum sodium to normal levels. In patients with acute hypernatremia, however, the treatment goal is to rapidly return the osmolality of the

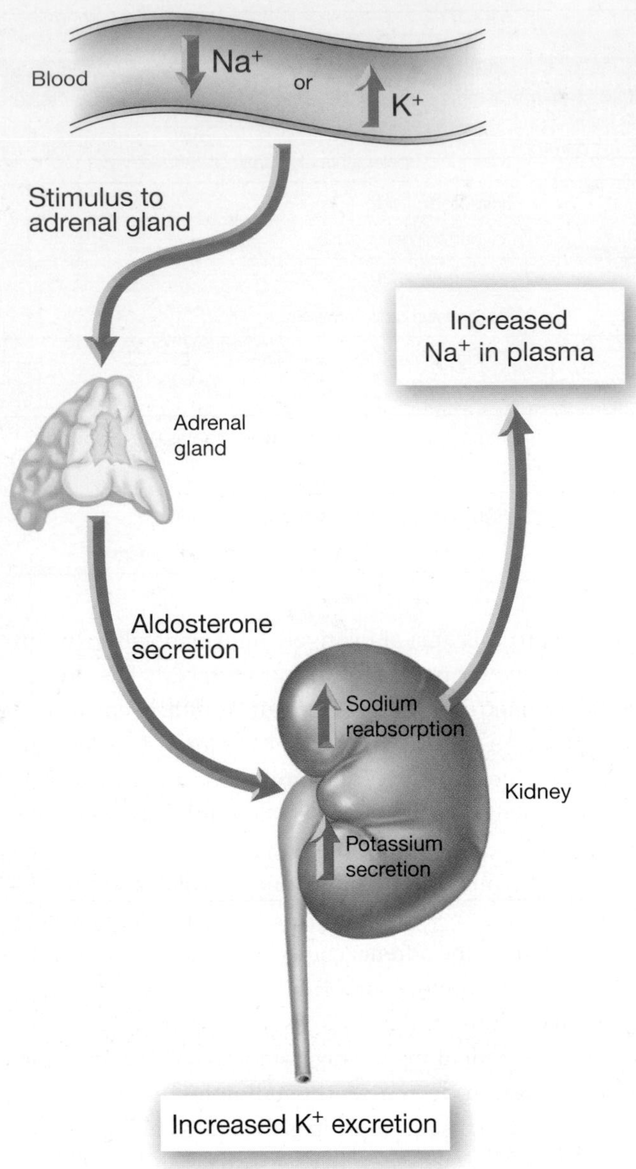

FIGURE 25.3 Renal regulation of sodium and potassium balance

plasma to normal. If the patient is hypovolemic, infusing hypotonic fluids such as 5% dextrose or 0.45% NaCl will increase plasma volume while at the same time reducing plasma osmolality. If the patient is hypervolemic, diuretics may be used to remove Na^+ and fluid from the body.

Hyponatremia

Sodium deficiency, or **hyponatremia,** is a serum sodium level less than 135 mEq/L. Hyponatremia may occur through *excessive dilution* of the plasma, caused by excessive ADH secretion or administration of hypotonic IV solutions. Hyponatremia may also result from *increased sodium loss* due to disorders of the skin, GI tract, or kidneys. Significant loss of sodium by the skin may occur in burn patients and in those experiencing excessive sweating or prolonged fever. GI sodium losses may occur from vomiting, diarrhea, or GI suctioning, and renal Na^+ loss may occur with diuretic use and in certain advanced kidney disorders. Early symptoms of hyponatremia include nausea, vomiting, anorexia, and abdominal cramping. Later signs include altered neurologic function such as confusion, lethargy, convulsions, coma, and muscle twitching or tremors.

Hyponatremia caused by excessive dilution is treated with loop diuretics (see chapter 24). These drugs will cause an isotonic diuresis, thus removing the fluid overload that caused the hyponatremia. Hyponatremia caused by Na^+ loss may be treated with oral or parenteral NaCl or with IV fluids containing salt, such as NS or lactated Ringer's. Tolvaptan (Samsca) is a newer drug approved to quickly raise serum sodium levels in patients experiencing symptoms of hyponatremia. Tolvaptan is a vasopressin (antidiuretic hormone) antagonist that enhances water excretion. As the amount of water in the blood is reduced, the serum sodium concentration increases. Therapy with the drug should only be conducted in a hospital where serum sodium levels can be monitored closely. Treatment is limited to 30 days due to the risk for liver injury.

25.7 Pharmacotherapy of Potassium Imbalances

Potassium ion (K^+), the most abundant intracellular cation, serves important roles in regulating intracellular osmolality and in maintaining acid–base balance. Potassium levels must be carefully balanced between adequate dietary intake and renal excretion. Like Na^+ excretion, K^+ excretion is influenced by the actions of aldosterone on the kidney. In fact, the renal excretion of Na^+ and K^+ ions is closely linked—for every sodium ion that is *reabsorbed,* one potassium ion is *secreted* into the renal tubules. Serum potassium levels must be maintained within narrow limits. Both hyper- and hypokalemia are associated with fatal dysrhythmias and serious neuromuscular disorders.

Hyperkalemia

Hyperkalemia is a serum potassium level greater than 5 mEq/L, which may be caused by high consumption of potassium-rich foods or dietary supplements, particularly when patients are taking potassium-sparing diuretics such as spironolactone (see chapter 24). Excess K^+ may also accumulate when renal excretion is diminished due to kidney pathology. The most serious consequences of hyperkalemia are related to cardiac function: dysrhythmias and heart block. Other symptoms are muscle twitching, fatigue, paresthesias, dyspnea, cramping, and diarrhea.

In mild cases of hyperkalemia, K^+ levels may be returned to normal by restricting primary dietary sources of potassium such as bananas, citrus and dried fruits, peanut butter, broccoli, and green leafy vegetables. If the patient is taking a potassium-sparing diuretic, the dose must be lowered, or a thiazide or loop diuretic must be substituted. In severe cases, serum K^+ levels may be temporarily lowered

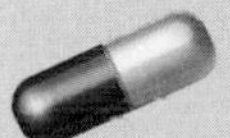

Prototype Drug | Sodium Chloride *(NaCl)*

Therapeutic Class: Drug for hyponatremia **Pharmacologic Class:** Electrolyte, sodium supplement

Actions and Uses

Sodium chloride is administered for hyponatremia when serum levels fall below 130 mEq/L. Normal saline consists of 0.9% NaCl, and it is used to treat mild hyponatremia. When serum sodium falls below 115 mEq/L, a highly concentrated 3% NaCl solution may be infused. Other concentrations include 0.45% and 0.22%, and both hypotonic and isotonic solutions are available. For less severe hyponatremia, 1 g tablets are available by the oral (PO) route.

Ophthalmic solutions of NaCl may be used to treat corneal edema, and an over-the-counter (OTC) nasal spray is available to relieve dry, inflamed nasal membranes. In conjunction with oxytocin, 20% NaCl may be used as an abortifacient late in pregnancy when instilled into the amniotic sac.

Administration Alerts

- Pregnancy category C.

Pharmacokinetics

Because sodium ion is a natural electrolyte, it is not possible to obtain accurate pharmacokinetic values.

Adverse Effects

Patients receiving NaCl infusions must be monitored frequently to prevent symptoms of hypernatremia, which include lethargy, confusion, muscle tremor or rigidity, hypotension, and restlessness. Because some of these symptoms are also common to hyponatremia, periodic laboratory assessments must be taken to be certain that sodium values lie within the normal range. When infusing 3% NaCl solutions, nurses should continuously check for signs of pulmonary edema.

Contraindications: This drug should not be administered to patients with hypernatremia, heart failure, or impaired renal function.

Interactions

Drug–Drug: There are no clinically significant drug interactions.

Lab Tests: NaCl increases the serum sodium level.

Herbal/Food: Unknown.

Treatment of Overdose: If fluid accumulation occurs due to excess sodium, diuretics may be administered to reduce pulmonary or peripheral edema.

Community-Oriented Practice

MAINTAINING FLUID BALANCE DURING EXERCISE

Hyponatremia from excessive fluid intake has been noted as a growing problem in athletes, particularly novice athletes who may have heard that they need to "keep drinking" to maintain hydration. Many sports drinks contain some electrolytes but are also high in fructose or other sugars. This creates a hypertonic solution that may paradoxically cause increased water loss. Unless exercise is extreme or prolonged, athletes, especially children, should be encouraged to drink when thirsty and maintain urine at a color of clear yellow, not dark yellow or colorless. Adequate fluid intake to match thirst will help ensure normal hydration and sodium levels and prevent complications such as exercise-associated hyponatremia.

by administering glucose and regular insulin IV, or aerosolized albuterol which cause K^+ to leave the extracellular fluid and enter cells. Calcium gluconate or calcium chloride may be administered to counteract K^+ toxicity to the heart. Sodium bicarbonate is sometimes infused to correct any acidosis that may be concurrent with the hyperkalemia. Excess K^+ may be eliminated by giving polystyrene sulfonate (Kayexalate) PO or rectally. This agent, which is not absorbed, exchanges Na^+ for K^+ as it travels through the intestine. The onset of action is 1 hour, and the dose may be repeated every 4 hours as needed. This drug is given concurrently with a laxative such as sorbitol to promote rapid evacuation of the potassium.

Hypokalemia

Hypokalemia occurs when the serum potassium level falls below 3.5 mEq/L. Hypokalemia is a frequent adverse effect resulting from high doses of loop diuretics such as furosemide (Lasix). In addition, strenuous muscular activity and severe vomiting or diarrhea can result in significant K^+ loss. Because the body does not have large stores of K^+, adequate daily intake is necessary. Neurons and muscle fibers are most sensitive to K^+ loss, and muscle weakness, lethargy, anorexia, dysrhythmias, and cardiac arrest are possible consequences.

Mild hypokalemia is treated by increasing the dietary intake of potassium-rich foods such as dried fruit, nuts, molasses, avocados, lima beans, and bran cereals. If increasing dietary intake is not possible, a large number of oral potassium supplements are available. Liquid preparations are very effective, although many must be diluted with water or fruit juices prior to administration. Extended release (K-Dur 20, Slow-K, Micro-K) and powders (Klor-Con) are also available. Severe deficiencies require doses of parenteral potassium supplements.

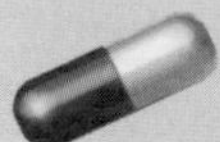

Prototype Drug | Potassium Chloride (KCl)

Therapeutic Class: Drug for hypokalemia **Pharmacologic Class:** Electrolyte, potassium supplement

Actions and Uses

Potassium chloride is the drug of choice for preventing or treating hypokalemia. It is also used to treat mild forms of alkalosis. Oral formulations include tablets, powders, and liquids, usually heavily flavored due to the unpleasant taste of the drug. Because potassium supplements can cause peptic ulcers, the drug should be diluted with plenty of water. When given IV, potassium must be administered slowly, since bolus injections can overload the heart and cause cardiac arrest. Because pharmacotherapy with loop or thiazide diuretics is the most common cause of K^+ depletion, patients taking these drugs are usually prescribed oral potassium supplements to prevent hypokalemia.

Administration Alerts

- Always give oral medication while the patient is upright to prevent esophagitis.
- Do not crush tablets or allow the patient to chew tablets.
- Dilute liquid forms before giving PO or through a nasogastric tube.
- Never administer IV push or in concentrated amounts, and do not exceed an IV rate of 10 mEq/h.
- Be extremely careful to avoid extravasation and infiltration.
- Pregnancy category A.

Pharmacokinetics

Because potassium ion is a natural electrolyte, it is not possible to obtain accurate pharmacokinetic values.

Adverse Effects

Nausea and vomiting are common, because potassium chloride irritates the GI mucosa when administered PO. The drug may be taken with meals or antacids to lessen gastric distress. When administered IV, phlebitis and venous irritation can occur. The drug should preferably be administered through a larger vessel to minimize this risk. The most serious adverse effects of potassium chloride are related to the possible accumulation of excess K^+. Hyperkalemia may occur if the patient takes potassium supplements concurrently with potassium-sparing diuretics. Because the kidneys perform more than 90% of the body's potassium excretion, reduced renal function can rapidly lead to hyperkalemia, particularly in patients taking potassium supplements.

Contraindications: Potassium chloride is contraindicated in patients with hyperkalemia, chronic renal failure, systemic acidosis, severe dehydration, extensive tissue breakdown as in severe burns, adrenal insufficiency, or the administration of a potassium-sparing diuretic.

Interactions

Drug–Drug: Potassium supplements interact with potassium-sparing diuretics and angiotensin-converting enzyme (ACE) inhibitors to increase the risk for hyperkalemia.

Lab Tests: Potassium chloride increases the serum potassium level.

Herbal/Food: Unknown.

Treatment of Overdose: When overdose is suspected, potassium-sparing diuretics and all foods and medications containing significant amounts of potassium should be withheld. Treatment includes IV administration of 50% dextrose solution containing 10–20 units of regular insulin. Sodium bicarbonate may be infused to correct acidosis. Polystyrene sulfonate may be administered to enhance potassium elimination.

☑ Check Your Understanding 25.1

What are the two most common causes of electrolyte imbalances? *Visit www.pearsonhighered.com/nursingresources for the answer.*

ACID–BASE IMBALANCE

Acidosis (excess acid) and alkalosis (excess base) are not diseases but are symptoms of an underlying disorder. Acidic and basic agents may be administered to rapidly correct pH imbalances in body fluids, supporting the patient's vital functions while the underlying disease is being treated. The correction of acid–base imbalance is illustrated in Figure 25.4.

25.8 Buffers and the Maintenance of Body pH

The degree of acidity or alkalinity of a solution is measured by its **pH.** A pH of 7.0 is defined as neutral, above 7.0 as basic or alkaline, and below 7.0 as acidic. To maintain homeostasis, the pH of plasma and most body fluids must be kept within the narrow range of 7.35 to 7.45. Nearly all proteins and enzymes in the body function optimally within this narrow range of pH values. A few enzymes, most notably those in the digestive tract, require pH values outside the 7.35 to 7.45 range to function properly.

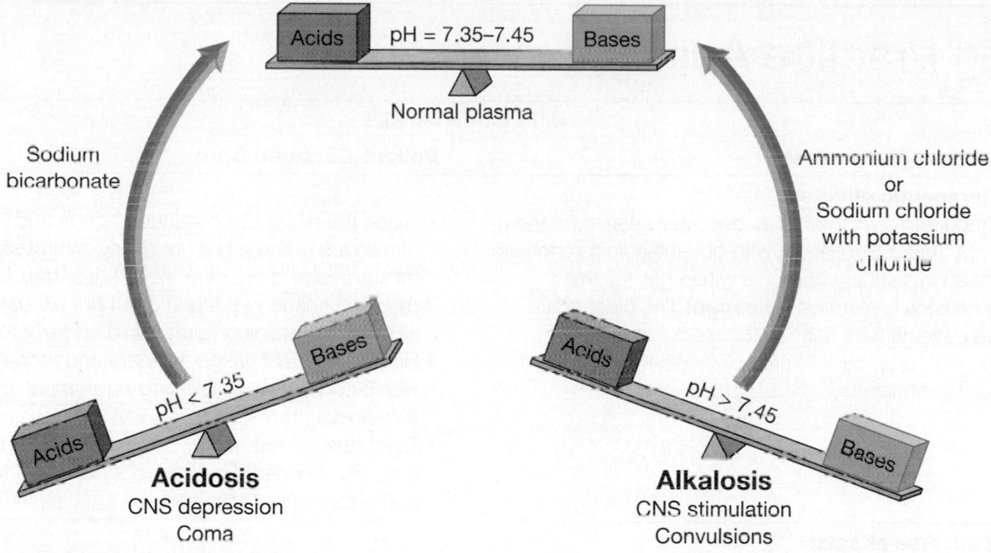

FIGURE 25.4 Acid–base imbalances

Nursing Practice Application

Intravenous Fluid and Electrolyte Replacement Therapy

ASSESSMENT	POTENTIAL NURSING DIAGNOSES*
Baseline assessment prior to administration: • Obtain a complete health history including cardiovascular (including HTN, myocardial infarction [MI]), neurologic (including cerebrovascular accident [CVA] or head injury), burns, endocrine, and hepatic or renal disease. Obtain a drug history including allergies, current prescription and OTC drugs, and herbal preparations. Be alert to possible drug interactions. • Obtain baseline weight and vital signs, level of consciousness (LOC), breath sounds, and urinary output as appropriate. • Evaluate appropriate laboratory findings (e.g., electrolytes, complete blood count [CBC], urine specific gravity and urinalysis, blood urea nitrogen [BUN] and creatinine, total protein and albumin levels, activated partial thromboplastin time (aPTT), antiprothrombin antibodies (aPT), or international normalized ratio (INR), renal and liver function studies).	• *Deficient Fluid Volume* • *Decreased Cardiac Output* • *Fatigue* • *Activity Intolerance* • *Deficient Knowledge* (drug therapy) • *Risk for Falls,* related to hypotension, dizziness associated with adverse effects • *Risk for Injury,* related to hypotension, dizziness associated with adverse effects • *Risk for Deficient Fluid Volume* • *Risk for Excessive Fluid Volume,* related to drug therapy • *Risk for Electrolyte Imbalance* • *Risk for Ineffective Health Management* *NANDA I © 2014
Assessment throughout administration: • Assess for desired therapeutic effects (e.g., electrolyte values return to within normal range, adequate urine output). • Continue monitoring of vital signs, urinary output, and LOC as appropriate. • Assess for and promptly report adverse effects: tachycardia, HTN, dysrhythmias, decreasing LOC, increasing dyspnea, lung congestion, pink tinged frothy sputum, decreased urinary output, muscle weakness or cramping, or allergic reactions.	

continued

Nursing Practice Application *continued*

IMPLEMENTATION	
Interventions and (Rationales)	**Patient-Centered Care**
Ensuring therapeutic effects: • Continue frequent assessments as described earlier for therapeutic effects. Assist the patient with obtaining fluids and with eating as needed. (Urinary output is within normal limits. Electrolyte balance is restored. **Lifespan:** The older adult, infants, and patients who cannot access fluids or eat by themselves, e.g., post-stroke, are at increased risk for fluid and electrolyte imbalance.)	• Teach the patient to continue to consume enough liquids to remain adequately, but not overly, hydrated. Drinking when thirsty, avoiding alcoholic beverages, maintaining a healthy diet, and ensuring adequate but not excessive salt intake will assist in maintaining normal fluid and electrolyte balance. • Have the patient weigh self daily and record weight along with blood pressure (BP) and pulse measurements as appropriate. • Teach the patient, family, or caregiver how to monitor pulse and BP if needed. Ensure proper use and functioning of any home equipment obtained.
Minimizing adverse effects: • Monitor for signs of fluid volume excess or deficit (e.g., increasing BP [excess], decreasing BP [deficit], tachycardia, changes in quality of pulse [bounding or thready]). Monitor for signs of potential electrolyte imbalance including nausea, vomiting, GI cramping, diarrhea, muscle weakness, cramping or twitching, paresthesias, and irritability. Confusion; decreasing LOC; increasing hypotension or HTN, especially if associated with tachycardia; decreased urine output; and seizures are reported immediately. (Many fluid and electrolyte imbalances have similar symptoms. When assessing the patient for adverse effects, consider past history, drug history, and current condition and medications to correlate symptoms to possible causes.)	• Instruct the patient to report changes in muscle strength or function; numbness and tingling in lips, fingers, arms, or legs; palpitations; dizziness; nausea or vomiting; GI cramping; or decreased urination. • Instruct patients with hypokalemia to consume foods high in potassium: fresh fruits such as strawberries and bananas, dried fruits such as apricots and prunes, vegetables and legumes such as tomatoes, beets, and beans, juices such as orange, grapefruit or prune, and fresh meats. Instruct patients with hyperkalemia to avoid the above foods as well as salt substitutes (which often contain potassium salts), and to consult with a health care provider before taking vitamin and mineral supplements or specialized sports beverages. Licorice should be avoided because it causes potassium loss and sodium retention.
• Frequently monitor CBC, electrolytes, aPTT, and aPT or INR levels. (Crystalloid solutions may cause electrolyte imbalances. Colloid solutions may reduce normal blood coagulation. Frequent monitoring of electrolyte levels while on replacement therapy may be needed to ensure therapeutic effects.)	• Instruct the patient on the need to return periodically for laboratory work.
• Continue to monitor vital signs. Take BP lying, sitting, and standing to detect orthostatic hypotension. **Lifespan:** Be cautious with older adults who are at increased risk for hypotension. (Dehydration and electrolyte imbalances may cause dizziness and hypotension. Orthostatic hypotension may increase the risk of injury.)	• **Safety:** Teach the patient to rise from lying or sitting to standing slowly to avoid dizziness or falls. If dizziness occurs, the patient should sit or lie down and not attempt to stand or walk until the sensation passes. • **Safety:** Instruct the patient to call for assistance prior to getting out of bed or attempting to walk alone, and to avoid driving or other activities requiring mental alertness or physical coordination if dizziness or lightheadedness occurs.
• Weigh the patient daily and report a weight gain or loss of 1 kg (2 lb) or more in a 24-hour period. (Daily weight is an accurate measure of fluid status and takes into account intake, output, and insensible losses. Weight gain or edema may signal excessive fluid volume or electrolyte imbalances.)	• Have the patient weigh self daily, ideally at the same time of day, and record weight along with BP and pulse measurements. Have the patient report significant weight loss or gain. • Teach the patient that excessive heat conditions contribute to excessive sweating and fluid and electrolyte loss, and extra caution is warranted in these conditions.
• **Safety:** Closely monitor for signs and symptoms of allergy if colloids are used. (Colloids may cause allergic and anaphylactic reactions.)	• Instruct the patient to immediately report dyspnea, itching, feelings of throat tightness, palpitations, chest pain or tightening, or headache.
• **Safety:** Closely monitor IV sites when infusing potassium or ammonium. Double-check doses with another nurse before giving. (Potassium and ammonium are irritating to the vessel and phlebitis may result. Potassium is a "high-alert" medication and double-checking doses before administering prevents medication errors.)	• Instruct the patient to report any irritation, pain, redness, or swelling at the IV site or in the arm where the drug is infusing.

Nursing Practice Application *continued*

IMPLEMENTATION

Interventions and (Rationales)	Patient-Centered Care
Patient understanding of drug therapy:	
• Use opportunities during administration of medications and during assessments to provide patient education. (Using time during nursing care helps to optimize and reinforce supportive drug treatment and care.)	• The patient, family, or caregiver should be able to state the reason for the drug; appropriate dose and scheduling; what adverse effects to observe for and when to report; and the anticipated length of medication therapy.
Patient self-administration of drug therapy:	
• When administering the medication, instruct the patient, family, or caregiver in proper self-administration of the drug (e.g., early in the day to prevent disruption of sleep from nocturia). (Proper administration will increase the effectiveness of the drug.)	• The patient, family, or caregiver are able to discuss appropriate dosing and administration needs. • **Lifespan:** Assess swallowing ability before the patient takes potassium chloride or ammonium chloride; they may cause mouth, esophageal, or gastric irritation. • Teach the patient that liquid forms should always be diluted with water or fruit juice and tablets swallowed whole.

See Tables 25.1, 25.2, and 25.4 for a list of the drugs to which these nursing actions apply.

The body generates significant amounts of acid during normal metabolic processes. Without sophisticated means of neutralizing these metabolic acids, the overall pH of body fluids would quickly fall below the normal range. **Buffers** are chemicals that help maintain normal body pH by neutralizing strong acids and bases. The two primary buffers in the body are bicarbonate ions and phosphate ions.

The body uses two mechanisms to remove acid. The carbon dioxide (CO_2) produced during body metabolism is an acid efficiently removed by the lungs during exhalation. The kidneys remove excess acid in the form of hydrogen ion (H^+) by excreting it in the urine. If retained in the body, CO_2 and/or H^+ would lower body pH. Thus, the lungs and the kidneys collaborate in the removal of acids to maintain normal acid–base balance.

25.9 Pharmacotherapy of Acidosis

Acidosis occurs when the pH of the plasma falls below 7.35, which is confirmed by measuring arterial pH, partial pressure of carbon dioxide (P_{CO_2}), and plasma bicarbonate levels. Diagnosis must differentiate between respiratory etiology and metabolic (renal) etiology. Occasionally, the cause has mixed respiratory and metabolic components. The most profound symptoms of acidosis affect the central nervous system (CNS) and include lethargy, confusion, and CNS depression leading to coma. A deep, rapid respiration rate indicates an attempt by the lungs to rid the body of excess acid. Common causes of acidosis are listed in Table 25.5.

In patients with acidosis, the therapeutic goal is to quickly reverse the level of acids in the blood. The preferred treatment for acute acidosis is to administer infusions of sodium bicarbonate. Bicarbonate ion acts as a base to quickly neutralize acids in the blood and other body fluids. The patient must be carefully monitored during infusions because this drug can "overcorrect" the acidosis, causing blood pH to turn alkaline. Sodium citrate, sodium lactate, and sodium acetate are alternative alkaline agents sometimes used in place of bicarbonate.

25.10 Pharmacotherapy of Alkalosis

Alkalosis develops when the plasma pH rises above 7.45. Like acidosis, alkalosis may have either respiratory or metabolic causes, as shown in Table 25.5. Also like acidosis, the CNS is greatly affected. Symptoms of CNS stimulation occur including nervousness, hyperactive reflexes, and convulsions. In metabolic alkalosis, slow, shallow breathing indicates that the body is attempting to compensate by retaining acid and lowering internal pH. Life-threatening dysrhythmias are the most serious adverse effects of alkalosis.

Table 25.5 Causes of Alkalosis and Acidosis

Acidosis	Alkalosis
RESPIRATORY ORIGINS OF ACIDOSIS	**RESPIRATORY ORIGINS OF ALKALOSIS**
Hypoventilation or shallow breathing	Hyperventilation due to asthma, anxiety, or high altitude
Airway constriction	
Damage to respiratory center in medulla	
METABOLIC ORIGINS OF ACIDOSIS	**METABOLIC ORIGINS OF ALKALOSIS**
Severe diarrhea	Constipation for prolonged periods
Kidney failure	Ingestion of excess sodium bicarbonate
Diabetes mellitus	Diuretics that cause potassium depletion
Excess alcohol ingestion	Severe vomiting
Starvation	

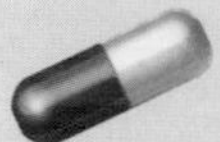

Prototype Drug | Sodium Bicarbonate

Therapeutic Class: Drug to treat acidosis or bicarbonate deficiency
Pharmacologic Class: Electrolyte, sodium and bicarbonate supplement

Actions and Uses

Sodium bicarbonate is a drug of choice for correcting metabolic acidosis. After dissociation, the bicarbonate ion directly raises the pH of body fluids. Sodium bicarbonate may be given orally, if acidosis is mild, or IV in cases of acute disease. IV concentrations range from 4.2% to 8.4%. Although sodium bicarbonate also neutralizes gastric acid, it is not used to treat peptic ulcers due to its tendency to cause uncomfortable gastric distention. The oral preparation of sodium bicarbonate is known as *baking soda*.

Sodium bicarbonate may also be used to alkalinize the urine and speed the excretion of acidic substances. This process is useful in the treatment of overdoses of acidic medications such as aspirin and phenobarbital, and as adjunctive therapy for certain chemotherapeutic drugs such as methotrexate.

Sodium bicarbonate may be used in chronic renal failure to neutralize the metabolic acidosis that occurs when the kidneys cannot excrete hydrogen ion. When IV sodium bicarbonate is given, it causes the urine to become more alkaline. Less acid is reabsorbed in the renal tubules, so more acid and acidic medicine is excreted. This process is known as ion trapping.

Administration Alerts

- Do not add oral preparation to calcium-containing solutions.
- Give oral sodium bicarbonate 2 to 3 hours before or after meals and other medications.
- Pregnancy category C.

PHARMACOKINETICS

Onset	Peak	Duration
15 min PO; immediate IV	2 h PO; unknown IV	1–3 h PO; 8–10 min IV

Adverse Effects

Most of the adverse effects of sodium bicarbonate therapy are the result of metabolic alkalosis caused by receiving *too much* bicarbonate ion. Symptoms may include confusion, irritability, slow respiration rate, and vomiting. Simply discontinuing the sodium bicarbonate infusion often reverses these symptoms; however, potassium chloride or ammonium chloride may be administered to reverse acute alkalosis. During sodium bicarbonate infusions, serum electrolytes should be carefully monitored, because sodium levels may give rise to hypernatremia and fluid retention. In addition, high levels of bicarbonate ion passing through the kidney tubules increase K^+ secretion, and hypokalemia is possible.

Contraindications: Patients who are vomiting or have continuous GI suctioning will lose acid and chloride and may be in a state of metabolic alkalosis; therefore, they should not receive sodium bicarbonate. Because of the sodium content of this drug, it should be used cautiously in patients with cardiac disease and renal impairment. Sodium bicarbonate is contraindicated in patients with hypertension, peptic ulcers, diarrhea, or vomiting.

Interactions

Drug–Drug: Sodium bicarbonate may decrease the absorption of ketoconazole and may decrease elimination of dextroamphetamine, ephedrine, pseudoephedrine, and quinidine. The elimination of lithium, salicylates, and tetracyclines may be increased.

Lab Tests: Urinary and serum pH increase with sodium bicarbonate administration. Urinary urobilinogen levels may increase.

Herbal/Food: Chronic use with milk or calcium supplements may cause milk–alkali syndrome, a condition characterized by serious hypercalcemia and possible kidney failure.

Treatment of Overdose: Overdose results in metabolic alkalosis, which is treated by administering acidic agents (see section 25.10).

Treatment of metabolic alkalosis is directed toward addressing the underlying condition that is causing the excess alkali to be retained. In mild cases, alkalosis may be corrected by administering NaCl concurrently with KCl. This combination increases the renal excretion of bicarbonate ion, which indirectly increases the acidity of the blood.

Patients with renal impairment or who have heart failure may not be able to tolerate the increased water load that follows NaCl infusions. For these acute patients, acidifying agents may be used. Hydrochloric acid and ammonium chloride are two drugs that can quickly lower the pH in patients with severe alkalosis.

Patient Safety: Concentrated Electrolyte Solutions

The student nurse is working with a clinical nurse preceptor and asks why they must wait for the pharmacy to deliver IV medications. "Wouldn't it just be faster to mix them ourselves? The patient in room 220 is supposed to have an IV with potassium and the IV is almost out." How should the nurse respond? *Visit www.pearsonhighered.com/nursingresources for the suggested answer.*

Chapter Review

KEY Concepts

The numbered key concepts provide a succinct summary of the important points from the corresponding numbered section within the chapter. If any of these points are not clear, refer to the numbered section within the chapter for review.

25.1 There is a continuous exchange of fluids across membranes separating the intracellular and extracellular fluid compartments. Large molecules and those that are ionized are less able to cross membranes.

25.2 Osmolality refers to the number of dissolved solutes (usually sodium, glucose, or urea) in a body fluid. Changes in the osmolality of body fluids can cause water to move to different compartments.

25.3 Overall fluid balance is achieved through complex mechanisms that regulate fluid intake and output. The greatest contributor to osmolality is sodium, which is controlled by the hormone aldosterone.

25.4 Intravenous fluid therapy using crystalloids and colloids replaces lost fluids. Crystalloids contain electrolytes and are distributed primarily to the interstitial spaces. Colloids are large molecules that stay in the intravascular space to rapidly expand plasma volume.

25.5 Electrolytes are charged inorganic molecules that are essential to nerve conduction, membrane permeability, water balance, and other critical body functions. Imbalances may lead to serious abnormalities.

25.6 Sodium is essential to maintaining osmolality, water balance, and acid–base balance. Hypernatremia may be corrected with hypotonic IV fluids or diuretics. Hyponatremia may be treated with infusions of sodium chloride. Dilutional hyponatremia is treated with diuretics.

25.7 Potassium is essential for proper nerve and muscle function as well as for maintaining acid–base balance. Hyperkalemia may be treated with glucose and insulin or by administration of polystyrene sulfonate. Hypokalemia is corrected with oral or IV potassium supplements.

25.8 Buffers in the body maintain overall pH within narrow limits. The kidneys and lungs work together to remove excess metabolic acid.

25.9 Pharmacotherapy of acidosis, a plasma pH below 7.35, includes the administration of sodium bicarbonate.

25.10 Pharmacotherapy of alkalosis, a plasma pH above 7.45, includes the administration of sodium chloride with potassium chloride. In acute cases, an acidifying agent such as hydrochloric acid or ammonium chloride may be infused.

REVIEW Questions

1. A patient is receiving intravenous sodium bicarbonate for treatment of metabolic acidosis. During this infusion, how will the nurse monitor for therapeutic effect?
   1. Blood urea nitrogen (BUN)
   2. White blood cell counts
   3. Serum pH
   4. Renal function laboratory values
2. Which of the following nursing interventions is most important when caring for a patient receiving dextran 40 (Gentran 40, LMD)?
   1. Assess the patient for deep venous thrombosis.
   2. Observe for signs of fluid overload.
   3. Encourage fluid intake.
   4. Monitor arterial blood gases.
3. The patient's serum sodium value is 152 mEq/L. Which of the following nursing interventions is most appropriate for this patient? (Select all that apply.)
   1. Assess for inadequate water intake or diarrhea.
   2. Administer a 0.45% NaCl intravenous solution.
   3. Hold all doses of glucocorticoids.
   4. Notify the health care provider.
   5. Have the patient drink as much water as possible.
4. A patient is receiving 5% dextrose in water (D_5W). Which of the following statements is correct?
   1. The solution may cause hypoglycemia in the patient who has diabetes.
   2. The solution may be used to dilute mixed intravenous drugs.
   3. The solution is considered a colloid solution.
   4. The solution is used to provide adequate calories for metabolic needs.
5. A patient will be sent home on diuretic therapy and has a prescription for liquid potassium chloride (KCl). What teaching will the nurse provide before the patient goes home?
   1. Do not dilute the solution with water or juice; drink the solution straight.
   2. Increase the use of salt substitutes; they also contain potassium.
   3. Report any weakness, fatigue, or lethargy immediately.
   4. Take the medication immediately before bed to prevent heartburn.
6. The nurse weighs the patient who is on an infusion of lactated Ringer's postoperatively and finds that there has been a weight gain of 1.5 kg since the previous day. What would be the nurse's next highest priority?
   1. Check with the patient to determine whether there have been any dietary changes in the last few days.
   2. Assess the patient for signs of edema and blood pressure for possible hypertension.
   3. Contact dietary to change the patient's diet to reduced sodium.
   4. Request a diuretic from the patient's provider.

PATIENT-FOCUSED Case Study

Sam Monzoni is a 72-year-old man with a history of heart failure. He is assessed in the emergency department after complaining of weakness and palpitations at work. Sam has been taking furosemide (Lasix) and potassium chloride (KCl) at home. His current ECG reveals atrial fibrillation, and serum electrolyte testing reveals a potassium level of 2.5 mEq/L. The health care provider orders an IV solution of 1,000 mL of lactated Ringer's with 40 mEq KCl to infuse over 8 hours.

1. What is the most likely cause of the change in serum potassium level?
2. What factors must the nurse consider to safely administer this drug?
3. What patient teaching should be given before sending this patient home?

CRITICAL THINKING Questions

1. An 18-year-old woman is admitted to the short stay unit for a minor surgical procedure. The nurse starts an IV line in the patient's left forearm and infuses D_5W at 15 mL/h. The patient asks why she needs the IV line since her provider told her that she will be returning home that afternoon. Why was an IV ordered for this patient, and what should the nurse explain to her?

2. A 24-year-old male is brought into the emergency department after collapsing at a local bike race. On admission, his serum sodium level is found to be 112 mEq/L. An IV infusion of 3% sodium chloride is ordered. What must the nurse monitor during this patient's infusion?

Visit www.pearsonhighered.com/nursingresources for answers and rationales for all activities.

REFERENCE

Herdman, T. H., & Kamitsuru, S. (2014). *NANDA International nursing diagnoses: Definitions and classification, 2015–2017*. Oxford, United Kingdom: Wiley-Blackwell.

SELECTED BIBLIOGRAPHY

Al-Absi, A., Gosmanova, E. O., & Wall, B. M. (2012). A clinical approach to the treatment of chronic hypernatremia. *American Journal of Kidney Diseases, 60*, 1032–1038. doi:10.1053/j.ajkd.2012.06.025

Bunn, F., & Trivedi, D. (2012). Colloid solutions for fluid resuscitation. *Cochrane Database of Systematic Reviews, 7*, Art. No.: CD001319. doi:10.1002/14651858.CD001319.pub4

Coyle, J. D., Joy, M. S., & Hladik, G. A. (2011). Disorders of sodium and water homeostasis. In J. T. DiPiro, R. L. Talbert, C. Y. Yee, G. R. Matzke, B. G. Wells, & L. M. Posey (Eds.), *Pharmacotherapy: A pathophysiologic approach* (8th ed.). New York, NY: McGraw-Hill.

Crawford, A., & Harris, H. (2011). Balancing act: Na^+ sodium K^+ potassium. *Nursing, 41*(7), 44–50. doi:10.1097/01.NURSE.0000397838.20260.12

Daly, K., & Farrington, E. (2013). Hypokalemia and hyperkalemia in infants and children: Pathophysiology and treatment. *Journal of Pediatric Health Care, 27*, 486–496. doi:10.1016/j.pedhc.2013.08.003

Huang, L. H. (2014). *Dehydration*. Retrieved from http://emedicine.medscape.com/article/906999-overview

Kraut, J. A. & Madias, N. E. (2012). Treatment of acute metabolic acidosis: A pathophysiologic approach. *Nature Reviews Nephrology, 8*, 589–601. doi:10.1038/nrneph.2012.186

Matzke, G. R., Devlin, J. W., & Palevsky, P. M. (2012). Acid-base disorders. In J. T. DiPiro, R. L. Talbert, C. Y. Yee, G. R. Matzke, B. G. Wells, & L. M. Posey (Eds.), *Pharmacotherapy: A pathophysiologic approach* (8th ed.). New York, NY. McGraw-Hill.

Myburgh, J. A., & Mythen, M. G. (2013). Resuscitation fluids. *New England Journal of Medicine, 369*, 1243–1251. doi:10.1056/NEJMra1208627

Palmer, B. F. (2012). Evaluation and treatment of respiratory alkalosis. *American Journal of Kidney Diseases, 60*, 834–838. doi:10.1053/j.ajkd.2012.03.025

Pepin, J., & Shields, C. (2012). Advances in diagnosis and management of hypokalemic and hyperkalemic emergencies. *Emergency Medicine Practice, 14*(2), 1–17.

Perel, P., Roberts, I., & Ker, K. (2013). Colloids versus crystalloids for fluid resuscitation in critically ill patients. *Cochrane Database of Systematic Reviews, 2*, Art. No.: CD000567. doi:10.1002/14651858.CD000567.pub6

Strickler, J. (2012). Halt the downward spiral of traumatic hypovolemic shock. *Nursing Critical Care, 7*(2), 42–47. doi:10.1097/01.CCN.0000398768.04355.4c

University of Maryland Medical Center. (2011). *Potassium*. Retrieved from http://umm.edu/health/medical/altmed/supplement/potassium

Verbalis, J. G., Goldsmith, S. R., Greenberg, A., Korzelius, C., Schrier, R. W., Sterns, R. H., & Thompson, C. J. (2013). Diagnosis, evaluation, and treatment of hyponatremia: Expert panel recommendations. *The American Journal of Medicine, 126*(10), S1–S42. doi:10.1016/j.amjmed.2013.07.006

Chapter 26

Drugs for Hypertension

Drugs at a Glance

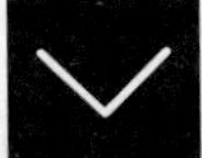

Learning Outcomes

After reading this chapter, the student should be able to:

1. Explain how hypertension is defined and classified.
2. Explain the effects of cardiac output, peripheral resistance, and blood volume on blood pressure.
3. Discuss how the vasomotor center, baroreceptors, chemoreceptors, emotions, and hormones influence blood pressure.
4. Summarize the long-term consequences of untreated hypertension.
5. Discuss the role of therapeutic lifestyle changes in the management of hypertension.
6. Differentiate between drug classes used for the primary treatment of hypertension and those secondary agents reserved for persistent hypertension.
7. Describe the nurse's role in the pharmacologic management of patients receiving drugs for hypertension.
8. For each of the drug classes listed in Drugs at a Glance, know representative drug examples, and explain their mechanisms of drug action, primary actions, and important adverse effects.
9. Use the nursing process to care for patients receiving pharmacotherapy for hypertension.

indicates a prototype drug, each of which is featured in a Prototype Drug box.

PharmFacts

STATISTICS OF HYPERTENSION

- High blood pressure affects more than 67 million U.S. adults, or approximately one in three Americans.
- About 7 of 10 persons with HTN have the condition treated with medications
- African Americans have the highest rate of HTN, and they develop the condition at an earlier age that Caucasians.
- For adults over age 65, HTN is more frequent in women than in men.
- Approximately 348,000 American deaths each year have HTN as a contributing cause.

Diseases affecting the heart and blood vessels are the most frequent causes of death in the United States. **Hypertension (HTN),** or high blood pressure, is defined as the consistent elevation of systemic arterial blood pressure. One of the most common of the cardiovascular diseases, chronic hypertension is associated with more than 348,000 deaths in the United States each year. Although mild HTN can often be controlled with lifestyle modifications, moderate to severe HTN requires pharmacotherapy.

Because nurses will encounter numerous patients with HTN, having an understanding of the underlying principles of antihypertensive therapy is essential. By improving public awareness of HTN and teaching the importance of early intervention, nurses can contribute significantly to reducing cardiovascular mortality.

26.1 Factors Responsible for Blood Pressure

Although many factors can influence blood pressure, the three factors responsible for creating the pressure are cardiac output, peripheral resistance, and blood volume. These are shown in Figure 26.1. An understanding of these factors is essential for relating the pathophysiology of HTN to its pharmacotherapy.

The volume of blood pumped per minute is the **cardiac output.** The higher the cardiac output, the higher the blood pressure. Cardiac output is determined by heart rate and **stroke volume,** the amount of blood pumped by a ventricle in one contraction. This is important to pharmacology because drugs that change the cardiac output, stroke volume, or heart rate have the potential to influence a patient's blood pressure.

As blood flows at high speeds through the vascular system, it exerts force against the walls of the vessels. Although the inner layer of the blood vessel lining, the endothelium, is extremely smooth, friction reduces the velocity of the blood. This friction in the arteries is called **peripheral resistance.** Arteries have smooth muscle in their walls that, when constricted, will cause the inside diameter or lumen to become smaller, thus creating more resistance and higher pressure. A large number of drugs affect vascular smooth muscle, causing vessels to constrict, thus raising blood pressure. Other drugs cause the smooth muscle to relax, thereby opening the lumen and lowering blood pressure. The role of the autonomic nervous system in regulating peripheral resistance is explained in chapters 12 and 13.

The third factor responsible for blood pressure is the total amount of blood in the vascular system, or blood volume. Although an average person maintains a relatively constant blood volume of approximately 5 L, this value can change due to many regulatory factors, certain disease states, and pharmacotherapy. More blood in the vascular system will exert additional pressure on the walls of the arteries and raise blood pressure. Drugs are frequently used to adjust blood volume. For example, infusion of

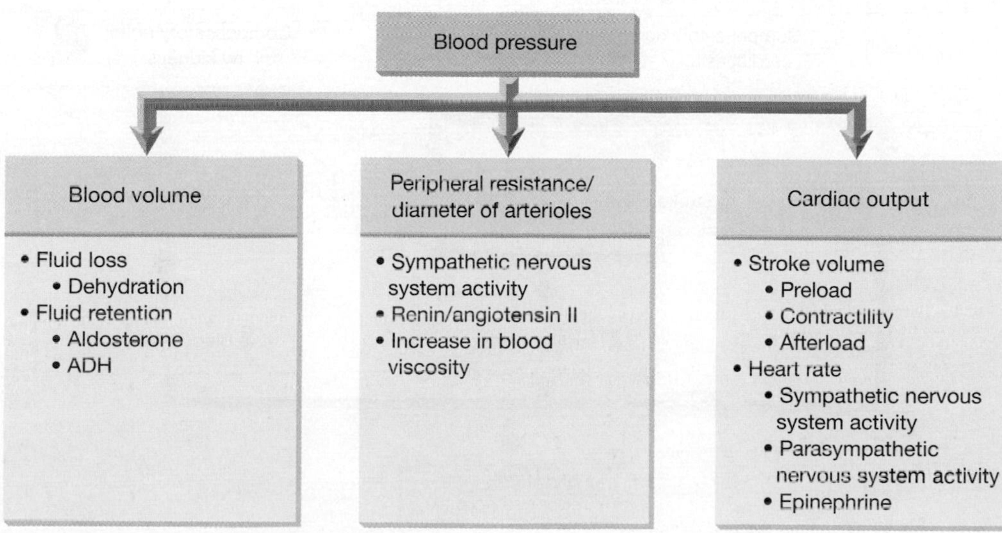

FIGURE 26.1 Primary factors affecting blood pressure

intravenous (IV) fluids increases blood volume and raises blood pressure. This factor is used to advantage when treating hypotension due to shock (see chapter 29). In contrast, substances known as **diuretics** cause fluid loss through urination, thus decreasing blood volume and lowering blood pressure.

26.2 Physiological Regulation of Blood Pressure

It is critical for the body to maintain a normal range of blood pressure and to have the ability to safely and rapidly change pressure as it proceeds through daily activities such as sleep and exercise. Hypotension can cause dizziness and lack of adequate urine formation, whereas extreme HTN can cause blood vessels to rupture, or restrict blood flow to critical organs. Figure 26.2 illustrates how the body maintains homeostasis during periods of blood pressure change.

The central and autonomic nervous systems are intimately involved in regulating blood pressure. On a minute-to-minute basis, a cluster of neurons in the medulla oblongata called the **vasomotor center** regulates blood pressure. Nerves travel from the vasomotor center to the arteries, where the smooth muscle is directed to either constrict (raise blood pressure) or relax (lower blood pressure). Sympathetic nerves from the vasomotor center stimulate alpha$_1$-adrenergic receptors on peripheral arterioles, causing vasoconstriction (see chapter 13).

Receptors in the aorta and the internal carotid artery act as sensors to provide the vasomotor center with vital information on conditions in the vascular system. **Baroreceptors** have the ability to sense pressure within blood vessels, whereas **chemoreceptors** recognize levels of oxygen and carbon dioxide and the pH in the blood. The vasomotor center reacts to information from baroreceptors and chemoreceptors by raising or lowering blood pressure accordingly. With aging or certain disease states such as diabetes, the baroreceptor response may be diminished.

Emotions can also have a profound effect on blood pressure. Anger and stress can cause blood pressure to rise, whereas mental depression and lethargy may cause it to fall. Strong emotions, if present for a prolonged time period, may become important contributors to chronic HTN.

A number of hormones and other agents affect blood pressure on a daily basis. When given as medications, some of these agents may have a profound effect on blood pressure. For example, injection of epinephrine or norepinephrine will immediately raise blood pressure. **Antidiuretic hormone (ADH)** is a potent vasoconstrictor that can also increase blood pressure by raising blood volume. ADH is available by parenteral administration as the drug vasopressin. The **renin–angiotensin–aldosterone system** is particularly important in the pharmacotherapy of HTN and is discussed in section 26.7. A summary of the various nervous and hormonal factors influencing blood pressure is shown in Figure 26.3.

26.3 Etiology and Pathogenesis of Hypertension

HTN is a complex disease that is caused by a combination of genetic and environmental factors. For the large majority of patients with HTN, no specific cause can be identified. HTN having no identifiable cause is called

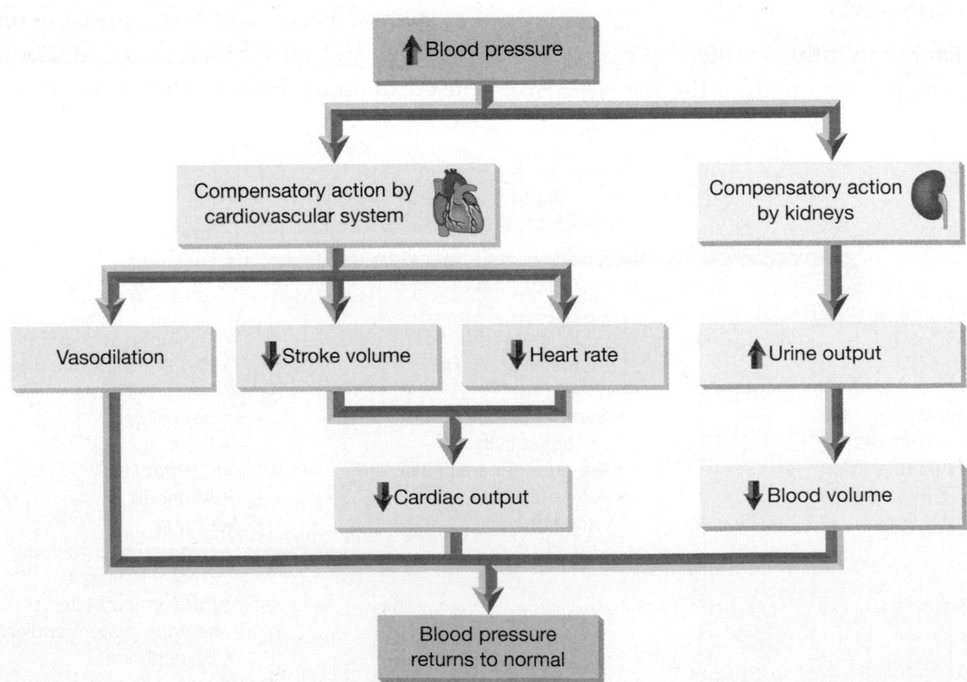

FIGURE 26.2 Blood pressure homeostasis

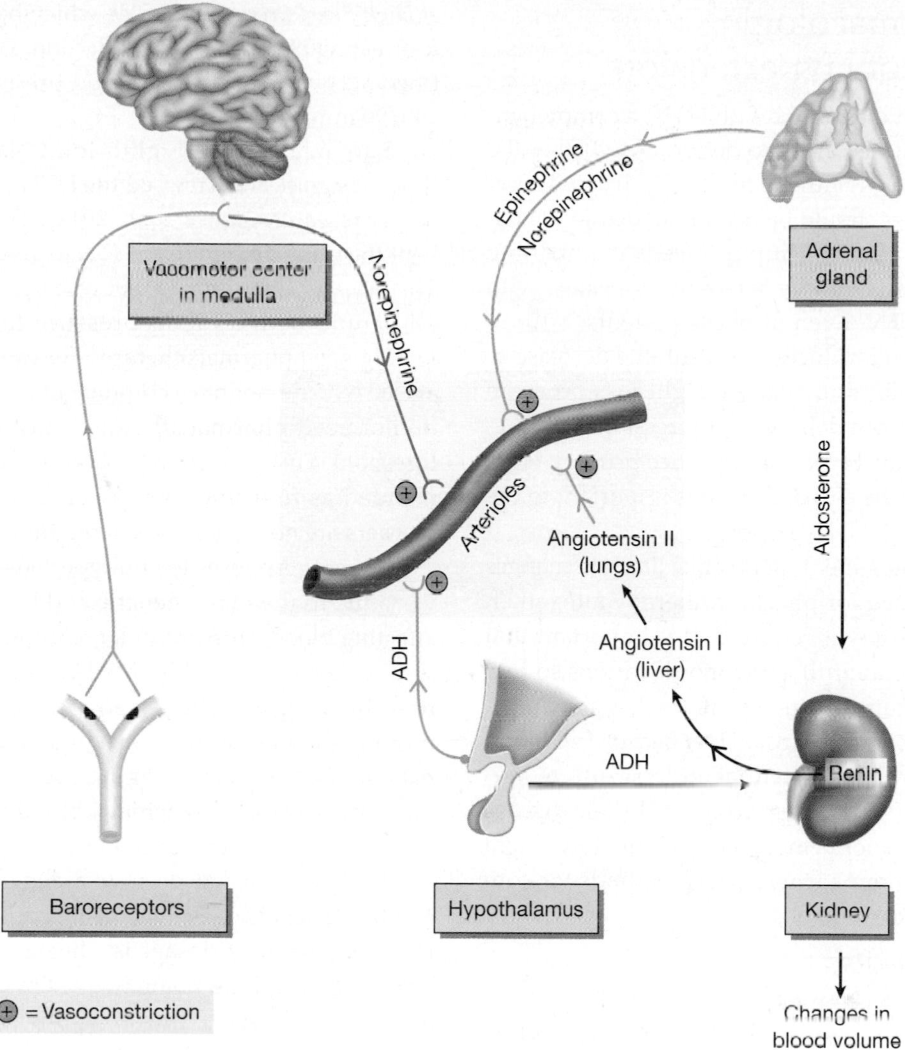

FIGURE 26.3 Hormonal and nervous factors influencing blood pressure

primary hypertension and accounts for 90% of all cases. This type is also referred to as idiopathic, or essential, HTN.

In some cases, a specific cause of the HTN *can* be identified. This is called **secondary hypertension.** Certain diseases—such as Cushing's syndrome, hyperthyroidism, and chronic renal disease—cause elevated blood pressure. Certain drugs are also associated with HTN, including corticosteroids, oral contraceptives, and erythropoietin (Epoetin alfa). The therapeutic goal for secondary HTN is to treat or remove the underlying condition that is causing the blood pressure elevation. In many cases, correcting the comorbid condition will cure the associated HTN.

Because chronic HTN may produce no identifiable symptoms, many people are not aware of their condition. Failure to control this condition, however, can result in serious consequences. Four target organs are most often affected by prolonged or improperly controlled HTN: the heart, brain, kidneys, and retina.

One of the most serious consequences of chronic HTN is that the heart must work harder to pump blood to the organs and tissues. The excessive cardiac workload can cause the heart to fail and the lungs to fill with fluid, a condition known as heart failure (HF). Drug therapy of HF is covered in chapter 27.

High blood pressure over a prolonged period adversely affects the vascular system. Damage to the blood vessels supplying blood and oxygen to the brain can result in transient ischemic attacks and strokes or cerebral vascular accidents. Chronic HTN damages arteries in the kidneys, leading to a progressive loss of renal function. Vessels in the retina can rupture or become occluded, resulting in visual impairment and even blindness.

The importance of treating this disorder at an early, prehypertensive stage cannot be overstated. If the disease is allowed to progress unchecked, the long-term damage to target organs caused by HTN may be irreversible. This is especially critical in patients with diabetes and those with chronic kidney disease, because these patients are particularly susceptible to the long-term consequences of HTN.

26.4 Nonpharmacologic Management of Hypertension

When a patient is first diagnosed with HTN, a comprehensive medical history is necessary to determine whether the disease can be controlled without the use of drugs. Therapeutic lifestyle changes should be recommended for all patients with HTN. Of greatest importance is maintaining optimal weight, because obesity is closely associated with dyslipidemia and HTN. Even in obese patients, a 10- to 20-lb weight loss often produces a measurable decrease in blood pressure. Combining a safe weight loss program with proper nutrition can delay the progression from prehypertension to chronic HTN. Indeed, once primary HTN develops it rarely can be cured; thus, it is important to delay or possibly prevent its development.

In many cases, implementing positive lifestyle changes may eliminate the need for pharmacotherapy altogether. Even if pharmacotherapy is required, it is important that the patients continue their lifestyle modifications so that dosages can be minimized. Nurses are the key to educating patients about how to control HTN. Because all blood pressure medications have potential adverse effects, it is important that patients attempt to control their disease through nonpharmacologic means to the greatest extent possible. Important nonpharmacologic methods for controlling HTN are as follows:

- Limit intake of alcohol
- Restrict sodium consumption
- Reduce intake of saturated fat and cholesterol and increase consumption of fresh fruits and vegetables
- Increase aerobic physical activity
- Discontinue use of tobacco products
- Reduce sources of stress and learn to implement coping strategies
- Maintain optimal weight.

26.5 Guidelines for the Management of Hypertension

The goal of antihypertensive therapy is to reduce the morbidity and mortality associated with chronic HTN. Research has confirmed that maintaining blood pressure within normal ranges reduces the risk of HTN-related diseases such as stroke and HF. Strategies that are used to achieve this goal are summarized in Pharmacotherapy Illustrated 26.1.

Several major attempts have been made to develop research-based guidelines for the treatment of HTN. In 2003, the National High Blood Pressure Education Program Coordinating Committee of the National Heart, Lung, and Blood Institute of the National Institutes of Health issued *The Seventh Report of the Joint National Committee on Prevention, Detection, Evaluation, and Treatment of High Blood Pressure (JNC-7)*, which became the standard for treating HTN for the next decade. The JNC-7 report defined HTN as a sustained blood pressure of greater than 140/90 mmHg.

Late in 2013, the Eighth Joint National Committee (JNC-8) significantly revised the HTN guidelines, based on newer research (James et al., 2014). The JNC-8 committee kept the same definition of HTN as JNC-7: 140/90 mmHg. The primary difference is that research has shown that not all people with a blood pressure higher than 140/90 mmHg need pharmacotherapy. For example, patients over age 60 who do not have chronic kidney disease or diabetes do not need pharmacotherapy until the 150/90 mmHg threshold. Furthermore, the classes of medications recommended as first-line therapy changed: Beta-adrenergic blockers are no longer considered first-line drugs.

Patient responses to antihypertensive medications can vary due to the many genetic and environmental factors affecting blood pressure. A large number of antihypertensive drugs are available. Medications recommended as first-line drugs by the JNC-8 are the most effective and provide the lowest incidence of adverse effects for most patients. Second-line drugs are used if additional medications are necessary to achieve blood pressure goals. The drug classes are summarized in Table 26.1.

In most cases, low doses of a single drug are prescribed and the patient is re-evaluated, after an appropriate time interval. If necessary, dosage is adjusted to maintain optimal blood pressure. Prescribing two antihypertensives from different drug classes results in additive or synergistic blood pressure reduction and is common practice when managing resistant HTN. This is often necessary when the patient has not responded to the initial medication, has a compelling condition, or has very high, sustained blood pressure. The advantage of using two drugs is that lower doses of each may be used, resulting in fewer side effects and better patient compliance with the therapy. For convenience, drug manufacturers have formulated multiple drugs into a single

Table 26.1 Drug Classes for Hypertension

Type	Class
First-line drugs	Angiotensin converting enzyme (ACE) inhibitors
	Angiotensin receptor blockers (ARBs)
	Calcium channel blockers (CCBs)
	Thiazide diuretics
Second-line drugs	$Alpha_2$-adrenergic agonists
	$Alpha_1$- adrenergic blockers
	Beta-adrenergic blockers
	Centrally acting alpha and beta blockers
	Direct-acting vasodilators
	Direct renin inhibitors
	Peripherally acting adrenergic neuron blockers

Pharmacotherapy Illustrated

26.1 | Mechanism of Action of Antihypertensive Drugs

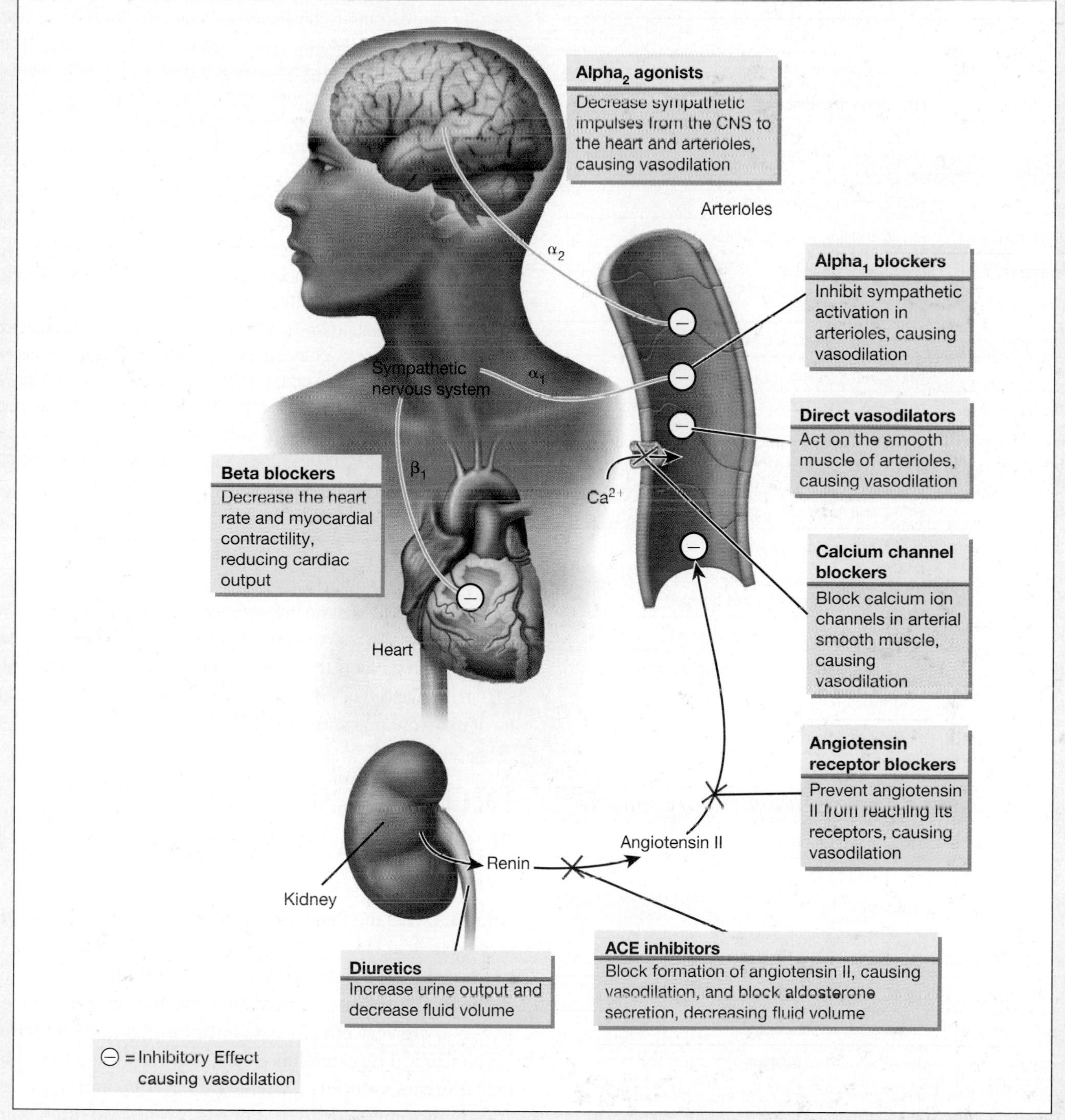

pill or capsule. The majority of these combinations include a thiazide diuretic, usually hydrochlorothiazide. Selected combination antihypertensives are listed in Table 26.2.

Convincing patients to change established lifestyle habits, spend money on medication, and take drugs on a regular basis when they feel well is often a difficult task for nurses. Patients with limited incomes or those who do not have health insurance are especially at risk for noncompliance. The health care provider should consider prescribing generic forms of these drugs to reduce cost and increase compliance with the therapeutic regimen.

Further reducing compliance is the occurrence of undesirable adverse effects. Some of the antihypertensive drugs cause embarrassing side effects such as impotence, which may go unreported. Others cause fatigue and generally make patients feel sicker than they were before therapy was initiated. Nurses

Table 26.2 Combination Drugs for Hypertension

THIAZIDE DIURETIC WITH ACE INHIBITOR	
Accuretic	HCTZ* and quinapril
Capozide	HCTZ and captopril
Lotensin HCT	HCTZ and benazepril
Uniretic	HCTZ and moexipril
Vaseretic	HCTZ and enalapril
Zestoretic	HCTZ and lisinopril
THIAZIDE DIURETIC WITH ANGIOTENSIN II BLOCKER	
Avalide	HCTZ and irbesartan
Atacand HCT	HCTZ and candesartan
Benicar HCT	HCTZ and olmesartan
Diovan HCT	HCTZ and valsartan
Edarbyclor	chlorthalidone and azilsartan
Hyzaar	HCTZ and losartan
Micardis HCT	HCTZ and telmisartan
Teveten HCT	HCTZ and eprosartan
THIAZIDE DIURETIC WITH AUTONOMIC DRUG	
Aldoril	HCTZ and methyldopa (alpha$_2$ agonist)
Corzide	HCTZ with bendroflumethiazide and nadolol (beta blocker)
Inderide	HCTZ and propranolol (beta blocker)
Lopressor HCT	HCTZ and metoprolol (beta blocker)
Minizide	polythiazide and prazosin (alpha blocker)
Tenoretic	chlorthalidone and atenolol (beta blocker)
Timolide	HCTZ and timolol (beta blocker)
Ziac	HCTZ and bisoprolol (beta blocker)
THIAZIDE DIURETIC WITH POTASSIUM-SPARING DIURETIC	
Aldactazide	HCTZ and spironolactone
Dyazide	HCTZ and triamterene
OTHER COMBINATIONS	
Amturnide	HCTZ with amlodipine (calcium channel blocker) and aliskiren (renin inhibitor)
Apresazide	HCTZ and hydralazine (direct vasodilator)
Azor	olmesartan and amlodipine
Exforge	valsartan and amlodipine
Lexxel	enalapril and felodipine (calcium channel blocker)
Lotrel	benazepril and amlodipine
Prestalia	perindopril and amlodipine
Tarka	trandolapril and verapamil (calcium channel blocker)
Tekamlo	amlodipine and aliskiren (renin inhibitor)
Tekturna HCT	HCTZ and aliskiren
Tribenzor	HCTZ with olmesartan and amlodipine

Note: *HCTZ = hydrochlorothiazide

Complementary and Alternative Therapies

GRAPE SEED EXTRACT FOR HYPERTENSION

Grapes and grape seed extract (GSE) have been used to maintain and improve health for thousands of years. Their primary use has been for cardiovascular conditions such as HTN, high blood cholesterol, and atherosclerosis, and to generally improve circulation. Some claim that GSE improves wound healing, prevents cancer, slows the progression of neurodegenerative diseases, and lowers the risk for the long-term consequences of diabetes.

The grape seeds, usually obtained from winemaking, are crushed and placed into tablet, capsule, or liquid forms. Typical doses are 50 to 300 mg/day. GSE contains polyphenols, which have antioxidant properties that have the potential to improve wound healing and repair cellular injury. Regular consumption of foods high in polyphenols has been shown to reduce the incidence of cancers of the breast, lung, digestive tract, and prostate (Dinicola et. al., 2014). A meta-analysis of studies that used randomized controls concluded that grape seed extract can significantly lower blood pressure and heart rate but has no effect on lipid or C-reactive protein levels (Feringa, Laskey, Dickson, & Coleman, 2011). GSE is well tolerated in most people, with the most common side effects being dry, itchy scalp; dizziness; headache; hives; indigestion; and nausea (National Center for Complementary and Integrative Health, 2012). It should not be used if taking anticoagulant drugs because increased bleeding may result.

should teach patients the importance of treating the disease to avoid serious long-term consequences. Furthermore, nurses should teach patients to report adverse drug effects promptly so that dosage can be adjusted, or the drug changed, and treatment may continue without interruption.

DIURETICS

26.6 Treating Hypertension With Diuretics

Diuretics were the first class of drugs that were widely prescribed to treat HTN in the 1950s. Despite many advances in pharmacotherapy, diuretics are still considered first-line drugs for this disease because they produce few adverse effects and are very effective at controlling mild to moderate HTN. Clinical research has clearly demonstrated that thiazide diuretics reduce HTN-related morbidity and mortality. Although sometimes used alone, diuretics are often combined with drugs from other antihypertensive classes to enhance their effectiveness. Diuretics are also used to treat kidney disorders (see chapter 24) and HF (see chapter 27). Doses for these medications are listed in Table 26.3.

Although many different diuretics are available for HTN, all produce a similar outcome: the reduction of blood volume through the urinary excretion of water and electrolytes. Electrolytes are ions such as sodium (Na^+), calcium (Ca^{2+}), chloride (Cl^-), and potassium (K^+). The mechanisms

Table 26.3 Diuretics for Hypertension

Drug	Route and Adult Dose (max dose where indicated)	Adverse Effects
POTASSIUM-SPARING DIURETICS		
amiloride (Midamor)	PO: 5–10 mg/day (max: 20 mg/day)	*Minor hyperkalemia, headache, fatigue, gynecomastia (spironolactone)*
eplerenone (Inspra)	PO: 25–50 mg once daily (max: 100 mg/day)	<u>Dysrhythmias (from hyperkalemia), dehydration, hyponatremia, agranulocytosis, and other blood dyscrasias</u>
spironolactone (Aldactone) (see page 351 for the Prototype Drug box)	PO: 25–100 mg one to two times/day (max: 400 mg/day)	
triamterene (Dyrenium)	PO: 50–100 mg bid (max: 300 mg/day)	
THIAZIDE AND THIAZIDE-LIKE DIURETICS		
chlorothiazide (Diuril)	PO: 250–500 mg/day (max: 2 g/day)	*Minor hypokalemia, fatigue*
chlorthalidone (Hygroton)	PO: 50–100 mg/day (max: 50 mg/day)	<u>Significant hypokalemia, electrolyte depletion,</u> dehydration, hypotension, hyponatremia, <u>hyperglycemia, coma, blood dyscrasias</u>
hydrochlorothiazide (Microzide) (see page 350 for the Prototype Drug box)	PO: 25–100 mg/day (max: 50 mg/day)	
indapamide (Lozol)	PO: 1.25–5 mg/day (max: 5 mg/day)	
methyclothiazide (Enduron)	PO: 2.5–5 mg once daily (max: 5 mg/day)	
metolazone (Zaroxolyn)	PO: 2.5–10 mg once daily (max: 20 mg/day)	
LOOP/HIGH-CEILING DIURETICS		
bumetanide (Bumex)	PO: 0.5–2.0 mg/day (max: 10 mg/day)	*Minor hypokalemia, postural hypotension, tinnitus, nausea, diarrhea, dizziness, fatigue*
furosemide (Lasix) (see page 348 for the Prototype Drug box)	PO: 20–80 mg/day (max: 600 mg/day)	<u>Significant hypokalemia, blood dyscrasias, dehydration, ototoxicity, electrolyte imbalances, circulatory collapse</u>
torsemide (Demadex)	PO/IV: 10–20 mg/day (max: 200 mg/day)	

Note: *Italics* indicate common adverse effects; <u>underlining</u> indicates serious adverse effects.

by which diuretics reduce blood volume differ among the various classes of diuretics and are discussed in chapter 24. When a drug changes urine composition or output, electrolyte depletion and dehydration are possible; the specific electrolyte lost is dependent on the mechanism of action of the particular drug. Potassium loss (hypokalemia) is of particular concern for loop and thiazide diuretics.

Thiazide and *thiazide-like* diuretics have been the mainstay for the pharmacotherapy of HTN for decades. The thiazide diuretics are inexpensive, and most are available in generic formulations. They are safe drugs, with urinary potassium loss being the primary adverse effect. The most frequently prescribed thiazide diuretic, hydrochlorothiazide, is presented in chapter 24 as the class prototype.

Although the *potassium-sparing diuretics* produce only a modest diuresis, their primary advantage is that they do not cause potassium depletion. Thus, they are beneficial when patients are at risk of developing hypokalemia due to their medical condition or the use of thiazide or loop diuretics. The primary concern when using potassium-sparing diuretics is the possibility of retaining *too much* potassium. Taking potassium supplements with potassium-sparing diuretics may result in dangerously high potassium levels in the blood (hyperkalemia) and lead to cardiac conduction abnormalities. Concurrent use with an **angiotensin-converting enzyme (ACE)** inhibitor or angiotensin II receptor blocker (ARB) significantly increases the potential for the development of hyperkalemia. Spironolactone (Aldactone) is featured as a prototype drug for this class in chapter 24.

The *loop diuretics* cause greater diuresis, and thus a greater reduction in blood pressure, than the thiazides or potassium-sparing diuretics. Although this makes them very effective at reducing blood pressure, they are not ideal drugs for HTN maintenance therapy. The risk of adverse effects such as hypokalemia and dehydration is greater than the thiazide or potassium-sparing diuretics because of their ability to remove large amounts of fluid from the body in a short time period. Loop diuretics are also ototoxic and may cause deafness. Because they have a higher potential for toxicity, loop diuretics are often reserved for more serious cases of HTN. Furosemide is the only loop diuretic in widespread use, and it is presented as a prototype in chapter 24. Refer also to the Nursing Process Application: Pharmacotherapy With Diuretics in chapter 24 for patients receiving these drugs.

DRUGS AFFECTING THE RENIN, ANGIOTENSIN, AND ALDOSTERONE SYSTEM

26.7 Treating Hypertension With Angiotensin-Converting Enzyme Inhibitors and Angiotensin Receptor Blockers

The renin–angiotensin–aldosterone system (RAAS) is one of the primary homeostatic mechanisms controlling blood

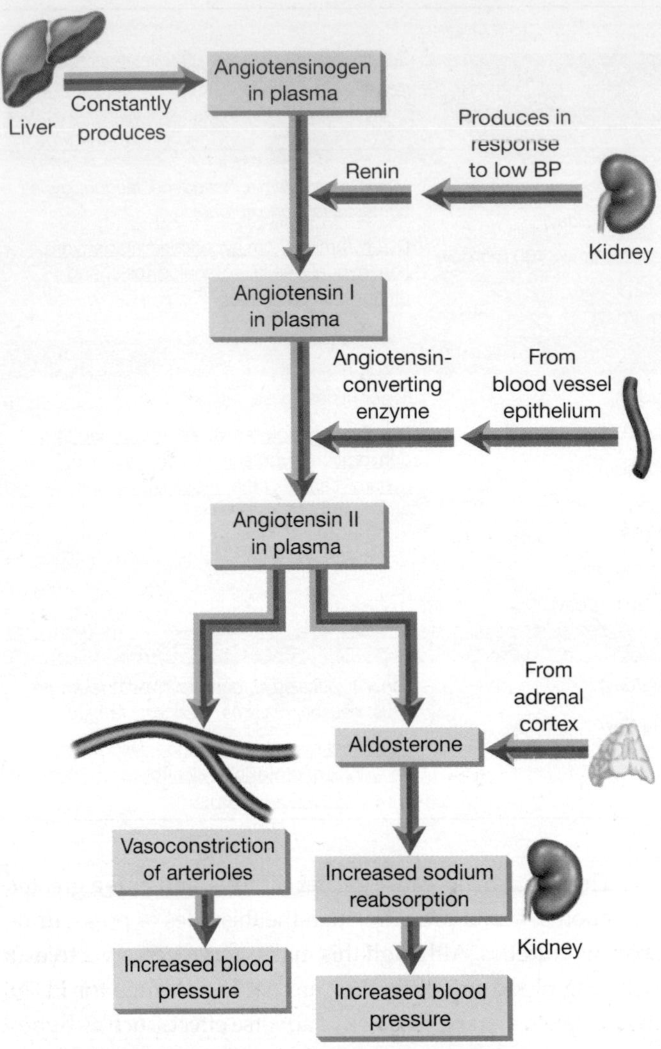

FIGURE 26.4 The renin–angiotensin–aldosterone pathway

pressure and fluid balance in the body. This mechanism is illustrated in Figure 26.4. Drugs that affect the RAAS decrease blood pressure and increase urine volume. They are widely used in the pharmacotherapy of HTN, HF, and myocardial infarction (MI). Doses for these drugs are listed in Table 26.4.

Renin is an enzyme secreted by specialized cells in the kidney when blood pressure falls, or when there is a decrease in sodium ion (Na^+) flowing through the kidney tubules. Once in the blood, renin converts the inactive liver protein angiotensinogen to angiotensin I. When it passes through the lungs, angiotensin I is converted to **angiotensin II**, one of the most potent natural vasoconstrictors known. The enzyme responsible for the final step in this system is **angiotensin-converting enzyme (ACE).** The intense vasoconstriction of arterioles caused by angiotensin II raises blood pressure by increasing peripheral resistance.

Angiotensin II also stimulates the secretion of **aldosterone,** a hormone from the adrenal cortex. The primary action of aldosterone is to increase Na^+ reabsorption in the kidney. The enhanced Na^+ reabsorption causes the body to retain water, increasing blood volume, and raising blood pressure. Thus, angiotensin II increases blood pressure through two distinct mechanisms: direct vasoconstriction and increased water retention.

First detected in the venom of pit vipers, ACE inhibitors have been approved for HTN since the 1980s. Since then, drugs in this class have become key medications in the treatment of HTN. ACE inhibitors block the effects of angiotensin II and decrease blood pressure through two mechanisms: lowering peripheral resistance and decreasing blood volume. ACE inhibitors and thiazide diuretics are often used concurrently in the management of HTN. Some ACE inhibitors have become primary drugs for the treatment of HF and MI, as discussed in chapters 27 and 28, respectively.

Adverse effects of ACE inhibitors are usually minor and include persistent cough and postural hypotension, particularly following the first few doses of the drug. The persistent, dry cough is believed to be caused by accumulation of bradykinin, a proinflammatory substance. Hyperkalemia may occur and can be a major concern for patients with diabetes, those with renal impairment, and patients taking potassium-sparing diuretics. Though rare, the most serious adverse effect of ACE inhibitors is the development of angioedema. Angioedema is swelling around the lips, eyes, throat, and other body regions. In advanced cases, angioedema may lead to airway closure, due to the intense swelling in the neck. When it does occur, angioedema most often develops within hours or days after beginning ACE inhibitor therapy. Late-onset angioedema has been reported after months and even years of treatment with these drugs.

A second mechanism for modifying the RAAS is to block the action of angiotensin II *after* it is formed. The angiotensin II receptor blockers (ARBs) block receptors for angiotensin II in arteriolar smooth muscle and in the adrenal gland, thus causing blood pressure to fall. Their effects of arteriolar dilation and increased sodium excretion by the kidneys are similar to those of the ACE inhibitors. ARBs have relatively few side effects, most of which are related to hypotension. Unlike the ACE inhibitors, they do not cause cough, and angioedema is even more rare with the ARBs. Drugs in this class are usually combined with drugs from other classes in the management of HTN.

A third method of blocking the RAAS is to block receptors for aldosterone. The two drugs available that block these receptors in the kidney are spironolactone (Aldactone) and eplerenone (Inspra). By preventing aldosterone from reaching its receptors in the kidneys, less Na^+ is reabsorbed and blood pressure falls. Because they act by this mechanism, these drugs are also classified as potassium-sparing diuretics. Spironolactone and eplenerone are approved to treat HTN, HF, and edema, and to reduce morbidity and mortality associated with post–MI in patients with left ventricular dysfunction.

The newest method of modifying the RAAS is to inhibit the effects of renin itself. The *direct renin inhibitors* prevent

Table 26.4 ACE Inhibitors and Angiotensin II Receptor Blockers for Hypertension

Drug	Route and Adult Dose (max dose where indicated)	Adverse Effects
ACE INHIBITORS		
benazepril (Lotensin)	PO: 10–40 mg in one dose or divided doses (max: 80 mg/day)	*Headache, dizziness, orthostatic hypotension, rash, cough* Angioedema, acute renal failure, first-dose phenomenon, fetal toxicity
captopril (Capoten)	PO: 12.5–25 mg bid or tid (max: 450 mg/day)	
enalapril (Vasotec)	PO: 2.5–40 mg in one dose or two divided doses (max: 40 mg/day)	
fosinopril (Monopril)	PO: 5–40 mg/day (max: 80 mg/day)	
lisinopril (Prinivil, Zestril) (see page 400 for the Prototype Drug box)	PO: 10 mg/day (max: 80 mg/day)	
moexipril (Univasc)	PO: 7.5–30 mg/day (max: 30 mg/day)	
perindopril (Aceon)	PO: 2–4 mg once daily (max: 16 mg/day)	
quinapril (Accupril)	PO: 10–20 mg/day (max: 80 mg/day)	
ramipril (Altace)	PO: 2.5–5 mg/day (max: 20 mg/day)	
trandolapril (Mavik)	PO: 1–4 mg/day (max: 8 mg/day)	
ANGIOTENSIN II RECEPTOR BLOCKERS		
azilsartan (Edarbi)	PO: 40–80 mg once daily	*Headache, dizziness, orthostatic hypotension, diarrhea, upper respiratory tract infection* Angioedema, acute renal failure, first-dose phenomenon, fetal toxicity and neonatal mortality, renal toxicity (aliskiren)
candesartan (Atacand)	PO: 8–32 mg/day (max: 32 mg/day)	
eprosartan (Teveten)	PO: 400–800 mg/day (max: 800 mg/day)	
irbesartan (Avapro)	PO: 150–300 mg/day (max: 300 mg/day)	
losartan (Cozaar)	PO: 25–50 mg in one dose or two divided doses (max: 100 mg/day)	
olmesartan (Benicar)	PO: 20–40 mg/day (max: 40 mg/day)	
telmisartan (Micardis)	PO: 40 mg/day (max: 80 mg/day)	
valsartan (Diovan)	PO: 80–160 mg/day (max: 320 mg/day)	

Note: *Italics* indicate common adverse effects; underlining indicates serious adverse effects.

the formation of angiotensin I and II. Aliskiren (Tekturna) was the first drug marketed in this class of antihypertensives. Pharmaceutical companies were quick to add aliskiren to fixed-dose combination drugs with HCTZ (Tekturna HCT), amlodipine (Tekamlo), and HCTZ with amlodipine (Amturnide). In 2012, the fixed dose combination of aliskirin and valsartan (Valturna) was removed from the market due to a high incidence of renal impairment and stroke. Aliskiren and its combination medications contain warnings that they should not be used in combination with ACE inhibitors, or in patients with moderate to severe kidney disease. The most common adverse effects of aliskiren are diarrhea, cough, flulike symptoms, and rash.

CALCIUM CHANNEL BLOCKERS

Calcium channel blockers (CCBs) exert beneficial effects on the heart and blood vessels by blocking calcium ion channels. They are used in the treatment of HTN and other cardiovascular diseases.

26.8 Treating Hypertension With Calcium Channel Blockers

CCBs comprise a group of drugs used to treat angina pectoris, dysrhythmias, and HTN. When CCBs were first approved for the treatment of angina in the early 1980s, it was quickly noted that a "side effect" was the lowering of blood pressure in patients with HTN. CCBs are usually not used as monotherapy for chronic HTN. They are, however, useful in treating certain populations such as the elderly and African Americans, who are sometimes less responsive to drugs in other antihypertensive classes. Doses for these drugs are listed in Table 26.5.

Contraction of muscle is regulated by the amount of calcium ion inside the cell. Muscular contraction occurs when calcium enters the cell through channels in the plasma membrane. CCBs block these channels and inhibit Ca^{2+} from entering the cell, limiting muscular contraction. At low doses, CCBs relax arterial smooth muscle, thus lowering peripheral resistance and decreasing blood pressure. Some CCBs such as nifedipine (Adalat CC, Procardia XL, others) are *selective* for calcium channels in arterioles, whereas others such as verapamil affect channels in *both* arterioles and cardiac muscle. CCBs vary in their potency and by the frequency and types of adverse effects produced. Verapamil (Calan, Isoptin, Verelan) is featured as a prototype antidysrhythmic in chapter 30, and diltiazem (Cardizem, Dilacor, Taztia XT, others) as an antianginal in chapter 28.

Two CCBs, clevidipine (Cleviprex) and nicardipine (Cardene), are used to treat patients who present with serious, life-threatening HTN. Clevidipine has an ultrashort half-life of 1 minute, which allows for rapid adjustments to blood pressure. Whereas clevidipine is indicated only by

Prototype Drug | Enalapril *(Vasotec)*

Therapeutic Class: Drug for hypertension and heart failure **Pharmacologic Class:** ACE inhibitor

Actions and Uses

Enalapril is one of the most frequently prescribed ACE inhibitors for HTN. Unlike captopril (Capoten), the first ACE inhibitor to be marketed, enalapril has a prolonged half-life, which permits administration once or twice daily. It is available as oral tablets and as an IV injection. Enalapril acts by reducing angiotensin II and aldosterone levels to produce a significant reduction in blood pressure with few serious adverse effects. Enalapril may be used as monotherapy or in combination with other antihypertensives. Enalapril is also indicated for symptomatic HF and to prevent the progression to HF in asymptomatic patients with left ventricular dysfunction. Vaseretic is a fixed-dose combination of enalapril and hydrochlorothiazide.

Administration Alerts

- This drug may produce a first-dose phenomenon, resulting in profound hypotension, which may result in syncope.
- Do not administer if the patient is pregnant.
- Pregnancy category D.

PHARMACOKINETICS

Onset	Peak	Duration
1 h PO; 15 min IV	4–8 h PO; 4 h IV	12–24 h PO; 4 h IV

Adverse Effects

Unlike diuretics, ACE inhibitors such as enalapril have little effect on electrolyte balance but may cause hyperkalemia. Unlike beta-adrenergic blockers, the ACE inhibitors cause few cardiac adverse effects. Enalapril may cause orthostatic hypotension when the patient moves quickly from a supine to an upright position. A rapid fall in blood pressure may occur following the first dose. Other adverse effects include headache and dizziness. ACE inhibitors can cause life-threatening angioedema, neutropenia, or agranulocytosis.

Black Box Warning: Fetal injury and death may occur when ACE inhibitors or ARBs are taken during pregnancy. If pregnancy is detected, they should be discontinued as soon as possible.

Contraindications: Enalapril is contraindicated in patients with prior hypersensitivity and should not be administered during pregnancy or lactation.

Interactions

Drug–Drug: When given concurrently, other antihypertensives have additive effects with enalapril on blood pressure. Thiazide diuretics increase potassium loss. Potassium supplements or potassium-sparing diuretics increase the risk of hyperkalemia. Enalapril and other ACE inhibitors should not be administered concurrently with aliskiren due to the potential for renal toxicity. Nonsteroidal anti-inflammatory drugs (NSAIDs) may reduce the hypotensive action of ACE inhibitors.

Lab Tests: May increase values of the following: blood urea nitrogen (BUN), alkaline phosphatase, serum potassium, serum creatinine, alanine aminotransferase (ALT), and aspartate aminotransferase (AST); may cause a positive antinuclear antibody titer.

Herbal/Food: Unknown.

Treatment of Overdose: The most likely sign of overdosage is hypotension, which may be treated with an IV infusion of normal saline solution.

Table 26.5 Calcium Channel Blockers for Hypertension

Drug	Route and Adult Dose (max dose where indicated)	Adverse Effects
SELECTIVE: FOR BLOOD VESSELS		
amlodipine (Norvasc)	PO: 5–10 mg once daily (max: 10 mg/day)	*Flushed skin, headache, dizziness, peripheral edema, light-headedness, nausea, constipation, fatigue, and sexual dysfunction* <u>Hepatotoxicity, MI, HF, confusion, mood changes, angioedema (particularly of the face)</u>
felodipine (Plendil)	PO: 5–10 mg once daily (max: 10 mg/day)	
isradipine (DynaCirc)	PO: (controlled release): 5–10 mg once daily (max: 10 mg/day)	
nicardipine (Cardene)	PO: 20–40 mg tid or 30–60 mg; Cardene SR bid (max: 120 mg/day)	
nifedipine (Adalat CC, Procardia XL, others)	PO: 10–20 mg tid (max: 180 mg/day) PO: (extended release): 17 mg once daily (max: 34 mg/day)	
nisoldipine (Sular)		
NONSELECTIVE: FOR BOTH BLOOD VESSELS AND HEART		
diltiazem (Cardizem, Dilacor, Taztia XT, others) (see page 423 for the Prototype Drug box)	PO: 30 mg four times daily (max: 480 mg/day) Extended-release: 120–240 mg once daily	
verapamil (Calan, Isoptin, Verelan) (see page 456 for the Prototype Drug box)	PO: 80–160 mg tid (max: 480 mg/day) PO: (Calan SR, Verelan): 100-200 mg once daily	

Note: *Italics* indicate common adverse effects; <u>underlining</u> indicates serious adverse effects.

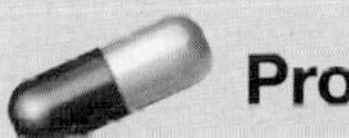

Prototype Drug | Nifedipine *(Adalat CC, Procardia XL)*

Therapeutic Class: Drug for hypertension and angina **Pharmacologic Class:** Calcium channel blocker

Actions and Uses

Nifedipine is a CCB generally prescribed for HTN and variant or vasospastic angina. It is occasionally used to treat Raynaud's phenomenon (off-label) and hypertrophic cardiomyopathy. Nifedipine acts by selectively blocking calcium channels in myocardial and vascular smooth muscle, including those in the coronary arteries. This results in less oxygen utilization by the heart, an increase in cardiac output, and a fall in blood pressure. It is available as immediate-release capsules and as extended-release tablets (XL).

Administration Alerts

- Do not administer immediate-release formulations of nifedipine if an impending MI is suspected or within 2 weeks following a confirmed MI.
- Administer nifedipine capsules or tablets whole. If capsules or extended-release tablets are chewed, divided, or crushed, the entire dose will be delivered at once.
- Pregnancy category C.

PHARMACOKINETICS

Onset	Peak	Duration
30–60 min (immediate release capsules); 6 h (extended release tablet)	30 min	4–8 h (24 h for extended release); half-life: 2–5 h

Adverse Effects

Adverse effects of nifedipine are generally minor and are related to vasodilation such as headache, dizziness, peripheral edema, and flushing. Immediate-acting forms of nifedipine can cause reflex tachycardia. To avoid rebound hypotension, the drug should be discontinued gradually. In rare cases, nifedipine may cause a paradoxical increase in anginal pain, possibly related to hypotension or HF.

Contraindications: The only contraindication is prior hypersensitivity to nifedipine.

Interactions

Drug–Drug: When given concurrently, other antihypertensives have additive effects with nifedipine on blood pressure. Concurrent use of nifedipine with a beta blocker increases the risk of HF. Nifedipine may increase serum levels of digoxin, leading to bradycardia and digoxin toxicity. Alcohol potentiates the vasodilating action of nifedipine and could lead to syncope caused by a severe drop in blood pressure.

Lab Tests: May increase values for the following: alkaline phosphatase, lactate dehydrogenase, ALT, creatine phosphokinase (CPK), and AST.

Herbal/Food: Grapefruit juice may enhance the absorption of nifedipine. Melatonin may increase blood pressure and heart rate.

Treatment of Overdose: The most likely sign of overdosage is hypotension, which is treated with vasopressors. Calcium infusions may be indicated.

Patient Safety: Risk of Falls Increases With Antihypertensive Daily Dose

Although HTN is occurring at earlier ages than before, the majority of patients who have it are in their middle to older adult years. Generally, the risk of falls may increase in the older adult which is particularly concerning when antihypertensives are used. Depending on the drug class, orthostatic hypotension, drowsiness, and dizziness may result. Callisaya, Sharman, Close, Lord, and Srikanth (2014) studied the association between the daily defined dose (DDD) of an antihypertensive drug and the risk of falls. The DDD is defined as the "assumed average maintenance dose per day for a drug used for its main indication in adults" (WHO Collaborating Centre for Drug Statistics Methodology, 2009). The DDD provides a method of comparing doses of different drug classifications in a standardized way. The research demonstrated that as the DDD increased, so did the risk of falls in older adults age 60–85. The risk for falls increased if the patient had a history of stroke. As the average daily maintenance dose is increased, or a second drug is added to the patient's medication regimen, nurses should be aware that the risk of falls also increases, regardless of the drug class's adverse effect profile.

the IV route for hypertensive emergencies, nicardipine is also available by the oral (PO) route for primary HTN and angina.

☑ Check Your Understanding 26.1

For most patients, what are the most common drug classes chosen for the initial treatment of hypertension? *Visit www.pearsonhighered.com/nursingresources for the answer.*

ADRENERGIC ANTAGONISTS

26.9 Treating Hypertension with Adrenergic Antagonists

The adrenergic receptor has been a site of pharmacologic action in the treatment of HTN since the first such drugs were developed for this disorder in the 1950s. Blockade of adrenergic receptors results in a number of therapeutic effects on the heart and vessels, and these autonomic drugs have been used for a wide variety of cardiovascular disorders. Table 26.6 lists the adrenergic antagonists used for HTN. Refer also to the Nursing Practice Application in chapter 13 for patients receiving therapy with adrenergic antagonists.

As discussed in chapters 12 and 13, the autonomic nervous system controls involuntary functions of the body such as heart rate, pupil size, and smooth muscle contraction, including that in the bronchi and arterial walls. Stimulation of the sympathetic division causes fight-or-flight responses such as faster heart rate, an increase in blood pressure, and bronchodilation.

Antihypertensive drugs have been developed that block the sympathetic fight-or-flight response through several distinct mechanisms, although all have in common the effect of lowering blood pressure. These mechanisms include blockade of beta$_1$-adrenergic receptors in the heart or alpha$_1$-adrenergic receptors in the arterioles, and activation of alpha$_2$-receptors in the brainstem (centrally acting). Some drugs are nonselective and act at multiple autonomic receptors.

Beta-Adrenergic Blockers

Of the subclasses of adrenergic antagonists, only the beta-adrenergic blockers are considered important drugs for the pharmacotherapy of HTN. By decreasing the heart rate and contractility, they reduce cardiac output and lower

Table 26.6 Adrenergic Antagonists for Hypertension

Drug	Route and Adult Dose (max dose where indicated)	Adverse Effects
BETA-ADRENERGIC ANTAGONISTS		
acebutolol (Sectral)	PO: 400–1200 mg/day (max: 1200 mg/day)	*Fatigue, insomnia, drowsiness, impotence or decreased libido, bradycardia, and confusion*
atenolol (Tenormin): (see page 422 for the Prototype Drug box)	PO: 25–50 mg/day (max: 100 mg/day)	<u>Agranulocytosis, laryngospasm, Stevens–Johnson syndrome, anaphylaxis; if the drug is abruptly withdrawn, palpitations, rebound HTN, dysrhythmias, MI</u>
betaxolol (Kerlone)	PO: 5–20 mg/day (max: 40 mg/day)	
bisoprolol (Zebeta)	PO: 2.5–5 mg/day (max: 20 mg/day)	
metoprolol (Lopressor, Toprol) (see page 404 for the Prototype Drug box)	PO: 50–100 mg once daily or bid (max: 450 mg/day)	
nadolol (Corgard)	PO: 40 mg/day (max: 320 mg/day)	
nebivolol (Bystolic)	PO: 5 mg once daily (max: 40 mg)	
pindolol (Visken)	PO: 5 mg bid (max: 60 mg/day)	
propranolol (Inderal, InnoPran XL) (see page 453 for the Prototype Drug box)	PO (extended release): 80–120 mg once daily at bedtime	
timolol (Blocadren) (see page 871 for the Prototype Drug box)	PO: 10 mg bid (max: 60 mg/day)	
ALPHA$_1$-ADRENERGIC ANTAGONISTS		
doxazosin (Cardura)	PO: (immediate release): 1–16 mg at bedtime	*Orthostatic hypotension, dizziness, headache, fatigue*
prazosin (Minipress) (see page 156 for the Prototype Drug box)	PO: 1 mg at bedtime; may increase to 1 mg bid–tid (max: 20 mg/day)	<u>First-dose phenomenon, tachycardia, dyspnea</u>
terazosin (Hytrin)	PO: 1 mg at bedtime; then 1–5 mg/day (max: 20 mg/day)	
ALPHA$_2$-ADRENERGIC AGONISTS (CENTRALLY ACTING)		
clonidine (Catapres)	PO: 0.1 mg bid–tid (max: 0.8 mg/day)	*Peripheral edema, sedation, depression, headache, dry mouth, decreased libido*
methyldopa (Aldomet)	PO: 250 mg bid or tid (max: 3 g/day)	<u>Hepatotoxicity, hemolytic anemia, granulocytopenia</u>
ALPHA$_1$- AND BETA BLOCKERS		
carvedilol (Coreg)	PO (immediate release): 3.125 mg bid (max: 50 mg/day) PO (extended release): 20-40 mg once daily (max: 80 mg/day)	*Dizziness, fatigue, weight gain, hyperglycemia, diarrhea* <u>Bradycardia, may worsen HF and mask symptoms of hypoglycemia</u>
labetalol (Trandate)	PO: 100 mg bid (max: 1200–2400 mg/day)	

Note: *Italics* indicate common adverse effects; <u>underlining</u> indicates serious adverse effects.

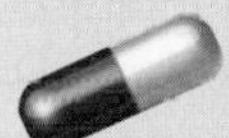

Prototype Drug | Doxazosin *(Cardura)*

Therapeutic Class: Drug for hypertension and benign prostatic hyperplasia
Pharmacologic Class: Alpha$_1$-adrenergic blocker

Actions and Uses

Doxazosin is a selective alpha$_1$-adrenergic blocker available as immediate release (Cardura) or extended release (Cardura XL) tablets. The extended release form is not indicated for HTN. Because it is selective for blocking alpha$_1$ receptors in vascular smooth muscle, it has few adverse effects on other autonomic organs and is preferred over nonselective beta blockers. Doxazosin dilates arteries and veins and is capable of causing a rapid fall in blood pressure. Doxazosin and several other alpha-adrenergic blockers also relax smooth muscle around the prostate gland. Patients who have benign prostatic hyperplasia (BPH) sometimes receive this drug to relieve symptoms of dysuria (see chapter 47).

Administration Alerts

- Monitor patients closely for profound hypotension and possible syncope 2–6 hours following the first few doses due to the first-dose phenomenon.
- The first-dose phenomenon can recur when the medication is resumed after a period of withdrawal and with dosage increases.
- Swallow Cardura XL whole: Do not crush, chew, or split the tablet.
- Pregnancy category B.

PHARMACOKINETICS

Onset	Peak	Duration
1–2 h (blood pressure) or 2 weeks (BPH)	2–6 h	24 h

Adverse Effects

The most common adverse effects of doxazosin are dizziness, dyspnea, asthenia, headache, hypotension, othostatic hypotension, and somnolence, although these effects are rarely severe enough to cause discontinuation of therapy. On starting doxazosin therapy, some patients experience serious orthostatic hypotension, although tolerance often develops to this side effect after a few doses.

Contraindications: Doxazosin is contraindicated in patients with prior hypersensitivity to alpha blockers.

Interactions

Drug–Drug: When given concurrently, other antihypertensives have additive effects with doxazosin on blood pressure. Oral cimetidine may cause a mild increase (10%) in the half-life of doxazosin. Concurrent administration of doxazosin with phosphodiesterase-5 inhibitors such as sildenafil (Viagra) can result in additive blood pressure lowering effects and symptomatic hypotension. Boceprevir increases the serum levels of doxazosin and the two drugs should not be given concurrently.

Lab Tests: Unknown.

Herbal/Food: Unknown.

Treatment of Overdose: The most likely sign of overdosage is hypotension, which is treated with a vasopressor and/or IV infusion of fluids.

systemic blood pressure. Some of their antihypertensive effect is also caused by blockade of beta$_1$-receptors in the juxtaglomerular apparatus, which inhibits the secretion of renin and the formation of angiotensin II.

Beta blockers have several other important therapeutic applications. By decreasing the cardiac workload, beta blockers can ease the symptoms of angina pectoris. By slowing conduction through the myocardium, beta blockers are able to treat certain types of dysrhythmias. Other therapeutic uses include the treatment of HF, MI, and migraines. Prototypes of beta-adrenergic antagonists can be found for metoprolol (Lopressor, Toprol) in chapter 27, atenolol (Tenormin) in chapter 28, propranolol (Inderal, InnoPranXL) in chapter 30, and timolol (Bocadren, Timoptic) in chapter 50. A Nursing Process Application for patients receiving beta adrenergic blockers is presented in chapter 13.

The adverse effects of beta blockers are predictable based on their inhibition of the fight-or-flight response. At low doses, the beta blockers are well tolerated, and serious adverse effects are uncommon. As the dosage is increased, beta blockers will slow the heart rate and cause bronchoconstriction; therefore, they should be used with caution in patients with asthma or HF. Many patients report fatigue and activity intolerance at higher doses, because the reduction in heart rate causes the heart to become less responsive to exertion. Less common, though sometimes a major cause of noncompliance, is the effect of beta blockers on male sexual function. These medications can cause decreased libido and erectile dysfunction (impotence). Because abrupt cessation of beta-blocker therapy can result in rebound HTN, angina, and MI, drug doses should be tapered over several weeks.

$Alpha_1$-Adrenergic Blockers

The $alpha_1$-adrenergic antagonists lower blood pressure directly by blocking sympathetic receptors in arterioles, causing the vessels to dilate. The alpha blockers are not first-line drugs for HTN because long-term clinical trials have shown them to be less effective at reducing the incidence of serious cardiovascular events than diuretics. When used to treat HTN, the alpha blockers are usually used concurrently with other classes of antihypertensives, such as the diuretics. Doxazosin (Cardura) is a prototype antihypertensive included in this chapter. Other prototypes for alpha blockers in this textbook include prazosin (Minipress) in chapter 13, and tamsulosin (Flomax) in chapter 47.

The $alpha_1$-adrenergic blockers tend to cause orthostatic hypotension when a person moves quickly from a supine to an upright position. Dizziness, nausea, nervousness, and fatigue are also common.

$Alpha_2$-Adrenergic Agonists

The $alpha_2$-adrenergic agonists decrease the outflow of sympathetic nerve impulses from the central nervous system (CNS) to the heart and arterioles. In effect, this produces the same responses as inhibition of the $alpha_1$ receptor: slowing of the heart rate and conduction velocity and dilation of the arterioles. The $alpha_2$ agonists cause sedation, dizziness, and other CNS effects. Abnormalities in sexual function may occur. Less common, though potentially severe, adverse effects include hemolytic anemia, leukopenia, thrombocytopenia, and lupus. With the exception of methyldopa (Aldomet), which is sometimes a preferred drug for treating HTN occurring during pregnancy, these drugs are rarely prescribed.

DIRECT VASODILATORS

26.10 Treating Hypertension With Direct Vasodilators

Many of the antihypertensive classes discussed thus far lower blood pressure through indirect means by affecting enzymes (ACE inhibitors), autonomic nerves (alpha and beta blockers), or fluid volume (diuretics). It would seem that a more efficient way to reduce blood pressure would be to cause a *direct* relaxation of vascular smooth muscle. Indeed, drugs that directly affect vascular smooth muscle are highly effective at lowering blood pressure, but they produce too many adverse effects to be drugs of first choice. These drugs are listed in Table 26.7.

Direct vasodilators produce **reflex tachycardia,** a compensatory response to the sudden decrease in blood pressure caused by the drug. Reflex tachycardia forces the heart to work harder and blood pressure increases, counteracting the effect of the antihypertensive drug. Patients with coronary artery disease could experience an acute angina attack. Fortunately, reflex tachycardia can be prevented by the concurrent administration of a beta-adrenergic blocker, such as propranolol.

A second potentially serious side effect of direct vasodilator therapy is sodium and water retention. As blood pressure drops, blood flow to the kidneys decreases and renin is released as the body activates the RAAS mechanism. Due to the vasodilation caused by the drug therapy, the angiotensin released does not cause vasoconstriction but *does* stimulate the release of aldosterone, causing the kidneys to reabsorb sodium and thus water. As the kidney retains more sodium and water, blood volume increases, thus raising blood pressure and canceling the antihypertensive action of the vasodilator. A diuretic may be administered concurrently with a direct vasodilator to prevent fluid retention but warrants extreme caution. Excessive diuresis and lowered blood volume may lead to excessive hypotension and circulatory collapse.

Check Your Understanding 26.2

Why is a diuretic sometimes needed along with some classes of antihypertensive medication? *Visit www.pearsonhighered.com/nursingresources for the answer.*

TREATMENT OF HYPERTENSIVE EMERGENCIES

A hypertensive emergency (HTN-E) is a condition in which systolic blood pressure is greater than 180 mmHg and diastolic blood pressure is greater than 120 mmHg with evidence of impending end-organ damage, usually to the heart, kidney, or brain. The most common cause of HTN-E is untreated or poorly controlled primary HTN.

Table 26.7 Direct-Acting Vasodilators for Hypertension

Drug	Route and Adult Dose (max dose where indicated)	Adverse Effects
hydralazine (Apresoline)	PO: 10–50 mg qid (max: 300 mg/day)	*Orthostatic hypotension, fluid retention, headache, palpitations*
minoxidil (Loniten)	PO: 5–40 mg/day (max: 100 mg/day)	<u>Lupus-like reaction (hydralazine), severe hypotension, MI, dysrhythmias, shock</u>
nitroprusside (Nitropress)	IV: 0.3–0.5 mcg/kg/min	

Note: *Italics* indicate common adverse effects; <u>underlining</u> indicates serious adverse effects.

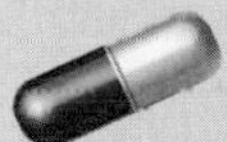

Prototype Drug | Hydralazine *(Apresoline)*

Therapeutic Class: Drug for hypertension and heart failure **Pharmacologic Class:** Direct-acting vasodilator

Actions and Uses

Hydralazine was one of the first oral antihypertensive drugs marketed in the United States. It acts through a direct vasodilation of arterial smooth muscle; it has no effect on veins. Therapy is begun with low doses, which are gradually increased until the desired therapeutic response is obtained. After several months of therapy, tolerance to the drug develops and a dosage increase may be necessary. Although hydralazine produces an effective reduction in blood pressure, drugs in other antihypertensive classes have largely replaced it due to safety concerns. The parenteral formulations of hydralazine are for the treatment of hypertensive emergency.

A relatively recent use of this drug is BiDil, a fixed-dose combination of hydralazine with isosorbide dinitrate. This combination is used to treat HF in African American patients, who appear to show an enhanced response to this medication.

Administration Alerts

- Abrupt withdrawal of the drug may cause rebound HTN and anxiety.
- Pregnancy category C.

PHARMACOKINETICS

Onset	Peak	Duration
20–30 min PO; 10–30 min IM; 5–20 min IV	1–2 h PO and IM; 30–45 min IV	3-8 h (PO); 1-4 h (IV)

Adverse Effects

Headache, reflex tachycardia, palpitations, flushing, nausea, and diarrhea are common but may resolve as therapy progresses. Patients taking hydralazine often receive a beta-adrenergic blocker to counteract reflex tachycardia. Rarely, the drug may produce a lupus-like syndrome that may persist for 6 months or longer. Sodium and fluid retention is a potentially serious adverse effect. Because of these adverse effects, the use of hydralazine is limited mostly to patients whose condition cannot be controlled with other, safer medications.

Contraindications: Because of its effects on the heart, hydralazine is contraindicated in patients with angina, rheumatic heart disease, MI, or tachycardia. Patients with lupus should not receive hydralazine, because the drug can worsen symptoms.

Interactions

Drug–Drug: Administering hydralazine with other antihypertensives may cause severe hypotension. This includes all drug classes used as antihypertensives. NSAIDs may decrease the antihypertensive action of hydralazine.

Lab Tests: May produce a false-positive Coombs tests.

Herbal/Food: Hawthorn should be avoided because it may cause additive hypotensive effects.

Treatment of Overdose: The most likely sign of overdosage is hypotension, which may be treated with a vasopressor and/or an IV infusion of fluids.

In some cases, the patient has abruptly discontinued use of prescribed antihypertensive medication. There are, however, a large number of possible secondary causes of HTN-E, including eclampsia or pre-eclampsia, head injuries, pheochromocytoma, substance abuse, and thyroid crisis.

Nitroprusside (Nitropress) is the traditional drug of choice for HTN-E. Nitroprusside, with a half-life of only 2 minutes, has the ability to lower blood pressure almost instantaneously on IV administration. Care must be taken not to decrease blood pressure too quickly, because overtreatment can result in hypotension and severe restriction of blood flow to the cerebral, coronary, or renal vascular capillaries. It is essential to continuously monitor patients receiving this drug because the drug is metabolized to cyanide (thiocyanate), which is very toxic to the body.

If blood pressure is significantly elevated but target organ damage has not yet developed, patients may be treated with oral antihypertensives because these have fewer adverse effects than nitroprusside. Oral drugs with a relatively rapid onset of action that may be used for hypertensive urgency include clonidine (Catapres), captopril (Capoten), furosemide (Lasix), or labetalol (Trandate).

Nursing Practice Application

Pharmacotherapy for Hypertension

ASSESSMENT	POTENTIAL NURSING DIAGNOSES*
Baseline assessment prior to administration: • Obtain a complete health history including cardiovascular (including MI, HF), renal, hepatic, musculoskeletal issues (pre-existing conditions that might result in fatigue, weakness, and muscle or joint pain), and the possibility of pregnancy. Obtain a drug history including allergies, current prescription and over-the-counter (OTC) drugs, herbal preparations, and alcohol use. Be alert to possible drug interactions. • Evaluate appropriate laboratory findings, electrolytes (especially potassium level), glucose, liver and renal function studies, and lipid profiles. • Obtain baseline weight, vital signs (especially blood pressure [BP] and pulse), breath sounds, pulse oximetry, and cardiac monitoring (e.g., ECG, cardiac output) if appropriate. Assess for location and character/amount of edema, if present.	• *Decreased Cardiac Output* • *Fatigue* • *Activity Intolerance,* related to adverse drug effects • *Impaired Tissue Perfusion,* related to adverse drug effects • *Sexual Dysfunction,* related to adverse drug effects • *Deficient Knowledge* (drug therapy) • *Risk for Falls,* related to adverse drug effects • *Risk for Injury,* related to adverse drug effects *NANDA I © 2014
Assessment throughout administration: • Assess for desired therapeutic effects (e.g., lowered BP within established limits; also lessened or absent angina and dysrhythmias if present). • Continue periodic monitoring of electrolytes, especially potassium. • Assess for adverse effects: nausea, headache, constipation, musculoskeletal fatigue or weakness, flushing, dizziness, or sexual dysfunction. For patients on ACE inhibitors or ARBs, angioedema, especially involving the facial area, should be immediately reported. For patients on CCBs, myalgia, arthralgia, peripheral or facial edema, significant constipation, inability to maintain activities of daily living (ADLs) due to musculoskeletal weakness or pain, and unexplained numbness or tingling of extremities should be reported immediately to the health care provider. For all antihypertensive drugs, immediately report bradycardia, hypotension, reflex tachycardia, decreased urinary output, severe hypotension, or seizures.	

IMPLEMENTATION

Interventions and (Rationales)	Patient-Centered Care
Ensuring therapeutic effects: • Continue frequent assessments as described earlier for therapeutic effects. (BP and pulse should be within normal limits or within parameters set by the health care provider. If the drug is given for angina and/or dysrhythmias, significant improvement in reports of pain, palpitations, or ECG demonstrates improvement.)	• Teach the patient, family, or caregiver how to monitor pulse and BP. Ensure proper use and functioning of any home equipment obtained.
Minimizing adverse effects: • Continue to monitor vital signs. Take BP lying, sitting, and standing to detect orthostatic hypotension. **Lifespan:** Be cautious with the older adult who is at increased risk for hypotension. (Vasodilation caused by some antihypertensive drugs may result in lowered BP. Orthostatic hypotension may increase the risk of falls and injury.)	• **Safety:** Teach the patient to rise slowly from lying or sitting to standing to avoid dizziness or falls. If dizziness occurs, the patient should sit or lie down and not attempt to stand or walk until the sensation passes. • Instruct the patient to stop taking the medication if BP is 90/60 mmHg or below (or according to parameters set by the health care provider) and promptly notify the provider.

Nursing Practice Application *continued*

IMPLEMENTATION	
Interventions and (Rationales)	**Patient-Centered Care**
• Continue to monitor periodic electrolyte levels (especially potassium), glucose, and ECG as appropriate, and hepatic and renal function laboratories. (Hypokalemia may increase the risk of dysrhythmias. Adrenergic blocking drugs may change the way a hypoglycemic reaction is perceived.)	• Instruct the patient on the need to return periodically for laboratory work or ECGs. • Advise the patient to carry a wallet identification card or wear medical identification jewelry indicating antihypertensive therapy. • Teach patients with diabetes to monitor blood glucose more frequently during early therapy to detect hypoglycemia and to be aware of subtle symptoms that hypoglycemia may be occurring (e.g., nervousness, irritability).
• **Safety and Lifespan:** Ensure patient safety, especially in the older adult. Give the first dose at bedtime and observe for excessive daytime drowsiness. Observe for dizziness and monitor ambulation. (Dizziness from orthostatic hypotension may occur. Many antihypertensives have a first-dose effect with a greater initial drop in BP than subsequent doses. Some adrenergic blocking drugs may cause excessive drowsiness.)	• **Safety:** Instruct the patient to call for assistance prior to getting out of bed or attempting to walk alone, and to avoid driving or other activities requiring mental alertness or physical coordination until the effects of the drug are known.
• Weigh the patient daily and report weight gain or loss of 1 kg (2 lb) or more in a 24-hour period. (Daily weight is an accurate measure of fluid status and takes into account intake, output, and insensible losses.)	• Have the patient weigh self daily, ideally at the same time of day, and record weight along with BP and pulse measurements. Have the patient report weight loss or gain of more than 1 kg (2 lb) in a 24-hour period.
• Observe for a paradoxical increase in chest pain or angina symptoms. (Severe hypotension may cause this and may indicate that BP has decreased too quickly or too substantially.)	• Instruct the patient to immediately report chest pain or other angina-like symptoms, especially if symptoms increase.
• Monitor for signs of HF, such as an increasing dyspnea or postural nocturnal dyspnea, rales or "crackles" in lungs, or frothy pink-tinged sputum. (CCBs and adrenergic blockers may decrease myocardial contractility, increasing the risk of HF.)	• Instruct the patient to immediately report any severe shortness of breath, frothy sputum, profound fatigue, or swelling of extremities as possible signs of HF.
• Assess the patient's mental status and mood. (Adrenergic blockers may cause depression or dysphoria.)	• Encourage the patient to report any unusual feelings of sadness, apathy, despondency, or depression.
• Observe for constipation. (CCBs may cause constipation due to decreased peristalsis.)	• Instruct the patient to increase fluid and fiber intake to facilitate stool passage. • If constipation persists, consider the use of a stool softener or laxative as recommended by the health care provider.
• Provide for eye comfort such as adequately lighted room. (Adrenergic blockers may cause miosis and difficulty seeing in low-light levels.)	• **Safety:** Caution the patient about driving or other activities in low-light conditions until effects of the drug are known.
• Monitor IV sites frequently. (Extravasation of vasoactive drugs may cause localized tissue injury.)	• Instruct the patient to report any burning or stinging pain, swelling, warmth, redness, or tenderness at the IV insertion site.
• Do not abruptly discontinue medication. (Rebound HTN and tachycardia may occur.)	• **Safety:** Teach the patient not to stop medication abruptly and to call the health care provider if unable to take the medication for more than one day due to illness.
Patient understanding of drug therapy:	
• Use opportunities during the administration of medications and during assessments to provide patient education. (Using time during nursing care helps to optimize and reinforce key teaching areas.)	• The patient should be able to state the reason for the drug, appropriate dose, and scheduling; what adverse effects to observe for and when to report; and the anticipated length of medication therapy.
Patient self-administration of drug therapy:	
• When administering the medication, instruct the patient and/or family in proper self-administration of the drug. (Proper administration improves the effectiveness of the drug.)	• The patient should be able to discuss appropriate dosing and administration needs.

See Tables 26.3, 26.4, 26.5, 26.6, and 26.7 for a list of drugs to which these nursing actions apply. See also the Nursing Process Application in chapter 13 for adrenergic antagonists and the Nursing Process Application in chapter 24 for diuretics.

Chapter Review

KEY Concepts

The numbered key concepts provide a succinct summary of the important points from the corresponding numbered section within the chapter. If any of these points are not clear, refer to the numbered section within the chapter for review.

26.1 The three primary factors controlling blood pressure are cardiac output, peripheral resistance, and blood volume.

26.2 Many factors help regulate blood pressure, including the vasomotor center; baroreceptors and chemoreceptors in the aorta and internal carotid arteries; and the renin–angiotensin system.

26.3 High blood pressure is classified as primary (idiopathic or essential) or secondary. Uncontrolled hypertension can lead to chronic and debilitating disorders such as stroke, heart attack, and heart failure.

26.4 Because antihypertensive medications may have adverse effects, lifestyle changes such as proper diet and exercise should be implemented prior to pharmacotherapy to attempt to prevent or slow development of hypertension and during pharmacotherapy to allow lower drug doses.

26.5 Pharmacotherapy of HTN often begins with low doses of a single medication. If this medication proves ineffective, a second drug from a different class may be added to the regimen.

26.6 Diuretics are first-line medications for HTN because they have few adverse effects and can effectively control minor to moderate hypertension.

26.7 Blocking the renin–angiotensin-aldosterone system prevents the intense vasoconstriction caused by angiotensin II. These drugs also decrease blood volume, which enhances their antihypertensive effect.

26.8 Calcium channel blockers (CCBs) block calcium ions from entering cells and cause smooth muscle in arterioles to relax, thus reducing blood pressure. CCBs have emerged as major drugs in the treatment of HTN.

26.9 Antihypertensive autonomic drugs are available that block alpha$_1$-adrenergic receptors, block beta$_1$- and/or beta$_2$-adrenergic receptors, or stimulate alpha$_2$-adrenergic receptors in the brainstem (centrally acting).

26.10 A few medications lower blood pressure by acting directly to relax arteriolar smooth muscle. However, these are not widely used due to their numerous adverse effects.

REVIEW Questions

1. The patient has been given a prescription of furosemide (Lasix) as an adjunct to treatment of hypertension and returns for a follow-up check. Which of the following is the most objective data for determining the therapeutic effectiveness of the furosemide?
   1. Absence of edema in lower extremities
   2. Weight loss of 13 kg (6 lb)
   3. Blood pressure log notes blood pressure 120/70 mmHg to 134/88 mmHg since discharge
   4. Frequency of voiding of at least six times per day

2. Nifedipine (Procardia) has been ordered for a patient with hypertension. In the care plan, the nurse includes the need to monitor for which adverse effect?
   1. Rash and chills
   2. Reflex tachycardia
   3. Increased urinary output
   4. Weight loss

3. The patient is taking atenolol (Tenormin) and doxazosin (Cardura). What is the rationale for combining two antihypertensive drugs?
   1. The blood pressure will decrease faster.
   2. Lower doses of both drugs may be given with fewer adverse effects.
   3. There is less daily medication dosing.
   4. Combination therapy will treat the patient's other medical conditions.
4. What health teaching should the nurse provide for the patient receiving nadolol (Corgard)?
   1. Increase fluids and fiber to prevent constipation.
   2. Report a weight gain of 1 kg per month or more.
   3. Immediately stop taking the medication if sexual dysfunction occurs.
   4. Rise slowly after prolonged periods of sitting or lying down.
5. The nurse is preparing to administer the first dose of enalapril (Vasotec). Identify the potential adverse effects of this medication. (Select all that apply.)
   1. Reflex hypertension
   2. Hyperkalemia
   3. Persistent cough
   4. Angioedema
   5. Hypotension
6. A patient with significant hypertension unresponsive to other medications is given a prescription for hydralazine (Apresoline). An additional prescription of propranolol (Inderal) is also given to the patient. The patient inquires why two drugs are needed. What is the nurse's best response?
   1. Giving the two drugs together will lower the blood pressure even more than just one alone.
   2. The hydralazine may cause tachycardia and the propranolol will help keep the heart rate within normal limits.
   3. The propranolol is to prevent lupus erythematosus from developing.
   4. Direct-acting vasodilators such as hydralazine cause fluid retention and the propranolol will prevent excessive fluid buildup.

PATIENT-FOCUSED Case Study

Leo Marshall is a 72-year-old with a history of HTN, mild renal failure, and angina. He is on a low-sodium, low-protein diet and has been adhering to his treatment plan. He has been admitted to the short-stay surgical unit for a minor procedure and will stay overnight. His blood pressure prior to discharge is 106/84.

1. What blood pressure parameters are commonly used to determine whether an antihypertensive dose is given or not?
2. Should the nurse give the patient benazepril (Lotensin) as scheduled in the morning after surgery?
3. What other patient data or assessments should the nurse check?

CRITICAL THINKING Questions

1. A patient with diabetes is on atenolol (Tenormin) for HTN. Identify a teaching plan for this patient.
2. A patient is having a hypertensive crisis (230/130), and the blood pressure needs to be lowered. The patient has an IV drip of nitroprusside (Nitropress) initiated. How much would the nurse want to lower this patient's blood pressure? Identify three nursing interventions that are crucial when administering this medication.

Visit www.pearsonhighered.com/nursingresources for answers and rationales for all activities.

REFERENCES

Callisaya, M. L., Sharman, J. E., Close, J., Lord, S. R., & Srikanth, V. K. (2014). Greater daily defined dose of antihypertensive medication increases the risk of falls in older people–A population-based study. *Journal of the American Geriatrics Society, 62*, 1527–1533. doi:10.1111/jgs.12925

Dinicola, S., Cucina, A., Antonacci, D., & Bizzarri, M. (2014). Anticancer effects of grape seed extract on human cancers: A review. *Journal of Carcinogenesis & Mutagenesis S8*(005), 60–70. doi:10.4172/2157-2518.S8-005

Feringa, H. H., Laskey, D. A., Dickson, J. E., & Coleman, C. I. (2011). The effect of grape seed extract on cardiovascular risk markers: A meta-analysis of randomized controlled trials. *Journal of the American Dietetic Association, 111*, 1173–1181. doi:10.1016/j.jada.2011.05.015

Herdman, T. H., & Kamitsuru, S. (2014). *NANDA International nursing diagnoses: Definitions and classification, 2015–2017*. Oxford, United Kingdom: Wiley-Blackwell.

James, P. A., Oparil, S., Carter, B. L., Cushman, W. C., Dennison-Himmelfarb, C., Handler, J., . . . Ortiz, E. (2014). 2014 Evidence-based guideline for the management of high blood pressure in adults: Report from the panel members appointed to the Eighth Joint National Committee (JNC 8). *JAMA: The Journal of the American Medical Association, 311*, 507–520. doi:10.1001/jama.2013.284427

National Center for Complementary and Integrative Health. (2012). *Grape seed extract*. Retrieved from https://nccih.nih.gov/health/grapeseed/ataglance.htm

WHO Collaborating Centre for Drug Statistics Methodology (2009). *Daily defined dose: Definition and general considerations*. Retrieved from http://www.whocc.no/ddd/definition_and_general_considera/

SELECTED BIBLIOGRAPHY

Centers for Disease Control and Prevention. (2014). *High blood pressure facts*. Retrieved from http://www.cdc.gov/bloodpressure/facts.htm

Colbert, B. J., & Mason, B. J. (2012). *Integrated cardiopulmonary pharmacology* (3rd ed.). Upper Saddle River, NJ: Pearson.

De Simoni, A., Hardeman, W., Mant, J., Farmer, A. J., & Kinmonth, A. L. (2013). Trials to improve blood pressure through adherence to antihypertensives in stroke/TIA: Systematic review and meta-analysis. *Journal of the American Heart Association, 2*, e000251. doi:10.1161/JAHA.113.000251

Hill, M. N., Miller, N. H., DeGeest, S., Materson, B. J., Black, H. R., Izzo, J. L. . . . Weber, M. A. (2011). Adherence and persistence with taking medication to control high blood pressure. *Journal of the American Society of Hypertension, 5*, 56–63. doi:10.1016/j.jash.2011.01.001

Hopkins, C. (2015). *Management of hypertensive emergencies*. Retrieved from http://emedicine.medscape.com/article/1952052-overview#a2

Krakoff, L. R., Gillespie, R. L., Ferdinand, K. C., Fergus, I. V., Akinboboye, O., Williams, K. A., . . . & Pepine, C. J. (2014). 2014 hypertension recommendations from the Eighth Joint National Committee panel members raise concerns for elderly black and female populations. *Journal of the American College of Cardiology, 64*, 394–402. doi:10.1016/j.jacc.2014.06.014

Madhur, M.S. (2014). *Hypertension practice essentials*. Retrieved from http://emedicine.medscape.com/article/241381-overview

Ramos, A. P., & Varon, J. (2014). Current and newer agents for hypertensive emergencies. *Current Hypertension Reports, 16*(7), 450. doi:10.1007/s11906-014-0450-z

Touyz, R. M. (2011). Advancement in hypertension pathogenesis: Some new concepts. *Current Opinion in Nephrology and Hypertension, 20*, 105–106. doi:10.1097/MNH.0b013e328343f526

Turgut, F., Yesil, Y., Balogun, R. A., & Abdel-Rahman, E. M. (2013). Hypertension in the elderly: Unique challenges and management. *Clinics in Geriatric Medicine, 29*, 593–609. doi:10.1016/j.cger.2013.05.002

Williams, H. (2013). An update on hypertension for nurse prescribers. *Nurse Prescribing, 11*, 70–75. doi:10.12968/npre.2013.11.2.70

Chapter 27

Drugs for Heart Failure

Drugs at a Glance

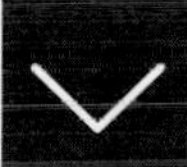

Learning Outcomes

After reading this chapter, the student should be able to:

1. Identify the major diseases that accelerate the progression of heart failure.
2. Relate how the symptoms associated with heart failure may be caused by weakened heart muscle and diminished cardiac output.
3. Explain how heart failure is classified.
4. Describe the nurse's role in the pharmacologic management of heart failure.
5. For each of the drug classes listed in Drugs at a Glance, know representative drug examples, and explain their mechanisms of action, primary actions, and important adverse effects.
6. Use the nursing process to care for patients who are receiving pharmacotherapy for heart failure.

indicates a prototype drug, each of which is featured in a Prototype Drug box.

Cardiovascular diseases are a group of disorders that include heart failure, coronary artery disease, stroke, deep vein thrombosis, peripheral artery disease, and congenital heart disease. Although there has been a dramatic decline in mortality from cardiovascular disease (CVD) over the past two decades, about 1 in 3 Americans die of CVD. This chapter examines the pharmacotherapy of heart failure, a condition that is associated with a significant decline in life expectancy. Historically, this condition was called congestive heart failure; however, because not all incidences of this disease are associated with congestion, the more appropriate name is heart failure.

PharmFacts

HEART FAILURE

- Heart failure (HF) affects 10% of those older than age 75.
- More than 277,000 deaths are caused by HF each year.
- Women tend to develop HF later in life than men.
- About 5.1 million Americans have HF.
- African Americans have one and a half to two times the incidence of HF as whites.
- About 50% of people who develop HF die within 5 years of diagnosis.

HEART FAILURE

27.1 The Etiology of Heart Failure

Heart failure (HF) is the inability of the ventricles to pump enough blood to meet the body's metabolic demands. HF can be caused by any disorder that affects the heart's ability to receive or eject blood. Although weakening of cardiac muscle is a natural consequence of aging, the process can be caused or accelerated by the following:

- Coronary artery disease (CAD)
- Mitral stenosis
- Myocardial infarction (MI)
- Chronic hypertension (HTN)
- Diabetes mellitus
- Hyperthyroidism or hypothyroidism.

Because there is no cure for HF, the treatment goals are to prevent or remove the underlying cause whenever possible and treat the symptoms of HF, so that the patient's quality of life can be improved. For many patients, HF is considered a preventable condition; controlling associated diseases will greatly reduce the risk of eventual HF. For example, controlling cholesterol levels and keeping blood pressure within normal limits reduces the incidences of CVD. Maintaining blood glucose within normal values reduces the cardiovascular consequences of uncontrolled diabetes. Therefore, the therapy of HF is no longer just focused on end stages of the disorder. Pharmacotherapy is now targeted at *prevention* and *slowing the progression* of HF. This change in emphasis has led to significant improvements in survival and the quality of life for patients with HF.

27.2 Cardiovascular Changes in Heart Failure

Although a number of diseases can lead to HF, the result is the same: The heart is unable to pump the volume of blood required to meet the metabolic needs of the body. To understand how medications act on the weakened myocardium, it is essential to understand the underlying cardiac physiology.

The right side of the heart receives blood from the venous system and pumps it to the lungs, where the blood receives oxygen and releases carbon dioxide. The blood returns to the left side of the heart, which pumps it to the rest of the body via the aorta. The amount of blood received by the right side should exactly equal that sent out by the left side. If the heart is unable to completely empty the left ventricle, HF may occur. The amount of blood pumped by each ventricle per minute is the **cardiac output.** The relationship between cardiac output and blood pressure is explained in chapter 26.

Although many variables affect cardiac output, the two most important factors are preload and afterload. Just before the chambers of the heart contract (systole), they are filled to their maximum capacity with blood. The degree to which the myocardial fibers are stretched just prior to contraction is called **preload.** The more these fibers are stretched, the more forcefully they will contract, a principle called the **Frank–Starling law.** This is somewhat similar to a rubber band; the more it is stretched, the more forcefully it will snap back. The strength of contraction of the heart is called **contractility.** Up to a physiological limit, drugs that increase preload and contractility will increase the cardiac output.

A change in contractility of the heart is called an **inotropic effect.** Drugs that increase contractility are called *positive inotropic agents.* Examples of positive inotropic drugs include epinephrine, norepinephrine, thyroid hormone, and dopamine. Drugs that decrease contractility are called *negative inotropic agents.* Examples include quinidine and beta-adrenergic antagonists such as propranolol.

The second important factor affecting cardiac output is **afterload,** the degree of pressure in the aorta that must be overcome for blood to be ejected from the left ventricle. As a simplified example, if the mean arterial pressure in the aorta is 80 mmHg, the left ventricle must generate a minimum of 81 mmHg to open the aortic valve, and even greater pressure to eject the blood from the ventricle and push along the pulse wave through the rest of the systemic circulation. The most common cause of increased afterload is an increase in peripheral resistance due to HTN. As blood pressure increases with HTN, the mean arterial pressure also increases, and the force the ventricle has to generate to eject the blood with each heartbeat increases. The greater afterload caused by chronic HTN creates a constant increased workload for the heart. This explains why patients with chronic HTN are more likely to experience HF. Lowering blood pressure creates less afterload, resulting in less workload for the heart.

In HF, the myocardium becomes weakened, and the heart cannot eject all the blood it receives. This impairment may occur on the left side, the right side, or both sides of the heart. If it occurs on the left side, excess blood accumulates in the left ventricle. The wall of the left ventricle thickens and enlarges (hypertrophy) in an attempt to compensate for the increased workload. Over time, changes in the size, shape, and structure of the myocardial cells (myocytes) occur, a process called **cardiac remodeling.** Myocytes are injured by the excessive workload and continually die; inflexible fibrotic tissue fills the spaces between the dead cells. Because the left ventricle has limits to its ability to compensate for the increased preload, blood "backs up" into the lungs, resulting in the classic symptoms of cough and shortness of breath. Left HF is sometimes called congestive heart failure (CHF). The pathophysiology of HF is shown in Figure 27.1.

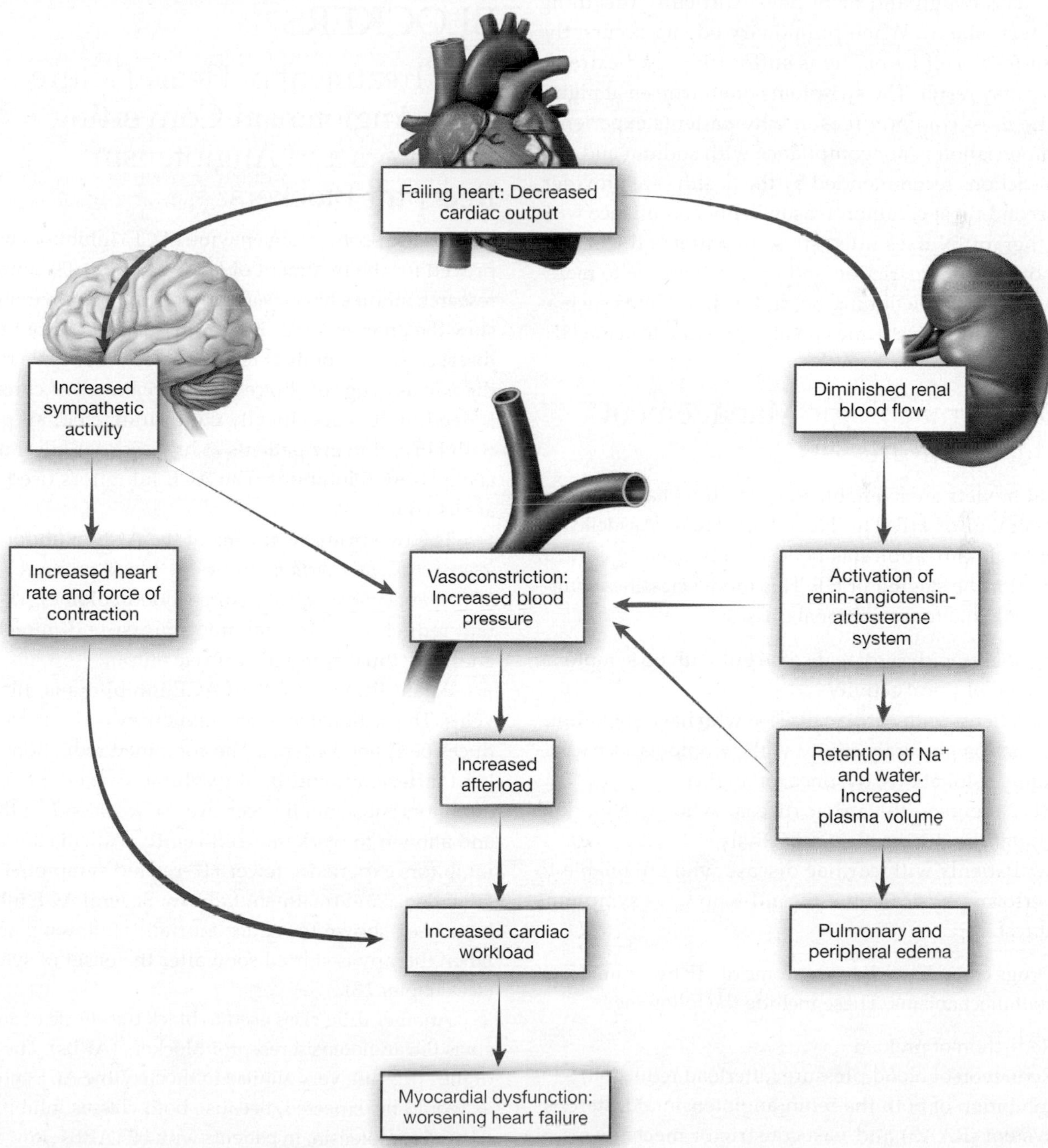

FIGURE 27.1 Pathophysiology of heart failure

Based on *Pharmacology: Connections to Nursing Practice* (3rd Ed.), by M. Adams and C. Urban, 2016. Reprinted and electronically reproduced by permission of Pearson Education, Inc., Upper Saddle River, New Jersey.

Although left HF is more common, the right side of the heart can also weaken, either simultaneously with the left side or independently. In right HF, the blood backs up into veins, resulting in **peripheral edema** and engorgement of organs such as the liver.

Through appropriate pharmacotherapy and lifestyle modifications, many patients with HF can be maintained in an asymptomatic state for years. When the heart reaches a stage at which it can no longer handle the workload, *cardiac decompensation* occurs and classic symptoms of HF appear such as dyspnea on exertion, fatigue, pulmonary congestion, and peripheral edema. Lung congestion causes cough and orthopnea (difficulty breathing when recumbent). When pulmonary edema occurs, the patient feels as if he or she is suffocating, and extreme anxiety may result. The symptoms often worsen at night.

The most common reason why patients experience decompensation is noncompliance with sodium and water restrictions recommended by the health care provider. The second most common reason is noncompliance with drug therapy. Nurses must stress to patients the importance of sodium restriction and drug adherence to maintain a properly functioning heart. Cardiac events such as MI or myocardial ischemia can also precipitate acute HF.

27.3 Pharmacologic Management of Heart Failure

Several models are available to guide the pharmacologic management of HF. The New York Heart Association (NYHA) classification has been widely used in clinical practice for the staging of HF. This model classifies symptomatic HF into four functional classes:

- I: Patients with cardiac disease but with no symptoms during physical activity
- II: Patients with cardiac disease who have slight limitations on physical activity, with symptoms such as fatigue, palpitations, dyspnea, or angina
- III: Patients with cardiac disease who have marked limitations during physical activity
- IV: Patients with cardiac disease who are unable to perform physical activity, and who have symptoms at rest.

Drugs can relieve the symptoms of HF by a number of different mechanisms. These include the following:

1. Reduction of preload
2. Reduction of blood pressure (afterload reduction)
3. Inhibition of both the renin-angiotensin-aldosterone-system (RAAS) and vasoconstrictor mechanisms of the sympathetic nervous system.

The first two mechanisms provide symptomatic relief but do not reverse the progression of the disease. Inhibition of the RAAS and vasoconstriction by the sympathetic nervous system can result in a significant reduction in morbidity and mortality from HF. These mechanisms are illustrated in Pharmacotherapy Illustrated 27.1.

ACE INHIBITORS AND ANGIOTENSIN RECEPTOR BLOCKERS

27.4 Treatment of Heart Failure With Angiotensin-Converting Inhibitors and Angiotensin Receptor Blockers

Angiotensin-converting enzyme (ACE) inhibitors were approved for the treatment of HTN in the 1980s. Since then, research studies have clearly demonstrated their ability to slow the progression of HF and reduce mortality from this disease. Because of their relative safety, they have replaced digoxin as drugs of choice for the treatment of chronic HF. Indeed, unless specifically contraindicated, all patients with HF and many patients at high risk for HF should receive an ACE inhibitor. The ACE inhibitors used for HF are listed in Table 27.1.

The two primary actions of the ACE inhibitors are to *lower peripheral resistance* (decrease blood pressure) and *inhibit aldosterone secretion* (reduce blood volume). The resultant reduction of arterial blood pressure diminishes the afterload, thus improving cardiac output.

An additional effect of ACE inhibitors is dilation of veins. This action decreases pulmonary congestion and reduces peripheral edema. The combined reductions in preload, afterload, and blood volume caused by the ACE inhibitors substantially decrease the workload on the heart and allow it to work more efficiently. Patients taking ACE inhibitors experience fewer HF-related symptoms, hospitalizations, and treatment failures. Several ACE inhibitors have been shown to reduce mortality following acute MI when therapy is started soon after the onset of symptoms (see chapter 28).

Another drug class used to block the effects of angiotensin is the angiotensin receptor blockers (ARBs). The actions of the ARBs are very similar to those of the ACE inhibitors, as would be expected, because both classes inhibit the actions of angiotensin. In patients with HF, ARBs show equivalent efficacy to the ACE inhibitors. Because they offer no

Pharmacotherapy Illustrated

27.1 | Mechanisms of Action of Drugs Used for Heart Failure

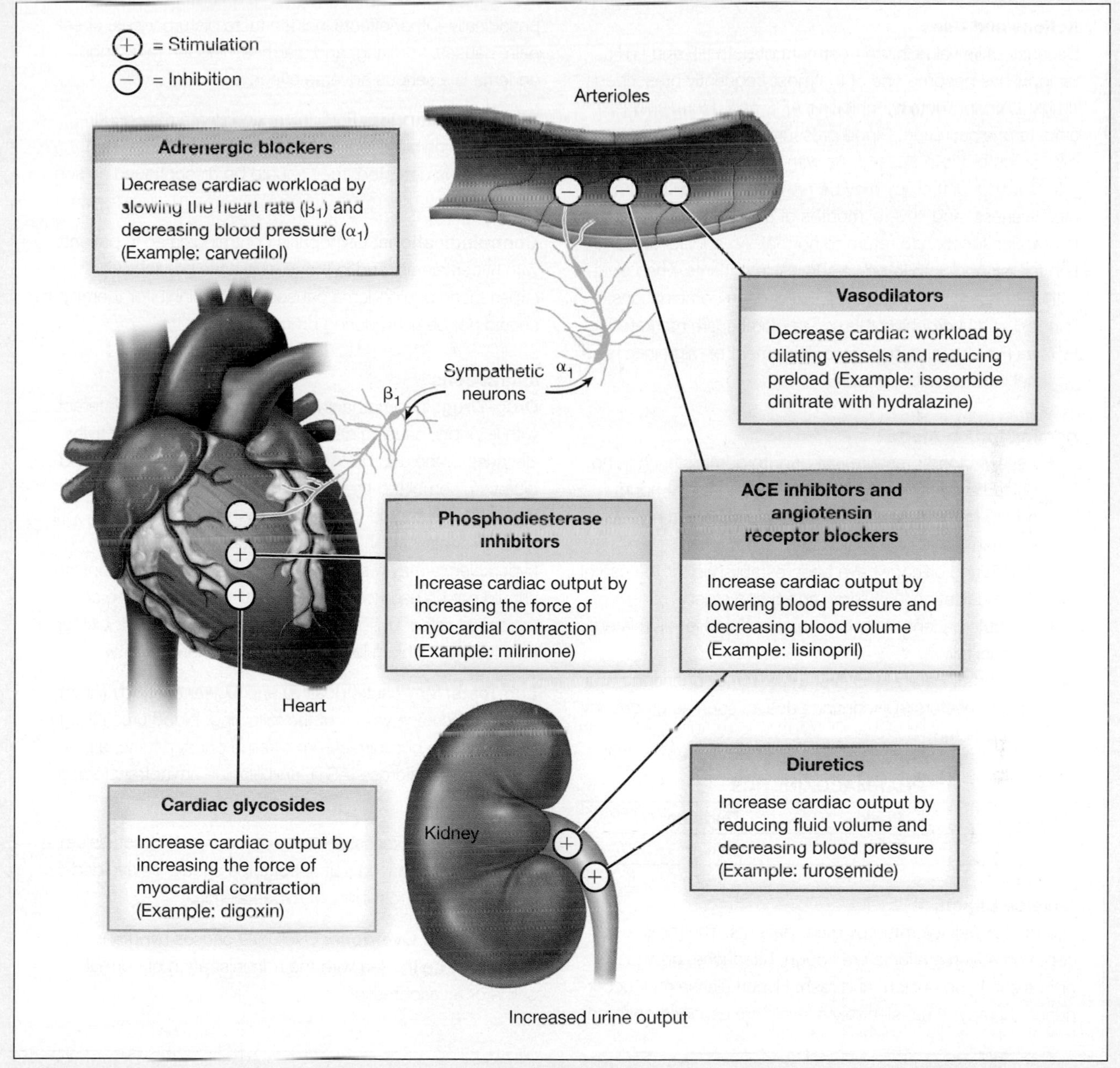

+ = Stimulation
− = Inhibition
Arterioles
Adrenergic blockers
Decrease cardiac workload by slowing the heart rate (β1) and decreasing blood pressure (α1) (Example: carvedilol)
Vasodilators
Decrease cardiac workload by dilating vessels and reducing preload (Example: isosorbide dinitrate with hydralazine)
Sympathetic neurons
β1
α1
Phosphodiesterase inhibitors
Increase cardiac output by increasing the force of myocardial contraction (Example: milrinone)
ACE inhibitors and angiotensin receptor blockers
Increase cardiac output by lowering blood pressure and decreasing blood volume (Example: lisinopril)
Heart
Diuretics
Increase cardiac output by reducing fluid volume and decreasing blood pressure (Example: furosemide)
Cardiac glycosides
Increase cardiac output by increasing the force of myocardial contraction (Example: digoxin)
Kidney
Increased urine output

clear advantage over ACE inhibitors, the use of ARBs in the treatment of HF is usually reserved for patients who are unable to tolerate the adverse effects of ACE inhibitors.

Refer to Nursing Practice Application: Pharmacotherapy for Hypertension in chapter 26, for additional information.

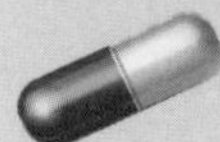

Prototype Drug | Lisinopril *(Prinivil, Zestril)*

Therapeutic Class: Drug for heart failure and HTN **Pharmacologic Class:** ACE inhibitor

Actions and Uses

Because of its value in the treatment of both HF and HTN, lisinopril has become one of the most frequently prescribed drugs. Lisinopril acts by inhibiting ACE and decreasing aldosterone secretion. Blood pressure is decreased and cardiac output is increased. As with other ACE inhibitors, 2 to 3 weeks of therapy may be required to reach maximum effectiveness, and several months of therapy may be needed for cardiac function to return to normal. An additional indication for lisinopril is to improve survival in patients when given within 24 hours of an acute MI. Fixed-dose combinations of lisinopril and hydrochlorothiazide (a diuretic) are marketed for HTN as Prinzide and Zestoretic. Treatment of migraines is an off-label indication for lisinopril.

Administration Alerts

- Assess blood pressure just prior to administering lisinopril to be certain that effects are lasting for 24 hours and to determine whether the patient's blood pressure is within the acceptable range.
- Safety and efficacy have been established for the use of this medication in children age 6 and older.
- Geriatric patients may have higher blood levels related to renal failure.
- Pregnancy category C (first trimester) or D (second and third trimesters). Discontinue use as soon as pregnancy is suspected.

PHARMACOKINETICS

Onset	Peak	Duration
1 h	6–8 h	24 h

Adverse Effects

Lisinopril is well tolerated by most patients. The most common adverse effects are cough, headache, dizziness, orthostatic hypotension, and rash. Hyperkalemia may occur during therapy; thus, electrolyte levels are usually monitored periodically. Other effects include taste disturbances, chest pain, nausea, vomiting, and diarrhea. Though rare, angioedema is a serious adverse effect.

Black Box Warning: Fetal injury and death may occur when ACE inhibitors are taken during pregnancy. When pregnancy is detected, they should be discontinued as soon as possible.

Contraindications: Lisinopril is contraindicated in patients with hyperkalemia and in those who have previously experienced angioedema caused by ACE inhibitor therapy. It should not be used during pregnancy.

Interactions

Drug–Drug: Indomethacin and other NSAIDs may interact with lisinopril, causing decreased antihypertensive activity. Because of the additive hypotensive action of lisinopril and diuretics, combined therapy with these or other antihypertensive drugs should be carefully monitored. When lisinopril is taken concurrently with potassium-sparing diuretics, hyperkalemia may result. Aliskirin (Tekturna), a renin inhibitor, should not be used concurrently with lisinopril due to an increased risk of hypotension and renal impairment. Lisinopril may increase lithium levels and cause lithium toxicity.

Lab Tests: May cause positive antinuclear antibody (ANA) titer and increase values of the following: blood urea nitrogen (BUN), serum bilirubin, serum alkaline phosphatase, aspartate aminotransferase (AST), and alanine aminotransferase (ALT).

Herbal/Food: Excessive intake of foods rich in potassium and potassium-based salt substitutes should be avoided because of the possibility of hyperkalemia.

Treatment of Overdose: Overdose causes hypotension, which may be treated with the administration of normal saline or a vasopressor.

DIURETICS

27.5 Treatment of Heart Failure With Diuretics

Diuretics are common drugs for the treatment of patients with HF because they produce few adverse effects and are effective at increasing urine flow and reducing blood volume, peripheral edema, and pulmonary congestion. When diuretics reduce fluid volume and lower blood pressure, the workload on the heart is reduced and cardiac output increases. Diuretics are rarely used alone but rather are prescribed in combination with ACE inhibitors or other HF drugs. Because clinical research has not demonstrated their effectiveness in slowing the progression of HF or in decreasing mortality associated with the disease, diuretics are indicated only when there is evidence of fluid retention. In patients presenting with fluid retention, especially with symptoms of severe pulmonary congestion or peripheral edema, diuretics are essential medications. Selected diuretics are listed in Table 27.1. Additional details on diuretics may be found in chapter 24.

Table 27.1 Drugs for Heart Failure

Drug	Route and Adult Dose (max dose where indicated)	Adverse Effects
ACE INHIBITORS AND ANGIOTENSIN RECEPTOR BLOCKERS		
candesartan (Atacand)	PO: 4 mg/day (max: 32 mg/day)	*Headache, dizziness, orthostatic hypotension, cough*
captopril (Capoten)	PO: 6.25–12.5 mg tid (max: 150 mg/day)	Severe hypotension (first dose phenomenon), syncope, angioedema, blood dyscrasias, angioedema, fetal toxicity
enalapril (Vasotec) (see page 384 for the Prototype Drug box)	PO: 2.5 mg qid–bid (max: 40 mg/day)	
fosinopril (Monopril)	PO: 5–40 mg/day (max: 40 mg/day)	
lisinopril (Prinivil, Zestril)	PO: 10 mg/day (max: 40 mg/day)	
quinapril (Accupril)	PO: 10–20 mg/day (max: 20 mg/day)	
ramipril (Altace)	PO: 2.5–5 mg bid (max: 10 mg/day)	
valsartan (Diovan)	PO: 40 mg bid (max: 320 mg/day)	
DIURETICS		
Loop or High Ceiling		Loop and thiazides:
bumetanide (Bumex)	PO: 0.5–2 mg/day (max: 10 mg/day)	*Electrolyte imbalances, orthostatic hypotension*
furosemide (Lasix) (see page 348 for the Prototype Drug box)	PO: 20–80 mg in one or more divided doses (max: 600 mg/day)	Severe hypotension, dehydration, hypokalemia, hyponatremia, ototoxicity (loop diuretics)
torsemide (Demadex)	PO: 10–20 mg/day (max: 200 mg/day)	
Thiazide and Thiazide-Like		
hydrochlorothiazide (Microzide) (see page 350 for the Prototype Drug box)	PO: 25–200 mg in a single dose or three divided doses (max: 200 mg/day)	
Potassium-Sparing (Aldosterone Antagonist)		Potassium-sparing: *Hyperkalemia, gynecomastia in males, fatigue*
eplerenone (Inspra)	PO: 25–50 mg once daily (max: 100 mg/day)	Dysrhythmias due to hyperkalemia
spironolactone (Aldactone) (see page 351 for the Prototype Drug box)	PO: 5–200 mg in divided doses (max: 200 mg/day)	
BETA-ADRENERGIC BLOCKERS		
carvedilol (Coreg)	PO: 3.125 mg bid for 2 wk (max: 25–50 mg bid)	*Fatigue, insomnia, drowsiness, impotence or decreased libido, bradycardia, confusion*
metoprolol extended release (Toprol-XL)	PO: 25 mg/day for 2 wk; 12.5 mg/day for severe cases (max: 200 mg/day)	Agranulocytosis, laryngospasm, Stevens–Johnson syndrome, anaphylaxis; if the drug is abruptly withdrawn, palpitations, rebound HTN, life-threatening dysrhythmias, or myocardial ischemia may occur
DIRECT VASODILATOR		
hydralazine with isosorbide dinitrate (BiDil)	PO: 1–2 tablets tid (each tablet contains 20 mg isosorbide dinitrate and 37.5 mg hydralazine) (max: 2 tablets/day)	*Headache, flushing of face, orthostatic hypotension, dizziness, reflex tachycardia* Fainting, severe headache, severe hypotension with overdose, lupus-like reaction (hydralazine)
nesiritide (Natrecor)	IV: 2 mcg/kg bolus followed by continuous infusion at 0.01 mcg/kg/min.	*Hypotension, increased serum creatinine, headache* Dysrhythmias
CARDIAC GLYCOSIDE		
digoxin (Lanoxin, Lanoxicaps)	PO: 0.125–0.5 mg/day	*Nausea, vomiting, headache, and visual disturbances such as seeing halos, a yellow-green tinge, or blurring* Dysrhythmias, atrioventricular block
PHOSPHODIESTERASE INHIBITORS		
inamrinone (Inocor)	IV: 0.75 mg/kg bolus given slowly over 2–3 min; then 5–10 mcg/kg/min (max: 10 mg/kg/day)	*Headache, hypotension* Dysrhythmias
milrinone (Primacor)	IV: 50 mcg over 10 min; then 0.375–0.75 mcg/kg/min	

Note: *Italics* indicate common adverse effects; underlining indicates serious adverse effects.

Of the diuretic classes, the loop diuretics such as furosemide are most commonly prescribed for HF because of their effectiveness in removing fluid from the body. Loop diuretics are also able to function in patients with renal impairment, an advantage for many patients with decompensated HF. Another major advantage in acute HF is that loop diuretics act quickly, especially IV formulations, which bring symptomatic relief to patients within minutes.

Thiazide diuretics are also used in the pharmacotherapy of HF. Because they are less effective than the loop diuretics, thiazides are generally reserved for patients with mild to moderate HF. They are sometimes combined with loop diuretics to achieve a more effective diuresis in patients with acute HF.

Potassium-sparing diuretics have limited roles in the treatment of HF because of their low efficacy. Spironolactone, however, is an exception. In addition to being a potassium-sparing diuretic, spironolactone is classified as an *aldosterone antagonist*. Clinical research has demonstrated that spironolactone blocks the deleterious effects of aldosterone on the heart. Spironolactone has been shown to decrease mortality due to sudden death as well as slow the progression to advanced HF.

Prototype features for furosemide, hydrochlorothiazide, and spironolactone are presented in chapter 24. Refer to Nursing Practice Application: Pharmacotherapy With Diuretics in chapter 24, for additional information.

CARDIAC GLYCOSIDES

27.6 Treatment of Heart Failure with Cardiac Glycosides

Once used as arrow poisons by African tribes and as medicines by the ancient Egyptians and Romans, the **cardiac glycosides** have been known to have value in treating heart disorders for over 2,000 years. Originally extracted from the beautiful flowering plants *Digitalis purpurea* (purple foxglove) and *Digitalis lanata* (white foxglove), drugs from this class are sometimes called digitalis glycosides. Until the discovery of ACE inhibitors, cardiac glycosides were the mainstay of HF treatment. Digoxin (Lanoxin) is the only drug in this class available in the United States. The routes and dose for digoxin are listed in Table 27.1.

The primary actions of digoxin are to cause the heart to beat more forcefully (positive inotropic effect) and more slowly, thus improving cardiac output. The reduced heart rate, combined with more forceful contractions, allows for much greater efficiency of the heart.

Although digoxin clearly produces symptomatic improvement in patients, it does not reduce mortality from HF. Because of the development of safer and more effective drugs such as ACE inhibitors, digoxin is now primarily used for more advanced stages of HF in combination with other medications.

The margin of safety between a therapeutic dose and a toxic dose of digoxin is narrow, and severe adverse effects may result from poorly monitored treatment. **Digitalization** refers to a procedure in which the dose of digoxin is gradually increased until tissues become saturated with the drug, and the symptoms of HF diminish. If the patient is critically ill, digitalization can be accomplished rapidly with intravenous (IV) doses in a controlled clinical environment in which potential adverse effects are carefully monitored. Patients who begin treatment outside the hospital may experience digitalization with digoxin over a period of 7 days, using oral (PO) dosing. In either case, the goal is to determine the proper dose of drug that may be administered without undue adverse effects. Frequent serum digoxin levels should be obtained during therapy, and the dosage should be adjusted based on the laboratory results and the patient's clinical response.

Check Your Understanding 27.1

Positive inotropic drugs increase the force of contraction of the heart muscle, improving cardiac output. What effects might a *negative* inotropic drug have in HF? *Visit www.pearsonhighered.com/nursingresources for answer.*

BETA-ADRENEGIC BLOCKERS (ANTAGONISTS)

27.7 Treatment of Heart Failure With Beta-Adrenergic Blockers (Antagonists)

Cardiac glycosides and other drugs that produce a positive inotropic effect increase the strength of myocardial contraction and are often used to reverse symptoms of HF. It may seem surprising, then, to find beta-adrenergic blockers—drugs that exhibit a *negative* inotropic effect—prescribed for this disease. Although this class of drugs does indeed have the potential to worsen HF, they have become standard therapy for many patients with this chronic disorder. Only two beta blockers are approved for the treatment of HF—carvedilol (Coreg) and metoprolol extended release (Toprol-XL). The doses for these drugs are listed in Table 27.1.

Patients with HF have excessive activation of the sympathetic nervous system, which damages the heart and leads to progression of the disease. Beta-adrenergic antagonists block the cardiac actions of the sympathetic nervous system, thus slowing the heart rate and reducing blood

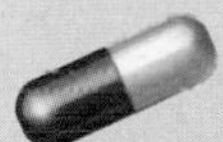

Prototype Drug | Digoxin *(Lanoxin, Lanoxicaps)*

Therapeutic Class: Drug for heart failure **Pharmacologic Class:** Cardiac glycoside

Actions and Uses

The primary benefit of digoxin is its ability to increase the contractility or strength of myocardial contraction—a positive inotropic action. Digoxin accomplishes this by inhibiting Na^+-K^+ ATPase, the critical enzyme responsible for pumping sodium ions out of the myocardial cell in exchange for potassium ions. As sodium accumulates, calcium ions are released from their storage areas in the cell. The release of calcium ions produces a more forceful contraction of the myocardial fibers.

By increasing myocardial contractility, digoxin directly increases cardiac output, thus alleviating symptoms of HF and improving exercise tolerance. The improved cardiac output results in increased urine production and a desirable reduction in blood volume, relieving distressing symptoms of pulmonary congestion and peripheral edema.

In addition to its positive inotropic effect, digoxin affects impulse conduction in the heart. Digoxin has the ability to suppress the sinoatrial (SA) node and slow electrical conduction through the atrioventricular (AV) node. Because of these actions, digoxin is sometimes used to treat dysrhythmias, as discussed in chapter 30.

Administration Alerts

- Take the apical pulse for 1 full minute, noting rate, rhythm, and quality before administering. If the pulse is below the parameter established by the health care provider (usually 60 beats per minute), withhold the dose and notify the provider.
- Check for recent serum digoxin level results before administering. If the level is higher than the parameter established by the health care provider (usually 1.8 ng/mL), withhold the dose and notify the provider.
- Use with caution in geriatric and pediatric patients because these populations may have inadequate renal and hepatic metabolic enzymes.
- Pregnancy category A.

PHARMACOKINETICS

Onset	Peak	Duration
30–60 min PO; 5–30 min IV	4–6 h PO; 1.5 h IV	6–8 days

Adverse Effects

The most dangerous adverse effect of digoxin is its ability to create dysrhythmias, particularly in patients who have hypokalemia or impaired renal function. Because diuretics can cause hypokalemia and are often used to treat HF, concurrent use of digoxin and diuretics must be carefully monitored. Other adverse effects of digoxin therapy include nausea, vomiting, fatigue, anorexia, and visual disturbances such as seeing halos, a yellow-green tinge, or blurring. Periodic serum drug levels should be obtained to determine whether the digoxin concentration is within the therapeutic range.

Contraindications: Patients with AV block or ventricular dysrhythmias unrelated to HF should not receive digoxin because the drug may worsen these conditions. Digoxin should be administered with caution to older adults because these patients experience a higher incidence of adverse effects. Patients with renal impairment should receive lower doses of digoxin, because the drug is excreted by this route. The drug should be used with caution in patients with MI, cor pulmonale, or hypothyroidism.

Interactions

Drug–Drug: Digoxin interacts with many drugs. Concurrent use of digoxin with diuretics can cause hypokalemia and increase the risk of dysrhythmias. Use with ACE inhibitors, spironolactone, or potassium supplements can lead to hyperkalemia and reduce the therapeutic action of digoxin. Administration of digoxin with other positive inotropic drugs can cause additive effects on heart contractility. Concurrent use with beta blockers may result in additive bradycardia. Antacids and cholesterol-lowering drugs can decrease the absorption of digoxin. If calcium is administered IV together with digoxin, it can increase the risk of dysrhythmias. Quinidine, verapamil, amiodarone, and alprazolam will decrease the distribution and excretion of digoxin, thus increasing the risk of digoxin toxicity.

Lab Tests: Unknown.

Herbal/Food: Ginseng may increase the risk of digoxin toxicity. Ma huang and ephedra may induce dysrhythmias.

Treatment of Overdose: Digoxin overdose can be fatal. Specific therapy involves IV infusion of digoxin immune fab (Digibind), which contains antibodies specific for digoxin.

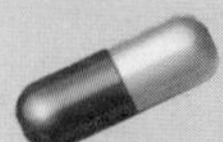

Prototype Drug | Metoprolol *(Lopressor, Toprol XL)*

Therapeutic Class: Drug for heart failure and HTN **Pharmacologic Class:** Beta-adrenergic blocker

Actions and Uses

Metoprolol is a selective $beta_1$-adrenergic blocker available in tablet, sustained-release tablet, and IV forms. At higher doses, it may also affect $beta_2$ receptors in bronchial smooth muscle. The drug acts by reducing sympathetic stimulation of the heart, thus decreasing cardiac workload. Metoprolol has been found to slow the progression of HF and to significantly reduce the long-term consequences of the disease. It is usually combined with other HF drugs such as ACE inhibitors. Metoprolol is also approved for angina, HTN, and for reducing cardiac complications following an MI.

Administration Alerts

- During IV administration, monitor the ECG, blood pressure, and pulse frequently.
- Assess the pulse and blood pressure before oral administration. Hold if the pulse is below 60 beats per minute or if the patient is hypotensive.
- Advise the patient not to crush or chew sustained-release tablets.
- Safety and efficacy in children under age 6 have not been established.
- Doses should be reduced for older patients because they are at risk for dizziness and falls.
- Pregnancy category C.

PHARMACOKINETICS

Onset	Peak	Duration
10–15 min; sustained release, unknown	1.5–4 h; 6–12 h sustained release	6 h (24 h sustained release)

Adverse Effects

Because it is selective for blocking $beta_1$ receptors in the heart, metoprolol has few adverse effects on other autonomic targets and thus is preferred over nonselective beta blockers such as propranolol for patients with respiratory disorders. Adverse effects are generally minor and relate to its autonomic activity, such as slowing of the heart rate and hypotension. Because of its multiple effects on the heart, patients with HF should be carefully monitored. Other frequent adverse effects include abnormal sexual function, drowsiness, fatigue, and insomnia.

Black Box Warning: Abrupt withdrawal is not advised in patients with angina or heart disease. Dosage should gradually be reduced over 1 to 2 weeks and the drug should be reinstituted if angina symptoms develop during this period.

Contraindications: This drug is contraindicated in patients with cardiogenic shock, sinus bradycardia, heart block greater than first degree, hypotension, and overt cardiac failure. Metoprolol should be used with caution in patients with asthma and those with a history of bronchospasm, because the drug may affect $beta_2$ receptors at high doses.

Interactions

Drug–Drug: Concurrent use with digoxin may result in bradycardia. Oral contraceptives may cause increased metoprolol effects. Use with alcohol or antihypertensives may result in additive hypotension. Metoprolol may enhance the hypoglycemic effects of insulin and oral hypoglycemic drugs. Concurrent use with verapamil increases the risk of heart block and bradycardia.

Lab Tests: Metoprolol may increase values for the following: uric acid, lipids, potassium, bilirubin, alkaline phosphatase, creatinine, and ANA.

Herbal/Food: Unknown.

Treatment of Overdose: Atropine or isoproterenol can be used to reverse bradycardia caused by metoprolol overdose. Hypotension may be reversed by a vasopressor such as parenteral dopamine or dobutamine.

pressure. Workload on the heart is decreased; after several months of therapy, heart size, shape, and function return to normal in some patients. Extensive clinical research has demonstrated that the proper use of beta blockers can dramatically reduce the number of HF-associated hospitalizations and deaths.

To benefit patients with HF beta blockers must be administered in a very specific manner. Initial doses must be 1/10 to 1/20 of the target dose. Doses are doubled every 2 to 4 weeks until the optimal dose is reached. If therapy is begun with too high a dose, or the dose is increased too rapidly, beta blockers can worsen HF. Beta blockers are rarely used as monotherapy for this disease, but instead are usually combined with other medications, especially ACE inhibitors.

A new drug was introduced in 2015 for patients in which beta blockers are contraindicated or when the maximum dose of the beta blocker fails to achieve therapeutic goals. Ivabradine (Corlanor) acts by a unique mechanism that slows ion (I_f) currents across the SA node, which slows the heart rate and reduces myocardial oxygen demand. The subscript "f" stands for "funny," so named because the original research determined this current had unusual properties, distinct from sodium, calcium, or potassium currents. Adverse effects include possible bradycardia, hypotension, and atrial fibrillation.

The basic pharmacology of the beta blockers is presented in chapter 13. Other uses of the beta-adrenergic blockers are discussed elsewhere in this text: for hypertension in chapter 26, for dysrhythmias in chapter 30, and for angina/MI in chapter 28.

Refer to Nursing Practice Application: Pharmacotherapy With Adrenergic Blockers in chapter 13 for additional information.

VASODILATORS

27.8 Treatment of Heart Failure With Vasodilators

The two primary drugs in this class, hydralazine (Apresoline) and isosorbide dinitrate (Isordil), act directly to relax blood vessels and lower blood pressure. Hydralazine acts on arterioles. It is an effective antihypertensive drug, although it is not a drug of first choice for this indication due to frequent side effects. Isosorbide dinitrate (Isordil) is an organic nitrate that acts on veins. The drug is not very effective as monotherapy, and tolerance to its actions develops with continued use.

Because the two drugs act synergistically, isosorbide dinitrate is combined with hydralazine in the treatment of HF. BiDil is a fixed-dose combination of 20 mg of isosorbide dinitrate with 37.5 mg of hydralazine. The high incidence of adverse effects, including reflex tachycardia and orthostatic hypotension, however, limits their use to patients who cannot tolerate ACE inhibitors. BiDil appears to be especially effective in treating HF in African American patients, who often exhibit resistance to standard therapies. Hydralazine is featured as a prototype drug in chapter 26. A third vasodilator used for HF is very different from hydralazine or isosorbide dinitrate. Nesiritide (Natrecor) is a small-peptide hormone, produced through recombinant DNA technology, that is structurally identical to human beta-type natriuretic peptide (hBNP). When HF occurs, the ventricles begin to secrete hBNP in response to the increased stretch on the ventricular walls. hBNP enhances diuresis and renal excretion of sodium.

In therapeutic doses, nesiritide causes vasodilation, which contributes to reduced preload. By reducing preload and afterload, the drug compensates for diminished cardiac function. The use of nesiritide is very limited because it can rapidly cause severe hypotension. The drug is given by IV infusion, and patients require continuous monitoring. It is approved only for patients with acute decompensated HF.

In 2015, the FDA approved Entresto, a combination drug containing valsartan and sacubitril. Sacubitril is a drug that increases the amount of atrial natriuretic peptide. Entresto is given PO.

Lifespan Considerations: Pediatric
Heart Failure in Children

Parents confronting a diagnosis of dilated cardiomyopathy (DCM) in their child must decide on treatment with the knowledge that 40% or more of children with DCM die or require heart transplantation within 5 years of diagnosis (Towbin et al., 2006). This fact has changed little over the past decade, despite newer treatment options (Rossano & Shaddy, 2014a). DCM is one of the most common causes of HF in children.

For adults with HF, there are well-established treatment algorithms although the cause of the condition is different than in children. Treatment algorithms have not been established for children to the extent that they have been for adults, and research is still ongoing. There are also differences in the way children respond to medications commonly used in adults. In an early, large, and randomized clinical trial assessing the use of carvedilol in children, no significant differences were noted between children treated with the drug and those who were not treated (Shaddy et al., 2007), despite the widespread and successful use of beta blockers in adults with HF. Since that time, much more has been discovered about the role that genetics plays in response to adrenergic blockers, not only by affecting the way a drug is metabolized, but also how it is used at the receptor site (Reddy et al., 2015; Rossano & Shaddy, 2014b). In a recent study, Molina et al. (2013) confirmed what had long been "conventional wisdom," that the diagnosis of DCM in late infancy and larger left ventricular size were predictors of disease progression and worsening condition. With the increase in knowledge about genetic risk markers, children with DCM may be able to receive earlier and more targeted drug therapy that will prevent or slow the progression of the disease.

PHOSPHODIESTERASE INHIBITORS AND OTHER INOTROPIC DRUGS

27.9 Treatment of Heart Failure With Phosphodiesterase Inhibitors and Other Inotropic Drugs

Advanced HF can be a medical emergency, and prompt, effective treatment is necessary to avoid organ failure or death. In addition to high doses of diuretics, use of positive inotropic drugs may be necessary. The two primary classes of inotropic agents used for decompensated HF are phosphodiesterase inhibitors and beta-adrenergic agonists.

In the 1980s, two drugs became available that block the enzyme **phosphodiesterase** in cardiac and smooth muscle. Blocking phosphodiesterase has the effect of increasing the amount of calcium available for myocardial contraction. The inhibition results in two main actions that benefit patients with HF: a positive inotropic action and vasodilation.

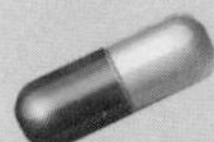

Prototype Drug | Milrinone *(Primacor)*

Therapeutic Class: Drug for heart failure **Pharmacologic Class:** Phosphodiesterase inhibitor

Actions and Uses

Of the two phosphodiesterase inhibitors available, milrinone is generally preferred because it has a shorter half-life and fewer side effects. It is given only IV and is primarily used for the short-term therapy of advanced HF. The drug has a rapid onset of action. Immediate effects of milrinone include an increased force of myocardial contraction and an increase in cardiac output.

Administration Alerts

- When this medication is administered IV, a microdrip set and an infusion pump should be used.
- Safety and efficacy have not been established in geriatric and pediatric patients.
- Pregnancy category C.

PHARMACOKINETICS

Onset	Peak	Duration
2–10 min	10 min	Variable

Adverse Effects

The most serious adverse effect of milrinone is ventricular dysrhythmia, which may occur in 1 of every 10 patients taking the drug. The patient's ECG should be monitored continuously during the infusion of the drug. Blood pressure is also continuously monitored during the infusion to prevent hypotension. Less serious side effects include headache, nausea, and vomiting.

Contraindications: The only contraindication to milrinone is previous hypersensitivity to the drug. Milrinone should be used with caution in patients with pre-existing dysrhythmias.

Interactions

Drug–Drug: Milrinone interacts with disopyramide, causing excessive hypotension. Caution should be used when administering milrinone with digoxin, dobutamine, or other inotropic drugs, because their positive inotropic effects on the heart may be additive.

Lab Tests: Unknown.

Herbal/Food: Unknown.

Treatment of Overdose: Overdose causes hypotension, which is treated with the administration of normal saline or a vasopressor.

Cardiac output is improved because of the increase in contractility and the decrease in left ventricular afterload. The phosphodiesterase inhibitors have a very brief half-life and are occasionally used for the short-term control of acute HF. The doses of these drugs are listed in Table 27.1. Prior to 2000, inamrinone was called amrinone. The name was changed to prevent medication errors: The name *amrinone* looked and sounded too similar to amiodarone, an antidysrhythmic drug.

Phosphodiesterase inhibitors have serious toxicity that limits their use to patients with resistant HF who have not responded to ACE inhibitors, digoxin, or other therapies. Therapy is limited to 2 to 3 days and the patient is continuously monitored for ventricular dysrhythmias. If the patient presents with hypokalemia, it should be corrected before administering phosphodiesterase inhibitors because it can increase the likelihood of dysrhythmias. These medications can also cause hypotension.

Complementary and Alternative Therapies

CARNITINE FOR HEART DISEASE

Carnitine is a natural substance structurally similar to amino acids. Its primary function in metabolism is to move fatty acids from the bloodstream into cells, where carnitine assists in the breakdown of lipids and the production of energy. The best food sources of carnitine are organ meats, fish, muscle meats, and milk products. Carnitine is available as a supplement in several forms, including L-carnitine, D-carnitine, and acetyl-L-carnitine. D-carnitine is associated with potential adverse effects and, therefore, should be avoided.

Carnitine has been claimed to enhance energy and sports performance, heart health, memory, immune function, and male fertility. It is sometimes marketed as a "fat burner" for weight reduction.

Carnitine has been extensively studied. There is solid evidence to support supplementation in patients who are deficient in carnitine. Although a normal diet supplies 300 mg per day, certain patients, such as vegetarians or those with heart disease, may need additional amounts. Carnitine supplementation has been shown to improve exercise tolerance in patients with angina. The use of carnitine may prevent the occurrence of dysrhythmias in the early stages of heart disease. Carnitine has also been shown to decrease triglyceride levels while increasing high-density lipoprotein (HDL) serum levels, thus helping to minimize one of the major risk factors associated with heart disease. Research has not shown carnitine supplementation to be of significant benefit in enhancing sports performance or weight loss.

Nursing Practice Application

Pharmacotherapy for Heart Failure

ASSESSMENT	POTENTIAL NURSING DIAGNOSES*
Baseline assessment prior to administration: • Obtain a complete health history including cardiovascular (including previous MI, HF, dysrhythmias, valvular disease), renal dysfunction, and pregnancy or lactation. Obtain a drug history including allergies, current prescription and over-the-counter (OTC) drugs, herbal preparations, and alcohol use. Be alert to possible drug interactions. • Obtain baseline weight, vital signs (especially pulse and blood pressure), breath sounds, and ECG. Assess for location and character of edema if present. • Evaluate appropriate laboratory findings; electrolytes, especially potassium level; renal function studies; and lipid profiles.	• *Decreased Cardiac Output* • *Excess Fluid Volume* • *Altered Tissue Perfusion* • *Fatigue* • *Activity Intolerance* • *Deficient Knowledge* (drug therapy) • *Risk for Reduced Cardiac Tissue Perfusion* • *Risk for Falls,* related to adverse drug effects • *Risk for Injury,* related to adverse drug effects *NANDA I © 2014
Assessment throughout administration: • Assess for desired therapeutic effects (e.g., heart rate and blood pressure return to, or remain within, normal limits; urine output returns to, or is within, normal limits; respiratory congestion (if present) is improved; peripheral edema (if present) is improved; level of consciousness, skin color, capillary refill, and other signs of adequate perfusion are within normal limits; fatigue lessens). • Continue periodic monitoring of electrolytes, especially potassium, renal function, and drug levels. • Assess for adverse effects: hypotension, bradycardia, nausea, vomiting, anorexia, visual changes, fatigue, dizziness, or drowsiness. A pulse rate below 60 or above 100, palpitations, significant dizziness or syncope, persistent anorexia or vomiting, or visual changes should be immediately reported to the health care provider. • **Lifespan:** Exercise caution when giving the drug to the older adult, pediatric patients, or patients with renal insufficiency. Immature or declines in renal function make these populations more susceptible to adverse effects.	

IMPLEMENTATION

Interventions and (Rationales)	Patient-Centered Care
Ensuring therapeutic effects: • Continue frequent assessments as described earlier for therapeutic effects. (Blood pressure and pulse should return to within normal limits or within parameters set by the provider; urine output returns to within normal limits; peripheral edema decreases; and lung sounds clear.)	• Teach the patient, family, or caregiver how to monitor pulse and blood pressure. Ensure the proper use and functioning of any home equipment obtained.
• **Collaboration:** Encourage appropriate lifestyle changes. Provide for dietitian consultation as needed. (Healthy lifestyle changes will support the benefits of drug therapy.)	• Encourage the patient to adopt a healthy lifestyle of low-fat food choices, increased exercise, decreased alcohol consumption, and smoking cessation. Provide educational materials on low-fat, low-sodium food choices. • Instruct the patient to increase intake of potassium rich foods such as bananas, apricots, kidney beans, sweet potatoes, and peanut butter.
Minimizing adverse effects: • Continue to monitor vital signs. Take an apical pulse for 1 full minute before giving the drug. Hold the drug and notify the provider if heart rate is below 60 or above 100. Monitor the ECG during infusion of milrinone or during the digitalization period for dysrhythmias and bradycardia. (Drugs that are positive inotropes increase myocardial contractility but may affect cardiac conduction. Milrinone is associated with serious and potentially life-threatening dysrhythmias. Digoxin slows the heart rate and may cause bradycardia.)	• Teach the patient, family, or caregiver how to take a peripheral pulse before taking the drug. Record daily pulse rates and bring the record to each health care visit. • Instruct patients receiving milrinone by infusion to immediately report any chest pain if it occurs.

continued

Nursing Practice Application *continued*

IMPLEMENTATION	
Interventions and (Rationales)	**Patient-Centered Care**
• Continue to monitor periodic electrolyte levels, especially potassium, renal function laboratories, drug levels, and ECG. (Hypokalemia increases the risk of dysrhythmias.)	• Instruct the patient on the need to return periodically for laboratory work. • Advise the patient to carry a wallet identification card or wear medical identification jewelry indicating drug therapy for HF.
• Weigh the patient daily and report a weight gain or loss of 1 kg (2 lb) or more in a 24-hour period. (Daily weight is an accurate measure of fluid status and takes into account intake, output, and insensible losses. Weight gain or edema may signal impending HF with reduced organ perfusion, stimulating renin release.)	• Have the patient weigh self daily, ideally at the same time of day, and record weight along with pulse measurements. Have the patient report a weight loss or gain of more than 1 kg (2 lb) in a 24-hour period.
• Monitor for signs of worsening HF (e.g., increasing dyspnea or postural nocturnal dyspnea, rales or "crackles" in the lungs, frothy pink-tinged sputum) and report immediately. (Positive inotropic drugs such as digoxin or phosphodiesterase inhibitors are usually reserved for patients with more advanced stages of HF. If signs and symptoms worsen, other treatment options may need to be considered.)	• Instruct the patient to immediately report any severe shortness of breath, frothy sputum, profound fatigue, or swelling of extremities as possible signs of HF.
• For patients taking digoxin, report signs of possible toxicity immediately to the provider and obtain a serum drug level. (Digoxin levels should remain less than 1.8 ng/mL. Signs and symptoms such as bradycardia, nausea and vomiting, anorexia, visual changes, depression or changes in level of consciousness, fatigue, dizziness, or syncope should be reported.) **Lifespan:** Digoxin is listed on the Beers list of potentially inappropriate drugs for the older adult and warrants careful monitoring. (Decreased excretion of digoxin and phosphodiesterase inhibitors due to age-related changes may increase the risk of adverse effects.)	• Instruct the patient or caregiver on signs to report to provider. Encourage the patient to promptly report any significant change in overall health or mental activity.
• **Lifespan:** Use extra caution when measuring the dose of medication ordered, and use extreme caution when measuring liquid doses, especially for pediatric patients. (For drugs such as digoxin with a long half-life and duration, toxic levels may result with only small amounts of additional drug.)	• Caution the patient on taking the precise dose of medication ordered, not doubling the dose if a dose is missed, and to use extreme caution when measuring liquid doses, especially for pediatric patients.
Patient understanding of drug therapy: • Use opportunities during administration of medications and during assessments to provide patient education. (Using time during nursing care helps to optimize and reinforce key teaching areas.)	• The patient should be able to state the reason for the drug; appropriate dose and scheduling; what adverse effects to observe for and when to report; and the anticipated length of medication therapy.
Patient self-administration of drug therapy: • When administering medications, instruct the patient, family, or caregiver in proper self-administration techniques. (Proper administration improves the effectiveness of the drug.)	• Instruct the patient in proper administration techniques, followed by teach-back. • The patient should be able to discuss appropriate dosing and administration needs. • The drug should be taken at the same time each day, and doses should not be skipped or doubled. • The brand of the drug prescribed should not be switched without consultation with the provider to ensure consistent effects.

See Table 27.1 for a list of drugs to which these nursing actions apply. See also the Nursing Practice Applications in chapter 13 for adrenergic antagonists and chapter 24 for diuretics.

Chapter Review

KEY Concepts

The numbered key concepts provide a succinct summary of the important points from the corresponding numbered section within the chapter. If any of these points are not clear, refer to the numbered section within the chapter for review.

27.1 Heart failure is closely associated with coronary artery disease, mitral stenosis, myocardial infarction, chronic HTN, diabetes mellitus, hyperthyroidism, and hypothyroidism.

27.2 The body attempts to compensate for HF by increasing cardiac output. Preload and afterload are two primary factors determining cardiac output.

27.3 Heart failure is often classified using the New York Heart Association (NYHA) model. This model classifies patients on the degree of physical limitation caused by the cardiac impairment.

27.4 ACE inhibitors reduce symptoms of HF by lowering blood pressure, reducing peripheral edema, and increasing cardiac output. They are drugs of choice for the treatment of HF. Use of ARBs is usually reserved for patients who cannot tolerate the adverse effects of ACE inhibitors.

27.5 Diuretics relieve symptoms of HF by reducing fluid overload and decreasing blood pressure.

27.6 Cardiac glycosides increase the force of myocardial contraction and were once drugs of choice for HF. Because of their narrow safety margin and the development of more effective drugs, their use has declined.

27.7 Beta-adrenergic blockers slow the heart rate and decrease blood pressure. They can dramatically reduce hospitalizations and increase the survival of patients with HF.

27.8 Vasodilators can relieve symptoms of HF by reducing preload and decreasing the cardiac workload.

27.9 Phosphodiesterase inhibitors and other inotropic drugs increase the force of myocardial contraction and improve cardiac output. They are used for the short-term therapy of acute HF.

REVIEW Questions

1. The patient is prescribed digoxin (Lanoxin) for treatment of HF. Which of the following statements by the patient indicates the need for further teaching?
   1. "I may notice my heart rate decrease."
   2. "I may feel tired during early treatment."
   3. "This drug should cure my heart failure."
   4. "My energy level should gradually improve."
2. The nurse reviews laboratory studies of a patient receiving digoxin (Lanoxin). Intervention by the nurse is required if the results include which of the following laboratory values?
   1. Serum digoxin level of 1.2 ng/dL
   2. Serum potassium level of 3 mEq/L
   3. Hemoglobin of 14.4 g/dL
   4. Serum sodium level of 140 mEq/L
3. A patient with heart failure has an order for lisinopril (Prinivil, Zestril). Which of the following conditions in the patient's history would lead the nurse to confirm the order with the provider?
   1. A history of hypertension previously treated with diuretic therapy
   2. A history of seasonal allergies currently treated with antihistamines
   3. A history of angioedema after taking enalapril (Vasotec)
   4. A history of alcoholism, currently abstaining

4. The teaching plan for a patient receiving hydralazine (Apresoline) should include which of the following points?
   1. Returning for monthly urinalysis testing
   2. Including citrus fruits, melons, and vegetables in the diet
   3. Decreasing potassium-rich food in the diet
   4. Rising slowly to standing from a lying or sitting position
5. Lisinopril (Prinivil) is part of the treatment regimen for a patient with heart failure. The nurse monitors the patient for the development of which of the following adverse effects of this drug? (Select all that apply.)
   1. Hyperkalemia
   2. Hypocalcemia
   3. Cough
   4. Dizziness
   5. Heartburn
6. The patient who has not responded well to other therapies has been prescribed milrinone (Primacor) for treatment of his heart failure. What essential assessment must the nurse make before starting this drug?
   1. Weight and presence of edema
   2. Dietary intake of sodium
   3. Electrolytes, especially potassium
   4. History of sleep patterns and presence of sleep apnea

PATIENT-FOCUSED Case Study

Juniata Meeks is a 62-year-old female who has a long history of Type 2 diabetes and HTN. She takes metformin (Glucophage) and occasional insulin injections for her diabetes, and has been taking chlorothiazide (Diuril) for HTN. She tells you, her nurse, that last month she suffered from a particularly "bad bout" of the flu and has been feeling extremely tired since that time. She has also noticed that her ankles have been swelling and she becomes "easily winded" doing her chores. In the health care provider's office, she is noted to have 1+ pitting ankle edema and has some fine crackles in the bases of her lungs bilaterally. She is started on lisinopril (Prinivil) for mild HF.

1. What is the drug classification of lisinopril (Prinvil) and why is it given in HF?
2. What other testing may be ordered for Ms. Meeks?
3. What teaching is important for this patient?

CRITICAL THINKING Questions

1. A patient is newly diagnosed with mild HF. The patient has been started on digoxin (Lanoxin). What objective evidence would indicate that this drug has been effective?
2. A 69-year-old patient has a sudden onset of acute pulmonary edema. The patient has no past cardiac history, is allergic to sulfa antibiotics, and routinely takes no medications. The health care provider orders furosemide (Lasix) to relieve the pulmonary congestion, along with digoxin (Lanoxin) to improve the patient's hemodynamic status. What interventions are essential in the care of this patient?

Visit www.pearsonhighered.com/nursingresources for answers and rationales for all activities.

REFERENCES

Herdman, T. H., and Kamitsuru, S. (2014). *NANDA International nursing diagnoses: Definitions and classification, 2015–2017*. Oxford, United Kingdom: Wiley-Blackwell

Molina, K. M., Shrader, P., Colan, S. D., Mital, S., Margossian, R., Sleeper, L. A., . . . Tani, L. Y. (2013). Predictors of disease progression in pediatric dilated cardiomyopathy. *Circulation: Heart Failure, 6*, 1214–1222. doi:10.1161/CIRCHEARTFAILURE.113.000125

Reddy, S., Fung, A., Manlhiot, C., Tierney, E. S., Chung, W. K., Blume, E., . . . Mital, S. (2015). Adrenergic receptor genotype influences heart failure severity and β-blocker response in children with dilated cardiomyopathy. *Pediatric Research, 77*, 363–369. doi:10.1038/pr.2014.183

Rossano, J. W., & Shaddy, R. E. (2014a). Heart failure in children: Etiology and treatment. *The Journal of Pediatrics, 165*, 228–233. doi:10.1016/j.jpeds. 2014.04.055

Rossano, J. W., & Shaddy, R. E. (2014b). Update on pharmacological heart failure therapies in children: Do adult medications work in children and if not, why not? *Circulation, 129*, 607–612. doi:10.1161/CIRCULATIONAHA.113.003615

Shaddy, R. E., Boucek, M. M., Hsu, D. T., Boucek, R. J., Canter, C. E., Mahony, L., . . . Tani, L. Y. (2007). Carvedilol for children and adolescents with heart failure: A randomized controlled trial. *JAMA, The Journal of the American Medical Association, 298*, 1171–1179. doi:10.1001/jama.298.10.1171

Towbin, J. A., Lowe, A. M., Colan, S. D., Sleeper, S. L., Orav, E. J, Clunie, S., . . . Lipshultz, S. E. (2006). Incidence, causes, and outcomes of dilated cardiomyopathy in children. *JAMA, 296*, 1867–1876. doi:10.1001/jama.296.15.1867

SELECTED BIBLIOGRAPHY

Al-Mohammad, A., & Mant, J. T. (2011). The diagnosis and management of chronic heart failure: Review following the publication of the NICE guidelines. *Heart, 97*, 411–416. doi:10.1136/hrt.2010.214999

Corotto, P. S., McCarey, M. M., Adams, S., Khazanie, P., & Whellan, D. J. (2013). Heart failure patient adherence: Epidemiology, cause, and treatment. *Heart Failure Clinics, 9*, 49–58. doi:10.1016/j.hfc.2012.09.004

Dumitru, I. (2014). *Heart failure*. Retrieved from http://emedicine.medscape.com/article/163062-overview

Go, A. S., Mozaffarian, D., Roger, V. L., Benjamin, E. J., Berry, J. D., Blaha, M. J., . . . Stroke, S. S. (2014). Executive summary: Heart disease and stroke statistics—2014 update: A report from the American Heart Association. *Circulation, 129*, 399. doi:10.1161/01.cir.0000442015.53336.12

Krum, H., & Driscoll, A. (2013). Management of heart failure. *The Medical Journal of Australia, 199*, 334–339. doi:10.5694/mja12.10993

Lam, C., & Smeltzer, S. C. (2013). Patterns of symptom recognition, interpretation, and response in heart failure patients: An integrative review. *Journal of Cardiovascular Nursing, 28*, 348–359. doi:10.1097/JCN.0b013e3182531cf7

Maron, B. A., & Rocco, T. P. (2011). Pharmacotherapy of congestive heart failure. In L. L. Brunton, B. A. Chabner, & B. C. Knollman (Eds.), *Goodman and Gilman's the pharmacological basis of therapeutics* (12th ed., pp. 789–814). New York, NY: McGraw-Hill.

Pahl, E., Sleeper, L. A., Canter, C. E., Hsu, D. T., Lu, M., Webber, S. A., . . . Lipshultz, S. E. (2012). Incidence of and risk factors for sudden cardiac death in children with dilated cardiomyopathy: A report from the Pediatric Cardiomyopathy Registry. *Journal of the American College of Cardiology, 59*, 607–615. doi:10.1016/jack.2011.10.878

Rich, M. W. (2012). Pharmacotherapy of heart failure in the elderly: Adverse events. *Heart Failure Reviews, 17*, 589–595. doi:10.1007/s10741-011-9263-1

Silva, J. N. A., & Canter, C. E. (2010). Current management of pediatric dilated cardiomyopathy. *Current Opinions in Cardiology, 25*, 80–87. doi:10.1097/HCO.0b013e328335b220

Stewart, S. (2013). What is the optimal place for heart failure treatment and care: Home or hospital? *Current Heart Failure Reports, 10*, 227–231. doi:10.1007/s11897-013-0144-x

Wakefield, B. J., Boren, S. A., Groves, P. S., & Conn, V. S. (2013). Heart failure care management programs: A review of study interventions and meta-analysis of outcomes. *Journal of Cardiovascular Nursing, 28*, 8–19. doi:10.1097/JCN.0b013e318239f9e1

Yancy, C. W., Jessup, M., Bozkurt, B., Butler, J., Casey, D. E., Jr., Drazner, M. H., . . . Wilkoff, B. L. (2013). 2013 ACCF/AHA guideline for the management of heart failure: A report of the American College of Cardiology Foundation/American Heart Association Task Force on Practice Guidelines. *Circulation, 128*, e240–e327. doi:10.1161/CIR.0b013e31829e8776

Chapter 28

Drugs for Angina Pectoris and Myocardial Infarction

Drugs at a Glance

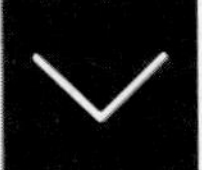

Learning Outcomes

After reading this chapter, the student should be able to:

1. Explain the pathogenesis of coronary artery disease.
2. Describe the signs and symptoms of angina pectoris.
3. Identify means by which angina may be managed without medications.
4. Explain mechanisms of drugs used to manage angina.
5. Identify the classes of drugs used to manage angina.
6. Describe the diagnosis of acute coronary syndrome.
7. Identify classes of drugs that are given to treat the symptoms and complications of myocardial infarction.
8. For each of the drug classes listed in Drugs at a Glance, know representative drug examples, and explain their mechanism of action, primary actions, and important adverse effects.
9. Use the nursing process to care for patients who are receiving pharmacotherapy for angina and myocardial infarction.

indicates a prototype drug, each of which is featured in a Prototype Drug box.

All tissues and organs of the body depend on a continuous arterial supply of oxygen and other vital nutrients to support life and health. With its high metabolic requirements, the heart is especially demanding of a steady source of oxygen. Should the blood supply to the myocardium become compromised, cardiovascular function may become impaired, resulting in angina pectoris, myocardial infarction (MI), and, possibly, death. This chapter focuses on the pharmacologic interventions related to angina pectoris and MI.

28.1 Pathogenesis of Coronary Artery Disease

The heart, from the moment it begins to function in utero until death, works to distribute oxygen and nutrients via its nonstop pumping action. It is the hardest working organ in the body, functioning continually during both activity and rest. Because the heart is a muscle, it needs a steady supply of nourishment to sustain itself and to maintain the systemic circulation in a balanced state of equilibrium. Any disturbance in blood flow to the vital organs or the myocardium itself—even for brief episodes—can result in life-threatening consequences.

The myocardium receives its blood supply via the right and left coronary arteries, which arise within the aortic sinuses at the base of the aorta. These arteries further diverge into smaller branches that encircle the heart.

Coronary artery disease (CAD), also called **coronary heart disease,** is a leading cause of death in the United States. The primary defining characteristic of CAD is narrowing or occlusion of a coronary artery. The narrowing deprives cells of needed oxygen and nutrients, a condition known as **myocardial ischemia.** If the ischemia develops over a long period, the heart may compensate for its inadequate blood supply, and the patient may experience no symptoms. Indeed, coronary arteries may be occluded 50% or more and cause no symptoms. As CAD progresses, however, the myocardium does not receive enough oxygen to meet the metabolic demands of the heart, and symptoms of angina begin to appear. Persistent myocardial ischemia may lead to myocardial infarction (heart attack).

The most common etiology of CAD in adults is **atherosclerosis,** the presence of **plaque**—a fatty, fibrous material within the walls of the coronary arteries. Plaque develops progressively over time, producing varying degrees of intravascular narrowing that limits the free flow of blood through the vessel. In addition, the plaque impairs normal vessel elasticity, and the coronary vessel is unable to dilate properly when the myocardium needs additional blood or oxygen, such as during periods of exercise. Plaque accumulation occurs gradually, over periods of 40 to 50 years in some individuals, but actually begins to accrue early in life. The development of atherosclerosis is illustrated in Figure 28.1.

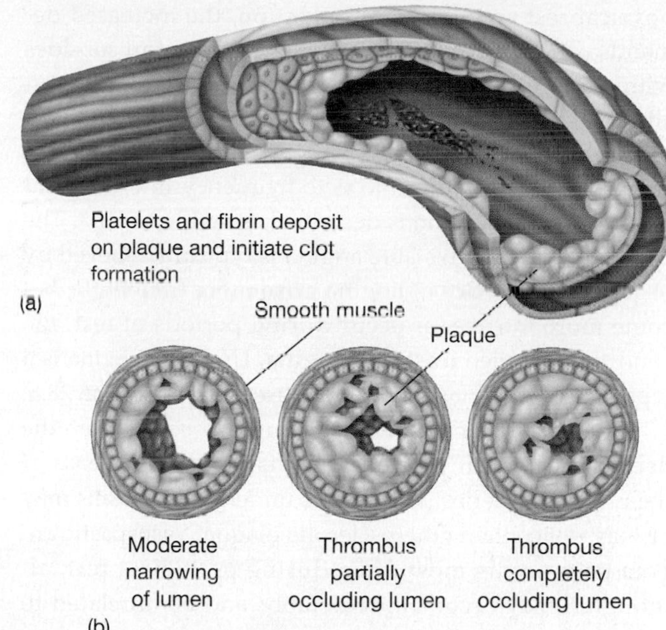

FIGURE 28.1 Atherosclerosis in the coronary arteries
Source: *Human Diseases: A Systemic Approach* (6th ed.), by M. L. Mulvihill, M. Zelman, P. Holdaway, E. Tompary, and J. Raymond, 2006. Reprinted and electronically produced by permission of Pearson Education, Inc., Upper Saddle River, NJ.

ANGINA PECTORIS

Angina pectoris is acute chest pain caused by insufficient oxygen to a portion of the myocardium. Nearly 10 million Americans have angina pectoris, with over 500,000 new cases occurring each year. It is most prevalent in those over 55 years of age.

28.2 Pathogenesis of Angina Pectoris

The classic presentation of angina pectoris is steady, intense pain in the anterior chest, sometimes accompanied by a crushing or constricting sensation. The discomfort may radiate to the left shoulder and proceed down the left arm and it may extend posterior to the thoracic spine or move upward to the jaw. In some patients, the pain is experienced in the mid-epigastric or abdominal area. Recent studies indicate that women do not always present with the classic symptoms of angina. In women, gastric distress, nausea and vomiting, a burning sensation in the chest or chest wall, overwhelming fatigue, and sweating may be more common symptoms. For most patients, the discomfort is accompanied by severe emotional distress—a feeling of panic with fear of impending death. There is usually pallor, dyspnea with cyanosis, diaphoresis, tachycardia, and elevated blood pressure.

Angina pain is usually preceded by physical exertion or emotional excitement—events associated with *increased myocardial oxygen demand*. Narrowed coronary arteries containing atherosclerotic deposits prevent the proper flow of oxygen and nutrients to the stressed cardiac muscle. With physical rest and/or stress reduction, the increased demands on the heart diminish, and the discomfort subsides within 5 to 10 minutes. Angina pectoris episodes are usually of short duration.

There are several types of angina. When angina occurrences are fairly predictable as to frequency, intensity, and duration, the condition is described as **stable angina.** The pain associated with stable angina is typically relieved by rest. When episodes of angina arise more frequently, become more intense, or occur during periods of rest, the condition is called **unstable angina.** Unstable angina is a type of acute coronary syndrome discussed in Section 28.8.

Vasospastic or **Prinzmetal's angina** occurs when the decreased myocardial blood flow is caused by *spasms* of the coronary arteries. The vessels undergoing spasms may or may not contain atherosclerotic plaque. Vasospastic angina pain occurs most often during periods of rest, although it may occur unpredictably, and be unrelated to rest or activity.

Silent angina is a form of the disease that occurs in the absence of chest pain. One or more coronary arteries are occluded, but the patient remains asymptomatic. Although the mechanisms underlying silent angina are not completely understood, the condition is associated with a high risk for acute MI and sudden death.

Angina pain closely resembles that of an MI. It is extremely important that the health care provider be able to accurately identify the characteristics that differentiate the two conditions, because the pharmacologic interventions related to angina differ considerably from those of MI. Angina, although painful and distressing, rarely leads to a fatal outcome, and the chest pain is usually immediately relieved by administering sublingual nitroglycerin. Myocardial infarction, however, carries a high mortality rate if appropriate treatment is delayed. Pharmacologic intervention must be initiated immediately and close patient follow-up must be maintained in the event of MI.

The nurse should understand that a number of conditions—many unrelated to cardiac pathology—may cause chest pain. These include gallstones, peptic ulcer disease, gastroesophageal reflux disease, biliary disease, pneumonia, musculoskeletal injuries, and certain cancers. When a person presents with chest pain, the foremost objective for the health care provider is to quickly determine the cause of the pain so that proper, effective interventions can be delivered.

28.3 Nonpharmacologic Management of Angina

A combination of variables influences the development and progression of CAD, including dietary patterns and lifestyle choices. The nurse is instrumental in teaching patients how to prevent CAD as well as how to reduce the recurrence of angina episodes. Such support includes the formulation of a comprehensive plan of care that incorporates psychosocial support and an individualized teaching plan. The patient needs to understand the causes of angina, identify the conditions and situations that trigger it, and develop motivation to modify behaviors associated with the disease.

Listing therapeutic lifestyle behaviors that modify the development and progression of cardiovascular disease (CVD) may seem repetitious because the student has encountered these same factors in chapters on hypertension, hyperlipidemia, and heart disease. However, the importance of prevention and management of CVD through nonpharmacologic means cannot be overemphasized. Practicing healthy lifestyle habits can *prevent* CAD in many individuals and *slow the progression* of the disease in those who have plaque buildup. The following factors have been shown to reduce the incidence of CAD:

- Limit alcohol consumption to small amounts.
- Eliminate foods high in cholesterol or saturated fats.
- Keep blood cholesterol and other lipid indicators within the normal ranges.
- Do not use tobacco.
- Keep blood pressure within the normal range.
- Exercise regularly and maintain optimal weight.
- Keep blood glucose levels within normal range.
- Limit salt (sodium) intake.

When the coronary arteries are significantly obstructed, **percutaneous coronary intervention (PCI)** is necessary. PCI may include atherectomy (removing the plaque) or angioplasty (compressing the plaque against the vessel wall). Because the artery may return to its original narrowed state after the procedure, a stent is often inserted following angioplasty. There are two different types of stents available, including bare metal stents (BMS) and drug-eluting stents (DES). Drug-eluting stents contain a

PharmFacts

PREVALENCE OF CARDIOVASCULAR DISEASE

- In every year since 1900 except 1918, CVD has accounted for more deaths than any other major cause of death in the United States.
- About 86 million Americans have CVD of which approximately half are 60 years of age or older.
- Over 8 million Americans have experienced anginal pain and about 7.6 million Americans have suffered at least one MI.
- By 2030, about 44% of the U.S. population is projected to have some form of CVD
- From 2001 to 2011, death rates attributable to CVD declined 30.8%.

Evidence-Based Practice: Sleep Duration and Angina

Clinical Question: Sleep apnea has been linked to vascular events such as stroke. Does the length of sleep (sleep duration) also play a role in cardiovascular disease?

Evidence: Recent clinical research suggests that not only sleep apnea, but the duration of sleep, may play a role in cardiovascular conditions, including angina. Several recent studies have noted an increased occurrence of angina and CVD, obesity, type 2 diabetes, hyperglycemia in pregnancy (gestational diabetes), and metabolic syndrome in patients who slept 6 hours or less, or more than 8 hours daily (Aggarwal, Loomba, Arora, & Molnar, 2013; Cooper, Westgate, Brage, Prevost, Griffin, & Simmons, 2014; Engeda, Mezuk, Ratliff, & Ning, 2013; Gutiérrez Repiso et al., 2014; Herring et al., 2014). The lowest occurrence seemed to be associated with between 6.5 and 7.5 hours of sleep (Aggarwal et al., 2013; Ohkuma et al., 2014). More research is needed to determine whether short- or long-duration sleep is a sign of CVD or whether it is a result of cardiovascular risk factors or other disease. In a recent study, Eguchi, Hoshide, Ishikawa, Shimada, & Kairo (2012) noted that the combination of short duration of sleep (less than 7.5 hours) and diabetes increased the risk of MI, stroke, and sudden death, more than having either diabetes or short duration of sleep alone. It has been postulated that sleep disturbances may be associated with derangements in endocrine or metabolic functions.

Nursing Implications: When taking the initial history and subsequent follow-up on a patient with known or suspected CVD, answers to questions about sleep duration or night-time awakening may be important data to gather. In addition, while nurses often teach patients to take antihypertensive medication at night to reduce the risk for dizziness and falls related to orthostatic hypotension, it may also be a strategy, even for once-daily medications, for reducing the occurrence of cardiovascular events.

medication such as sirolimus, everolimus, or paclitaxel, which inhibit tissue growth on the stent. Angioplasty with stenting typically relieves 90% of the original blockage in the artery.

Coronary artery bypass graft (CABG) surgery is reserved for severe cases of coronary obstruction that cannot be effectively removed by PCI. A portion of a vein from the leg or chest is used to create a "bypass artery." One end of the graft is sewn to the aorta and the other end to the coronary artery beyond the narrowed area. Blood from the aorta then flows through the new grafted vessel to the heart muscle, bypassing the blockage in the coronary artery. The result is increased blood flow to the heart muscle, which reduces angina and the risk of MI.

28.4 Pharmacologic Management of Angina

There are several desired therapeutic goals for a patient receiving pharmacotherapy for angina. A primary goal is to reduce the intensity and frequency of angina episodes. Additionally, successful pharmacotherapy should improve exercise tolerance and allow the patient to actively participate in activities of daily living. Long-term goals include extending the patient's life span by preventing serious consequences of ischemic heart disease such as dysrhythmias, heart failure, and MI. To be most effective, pharmacotherapy must be accompanied by therapeutic lifestyle changes that promote a healthy heart.

Although various drug classes are used to treat the disease, antianginal medications may be placed into two basic categories: those that *terminate* an acute angina episode in progress, and those that decrease the *frequency* of angina episodes. The primary means by which antianginal drugs accomplish these goals is to reduce the myocardial demand for oxygen. This may be accomplished by the following mechanisms:

- Slowing the heart rate
- Dilating veins so the heart receives less blood (reduced preload)
- Causing the heart to contract with less force (reduced contractility)
- Lowering blood pressure, thus offering the heart less resistance when ejecting blood from its chambers (reduced afterload).

The pharmacotherapy of angina consists of three primary classes of drugs: organic nitrates, beta-adrenergic antagonists, and calcium channel blockers (CCBs). Rapid-acting organic nitrates are drugs of choice for *terminating* an acute angina episode. Beta-adrenergic blockers are first-line drugs for preventing angina pain. Calcium channel blockers are used when beta blockers are not tolerated well by a patient. Long-acting nitrates, given by the oral (PO) or transdermal routes, are effective alternatives for prophylaxis. Persistent angina requires drugs from two or more classes, such as a beta-adrenergic blocker combined with a long-acting nitrate or CCB. Pharmacotherapy Illustrated 28.1 illustrates the mechanisms of action of drugs used to prevent and treat CAD.

Ranolazine (Ranexa) is a newer drug for angina that is believed to act by shifting the metabolism of cardiac muscle cells so that they use glucose as the primary energy source rather than fatty acids. This decreases the metabolic rate and oxygen demands of myocardial cells. Thus, this is the only antianginal that acts through its *metabolic* effects, rather than *hemodynamic* effects. Ranolazine does not change heart rate or blood pressure. The drug is well tolerated with dizziness, nausea, constipation, and headache being the most frequently reported adverse effects. It is

Pharmacotherapy Illustrated

28.1 | Mechanisms of Action of Drugs Used to Treat Angina

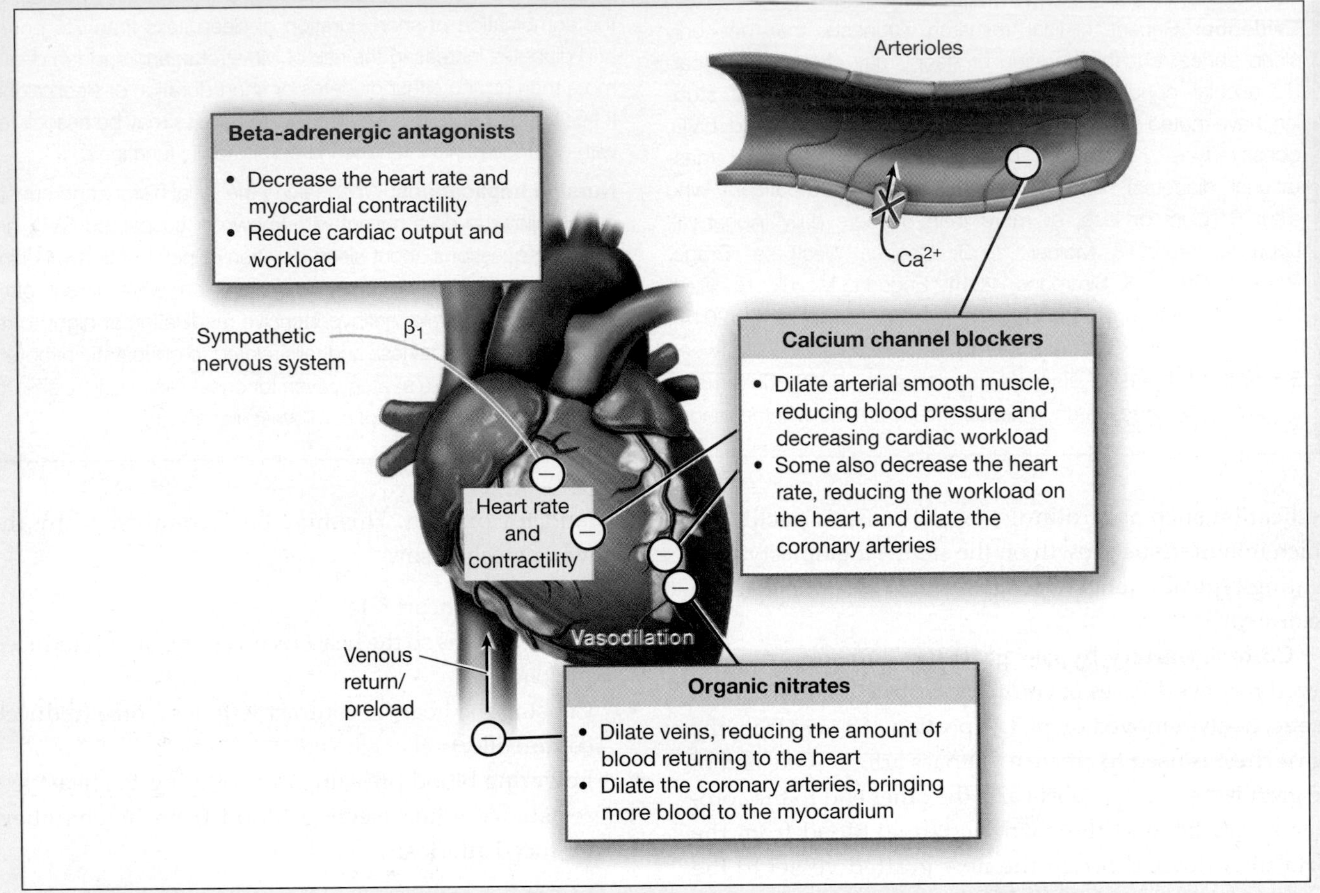

used to prevent anginal episodes. It will not terminate an acute attack. The drug is approved only for chronic angina that has not responded to other drugs, and it is usually prescribed concurrently with other antianginal drugs.

Cholesterol-lowering drugs such as the statins are often prescribed as a component of angina pharmacotherapy. Reduction of LDL-cholesterol in patients with CAD slows the progression of the disease, reduces the number of acute angina episodes, and lowers the incidence of MI. Pharmacotherapy with statins was presented in chapter 23.

ORGANIC NITRATES

After their medicinal properties were discovered in 1857, the organic nitrates became the mainstay for the treatment of angina for many decades. Their mechanism of action is the result of the formation of nitric acid, a potent vasodilator, in vascular smooth muscle.

28.5 Treating Angina With Organic Nitrates

The primary therapeutic action of the organic nitrates is their ability to relax both arterial and venous smooth muscle. Dilation of veins reduces the amount of blood returning to the heart (preload), so the chambers contain a smaller volume. With less blood for the ventricles to pump, cardiac output is reduced and the workload on the heart is decreased, thereby lowering myocardial oxygen demand. The therapeutic outcome is that chest pain is alleviated and episodes of angina become less frequent. The organic nitrates are shown in Table 28.1.

Organic nitrates also have the ability to dilate the coronary arteries, which was once thought to be their primary mechanism of action. It seems logical that dilating a partially occluded coronary artery would allow more oxygen to reach the ischemic tissue. Although this effect does indeed occur, it is no longer considered the primary mechanism of

Table 28.1 Selected Drugs for Angina and Myocardial Infarction

Drug	Route and Adult Dose (max dose where indicated)	Adverse Effects
ORGANIC NITRATES		
isosorbide dinitrate (Dilatrate SR, Isordil)	PO (regular release): 2.5–30 mg qid (max: 480 mg/day) PO (sustained release): 40 mg 2–4 times/day	*Headache, postural hypotension, flushing of face, dizziness, rash (transdermal patch), tolerance* Anaphylaxis, circulatory collapse due to hypotension, syncope due to orthostatic hypotension
isosorbide mononitrate (Imdur, Ismo, Monoket)	PO (regular release: ISMO, Monoket): 20 mg bid (max: 240 mg/day with sustained release) PO (sustained release: Imdur): 30–60 mg once daily	
nitroglycerin (Nitrostat, Nitro-Dur, Nitro-Bid, others)	SL: 1 tablet (0.3–0.6 mg) or 1–2 sprays (0.4–0.8 mg) every 3–5 min (max: three doses in 15 min) Transdermal: 1 patch daily (leave on for 12 hours, then remove for 12 hours)	
BETA-ADRENERGIC BLOCKERS		
atenolol (Tenormin)	PO: 25–50 mg/day (max: 100 mg/day)	*Fatigue, insomnia, drowsiness, impotence or decreased libido, bradycardia, confusion* Agranulocytosis, laryngospasm, Stevens–Johnson syndrome, anaphylaxis; if the drug is abruptly withdrawn, palpitations, rebound hypertension, life-threatening dysrhythmias, or MI may occur
metoprolol (Lopressor, Toprol XL) (see page 404 for the Prototype Drug box)	PO: 100 mg bid (max: 400 mg/day)	
nadolol (Corgard)	PO: 40 mg once daily (max: 240 mg/day)	
propranolol (Inderal, Innopran XL, Inderal LA) (see page 453 for the Prototype Drug box)	PO (immediate release): 10–20 mg bid–tid (max: 320 mg/day) PO (extended release): 80–160 mg/day (max: 320 mg/day)	
timolol (Betimol) (see page 871 for the Prototype Drug box)	PO (for MI): 10 mg once daily	
CALCIUM CHANNEL BLOCKERS		
amlodipine (Norvasc)	PO: 5–10 mg/day (max: 10 mg/day)	*Flushed skin, headache, dizziness, peripheral edema, light-headedness, nausea, constipation* Hepatotoxicity, MI, HF, confusion, mood changes
diltiazem (Cardizem, Cartia XT, Dilacor XR,others)	PO (regular release): 30 mg tid–qid (max: 480 mg/day) PO (extended release): 20–240 mg bid (max: 540 mg/day)	
nicardipine (Cardene)	PO: 20–40 mg tid or 30–60 mg SR bid (max: 120 mg/day)	
nifedipine (Adalat CC, Procardia XL, others) (see page 385 for the Prototype Drug box)	PO (regular release): 10–20 mg tid (max: 180 mg/day) PO (extended release): 30–60 mg/day	
verapamil (Calan, Covera-HS) (see page 456 for the Prototype Drug box)	PO: 80 mg tid–qid (max: 48 mg/day) PO (Covera-HS): 180–540 mg once daily at bedtime	
MISCELLANEOUS DRUGS		
ranolazine (Ranexa)	PO: 500–1000 mg bid (max: 2000 mg/day)	*Dizziness, headache, constipation, nausea* Prolongation of QT interval, bradycardia, palpitations, hypotension

Note: *Italics* indicate common adverse effects; underlining indicates serious adverse effects.

nitrate action in *stable* angina. This action, however, is crucial in treating *vasospastic* angina, in which the chest pain is caused by coronary artery spasm. The organic nitrates can relax these spasms, allowing more oxygen to reach the myocardium, thereby terminating the pain.

Organic nitrates are of two types, short acting and long acting. The short-acting nitrates, such as nitroglycerin, are taken sublingually to quickly terminate an acute angina episode. Long-acting nitrates, such as isosorbide dinitrate (Dilatate, Isordil), are taken orally or delivered through a transdermal patch to decrease the frequency and severity of angina episodes. Long-acting organic nitrates are also occasionally used to treat symptoms of heart failure, and their role in the treatment of this disease is discussed in chapter 26.

Tolerance is a common and potentially serious problem with the long-acting organic nitrates. The magnitude of the tolerance depends on the dosage and the frequency of drug administration. Although tolerance develops rapidly, after only 24 hours of therapy in some patients, it also disappears rapidly when the drug is withheld. Daily use of nitrates often warrants a nitrate-free interval. Transdermal patches should be removed for 6 to 12 hours a day and oral nitrates should only be dosed to cover a duration of 12 to 18 hours a day. Because the oxygen demands on the heart during sleep are diminished, the patient with stable angina experiences few angina episodes during this drug-free interval. The long-acting nitrates have not been shown to reduce mortality in patients with CAD; therefore, they are no longer considered first-line drugs for angina prophylaxis.

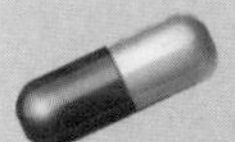

Prototype Drug | Nitroglycerin *(Nitrostat, Nitro-Bid, Nitro-Dur, others)*

Therapeutic Class: Antianginal drug **Pharmacologic Class:** Organic nitrate, vasodilator

Actions and Uses

Nitroglycerin, the oldest and most widely used organic nitrate, can be delivered by a number of different routes: sublingual, PO, intravenous (IV), transmucosal, transdermal, topical, and extended-release PO forms. It is taken while an acute angina episode is in progress or just prior to physical activity. When given sublingually, it reaches peak plasma levels in 2 to 4 minutes, thus terminating angina pain rapidly. Chest pain that does not respond within 10 to 15 minutes after a single dose of sublingual nitroglycerin may indicate MI, and emergency medical services (EMS) should be contacted. The transdermal and oral extended-release forms are for prophylaxis only because they have a relatively slow onset of action.

Administration Alerts

- For IV administration, use a glass IV bottle and special IV tubing because plastic absorbs nitrates significantly, thus reducing the patient dose.
- Cover the IV bottle to reduce the degradation of nitrates due to light exposure.
- Use gloves when applying nitroglycerin paste or ointment to prevent self-administration.
- Pregnancy category C.

PHARMACOKINETICS

Onset	Peak	Duration
1–3 min sublingual; 2–5 min buccal; 40–60 min transdermal patch; 15-30 min topical ointment	4–8 min sublingual; 4–10 min buccal; 1–2 h transdermal patch; topical ointment 1 h	30–60 min sublingual; 2 h buccal; 18–24 h transdermal patch; topical ointment 7 h

Adverse Effects

The adverse effects of nitroglycerin are usually cardiovascular in nature and rarely life threatening. Because nitroglycerin can dilate cerebral vessels, headache is a common side effect and may be severe. Occasionally, the venous dilation caused by nitroglycerin produces reflex tachycardia. Some health care providers prescribe a beta-adrenergic blocker to diminish this undesirable increase in heart rate. Many of the side effects of nitroglycerin diminish after a few doses.

Contraindications: Nitroglycerin should not be given to patients with pre-existing hypotension or with high intracranial pressure or head trauma. Drugs in this class are contraindicated in pericardial tamponade and constrictive pericarditis because the heart cannot increase cardiac output to maintain blood pressure when vasodilation occurs. Sustained-release forms should not be given to patients with glaucoma because they may increase intraocular pressure. Dehydration or hypovolemia should be corrected before nitroglycerin is administered; otherwise, serious hypotension may result.

Interactions

Drug–Drug: Concurrent use with phosphodiesterase-5 inhibitors such as sildenafil (Viagra), vardenafil (Levitra), or tadalafil (Cialis) may cause life-threatening hypotension and cardiovascular collapse. Use with alcohol and antihypertensive drugs may cause additive hypotension.

Lab Tests: Nitroglycerin may increase values of urinary catecholamines and vanillylmandelic acid (VMA) concentrations.

Herbal/Food: Use with hawthorn may result in additive hypotension.

Treatment of Overdose: Hypotension may be reversed with administration of IV normal saline. If methemoglobinemia is suspected, methylene blue may be administered.

BETA-ADRENERGIC BLOCKERS (ANTAGONISTS)

28.6 Treating Angina With Beta-Adrenergic Blockers

Beta-adrenergic antagonists or blockers reduce the cardiac workload by slowing the heart rate and reducing contractility. These drugs are as effective as the organic nitrates in decreasing the frequency and severity of angina episodes caused by exertion. Unlike the organic nitrates, tolerance does not develop to the antianginal effects of the beta blockers. They are ideal for patients who have both hypertension *and* CAD because of their antihypertensive action. They have been shown to reduce the incidence of MI.

Beta-adrenergic blockers are drugs of choice for the prophylaxis of stable angina. However, they are not effective for treating vasospastic angina and may, in fact, worsen this condition. The beta blockers used for angina are listed in Table 28.1. Beta blockers are widely used in medicine, and additional details may be found in chapters 13, 26, 27, and 30.

Refer to Nursing Practice Application: Pharmacotherapy With Adrenergic-Blockers in chapter 13 for additional information.

Nursing Practice Application

Pharmacotherapy With Organic Nitrates

ASSESSMENT	POTENTIAL NURSING DIAGNOSES*
Baseline assessment prior to administration: • Obtain a complete health history including cardiovascular (including previous MI, heart failure, valvular disease), cerebrovascular and neurologic (including level of consciousness, stroke, head injury, increased intracranial pressure), renal or hepatic dysfunction, dysrhythmias, and pregnancy or lactation. Obtain a drug history including allergies, current prescription and over-the-counter (OTC) drugs, herbal preparations, and alcohol use. Be aware that use of erectile dysfunction drugs (e.g., sildenafil [Viagra]) within the past 24 to 48 hours may cause profound and prolonged hypotension when nitrates are administered. Be alert to possible drug interactions. • Obtain baseline weight, vital signs (especially blood pressure [BP] and pulse), and ECG. Assess for location and character of angina if currently present. • Evaluate appropriate laboratory findings, electrolytes, renal function studies, and lipid profiles. Troponin and/or CK-MB laboratory values may be ordered to rule out MI.	• *Decreased Cardiac Output* • *Acute Pain* • *Fatigue* • *Activity Intolerance* • *Deficient Knowledge* (drug therapy) • *Risk for Decreased Cardiac Tissue Perfusion,* related to adverse drug effects • *Risk for Falls,* related to adverse drug effects • *Risk for Injury,* related to adverse drug effects *NANDA I © 2014
Assessment throughout administration: • Assess for desired therapeutic effects (e.g., chest pain has subsided or has significantly lessened), heart rate and BP remain within normal limits, and ECG remains within normal limits without signs of ischemia or infarction. • Continue periodic monitoring of ECG for ischemia or infarction.	
• Continue frequent monitoring of BP and pulse whenever IV nitrates are used or when giving rapid-acting (e.g., sublingual) nitrates. With sublingual nitrates, take BP before and 5 minutes after giving the dose. Hold the drug if BP is less than 90/60, pulse is over 100, or parameters as ordered, and consult with the health care provider before continuing to give the drug. • Assess for and promptly report adverse effects: excessive hypotension, dysrhythmias, reflex tachycardia (from too-rapid decrease in BP or significant hypotension), headache that does not subside within 15–20 minutes or when accompanied by neurologic changes, or decreased urinary output. Immediately report severe hypotension, seizures, or dysrhythmias. Chest pain that remains present after one sublingual nitroglycerin tablet is given should be reported immediately, even if the pain has lessened, because this may be a sign of an impending ischemia or infarction.	

IMPLEMENTATION

Interventions and (Rationales)	Patient-Centered Care
Ensuring therapeutic effects: • Continue frequent assessments as above for therapeutic effects. (Because nitrates cause vasodilation, preload and afterload diminish, decreasing myocardial oxygenation needs, and chest pain diminishes.)	• Ask the patient to briefly describe the location and character of pain (use a pain rating scale for rapid assessment) prior to and after giving nitrates to assess for the extent of relief. Correlate with objective findings. **Lifespan and Diverse Patients:** Due to differences in reporting pain, use subjective and objective data in evaluating pain relief in ethnically diverse and older adult patients.
• Continue to monitor ECG, BP, and pulse. (Nitrates cause vasodilation and possible hypotension. BP assessment aids in determining drug frequency and dose. ECG monitoring helps detect adverse effects such as reflex tachycardia, ischemia, or infarction.)	• Teach the patient, family, or caregiver how to monitor pulse and BP. Ensure the proper use and functioning of any home equipment obtained.

continued

Nursing Practice Application *continued*

IMPLEMENTATION	
Interventions and (Rationales)	**Patient-Centered Care**
• Evaluate the need for adjunctive treatment with the health care provider for angina prevention and treatment (e.g., beta blockers, aspirin therapy) or further cardiac studies. (Patients with unstable angina may require adjunctive drug therapy or definitive cardiac studies to determine the need for other treatment options.)	• Encourage the patient to discuss any changes in character, severity, or frequency of angina episodes with the provider. Instruct the patient not to take daily aspirin without discussing it with the health care provider first, because the drug may be contraindicated depending on other conditions or medications.
• For patients on transdermal nitroglycerin patches, remove the patch for 6–12 hours at night, or as directed by the health care provider. (Removing the patch at night helps to prevent or delay the development of tolerance to nitrates.)	• Instruct the patient on the proper use of nitroglycerin and rationale for removing transdermal patches. • Instruct the patient to always remove the old patch, cleanse the skin underneath gently, and to rotate sites before applying a new patch. Use hair-free areas of the torso to apply the patch, not on arms or legs. Increased muscle activity of the limbs may increase drug absorption.
• **Collaboration:** Encourage appropriate lifestyle changes. Provide for dietitian consultation as needed. (Healthy lifestyle changes will support the benefits of drug therapy.)	• Encourage the patient to adopt a healthy lifestyle of low-fat food choices, increased exercise, decreased alcohol consumption, and smoking cessation. Provide educational materials on low-fat, low-sodium food choices.
Minimizing adverse effects: • Continue to monitor vital signs frequently. **Lifespan:** Be cautious with older adults who are at increased risk for hypotension, patients with a pre-existing history of cardiac or cerebrovascular disease, or patients with a recent head injury, which may be worsened by vasodilation. Notify the health care provider immediately if the angina remains unrelieved or if BP or pulse decrease beyond established parameters, or if hypotension is accompanied by reflex tachycardia. (Nitrates may cause vasodilation, resulting in the potential for hypotension accompanied by reflex tachycardia. Reflex tachycardia increases myocardial oxygen demand, worsening angina.)	• Instruct the patient to report dizziness, faintness, palpitations, or headache unrelieved after taking nonnarcotic analgesics (e.g., acetaminophen). • **Safety:** Instruct the patient on nitrates to rise slowly from lying or sitting to standing to avoid dizziness or falls, especially if taking sublingual nitrates, or until the drug effects are known. If dizziness occurs, the patient should sit or lie down and not attempt to stand or walk until the sensation passes.
• Continue cardiac monitoring (e.g., ECG) if IV nitrates are administered. (Monitoring devices assist in detecting early signs of adverse effects of drug therapy and myocardial ischemia or infarction, as well as therapeutic effects.)	• To allay possible anxiety, teach the patient the rationale for all equipment used and the need for frequent monitoring.
• Continue frequent physical assessments, particularly neurologic, cardiac, and respiratory. Immediately report any changes in level of consciousness, headache, or changes in heart or lung sounds. (Nitrate therapy may worsen pre-existing neurologic, cardiac, or respiratory conditions as BP drops and perfusion to vital organs diminishes. Lung congestion may signal an impending heart failure.)	• When on PO therapy at home, instruct the patient to immediately report changes in mental status or level of consciousness, palpitations, dizziness, dyspnea, or increasing productive cough, especially if frothy sputum is present, and to seek medical attention.
• Review the medications taken by the patient before discharge, and review all prescription as well as OTC medications with the patient. Current use of erectile dysfunction drugs is contraindicated with nitrates. (Erectile dysfunction drugs lower BP and, when combined with nitrates, can result in severe and prolonged hypotension.)	• Instruct the patient to not take erectile dysfunction drugs (e.g., sildenafil [Viagra]) while taking nitrates and to discuss treatment options for erectile dysfunction with the health care provider.
Patient understanding of drug therapy: • Use opportunities during administration of medications and during assessments to provide patient education. (Using time during nursing care helps to optimize and reinforce key teaching areas.)	• The patient should be able to state the reason for the drug; appropriate dose and scheduling; what adverse effects to observe for and when to report; equipment needed as appropriate and how to use that equipment; and the required length of medication therapy needed with any special instructions regarding renewing or continuing the prescription as appropriate.

Nursing Practice Application *continued*

IMPLEMENTATION

Interventions and (Rationales)	Patient-Centered Care
Patient self-administration of drug therapy: • When administering medications, instruct the patient, family, or caregiver in proper self-administration of the drugs and when to contact the provider. (Proper administration increases the effectiveness of the drug.)	• The patient should be able to state how to use sublingual nitroglycerin at home: • Take one nitroglycerin tablet under the tongue for angina/chest pain. Remain seated or lie down to avoid dizziness or falls. • If chest pain continues call EMS. • If chest pain continues, even if reduced, do not take further nitroglycerin unless specifically directed by the health care provider. Call EMS system (e.g., 911) for assistance. Do *not* drive self to the emergency department. • If BP monitoring equipment is available at home, have the patient, family, or caregiver take BP after the first nitroglycerin dose. Hold the drug and contact EMS if BP is less than 90/60 mmHg. • Remind the patient to store SL nitroglycerin in its original container to protect from light degradation

See Table 28.1 for a list of the drugs to which these nursing actions apply.

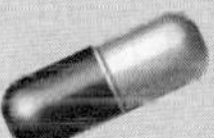

Prototype Drug | Atenolol *(Tenormin)*

Therapeutic Class: Antianginal drug **Pharmacologic Class:** Beta-adrenergic blocker

Actions and Uses

Atenolol is one of the most frequently prescribed drugs in the United States due to its relative safety and effectiveness in treating a number of chronic disorders, including heart failure, hypertension, angina, and MI. The drug selectively blocks $beta_1$-adrenergic receptors in the heart. Its effectiveness in treating angina is attributed to its ability to slow heart rate and reduce contractility, both of which lower myocardial oxygen demand. As with other beta blockers, therapy generally begins with low doses, which are gradually increased until the therapeutic effect is achieved. Because of its 7- to 9-hour half-life, it may be taken once daily.

Administration Alerts

- Blood pressure and pulse should be assessed before, during, and after the dose is administered.
- Assess pulse and blood pressure before oral administration. Hold if the pulse is below 60 beats per minute or if the patient is hypotensive.
- Pregnancy category D.

PHARMACOKINETICS

Onset	Peak	Duration
1 h	2–4 h	12–24 h

Adverse Effects

Being a cardioselective $beta_1$-adrenergic blocker, atenolol has few adverse effects on the lung. The most frequently reported adverse effects of atenolol include fatigue, weakness, bradycardia, and hypotension.

Black Box Warning: Abrupt discontinuation should be avoided in patients with ischemic heart disease; doses should be gradually reduced over a 1- to 2-week period. If angina worsens during the withdrawal period, the drug should be reinstituted.

Contraindications: Because atenolol slows heart rate, it should not be used in patients with severe bradycardia, atrioventricular (AV) heart block, cardiogenic shock, or decompensated HF. Due to its vasodilation effects, it is contraindicated in patients with severe hypotension.

Interactions

Drug–Drug: Concurrent use with CCBs may result in excessive cardiac suppression. Use with digoxin may slow AV conduction, leading to heart block. Concurrent use of atenolol with other antihypertensives may result in additive hypotension. Anticholinergics may cause decreased absorption from the gastrointestinal (GI) tract.

Lab Tests: Atenolol may increase values of the following blood tests: uric acid, lipids, potassium, creatinine, and antinuclear antibody.

Herbal/Food: Unknown.

Treatment of Overdose: The most serious symptoms of atenolol overdose are hypotension and bradycardia. Atropine or isoproterenol may be used to reverse bradycardia. Atenolol can be removed from the systemic circulation by hemodialysis.

CALCIUM CHANNEL BLOCKERS

28.7 Treating Angina With Calcium Channel Blockers

Blockade of calcium channels has a number of effects on the heart, most of which are similar to those of beta blockers. Like beta blockers, CCBs are used for a number of cardiovascular conditions, including hypertension (see chapter 26) and dysrhythmias (see chapter 30). The CCBs used for angina are shown in Table 28.1.

CCBs have several cardiovascular actions that benefit the patient with angina. Most important, CCBs relax arteriolar smooth muscle, thus lowering blood pressure. This reduction in afterload decreases myocardial oxygen demand. Some of the CCBs also slow conduction velocity through the heart, decreasing heart rate and contributing to the reduced cardiac workload. An additional effect of the CCBs is their ability to dilate the coronary arteries and bring more oxygen to the myocardium. This is especially important in patients with vasospastic angina. Because they are able to relieve the acute spasms of vasospastic angina, CCBs are preferred drugs for this condition. For stable angina, they are generally used in patients who are unable to tolerate beta blockers. In patients with persistent symptoms, CCBs may be combined with organic nitrates or beta blockers.

Refer to Nursing Practice Application: Pharmacotherapy With Antihypertensives in chapter 26 for the complete nursing process applied to patients receiving CCBs.

Check Your Understanding 28.1

Considering the three main classifications of drugs used to prevent or treat angina, what are the main mechanisms by which these drugs exert their effects? *Visit www.pearsonhighered.com/nursingresources for answers.*

MYOCARDIAL INFARCTION

Heart attacks or **myocardial infarctions (MIs)** are responsible for a substantial number of deaths each year. Some patients die before reaching a medical facility for treatment, and many others die within 48 hours following the initial MI. Clearly, MI is a serious and frightening disease and one responsible for a large percentage of sudden deaths.

28.8 Diagnosis of Acute Coronary Syndrome

An **acute coronary syndrome** is a collection of symptoms that occur when a coronary artery is suddenly blocked, usually by a piece of plaque that has broken off and occluded a portion of the coronary artery. Exposed plaque activates the coagulation cascade, resulting in platelet aggregation and adherence. A new clot quickly builds on the existing plaque, making obstruction of the vessel imminent.

The two primary types of acute coronary syndromes are unstable angina and MI. Both are caused by the same pathophysiology and have the same patient presentation. Early management of the two is the same. It is essential, however, for the health care provider to quickly distinguish the cause of the acute coronary syndrome because the medical intervention options differ.

Unstable angina gives the same extreme chest pain as MI. The thrombus causing the pain, however, has not completely occluded the coronary artery. Initial management should include MONA: morphine, oxygen, nitroglycerin, and high dose aspirin.

An MI occurs when a coronary artery becomes completely occluded. Deprived of its oxygen supply, the affected area of myocardium becomes ischemic, and myocytes begin to die in about 20 minutes unless the blood supply is quickly restored. Ischemia to the myocardial tissue, which may cause irreversible myocardial tissue necrosis, releases certain enzyme markers, which can be measured in the blood to confirm that the patient has experienced an MI versus unstable angina. Table 28.2 describes some of these important laboratory values.

An ECG can give important clues as to the extent and location of the MI. The infarcted region of the myocardium is nonconducting and usually produces abnormalities of Q waves, T waves, and S-T segments (see chapter 30). When the ST segment is elevated (STEMI), the MI must be treated aggressively because mortality is very high in this group of patients.

Refer to Nursing Practice Application: Pharmacotherapy With Thrombolytics in chapter 31 for the complete nursing process applied to patients receiving thrombolytic therapy.

Early diagnosis of MI and prompt initiation of pharmacotherapy can significantly reduce mortality and the long-term disability associated with MI. The pharmacologic goals for treating a patient with an acute MI are as follows:

- Restore blood supply (reperfusion) to the damaged myocardium as quickly as possible through the use of thrombolytics or PCI.
- Reduce myocardial oxygen demand with organic nitrates, beta blockers, or angiotensin-converting enzyme (ACE) inhibitors to prevent additional infarctions.
- Control or prevent MI-associated dysrhythmias with beta blockers or other antidysrhythmics.
- Reduce post-MI mortality with aspirin, beta blockers, and ACE inhibitors.
- Manage severe MI pain and associated anxiety with narcotic analgesics.
- Prevent enlargement of the thrombus with anticoagulants and antiplatelet drugs.

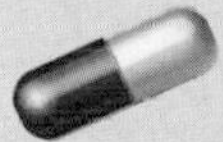

Prototype Drug | Diltiazem *(Cardizem, Cartia XT, Dilacor XR, others)*

Therapeutic Class: Antianginal drug **Pharmacologic Class:** Calcium channel blocker

Actions and Uses

Like other CCBs, diltiazem inhibits the transport of calcium into myocardial cells. It has the ability to relax both coronary and peripheral blood vessels, bringing more oxygen to the myocardium and reducing cardiac workload. It is useful in the treatment of atrial dysrhythmias and hypertension as well as stable and vasospastic angina. Diltiazem is available by the IV route and as immediate and extended-release PO forms. When given as sustained-release capsules, it is usually administered once daily.

Administration Alerts

- During IV administration, the patient must be continuously monitored, and cardioversion equipment must be available.
- Extended release tablets and capsules should not be crushed or split.
- Pregnancy category C.

PHARMACOKINETICS

Onset	Peak	Duration
30–60 min (immediate release); 2–3 h (extended release); IV: 3 min	2–3 h (immediate release); 6–11 h (extended release)	6–8 h (immediate release); 12 h (extended release); continuous infusion (after discontinuation): 0.5–10 h

Adverse Effects

Adverse effects of diltiazem are generally not serious and are related to vasodilation: headache, dizziness, and edema of the ankles and feet. Abrupt withdrawal may precipitate an acute anginal episode.

Contraindications: Diltiazem is contraindicated in patients with AV heart block, sick sinus syndrome, severe hypotension, bleeding aneurysm, or those undergoing intracranial surgery. This drug should be used with caution in patients with renal or hepatic impairment.

Interactions

Drug–Drug: Concurrent use of diltiazem with other cardiovascular drugs, particularly digoxin or beta-adrenergic blockers, may cause partial or complete heart block, heart failure, or dysrhythmias. Diltiazem may increase digoxin or quinidine levels when taken concurrently. Additive hypotension may occur if used with ethanol, beta blockers, or antihypertensives. Diltiazem and dantrolene should never be used in combination because cardiovascular collapse may result. Diltiazem is a moderate cytochrome p-450 3A4 inhibitor and may inhibit the metabolism of drugs that utilize this pathway.

Lab Tests: Unknown.

Herbal/Food: St. John's wort and ginseng may decrease the effectiveness of diltiazem. Garlic, hawthorn, and goldenseal may increase the antihypertensive effect of diltiazem.

Treatment of Overdose: Atropine or isoproterenol may be used to reverse bradycardia caused by diltiazem overdose. Hypotension may be reversed by a vasopressor such as dopamine or dobutamine. Calcium chloride can be administered by slow IV push to reverse hypotension or heart block induced by CCBs.

Table 28.2 Changes in Blood Test Values Following Acute Myocardial Infarction

Blood Test	Initial Elevation After MI	Peak Elevation After MI	Duration of Elevation	Normal Range
CK: Total creatine kinase (also called creatine phosphokinase)	3–8 h	12–24 h	2–4 days	Males: 5–35 mcg/L Females: 5–25 mcg/L
CK-MB	4–6 h	10–24 h	3–4 days	Greater than 3–5% of total CK
ESR (erythrocyte sedimentation rate)	2–3 days	4–5 days	Several weeks	Males: 15–20 mm/h Females: 20–30 mm/h
LDH: Total (lactate dehydrogenase)	12–42 h	2–5 days	6–12 days	70–250 units/L
Myoglobin	2–6 h	8–12 h	1–2 days	12–90 ng/mL
Troponin I	1–3 h	24–36 h	5–9 days	12–90 mcg/L
Troponin T	1–3 h	24–36 h	10–14 days	less than 0.2 mcg/L

THROMBOLYTICS

In treating MI, thrombolytic therapy is administered to dissolve clots obstructing the coronary arteries, thus restoring circulation to the myocardium. Dosages and descriptions of the various thrombolytics are given in chapter 31.

28.9 Treating Myocardial Infarction With Thrombolytics

Quick restoration of cardiac circulation (reperfusion) with thrombolytic therapy reduces mortality caused by acute MI. After the clot is successfully dissolved, anticoagulant therapy is initiated to prevent the formation of additional clots. Figure 28.2 illustrates the pathogenesis and treatment of MI.

Thrombolytics are most effective when administered from 20 minutes to 12 hours after the onset of MI symptoms. The American Heart Association recommends that a PCI be performed within 90 minutes after hospital arrival. If that is not possible, thrombolytics should be given within 30 minutes of arrival. If administered after 24 hours, the drugs are mostly ineffective. In addition, research has suggested that patients older than age 75 do not experience reduced mortality from these drugs. Because thrombolytic therapy is expensive and has the potential to produce serious adverse effects, it is important to identify circumstances that contribute to successful therapy. The development of clinical practice guidelines to identify those patients who benefit most from thrombolytic therapy is an ongoing process.

Thrombolytics have a narrow margin of safety between dissolving clots and producing serious adverse effects. Although therapy is usually targeted to a single thrombus in a specific artery, once infused in the blood, the drugs travel to all vessels and may cause adverse effects anywhere in the body. The primary risk of thrombolytics is excessive bleeding due to interference with the normal clotting process. Vital signs must be monitored continuously; signs of bleeding call for discontinuation of therapy. Because these drugs are rapidly destroyed in the blood, stopping the infusion normally results in the rapid termination of adverse effects.

ADJUNCT DRUGS FOR TREATMENT OF ACUTE MYOCARDIAL INFARCTION

28.10 Drugs for Symptoms and Complications of Acute Myocardial Infarction

The most immediate needs of the patient with MI are to ensure that the heart continues functioning and that permanent damage from the infarction is minimized. In addition to thrombolytic therapy to restore perfusion to the myocardium, drugs from several other classes are administered soon after the onset of symptoms to prevent reinfarction and, ultimately, to reduce mortality from the episode.

Antiplatelet and Anticoagulant Drugs

Unless contraindicated, 160 to 325 mg of aspirin is given as soon as an MI is suspected. Aspirin use in the weeks following an acute MI dramatically reduces mortality, probably due to its antiplatelet action. The low doses used in maintenance therapy (75–150 mg/day) rarely cause GI bleeding.

The adenosine diphosphate (ADP)–receptor blocker clopidogrel (Plavix), prasugrel (Effient), and ticagrelor (Brilinta) are effective antiplatelet medications approved to reduce the risk of reinfarction in patients with an MI. For high-risk patients, a loading dose of clopidogrel is administered as soon as the diagnosis of acute coronary syndrome is confirmed and prior to PCI. These agents are administered as a loading dose prior to PCI or fibrinolytic therapy and then maintenance therapy.

Glycoprotein IIb/IIIa inhibitors are antiplatelet drugs with a mechanism of action distinct from that of aspirin. These medications are sometimes indicated for unstable angina or MI, or for patients undergoing PCI. The agents include eptifibatide (Integrilin), abciximab (ReoPro), and tirofiban (Aggrestat). Infusion is usually initiated at the time of PCI and may be continued for several hours after.

On diagnosis of MI in the emergency department, patients are immediately placed on the anticoagulant heparin to prevent additional thrombi from forming. Heparin therapy is generally continued for 48 hours, or until PCI is completed. Refer to chapter 31 for a comparison of the different coagulation modifiers and the dosages for these medications.

Nitrates

The value of organic nitrates in treating angina is discussed in Section 28.5. Nitrates have additional uses in the patient with a suspected MI. At the initial onset of chest pain, sublingual nitroglycerin is administered to assist in the diagnosis. Pain that persists 5 to 10 minutes after the initial dose may indicate an MI, and the patient should seek immediate medical assistance.

Patients with persistent pain, heart failure, or severe hypertension may receive IV nitroglycerin for 24 hours following the onset of pain. The arterial and venous dilation produced by the drug reduces myocardial oxygen demand. Organic nitrates also relieve coronary artery vasospasm, which may be present during the acute stage of MI.

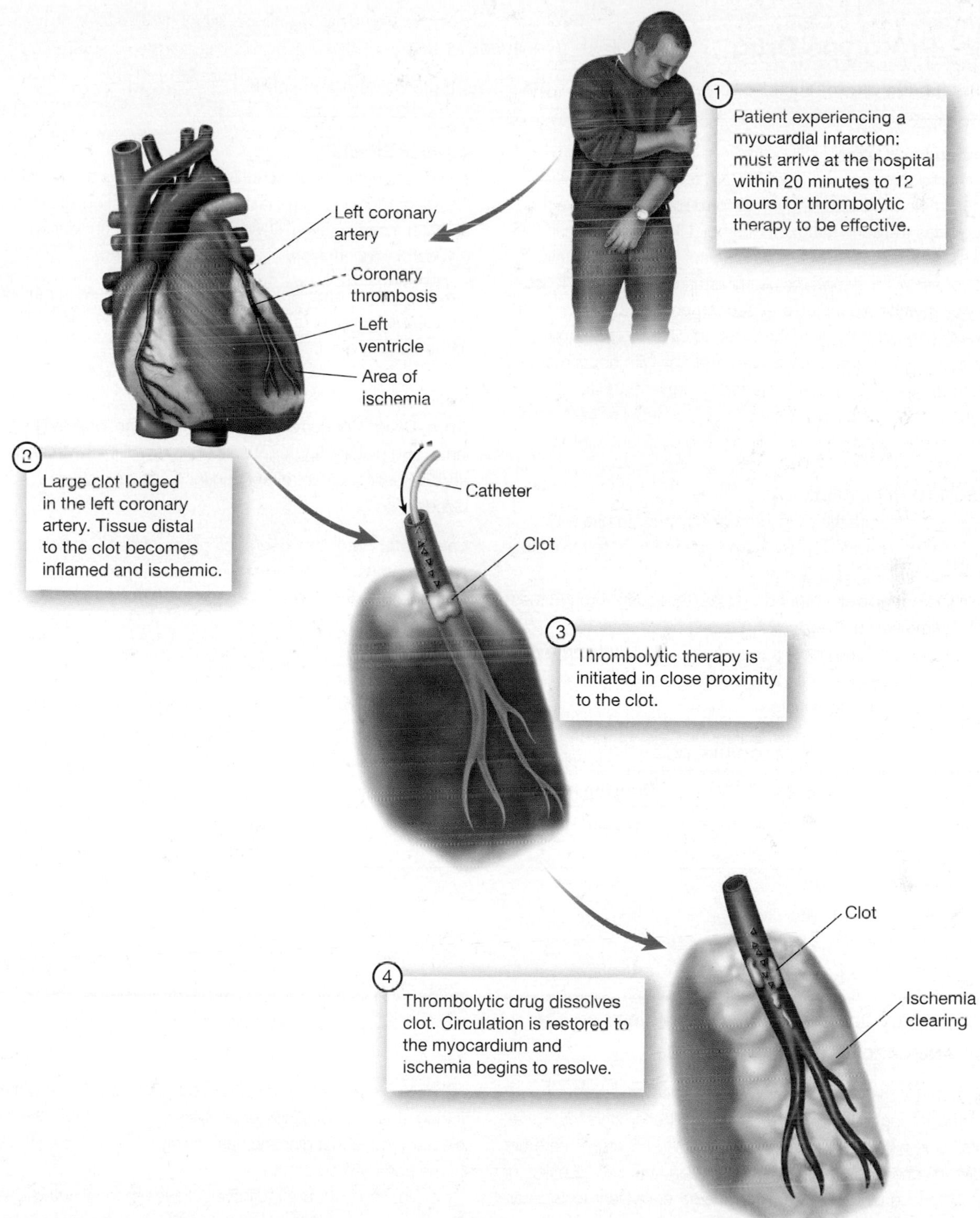

FIGURE 28.2 Blockage and reperfusion following myocardial infarction: (1) blockage of left coronary artery with myocardial ischemia; (2) infusion of thrombolytics; (3) blood supply returning to myocardium; (4) thrombus dissolving and ischemia clearing

On the patient's discharge from the hospital, organic nitrates are discontinued, unless they are needed for relief of stable angina pain.

Beta-Adrenergic Blockers

Beta blockers reduce myocardial oxygen demand, which is critical for patients experiencing a recent MI. In addition, they slow impulse conduction through the heart, thereby suppressing dysrhythmias, which are serious and sometimes fatal complications following an MI. Research has clearly demonstrated that beta blockers can reduce MI-associated mortality if they are administered within 8 hours of MI onset. These drugs may initially be administered IV in the hospital, and later switched to oral dosing

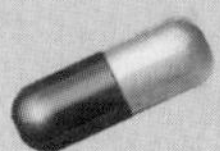

Prototype Drug | Reteplase *(Retavase)*

Therapeutic Class: Drug for dissolving blood clots **Pharmacologic Class:** Thrombolytic

Actions and Uses

Prepared through recombinant DNA technology, reteplase acts by cleaving plasminogen to form plasmin. Plasmin then degrades the fibrin matrix of thrombi. Like other drugs in this class, reteplase should be given as soon as possible after the onset of MI symptoms. Administered by IV bolus, it usually acts within 20 minutes. A second bolus may be injected 30 minutes after the first, if needed to clear the thrombus. After the clot has been dissolved, therapy with heparin or an alternative anticoagulant is started to prevent additional clots from forming. Reteplase may be used off-label to treat acute and chronic deep vein thrombosis and occluded catheters.

Administration Alerts

- Reconstitute the drug immediately prior to use with diluent provided by the manufacturer; swirl to mix—do not shake.
- Do not give any other drug simultaneously through the same IV line.
- Reteplase and heparin are incompatible and must never be combined in the same solution.
- Pregnancy category C.

PHARMACOKINETICS

Onset	Peak	Duration
Immediate	Unknown	Unknown

Adverse Effects

The most serious adverse effect of reteplase is abnormal bleeding. Bleeding may be prolonged at injection sites and catheter insertion sites. Dysrhythmias may occur during myocardial reperfusion.

Contraindications: Reteplase is contraindicated in patients with active bleeding or history of sroke or who have had recent surgical procedures.

Interactions

Drug–Drug: Concurrent therapy with aspirin, anticoagulants, and platelet aggregation inhibitors will produce an additive anticoagulant effect and increase the risk of bleeding.

Lab Tests: Reteplase degrades plasminogen in blood samples, thus decreasing serum plasminogen and fibrinogen levels.

Herbal/Food: Ginkgo biloba should be avoided because it may increase the risk of bleeding.

Treatment of Overdose: There is no specific treatment for overdose.

Complementary and Alternative Therapies

GINSENG AND CARDIOVASCULAR DISEASE

Ginseng is one of the oldest known herbal remedies. *Panax ginseng* is distributed throughout China, Korea, and Siberia, whereas *Panax quinquefolius* is native to Canada and the United States. There are differences in chemical composition between the two species of ginseng; American ginseng is not considered equivalent to Siberian ginseng. The plant's popularity has led to its extinction from certain regions, and much of the available ginseng is now grown commercially.

Ginseng has been used for centuries to promote general wellness, boost immune function, increase mental performance, and reduce fatigue. There are some claims that the herb lowers blood glucose in patients with type 2 diabetes and can help in the management of erectile dysfunction.

An analysis of five clinical trials with ginseng concluded that there is no convincing evidence that the herb has a cognitive-enhancing effect either in healthy subjects or in those with dementia (Geng et al., 2010). Another analysis concluded that there is insufficient evidence that ginseng has any effect on reducing the incidence of the common cold.

Ginseng is thought to have calcium channel antagonist actions. The herb may improve blood flow to the heart in times of low oxygen supply, such as with myocardial ischemia. Some research suggests that ginseng may have effectiveness equal or greater to that of nitrates when treating angina (Seida, Durec, & Kuhle, 2011). Caution must be used when concurrently taking ginseng and anticoagulants because bleeding time may be affected. A common theme among all ginseng research is that additional randomized, controlled studies must be done before definitive conclusions may be reached regarding the effectiveness of ginseng.

for continued therapy. Unless contraindicated, beta-blocker therapy continues for the remainder of the patient's life. For patients who are unable to tolerate beta blockers, CCBs are an alternative.

Angiotensin-Converting Enzyme Inhibitors

Clinical research has demonstrated increased survival for patients administered the ACE inhibitors captopril (Capoten) or lisinopril (Prinivil, Zestoretic) following an acute MI. These drugs are most effective when therapy is started within 24 hours after the onset of symptoms. Oral doses are normally begun after thrombolytic therapy is completed and the patient's condition has stabilized. IV therapy may be used during the early stages of MI pharmacotherapy.

Pain Management

The pain associated with an MI can be debilitating. Pain control is essential to ensure patient comfort and to reduce stress. Opioids such as morphine or fentanyl are given to ease extreme pain and to sedate the anxious patient. Pharmacology of the opioids was presented in chapter 18.

Chapter Review

KEY Concepts

The numbered key concepts provide a succinct summary of the important points from the corresponding numbered section within the chapter. If any of these points are not clear, refer to the numbered section within the chapter for review.

28.1 Myocardial ischemia develops when there is inadequate blood supply to meet the metabolic demands of cardiac muscle. The most common cause of myocardial ischemia is atherosclerotic plaque.

28.2 Angina pectoris is the narrowing of a coronary artery, resulting in lack of sufficient oxygen to the heart muscle. Chest pain on emotional or physical exertion is the most characteristic symptom, although some forms of angina do not cause pain.

28.3 Angina management may include nonpharmacologic therapies such as diet and lifestyle modifications, angioplasty, or surgery.

28.4 Goals for the pharmacotherapy of angina are to reduce the intensity and frequency of attacks, improve the ability to participate in activities of daily living, and extend the patient's life span by preventing consequences of ischemic heart disease. They are usually achieved by including lifestyle changes along with pharmacotherapy.

28.5 The organic nitrates relieve angina by dilating veins and coronary arteries. They are drugs of choice for terminating acute episodes of stable angina.

28.6 Beta-adrenergic blockers relieve anginal pain by decreasing the oxygen demands on the heart. They are often preferred drugs for prophylaxis of stable angina.

28.7 Calcium channel blockers relieve angina by dilating the coronary vessels and reducing the workload on the heart. They are drugs of first choice for treating vasospastic angina.

28.8 The early diagnosis of MI increases chances of survival.

28.9 If given within hours after the onset of MI, thrombolytic drugs can dissolve clots and restore perfusion to affected regions of the myocardium.

28.10 A number of additional drugs are used to treat the symptoms and complications of acute MI. These include antiplatelet and anticoagulant drugs, nitrates, beta blockers, analgesics, and ACE inhibitors.

REVIEW Questions

1. The patient is being discharged with nitroglycerin (Nitrostat) for sublingual use. While planning patient education, what instruction will the nurse include?
   1. "Swallow three tablets immediately for pain and call 911."
   2. "Put one tablet under your tongue for chest pain. If pain does not subside, call 911."
   3. "Call your health care provider when you have chest pain. He will tell you how many tablets to take."
   4. "Place three tablets under your tongue and call 911."
2. Nitroglycerin patches have been ordered for a patient with a history of angina. What teaching will the nurse give to this patient?
   1. Keep the patches in the refrigerator.
   2. Use the patches only if the chest pain is severe.
   3. Remove the old patch and wait 6–12 hours before applying a new one.
   4. Apply the patch only to the upper arm or thigh areas.
3. Which of the following assessment findings in a patient who is receiving atenolol (Tenormin) for angina would be cause for the nurse to hold the drug and contact the provider? (Select all that apply.)
   1. Heart rate of 50 beats/minute
   2. Heart rate of 124 beats/minute
   3. Blood pressure 86/56
   4. Blood pressure 156/88
   5. Tinnitus and vertigo
4. The nurse is caring for a patient with chronic stable angina who is receiving isosorbide dinitrate (Isordil). Which of the following are common adverse effects of isosorbide?
   1. Flushing and headache
   2. Tremors and anxiety
   3. Sleepiness and lethargy
   4. Light-headedness and dizziness
5. Place the following nursing interventions in order for a patient who is experiencing chest pain.
   1. Administer nitroglycerin sublingually.
   2. Assess heart rate and blood pressure.
   3. Assess the location, quality, and intensity of pain.
   4. Document interventions and outcomes.
   5. Evaluate the location, quality, and intensity of pain.
6. Erectile dysfunction drugs such as sildenafil (Viagra) are contraindicated in patients taking nitrates for angina. What is the primary concern with concurrent administration of these drugs?
   1. They contain nitrates, resulting in an overdose.
   2. They also decrease blood pressure through vasodilation and may result in prolonged and severe hypotension when combined with nitrates.
   3. They will adequately treat the patient's angina as well as erectile dysfunction.
   4. They will increase the possibility of nitrate tolerance developing and should be avoided unless other drugs can be used.

PATIENT-FOCUSED Case Study

Sharad Patel is a 43-year-old computer systems engineer. He has a history of hypertension and angina of two year's duration, and has been admitted to the medical unit for a gastrointestinal illness. He is complaining of chest pain (4 on a scale of 0–10), and is requesting his PRN sublingual nitroglycerin tablet. His blood pressure is 96/60.

1. As the nurse, what will you do first?
2. Should Mr. Patel be given his sublingual nitroglycerin tablet he has ordered for PRN use? Why or why not?
3. What additional follow-up will be needed?

CRITICAL THINKING Questions

1. A patient is recovering from an acute MI and has been put on atenolol (Tenormin). What teaching should the patient receive prior to discharge from the hospital?
2. A patient with chest pain has been given the CCB diltiazem (Cardizem) IV for a heart rate of 118 beats per minute. Blood pressure at this time is 100/60 mmHg. What precautions should the nurse take?

Visit www.pearsonhighered.com/nursingresources for answers and rationales for all activities.

REFERENCES

Aggarwal, S., Loomba, R. S., Arora, R. R., & Molnar, J. (2013). Associations between sleep duration and prevalence of cardiovascular events. *Clinical Cardiology, 36,* 671–676. doi:10.1002/clc.22160

Cooper, A. J., Westgate, K., Brage, S., Prevost, A. T., Griffin, S. J., & Simmons, R. K. (2015). Sleep duration and cardiometabolic risk factors among individuals with type 2 diabetes. *Sleep Medicine, 16,* 119–125. doi:10.1016/j.sleep.2014.10.006

Eguchi, K., Hoshide, S., Ishikawa, S., Shimada, K., & Kario, K. (2012). Short sleep duration and type 2 diabetes enhance the risk of cardiovascular events in hypertensive patients. *Diabetes Research and Clinical Practice, 98,* 518–523. doi:10.1016/j.diabres.2012.09.014

Engeda, J., Mezuk, B., Ratliff, S., & Ning, Y. (2013). Association between duration and quality of sleep and the risk of pre-diabetes: Evidence from NHANES. *Diabetic Medicine, 30,* 676–680. doi:10.1111/dme.12165

Geng, J., Dong, J., Ni, H., Lee, M. S., Wu, T., Jiang, K., . . . Malouf, R. (2010). Ginseng for cognition. *Cochrane Database of Systematic Reviews, 12.* Art. No.: CD007769. doi:10.1002/14651858.CD007769.pub2

Gutiérrez-Repiso, C., Soriguer, F., Rubio-Martin, E., Esteva de Antonio, I., Ruiz de Adana, M. S., Almaraz, M. C., . . . Rojo-Martinez, G. (2014). Night-time sleep duration and the incidence of obesity and type 2 diabetes: Findings from the prospective Pizarra study. *Sleep Medicine, 15,* 1398–1404. doi:10.1016/j.sleep.2014.06.014

Herdman, T. H., & Kamitsuru, S. (2014). *NANDA International nursing diagnoses: Definitions and classification, 2015–2017.* Oxford, United Kingdom: Wiley-Blackwell.

Herring, S. J., Nelson, D. B., Pien, G. W., Goetzl, L. M., Davey, A., & Foster, G. D. (2014). Objectively measured sleep duration and hyperglycemia in pregnancy. *Sleep Medicine, 15,* 51–55. doi: 10.1016/j.sleep.2013.07.018

Ohkuma, T., Fujii, H., Ogata-Kaizu, S., Ide, H., Kikuchi, Y., Idewaki, Y., . . . Kitazono, T. (2014). U-shaped association of sleep duration with metabolic syndrome and insulin resistance in patients with type 2 diabetes: The Fukuoka diabetes registry. *Metabolism: Clinical and Experimental, 63,* 484–491. doi:10.1016/j.metabol.2013.12.001

Seida, J. K., Durec, T., & Kuhle, S. (2011). North American (*Panax quinquefolius*) and Asian ginseng (*Panax ginseng*) preparations for prevention of the common cold in healthy adults: A systematic review. *Evidence-Based Complementary and Alternative Medicine,* Article ID 282151. doi:10.1093/ecam/nep068

SELECTED BIBLIOGRAPHY

Alaeddini, J. (2014). *Angina pectoris.* Retrieved from http://emedicine.medscape.com/article/150215-overview

Amsterdam, E. A., Kirk, J. D., Bluemke, D. A., Diercks, D., Farkouh, M. E., Garvey, J. L., . . . Thompson, P. D. (2010). Testing of low-risk patients presenting to the emergency department with chest pain: A scientific statement from the American Heart Association. *Circulation, 122,* 1756–1776. doi:10.1161/CIR.0b013e3181ec61df

Casey, D. E., Ettinger, S. M., Fesmire, F. M., Ganiats, T. G., Lincoff, A. M., Anderson, J. L., . . . Wright, R. S. (2012). 2012 ACCF/AHA focused update of the guideline for the management of patients with unstable angina/non–ST-elevation myocardial infarction (Updating the 2007 guideline and replacing the 2011 focused update). *Circulation, 126,* 875–910. doi:10.1161/CIR.0b013e318256f1e0

Gupta, A. K., Winchester, D., & Pepine, C. J. (2013). Antagonist molecules in the treatment of angina. *Expert Opinion on Pharmacotherapy, 14,* 2323–2342. doi:10.1517/14656566.2013.834329

Hermida, R. C., Ayala, D. E., Mojón, A., & Fernández, J. R. (2011). Bedtime dosing of antihypertensive medications reduces cardiovascular risk in CKD. *Journal of the American Society of Nephrology, 22,* 2313–2321. doi:10.1681/ASN.2011040361

Jones, D. A., Timmis, A., & Wragg, A. (2013). Novel drugs for treating angina. *BMJ, 347,* f4726. doi:10.1136/bmj.f4726

Kee, J. L. (2014). *Laboratory and diagnostic tests with nursing implications* (9th ed.). Upper Saddle River, NJ: Pearson.

Mozaffarian, D., Benjamin, E. J., Go, A. S., Arnett, D. K., Blaha, M. J., Cushman, M., . . . Turner, M. B. (2014). AHA statistical update: Heart disease and stroke statistics—2015 update: A report from the American Heart Association. *Circulation, 131, e29–e322.* doi:10.1161/CIR.0000000000000152

Pedrinelli, R., Ballo, P., Fiorentini, C., Galderisi, M., Ganau, A., Germanò, G., . . . Zacà, V. (2013). Hypertension and stable coronary artery disease: An overview. *Journal of Cardiovascular Medicine, 14,* 545–552. doi:10.2459/JCM.0b013e3283609332

Shah, A., & Fox, K. (2013). Stable angina: Current guidelines and advances in management. *Prescriber, 24* (17), 35–44. doi:10.1002/psb.1095

Tisminetzky, M., Joffe, S., McManus, D. D., Darling, C., Gore, J. M., Yarzebski, J., . . . Goldberg, R. J. (2014). Decade-long trends in the characteristics, management and hospital outcomes of diabetic patients with ST-segment elevation myocardial infarction. *Diabetes and Vascular Disease Research, 11,* 182–189. doi:10.1177/1479164114524235

Valgimigli, M., & Biscaglia, S. (2014). Stable Angina Pectoris. *Current Atherosclerosis Reports, 16* (7), 1–10. doi:10.1007/s11883-014-0422-4

Wright, R. S., Anderson, J. L., Adams, C. D., Bridges, C. R., Casey, D. E., Ettinger, S. M., . . . Zidar, J. P. (2011). 2011 ACCF/AHA focused update of the guidelines for the management of patients with unstable angina/non–ST-elevation myocardial infarction (updating the 2007 guideline): A report of the American College of Cardiology Foundation/American Heart Association Task Force on Practice Guidelines. *Journal of the American College of Cardiology, 57,* 1929–1959. doi:10.1016/j.jacc.2011.02.009

Young, J. W., & Melander, S. (2013). Evaluating symptoms to improve quality of life in patients with chronic stable angina. *Nursing Research and Practice,* Article ID 504915. doi:10.1155/2013/504915

Zafari, A. M. (2015). *Myocardial infarction.* Retrieved from http://emedicine.medscape.com/article/155919-overview

Chapter 29

Drugs for Shock

Drugs at a Glance

- **FLUID REPLACEMENT AGENTS** page 433
  - **Blood and Blood Products** page 433
  - **Colloid Solutions** page 433
  - **Crystalloid Solutions** page 433
    - *normal serum albumin (Albuminar, Plasbumin, others)* page 434
- **VASOCONSTRICTORS/VASOPRESSORS** page 433
  - *norepinephrine (Levophed)* page 439
- **INOTROPIC DRUGS** page 435
  - *dopamine (Intropin)* page 435
- **ANAPHYLAXIS** page 437
  - *epinephrine (Adrenalin)* page 440

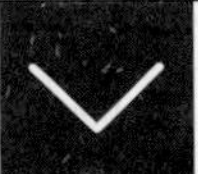

Learning Outcomes

After reading this chapter, the student should be able to:

1. Compare and contrast the different types of shock.
2. Relate the general symptoms of shock to their physiological causes.
3. Explain the initial treatment priorities for a patient who is in shock.
4. Compare and contrast the use of blood products, colloids, and crystalloids in fluid replacement therapy.
5. Explain the rationale for using vasoconstrictors and inotropic drugs to treat shock.
6. List the drugs used in the pharmacotherapy of anaphylaxis and discuss their indications.
7. For each of the classes shown in Drugs at a Glance, know representative drug examples, and explain their mechanism of action, primary actions, and important adverse effects.
8. Use the steps of the nursing process to care for patients who are receiving pharmacotherapy for shock.

(prototype drug icon) indicates a prototype drug, each of which is featured in a Prototype Drug box.

Shock is a condition in which vital tissues and organs are not receiving enough blood flow to function properly. Without adequate oxygen and nutrients, cells cannot carry out normal metabolic processes. Shock is a medical emergency; failure to reverse the causes and symptoms of shock may lead to irreversible organ damage and death. This chapter examines how drugs are used to aid in the treatment of different types of shock.

SHOCK

29.1 Characteristics of Shock

Although symptoms vary among the different kinds of shock, some similarities exist. The patient appears pale and may claim to feel sick or weak without reporting specific complaints. Behavioral changes are often some of the earliest symptoms and may include restlessness, anxiety, confusion, depression, and apathy. Lack of sufficient blood flow to the brain may cause unconsciousness. Thirst is a common complaint. The skin may feel cold or clammy. Without immediate treatment, multiple body systems will be affected and respiratory or renal failure may result. Figure 29.1 shows common symptoms of a patient in shock.

The central problem in most types of shock is the inability of the cardiovascular system to send sufficient blood to the vital organs, with the heart and brain being affected early in the progression of the condition. Assessment of the patient's cardiovascular status provides important clues for a diagnosis of shock. Blood pressure is usually low and cardiac output is diminished. Heart rate may be rapid with a weak, thready pulse. Breathing is usually rapid and shallow. Figure 29.2 illustrates the physiological changes that occur during circulatory shock.

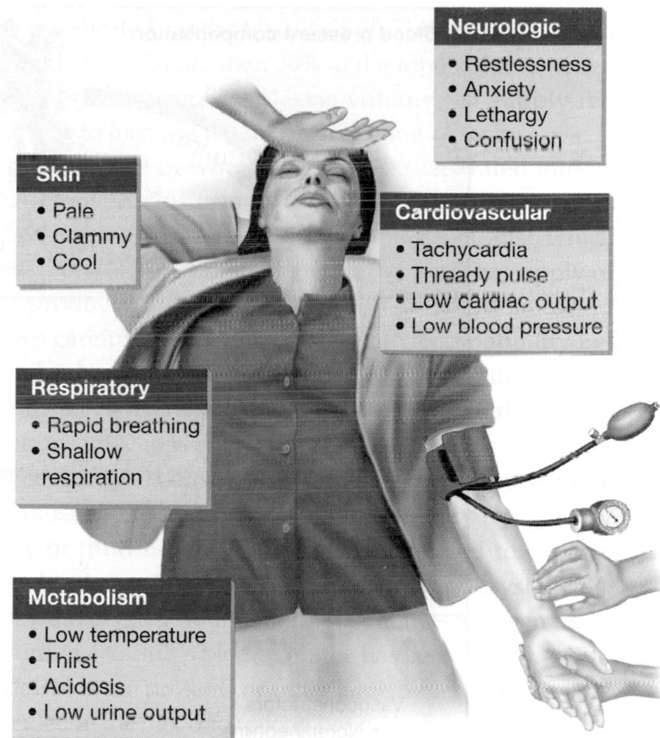

FIGURE 29.1 Symptoms of a patient in shock

Based on *Core Concepts in Pharmacology* (4th Ed.), by N. Holland, M. Adams, & C. Urban, 2015. Reprinted and electronically reproduced by permission of Pearson Education, Inc., Upper Saddle River, New Jersey.

29.2 Causes of Shock

Shock is often classified by naming the underlying pathologic process or organ system causing the disease. Table 29.1 describes the different types of shock and their primary causes.

The diagnosis of shock is rarely based on nonspecific symptoms. A careful medical history, however, may give the nurse valuable clues as to what type of shock may be present. For example, obvious trauma or bleeding would suggest **hypovolemic shock** related to blood loss. If trauma to the brain

Table 29.1 Common Types of Shock

Type of Shock	Definition	Underlying Pathology
Anaphylactic	Acute allergic reaction	Severe reaction to an allergen such as penicillin, nuts, shellfish, or animal proteins
Cardiogenic	Failure of the heart to pump sufficient blood to tissues	Left heart failure, myocardial ischemia, myocardial infarction (MI), dysrhythmias, pulmonary embolism, or myocardial or pericardial infection
Hypovolemic	Loss of blood volume	Hemorrhage, burns, excessive diuresis, or severe vomiting or diarrhea
Neurogenic	Vasodilation due to overstimulation of the parasympathetic nervous system or understimulation of the sympathetic nervous system	Trauma to the spinal cord or medulla, severe emotional stress or pain, or drugs that depress the central nervous system
Septic	Multiple organ dysfunction as a result of pathogenic organisms in the blood; often a precursor to acute respiratory distress syndrome and disseminated intravascular coagulation	Widespread inflammatory response to bacterial, fungal, or parasitic infection

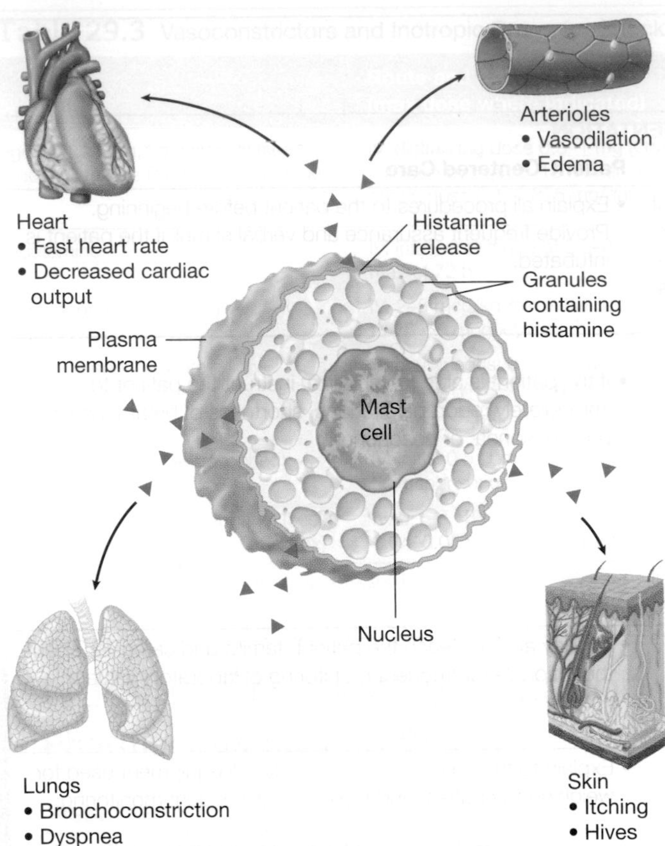

FIGURE 29.3 Symptoms of anaphylaxis

It is always preferable to *prevent* anaphylaxis than to *treat* it. Prevention measures include obtaining a thorough health history regarding drugs and environmental substances that have triggered past allergy attacks. Patients with serious allergies may be advised to carry a portable form of epinephrine such as an EpiPen or Auvi-Q, a newer self-administration device that has built-in verbal instructions.

Once anaphylaxis has begun, epinephrine, 1:1000, given subcutaneously or intramuscularly (IM), is considered a first-line drug because it causes vasoconstriction and can rapidly relieve symptoms of bronchoconstriction. If necessary, the dose may be repeated up to three times at 10- to 15-minute intervals. Crystalloids or colloids may be needed to prevent shock if the patient presents with volume depletion. Antihistamines such as diphenhydramine (Benadryl) may be administered IM or IV to prevent further release of histamine. A bronchodilator such as albuterol (Proventil, Ventolin, VoSpire) is often administered by inhalation to relieve the acute shortness of breath caused by histamine release. High-flow oxygen is usually administered. Systemic corticosteroids such as hydrocortisone are given to dampen the *delayed* inflammatory response that may occur several hours after the initial event.

Evidence-Based Practice: Toxic Shock Syndrome and Superantigens

Clinical Question: How is toxic shock different from other forms of septic shock, and does the treatment differ?

Evidence: Toxic shock syndrome (TSS) is a shock state often caused by *Staphylococcus aureus*. It has also been associated with *Streptococcus pyogenes* (group A beta haemolytic strep) and even methicillin-resistant Staphylococcus aureus (MRSA) (Kulhankova, King, & Salgad-Pabón, 2014; Low, 2013; Rostad, Phillipsborn, & Berkowitz, 2014). Identified in the 1970s, TSS was initially associated with the superabsorbent tampons that were new on the market. It is known that TSS is also associated with infections attributed to *Staph* or *Strep* bacteria such as pharyngitis, burns, or simple skin infections. It is sometimes labeled as "menstrual TSS" or "non-menstrual TSS" to denote the suspected original site of infection (Shalaby Anandappa, Pocock, Keough, & Turner, 2014). TSS is a rapidly progressing form of septic shock, although blood cultures may be negative, and multi-organ failure rapidly ensues (Shalaby et al., 2014). Mortality rate is high, up to 70% in some cases, and patients who survive may have recurrent TSS, even after discontinuing tampon use (Dixit, Fischer, & Wittekind, 2012; Tremlett, Michie, Kenol, & van der Bijl, 2014). It has also been noted that approximately 20% of survivors do not create antibodies to the causative organism (Kulhankova, King, & Salgad-Pabón, 2014). One study found that TSS is possibly underreported or unrecognized as the cause for shock, and TSS may account for 27% or more of all cases of infectious shock (Smit, Nyquist, & Todd, 2013).

TSS appears to differ from other forms of infectious/septic shock by the formation of "superantigens" by the *Staph* organism (Courjon et al., 2013). *Staph* organisms are known to be able to secrete antigens of varying virulence, and it is unknown why sometimes superantigens are produced. These superantigens quickly overwhelm the body's defense mechanisms and appear to even interfere with the formation of antibodies, allowing the infection to rapidly multiply (Kulhankova, King, & Salgad-Pabón, 2014). The treatment of TSS is similar to the treatment of other forms of shock and includes fluid resuscitation and vasopressors. Because TSS is an infectious shock, it is also treated with antibiotics. Clindamycin is currently the drug of choice, although rifampicin has also been used (Dixit, Fischer, & Wittekind, 2012; Shallaby et al., 2014). Newer investigative therapies include the use of immunoglobulins and nasal decontamination with mupirocin. The latter therapy was effective in one case of recurrent TSS after tampon use was discontinued following negative vaginal swabs (Tremlett et al., 2014). This suggests that TSS resides elsewhere and that tampons are only part of the picture.

Nursing Implications: *S. aureus* is a ubiquitous organism and the causative factor in both minor and major infections. Nurses should be vigilant whenever signs and symptoms of an infection are present, even if they appear minor. If *Staph* is the suspected organism, signs and symptoms of increasing infection may occur rapidly if TSS develops. Symptoms include anorexia, headache, myalgias and arthralgias, and skin rash or erythema, particularly involving the palms and soles of the feet and spreading outward. Hypotension and true shock symptoms may be exhibited within hours, and time-to-treatment is crucial. Because nurses so often are with the patient most often throughout the day, they may be the first to notice the development of TSS and alert the provider so that treatment can be started.

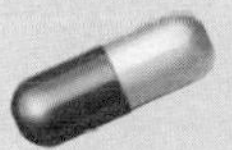

Prototype Drug | Norepinephrine *(Levophed)*

Therapeutic Class: Drug for shock **Pharmacologic Class:** Nonselective adrenergic agonist: vasopressor

Actions and Uses

Norepinephrine is a sympathomimetic that acts directly on alpha-adrenergic receptors in vascular smooth muscle to immediately raise blood pressure. To a lesser degree, it also stimulates beta$_1$-receptors in the heart, thus producing a positive inotropic response that may increase cardiac output. Its primary indications are acute shock and cardiac arrest. Norepinephrine is the vasopressor of choice for septic shock because research has demonstrated that it significantly decreases mortality. It is given by the IV route and has a duration of only 1 to 2 minutes after the infusion is terminated.

Administration Alerts

- Start an infusion only after ensuring the patency of the IV. Monitor the flow rate continuously.
- If extravasation occurs, administer phentolamine to the area of infiltration as soon as possible.
- Do not abruptly discontinue infusion.
- Pregnancy category D.

PHARMACOKINETICS

Onset	Peak	Duration
Immediate	1–2 min	1–2 min

Adverse Effects

Norepinephrine is a powerful vasoconstrictor; thus, continuous monitoring of the patient's blood pressure is required to prevent the development of hypertension. When first administered, reflex bradycardia is sometimes experienced. It also has the ability to produce various types of dysrhythmias, although less so than other vasopressors. If extravasation occurs, the drug may cause serious skin and soft tissue injury. Blurred vision and photophobia are signs of overdose.

Black Box Warning: Following extravasation, the affected area should be infiltrated immediately with 5 mg to 10 mg of phentolamine, an adrenergic blocker.

Contraindications: Norepinephrine should not be administered to patients who are experiencing hypotension due to blood volume deficits because vasoconstriction already exists in such patients. Norepinephrine may cause additional, severe peripheral and visceral vasoconstriction with decreased urine output. Norepinephrine is not usually given to patients with mesenteric or peripheral vascular thrombosis, because there is an increased risk of increasing ischemia and worsening the infarction.

Interactions

Drug–Drug: Alpha and beta blockers may antagonize the drug's vasopressor effects. Conversely, ergot alkaloids and tricyclic antidepressants may potentiate vasopressor effects. Digoxin, halothane, and cyclopropane may increase the risk of dysrhythmias.

Lab Tests: Unknown.

Herbal/Food: Unknown.

Treatment of Overdose: Discontinuing the infusion usually results in a rapid reversal of adverse effects such as hypertension.

Nearly all drugs have the capability to cause anaphylaxis. Although this is a rare adverse drug effect, the nurse must be prepared to quickly deal with anaphylaxis by understanding the indications and doses of the various drugs on the emergency cart. The most common drugs causing anaphylaxis include the following:

- Antibiotics, especially penicillins, cephalosporins, and sulfonamides
- Nonsteroidal anti-inflammatory drugs (NSAIDs), such as aspirin, ibuprofen, and naproxen
- Angiotensin-converting enzyme (ACE) inhibitors.
- Opioid analgesics
- Iodine-based contrast media used for radiographic exams.

Although obtaining a patient history of drug allergy is helpful in predicting some adverse drug reactions, anaphylaxis may occur without a previously reported incident. However, previous severe hypersensitivity to a drug is always a contraindication to the future use of that or closely related drugs in the same class. Unless the drug is the only one available to treat the patient's condition, it should not be administered.

If a drug must be given for which the patient has a known allergy, the patient may be *pretreated* with antihistamines or glucocorticoids to suppress the inflammatory response. If time permits, patients may be desensitized. Desensitization for penicillin and cephalosporin allergy, which takes about 6 hours, has been shown to be effective in preventing severe allergic reactions to these antibiotics. A typical desensitization regimen would involve administering an initial dose of 0.01 mg of the antibiotic and observing the patient for allergy. The dose may then be doubled every 15 to 20 minutes until the full dose has been achieved. Desensitization has also been achieved for patients with aspirin-induced asthma who require aspirin therapy for another condition.

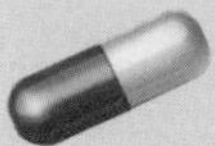

Prototype Drug | Epinephrine *(Adrenalin)*

Therapeutic Class: Drug for anaphylaxis and shock **Pharmacologic Class:** Nonselective adrenergic agonist; vasopressor

Actions and Uses

Subcutaneous or IV epinephrine is a preferred drug for anaphylaxis because it can reverse many of the distressing symptoms within minutes. Epinephrine is a nonselective adrenergic agonist, stimulating both alpha- and beta-adrenergic receptors. Almost immediately after injection, blood pressure rises due to stimulation of alpha$_1$ receptors. Activation of beta$_2$ receptors in the bronchi opens the airways and relieves the patient's shortness of breath. Cardiac output increases due to stimulation of beta$_1$ receptors in the heart. In addition to the subcutaneous and IM routes, topical, inhalation, and ophthalmic preparations are available. The intracardiac route is used for cardiopulmonary resuscitation under extreme conditions, usually during open cardiac massage, or when no other route is possible.

Administration Alerts

- Parenteral epinephrine is an irritant that may cause tissue damage if extravasation occurs.
- Pregnancy category C.

PHARMACOKINETICS

Onset	Peak	Duration
3–5 min (subcutaneous); 5–10 min (IM)	20 min	1–4 h

Adverse Effects

The most common adverse effects of epinephrine are nervousness, tremors, palpitations, tachycardia, dizziness, headache, and stinging/burning at the site of application. When administered parenterally, hypertension and dysrhythmias may occur rapidly; therefore, the patient should be monitored carefully following injection.

Contraindications: In life-threatening conditions such as anaphylaxis, there are no absolute contraindications for the use of epinephrine. The drug must be used with caution, however, in patients with dysrhythmias, cerebrovascular insufficiency, hyperthyroidism, narrow-angle glaucoma, hypertension, or coronary ischemia, because epinephrine may worsen these conditions.

Interactions

Drug–Drug: Epinephrine may result in hypotension if used with phenothiazines or oxytocin. There may be additive cardiovascular effects with other sympathomimetics. MAOIs, tricyclic antidepressants, and alpha- and beta-adrenergic drugs inhibit the actions of epinephrine. Epinephrine will decrease the effects of beta blockers. Some general anesthetics may sensitize the heart to the effects of epinephrine.

Lab Tests: Epinephrine may decrease serum potassium level and increase blood glucose levels.

Herbal/Food: Unknown.

Treatment of Overdose: Overdose may be serious, and alpha- and beta-adrenergic blockers are indicated. If blood pressure remains high, a vasodilator may be administered.

Chapter Review

KEY Concepts

The numbered key concepts provide a succinct summary of the important points from the corresponding numbered section within the chapter. If any of these points are not clear, refer to the numbered section within the chapter for review.

29.1 Shock is a clinical syndrome characterized by the inability of the cardiovascular system to pump enough blood to the vital organs.

29.2 Shock is often classified by the underlying pathologic process or by the organ system that is primarily affected, including anaphylactic, cardiogenic, hypovolemic, neurogenic, and septic shock.

29.3 The initial treatment of shock involves administration of basic life support, replacement of lost fluid, and maintenance of blood pressure.

29.4 During hypovolemic shock, colloids expand plasma volume and maintain blood pressure; crystalloids replace lost fluids and electrolytes. Whole blood may be indicated in cases of massive hemorrhage.

29.5 Vasopressors are critical care drugs sometimes needed during severe shock to maintain blood pressure. These drugs are sympathomimetics that strongly constrict the arteries and immediately raise blood pressure.

29.6 Inotropic drugs are useful in reversing the decreased cardiac output resulting from shock by increasing the strength of myocardial contraction.

29.7 Anaphylaxis is a serious hypersensitivity response to an allergen that is treated with a large number of different drugs, including sympathomimetics, antihistamines, and glucocorticoids. Common drugs such as penicillins, cephalosporins, NSAIDs, and ACE inhibitors may cause anaphylaxis.

REVIEW Questions

1. The patient in hypovolemic shock is prescribed an infusion of lactated Ringer's. What is the purpose for infusing this solution in shock? (Select all that apply.)
   1. The solution will help to replace fluid and promote urine output.
   2. The solution will draw water into cells.
   3. The solution will draw water from cells to blood vessels.
   4. The solution will help to maintain vascular volume.
   5. The solution is used to provide adequate calories for metabolic needs.

2. The nurse evaluates the effectiveness of dopamine therapy for a patient in shock. Which of the following may indicate treatment is successful? (Select all that apply.)
   1. Improved urine output
   2. Increased blood pressure
   3. Breath sounds are diminished
   4. Slight hypotension occurs
   5. Peripheral pulses are intact

3. A patient who is experiencing shock is started on norepinephrine (Levophed) by intravenous drip. Why must the nurse conduct frequent inspections of the intravenous insertion site while the patient remains on this drug?
   1. The patient's blood pressure may rise if the site is occluded.
   2. Extravasation and leakage at the intravenous site may cause local tissue damage.
   3. Bleeding may occur from the site due to localized drug effects.
   4. The patient's blood pressure may drop precipitously if the intravenous runs too quickly.

4. While planning care for a patient receiving plasma protein fraction (Plasmanate), the nurse will include frequent assessments for which of the following possible adverse reactions?
   1. Electrolyte imbalance
   2. Hyperglycemia
   3. Anaphylactic reaction
   4. Hypotension

5. Nursing assessment of a patient receiving normal serum albumin for treatment of shock should include which of the following assessments?
   1. Breath sounds
   2. Serum glucose levels
   3. Potassium level
   4. Hemoglobin and hematocrit

6. A patient is receiving PlasmaLyte for treatment of hypovolemic shock. When monitoring for therapeutic effects, which of the following will the nurse expect to occur?
   1. Breath sounds are clear.
   2. Potassium, glucose, and sodium levels remain within normal range.
   3. Blood pressure returns to within normal range and urine output increases.
   4. The pulse rate and ECG return to normal rate and pattern.

PATIENT-FOCUSED Case Study

A 48-year-old male is admitted to the ICU with a diagnosis of cardiogenic shock, secondary to a massive MI. His blood pressure is 84/40 mmHg, his heart rate is 108, and he is intubated and on a ventilator. He is currently on a dobutamine drip.

1. Why is this patient on this medication?
2. What nursing assessments should occur?
3. When and how should the dobutamine drip be discontinued?

CRITICAL THINKING Questions

1. The health care provider orders 3 L of 0.9% normal saline (NS) for a 22-year-old patient with vomiting and diarrhea, dry mucous membranes, poor skin turgor, heart rate of 122 beats/min, and blood pressure of 92/54 mmHg. Is this an appropriate IV solution for this patient? Why or why not?
2. A patient in shock is started on a dopamine drip starting at 10 mcg/kg/min and titrated to maintain a blood pressure of 90/50. What are key nursing interventions that are required while the patient remains on this drug?

Visit www.pearsonhighered.com/nursingresources for answers and rationales for all activities.

REFERENCES

Courjon, J., Hubiche, T., Phan, A., Tristan, A., Bès, M., Vandenesch, F., . . . Gillet, Y. (2013). Skin findings in *Staphylococcus aureus* toxin-mediated infection in relation to toxin encoding genes. *The Pediatric Infectious Disease Journal, 32*, 727–730. doi:10.1097/INF.0b013e31828e89f5

Dixit, S., Fischer, G., & Wittekind, C. (2013). Recurrent menstrual toxic shock syndrome despite discontinuation of tampon use: Is menstrual toxic shock syndrome really caused by tampons? *Australasian Journal of Dermatology, 54*, 283–286. doi:10.1111/j.1440-0960.2012.00938.x

Herdman, T. H., & Kamitsuru, S. (2014). *NANDA International nursing diagnoses: Definitions and classification, 2015–2017*. Oxford, United Kingdom: Wiley-Blackwell.

Kulhankova, K., King, J., & Salgado-Pabón, W. (2014). Staphylococcal toxic shock syndrome: Superantigen-mediated enhancement of endotoxin shock and adaptive immune suppression. *Immunologic Research, 59*, 182–187. doi:10.1007/s12026-014-8538-8

Low, D. E. (2013). Toxic shock syndrome: Major advances in pathogenesis, but not treatment. *Critical Care Clinics, 29*, 651–675. doi:10.1016/j.ccc.2013.03.012

Rostad, C. A., Phillipsborn, R. P., & Berkowitz, F. E. (2014). Evidence of Stapholococcal toxic shock. *The Pediatric Infectious Disease Journal, 34*, 450–452. doi:10.1097/INF.0000000000000580

Shalaby, T., Anandappa, S., Pocock, N. J., Keough, A., & Turner, A. (2014). Lesson of the month 2: Toxic shock syndrome. *Clinical Medicine, 14*, 316–318. doi:10.7861/clinmedicine.14-3-316

Smit, M. A., Nyquist, A. C., & Todd, J. K. (2013). Infectious shock and toxic shock syndrome diagnoses in hospitals, Colorado, USA. *Emerging Infectious Diseases, 19*, 1855–1858. doi:10.3201/eid1011.121547

Tremlett, W., Michie, C., Kenol, B., & van der Bijl, S. (2014). Recurrent menstrual toxic shock syndrome with and without tampons in an adolescent. *The Pediatric Infectious Disease Journal, 33*, 783–785. doi:10.1097/INF.0000000000000290

SELECTED BIBLIOGRAPHY

Bockenstedt, T. L., Baker, S. N., Weant, K. A., & Mason M. A. (2012). Review of vasopressor therapy in the setting of vasodilatory shock. *Advanced Emergency Nursing Journal, 34*(1), 16–23. doi:10.1097/TME.0b013e31824371d3

Bracht, H., Calzia, E., Georgieff, M., Singer, J., Radermacher, P., & Russell, J. A. (2012). Inotropes and vasopressors: More than haemodynamics! *British Journal of Pharmacology, 165*, 2009–2011. doi:10.1111/j.1476-5381.2011.01776.x

Crawford, A., & Harris, H. (2011). I.V. fluids: What nurses need to know. *Nursing 2012, 41*(5), 30–38. doi:10.1097/01.NURSE.0000396282.43928.40

De Backer, D., Aldecoa, C., Njimi, H., & Vincent, J. L. (2012). Dopamine versus norepinephrine in the treatment of septic shock: A meta-analysis. *Critical Care Medicine, 40*, 725–730. doi:10.1097/CCM.0b013e31823778ee

Delaney, A. P., Dan, A., McCaffrey, J., & Finfer, S. (2011). The role of albumin as a resuscitation fluid for patients with sepsis: A systematic review and meta-analysis. *Critical Care Medicine, 39*, 386–391. doi:10.1097/CCM.0b013e3181ffe217

Han, J. & Martin, G. S. (2011). Does albumin fluid resuscitation in sepsis save lives? *Critical Care Medicine, 39*, 418–419. doi:10.1097/CCM.0b013e318206b0ff

Havel, C., Arrich, J., Losert, H., Gamper, G., Müllner, M., & Herkner, H. (2011). Vasopressors for hypotensive shock. *Cochrane Database of Systematic Reviews, 5*. Art. No.: CD003709. doi:10.1002/14651858.CD003709.pub3

Kalil, A. (2014). *Septic shock*. Retrieved from http://emedicine.medscape.com/article/168402-overview

Mustafa, S. S. (2014). *Anaphylaxis*. Retrieved from http://emedicine.medscape.com/article/135065-overview

Xiushui, M. (2014). *Cardiogenic shock*. Retrieved from http://emedicine.medscape.com/article/152191-overview

Chapter 30

Drugs for Dysrhythmias

Drugs at a Glance

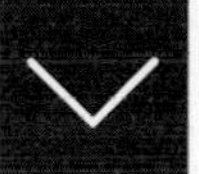

Learning Outcomes

After reading this chapter, the student should be able to:

1. Explain how rhythm abnormalities can affect cardiac function.
2. Illustrate the flow of electrical impulses through the normal heart.
3. Classify dysrhythmias based on their location and type of rhythm abnormality.
4. Explain how an action potential is controlled by the flow of sodium, potassium, and calcium ions across the myocardial membrane.
5. Identify the importance of nonpharmacologic therapies in the treatment of dysrhythmias.
6. Identify the general mechanisms of action of antidysrhythmic drugs.
7. Describe the nurse's role in the pharmacologic management of patients with dysrhythmias.
8. Know representative drug examples for each of the drug classes listed in Drugs at a Glance, and explain their mechanisms of action, primary actions, and important adverse effects.
9. Use the nursing process to care for patients receiving pharmacotherapy for dysrhythmias.

(prototype drug icon) indicates a prototype drug, each of which is featured in a Prototype Drug box.

Dysrhythmias are abnormalities of electrical conduction that may result in alterations in heart rate or cardiac rhythm. Sometimes called *arrhythmias,* they encompass a number of different disorders that range from harmless to life threatening. Diagnosis is often difficult because patients often must be connected to an electrocardiograph (ECG) and be experiencing symptoms in order to determine the exact type of rhythm disorder. Proper diagnosis and optimal pharmacotherapy can significantly affect the frequency of dysrhythmias and the patient's prognosis.

Table 30.1 Types of Dysrhythmias

Name of Dysrhythmia	Description
Atrial or ventricular tachycardia	Rapid heartbeat greater than 100 beats/min in adults; ventricular tachycardia is more serious than atrial tachycardia
Atrial or ventricular flutter	Rapid, regular heartbeats; may range between 200 and 300 beats/min; atrial flutter may require treatment but is not usually fatal; ventricular flutter requires immediate treatment
Atrial or ventricular fibrillation	Very rapid, uncoordinated contractions with complete disorganization of rhythm; ventricular fibrillation requires immediate treatment
Heart block	Blockage in the electrical conduction system of the heart; may be partial or complete; classified as first, second, or third degree
Premature atrial or premature ventricular contractions (PVCs)	An extra beat often originating from a source other than the SA node; only considered serious if it occurs in high frequency; may be a precursor of more serious dysrhythmias.
Sinus bradycardia	Slow heartbeat, less than 60 beats per minute, originating in the sinoatrial (SA) node; may require a pacemaker

DYSRHYTHMIAS

30.1 Etiology and Classification of Dysrhythmias

Whereas some dysrhythmias produce no symptoms and have negligible effects on cardiac function, others are life threatening and require immediate treatment. Typical symptoms include dizziness, weakness, decreased exercise tolerance, shortness of breath, and fainting. Patients may report palpitations or a sensation that their heart has skipped a beat. Persistent dysrhythmias are associated with increased risk of stroke and heart failure (HF). Severe dysrhythmias may result in sudden death. Because asymptomatic patients may not seek medical attention, it is difficult to estimate the frequency of the disease, although it is likely that dysrhythmias are quite common in the population.

Dysrhythmias are classified by a number of different methods. The simplest method is to name dysrhythmias according to the *type* of rhythm abnormality produced and its *location*. Dysrhythmias that originate in the atria are sometimes referred to as *supraventricular*. Atrial **fibrillation,** a complete disorganization of rhythm, is the most common type of dysrhythmia. Dysrhythmias that originate in the ventricles are generally more serious, because they are more likely to interfere with the normal function of the heart. For example, ventricular fibrillation is a total disorganization of cardiac contractions that requires immediate reversal or the initiation of basic life support. A summary of common dysrhythmias and a brief description of each abnormality are given in Table 30.1. Although a correct diagnosis of the type of dysrhythmia is sometimes difficult, it is essential for effective treatment.

Dysrhythmias can occur in both healthy and diseased hearts. Although the actual cause of most dysrhythmias is elusive, they are closely associated with certain conditions, primarily heart disease and myocardial infarction (MI). The following are diseases and conditions associated with dysrhythmias:

- Hypertension (HTN)
- Cardiac valve disease such as aortic stenosis
- Coronary artery disease
- Medications such as digoxin
- Low potassium or magnesium levels in the blood
- Myocardial infarction
- Stroke
- Diabetes mellitus
- Heart failure.

30.2 Conduction Pathways in the Myocardium

Although there are many types of dysrhythmias, all have in common a defect in the *generation* or *conduction* of electrical impulses across the myocardium. These electrical impulses, or **action potentials,** carry the signal for cardiac muscle cells to contract and are precisely coordinated for the chambers to beat in a synchronized manner. For the heart to function properly, the atria must contract simultaneously, sending their blood into the ventricles. Following atrial contraction, the right and left ventricles then must contract simultaneously. Lack of synchronization of the atria and ventricles or of the right and left sides of the heart may have profound consequences. The total time for the electrical impulse to travel across the heart is about 0.22 second. The normal conduction pathway in the heart is illustrated in Figure 30.1.

Control of synchronization begins in a small area of tissue in the wall of the right atrium known as the **sinoatrial (SA) node.** The SA node or pacemaker of the heart has a property called **automaticity,** the ability of certain cells to spontaneously generate an action potential. The SA node generates a new action potential approximately

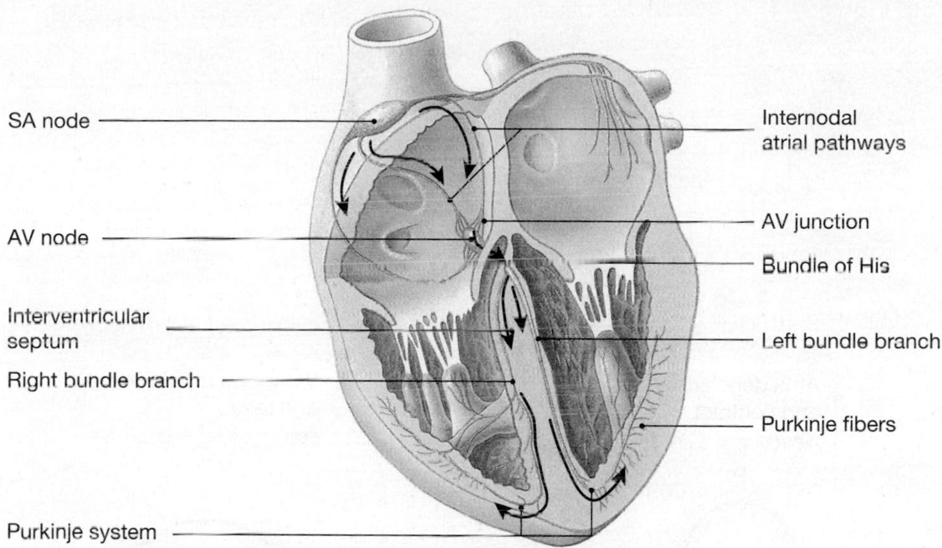

FIGURE 30.1 Normal conduction pathway in the heart

PharmFacts

DYSRHYTHMIAS

- If someone suffers an acute MI dysfunction, the risk of mortality from the event is increased 40% if they also have atrial fibrillation.
- The incidence of ventricular fibrillation is three times higher in men than in women, which reflects the higher incidence of coronary artery disease in men.
- The incidence of atrial dysrhythmias increases with age. They affect:
  - 0.1% of those younger than age 55.
  - 4% of those age 60–79.
  - 8% of those over age 80.
- Sudden cardiac death accounts for approximately 300,000 deaths per year in the United States; a large majority of these deaths are caused by ventricular dysrhythmias.
- Atrial fibrillation affects about 2.2 million people in the United States.
- Up to 30% of survivors of cardiac arrest may experience recurrent ventricular fibrillation in the first year afterward.

75 times per minute under resting conditions, with a normal range of 60 to 100 beats per minute. This is referred to as the normal **sinus rhythm.** The SA node is greatly influenced by the activity of the sympathetic and parasympathetic divisions of the autonomic nervous system.

On leaving the SA node, the action potential travels quickly across both atria to the **atrioventricular (AV) node.** The AV node also has the property of automaticity, although less so than the SA node. Should the SA node malfunction, the AV node has the ability to spontaneously generate action potentials and continue the heart's contraction at a rate of 40 to 60 beats per minute. Impulse conduction through the AV node, compared with other areas in the heart, is slow. This allows the atrial contraction enough time to completely empty blood into the ventricles, thereby optimizing cardiac output.

As the action potential leaves the AV node, it travels rapidly to the **atrioventricular bundle,** or bundle of His. The impulse is then conducted down the right and left **bundle branches** to the **Purkinje fibers,** which carry the action potential to all regions of the ventricles almost simultaneously. Should the SA and AV nodes become nonfunctional, cells in the AV bundle and Purkinje fibers can continue to generate myocardial contractions at a rate of about 30 beats per minute.

Although action potentials normally begin at the SA node and spread across the myocardium in a coordinated manner, other regions of the heart may begin to initiate beats. These areas, known as **ectopic foci** or **ectopic pacemakers,** may send impulses across the myocardium that compete with those from the normal conduction pathway. Although healthy hearts often experience an extra beat without incident, ectopic foci in diseased hearts have the potential to cause the types of dysrhythmias noted in Table 30.1.

It is important to understand that the underlying purpose of this conduction system is to keep the heart beating in a regular, synchronized manner so that cardiac output can be maintained. Some dysrhythmias occur sporadically, elicit no symptoms, and do not affect cardiac output. These types of abnormalities usually go unnoticed by the patient, and rarely require treatment. Others, however, profoundly affect cardiac output, result in patient symptoms, and have the potential to produce serious if not mortal consequences. It is these types of dysrhythmias that require pharmacotherapy.

30.3 The Electrocardiograph

The wave of electrical activity across the myocardium can be measured using the electrocardiograph. The graphic recording from this device, or **electrocardiogram (ECG),** is

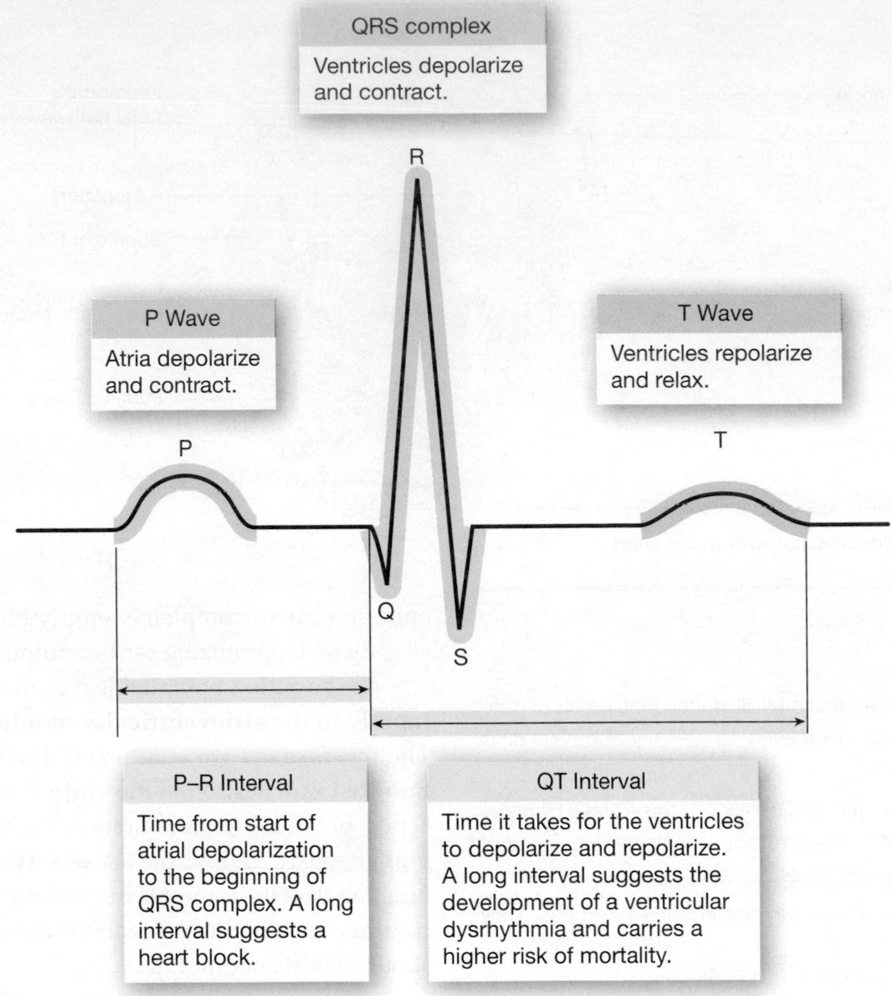

FIGURE 30.2 Relationship of the electrocardiogram to electrical conduction in the heart

useful in diagnosing many types of heart conditions, including dysrhythmias.

Three distinct waves are produced by a normal ECG: the P wave, the QRS complex, and the T wave. Changes to the wave patterns or in their timing can reveal certain pathologies. For example, a long PR interval suggests a heart block, and a flat T wave indicates ischemia to the myocardium. Elevated ST segments are used to guide the pharmacotherapy of MI (see chapter 28). A normal ECG and its relationship to impulse conduction in the heart is shown in Figure 30.2.

30.4 Nonpharmacologic Therapy of Dysrhythmias

The therapeutic goals of antidysrhythmic pharmacotherapy are to prevent or terminate dysrhythmias in order to reduce the risks of sudden death, stroke, or other complications resulting from the disease. Because these drugs can cause serious adverse effects, antidysrhythmics are normally reserved for patients experiencing symptoms of dysrhythmia or for those whose condition cannot be controlled by other means. Treating asymptomatic dysrhythmias with medications provides little or no benefit to the patient. Health care providers use several nonpharmacologic strategies to eliminate dysrhythmias.

The more serious types of dysrhythmias are corrected through electrical shock of the heart, with treatments such as elective **cardioversion** and **defibrillation.** The electrical shock momentarily stops all electrical impulses in the heart, both normal and abnormal. The temporary cessation of electrical activity often allows the SA node to automatically return conduction to a normal sinus rhythm.

Other types of nonpharmacologic treatment include identification and destruction of the myocardial cells responsible for the abnormal conduction through a surgical procedure called catheter ablation. Cardiac pacemakers are sometimes implanted to correct the types of dysrhythmias that cause the heart to beat too slowly. **Implantable cardioverter defibrillators (ICD)** are placed in patients to restore normal rhythm by either pacing the heart or giving it an electric shock when dysrhythmias occur. In addition, the ICD is capable of storing information regarding the heart rhythm for the health care provider to evaluate.

30.5 Phases of the Myocardial Action Potential

Because most antidysrhythmic drugs act by interfering with myocardial action potentials, a firm grasp of this phenomenon is necessary for understanding drug mechanisms. Action potentials occur in both neurons and cardiac muscle cells due to differences in the concentration of certain ions found inside and outside the cell. Under resting conditions, sodium ion (Na^+) and calcium ion (Ca^{2+}) are found in higher concentrations *outside* myocardial cells, and potassium ion (K^+) is found in higher concentration *inside* these cells. These imbalances are, in part, responsible for the slight negative charge (80 to 90 mV) inside a myocardial cell membrane relative to the outside of the membrane. A cell having this negative membrane potential is called **polarized.**

An action potential begins when **sodium ion channels** located in the plasma membrane open and Na^+ rushes *into* the cell, producing a rapid **depolarization,** or loss of membrane potential. During this period, Ca^{2+} also enters the cell through **calcium ion channels,** although the influx is slower than that of sodium. The entry of Ca^{2+} into the cells is a signal for the release of additional intracellular calcium that is held in storage inside the sarcoplasmic reticulum. It is this large increase in intracellular Ca^{2+} that is responsible for the contraction of cardiac muscle.

During depolarization, the inside of the plasma membrane temporarily reverses its charge, becoming positive. The cell returns to its polarized state by the removal of Na^+ from the cell via the sodium pump and movement of K^+ back into the cell through **potassium ion channels.** In cells located in the SA and AV nodes, it is the influx of Ca^{2+}, rather than Na^+, that generates the rapid depolarization of the membrane.

Although it may seem complicated to learn the different ions involved in an action potential, understanding the process is very important to cardiac pharmacology. Blocking potassium, sodium, or calcium ion channels is the primary pharmacologic strategy used to prevent or terminate dysrhythmias. Figure 30.3 illustrates the flow of ions during the action potential.

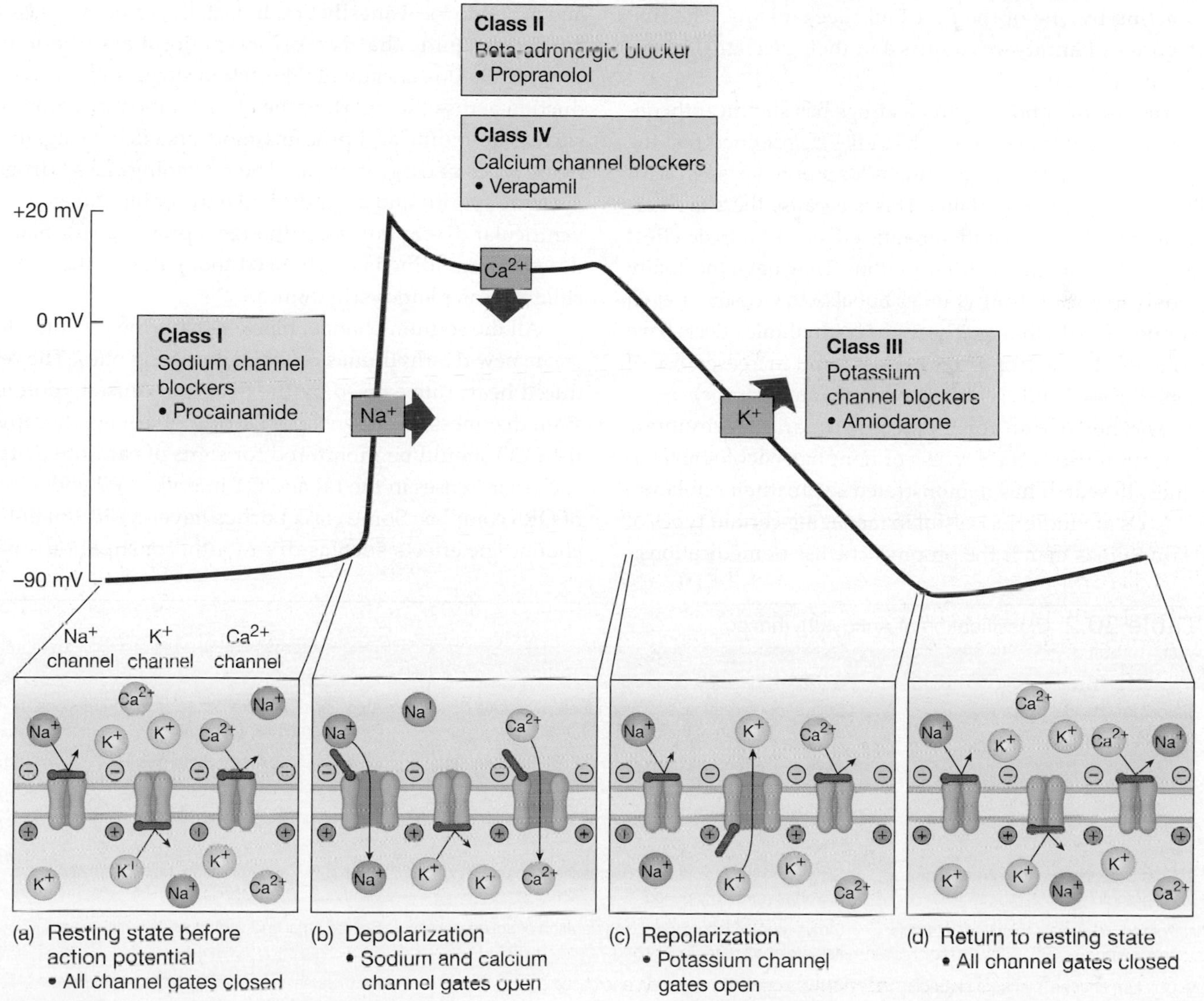

FIGURE 30.3 Ion channels in myocardial cells

The pumping action of the heart requires alternating periods of contraction and relaxation. There is a brief period following depolarization, and most of repolarization, during which the cell cannot initiate another action potential. This time, known as the **refractory period,** ensures that the myocardial cell finishes contracting before a second action potential begins. Some antidysrhythmic drugs produce their effects by prolonging the refractory period.

30.6 Mechanisms and Classification of Antidysrhythmic Drugs

Antidysrhythmic drugs act by altering specific electrophysiological properties of the heart. They do this through two basic mechanisms: blocking flow through ion channels (conduction) or altering autonomic activity (automaticity).

Antidysrhythmic drugs are grouped according to the stage in which they affect the action potential. These drugs fall into four primary classes, referred to as classes I, II, III, and IV, and a fifth group that includes miscellaneous drugs not acting by one of the first four mechanisms. The five categories of antidysrhythmics and their mechanisms are listed in Table 30.2.

The use of antidysrhythmic drugs has significantly declined in recent years. Research studies determined that the use of antidysrhythmic medications for prophylaxis can actually *increase* patient mortality. This is because there is a narrow margin between a therapeutic effect and a toxic effect with drugs that affect cardiac rhythm. They have the ability not only to *correct* dysrhythmias but also to worsen or even *create* new dysrhythmias. These prodysrhythmic effects have resulted in less use of drugs in class I and increased use of drugs in class II and class III (specifically, amiodarone).

Another reason for the decline in antidysrhythmic medication use is the success of nonpharmacologic techniques. Research has demonstrated that catheter ablation and ICDs are more successful in managing certain types of dysrhythmias than is the prophylactic use of medications.

SODIUM CHANNEL BLOCKERS (CLASS I)

The first medical use of quinidine, a sodium channel blocker, was recorded in the 18th century. Doses for the sodium channel blockers, the largest class of antidysrhythmics, are listed in Table 30.3.

30.7 Treating Dysrhythmias With Sodium Channel Blockers

Sodium channel blockers, the class I drugs, are divided into three subgroups, IA, IB, and IC, based on subtle differences in their mechanism of action. Because the action potential is dependent on the opening of sodium ion channels, a blockade of these channels will prevent depolarization. The spread of the action potential across the myocardium will slow, and areas of ectopic pacemaker activity will be suppressed.

The sodium channel blockers are similar in structure and action to local anesthetics. In fact, lidocaine is a class I antidysrhythmic that is a prototype local anesthetic in chapter 19. This anesthetic-like action slows impulse conduction across the heart. Some class I antidysrhythmics, such as quinidine and procainamide, are effective against many types of dysrhythmias. The remaining class I drugs are more specific and are indicated only for life-threatening ventricular dysrhythmias. Although a prototype for many decades, quinidine is rarely used today due to the availability of safer antidysrhythmics.

All the sodium channel blockers have the potential to create new dysrhythmias or worsen existing ones. The reduced heart rate caused by the drug can cause hypotension, dizziness, and syncope. During pharmacotherapy, the ECG should be monitored for signs of cardiotoxicity, such as increases in the PR and QT intervals and widening of QRS complex. Some class I drugs have significant anticholinergic effects such as dry mouth, constipation, and

Table 30.2 Classification of Antidysrhythmics

Class	Actions	Indications
I: Sodium channel blockers IA example: procainamide	Delays repolarization; slows conduction velocity; increases duration of the action potential	Atrial fibrillation, premature atrial contractions, PVCs, ventricular tachycardia
IB example: lidocaine	Accelerates repolarization; slows conduction velocity; decreases duration of action potential	Severe ventricular dysrhythmias
IC example: flecainide	No significant effect on repolarization; slows conduction velocity	Severe ventricular dysrhythmias
II: Beta-adrenergic antagonists example: propranolol	Slows conduction velocity; decreases automaticity; prolongs refractory period	Atrial flutter and fibrillation, tachydysrhythmia, ventricular dysrhythmias
III: Potassium channel blockers example: amiodarone	Slows repolarization; increases duration of action potential; prolongs refractory period	Severe atrial and ventricular dysrhythmias
IV: Calcium channel blockers example: verapamil	Slows conduction velocity; decreases contractility; prolongs refractory period	Paroxysmal supraventricular tachycardia, supraventricular tachydysrhythmia

Table 30.3 Antidysrhythmic Drugs

Drug	Route and Adult Dose (max dose where indicated)	Adverse Effects
CLASS IA: SODIUM CHANNEL BLOCKERS		
disopyramide (Norpace)	PO: (immediate release): 100–200 mg q6h PO: (controlled release): 300 mg bid	*Nausea, vomiting, diarrhea, dry mouth, urinary retention* May produce new dysrhythmias or worsen existing ones; hypotension, blood dyscrasias (procainamide, quinidine), and lupus-like syndrome (procainamide)
procainamide	IV: 100 mg q5min at a rate of 25-50 mg/min (max: 1 g)	
quinidine gluconate	PO: 400–600 mg tid–qid (max: 3–4 g/day) IV: 0.25 mg/kg/min (max: 5–10 mg/kg)	
quinidine sulfate	PO: 200–300 mg tid–qid (max: 3–4 g/day); therapeutic serum drug level is 2–5 mcg/mL	
CLASS IB: SODIUM CHANNEL BLOCKERS		
lidocaine (Xylocaine) (see page 267 for the Prototype Drug box)	IV: 1–4 mg/min infusion rate (max: 3 mg/kg per 5–10 min)	*Nausea, vomiting, drowsiness, dizziness, lethargy* May produce new dysrhythmias or worsen existing ones; hypotension, bradycardia, central nervous system (CNS) toxicity (lidocaine), malignant hyperthermia (lidocaine), status epilepticus if abruptly withdrawn (phenytoin)
mexiletine (Mexitil)	PO: 200–300 mg tid (max: 1,200 mg/day)	
phenytoin (Dilantin) (see page 191 for the Prototype Drug box)	PO: 100–200 mg tid (max: 625 mg/day) IV: 50–100 mg every 10–15 min until dysrhythmia is terminated (max: 1 g/day)	
CLASS IC: SODIUM CHANNEL BLOCKERS		
flecainide (Tambocor)	PO: 50–100 mg bid (max: 300-400 mg/day)	*Visual disturbances, nausea, vomiting, dizziness, headache, palpitations* May produce new dysrhythmias or worsen existing ones; hypotension, bradycardia
propafenone (Rythmol)	PO: (immediate release): 150–300 mg tid PO: (sustained release): 225 mg bid	
CLASS II: BETA-ADRENERGIC BLOCKERS		
acebutolol (Sectral)	PO: 200–600 mg bid (max: 1,200 mg/day)	*Fatigue, insomnia, drowsiness, impotence or decreased libido, bradycardia, confusion* Agranulocytosis, laryngospasm, Stevens–Johnson syndrome, anaphylaxis; if the drug is abruptly withdrawn, palpitations, rebound hypertension, life-threatening dysrhythmias, or myocardial ischemia
esmolol (Brevibloc)	IV: 50 mcg/kg/min maintenance dose (max: 200 mcg/kg/min)	
propranolol (Inderal, InnoPran XL)	PO: 10–30 mg tid–qid (max: 480 mg/day) IV: 0.5–3.1 mg q4h	
CLASS III: POTASSIUM CHANNEL BLOCKERS		
amiodarone (Cordarone, Pacerone)	PO: 400–600 mg/day (max: 2.2 g/day as loading dose)	*Blurred vision (amiodarone), photosensitivity, nausea, vomiting, anorexia* May produce new dysrhythmias or worsen existing ones; hypotension, bradycardia, pneumonia-like syndrome (amiodarone), angioedema (dofetilide), CNS toxicity (ibutilide)
dofetilide (Tikosyn)	PO: 125–500 mcg bid based on creatinine clearance	
dronedarone (Multaq)	PO: 400 mg bid	
ibutilide (Corvert)	IV: 1 mg infused over 10 min	
sotalol* (Betapace, Betapace AF, Sorine)	PO: 80 mg bid (max: 320 mg/day)	
CLASS IV: CALCIUM CHANNEL BLOCKERS		
diltiazem (Cardizem, Dilacor, Taztia XT, Tiazac) (see page 423 for the Prototype Drug box)	IV: 5–10 mg/h continuous infusion for a maximum of 24 h (max: 15 mg/h)	*Flushed skin, headache, dizziness, peripheral edema, light-headedness, nausea, diarrhea* Hepatotoxicity, MI, HF, confusion, mood changes
verapamil (Calan, Covera-HS, Verelan)	PO: 240–480 mg/day IV: 5–10 mg direct; may repeat in 15–30 min if needed	
MISCELLANEOUS ANTIDYSRHYTHMICS		
adenosine (Adenocard, Adenoscan)	IV: 6–12 mg given as a bolus injection every 1–2 min as needed (max: 12 mg/dose)	*Facial flushing, dyspnea, chest warmth* May produce new dysrhythmias or worsen existing ones
digoxin (Lanoxin, Lanoxicaps) (see page 403 for the Prototype Drug box)	PO: 0.125–0.5 mg qid; therapeutic serum drug level is 0.8–2 ng/mL	*Nausea, vomiting, headache, and visual disturbances* May produce new dysrhythmias or worsen existing ones

Note: *Italics* indicate common adverse effects, underlining indicates serious adverse effects.
*Sotalol is a beta blocker, but because its cardiac effects are similar to those of amiodarone, it is considered a class III drug.

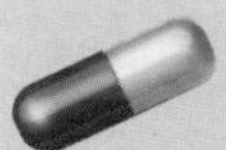

Prototype Drug | Procainamide

Therapeutic Class: Class IA antidysrhythmic **Pharmacologic Class:** Sodium channel blocker

Actions and Uses

Procainamide is an older drug, approved in 1950, that is chemically related to the local anesthetic procaine. Procainamide blocks sodium ion channels in myocardial cells, thus reducing automaticity and slowing conduction of the action potential across the myocardium. This slight delay in conduction velocity prolongs the refractory period and can suppress dysrhythmias. Procainamide is referred to as a broad-spectrum drug because it has the ability to correct many different types of atrial and ventricular dysrhythmias. The most common dosage form is the extended-release tablet; however, procainamide is also available in intravenous (IV) and intramuscular (IM) formulations. The therapeutic serum drug level is 4 to 8 mcg/mL. The use of procainamide has declined significantly due to the development of more specific and safer drugs.

Administration Alerts

- Use the supine position during IV administration because severe hypotension may occur.
- Pregnancy category C.

PHARMACOKINETICS

Onset	Peak	Duration
immediate IV; 10–30 min IM	1–1.5 h	3–4 h

Adverse Effects

Nausea, vomiting, abdominal pain, hypotension, and headache are common during procainamide therapy. High doses may produce CNS effects such as confusion or psychosis.

Black Box Warning: Prolonged administration may result in an increased titer of antinuclear antibodies (ANAs). A lupus-like syndrome may occur in 30% to 50% of patients who are taking the drug for more than a year. Procainamide should be reserved for life-threatening dysrhythmias because it has the ability to produce new dysrhythmias or worsen existing ones. Agranulocytosis, bone marrow depression, neutropenia, hypoplastic anemia, and thrombocytopenia have been reported, usually within the first 3 months of therapy. Complete blood counts should be monitored carefully and the drug discontinued at the first sign of potential blood dyscrasia.

Contraindications: Procainamide is contraindicated in patients with complete AV block, severe HF, blood dyscrasias, and myasthenia gravis.

Interactions

Drug–Drug: Additive cardiac depressant effects may occur if procainamide is administered with other antidysrhythmics. Additive anticholinergic side effects will occur if procainamide is used concurrently with anticholinergic drugs.

Lab Tests: Procainamide may increase values for the following: aspartate aminotransferase (AST), alanine aminotransferase (ALT), serum alkaline phosphatase (ALP), lactate dehydrogenase (LDH), and serum bilirubin. False-positive Coombs test and ANA titers may occur.

Herbal/Food: Unknown.

Treatment of Overdose: Supportive treatment is targeted to reversing hypotension with vasopressors and preventing or treating procainamide-induced dysrhythmias.

urinary retention. Special precautions should be taken with older adults, because anticholinergic side effects can cause mental status changes and may worsen urinary hesitancy in patients with prostate enlargement. Lidocaine can cause CNS toxicity such as drowsiness, confusion, and convulsions.

BETA-ADRENERGIC ANTAGONISTS (CLASS II)

Beta-adrenergic antagonists, also called beta blockers, are widely used for cardiovascular disorders, including HTN, MI, HF, and dysrhythmias. Their ability to slow the heart rate and conduction velocity can suppress several types of dysrhythmias. The beta blockers are listed in Table 30.3.

30.8 Treating Dysrhythmias With Beta-Adrenergic Antagonists

As expected from their effects on the autonomic nervous system, beta-adrenergic blockers slow the heart rate and decrease conduction velocity through the AV node. Myocardial automaticity is reduced, and many types of dysrhythmias are stabilized. These effects are primarily caused by blockade of calcium ion channels in the SA and AV nodes, although these drugs also block sodium ion channels in the atria and ventricles.

The main value of beta blockers as antidysrhythmic drugs is to treat atrial dysrhythmias associated with HF. In post-MI patients, beta blockers decrease the likelihood of sudden death due to their antidysrhythmic effects. The basic pharmacology of beta-adrenergic antagonists is explained in chapter 13.

Nursing Practice Application

Pharmacotherapy With Antidysrhythmic Drugs

ASSESSMENT	POTENTIAL NURSING DIAGNOSES*
Baseline assessment prior to administration: • Obtain a complete health history including cardiovascular (including previous dysrhythmias, HTN, MI, HF), and the possibility of pregnancy. Obtain a drug history including allergies, current prescription and over-the-counter (OTC) drugs, herbal preparations, and alcohol use. Be alert to possible drug interactions. • Obtain baseline weight, vital signs (especially blood pressure [BP] and pulse), ECG (rate and rhythm), cardiac monitoring (such as cardiac output if appropriate), and breath sounds. Assess for location and character/amount of edema, if present. • Evaluate appropriate laboratory findings; electrolytes, especially potassium level; renal and liver function studies; and lipid profiles.	• *Decreased Cardiac Output* • *Anxiety* • *Fatigue,* related to adverse drug effects • *Activity Intolerance,* related to adverse drug effects • *Sexual Dysfunction,* related to adverse drug effects • *Deficient Knowledge* (drug therapy) • *Risk for Decreased Cardiac Tissue Perfusion* • *Risk for Falls,* related to hypotension or dizziness associated with dysrhythmias or adverse drug effects • *Risk for Injury,* related to hypotension or dizziness associated with dysrhythmias or to adverse drug effects *NANDA I © 2014
Assessment throughout administration: • Assess for desired therapeutic effects (e.g., control or elimination of dysrhythmia, BP and pulse within established limits). • Continue frequent monitoring of the ECG. Check pulse quality, volume, and regularity along with the ECG. Assess for complaints of palpitations, and correlate symptoms with the ECG findings. • Continue periodic monitoring of electrolytes, especially potassium and magnesium. • Assess for adverse effects: dizziness, hypotension, nausea, vomiting, headache, fatigue or weakness, flushing, or sexual dysfunction. Bradycardia, tachycardia, or new or different dysrhythmias should be reported to the health care provider immediately.	

IMPLEMENTATION

Interventions and (Rationales)	Patient-Centered Care
Ensuring therapeutic effects: • Continue frequent assessments as above for therapeutic effects. (Dysrhythmias have diminished or are eliminated. BP and pulse should be within normal limits or within the parameters set by the health care provider.)	• To allay possible anxiety, teach the patient, family, or caregiver the rationale for all equipment used and the need for frequent monitoring.
• Encourage appropriate lifestyle changes. **Collaboration:** Provide for dietitian consultation as needed. (Healthy lifestyle changes will support and minimize the need for drug therapy.)	• Encourage the patient to adopt a healthy lifestyle of low-fat food choices, increased exercise, decreased caffeine and alcohol consumption, and smoking cessation.
Minimizing adverse effects: • Continue to monitor the ECG and pulse for quality and volume. Take pulse for 1 full minute to assess for regularity. Continue to assess for complaints of palpitations, correlating palpitations or pulse irregularities with the ECG. (Not all dysrhythmias are symptomatic. Correlating symptoms with the ECG may help determine the need for further symptom management. **Diverse Patients:** Because of differences in metabolism and because some antidysrhythmics metabolize through the P450 pathways, monitor ethnically diverse patients frequently to ensure optimal therapeutic effects and to minimize adverse effects.)	• Teach the patient, family, or caregiver how to take a peripheral pulse for 1 full minute before taking the drug. Assist the patient to find the pulse area that is most convenient and easily felt. Record daily pulse rates and regularity and bring the record to each health care visit. Instruct the patient to notify the health care provider if pulse is below 60 or above 100, there is a noticeable change in regularity from previously felt, or if palpitations develop or worsen.

Nursing Practice Application *continued*

IMPLEMENTATION	
Interventions and (Rationales)	**Patient-Centered Care**
• Take BP lying, sitting, and standing to detect orthostatic hypotension. **Lifespan:** Be cautious with the first few doses of the drug and with the older adult who is at increased risk for hypotension. (Antidysrhythmic drugs may cause hypotension. A first-dose effect may occur with a significant drop in BP with the first few doses. Orthostatic hypotension may increase the risk of falls and injury.)	• **Safety:** Teach the patient to rise slowly from lying or sitting to standing to avoid dizziness or falls. If dizziness occurs, the patient should sit or lie down and not attempt to stand or walk, until the sensation passes. • Instruct the patient to take the first dose of the new prescription before bedtime and to be cautious during the next few doses until drug effects are known. • Teach the patient, family, or caregiver how to monitor BP if required. Ensure proper use and functioning of any home equipment obtained. • Instruct the patient to notify the health care provider if BP is 90/60 mmHg or below, or per parameters set by the health care provider.
• Continue to monitor periodic electrolyte levels, especially potassium and magnesium, renal function labs, and drug levels as needed. (Hypokalemia or hypomagnesia increases the risk of dysrhythmias. Inadequate, or high, levels of an antidysrhythmic drug may lead to increased or more lethal dysrhythmias.)	• Instruct the patient on the need to return periodically for laboratory work. • Advise the patient to carry a wallet identification card or wear medical identification jewelry indicating antidysrhythmic therapy.
• Weigh the patient daily and report a weight gain or loss of 1 kg (2 lb) or more in a 24-hour period. Continue to assess for edema, noting location and character. (Daily weight is an accurate measure of fluid status and takes into account intake, output, and insensible losses. Weight gain or edema may indicate adverse drug effects or worsening cardiovascular disease processes.)	• Have the patient weigh self daily, ideally at the same time of day, and record weight along with pulse measurements. Have the patient report a weight loss or gain of more than 1 kg (2 lb) in a 24-hour period.
• Monitor for breath sounds and heart sounds (e.g., increasing dyspnea or postural nocturnal dyspnea, rales or "crackles" in lungs, frothy pink-tinged sputum, murmurs or extra heart sounds) and report immediately. (Increasing lung congestion or new or worsening heart murmurs may indicate impending HF. Potassium-channel blockers are associated with pulmonary toxicity.)	• Instruct the patient to immediately report any severe shortness of breath, frothy sputum, profound fatigue, or swelling of extremities as possible signs of HF or pulmonary toxicity.
• Report any visual changes, skin rashes, and sunburning to the health care provider. (Potassium-channel blockers may cause photosensitivity, skin rashes, and blurred vision.)	• Teach the patient to report any vision changes promptly and to maintain regular eye examinations. • Teach the patient the importance of wearing protective clothing and applying sunscreen regularly during periods of sun exposure.
Patient understanding of drug therapy: • Use opportunities during administration of medications and during assessments to provide patient education. (Using time during nursing care helps to optimize and reinforce key teaching areas.)	• The patient, family, or caregiver should be able to state the reason for the drug; appropriate dose and scheduling; what adverse effects to observe for and when to report; equipment needed as appropriate and how to use that equipment; and the required length of medication therapy needed with any special instructions regarding renewing or continuing the prescription as appropriate.
Patient self-administration of drug therapy: • When administering medications, instruct the patient, family, or caregiver in proper self-administration techniques. (Proper administration increases the effectiveness of the drug.)	• Teach the patient to take drugs as evenly spaced apart as possible and not to double dose if a dose is missed. • Teach the patient not to discontinue the medication abruptly and to call the health care provider if the patient is unable to take medication for more than 1 day due to illness. • The patient is able to discuss appropriate dosing and administration needs.

See Table 30.3 for a list of drugs to which these nursing actions apply. See also the Nursing Practice Applications in chapter 26 for information related to specific categories of antidysrhythmic drugs (e.g., calcium channel blockers).

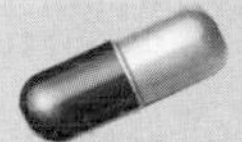

Prototype Drug | Propranolol *(Inderal, InnoPran XL)*

Therapeutic Class: Class II antidysrhythmic **Pharmacologic Class:** Beta-adrenergic antagonist

Actions and Uses

Propranolol is a nonselective beta-adrenergic blocker, affecting $beta_1$ receptors in the heart and $beta_2$ receptors in pulmonary and vascular smooth muscle. Propranolol reduces heart rate, slows myocardial conduction velocity, and lowers blood pressure. Propranolol is most effective in treating tachycardia that is caused by excessive sympathetic stimulation. It is approved to treat a wide variety of diseases, including HTN, angina, and migraine headaches, and for the prevention of MI.

Propranolol has several off-label indications, including reducing portal HTN and bleeding due to esophageal varices, reducing the tachycardia, tremor, and nervousness associated with thyroid crisis (storm), panic attacks, post-traumatic stress disorder (PTSD), chronic agitation, aggressive behavior, and involuntary movements of essential tremor. The drug is available in tablet, extended-release capsules, and IV formulations. InnoPran XL is a long-acting form of the drug that has a timed delivery system designed for bedtime dosing, with a peak effect in the morning.

Administration Alerts

- Abrupt discontinuation may cause MI, severe HTN, and ventricular dysrhythmias.
- Swallow extended-release tablets whole: Do not crush or chew contents.
- If pulse is less than 60 beats per minute, notify the health care provider.
- Pregnancy category C.

PHARMACOKINETICS

Onset	Peak	Duration
30–60 min PO	1–2 h (6 h extended release)	6–12 h (immediate release) 24–27 h (extended release)

Adverse Effects

Common adverse effects of propranolol include fatigue, hypotension, and bradycardia. Because of the ability of propranolol to slow the heart rate, patients with serious cardiac disorders such as HF must be carefully monitored. Adverse effects such as diminished libido and impotence may result in noncompliance in male patients. Propranolol should be used cautiously in patients with diabetes due to its hypoglycemic effects and because it may mask the symptoms of hypoglycemia as the adrenergic "fight-or-flight" response to hypoglycemia is blocked. This drug should be used with caution in patients with reduced renal output, because the drug may accumulate to toxic levels in the blood and cause dysrhythmias.

Black Box Warning: Abrupt withdrawal is not advised in patients with angina or heart disease. Dosage should gradually be reduced over 1 to 2 weeks and the drug should be reinstituted if angina symptoms develop during this period.

Contraindications: Because of its depressive effects on the heart, propranolol is contraindicated in patients with cardiogenic shock, sinus bradycardia, greater than first-degree heart block, and HF. Because it constricts smooth muscle in the airways, the drug is contraindicated in patients with COPD or asthma.

Interactions

Drug–Drug: Concurrent administration with other beta blockers may produce additive effects on the heart, and bradycardia or hypotension may result. Because both propranolol and calcium channel blockers (CCBs) suppress myocardial contractility, their concurrent use may lead to additive bradycardia. Phenothiazines can add to the hypotensive effects of propranolol. Propranolol should not be given within 2 weeks of a monoamine oxidase inhibitor (MAOI), because severe bradycardia and hypotension could result. Use of ethanol or antacids containing aluminum hydroxide gel will slow the absorption of propranolol and reduce its therapeutic effects. Administration of beta-adrenergic agonists such as albuterol will antagonize the actions of propranolol.

Lab Tests: Propranolol may give a false increase for urinary catecholamines.

Herbal/Food: Unknown.

Treatment of Overdose: Treatment is targeted to reversing hypotension with vasopressors, and bradycardia with atropine or isoproterenol. Intravenous glucagon reverses the cardiac depression caused by beta blocker overdose by enhancing myocardial contractility, increasing heart rate, and improving AV node conduction.

Only a few beta blockers are approved for dysrhythmias because of the potential for serious adverse effects. Blockade of beta receptors in the heart may result in bradycardia, and hypotension may cause dizziness and possible syncope. Those beta blockers that affect $beta_2$-adrenergic receptors will also affect the lung, possibly causing bronchospasm. This is of particular concern in patients with asthma or in older patients with chronic obstructive pulmonary disease (COPD). Unless a functioning pacemaker is present, these drugs are contraindicated in patients with severe bradycardia, sick sinus syndrome, or advanced AV block because they depress conduction through the AV node. Abrupt discontinuation of beta blockers can lead to dysrhythmias and HTN.

POTASSIUM CHANNEL BLOCKERS (CLASS III)

Although a small class of drugs, the potassium channel blockers have important applications in the treatment of dysrhythmias. These drugs prolong the duration of the action potential and reduce automaticity. The potassium channel blockers are listed in Table 30.3.

30.9 Treating Dysrhythmias With Potassium Channel Blockers

After the action potential has passed and the myocardial cell is in a depolarized state, repolarization depends on restoring potassium ions inside the cell. By blocking potassium channels, the class III antidysrhythmics delay repolarization of the myocardial cells and lengthen the refractory period, which tends to stabilize dysrhythmias. Most drugs in this class have multiple actions and also affect adrenergic receptors or sodium channels. For example, in addition to blocking potassium channels, sotalol (Betapace, Betapace AF, Sorine) is considered a beta-adrenergic blocker.

The potassium channel blockers are reserved for serious dysrhythmias. Amiodarone (Cordarone, Pacerone) is one of the more frequently used drugs in this class and is featured as the class III antidysrhythmic. It may be used to treat many different types of atrial and ventricular dysrhythmias. Dofetilide (Tikosyn) and ibutilide (Corvert) are given to terminate atrial flutter or fibrillation. Sotalol is approved for specific types of atrial and ventricular dysrhythmias, when safer drugs have failed to terminate the dysrhythmia.

Drugs in this class have limited uses because of potentially serious adverse effects. Like other antidysrhythmics, potassium channel blockers slow the heart rate, resulting in serious bradycardia and possible hypotension. These adverse effects occur in a significant number of patients. These drugs can worsen dysrhythmias, especially following the first few doses. Older adults with pre-existing HF must be carefully monitored because they are particularly at risk for adverse cardiac effects of potassium channel blockers.

Amiodarone can produce liver toxicity and thyroid dysfunction in a significant number of patients. Pulmonary toxicity is a rare though serious adverse effect. All the antidysrhythmic drugs can produce torsades de pointes, a type of ventricular tachycardia that can become rapidly fatal if not recognized and treated. Treatment of torsades de pointes includes IV magnesium sulfate or potassium chloride. Notify the prescriber if the QTC is greater than 500 ms.

Approved in 2009, dronedarone (Multaq) is chemically similar to amiodarone but is claimed to have a reduced incidence of adverse effects. Like sotalol, dronedarone has multiple actions on the heart. Dronedarone is approved for the treatment of paroxysmal or persistent atrial fibrillation or flutter. The labeling includes a boxed warning stating that dronedarone increases the risk of death and is contraindicated in patients with serious HF. Therefore, amiodarone is still much more widely used than dronederone.

CALCIUM CHANNEL BLOCKERS (CLASS IV)

Like beta blockers, the CCBs are widely prescribed for various cardiovascular disorders. By slowing conduction

Evidence-Based Practice: Do Asthma Inhalers Cause Dysrhythmias?

Clinical Question: Do inhalers for asthma that contain a long-acting beta agonist drug cause dysrhythmias?

Evidence: Beta agonist drugs are used as bronchodilators. Inhalers with long-acting beta agonists (LABA) combined with inhaled corticosteroids (ICS) are effective maintenance inhalers to prevent acute asthma attacks in adults. Because adults may use these inhalers for years, there is a concern that the beta adrenergic drug contained in the inhaler has the potential to cause cardiac dysrhythmias. Short-term beta adrenergic agonist inhalers such as albuterol may cause adverse effects such as tachycardia, increased blood pressure, and dysrhythmias in some patients; however, little is known about the use of LABA inhalers.

Iftikhar, Imtiaz, Brett, and Amrol (2014) conducted a systematic review and analysis of published studies and clinical trials where a LABA-ICS combination inhaler was used. Out of 17 studies (5,440 participants), three studies reported the development of dysrhythmias that began after the use of the LABA-ICS inhaler. Based on their analysis, the authors concluded that there was no statistically significant support for the conclusion that a LABA-ICS inhaler causes dysrhythmias.

Nursing Implications: Adult patients with asthma may be concerned about the side effect profiles of their medications. Results from this systematic review suggest that LABA-ICS inhalers have a good safety profile and are not linked to dysrhythmia development. As with any drug, individual patients may experience different results. The nurse should take a thorough drug history on patients who complain of tachycardia, "skipped beats," or other signs and symptoms of dysrhythmias. If the patient is on a LABA-ICS inhaler, questions about pulse rate and any cardiovascular symptoms should be included in the patient's history taking.

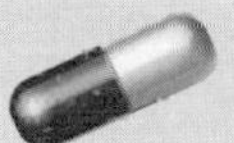

Prototype Drug | Amiodarone (*Cordarone, Pacerone*)

Therapeutic Class: Class III antidysrhythmic **Pharmacologic Class:** Potassium channel blocker

Actions and Uses

Amiodarone is structurally similar to thyroid hormone. It is approved for the treatment of resistant ventricular tachycardia that may prove life threatening, and it has become a preferred medication for the treatment of atrial dysrhythmias in patients with HF. In addition to blocking potassium ion channels, some of this drug's actions on the heart relate to its blockade of sodium ion channels. Amiodarone is available as oral tablets and as an IV infusion. IV infusions are limited to short-term therapy, normally only 2 to 4 days. This drug requires a 10-gram loading dose to achieve a steady concentration in the blood, so doses are usually higher in the first 2–3 weeks. Its effects, however, can last 4 to 8 weeks after the drug is discontinued because it has an extended half-life that may exceed 50 days. The therapeutic serum level of amiodarone is 0.8 to 2.8 mcg/mL.

Administration Alerts

- Hypokalemia and hypomagnesemia should be corrected prior to initiating therapy.
- Pregnancy category D.

PHARMACOKINETICS

Onset	Peak	Duration
2-3 d PO, 2 hr IV	3–7 h	10–50 days

Adverse Effects

The most serious adverse effect is pulmonary toxicity. Amiodarone may also cause elevated liver enzymes, thyroid dysfunction, blue-gray skin discoloration, blurred vision, rashes, photosensitivity, nausea, vomiting, anorexia, fatigue, dizziness, and hypotension. Because this medication is concentrated by certain tissues and has a prolonged half-life, adverse effects may be slow to resolve.

Black Box Warning (oral form only): Amiodarone causes a pneumonia-like syndrome in the lungs. Because the pulmonary toxicity may be fatal, baseline and periodic assessment of lung function is essential. Amiodarone has prodysrhythmic action and may cause bradycardia, cardiogenic shock, or AV block. Mild liver injury is frequent with amiodarone.

Contraindications: Amiodarone is contraindicated in patients with severe bradycardia, cardiogenic shock, sick sinus syndrome, severe sinus node dysfunction, or third-degree AV block.

Interactions

Drug–Drug: Amiodarone can increase serum digoxin levels by as much as 70%. Amiodarone can block the metabolism of warfarin, thus requiring lower doses of the anticoagulant. Use with beta-adrenergic blockers or CCBs may cause or worsen sinus bradycardia, sinus arrest, or AV block. Amiodarone may increase phenytoin levels two- to threefold.

Lab Tests: Amiodarone may increase values for the following tests: ANA, ALT, AST, ALP, thyroid-stimulating hormone (TSH), and T_4.

Herbal/Food: Use with echinacea may cause an increased risk of hepatotoxicity. Aloe may cause an increased effect of amiodarone.

Treatment of Overdose: Treatment of amiodarone overdose is targeted to reversing hypotension with vasopressors, and bradycardia with atropine or isoproterenol.

velocity, they are able to stabilize certain dysrhythmias. Doses for the antidysrhythmic CCBs are listed in Table 30.3.

30.10 Treating Dysrhythmias With Calcium Channel Blockers

Although about 10 CCBs are available to treat cardiovascular diseases, only a limited number have been approved for dysrhythmias. A few CCBs, such as diltiazem (Cardizem, Dilacor, others) and verapamil (Calan, Isoptin, Verelan), block calcium ion channels in both the heart and arterioles; the remaining CCBs are specific to calcium channels in vascular smooth muscle. Diltiazem is a prototype drug for the treatment of angina, as discussed in chapter 28. The basic pharmacology of this drug class is presented in chapter 26.

Blockade of calcium ion channels has a number of effects on the heart, most of which are similar to those of beta-adrenergic blockers. Effects include reduced automaticity in the SA node and slowed impulse conduction through the AV node. This slows the heart rate and prolongs the refractory period. CCBs are only effective against supraventricular dysrhythmias.

CCBs are well tolerated by most patients. As with other antidysrhythmics, bradycardia and hypotension are frequent adverse effects. Because the cardiac effects of CCBs are almost identical with those of beta-adrenergic blockers, patients concurrently taking drugs from both classes are

Chapter 31

Drugs for Coagulation Disorders

Drugs at a Glance

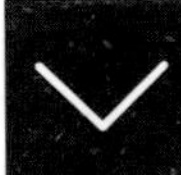

Learning Outcomes

After reading this chapter, the student should be able to:

1. Illustrate the major steps of hemostasis and fibrinolysis.
2. Describe thromboembolic disorders that are indications for coagulation modifiers.
3. Identify the primary mechanisms by which coagulation modifier drugs act.
4. Explain how laboratory testing of coagulation parameters is used to monitor anticoagulant pharmacotherapy.
5. Describe the nurse's role in the pharmacologic management of coagulation disorders.
6. For each of the classes listed in Drugs at a Glance, know representative drug examples, and explain the mechanism of drug action, primary actions, and important adverse effects.
7. Use the nursing process to care for patients receiving pharmacotherapy for coagulation disorders.

(pill icon) indicates a prototype drug, each of which is featured in a Prototype Drug box.

Hemostasis, or the stopping of blood flow, is an essential mechanism that protects the body from both external and internal injury. Without efficient hemostasis, bleeding from wounds or internal injuries would lead to shock and perhaps death. Too much clotting, however, can also be dangerous. The physiological processes of hemostasis must maintain a delicate balance between blood fluidity and coagulation.

Many common diseases affect hemostasis, including myocardial infarction (MI), stroke, venous or arterial thrombosis, valvular heart disease, and indwelling catheters. Because these conditions are so prevalent in clinical practice, the nurse will have frequent occasions to administer and monitor coagulation modifier drugs.

31.1 The Process of Hemostasis

Hemostasis is a complex process involving a large number of **clotting factors** that are activated in a series of sequential steps. Drugs may be used to modify several of these steps.

When a blood vessel is injured, a series of events initiate the clotting process. The vessel spasms and constricts, which limits the flow of blood to the injured area. Platelets become sticky, adhering to each other and to the damaged vessel. Aggregation is facilitated by adenosine diphosphate (ADP), the enzyme thrombin, and thromboxane A_2. Adhesion is made possible by platelet receptor sites (glycoprotein IIb/IIIa) and von Willebrand's factor. As the bound platelets break down, they release substances that attract more platelets to the area. The flow of blood is reduced, thus allowing the process of **coagulation,** the formation of an insoluble clot, to occur. The basic steps of hemostasis are shown in Figure 31.1.

When collagen is exposed at the site of injury, the damaged cells initiate a series of complex reactions called the **coagulation cascade.** Coagulation occurs when fibrin threads create a meshwork that traps blood constituents so that they develop a clot. During the cascade, various plasma proteins circulating in an inactive state are converted to their active forms. Two separate pathways, along with numerous biochemical processes, lead to coagulation. The *intrinsic* pathway is activated in response to injury. The *extrinsic* pathway is activated when blood leaks out of a vessel and enters tissue spaces. The two pathways have common steps, and the outcome is the same—the formation of the fibrin clot. The steps in each coagulation cascade are shown in Figure 31.2.

Near the end of the cascade, a chemical called **prothrombin activator** or prothrombinase is formed. Prothrombin activator converts the clotting factor **prothrombin** to an enzyme called **thrombin.** Thrombin then converts **fibrinogen,** a plasma protein, to long strands of **fibrin.** The fibrin strands provide a framework for the clot. Thus, two of the factors essential to clotting, thrombin and fibrin, are formed only *after* injury to the vessels. The fibrin strands form an insoluble web over the injured area to stop blood loss. Normal blood clotting occurs in approximately 6 minutes.

It is important to note that several clotting factors, including fibrinogen, are proteins made by the liver that constantly circulate through the blood in an *inactive* form. Vitamin K is required for the liver to make four of the clotting factors. Because of the crucial importance of the liver

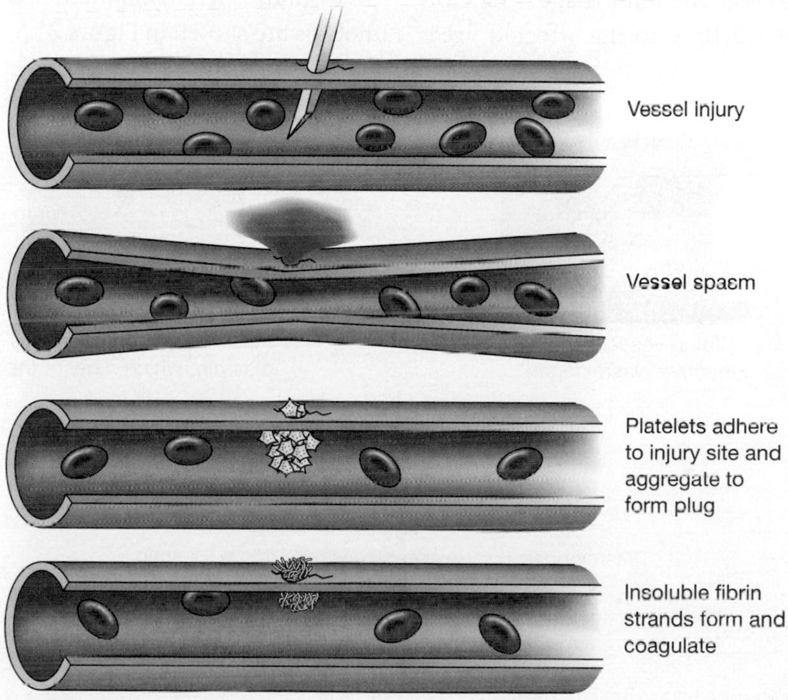

FIGURE 31.1 Basic steps in hemostasis

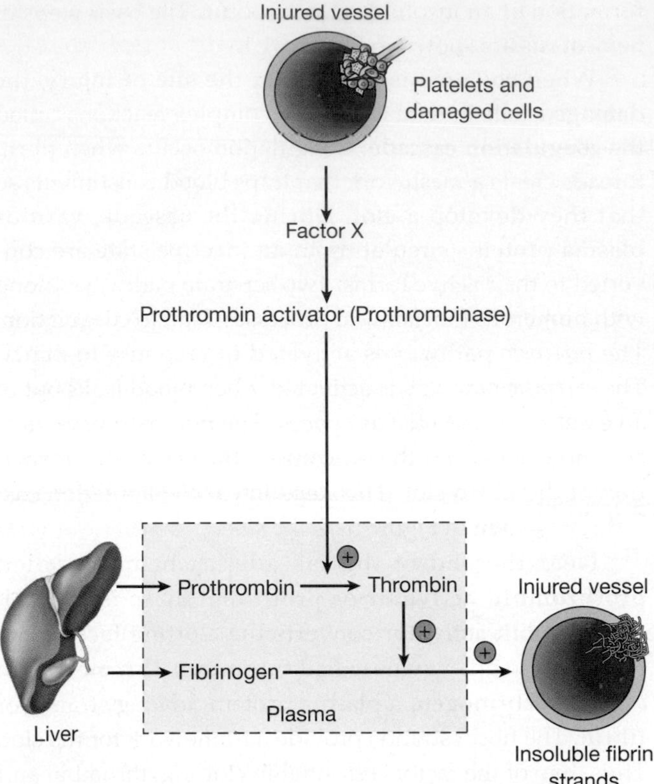

FIGURE 31.2 Major steps in the coagulation cascade: common pathway

in creating these clotting factors, patients with serious hepatic impairment usually have abnormal coagulation.

31.2 Removal of Blood Clots

Hemostasis is achieved once a blood clot is formed and the body is protected from excessive hemorrhage. The clot, however, may restrict blood flow to the affected area; circulation must eventually be restored so that the tissue can resume normal function. The process of clot removal is called **fibrinolysis.** It is initiated within 24 to 48 hours of clot formation and continues until the clot is dissolved.

Fibrinolysis also involves several sequential steps. When the fibrin clot is formed, nearby blood vessel cells secrete the enzyme **tissue plasminogen activator (TPA).** TPA converts the inactive protein **plasminogen,** which is present in the fibrin clot, to its active enzymatic form, **plasmin.** Plasmin then digests the fibrin strands to remove the clot. The body normally regulates fibrinolysis such that *unwanted* fibrin clots are removed, whereas fibrin present in wounds is left to maintain hemostasis. The steps of fibrinolysis are shown in Figure 31.3.

PharmFacts

CLOTTING DISORDERS

- von Willebrand's disease (vWD), the most common hereditary bleeding disorder, is caused by a deficiency of the protein von Willebrand factor (vWF). This factor plays a role in platelet aggregation and acts as a carrier for factor VIII.
- More than 2 million patients each year develop a deep vein thrombosis (DVT).
- DVT-associated pulmonary emboli are responsible for as many as 300,000 deaths annually in the United States.
- Hemophilia A, or classic hemophilia, is a hereditary condition in which a person lacks clotting factor VIII; it accounts for 80% of all hemophilia cases.
- Hemophilia B, or "Christmas disease," is a hereditary absence of clotting factor IX.
- About 20,000 people in the United States have hemophilia A or B.

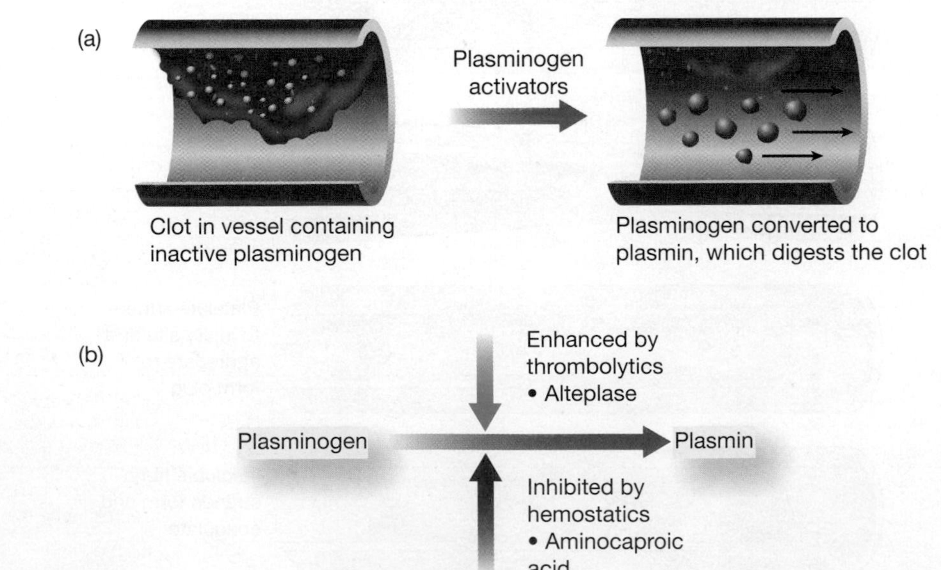

FIGURE 31.3 Primary steps in fibrinolysis

31.3 Alterations of Hemostasis

To diagnose a bleeding disorder, a thorough health history and physical examination is necessary. Laboratory tests measuring coagulation must be obtained. These may include prothrombin time (PT), thrombin time, activated partial thromboplastin time (aPTT), and, in some instances, a bleeding time. Platelet count is also important when assessing bleeding disorders. Additional tests may be indicated, based on the results of initial laboratory analyses. A summary of these tests is shown in Table 31.1.

Hemostasis is a delicate balance regulated by a large number of natural substances in the blood. Some of these substances, called procoagulants, promote the formation of clots. Natural procoagulants are essential to protecting the body by causing clot formation following vessel injury. The other natural substances that regulate hemostasis, the anticoagulants, restrain the clotting cascade and prevent it from becoming overactive. Effective hemostasis requires that procoagulants and anticoagulants become activated (and inactivated) at very specific times. Alterations in hemostasis occur when there is too much clotting or too little clotting.

Thromboembolic Disorders

The term **thromboembolic disorders** is used to describe conditions in which the body forms undesirable clots. Thromboembolic disorders may arise in both arteries and veins. Once a stationary clot, called a **thrombus,** forms in a vessel, it often grows larger as more fibrin is added. Arterial thrombi are particularly problematic because they deprive an area of adequate blood flow, causing tissue ischemia. Cessation of blood flow may result in infarction or tissue death. This is the case in MIs and many strokes.

Pieces of a thrombus may break off and travel through the bloodstream to affect other vessels. A traveling clot is called an **embolus**. Thrombi in the venous system usually form in the veins of the legs in susceptible patients due to sluggish blood flow, a condition called **deep vein thrombosis (DVT).** Thrombi can also form in the atria during atrial fibrillation. An embolus from the right atrium will cause pulmonary emboli, whereas an embolus from the left atrium will cause a stroke or an arterial infarction elsewhere in the body. Arterial thrombi and emboli can also occur following surgical procedures and following arterial punctures such as angiography. Patients with indwelling catheters and mechanical heart valves are susceptible to thrombi formation and frequently receive prophylactic anticoagulant therapy. Thromboembolic disorders are the most common indications for pharmacotherapy with coagulation modifiers.

Coagulation Disorders

Whereas thromboembolic disorders are caused by too much clotting, coagulation disorders result from too little clotting. The two most common causes of coagulation disorders are decreased numbers of platelets and deficiencies in one or more clotting factors.

Table 31.1 Laboratory Testing for Coagulation Disorders

Test	Description	Normal Values*	Significance
Activated clotting time	Used to monitor high-dose heparin pharmacotherapy; also used before, during, and after surgery or medical procedures	70–180 seconds; 400–500 seconds during coronary bypass surgery	High values indicate a risk for bleeding and that heparin dose may need to be reduced
Activated partial thromboplastin time (aPTT)	Used to monitor heparin pharmacotherapy	25–35 seconds; 1.5–2 times higher than the pretreatment value	High values indicate a risk for bleeding and that heparin dose may need to be reduced
Bleeding time	Used for general diagnosis of coagulation disorders	2–9 minutes (forearm)	Long bleeding time may indicate a low platelet count or anticoagulant therapy
Heparin anti-Xa	Used to monitor heparin or low-molecular-weight heparin (LMWH) pharmacotherapy in patients with heparin resistance	0.3–0.7 international units/mL for heparin; 0.4–1.1 international units/mL for LMWH	High values indicate a risk for bleeding and that heparin or LMWH dose may need to be reduced
Platelet count	Part of a complete blood count	150,000–350,000	Values below 50,000 indicate thrombocytopenia
Prothrombin time (PT)	Used to monitor warfarin therapy	International normalized ratio (INR) should be 2–3 to prevent DVT; 2.5–3.5 to prevent arterial thrombosis	High values indicate a risk for bleeding and that anticoagulant dose may need to be reduced
Thrombin time	Used to assess for fibrinogen deficiency; may be used to monitor effectiveness of heparin pharmacotherapy	13–15 seconds	Prolonged values may occur with heparin pharmacotherapy

Note: *Coagulation values are always individualized for each patient.

Complementary and Alternative Therapies

GARLIC FOR CARDIOVASCULAR HEALTH

Garlic (*Allium sativum*) is one of the best-studied herbs. Several substances, known as *alliaceous oils,* have been isolated from garlic and shown to have pharmacologic activity. Dosage forms include eating prepared garlic oil or the fresh bulbs from the plant.

Modern claims for garlic uses have focused on the cardiovascular system: treatment of high blood lipid levels, atherosclerosis, and hypertension (HTN). Other modern claims are that garlic reduces blood glucose levels and has antibacterial and antiviral properties.

Like many other supplements, garlic likely has some health benefits, but controlled, scientific studies are often lacking and the results are mixed. Garlic has been shown to decrease the aggregation or "stickiness" of platelets, thus producing an anticoagulant effect. There is some research to show that the herb has a small effect on lowering blood cholesterol (Ried, Toben, & Fakler, 2013). Evidence regarding the effects of the herb on blood pressure is mixed. An analysis of the research of the effect of garlic on the common cold concluded that there is insufficient clinical evidence to show any benefit (Lissiman, Bhasale, & Cohen, 2012).

Garlic is safe for consumption in moderate amounts. Patients taking anticoagulant medications should limit their intake of garlic to avoid bleeding complications. Patients with diabetes should monitor their blood glucose levels closely if taking high doses of garlic.

The most common coagulation disorder is a deficiency of platelets known as **thrombocytopenia,** which occurs when platelet counts fall significantly below normal levels. Thrombocytopenia is the result of either decreased platelet production or increased platelet destruction. This may occur from any condition that suppresses bone marrow function and from the administration of immunosuppressant drugs and most of the medications used for cancer chemotherapy. Other common causes of decreased platelet production are folic acid or vitamin B_{12} deficiencies and hepatic failure.

Deficiencies in specific clotting factors may prolong coagulation and lead to excess bleeding. Deficiencies in multiple coagulation factors occur frequently in patients with serious hepatic impairment, because the liver synthesizes most clotting factors. Deficiency in a single coagulation factor suggests hemophilia which is a genetic deficiency in a specific clotting factor. The pharmacotherapy of hemophilia disorders is discussed in section 31.9.

31.4 Mechanisms of Coagulation Modification

Drugs can modify hemostasis by five basic mechanisms, as summarized in Table 31.2. The most commonly prescribed coagulation modifiers are the **anticoagulants,** which are used to prevent the formation of clots. Anticoagulants usually act by inhibiting specific clotting factors in the coagulation cascade. A second widely used drug class is the antiplatelet medications, which act by inhibiting the clotting action of platelets. Regardless of the mechanism, all anticoagulant drugs will increase the normal clotting time.

Table 31.2 Overview of Coagulation Modifiers

Type of Modification	Mechanism of Drug Action	Drug Classification
Prevention of clot formation	Inhibition of specific clotting factors	Anticoagulants
	Inhibition of platelet actions	Antiplatelet drugs
Removal of an existing clot	Clot dissolved by the drug	Thrombolytics
Promotion of clot formation	Inhibition of fibrin destruction	Hemostatics
	Administration of missing clotting factors	Clotting factor concentrates

Once an abnormal clot has formed in a blood vessel, it may be critical to remove it quickly to restore normal tissue function. This is particularly important for vessels serving the heart, lungs, and brain. A specific class of drugs, the **thrombolytics,** are used to dissolve such life-threatening clots.

Occasionally, it is necessary to *promote* the formation of clots with drugs called **hemostatics.** These drugs inhibit the normal removal of fibrin, thus keeping the clot in place for a longer period. Hemostatics are used to speed clot formation, thereby limiting bleeding from a surgical site.

To prevent serious adverse effects, pharmacotherapy with coagulation modifiers is individualized to each patient. Drug–drug interactions are common with anticoagulants and can either increase or diminish the anticoagulant effect. Kidney or liver disease can contribute to drug toxicity. Patients who are taking coagulation modifiers require regular physical assessment and laboratory monitoring.

ANTICOAGULANTS

Anticoagulants are drugs used to prolong bleeding time and thereby prevent blood thrombi from forming or growing larger. They are widely used in the treatment of thromboembolic disease. Table 31.3 lists the primary anticoagulants.

31.5 Pharmacotherapy With Anticoagulants

Anticoagulants act by a number of different mechanisms, as illustrated in Figure 31.4. These drugs are often referred

Table 31.3 Anticoagulants

Drug	Route and Adult Dose (max dose where indicated)	Adverse Effects
antithrombin, recombinant (ATryn)	IV infusion: Dose is individualized based on pretreatment antithrombin level and body weight	*Nausea, vomiting, transient thrombocytopenia (heparin), anemia (fondaparinux)*
fondaparinux (Arixtra)	Subcutaneous: 2.5 mg/day starting at least 6 h postop for 5–9 days	Hemorrhage, anaphylaxis (antithrombin, heparin)
heparin	IV: 5,000 unit bolus dose, then 20,000-40,000 units infused over 24 h (use agency-specific heparin nomogram)	
	Subcutaneous: 10,000–20,000 units followed by 8,000–20,000 units q8–12h	
warfarin (Coumadin)	PO: Dose varies based on target INR, which is usually within the range of 2–3	
LOW-MOLECULAR-WEIGHT HEPARINS (LMWHS)		
dalteparin (Fragmin)	Subcutaneous (prevention of DVT following surgery): 2,500–5,000 units/day for 5–10 days (max: 18,000 international units/day)	*Minor bleeding, nausea, vomiting, hematoma, local pain, fever*
	Subcutaneous (thromboembolism): 120 international units/kg bid for at least 5 days	Hemorrhage, thrombocytopenia, pancytopenia, anaphylaxis
enoxaparin (Lovenox)	Subcutaneous (prevention of DVT after surgery): 30 mg bid for 7–10 days	
	Subcutaneous (treatment of DVT): 1 mg/kg q12h or 1.5 mg/kg/day	
	IV (acute STEMI): 30 mg bolus followed by subcutaneous doses	
tinzaparin (Innohep)	Subcutaneous (treatment of DVT): 175 units/kg daily for at least 6 days	
DIRECT THROMBIN INHIBITORS		
argatroban (Acova, Novastan)	IV: 2 mcg/kg/min (max: 10 mcg/kg/min)	*Fever, nausea, allergic skin reactions, hepatic impairment, minor bleeding, back pain (bivalirudin)*
bivalirudin (Angiomax)	IV: 0.75 mg/kg initial bolus followed by 1.75 mg/kg/h for 4 h	
dabigatran (Pradaxa)	PO: 75–150 mg bid	Serious internal hemorrhage, hemoptysis, hematuria, sepsis, heart failure
desirudin (Iprivask)	Subcutaneous: 15 mg bid for 9–12 days (max: 80 mg/day)	
FACTOR Xa INIBITORS		
apixaban (Eliquis)	PO: 2.5–10 mg bid	*Minor bleeding,*
edoxaban (Savaysa)	PO: 30–60 mg once daily	Major bleeding including stroke; hypersensitivity reactions
rivaroxaban (Xarelto)	PO: 10–20 mg once daily	

Note: *Italics* indicate common adverse effects; underlining indicates serious adverse effects.

to as blood thinners, which is a misnomer, because they do not change the thickness of the blood. Instead, anticoagulants impart a negative charge to the surface of the platelets, which inhibits the clumping action or aggregation of these cells.

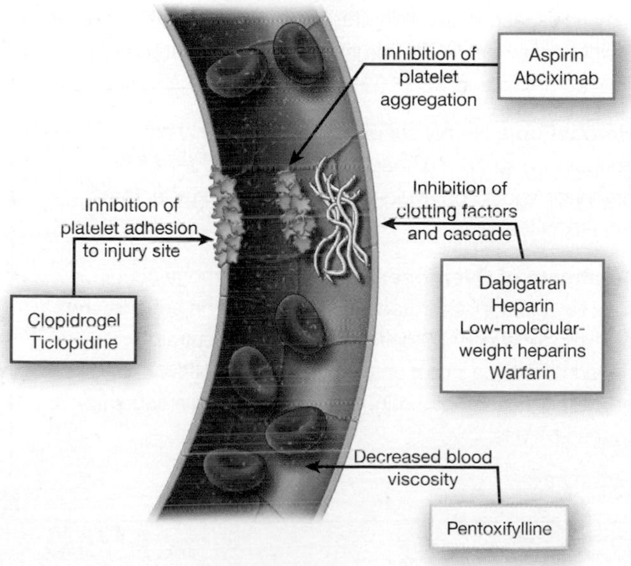

FIGURE 31.4 Mechanisms of action of coagulation modifiers

By inhibiting certain clotting factors, anticoagulants lengthen clotting time and prevent thrombi from forming or growing larger. Thromboembolic disease can be life threatening; thus, therapy is often begun by administering anticoagulants intravenously or subcutaneously to achieve a rapid onset of action. The patient is then switched to oral anticoagulants with careful monitoring of appropriate coagulation laboratory studies.

Parenteral Anticoagulants

The traditional drug of choice for parenteral anticoagulation is heparin. Heparin acts by enhancing actions of antithrombin III. **Antithrombin III** is a protein in plasma that inactivates thrombin (and several other procoagulant enzymes) and inhibits coagulation. Within minutes after intravenous (IV) administration of heparin, the loss of activated clotting factors slows the formation and growth of fibrin clots.

Although heparin was the drug of choice for many decades, several effective alternatives are now available.

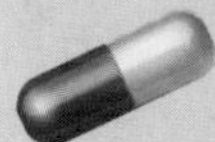

Prototype Drug | Heparin

Therapeutic Class: Anticoagulant *(Parenteral)* **Pharmacologic Class:** Indirect thrombin inhibitor

Actions and Uses

Heparin is a natural substance found in the liver and in the lining of blood vessels. Its normal function is to prolong coagulation time, thereby preventing excessive clotting within blood vessels. As a result, heparin prevents the enlargement of existing clots and the formation of new ones. It has no ability to *dissolve* existing clots.

The binding of heparin to antithrombin III inactivates several clotting factors and inhibits thrombin activity. The onset of action for IV heparin is immediate, whereas subcutaneous heparin may take up to 1 hour to achieve a therapeutic effect. This drug is also called *unfractionated* heparin to distinguish it from the LMWHs.

Heparin has both prophylactic and treatment indications. It is used at low doses to *prevent* thromboembolic events arising from open heart and vascular surgery, dialysis procedures, or in patients with unstable angina or in the acute stages of MI. It is used at higher doses to *treat* conditions in which immediate anticoagulation is necessary, such as confirmed DVT and pulmonary embolism. Dosing is highly variable depending upon the indication and is often based on a weight-based nomogram and aPTT values.

Administration Alerts

- Heparin is poorly absorbed by the gastrointestinal (GI) mucosa because of rapid metabolism by the hepatic enzyme heparinase. Therefore, it must be given either subcutaneously or through IV bolus injection or continuous infusion.
- When giving IV heparin, a weight-based nomogram may be used. The heparin nomogram system calculates the appropriate heparin dose using patient weight, aPTT value, and clinical indication for the drug (e.g., DVT, acute coronary syndrome). The use of the nomogram decreases the chance of medication calculation errors and for over- or under-therapeutic doses.
- When administering heparin subcutaneously, never draw back the syringe plunger once the needle has entered the skin, and never massage the site after injection. Doing either can contribute to bleeding or tissue damage.
- Intramuscular (IM) administration is contraindicated due to bleeding risk.
- Pregnancy category C.

PHARMACOKINETICS (SUBCUTANEOUS)

Onset	Peak	Duration
30–60 min	2 h	8–12 h

Adverse Effects

Abnormal bleeding may occur during heparin therapy. Should aPTT become prolonged or toxicity be observed, stopping the infusion will result in diminished anticoagulant activity within hours. Heparin-induced thrombocytopenia (HIT) is a serious complication that occurs in up to 30% of patients taking the drug. More severe symptoms usually appear after 5 to 10 days of therapy; thus, frequent blood laboratory testing should be conducted during this period. Although thrombocytopenia usually leads to excessive bleeding, HIT causes the opposite effect: an *increase* in adverse thromboembolic events. The patient may experience serious and even life-threatening thrombosis. Although the half-life of heparin is brief, it may take a week after the drug is discontinued for platelets to completely recover.

Black Box Warning: Epidural or spinal hematomas may occur when heparin or LMWHs are used in patients receiving spinal anesthesia or lumbar puncture. Because these can result in long-term or permanent paralysis, frequent monitoring for neurologic impairment is essential.

Contraindications: Heparin should not be administered to patients with active internal bleeding, bleeding disorders, severe HTN, recent trauma, intracranial hemorrhage, or bacterial endocarditis.

Interactions

Drug–Drug: Oral anticoagulants, including warfarin, potentiate the action of heparin. Drugs that inhibit platelet aggregation, such as aspirin, indomethacin, and ibuprofen, may induce bleeding. Nicotine, digoxin, tetracyclines, or antihistamines may inhibit anticoagulation.

Lab Tests: Heparin may increase the following values: free fatty acids, aspartate aminotranferase (AST), and alanine aminotransferase (ALT). Serum cholesterol and triglycerides may be decreased.

Herbal/Food: Herbal supplements that may affect coagulation such as ginger, garlic, green tea, feverfew, or ginkgo should be avoided because they may increase the risk of bleeding.

Treatment of Overdose: If serious hemorrhage occurs, a specific antagonist, protamine sulfate, may be administered IV (1 mg for every 100 units of heparin) to neutralize heparin's anticoagulant activity. Protamine sulfate has an onset of action of 5 minutes and is also an antagonist to the LMWHs.

The heparin molecule has been shortened and modified to create a newer class of drugs called **low-molecular-weight heparins (LMWHs).** The mechanism of action of these drugs is similar to that of heparin, except their inhibition is more specific to active Factor X (see Figure 31.2). LMWHs are parenteral anticoagulants that possess the same degree of anticoagulant activity as heparin but have several advantages. Their duration of action is two to four times longer than that of heparin. The LMWHs also produce a more stable response than heparin; thus, fewer follow-up laboratory tests are needed, and family members, caregivers, or the patient can be trained to give the necessary subcutaneous injections at home. These anticoagulants are less likely than heparin to cause thrombocytopenia. Like heparin, however, bleeding is a potentially serious adverse effect of the LMWHs. LMWHs have become the preferred drugs for a number of clotting disorders, including the prevention of DVT following surgery.

A third class of anticoagulants includes direct thrombin inhibitors such as dabigatran (Pradaxa). These drugs bind to the active site of thrombin, preventing the formation of fibrin clots. They act on circulating thrombin as well as on thrombin that has already bound to a clot. These drugs are administered until a therapeutic aPTT value is obtained, usually one and a half to three times the control value. The thrombin inhibitors have limited therapeutic application. Bivalirudin (Angiomax) and argatroban (Acova, Novastan) are administered in combination with aspirin to prevent thrombi in patients undergoing percutaneous coronary intervention and for the prevention or treatment of thrombocytopenia induced by heparin therapy. Desirudin (Iprivask) is given subcutaneously 15 minutes prior to hip replacement surgery for prophylaxis of DVT. The newest of the drugs in this class, dabigatran (Pradaxa), is the only one that is given orally (PO). It is approved to reduce the risk of stroke and embolism in patients with atrial fibrillation. Initially approved for stroke prevention in patients with nonvalvular atrial fibrillation, its indications were extended in 2014 to include treatment of DVT and pulmonary embolus in patients who have been treated with a parenteral anticoagulant for 5 to 10 days.

The final parenteral anticoagulant is antithrombin (ATryn), which is unusual because it is obtained from genetically engineered goats. The goats are engineered through recombinant DNA technology to secrete human antithrombin in their milk. The drug is then purified and powdered for reconstitution as an IV infusion. It is approved to treat patients with a congenital deficiency of antithrombin III, who experience a high incidence of blood clots, especially DVTs. The drug is indicated for the prevention of perioperative and peripartum thromboembolic events in patients with hereditary antithrombin deficiency.

Oral Anticoagulants

Although parenteral anticoagulants have the advantage of an almost immediate onset of action, drugs given by this route require close medical supervision because adverse effects such as bleeding can rapidly ensue. When the patient's condition allows, oral anticoagulants are used due to their convenience and greater safety.

The most commonly prescribed oral anticoagulant is warfarin (Coumadin). Warfarin acts by inhibiting the hepatic synthesis of coagulation Factors II, VII, IX, and X. Because warfarin has a delayed onset of several days, it is not suitable for emergency anticoagulation. For these patients rapid anticoagulation is achieved with heparin. When transitioning, the two drugs are administered concurrently until laboratory values indicate that target anticoagulation values have been achieved.

Pentoxifylline (Trental) is another oral anticoagulant that works by a different mechanism than heparin. Pentoxifylline reduces the viscosity (thickness) of red blood cells (RBCs) and increases their flexibility. It is given to increase the microcirculation in patients with intermittent claudication.

Several newer drugs have emerged as significant alternatives to warfarin for stroke prevention. Rivaroxaban (Xarelto), apixaban (Eliquis), and edoxaban (Savaysa) are the first anticoagulants available by the oral (PO) route that *directly* inhibit Factor Xa in the clotting cascade. The other drugs that inhibit Factor Xa, heparin and the LMWHs, inhibit Factor Xa indirectly and must be administered parenterally. The oral Factor Xa inhibitors are indicated for the prophylaxis and treatment of DVT and the reduction of stroke risk and systemic embolism in patients with atrial fibrillation. These alternatives appear to be as effective as warfarin in preventing strokes and they do not require INR monitoring or exhibit extensive drug interactions compared to warfarin. Rivaroxaban, apixaban, and edoxaban carry black box warnings that extreme care must be taken not to discontinue them quickly unless another anticoagulant has been substituted. Failure to provide adequate anticoagulant following discontinuation may result in serious ischemic events. The black box warning also states that they should not be used in patients undergoing neuraxial anesthesia or spinal puncture due to a risk for the development of epidural or spinal hematomas resulting in long term paralysis.

The most frequent, and potentially serious, adverse effect of all the anticoagulant drugs is bleeding. Patients who have recently experienced a traumatic injury or surgery are especially at risk. Specific antagonists may be administered to reverse the anticoagulant effects: Protamine sulfate is used for heparin, and vitamin K is administered for warfarin (see the drug prototype features in this chapter).

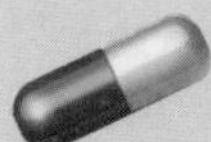

Prototype Drug | Warfarin *(Coumadin)*

Therapeutic Class: Anticoagulant (oral) **Pharmacologic Class:** Vitamin K antagonist

Actions and Uses

Indications for warfarin therapy include the prevention of stroke, MI, DVT, and pulmonary embolism in patients undergoing hip or knee surgery or in those with long-term indwelling central venous catheters or prosthetic heart valves. The drug may be given to prevent thromboembolic events in high-risk patients following an MI or an atrial fibrillation episode.

Unlike with heparin, the anticoagulant activity of warfarin can take several days to reach its maximum effect. This explains why heparin and warfarin therapy are overlapped. Warfarin inhibits the action of vitamin K. Without adequate vitamin K, the synthesis of clotting Factors II, VII, IX, and X is diminished. Because these clotting factors are normally circulating in the blood, it takes several days for their plasma levels to fall and for the anticoagulant effect of warfarin to appear. Another reason for the slow onset is that 99% of the warfarin is bound to plasma proteins and is thus unavailable to produce its effect. The therapeutic range of serum warfarin levels varies from 1 to 10 mcg/mL to achieve an INR value of 2 to 3.

Administration Alerts

- If life-threatening bleeding occurs during therapy, the anticoagulant effects of warfarin can be reduced by IM or subcutaneous administration of its antagonist, vitamin K_1.
- Pregnancy category X.

PHARMACOKINETICS (PO)

Onset	Peak	Duration
2–7 days	0.5–3 days	3–5 days

Adverse Effects

The most serious adverse effect of warfarin is abnormal bleeding. On discontinuation of therapy, the anticoagulant activity of warfarin may persist for up to 10 days.

Black Box Warning: Warfarin can cause major or fatal bleeding, and regular monitoring of INR is required. Patients should be instructed about prevention measures to minimize bleeding risk and to immediately notify health care providers of signs and symptoms of bleeding.

Contraindications: Patients with recent trauma, active internal bleeding, bleeding disorders, intracranial hemorrhage, severe HTN, bacterial endocarditis, or severe hepatic or renal impairment should not take warfarin.

Interactions

Drug–Drug: Extensive protein binding is responsible for numerous drug–drug interactions, including an increased effect of warfarin with alcohol, nonsteroidal anti-inflammatory drugs (NSAIDs), diuretics, selective serotonin reuptake inhibitors (SSRIs) and other antidepressants, steroids, antibiotics and vaccines, and vitamins (e.g., vitamin K). During warfarin therapy, the patient should not take any other prescription or over-the-counter (OTC) drugs unless approved by the health care provider.

Lab Tests: Unknown.

Herbal/Food: Use of warfarin with herbal supplements such as green tea, ginkgo, feverfew, garlic, cranberry, chamomile, and ginger may increase the risk of bleeding. Consumption of foods rich in vitamin K, such as kale, spinach, turnip or mustard greens, broccoli, Brussels sprouts, or cabbage may reduce the therapeutic effects of warfarin.

Treatment of Overdose: The specific treatment for overdose is PO or parenteral administration of vitamin K_1. When administered IV, vitamin K_1 can reverse the anticoagulant effects of warfarin within 6 hours.

☑ Check Your Understanding 31.1

Will an anticoagulant drug prevent emboli? *Visit www.pearsonhighered.com/nursingresources for the answer.*

ANTIPLATELET DRUGS

Antiplatelet drugs produce an anticoagulant effect by interfering with platelet aggregation. Unlike the anticoagulants, which are used primarily to prevent thrombosis in veins, antiplatelet drugs are used to prevent clot formation in arteries. The antiplatelet medications are listed in Table 31.4.

31.6 Pharmacotherapy With Antiplatelet Drugs

Platelets are a key component of hemostasis: too few platelets or diminished platelet function can profoundly increase bleeding time. Antiplatelet medications include the following:

1. Aspirin
2. Adenosine diphosphate (ADP) receptor blockers
3. Glycoprotein IIb/IIIa receptor antagonists
4. Drugs for intermittent claudication.

Table 31.4 Antiplatelet Drugs

Drug	Route and Adult Dose (max dose where indicated)	Adverse Effects
anagrelide (Agrylin)	PO: 0.5 mg qid or 1 mg bid (max: 10 mg/day)	*Nausea, vomiting, diarrhea, abdominal pain, headache (anagrelide)*
aspirin (acetylsalicylic acid, ASA) (see page 252 for the Prototype Drug box)	PO: 80 mg/day to 650 mg bid	Increased clotting time, GI bleeding (aspirin), central nervous system (CNS) effects (dipyridamole), anaphylaxis (aspirin), cardiac toxicity (anagrelide)
dipyridamole (Persantine)	PO: 75–100 mg qid	
vorapaxar (Zontivity)	PO: 2.08 mg/day	
ADP RECEPTOR BLOCKERS		
clopidogrel (Plavix)	PO: 75 mg/day	*Minor bleeding, dyspepsia, abdominal pain, dizziness, headache*
prasugrel (Effient)	PO: 60 mg loading dose followed by 10 mg/day	Increased clotting time, GI bleeding, blood dyscrasias, angina
ticagrelor (Brilinta)	PO: 180 mg loading dose followed by 90 mg bid	
ticlopidine (Ticlid)	PO: 250 mg bid (max: 500 mg/day)	
GLYCOPROTEIN IIB/IIIA RECEPTOR ANTAGONISTS		
abciximab (ReoPro)	IV: 0.25 mg/kg initial bolus over 5 min; then 10 mcg/kg/min for 12 h (max: 10 mcg/min)	*Dyspepsia, dizziness, pain at injection site, hypotension, bradycardia, minor bleeding*
eptifibatide (Integrilin)	IV: 180 mcg/kg initial bolus over 1–2 min; then 2 mcg/kg/min for 24–72 h	Hemorrhage, thrombocytopenia
tirofiban (Aggrastat)	IV: 0.4 mcg/kg/min for 30 min; then 0.1 mcg/kg/min for 12–24 h	
AGENTS FOR INTERMITTENT CLAUDICATION		
cilostazol (Pletal)	PO: 100 mg bid	*Dyspepsia, nausea, vomiting, dizziness, myalgia, headache*
pentoxifylline (Trental)	PO: 400 mg tid	Tachycardia and palpitations (cilostazol), CNS effects (pentoxifylline), heart failure, MI

Note: *Italics* indicate common adverse effects; underlining indicates serious adverse effects.

Nursing Practice Application

Pharmacotherapy With Anticoagulant and Antiplatelet Drugs

ASSESSMENT	POTENTIAL NURSING DIAGNOSES*
Baseline assessment prior to administration: • Obtain a complete health history including cardiovascular (including HTN, MI, heart failure) and peripheral vascular disease (including thrombophlebitis), respiratory (including previous pulmonary embolism), neurologic (including recent head injury, stroke), hepatic or renal disease, diabetes, peptic ulcer disease, hypercholesterolemia, and the possibility of alcoholism or pregnancy. **Lifespan:** Ask women of menstrual age about length and heaviness of usual menstrual flow. Obtain a drug history including allergies, current prescription and OTC drugs, herbal preparations, and alcohol use. Be alert to possible drug interactions. • Obtain baseline weight, vital signs, ECG (if appropriate), and breath sounds. Assess for presence, quality, location of angina, and for presence of dyspnea or chest pain. Assess extremities for symptoms of thrombophlebitis (e.g., warmth, swelling, tenderness in calf) and for location and character/amount of edema, if present. • Evaluate appropriate laboratory findings (e.g., aPTT, antiprothrombin antibodies (aPT), or INR), complete blood count (CBC), renal and liver function studies, arterial blood gases (ABGs) as appropriate, and lipid profiles.	• *Acute Pain* • *Ineffective Tissue Perfusion* • *Impaired Skin Integrity* • *Anxiety* • *Deficient Knowledge* (drug therapy) • *Risk for Injury,* related to adverse effects of anticoagulant therapy *NANDA I © 2014

continued

Nursing Practice Application *continued*

ASSESSMENT	POTENTIAL NURSING DIAGNOSES*
Assessment throughout administration: • Assess for desired therapeutic effects (e.g., area of phlebitis exhibits signs of improvement with no symptoms of thrombosis formation; signs and symptoms of existing thrombosis show gradual improvement: e.g., previous anginal or peripheral extremity pain has diminished or is eliminated; peripheral pulses are improving in quality and volume). • Continue periodic monitoring of appropriate laboratory values (e.g., aPTT, PT, or INR).	
• Assess for adverse effects: bleeding at IV sites, wounds, excessive ecchymosis, petechiae, hematuria, black/tarry stools, rectal bleeding, "coffee-ground" emesis, epistaxis, bleeding from gums, hemoptysis, prolonged or heavy menstrual flow, and for symptoms of occult bleeding, such as pallor, dizziness, hypotension, tachycardia, abdominal pain, areas of abdominal wall swelling or firmness, lumbar pain, or decreased level of consciousness.	

IMPLEMENTATION

Interventions and (Rationales)	Patient-Centered Care
Ensuring therapeutic effects: • Continue frequent assessments as described earlier for therapeutic effects (e.g., existing area of phlebitis exhibits signs of improvement; signs and symptoms of existing thrombosis show gradual improvement; and peripheral pulses are improving in quality and volume). (Anticoagulants help prevent the formation of thrombi or prevent existing thrombi from increasing in size.)	• To allay possible anxiety, teach the patient, family, or caregiver the rationale for all equipment used (e.g., antiembolic stockings, intermittent pneumatic sequential compression devices) and the need for frequent monitoring.
• Encourage early ambulation postoperatively in the hospitalized patient and active range of motion (ROM) if the patient is on bed rest or has limited mobility. Perform passive ROM in patients who are unable to perform active ROM. (Early ambulation and ROM prevents venous stasis and thrombosis formation, lessening the need for anticoagulant therapy.)	• Assist the patient with ambulation postoperatively and teach active ROM. Teach the patient, family, or caregiver how to perform passive ROM exercises for patients who are unable to perform active ROM.
• Assess the patient's lifestyle and occasions of travel over extended lengths of time. (Prolonged sitting during air or car travel may limit blood flow to lower extremities and venous return, promoting the formation of thrombi.)	• Educate patients and consumers about thrombosis prevention during travel: periodic stretching, short periods of ambulation, avoiding sitting for prolonged periods, and increasing fluid intake.
• Encourage appropriate lifestyle changes. Provide for dietitian consultation as needed. (Smoking increases platelet aggregation and promotes the formation of thrombi.)	• Encourage the patient to adopt a healthy lifestyle of low-fat food choices, increased exercise, decreased caffeine and alcohol consumption, and smoking cessation. Provide for appropriate consultation (e.g., dietitian) as needed.
Minimizing adverse effects: • Monitor for signs and symptoms of increased or excessive visible bleeding and for occult bleeding. (Frequent assessment for both visible and occult bleeding is necessary to prevent hemorrhage and to start early corrective treatment as appropriate. **Diverse Patients:** Because some drugs such as clopidogrel [Plavix] metabolize through the P450 system pathways, monitor ethnically diverse patients to ensure optimal therapeutic effects and to minimize adverse effects.)	• **Safety:** Anticoagulant use is a high-risk safety concern and is included in The Joint Commission's National Patient Safety Goals. • Teach the patient, family, or caregiver signs and symptoms of excessive bleeding, including occult bleeding. If external bleeding occurs, pressure over the site should be held up to 15 minutes. If bleeding continues, is severe, or is accompanied by dizziness or syncope, immediate medical attention (e.g., 911) should be obtained. • **Lifespan:** Women of menstrual age should report excessively heavy or prolonged menstrual bleeding and should keep a "pad count" and report to the health care provider.

Nursing Practice Application *continued*

IMPLEMENTATION	
Interventions and (Rationales)	**Patient-Centered Care**
• Continue to monitor frequent labs (aPTT, aPT, or INR), CBC, and platelets. (Therapeutic aPTT and aPT levels are usually 1.5–2.5 times the normal control value. INR is usually 2–3.5 or 4. Values below the norm indicate below-therapeutic levels of the drug; values above the norm indicate a high potential for bleeding and hemorrhage. CBC, especially RBC, Hgb and Hct, and platelet levels should remain within normal limits. Decreasing values on the CBC may indicate excessive bleeding and the need to assess for location. **Lifespan:** Be especially cautious with the older adult as age-related hepatic changes may increase the risk of bleeding.)	• Instruct the patient on the need to return periodically for laboratory work and to alert laboratory personnel that anticoagulant therapy is being used. • Instruct the patient to carry a wallet identification card or wear medical identification jewelry indicating anticoagulant therapy.
• Continue to monitor peripheral pulses for quality and volume, and complaints of angina or chest pain, especially if new or sudden onset or accompanied by dyspnea. (Anticoagulants prevent thrombus formation or extension; they do not prevent emboli from occurring. Monitoring for new or sudden onset of pain is necessary to ensure prompt treatment of possible emboli.)	• Teach the patient to immediately report any sudden pain in chest, legs or calves, dyspnea, or new-onset anginal pain.
• Minimize opportunities for injury or bleeding where possible, including avoiding IM injections. **Lifespan:** Be cautious when providing care, especially with the older adult who may have fragile skin. (The risk of bleeding with antiplatelet drugs is not as severe as with anticoagulants, but it is still possible. Anticoagulants significantly raise the risk of bleeding, and causes of even minor bleeding should be avoided when possible. Warfarin and antiplatelet drugs may continue to have effects after the drug is stopped. Older adults with fragile skin may experience skin tears or ecchymosis more frequently)	• Instruct the patient on ways to minimize opportunities for injury or bleeding where possible: • Switch to a soft toothbrush and inspect gums after brushing. • Use an electric razor if possible or be cautious with a safety razor, holding prolonged pressure over small nicks. • Be cautious with food preparation, especially when cutting food. • Avoid contact sports, amusement park rides, or other physical activities that may cause intense or violent bumping, jostling, or injury. These safety precautions should be continued for up to one month following discontinuation of oral anticoagulants such as warfarin. • **Lifespan:** Frequently assess older adult family members who are on anticoagulant therapy for fragile skin.
• Closely evaluate all new prescriptions or use of OTC medications for drug interactions. (Many drugs interact with anticoagulants, increasing the chance for bleeding. All OTC medications containing salicylates, e.g., aspirin, and NSAIDs are contraindicated.)	• Instruct the patient to consult the health care provider before taking any new prescription or OTC medication, including herbal preparations.
• Maintain a normal diet, avoiding increases or decreases in vitamin K–rich foods (e.g., asparagus, broccoli, cabbage, cauliflower, kale) and limit or eliminate alcohol intake. (Vitamin K is necessary for the synthesis of clotting agents. Sudden increases or decreases in dietary intake of vitamin K–rich foods may increase or decrease the effectiveness of anticoagulants, particularly oral anticoagulant therapy. Excessive intake of alcohol, over two drinks per day in men or one in women, may alter the effectiveness of oral anticoagulants.)	• Teach the patient to maintain a normal diet, avoiding increases or decreases in vitamin K–rich foods and limit or eliminate alcohol intake. Vitamin K supplements and protein supplement drinks (e.g., Ensure, or Boost) that often have vitamin K added should also be avoided. • Advise patients to avoid excessive intake of alcohol while on oral anticoagulants.
• Assess for any symptoms of hepatitis (e.g., darkening urine, light or clay-colored stools, itchy skin, jaundice of sclera or skin, abdominal pain especially in the right upper quadrant [RUQ]) in patients receiving oral anticoagulant therapy. (Drug-induced hepatitis is a possible adverse effect of oral anticoagulant therapy.)	• Instruct the patient to report any signs of possible hepatitis immediately, especially abdominal discomfort that localizes to the RUQ.
Patient understanding of drug therapy:	
• Use opportunities during administration of medications and during assessments to provide patient education. (Using time during nursing care helps to optimize and reinforce key teaching areas.)	• The patient should be able to state the reason for the drug; appropriate dose and scheduling; what adverse effects to observe for and when to report; equipment needed as appropriate and how to use that equipment; and the required length of medication therapy needed with any special instructions regarding renewing or continuing the prescription as appropriate.

continued

Nursing Practice Application *continued*

IMPLEMENTATION	
Interventions and (Rationales)	**Patient-Centered Care**
Patient self-administration of drug therapy: • When administering medications, instruct the patient, family, or caregiver in proper self-administration techniques followed by teach-back. (Proper drug administration increases the effectiveness of the drug.)	• Teach the patient, family, or caregiver in proper self-administration techniques: • Injections of heparin or LMWH should be administered in the fatty layers of the abdomen or just above the iliac crest, avoiding the periumbilical area by 5 cm (2 in.). • Skin is drawn up ("pinched") and the needle is inserted at a 90-degree angle. • Injection is given without aspirating for blood return. • Release the skin and hold slight pressure to the site but do not massage the area. • Have the patient, family, or caregiver perform teach-back until the proper technique is used and they are comfortable giving the injection. • Teach the patient on oral anticoagulants to take the medication at the same time each day.

See Tables 31.3 and 31.4 for a list of drugs to which these nursing actions apply.

Aspirin deserves special mention as an antiplatelet drug. Because it is available OTC, patients may not consider aspirin a potent medication; however, its anticoagulant activity is well documented. Aspirin acts by binding irreversibly to the enzyme cyclooxygenase in platelets. This binding inhibits the formation of thromboxane A_2, a powerful inducer of platelet aggregation. The anticoagulant effect of a single dose of aspirin may persist for as long as a week. Concurrent use of aspirin with other coagulation modifiers should be avoided, unless approved by the prescriber. Aspirin is featured as a drug prototype for pain relief in chapter 18, and it is also indicated for prevention of strokes and MI in chapter 28, and reduction of inflammation in chapter 33.

Following vessel injury, platelets become "sticky," bind to the injury site, and release substances that recruit additional platelets. One of these chemicals is adenosine diphosphate (ADP), whose function is to promote platelet aggregation. The ADP receptor blockers are medications that irreversibly block the ADP receptor sites thus altering the plasma membrane of platelets. For the remainder of their life spans, the affected platelets are unable to recognize the chemical signals required for them to aggregate.

There are four ADP receptor blockers. Ticlopidine (Ticlid) and clopidogrel (Plavix) are given PO to prevent thrombi formation in patients who have experienced a recent thromboembolic event such as a stroke or MI. Ticlopidine can cause life-threatening neutropenia and agranulocytosis. Clopidogrel is considerably safer, having adverse effects comparable to those of aspirin. Prasugrel (Effient) and ticagrelor (Brilinta) are newer ADP receptor blockers indicated to prevent thrombotic events in patients with acute coronary syndromes who undergo percutaneous coronary intervention (PCI). Like other antiplatelet drugs, the ADP receptor blockers can cause excessive bleeding in patients who sustain trauma or are undergoing dental procedures. These drugs should be discontinued at least 5 days prior to an expected medical-surgical procedure.

Glycoprotein IIb/IIIa is a receptor on the surface of platelets that is necessary for platelet aggregation. These receptors serve as docking stations, waiting for signals from chemical messengers that indicate injury may have occurred. Substances that may bind to and activate glycoprotein IIb/IIIa receptors include thrombin, von Willebrand factor, ADP, and thromboxane A2. Following activation of the surface glycoprotein, the platelets change shape and become sticky.

The glycoprotein IIb/IIIa receptor antagonists are medications that block this receptor, thus preventing platelet activation. Their primary indications are to prevent thrombi in patients experiencing a recent MI, stroke, or PCI. Although these drugs are very effective antiplatelet agents, they are expensive and can be administered only by the IV route.

Intermittent claudication (IC) is pain or cramping in the lower legs that worsens with walking or exercise. IC is the primary symptom of peripheral vascular disease, in which progressive atherosclerosis of vessels causes a lack of sufficient oxygen to major muscles of the legs. Although some of the therapies for myocardial ischemia are beneficial in treating IC, two drugs are approved *only* for this disorder. Pentoxifylline (Trental) acts on RBCs to reduce their viscosity and increase their flexibility, thus

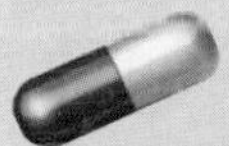

Prototype Drug | Clopidogrel *(Plavix)*

Therapeutic Class: Antiplatelet drug **Pharmacologic Class:** ADP receptor blocker

Actions and Uses

Clopidogrel is indicated for the prevention of thromboembolic events in patients with a recent history of MI, stroke, or peripheral artery disease. It is also approved for thrombi prophylaxis in patients with unstable angina, including those who are receiving vascular bypass procedures or PCI. It may be given off-label to prevent thrombi formation in patients with coronary artery stents, and to prevent postoperative DVTs. Because the drug is expensive, it is usually prescribed for patients who are unable to tolerate aspirin, which has similar anticoagulant activity. It is given PO and has the advantage of once-daily dosing.

Clopidogrel prolongs bleeding time by inhibiting platelet aggregation, directly inhibiting ADP binding to its receptor. This binding is irreversible and the platelet will be affected for the remainder of its life span.

Administration Alerts

- Tablets should not be crushed or split.
- Discontinue drug at least 5 days prior to surgery.
- Pregnancy category B.

PHARMACOKINETICS (PO)

Onset	Peak	Duration
1–2 h	2 h	5 days

Adverse Effects

Clopidogrel is generally well tolerated. Frequent adverse effects include flulike syndrome, headache, dizziness, bruising, and rash or pruritus. Like other coagulation modifiers, bleeding is a potential adverse event.

Black Box Warning: Because the effectiveness of clopidogrel is dependent on its metabolic activation by CYP 450 enzymes, poor metabolizers will exhibit less therapeutic effect and more adverse cardiovascular events.

Contraindications: Clopidogrel is contraindicated in patients with active bleeding.

Interactions

Drug–Drug: Use with anticoagulants, other antiplatelet agents, thrombolytic agents, or NSAIDs, including aspirin, will increase the risk of bleeding. Barbiturates, rifampin, or carbamazepine may increase the anticoagulant activity of clopidogrel. The azole antifungals, protease inhibitors, erythromycin, verapamil, zafirlukast, fluoxetine, and proton pump inhibitors such as omeprazole may diminish the antiplatelet actions of clopidogrel.

Lab Tests: Clopidogrel prolongs bleeding time.

Herbal/Food: Herbal supplements that affect coagulation such as feverfew, green tea, ginkgo, fish oil, ginger, or garlic may increase the risk of bleeding.

Treatment of Overdose: In cases of poisoning, platelet transfusions may be necessary to prevent hemorrhage.

allowing them to enter vessels that are partially occluded and reduce hypoxia and pain in the muscle. Pentoxifylline also has antiplatelet action. Cilostazol (Pletal) inhibits platelet aggregation and promotes vasodilation, which brings additional blood to ischemic muscles. Both drugs are given PO and show only modest improvement in IC symptoms. Exercise and therapeutic lifestyle changes are necessary for maximum benefit.

THROMBOLYTICS

It is often mistakenly believed that the purpose of anticoagulants such as heparin or warfarin is to digest and remove pre-existing clots, but this is not the case. A totally different class of drugs, the thrombolytics, is needed for this purpose. The thrombolytics are listed in Table 31.5.

Patient Safety: The Importance of Patient Education

A 35-year old male develops thrombophlebitis after extensive travel for his job. He is started on warfarin (Coumadin) and is to remain on the drug for one month. The nurse provides the patient with education about returning for laboratory work weekly, dietary needs, and exercising caution with sharp objects such as knives. A week after stopping the drug, the patient is admitted to the emergency department with abdominal pain, abdominal swelling, and hypotension after collapsing in the evening following playing soccer that afternoon with friends. An intra-abdominal bleed is suspected. What is a possible explanation for this diagnosis? How could it have been prevented? *Visit www.pearsonhighered.com/nursingresources for the suggested answer.*

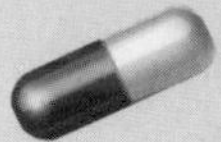

Prototype Drug | Alteplase *(Activase)*

Therapeutic Class: Drug for dissolving clots **Pharmacologic Class:** Thrombolytic

Actions and Uses

Produced through recombinant DNA technology, alteplase is identical to human TPA. As with other thrombolytics, the primary action of alteplase is to convert plasminogen to plasmin, which then dissolves fibrin clots. To achieve maximum effect, therapy should begin immediately after the onset of symptoms. Alteplase does not exhibit the allergic reactions seen with streptokinase. Alteplase is a preferred drug for the treatment of stroke due to thrombus and is used off-label to restore the patency of IV catheters.

Administration Alerts

- Alteplase must be given within 12 hours of onset of symptoms of MI and within 3 hours of thrombotic stroke for maximum effectiveness.
- Avoid parenteral injections during alteplase infusion to decrease risk of bleeding.
- Pregnancy category C.

PHARMACOKINETICS

Onset	Peak	Duration
Immediate	5–10 min	3 h

Adverse Effects

The most common adverse effect of alteplase is bleeding, which may occur superficially at needle puncture sites or internally. Intracranial bleeding is a rare, though possible, adverse effect. Signs of bleeding such as spontaneous ecchymoses, hematomas, or epistaxis should immediately be reported to the health care provider.

Contraindications: Alteplase is contraindicated in active internal bleeding, history of stroke or head injury within the past 3 months, recent trauma or surgery, severe uncontrolled HTN, intracranial neoplasm, or arteriovenous malformation.

Interactions

Drug–Drug: Concurrent use with anticoagulants, antiplatelet agents, or NSAIDs, including aspirin, may increase the risk of bleeding.

Lab Tests: Alteplase will increase PT and aPTT.

Herbal/Food: Use with supplements that may affect coagulation such as feverfew, green tea, ginkgo, fish oil, ginger, or garlic should be avoided, because they may increase the risk of bleeding.

Treatment of Overdose: There is no specific treatment for overdose.

31.7 Pharmacotherapy With Thrombolytics

Thrombolytics promote the process of fibrinolysis, or clot destruction, by converting plasminogen to plasmin. The enzyme plasmin digests fibrin and breaks it down into small soluble fragments. Unlike the anticoagulants that can only *prevent* clots, thrombolytics actually *dissolve* the insoluble fibrin within the clot. These agents are administered for disorders in which an intravascular clot has already formed, such as in acute MI, pulmonary embolism, acute ischemic stroke, and DVT.

The goal of thrombolytic therapy is to quickly restore blood flow to the tissue served by the blocked vessel. Delays in reestablishing circulation may result in ischemia and permanent tissue damage. The therapeutic effect of thrombolytics is greater when they are administered no later than 4 hours after clot formation occurs.

Because clotting is a natural and desirable process to prevent excessive bleeding, thrombolytics have a narrow

Table 31.5 Thrombolytics

Drug	Route and Adult Dose (max dose where indicated)	Adverse Effects
alteplase (Activase, TPA)	IV: 60 mg initially then 20 mg/h infused over next 2 h	*Superficial bleeding at injection sites, allergic reactions*
reteplase (Retavase) (see page 426 for the Prototype Drug box)	IV: 10 units over 2 min; repeat dose in 30 min	<u>Serious internal bleeding, intracranial hemorrhage, HTN</u>
streptokinase (Kabikinase)	IV: 250,000–1.5 million units over 60 min	
tenecteplase (TNKase)	IV: 30–50 mg infused over 5 seconds	

Note: *Italics* indicate common adverse effects; <u>underlining</u> indicates serious adverse effects.

Nursing Practice Application

Pharmacotherapy With Thrombolytics

ASSESSMENT	POTENTIAL NURSING DIAGNOSES*
Baseline assessment prior to administration: • Obtain a complete health history including cardiovascular, peripheral vascular disease, respiratory, neurologic (including recent head injury), recent surgeries or injuries, hepatic or renal disease, diabetes, peptic ulcer disease, recent childbirth (within 10 days), or the possibility of pregnancy. **Lifespan:** Ask women of menstrual age about length and heaviness of their usual menstrual flow. Obtain a drug history including allergies, current prescription and OTC drugs, herbal preparations, and alcohol use. Be alert to possible drug interactions. • Obtain baseline weight, vital signs, ECG, and breath sounds. Assess the presence, quality, and location of angina, and for the presence of dyspnea or chest pain. Assess neurologic status. • Evaluate laboratory findings (aPTT, aPT, INR, bleeding time), CBC and platelets, renal and liver function studies, ABGs as appropriate, and lipid profiles. Support the patient during other required tests (e.g., CT or MRI prior to thrombolytic therapy for stroke). • Establish all monitoring equipment and necessary lines or arrange for their insertion (e.g., ECG monitoring, IV, Foley catheter, arterial line).	• *Acute Pain* • *Ineffective Tissue Perfusion* • *Impaired Gas Exchange* • *Impaired Skin Integrity* • *Anxiety* • *Deficient Knowledge* (drug therapy) • *Risk for Injury,* related to adverse effects of thrombolytic therapy *NANDA I © 2014
Assessment throughout administration: • Continue frequent assessments for therapeutic effects (e.g., angina has diminished significantly or is eliminated and ECG findings within normal limits, respiratory effort and ABGs significantly improved). • Continue frequent monitoring of appropriate laboratory values (e.g., Hgb, Hct, platelets, RBC, urinalyis, ABGs). • Monitor vital signs and ECG every 15 minutes during the first hour of infusion, and then every 30 minutes during the remainder of the infusion and for the first 8 hours. • Assess for adverse effects: bleeding at the IV sites, wounds, excessive ecchymosis, petechiae, hematuria, black/tarry stools, rectal bleeding, "coffee-ground" emesis, epistaxis, bleeding from gums, hemoptysis, dysrhythmias, and for symptoms of occult bleeding, such as pallor, dizziness, hypotension, tachycardia, abdominal pain, areas of abdominal wall swelling or firmness, lumbar pain, or decreased level of consciousness. • Monitor neurologic status frequently, especially if thrombolytics are used for stroke.	

IMPLEMENTATION

Interventions and (Rationales)	Patient-Centered Care
Ensuring therapeutic effects: • Continue frequent assessments as above for therapeutic effects (e.g., previous angina has diminished significantly or is eliminated and ECG findings show decrease in ischemia). (Thrombolytics rapidly dissolve existing clots to allow reperfusion of the affected area.)	• Teach the patient about all procedures and their necessity prior to beginning thrombolytic therapy. • To allay anxiety, teach the patient, family, or caregiver the rationale for all equipment used.
• Post-therapy, encourage appropriate lifestyle changes. **Collaboration:** Provide for dietitian consultation as needed. (Smoking increases platelet aggregation and promotes the formation of thrombi. Healthy lifestyle changes will support and minimize the need for future drug therapy.)	• Encourage the patient to adopt a healthy lifestyle of low-fat food choices, increased exercise, decreased caffeine and alcohol consumption, and smoking cessation.

continued

Nursing Practice Application *continued*

IMPLEMENTATION	
Interventions and (Rationales)	**Patient-Centered Care**
Minimizing adverse effects: • Monitor frequently for signs and symptoms of excessive bleeding, such as pallor, hypotension, tachycardia, dizziness, sudden severe headache, lumbar pain, or decreased level of consciousness. (Frequent assessment for both visible and occult bleeding is necessary to prevent extensive hemorrhage and to start corrective treatment as early as possible. Bleeding risk is elevated up to 2 to 4 days post-treatment and if the patient is maintained on anticoagulant or antiplatelet therapy post-thrombolytics.)	• Allay anxiety by reassuring the patient and explaining the rationale for frequent monitoring. Provide adequate pain relief as appropriate.
• Monitor vital signs and ECG every 15 minutes during the first hour of infusion, and then every 30 minutes during the remainder of the infusion and for the first 8 hours. Report any dysrhythmias immediately. (Obtaining vital signs frequently will assess for adverse effects of the drug including hypotension and tachycardia associated with bleeding and for dysrhythmias. Dysrhythmias may occur after re-perfusion of the coronary arteries or may be associated with adverse effects.)	• To allay possible anxiety, teach the patient, family, or caregiver the rationale for all equipment used and the need for frequent monitoring. • Teach the patient to report any palpitations, dyspnea, or angina postinfusion.
• Maintain the patient on bed rest and with limited activity during the infusion. (Limited physical activity and bed rest decrease the chance for bruising, injury, and bleeding.)	• Provide an explanation and rationale that activity will be limited during infusion and for up to 8 hours post-treatment.
• Monitor neurologic status frequently, especially if thrombolytics are used for stroke. (A sudden change in neurologic status or sudden severe headache is a possible sign of an intracranial bleed with increased intracranial pressure.)	• To allay possible anxiety, teach the patient the rationale for the frequent assessments and provide reassurance. • Instruct the family or caregiver to report any change in the patient's mental status or level of consciousness during the postinfusion period immediately.
• Avoid invasive procedures during the infusion and up to 8 hours postinfusion. (Any puncture site or site of invasive procedure will create an additional site for bleeding. Whenever an invasive procedure must be used, the site must be maintained under pressure for 30 minutes or longer to prevent hemorrhage.)	• Teach the patient that after any required procedures, pressure will be maintained to the site for a prolonged period.
• Continue to monitor laboratory work (Hgb, Hct, platelet counts, and bleeding time) frequently post-treatment. Periodic CBC and ABGs may also be monitored. Activity may be limited during this postinfusion time period. (The risk of bleeding remains high for 2 to 4 days postinfusion.)	• Explain the need for activity restriction and frequent monitoring during this time.
Patient understanding of drug therapy: • Use opportunities during administration of thrombolytic therapy to provide patient education about precautions that will be taken during the infusion and in the immediate postinfusion time period. (Using time during nursing care helps to reassure the patient and allay anxiety.)	• The patient should have an understanding of the rationale behind thrombolytic therapy, equipment, and monitoring that will be used, and the care required in the postinfusion period.
• Provide support and reassurance to the family and caregivers during the time of treatment. (Providing support, reassurance, and appropriate referrals, e.g., pastoral care or social service support, assists family members in a stressful situation.)	• Allow family members time to discuss fears or concerns, and provide referral to appropriate support and ancillary providers as appropriate.
Patient self-administration of drug therapy: • Provide education during the postinfusion period about required medical care follow-up, postinfusion drug therapy (e.g., anticoagulants or antiplatelet drugs), and lifestyle changes. (Using time during nursing care helps to reinforce teaching and assess for any questions or concerns the patient, family, or caregiver may have.)	• Teach the patient, family, or caregiver in proper self-administration techniques of anticoagulants or antiplatelet drugs as ordered post-thrombolytic therapy.

See Table 31.5 for a list of drugs to which these nursing actions apply.

margin of safety between dissolving "normal" and "abnormal" clots. Vital signs must be monitored continuously, and signs of bleeding call for discontinuation of therapy. Because these drugs are rapidly destroyed in the bloodstream, discontinuation of the infusion normally results in the immediate termination of thrombolytic activity. After the clot is successfully dissolved with the thrombolytic, therapy with a coagulation modifier is generally initiated to prevent the re-formation of clots.

Since the discovery of streptokinase, the first drug in this class, there have been a number of subsequent generations of thrombolytics. The newer drugs such as tenecteplase (TNKase) have a more rapid onset and longer duration and are reported to have fewer side effects than older drugs in this class. TPA, marketed as alteplase (Activase), has replaced urokinase as the preferred thrombolytic in clearing thrombosed central IV lines. Because urokinase was obtained from pooled human donors and had a small risk for being contaminated with viruses, it was removed from the market.

HEMOSTATICS

Hemostatics, also called *antifibrinolytics*, have an action opposite to that of anticoagulants: They shorten bleeding time. The class name hemostatics comes from the drugs' ability to slow blood flow. They are used to prevent excessive bleeding following surgical procedures.

31.8 Pharmacotherapy With Hemostatics

The final class of coagulation modifiers, the hemostatics, is a small group of drugs used to prevent and treat excessive bleeding from surgical sites. All the hemostatics have very specific indications for use, and none are commonly prescribed. Aminocaproic acid is administered IV to prevent bleeding in patients who have systemic clotting disorders. Tranexamic acid (Cyklokapron) was first approved as an IV medication to reduce or prevent bleeding in patients with hemophilia who were undergoing dental procedures. Later, a PO form of the drug (Lysteda) was approved for the treatment of excessive menstrual bleeding. Thrombin (Evithrom, Recothrom, Thrombinar) is approved as a topical drug to prevent minor oozing and bleeding from surgical sites. Although their mechanisms differ, all drugs in this class prevent fibrin from dissolving, thus enhancing the stability of the clot. The hemostatics are listed in Table 31.6.

CLOTTING FACTOR CONCENTRATES

Some patients experience bleeding disorders because they are missing specific components of the clotting cascade. Patients with these genetic disorders require replacement therapy with the missing factor through periodic infusions of clotting factor concentrates.

31.9 Pharmacotherapy of Hemophilia

Hemophilias are bleeding disorders caused by genetic deficiencies in specific clotting factors. Hereditary disorders of coagulation are relatively rare and may be caused by deficiency in any blood factor in the coagulation cascade. Symptoms of congenital coagulation disorders manifest as bleeding in muscles or weight-bearing joints, epistaxis, gingival bleeding, and abnormally long bleeding times following trauma or surgery. Joint bleeding causes chronic inflammation and may result in permanent deformity and loss of mobility. Some patients have mild forms of hemophilia, exhibiting no symptoms of excessive bleeding until they experience major trauma or surgery. The most severe forms of these disorders, however, are diagnosed shortly after birth and require a lifetime of lifestyle adjustment and pharmacotherapy. Diagnosis requires laboratory assays for each of the clotting factors to determine which deficiency is causing the disorder.

The classic treatment for hemophilia was transfusions of fresh frozen plasma obtained from human donors. Plasma contains the missing clotting factor(s) but carries the risk for transmission of the human immunodeficiency virus (HIV) and the hepatitis virus. Technology has allowed scientists to synthesize each clotting factor individually and produce products without the risk of pathogen transmission. This change in the pharmacotherapy of hereditary coagulation disorders has resulted in a remarkable change in the life spans of afflicted patients.

The classic form, hemophilia A, is caused by a lack of clotting Factor VIII and accounts for approximately 80% of all cases of hemophilia. A large number of Factor VIII

Table 31.6 Hemostatics

Drug	Route and Adult Dose (max dose where indicated)	Adverse Effects
aminocaproic acid (Amicar)	IV/PO: 4–5 g for 1 h, then 1–1.25 g/h for 8 h or until bleeding is controlled	*Allergic skin reactions, headache*
thrombin (Evithrom, Recothrom, Thrombinar)	Topical: amounts vary based on the size of the treated area	
tranexamic acid (Cyklokapron, Lysteda)	IV: 10 mg/kg, tid to qid for 2 to 8 days PO: two 650 mg tablets, tid for a maximum of 5 days	Anaphylaxis, thrombosis, bronchospasm, nephrotoxicity

Note: *Italics* indicate common adverse effects; underlining indicates serious adverse effects.

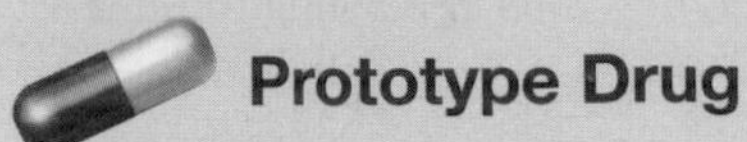

Prototype Drug | Aminocaproic Acid *(Amicar)*

Therapeutic Class: Clot stabilizer **Pharmacologic Class:** Hemostatic/antifibrinolytic

Actions and Uses

Aminocaproic acid is prescribed in situations in which there is excessive bleeding because clots are being dissolved prematurely. The drug acts by inactivating plasminogen, the precursor of the enzyme plasmin that digests the fibrin clot. During acute hemorrhage, the drug can be given IV to reduce bleeding in 1 to 2 hours. It is also available in tablet form. It is most commonly prescribed following surgery to reduce postoperative bleeding. Patients with hemophilia A may receive aminocaproic acid immediately following dental procedures to control bleeding. The therapeutic serum level is 100 to 400 mcg/mL.

Administration Alerts

- Aminocaproic acid may cause hypotension and bradycardia when given IV. Assess vital signs frequently and place the patient on a cardiac monitor to assess for dysrhythmias.
- Pregnancy category C.

PHARMACOKINETICS (PO)

Onset	Peak	Duration
1 h	2 h	3–4 h

Adverse Effects

Because aminocaproic acid tends to stabilize clots, it should be used cautiously in patients with a history of thromboembolic disease. Rapid IV administration may cause hypotension or bradycardia. Side effects are generally mild.

Contraindications: Aminocaproic acid is contraindicated in patients with disseminated intravascular clotting or severe renal impairment.

Interactions

Drug–Drug: Hypercoagulation may occur with concurrent use of estrogens or oral contraceptives.

Lab Tests: Serum potassium may be elevated.

Herbal/Food: Unknown.

Treatment of Overdose: There is no treatment for overdose.

products are available, and some trade names include Advate, Eloctate, Helixate, Humate, Kogenate, Monoclate, NovoEight, Obizur, Recombinate, ReFacto, and Xyntha. These products are not interchangeable, and care must be taken to infuse the correct dose using the recommended dosing schedule. Some patients receive prophylactic therapy, with infusions normally done 3 times weekly. Should a bleeding episode occur, prompt therapy is required which may include doses every 8–12 hours until the target dose is reached.

Hemophilia B is caused by a deficiency of Factor IX; about 20% of those afflicted with hemophilia have this type. Factor IX, in conjunction with activated Factor VIII, is required for the activation of Factor X in the coagulation cascade. Products containing recombinant Factor IX include Alprolix, BeneFIX, and Rixubis.

Chapter Review

KEY Concepts

The numbered key concepts provide a succinct summary of the important points from the corresponding numbered section within the chapter. If any of these points are not clear, refer to the numbered section within the chapter for review.

31.1 Hemostasis is a complex process involving multiple steps and a large number of enzymes and clotting factors. The final product is a fibrin clot that stops blood loss.

31.2 Fibrinolysis, or removal of a blood clot, is an enzymatic process initiated by the release of TPA. Plasmin digests the fibrin strands, thus restoring circulation to the injured area.

31.3 Diseases of hemostasis include thromboembolic disorders caused by thrombi and emboli, thrombocytopenia, and bleeding disorders such as hemophilia.

31.4 The normal coagulation process can be modified by a number of different mechanisms, including inhibiting specific clotting factors, inhibiting platelet function, and destroying fibrin.

31.5 Anticoagulants are used to prevent thrombi from forming or enlarging. The primary drugs in this category are heparin (parenteral) and warfarin (oral), although low-molecular-weight heparins and thrombin inhibitors are also available.

31.6 Several drugs prolong bleeding time by interfering with the aggregation of platelets. Antiplatelet drugs include aspirin, ADP blockers, glycoprotein IIb/IIIa receptor antagonists, and miscellaneous agents for treating intermittent claudication.

31.7 Thrombolytics are used to dissolve existing intravascular clots in patients with MI or stroke.

31.8 Hemostatics or antifibrinolytics are used to promote the formation of clots in patients with excessive bleeding from surgical sites.

31.9 Hemophilia is an inherited deficiency in a specific clotting factor. Pharmacotherapy includes replacing the missing clotting factor through periodic infusions.

REVIEW Questions

1. A patient with deep vein thrombosis is receiving an infusion of heparin and will be started on warfarin (Coumadin) soon. While the patient is receiving heparin, what laboratory test will provide the nurse with information about its therapeutic effects?
   1. Prothrombin time (PT)
   2. International Normalized Ratio (INR)
   3. Activated partial thromboplastin time (aPTT)
   4. Platelet count
2. The patient receiving heparin therapy asks how the "blood thinner" works. What is the best response by the nurse?
   1. "Heparin makes the blood less thick."
   2. "Heparin does not thin the blood but prevents clots from forming as easily in the blood vessels."
   3. "Heparin decreases the number of platelets so that blood clots more slowly."
   4. "Heparin dissolves the clot."
3. What patient education should be included for a patient receiving enoxaparin (Lovenox)? (Select all that apply.)
   1. Teach the patient or family to give subcutaneous injections at home.
   2. Teach the patient or family not to take any over-the-counter drugs without first consulting with the health care provider.
   3. Teach the patient to observe for unexplained bleeding such as pink, red, or dark brown urine or bloody gums.
   4. Teach the patient to monitor for the development of deep vein thrombosis.
   5. Teach the patient about the importance of drinking grapefruit juice daily.

4. A patient with a congenital coagulation disorder is given aminocaproic acid (Amicar) to stop bleeding following surgery. The nurse will carefully monitor this patient for development of which of the following adverse effects? (Select all that apply.)
   1. Anaphylaxis
   2. Hypertension
   3. Hemorrhage
   4. Headache
   5. Hypotension
5. A patient is receiving a thrombolytic drug, alteplase (Activase), following an acute myocardial infarction. Which of the following effects is most likely attributed to this drug?
   1. Skin rash with urticaria
   2. Wheezing with labored respirations
   3. Bruising and epistaxis
   4. Temperature elevation of 38.2°C (100.8°F)
6. A patient has started clopidogrel (Plavix) after experiencing a transient ischemic attack. What is the desired therapeutic effect of this drug?
   1. Anti-inflammatory and antipyretic effects
   2. To reduce the risk of a stroke from a blood clot
   3. Analgesic as well as clot-dissolving effects
   4. To stop clots from becoming emboli

PATIENT-FOCUSED Case Study

Caroline Roberts is a 59-year-old woman who has just flown home from visiting her children and grandchildren on the opposite coast from where she currently lives. She noticed soreness in her left calf muscle, and when she noticed increased pain and swelling in her leg, she made an appointment with her provider. A diagnosis of DVT is made and the treatment plan is to admit her into the hospital for anticoagulant therapy.

1. Mrs. Roberts asks, "How soon will the heparin dissolve my blood clot?" How would you respond to this question?
2. What patient education should you provide Mrs. Roberts about anticoagulation therapy?
3. What factors predisposed this patient to DVT?

CRITICAL THINKING Questions

1. A patient has had an acute MI and has received alteplase (Activase) to dissolve the clot. What nursing actions should have been taken prior to administering the medication to the patient?
2. A patient is receiving enoxaparin subcutaneously after being diagnosed with thrombophlebitis. What precautions should be taken when giving this medication?

Visit www.pearsonhighered.com/nursingresources for answers and rationales for all activities.

REFERENCES

Herdman, T. H., & Kamitsuru, S. (2014). *NANDA International nursing diagnoses: Definitions and classification, 2015–2017*. Oxford, United Kingdom: Wiley-Blackwell.

Lissiman, E., Bhasale, A. L., & Cohen, M. (2012). Garlic for the common cold. *Cochrane Database of Systematic Reviews, 3*, Art. No.: CD006206. doi:10.1002/14651858.CD006206.pub3

Ried, K., Toben, C., & Fakler, P. (2013). Effect of garlic on serum lipids: An updated meta-analysis. *Nutrition Reviews, 71*, 282–299. doi:10.1111/nure,12012

SELECTED BIBLIOGRAPHY

Angiolillo, D. J., & Ferreiro, J. L. (2013). Antiplatelet and anticoagulant therapy for atherothrombotic disease: The role of current and emerging agents. *American Journal of Cardiovascular Drugs, 13*, 233–250. doi:10.1007/s40256-013-0022-7

Berra, K. (2014). Antithrombotics for stroke prevention in nonvalvular atrial fibrillation: An update. *European Journal of Cardiovascular Nursing, 13*, 32–40. doi:10.1177/1474515113477957

Fareed, J., Hoppensteadt, D., & Jeske, W. P. (2014). An update on low-molecular-weight heparins. In H. I. Saba & H. R. Roberts (Eds.), *Hemostasis and thrombosis* (pp. 296–313). Oxford, United Kingdom: John Wiley & Sons, Ltd. doi:10.1002/9781118833391.ch31

Patel, K. (2014). *Deep venous thrombosis*. Retrieved from http://emedicine.medscape.com/article/1911303-overview

Pollack, C. V., Jr. (2013). Current and future options for anticoagulant therapy in the acute management of ACS. *Current Treatment Options in Cardiovascular Medicine, 15*, 21–32. doi:10.1007/s11936-012-0216-3

Srivastava, A., Brewer, A. K., Mauser-Bunschoten, E. P., Key, N. S., Kitchen, S., Llinas, A., . . . Street, A. (2013). Guidelines for the management of hemophilia. *Haemophilia, 19*, e1–e47. doi:10.1111/j.1365-2516.2012.02909.x

Zalden, R. A. (2014). *Hemophilia A*. Retrieved from http://emedicine.medscape.com/article/779322-overview#a0101

Chapter 32

Drugs for Hematopoietic Disorders

Drugs at a Glance

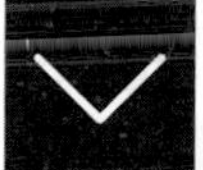

Learning Outcomes

After reading this chapter, the student should be able to:

1. Describe the process of hematopoiesis.
2. Explain how aspects of hematopoiesis can be modified by the administration of drugs that stimulate the production of erythrocytes, leukocytes, and platelets.
3. Explain why hematopoietic enhancers are often administered to patients following chemotherapy or organ transplant.
4. Classify types of anemia based on their causes.
5. Identify medications that are used to treat anemias.
6. Describe the nurse's role in the pharmacologic management of hematologic disorders.
7. For each of the drug classes listed in Drugs at a Glance, know representative drugs, and explain their mechanism of drug action, primary actions, and important adverse effects.

6\. Use the nursing process to care for patients who are receiving pharmacotherapy for hematologic disorders.

indicates a prototype drug, each of which is featured in a Prototype Drug box.

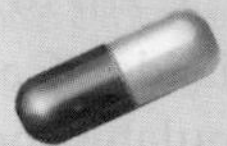

Prototype Drug | Epoetin Alfa *(Epogen, Procrit)*

Therapeutic Class: Erythropoiesis-stimulating drug **Pharmacologic Class:** Erythropoietin

Actions and Uses

Epoetin alfa is made through recombinant DNA technology and is functionally identical to human erythropoietin. Because of its ability to stimulate erythropoiesis, epoetin alfa is effective in treating disorders caused by a deficiency in RBC formation. Patients with chronic renal failure often cannot secrete enough endogenous erythropoietin and benefit from epoetin alfa administration. Epoetin alfa is sometimes given to patients undergoing cancer chemotherapy to counteract the anemia caused by antineoplastic drugs. It is occasionally prescribed for patients prior to blood transfusions or surgery, and to treat anemia in patients infected with human immunodeficiency virus (HIV). Epoetin alfa is usually administered by the subcutaneous route three times per week until a therapeutic response is achieved (usually 2 to 6 weeks).

Administration Alerts

- The subcutaneous route is generally preferred over intravenous (IV), because lower doses are needed and absorption is slower.
- Do not shake the vial, because this may deactivate the drug. Visibly inspect the solution for particulate matter.
- Pregnancy category C.

PHARMACOKINETICS (SUBCUTANEOUS)

Onset	Peak	Duration
1–2 wk	Unknown	2 wk

Adverse Effects

Hypertension may occur in as many as 30% of patients receiving the drug, and a concurrent antihypertensive drug may be indicated. Other frequent adverse effects include headache, fever, nausea, diarrhea, and edema.

Black Box Warning: The risk of serious cardiovascular and thromboembolic events is increased with epoetin alfa therapy. Transient ischemic attacks (TIAs), myocardial infarctions (MIs), and strokes have occurred in patients with chronic renal failure who are on dialysis and being treated with epoetin alfa. Epoetin alfa increased the rate of deep vein thrombosis in patients not receiving concurrent anticoagulation. The lowest dose possible should be used in patients with cancer because the drug can promote tumor progression and shorten overall survival in some patients.

Contraindications: Contraindications include uncontrolled hypertension and known hypersensitivity to mammalian cell products. Care must be taken not to administer epoetin alfa to patients with *myeloid* malignancies such as myelogenous leukemia because the drug may increase tumor growth.

Interactions

Drug–Drug: Androgens can increase blood viscosity, resulting in an increased response from epoetin alfa. The effectiveness of epoetin alfa will be greatly reduced in patients with iron deficiency or other vitamin-depleted states. Most patients receive iron supplements during therapy to compensate for the increased RBC production.

Lab Tests: Unknown.

Herbal/Food: Unknown.

Treatment of Overdose: Overdose may lead to polycythemia (too many erythrocytes), which can be corrected by phlebotomy.

32.2 Pharmacotherapy With Erythropoiesis-Stimulating Drugs

The process of RBC formation, or erythropoiesis, is regulated primarily by the hormone **erythropoietin.** Secreted by the kidneys, erythropoietin travels to the bone marrow, where it interacts with receptors on hematopoietic stem cells with the message to increase erythrocyte production. Erythropoietin also stimulates the production of hemoglobin, which is required for a functional erythrocyte.

The primary signal for the increased secretion of erythropoietin is a reduction in oxygen reaching the kidneys. Serum levels of erythropoietin may increase as much as 1,000-fold in response to severe hypoxia. Hemorrhage, chronic obstructive pulmonary disease, anemia, or high altitudes may cause this hypoxia.

Erythropoietin is marketed as epoetin alfa (Epogen, Procrit). Darbepoetin alfa (Aranesp) is closely related to epoetin alfa. It has the same action, effectiveness, and safety profile; however, it has a longer duration of action that allows it to be administered once weekly or once every two weeks. Darbepoetin alfa is approved for the treatment of anemia associated with chemotherapy or chronic renal failure. It should be noted that when the drug is given as an adjunctive agent in cancer treatment, the anemia must be secondary to the *chemotherapy*, not the *cancer* itself. Research has shown that the administration of these drugs does not benefit patients when the anemia is caused by the malignancy; in fact, mortality is *increased* in these patients by the administration of the drug.

Nursing Practice Application

Pharmacotherapy With Erythropoiesis-Stimulating Drugs

ASSESSMENT	POTENTIAL NURSING DIAGNOSES*
Baseline assessment prior to administration: • Obtain a complete health history including cardiovascular (including hypertension [HTN], MI) and peripheral vascular disease, respiratory (including previous pulmonary embolism), neurologic (including stroke), or hepatic or renal disease. Obtain a drug history including allergies, current prescription and over-the-counter (OTC) drugs, herbal preparations, and alcohol use. Be alert to possible drug interactions. • Obtain baseline weight and vital signs, especially blood pressure. • Evaluate appropriate laboratory findings (e.g., complete blood count (CBC), activated partial thromboplastin time (aPTT), international normalized ratio (INR), transferrin and serum ferritin levels, renal and liver function studies).	• *Ineffective Tissue Perfusion* • *Activity Intolerance* • *Fatigue* • *Deficient Knowledge* (drug therapy) • *Risk for Injury,* related to adverse drug effects *NANDA I © 2014
Assessment throughout administration: • Continue assessment for therapeutic effects (e.g., hematocrit (Hct), RBC count significantly improved, patient's activity level and ability to carry out activities of daily living (ADLs) have improved). • Continue frequent monitoring of appropriate laboratory values (e.g., CBC, aPTT, INR). • Monitor vital signs frequently, especially blood pressure, during the first 2 weeks of therapy. • Assess for adverse effects: HTN, headache, neurologic changes in level of consciousness or premonitory signs and symptoms of seizure activity, angina, and signs of thrombosis development in peripheral extremities.	

IMPLEMENTATION

Interventions and (Rationales)	Patient-Centered Care
Ensuring therapeutic effects: • Continue frequent assessments as above for therapeutic effects. (RBC count increases rapidly in first 2 weeks of therapy. CBC and platelet count should show continued improvement. Blood pressure and pulse should remain within normal limits or within parameters set by the health care provider.)	• Instruct the patient on the need to return frequently for follow-up laboratory work.
• Encourage adequate rest periods and adequate fluid intake. (The patient may be significantly fatigued due to low hemoglobin (Hgb) and Hct. Adequate fluid intake helps maintain adequate fluid balance as Hct levels rise.)	• Encourage the patient to rest when fatigued and to space activities throughout the day to allow for adequate rest periods. • Encourage intake of water and non-hyperosmolar beverages.
Minimizing adverse effects: • Continue to monitor for adverse effects, especially HTN, peripheral thrombosis, or seizure activity. (As Hct rapidly increases during the first 2 weeks of therapy, HTN or seizures may occur. Peripheral thrombosis, including coronary or cerebral, may also occur. **Lifespan:** Be especially cautious with the older adult who may be at greater risk for thromboembolic events due to age-related vascular changes.)	• Teach the patient, family, or caregiver how to monitor pulse and blood pressure as appropriate. Ensure the proper use and functioning of any home equipment obtained. • Instruct the patient, family, or caregiver to immediately report headache (especially if sudden onset or severe), changes in level of consciousness, weakness or numbness in the extremities, or premonitory signs of seizure activity (e.g., aura), angina, or symptoms of peripheral thrombosis (e.g., leg pain, pale extremity, diminished peripheral pulses).
• Assess the transportation needs of the patient and refer to appropriate resources as needed. (Driving may be restricted up to 90 days after initiation of drug therapy because of the potential for seizure activity.)	• Advise the patient to consult with the health care provider about driving or other hazardous activities during the first several months of drug therapy.

continued

Nursing Practice Application *continued*

IMPLEMENTATION	
Interventions and (Rationales)	**Patient-Centered Care**
• Continue to monitor aPTT prior to dialysis in patients with chronic renal failure. (The heparin dose during dialysis may need to be increased as the Hct increases.)	• Explain any changes in medication routine to the patient and provide a rationale.
• Encourage adequate dietary intake of iron, folic acid, and vitamin B_{12}. **Collaboration:** Provide dietary consult as needed. Consider nutritional supplements of these nutrients if the diet is inadequate. (The response to erythropoiesis-stimulating therapy may be decreased if blood levels of iron, folic acid, and vitamin B_{12} are deficient.)	• Teach the patient to maintain a healthy diet with adequate amounts of iron, folic acid, and vitamin B_{12} (e.g., found in meats, dairy, eggs, fortified cereals and breads, leafy green vegetables, citrus fruits, dried beans, and peas).
• **Lifespan:** When administering epoetin alfa to premature infants, use preservative-free formulations. (Epoetin alfa may contain preservatives such as benzyl alcohol. Benzyl alcohol may cause fetal gasping syndrome.)	• To allay anxiety, offer parents rationales for all treatments provided for the infant.
Patient understanding of drug therapy: • Use opportunities during administration of medications and during assessments to provide patient education. (Using time during nursing care helps to optimize and reinforce key teaching areas.)	• The patient should be able to state the reason for the drug, appropriate dose and scheduling; what adverse effects to observe for and when to report; and the anticipated length of medication therapy.
Patient self-administration of drug therapy: • When administering medications, instruct the patient, family, or caregiver in proper self-administration techniques followed by teach-back. (Proper administration increases the effectiveness of the drug.)	• Teach the patient, family, or caregiver in proper self-administration techniques. Proper technique includes: • The vial should be gently rotated to mix contents and never shaken. Vials are kept under refrigeration and should be gently warmed in the hand. • All vials are for one-time use only and any remaining amount should be discarded. • If indwelling subcutaneous soft catheter (e.g., Insuflon soft catheter) is left in place for injections, teach the patient the proper care of the site and catheter, and any schedule for rotating sites. • Have the patient, family, or caregiver perform the teach-back technique until the proper technique is used and they are comfortable giving the injection.

See Table 32.1 for a list of drugs to which these nursing actions apply.

Treating the Diverse Patient: Epoetin Use by Athletes

Blood doping, withdrawing blood and then retransfusing it before a competitive sporting event, has been used by some athletes in an attempt to gain a competitive edge. With increased RBCs and higher Hgb, oxygen-carrying capacity is thought to increase, boosting endurance. With the advent of epoetin alfa, blood doping took on new meaning. Some athletes found that the use of epoetin alfa well before an athletic meet achieved the same effects without the ability (through testing) to detect the dramatic increase in RBCs that was apparent immediately following a transfusion. Charges of blood doping with epoetin alfa were initially difficult to prove. However, as more sophisticated tests became available, detection of the presence of the drug was possible. Blood doping with epoetin alfa even occurs among olympic and paralympic athletes (Sobolevsky et al., 2014). Urine testing for epoetin alfa has been standard, but there are newer, more rapid blood tests available (Dehnes, Myrvold, Ström, Ericsson, & Hemmersbach, 2014). Newer drugs, without new tests to detect them initially, are on the horizon, and the race against cheating in sports continues.

Blood doping is not without a price to the user, however. Increased blood volume and viscosity have led to hypertension, thrombosis, and death. Undeterred, some athletes, desperate for a competitive edge, continue to use it. Adolescents involved in competitive sports activities may have heard about epoetin alfa and may question its advantages. The nurse plays a key role in providing accurate information about epoetin alfa and related drugs, and counseling adolescents about the risks and adverse effects of sports-enhancing drugs.

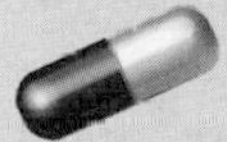

Prototype Drug | Filgrastim *(Granix, Neupogen)*

Therapeutic Class: Drug for increasing neutrophil production **Pharmacologic Class:** Colony-stimulating factor

Actions and Uses

Filgrastim is human G-CSF produced through recombinant DNA technology. Its two primary actions are to increase neutrophil production in the bone marrow and to enhance the phagocytic and cytotoxic functions of existing neutrophils. This is particularly important for patients with neutropenia, which often is associated with severe bacterial and fungal infections. Administration of filgrastim will shorten the length of time of neutropenia in patients with cancer whose bone marrow has been suppressed by antineoplastic drugs or in patients following bone marrow or stem cell transplants. It may also be used in patients with AIDS-related immunosuppression. It is administered subcutaneously or by slow IV infusion. The dose is based on absolute neutrophil counts (ANCs): The target range is 1,500 to 10,000 cells/mm^3.

In 2012 a new form of the drug, TBO-filgrastim (Granix), was approved by the FDA to reduce severe neutropenia in adults with certain malignancies. A self-administration kit for Granix has also been approved so the drug may be injected at home. While technically not identical, Granix and Neupogen have the same pharmacologic actions and adverse effects.

Administration Alerts

- Do not administer within 24 hours before or after chemotherapy with cytotoxic drugs because this will greatly decrease the effectiveness of filgrastim.
- Pregnancy category C.

PHARMACOKINETICS (SUBCUTANEOUS)

Onset	Peak	Duration
4 h	2–8 h	Up to 1 wk

Adverse Effects

Common adverse effects include fatigue, rash, epistaxis, decreased platelet counts, neutropenic fever, nausea, and vomiting. Filgrastim is associated with potentially serious adverse effects, and close monitoring is required. Bone pain may occur in up to 33% of patients receiving filgrastim. A small percentage of patients may develop an allergic reaction. Frequent laboratory tests are necessary to ensure that excessive numbers of neutrophils, or leukocytosis, does not occur. Leukocyte counts higher than 100,000 cells/mm^3 increase the risk of serious adverse effects such as respiratory failure, intracranial hemorrhage, retinal hemorrhage, and MI. Fatal rupture of the spleen has occurred in a small number of patients.

Contraindications: The only contraindication is hypersensitivity to *E. coli* proteins because this microbe is used to produce the recombinant drug.

Interactions

Drug–Drug: Because antineoplastic drugs and CSFs produce opposite effects, filgrastim is not administered until at least 24 hours after a chemotherapy session.

Lab Tests: Values for the following may be increased: leukocyte alkaline phosphatase, serum alkaline phosphatase, uric acid, and lactate dehydrogenase (LDH).

Herbal/Food: Unknown.

Treatment of Overdose: There is no treatment for overdose.

32.3 Pharmacotherapy With Colony-Stimulating Factors

Regulation of WBC production, or leukopoiesis, is more complicated than erythropoiesis because there are different types of leukocytes in the blood. Pharmacologically, the most important substances controlling production are **colony-stimulating factors (CSFs).** Also called leukopoietic growth factors, the CSFs comprise a small group of drugs that stimulate the growth and differentiation of one or more types of leukocytes. Doses for these medications are listed in Table 32.1.

When the body receives a bacterial challenge, the production of CSFs increases rapidly. The CSFs are active at very low concentrations; each stem cell stimulated by these growth factors is capable of producing as many as 1,000 mature leukocytes. The CSFs not only increase the production of *new* leukocytes, they also activate *existing* WBCs. Examples of enhanced functions include increased migration of leukocytes to the bacteria, increased antibody toxicity, and increased phagocytosis.

CSFs are named according to the types of blood cells they stimulate. For example, granulocyte colony-stimulating factor (G-CSF) increases the production of neutrophils, the most common type of granulocyte. Granulocyte/macrophage colony-stimulating factor (GM-CSF) stimulates both neutrophil and macrophage production. The process of identifying the many endogenous CSFs, determining their normal functions, and discovering their potential value as therapeutic agents is an emerging area of pharmacology.

The goal of CSF pharmacotherapy is to produce a rapid increase in the number of neutrophils in patients who have suppressed immune systems. CSF therapy shortens the length of time patients are susceptible to life-threatening infections due to low numbers of neutrophils (neutropenia). Indications include patients undergoing chemotherapy or receiving bone marrow or stem cell transplants or who have certain malignancies. By raising neutrophil counts, CSFs can assist in keeping antineoplastic dosing regimens on schedule and thus, more effective.

Filgrastim (Granix, Neupogen) is similar to natural G-CSF and is primarily used for chronic neutropenia or neutropenia secondary to chemotherapy. Pegfilgrastim (Neulasta) is a form of filgrastim bonded to a molecule of polyethylene glycol (PEG). The PEG decreases the renal excretion of the molecule, allowing it to remain in the body with a sustained duration of action. Sargramostim (Leukine) is similar to natural GM-CSF and is used to treat neutropenia in patients treated for acute myelogenous leukemia and patients who are having autologous bone marrow transplantation.

Nonspecific adverse effects of CSFs include nausea, vomiting, fatigue, fever, and flushing. CSF therapy requires careful laboratory monitoring to avoid producing too many neutrophils. The risk of developing acute myeloid leukemia or myelodysplastic syndrome may be increased when CSFs are administered to patients undergoing chemotherapy for breast cancer.

32.4 Pharmacotherapy With Platelet Enhancers

The production of platelets, or thrombocytopoiesis, begins when megakaryocytes in the bone marrow start shedding membrane-bound packets. These packets enter the bloodstream and become platelets. A single megakaryocyte can produce thousands of platelets.

Megakaryocyte activity is controlled by the hormone **thrombopoietin,** which is produced by the liver. Thrombopoietin is not available as a medication. The drug most frequently used to enhance platelet production is oprelvekin (Neumega). Produced through recombinant DNA technology, oprelvekin stimulates the production of

Nursing Practice Application

Pharmacotherapy With Colony-Stimulating Factors

ASSESSMENT	POTENTIAL NURSING DIAGNOSES*
Baseline assessment prior to administration: • Obtain a complete health history including recent or current infections, recent surgeries, injuries or wounds, yeast infections (e.g., thrush), vaccination history, cardiac conditions (e.g., dysrhythmias, heart failure), or respiratory, renal, and hepatic conditions. Obtain a drug history including allergies, current prescription and OTC drugs, herbal preparations, and alcohol use. Be alert to possible drug interactions. • Obtain baseline weight and vital signs. Assess level of fatigue. • Evaluate appropriate laboratory findings (e.g., CBC, WBC, or ANC), renal and liver function studies, uric acid levels, and ECG. (ANC = Total WBC count multiplied by the total percentage of neutrophils [segmented neutrophils plus banded neutrophils]).	• *Anxiety* • *Activity Intolerance* • *Fatigue* • *Deficient Knowledge* (drug therapy) • *Risk for Infection* • *Risk for Caregiver Role Strain* *NANDA I © 2014
Assessment throughout administration: • Continue assessment for therapeutic effects (e.g., CBC and WBC or ANC has increased, no signs or symptoms of infection). • Continue frequent monitoring of appropriate laboratory values (e.g., CBC, WBC or ANC, Hct, platelet count, renal and hepatic labs, uric acid levels). • Monitor vital signs and level of fatigue. • Assess for adverse effects: bone pain (especially lower back, posterior iliac crests, and sternum), fever, nausea, anorexia, hyperuricemia, anemia, ST depression on ECG, angina, respiratory distress, and allergic reaction. Continue to assess for infection and fatigue related to drug treatment (e.g., chemotherapy).	

Nursing Practice Application *continued*

IMPLEMENTATION	
Interventions and (Rationales)	**Patient-Centered Care**
Ensuring therapeutic effects: • Continue frequent assessments as described earlier for therapeutic effects. (Rise in WBC and/or ANC counts will depend on the condition treated, e.g., depth and length of nadir from cytotoxic chemotherapy.)	• Instruct the patient on the need to return frequently for follow-up laboratory work.
• Encourage adequate rest periods and adequate fluid intake. (The patient may be significantly fatigued due to the drug therapy for the disease condition. Adequate fluid intake helps maintain adequate urinary output and prevent urinary tract infections.)	• Encourage the patient to rest when fatigued and to space activities throughout the day to allow for adequate rest periods. • Encourage the intake of water and non-hyperosmolar beverages and drinking whenever thirsty.
Minimizing adverse effects: • Continue to monitor for adverse effects: bone pain (especially lower back, posterior iliac crests, and sternum), fever, nausea, anorexia, hyperuricemia, anemia, ST depression on ECG, angina, respiratory distress, and allergic reaction. Continue to assess for infection and fatigue related to drug treatment, (e.g., chemotherapy). (Bone pain tends to occur 2 to 3 days prior to rise in circulating WBC due to the production of WBCs in bone marrow. ST segment depression on ECG may occur with potential for serious dysrhythmias. Respiratory distress may develop after the administration of sargramostim and should be reported immediately. Hyperuricemia may cause goutlike conditions.)	• Instruct the patient to report any severe bone pain not relieved by nonnarcotic analgesics. • Teach the patient to immediately report any palpitations, dizziness, angina, or dyspnea. • Patients who are prone to gout should report signs and symptoms of gout and increase fluid intake to enhance the renal elimination of uric acid.

• Maintain meticulous infection control measures. Report any signs and symptoms of infections or fever immediately. (The patient will continue to be at risk for infections until WBC/ANC levels rise. Opportunistic infections, such as yeast, and viruses, such as herpes simplex, may occur. Parameters will be set by the health care provider for reporting fever, e.g., any temperature over 100.5°F, depending on the underlying disease condition and drug therapy.)	• Instruct the patient in hygiene and infection control measures such as:
	  • Frequent hand washing.
	  • Avoiding crowded indoor places.
	  • Avoiding people with known infections or young children who have a higher risk of having an infection.
	  • Cooking food thoroughly, allowing the family or caregiver to prepare raw foods prior to cooking, and to clean up, but the patient should not consume raw fruits or vegetables.
	• Teach the patient to report any fever and symptoms of infection such as wounds with redness or drainage, increasing cough, increasing fatigue, white patches on oral mucous membranes, white and itchy vaginal discharge, or itchy blister-like vesicles on the skin.

• Monitor the ECG periodically for ST segment depression or dysrhythmias and report immediately. (Sargramostim may cause significant ST depression with potential for serious dysrhythmias, especially in patients with previous cardiac conditions.)	• Teach the patient to immediately report any palpitations, dizziness, or angina.
• Monitor for signs of dyspnea or respiratory distress, especially when accompanied by tachycardia and hypotension, and report immediately. (Sargramostim may cause respiratory distress as granulocyte counts rise, especially in patients with pre-existing respiratory disorders.)	• Teach the patient to immediately report any dyspnea, respiratory distress, palpitations, or dizziness.
• Monitor for signs and symptoms of allergic-type reactions. (The patient may be hypersensitive to proteins from *E. coli* used to develop the drug.)	• Teach the patient to immediately report symptoms of allergic reaction such as rash, urticaria, wheezing, and dyspnea.
• Monitor hepatic status during the drug administration period. (Filgrastim may cause an elevation in liver enzymes.)	• Instruct the patient to report any significant itching, yellowing of the sclera or skin, darkened urine, or light or clay-colored stools.
• Assess for spleen enlargement periodically and report. (Filgrastim has been associated with rare but potentially fatal cases of splenomegaly and rupture.)	• Instruct the patient, family, or caregiver to report any symptoms of left upper abdominal pain or left shoulder pain, which may indicate spleen enlargement or rupture.

continued

Nursing Practice Application *continued*

IMPLEMENTATION	
Interventions and (Rationales)	**Patient-Centered Care**
• **Lifespan:** Monitor laboratory results for pediatric patients with forms of congenital neutropenia (e.g., congenital agranulocytosis) more frequently. (Patients with these disorders are at greater risk for developing acute myelogenous leukemia and myelodysplastic neutropenia related to drug therapy.)	• Teach the patient, family, or caregivers that frequent laboratory studies may be needed.
• Stop administration when WBC counts reach the level determined by the health care provider. (Filgrastim may be stopped when neutrophil counts reach 10,000/mm^3; sargramostim may be stopped when neutrophil counts reach 20,000/mm^3 or as ordered by the health care provider.)	• Teach the patient about the importance of returning regularly for laboratory work.
Patient understanding of drug therapy: • Use opportunities during administration of medications and during assessments to provide patient education. (Using time during nursing care helps to optimize and reinforce key teaching areas.)	• The patient, family, or caregiver should be able to state the reason for the drug, appropriate dose and scheduling; what adverse effects to observe for and when to report; and the anticipated length of medication therapy.
Patient self-administration of drug therapy: • When administering medications, instruct the patient, family, or caregiver in proper self-administration techniques followed by teach-back. (Proper administration increases the effectiveness of the drug.)	• Teach the patient, family, or caregiver in proper self-administration techniques. Proper technique includes: • Vial should be gently rotated to mix contents and never shaken. Vials are kept under refrigeration and should be gently warmed in the hand. • All vials are for one-time use only and any remaining amount should be discarded. • If indwelling subcutaneous soft catheter (e.g., Insuflon soft catheter) is used, the patient should be taught appropriate site care, insertion technique as appropriate, or schedule for rotating sites. • Have the patient, family, or caregiver teach-back the technique until the proper technique is used and they are comfortable giving the injection.

See Table 32.1 for a list of drugs to which these nursing actions apply.

megakaryocytes and thrombopoietin. Oprelvekin is functionally equivalent to interleukin-11 (IL-11), a substance secreted by monocytes and lymphocytes that signals cells in the immune system to respond to an infection.

Oprelvekin is used to enhance the production of platelets in patients who are at risk for thrombocytopenia caused by cancer chemotherapy. The drug shortens the time that the patient is thrombocytopenic and very susceptible to adverse bleeding events. The onset of action is 5 to 9 days, and therapy generally continues until the platelet count returns to greater than 50,000/mm^3. Platelet counts will remain elevated for about 7 days after the last dose. Oprelvekin is given only by the subcutaneous route. The primary adverse effect is fluid retention, which occurs in about 60% of patients and can be a concern for patients with pre-existing cardiovascular or renal disease. Visual impairment may occur during therapy. Nursing care for patients receiving treatment with oprelvekin is similar to care for patients receiving the CSFs for WBCs.

Two other platelet enhancers are available but have more limited application. Romiplostim (Nplate) and eltrombopag (Promacta) are approved to improve platelet function in patients with chronic immune (idiopathic) thrombocytopenic purpura (ITP). Chronic ITP is a disorder characterized by inadequate platelet production and/or increased platelet destruction. Patients with ITP experience a high risk for bruising and bleeding, which may occur anywhere in the body. Both drugs increase the number of platelets by activating the natural receptor for thrombopoietin. Eltrombopag is an oral (PO) drug, whereas romiplostim is given by the subcutaneous route.

☑ Check Your Understanding 32.1

While the patient is receiving CSF drugs such as filgrastim (Granix, Neupogen) and pegfilgrastim (Neumega), neutropenia continues to present a risk to the patient until blood counts increase. What infection control measures will the nurse follow and teach the patient to avoid risks associated with neutropenia? *Visit www.pearsonhighered.com/nursingresources for the answer.*

Table 32.2 Classification of Anemia

Morphology	Description	Examples
Macrocytic–normochromic	Large, abnormally shaped erythrocytes with normal hemoglobin concentration	Pernicious anemia, folate-deficiency anemia
Microcytic–hypochromic	Small, abnormally shaped erythrocytes with decreased hemoglobin concentration	Iron-deficiency anemia, thalassemia
Normocytic–normochromic	Destruction or depletion of normal erythroblasts or mature erythrocytes	Aplastic anemia, hemorrhagic anemia, sickle-cell anemia, hemolytic anemia

ANEMIAS

Anemia is a condition in which RBCs have a diminished capacity to deliver oxygen to tissues. Although there are many different causes of anemia, they fall into one of the following categories:

- Blood loss due to hemorrhage.
- Increased erythrocyte destruction.
- Decreased erythrocyte production.

Anemia is considered a sign of an underlying disorder, rather than a distinct disease. For therapy to be successful, the underlying pathology must be identified and treated.

32.5 Classification of Anemias

Classification of anemia is generally based on a description of the erythrocyte's size and color. Sizes are described as normal (normocytic), small (microcytic), or large (macrocytic). Color is based on the amount of hemoglobin present and is described as normal red (normochromic) or light red (hypochromic). This classification is shown in Table 32.2.

Although each type of anemia has specific characteristics, all have common signs and symptoms. If the anemia occurs gradually, the patient may remain asymptomatic, except during periods of physical exercise. As the condition progresses, the patient often exhibits pallor, which is a paleness of the skin and mucous membranes due to hemoglobin deficiency. Decreased exercise tolerance, fatigue, and lethargy occur because insufficient oxygen reaches muscles. Dizziness and fainting are common as the brain does not receive enough oxygen to function properly. The respiratory and cardiovascular systems compensate for the oxygen depletion by increasing respiration rate and heart rate. Chronic or severe disease can result in heart failure.

ANTIANEMIC DRUGS

Depending on the type of anemia, several vitamins and minerals may be given to enhance the oxygen-carrying capacity of blood. The most common antianemic drugs are cyanocobalamin (Nascobal), folic acid, and ferrous sulfate (Feosol, others). These drugs are listed in Table 32.3.

Table 32.3 Antianemic Drugs

Drug	Route and Adult Dose (max dose where indicated)	Adverse Effects
VITAMIN SUPPLEMENTS		
cyanocobalamin (Nascobal)	IM/deep subcutaneous: 30 mcg/day for 5–10 days; then 100–200 mcg/month Intranasal: one spray (500 mcg) in one nostril once weekly	*Arthralgia, dizziness, headache, nasopharyngitis* <u>Anaphylaxis, hypokalemia</u>
folic acid	PO/IM/subcutaneous/IV: less than 1 mg/day	*Flushing, rash* <u>Hypersensitivity</u>
IRON SALTS		
ferrous fumarate (Feostat, others)	PO: 200 mg tid or qid	*Nausea, heartburn, constipation, diarrhea, dark stools, hypotension* <u>Cardiovascular collapse, aggravation of peptic ulcers or ulcerative colitis, hepatic necrosis, anaphylaxis (ferumooxytol, iron dextran)</u>
ferrous gluconate (Fergon, Ferralet)	PO: 325–600 mg qid; may be gradually increased to 650 mg qid as needed and tolerated	
ferrous sulfate (Feosol, others)	PO: 750–1,500 mg/day in 1–3 divided doses	
ferumoxytol (Feraheme)	IV: single dose of 510 mg followed by a second 510 mg dose 3 to 8 days later	
iron dextran (Dexferrum)	IM/IV: dose is individualized and determined from a table supplied by the drug manufacturer that correlates body weight to hemoglobin values (max: 100 mg within 24 h)	
iron sucrose (Venofer)	IV: 100–200 mg by slow injection or infusion	

Note. *Italics* indicate common adverse effects; <u>underlining</u> indicates serious adverse effects.

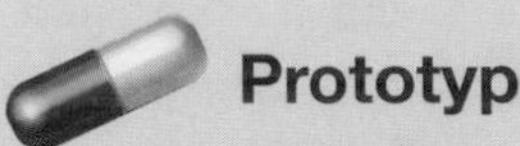

Prototype Drug | Cyanocobalamin *(Nascobal)*

Therapeutic Class: Drug for anemia **Pharmacologic Class:** Vitamin supplement

Actions and Uses

Cyanocobalamin is a purified form of vitamin B_{12} that is indicated for patients with vitamin B_{12} deficiency anemia. Treatment is most often by weekly, biweekly, or monthly intramuscular (IM) or subcutaneous injections. Oral vitamin B_{12} formulations are available primarily as vitamin supplementation, although they are only effective in patients who have sufficient amounts of intrinsic factor. An intranasal spray formulation is available that provides for once-weekly (Nascobal) dosage. The intranasal formulation is used for maintenance therapy after normal vitamin B_{12} levels have been restored by parenteral preparations.

Parenteral administration rapidly reverses most signs and symptoms of B_{12} deficiency, usually within a few days or weeks. If the disease has been prolonged, symptoms may take longer to resolve, and some neurologic damage may be permanent. In most cases, treatment must often be maintained for the remainder of the patient's life.

Administration Alerts

- If PO preparations are mixed with fruit juices, administer quickly because ascorbic acid affects the stability of vitamin B_{12}.
- Pregnancy category A (C when used parenterally).

PHARMACOKINETICS

Onset	Peak	Duration
Days to weeks	8–12 h PO; 1–2 h intranasal; 1 h IV	Unknown

Adverse Effects

Adverse effects from cyanocobalamin are uncommon. Hypokalemia is possible; thus, serum potassium levels are monitored periodically. A small percentage of patients receiving B_{12} exhibit arthralgia, dizziness, or headache. Anaphylaxis is possible, though rare.

Contraindications: Contraindications include sensitivity to cobalt and folic acid–deficiency anemia. Cyanocobalamin is contraindicated in patients with severe pulmonary disease and should be used cautiously in patients with heart disease because of the potential for sodium retention caused by the drug.

Interactions

Drug–Drug: Drug interactions with cyanocobalamin include a decrease in absorption when given concurrently with alcohol, aminosalicylic acid, neomycin, and colchicine. Chloramphenicol may interfere with therapeutic response to cyanocobalamin.

Lab Tests: Unknown.

Herbal/Food: Unknown.

Treatment of Overdose: No overdosage has been reported.

32.6 Pharmacotherapy With Vitamin B_{12} and Folic Acid

Vitamin B_{12} is an essential component of two coenzymes that are required for actively growing and dividing cells. Vitamin B_{12} is not synthesized by either plants or animals; only bacteria can make this substance. Because only minuscule amounts of vitamin B_{12} are required (3 mcg/day), deficiency of this vitamin is usually not due to insufficient dietary intake. Instead, the most common cause of vitamin B_{12} deficiency is absence of **intrinsic factor,** a protein secreted by stomach cells. Intrinsic factor is required for vitamin B_{12} to be absorbed from the intestine. Figure 32.2 illustrates the metabolism of vitamin B_{12}. Inflammatory diseases of the stomach or surgical removal of the stomach may result in deficiency of intrinsic factor. Inflammatory diseases of the small intestine that affect food and nutrient absorption may also cause vitamin B_{12} deficiency. Because vitamin B_{12} is found primarily in foods of animal origin, strict vegetarians may require careful meal planning or a vitamin supplement to prevent deficiency.

The most profound consequence of vitamin B_{12} deficiency is a condition called **pernicious** or **megaloblastic anemia,** which affects both the hematologic and nervous systems. The hematopoietic stem cells produce abnormally large erythrocytes that do not fully mature. Red blood cells are most affected, though lack of maturation of all blood cell types may occur in severe disease. The symptoms of pernicious anemia are often nonspecific and develop slowly, sometimes over decades. Nervous system symptoms may include memory loss, confusion, unsteadiness, tingling or numbness in the limbs, delusions, mood disturbances, and even hallucinations in severe deficiencies. Permanent nervous system damage may result if the disease remains untreated. Pharmacotherapy includes the administration of cyanocobalamin, a form of vitamin B_{12} (see the prototype drug feature in this chapter).

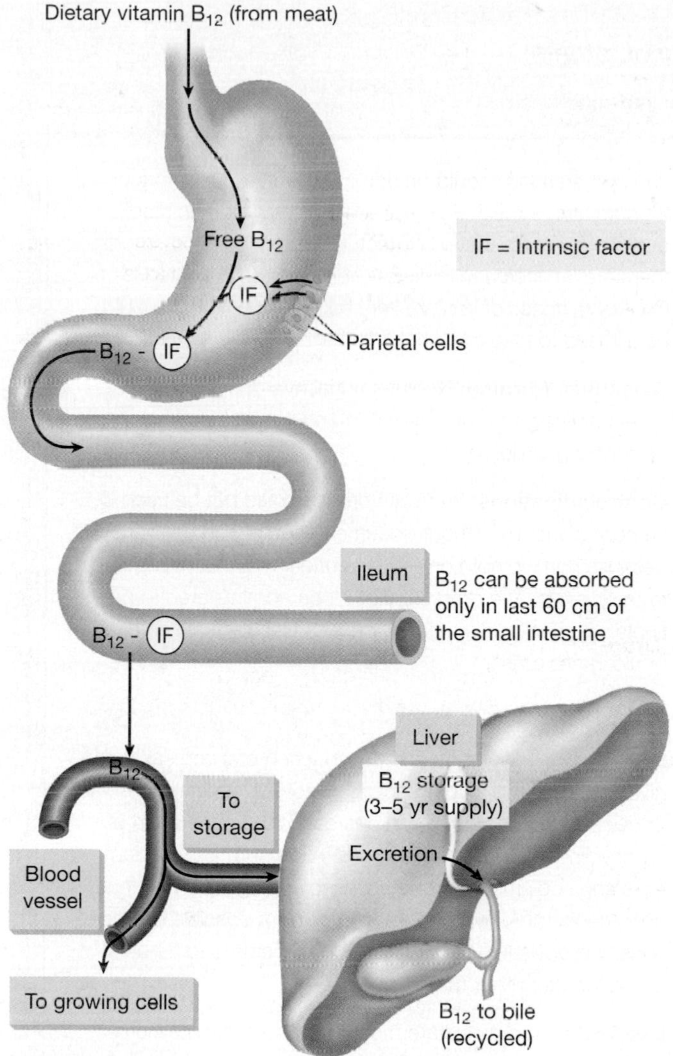

FIGURE 32.2 Metabolism of vitamin B_{12}

Folic acid, or **folate,** is a B-complex vitamin that is essential for normal DNA and RNA synthesis. As with B_{12} deficiency, insufficient folic acid can manifest itself as anemia. In fact, the metabolism of vitamin B_{12} and folic acid are intricately linked; a B_{12} deficiency will create a lack of activated folic acid.

Folic acid does not require intrinsic factor for intestinal absorption, and the most common cause of folate deficiency is insufficient dietary intake. This is often observed in patients with chronic alcoholism because their diets are often deficient in this nutrient, and alcohol interferes with folate metabolism in the liver. Fad diets and malabsorption disorders of the small intestine can also result in folate anemia. Hematopoietic signs of folate deficiency are the same as those for B_{12} deficiency; however, no neurologic signs are present. Folate deficiency during pregnancy has been linked to neural birth defects such as spina bifida.

Treatment of mild deficiency or prophylaxis of folate deficiency is accomplished by increasing the dietary intake of folic acid by including fresh green vegetables, dried beans, and wheat products. In cases when adequate dietary intake cannot be achieved, therapy with folate sodium (Folvite) or folic acid is warranted. Folic acid is discussed further in chapter 43, where it is a drug prototype for water-soluble vitamins.

32.7 Pharmacotherapy With Iron

Iron is a mineral essential to the function of several mitochondrial enzymes involved in metabolism and energy production in the cell. Most iron in the body, 60% to 80%, is associated with hemoglobin inside erythrocytes. Because free iron is toxic, the body binds the mineral to the protein complexes **ferritin, hemosiderin,** and **transferrin.** Ferritin and hemosiderin maintain iron stores *inside* cells, whereas transferrin *transports* iron to sites in the body where it is needed.

After erythrocytes die, nearly all the iron in their hemoglobin is incorporated into transferrin and recycled for later use. Because of this efficient recycling, only about 1 mg of iron is excreted from the body per day, making daily dietary iron requirements in most individuals quite small. Iron balance is maintained by the increased absorption of the mineral from the proximal small intestine during periods of deficiency. Because iron is found in greater quantities in meat products, vegetarians are at higher risk of iron-deficiency anemia.

Iron deficiency is the most common cause of anemia. More than 50% of patients diagnosed with iron deficiency anemia have gastrointestinal (GI) bleeding, such as may occur from GI malignancies or chronic peptic ulcer disease. In the United States and Canada, iron deficiency most commonly occurs in women of child-bearing age due to blood losses during menses and pregnancy. These conditions may require more than the recommended daily allowance (RDA) of iron (see chapter 43). The most significant effect of iron deficiency is a reduction in erythropoiesis, resulting in symptoms of anemia.

Mild iron-deficiency anemia may be prevented or corrected by increasing the intake of iron-rich foods, such as fish, red meat, fortified cereal, and whole-grain breads. For more severe deficiencies, ferrous sulfate (Feosol, others), ferrous gluconate (Fergon), and ferrous fumarate (Feostat, others) are used as iron supplements. Slow-release products, called iron carbonyl (Feosol-caps, Ferronyl), are more expensive but may give fewer GI side effects. They are also less dangerous following accidental exposure in children because there is a longer period for intervention before toxic effects materialize. Iron dextran (Dexferrum) is a parenteral supplement that may be used when the patient is unable to take PO preparations. Because iron oxidizes vitamin C, many iron supplements contain this vitamin. Vitamin C also is believed to enhance iron absorption. Depending on the degree of iron depletion and the amount of iron supplement that can be tolerated by the patient

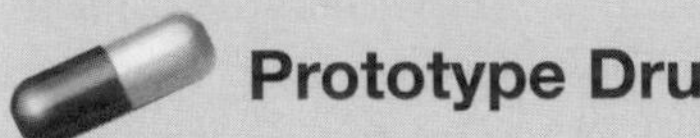

Prototype Drug | Ferrous Sulfate *(Feosol, others)*

Therapeutic Class: Antianemic drug **Pharmacologic Class:** Iron supplement

Actions and Uses

Ferrous sulfate is an iron supplement containing 20% to 30% elemental iron. It is available in a wide variety of dosage forms to prevent or rapidly reverse symptoms of iron-deficiency anemia. Other forms of iron include ferrous fumarate, which contains 33% elemental iron, and ferrous gluconate, which contains 12% elemental iron. The doses of these various preparations are based on their iron content. In general, patients with iron deficiency respond rapidly to the administration of ferrous sulfate. Although a positive therapeutic response may be achieved in 48 hours, therapy may continue for several months to replenish the storage depots for iron.

Laboratory evaluation of hemoglobin (Hgb) or hematocrit (Hct) values is conducted regularly, as excess iron is toxic. Although a positive therapeutic response may be achieved in 48 hours, therapy may continue for several months.

Administration Alerts

- When administering IV be careful to prevent infiltration because iron is highly irritating to tissues.
- Use the Z-track method (deep muscle) when giving IM.
- Do not crush tablets or empty contents of capsules when administering.
- Do not give tablets or capsules within 1 hour of bedtime.
- Pregnancy category A.

PHARMACOKINETICS

Because iron is a natural substance, it is difficult to obtain pharmacokinetic values.

Adverse Effects

The most frequent adverse effect of ferrous sulfate is GI upset. Taking the drug with food will diminish GI symptoms but can decrease the absorption of iron by 50% to 70%. In addition, antacids should not be taken with ferrous sulfate because they also reduce absorption of the mineral. Ideally, iron preparations should be administered 1 hour before or 2 hours after a meal. Iron preparations may darken stools, but this is a harmless side effect. Constipation is common; therefore, an increase in dietary fiber may be indicated. Excessive doses of iron are very toxic, and patients should be advised to take the medication exactly as directed.

Black Box Warning: Nonintentional overdoses of iron-containing products are a leading cause of fatal poisoning of children.

Contraindications: Iron salts drugs should not be used in hemolytic anemia without documentation of iron deficiency because iron will not correct this condition and it may build to toxic levels. The drug should not be administered to patients with hemochromatosis, peptic ulcer, regional enteritis, or ulcerative colitis.

Interactions

Drug–Drug: Absorption is reduced when oral iron salts are given concurrently with antacids, proton-pump inhibitors, or calcium supplements. Iron decreases the absorption of tetracyclines and fluoroquinolones. Aluminum and calcium salts and sodium bicarbonate will increase gastric pH, thus delaying the absorption of iron. To prevent possible interactions, it is advisable to take iron supplements 1 to 2 hours before or after other medications.

Lab Tests: Ferrous sulfate may decrease serum calcium level and increase serum bilirubin.

Herbal/Food: Food, especially dairy products, will inhibit absorption of ferrous sulfate. Foods high in vitamin C such as orange juice and strawberries can increase the absorption of iron.

Treatment of Overdose: The antidote for acute iron intoxication is deferoxamine (Desferal). This parenteral agent binds iron, which is subsequently removed by the kidneys, turning the urine a reddish brown color.

without significant side effects, 3 to 6 months of therapy may be required.

A newer and unique form of iron is ferumoxytol (Feraheme), which is indicated to treat iron deficiency associated with chronic kidney disease (with or without dialysis). The drug consists of iron oxide protected by a carbohydrate shell. The shell remains intact until the drug enters macrophages, whereby the iron is released to its storage depots. The advantage of ferumoxytol over existing iron salts is that it can be administered safely by the IV route and can raise iron levels more rapidly.

Nursing Practice Application

Pharmacotherapy for Anemia (Folic Acid, Vitamin B_{12}, Ferrous Sulfate)

ASSESSMENT	POTENTIAL NURSING DIAGNOSES*
Baseline assessment prior to administration: • Obtain a complete health history including cardiovascular, GI, hepatic, or renal disease. Obtain a drug history including allergies, current prescription and OTC drugs, and herbal preparations. Be alert to possible drug interactions. Obtain a dietary history, including alcohol use. • Obtain baseline weight and vital signs. Assess fatigue level. • Evaluate appropriate laboratory findings (e.g., CBC, electrolytes, transferrin and serum ferritin levels, renal and liver function studies.)	• *Activity Intolerance* • *Fatigue* • *Imbalanced Nutrition, Less Than Body Requirements* • *Deficient Knowledge* (drug therapy) • *Risk for Injury,* related to underlying disorder or adverse drug effects *NANDA I © 2014
Assessment throughout administration: • Continue assessment for therapeutic effects (e.g., Hct, RBC count improved, patient's activity level, and general sense of well-being). • Continue monitoring of appropriate laboratory values (e.g., CBC, electrolytes, hepatic, and renal function). • Assess for adverse effects: itching, skin rash, hypokalemia, nausea, vomiting, heartburn, constipation, black stools (iron preparations), or allergic reactions.	

IMPLEMENTATION

Interventions and (Rationales)	Patient-Centered Care
Ensuring therapeutic effects: • Continue assessments as described earlier for therapeutic effects. (RBC and Hct counts may rise over 3 to 6 months. Note gradually increasing levels of activity and fewer complaints of fatigue as counts rise.)	• Instruct the patient on the need to return for periodic laboratory work.
• Encourage adequate dietary intake of nutrient whenever possible. Consider long-term supplementation as appropriate. (Maintaining a healthy diet may decrease the need for long-term supplementation or will enhance therapeutic effects.)	• Teach the patient to increase intake of folic acid, vitamin B_{12}, and iron-rich foods such as: • Folic acid: leafy green vegetables, citrus fruits, and dried beans and peas • Vitamin B_{12}: fish, meat, poultry, eggs, milk and milk products, and fortified breakfast cereals • Iron: meats, fish, poultry, lentils, and beans
• Follow appropriate administration guidelines. (Following appropriate administration techniques maximizes absorption for enhanced therapeutic effect. Oral formulations may require special administration requirements.)	• Teach the patient specific administration guidelines, including: • Folic acid: May be taken on empty stomach or with food. • Vitamin B_{12}: Must be given IM in cases of pernicious anemia until therapeutic levels are reached, and then may be prescribed by nasal spray. Take oral formulations with meals. • Iron: Take on empty stomach when possible. Liquid preparations should be sipped through a straw with the straw held toward the back of the mouth to avoid staining teeth. Increasing intake of vitamin C rich foods may also enhance iron absorption.
Minimizing adverse effects: • Continue to monitor for adverse effects, including skin rash, hypokalemia, nausea, vomiting, constipation, heartburn, staining of teeth, black stools (iron preparations), or allergic reactions. (Hypokalemia and subsequent significant dysrhythmias may occur with vitamin B_{12} administration. Staining of the teeth from liquid oral preparations and black stools may occur with iron.)	• Instruct the patient to monitor for signs and symptoms of hypokalemia (e.g., muscle weakness or cramping, palpitations) and to report promptly. • Teach the patient to increase fluid and fiber intake as part of a healthy diet while on iron preparations and to dilute oral liquid formulations and sip through a straw placed in the back of the mouth.
• Plan activities to allow for periods of rest to help the patient conserve energy. (Fatigue from anemia due to decreased Hgb levels is common.)	• Encourage the patient to rest when fatigued and to space activities throughout the day to allow for adequate rest periods.

continued

Nursing Practice Application *continued*

IMPLEMENTATION	
Interventions and (Rationales)	**Patient-Centered Care**
Patient understanding of drug therapy: • Use opportunities during administration of medications and during assessments to provide patient education. (Using time during nursing care helps to optimize and reinforce key teaching areas.)	• The patient, family, or caregiver should be able to state the reason for the drug; appropriate dose and scheduling; what adverse effects to observe for and when to report; and the anticipated length of medication therapy.
Patient self-administration of drug therapy: • When administering medications, instruct the patient, family, or caregiver in proper self-administration techniques as described earlier and of proper IM injection technique for vitamin B_{12} followed by teach-back. (Proper administration will increase the effectiveness of the drug.)	• The patient should be able to discuss appropriate dosing and any special administration techniques required related to the drug taken. • Teach the patient specific administration guidelines, including: • Folic acid: May be taken on an empty stomach or with food. • Vitamin B_{12}: Must be given IM in cases of pernicious anemia until therapeutic levels are reached, and then may be prescribed by nasal spray. Take oral formulations with meals. • Iron: Take on an empty stomach. Liquid preparations should be sipped through a straw with the straw held toward the back of the mouth to avoid staining the teeth. Increasing intake of vitamin C–rich foods may also enhance iron absorption. • Have the patient, family, or caregiver teach-back the technique until the proper technique is used and they are comfortable giving the injection.
• Keep all vitamins and iron preparations out of the reach of young children. (Iron poisoning may be fatal in young children.)	• Teach the patient to keep iron preparations and vitamins containing iron in a secure place if young children are present in the home.

See Table 32.3 for a list of drugs to which these nursing actions apply.

Chapter Review

KEY Concepts

The numbered key concepts provide a succinct summary of the important points from the corresponding numbered section within the chapter. If any of these points are not clear, refer to the numbered section within the chapter for review.

32.1 Hematopoiesis is the process of blood cell production that begins with primitive stem cells that reside in bone marrow. Homeostatic control of hematopoiesis is maintained through hormones and growth factors.

32.2 Erythropoietin is a hormone that stimulates the production of red blood cells when the body experiences hypoxia. Epoetin alfa is a synthetic form of erythropoietin used to treat specific anemias.

32.3 Colony-stimulating factors (CSFs) are growth factors that stimulate the production of leukocytes. They are used to reduce the duration of neutropenia in patients undergoing chemotherapy or organ transplantation.

32.4 Platelet enhancers stimulate the activity of megakaryocytes and thrombopoietin and increase the production of platelets. Oprelvekin, the only drug in this class, is prescribed for patients at risk for or with thrombocytopenia.

32.5 Anemias are classified based on a description of the size and color of the erythrocyte. All types of anemias have similar patient symptoms such as fatigue, pallor, dizziness and fainting.

32.6 Deficiencies in either vitamin B_{12} or folic acid can lead to pernicious anemia. Treatment with cyanocobalamin can reverse symptoms of pernicious anemia in many patients, although some degree of nervous system damage may be permanent.

32.7 Iron deficiency is the most common cause of nutritional anemia. Severe anemia can be successfully treated with iron supplements.

REVIEW Questions

1. An older adult patient diagnosed with iron-deficiency anemia will be taking ferrous sulfate (Feosol). The nurse will teach which of the required administration guidelines to the patient? (Select all that apply.)
   1. Take the tablets on an empty stomach if possible.
   2. Increase fluid intake and increase dietary fiber while taking this medication.
   3. If liquid preparations are used, dilute with water or juice and sip through a straw placed in the back of the mouth.
   4. Crush or dissolve sustained-release tablets in water if they are too big to swallow.
   5. Take the drug at bedtime for best results.
2. When planning to teach the patient about the use of epoetin alfa (Epogen, Procrit), the nurse would give which of the following instructions?
   1. Eating raw fruits and vegetables must be avoided.
   2. Frequent rest periods should be taken to avoid excessive fatigue.
   3. Skin and mucous membranes should be protected from traumatic injury.
   4. Exposure to direct sunlight must be minimized and sunscreen used when outdoors.
3. Darbepoetin (Aranesp) is ordered for each of the following patients. The nurse would question the order for which condition?
   1. A patient with chronic renal failure
   2. A patient with AIDS who is receiving anti-AIDS drug therapy
   3. A patient with hypertension
   4. A patient on chemotherapy for cancer
4. The nursing plan of care for a patient receiving oprelvekin (Neumega) should include careful monitoring for symptoms of which adverse effect?
   1. Fluid retention
   2. Severe hypotension
   3. Impaired liver function
   4. Severe diarrhea
5. To best monitor for therapeutic effects from filgrastim (Granix, Neupogen), the nurse will assess which laboratory finding?
   1. Hemoglobin and hematocrit
   2. White blood cell or absolute neutrophil counts
   3. Serum electrolytes
   4. Red blood cell count
6. A patient diagnosed with pernicious anemia is to start cyanocobalamin (Nascobal) injections. Which of the following patient statements demonstrates an understanding of the nurse's teaching? (Select all that apply.)
   1. "I need to be careful to avoid infections."
   2. "I will need to take this drug for the rest of my life."
   3. "I should increase my intake of foods that contain vitamin B_{12}."
   4. "I need to take the liquid preparation through a straw."
   5. "I may be able to switch over to nasal sprays once my vitamin B_{12} levels are normal."

PATIENT-FOCUSED Case Study

Dave Sweeney is a 59-year-old patient with chronic kidney disease and has been on dialysis for one year while awaiting a kidney transplant. He has begun to receive injections of epoetin alfa (Epogen, Procrit) and asks the nurse why he must receive the injections.

1. As the nurse, how would you answer Mr. Sweeney's question?
2. What teaching points would you include about this drug when providing education for Mr. Sweeney?

CRITICAL THINKING Questions

1. A patient is receiving filgrastim (Granix, Neupogen). What nursing interventions are appropriate to safely administer this drug and provide patient safety throughout therapy?
2. A patient is receiving ferrous sulfate (Feosol, others). What teaching should the nurse provide to this patient?

Visit www.pearsonhighered.com/nursingresources for answers and rationales for all activities.

REFERENCES

Dehenes, Y., Myrvold, L., Ström, H., Ericsson, M., & Hemmersbach, P. (2014). MAIIA EPO SeLect–a rapid screening kit for the detection of recombinant EPO analogues in doping control: Inter-laboratory prevalidation and normative study of athlete urine and plasma samples. *Drug Testing and Analysis, 6,* 1144–1150. doi:10.1002/dta.1752

Herdman, T. H., & Kamitsuru, S. (2014). *NANDA International nursing diagnoses: Definitions and classification, 2015–2017.* Oxford, United Kingdom: Wiley-Blackwell.

Sobolevsky, T., Krotov, G., Dikunets, M., Nikitina, M., Mochalova, E., & Rodchenkov, G. (2014). Anti-doping analysis at the Sochi Olympic and Paralympic games 2014. *Drug Testing and Analysis, 6,* 1087–1101. doi:10.1002/dta.1734

SELECTED BIBLIOGRAPHY

Foster, M. (2014). Reevaluating the neutropenic diet: Time to change. *Clinical Journal of Oncology Nursing, 18,* 239–241. doi:10.1188/14.CJON.239-241

Hörl, W. H. (2013). Differentiating factors between erythropoiesis-stimulating agents: An update to selection for anaemia of chronic kidney disease. *Drugs, 73,* 117–130. doi:10.1007/s40265-012-0002-2

Kaushansky, K., & Kipps, T. J. (2012). Hematopoietic agents: Growth factors, minerals and vitamins. In L. L. Brunton, B. A. Chabner, & B. C. Knollman (Eds.), *Goodman and Gilman's the pharmacological basis of therapeutics* (12th ed., pp. 1067–1100). New York, NY: McGraw-Hill.

Lambing, A., Kachalsky, E., & Mueller, M. L. (2012). The dangers of iron overload: Bring in the iron police. *Journal of the American Academy of Nurse Practitioners, 24,* 175–183. doi:10.1111/j.1745-7599.2011.00680.x

National Institutes of Health, Office of Dietary Supplements. (2011). *Vitamin B12: Dietary supplement fact sheet.* Retrieved from http://ods.od.nih.gov/factsheets/VitaminB12-HealthProfessional/

National Institutes of Health, Office of Dietary Supplements. (2014). *Iron: Dietary supplement fact sheet.* Retrieved from http://ods.od.nih.gov/factsheets/Iron-HealthProfessional/#h2

Unit 5

The Immune System

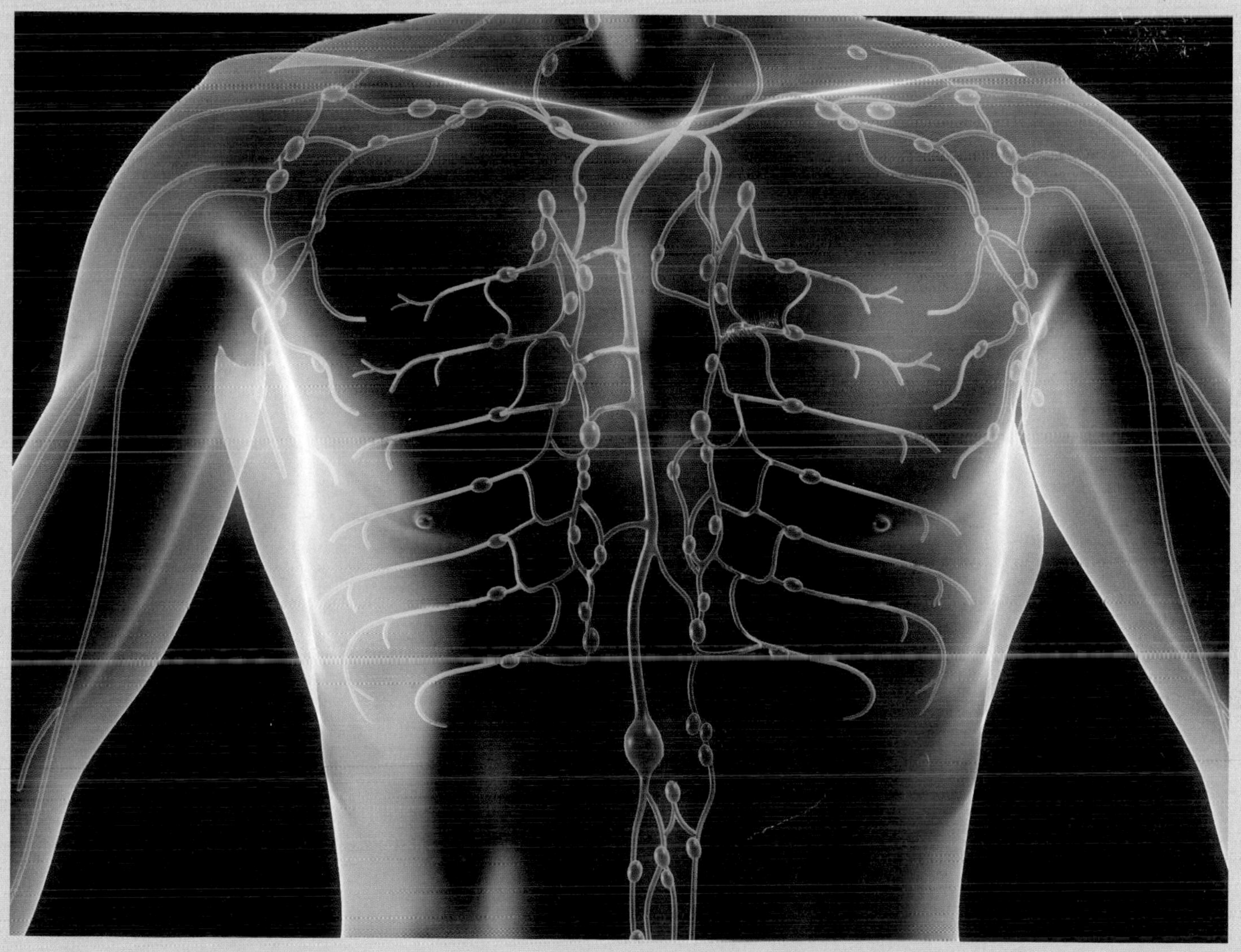

The Immune System

Chapter 33

Drugs for Inflammation and Fever

Drugs at a Glance

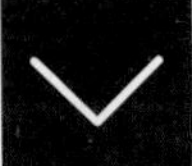

Learning Outcomes

After reading this chapter, the student should be able to:

1. Explain the pathophysiology of inflammation and fever.
2. Outline the basic steps in the acute inflammatory response.
3. Explain the role of chemical mediators in the inflammatory response.
4. Outline the general strategies for treating inflammation.
5. Compare and contrast the actions and adverse effects of the different nonsteroidal anti-inflammatory drugs.
6. Explain the role of corticosteroids in the pharmacologic management of inflammation.
7. For each of the classes listed in Drugs at a Glance, know representative drugs, and explain their mechanisms of drug action, primary actions related to inflammation and fever, and important adverse effects.
8. Use the nursing process to care for patients receiving pharmacotherapy for inflammation or fever.

(capsule icon) indicates a prototype drug, each of which is featured in a Prototype Drug box.

The pain and redness of inflammation following minor abrasions and cuts is something everyone has experienced. Although there is discomfort from such scrapes, inflammation is a normal and expected part of our body's defense against injury. For some diseases, however, inflammation can rage out of control, producing severe pain, fever, and other distressing symptoms. It is these sorts of conditions for which pharmacotherapy may be needed.

INFLAMMATION

Inflammation is a nonspecific defense system of the body. Through the process of inflammation, a large number of potentially damaging chemicals and microorganisms may be neutralized.

33.1 The Function of Inflammation

Inflammation is a body defense mechanism that occurs in response to many different stimuli, including physical injury, exposure to toxic chemicals, extreme heat, invading microorganisms, or death of cells. It is considered an innate (nonspecific) defense mechanism because inflammation proceeds in the same manner, regardless of the cause that triggered it. Only innate immunity will be presented in this chapter as it is more commonly associated with acute inflammation. The adaptive (specific) immune defenses of the body are presented in chapter 34.

The central purpose of inflammation is to contain the injury or destroy the microorganism. By neutralizing the foreign agent and removing cellular debris and dead cells, repair of the injured area is able to proceed at a faster pace. Signs of inflammation include swelling, pain, warmth, and redness of the affected area.

Inflammation may be classified as acute or chronic. Acute inflammation has an immediate onset and 8 to 10 days are normally needed for the symptoms to resolve and for repair to begin. If the body cannot contain or neutralize the damaging agent, inflammation may continue for long periods and become chronic.

Chronic inflammation has a slower onset and may continue for prolonged periods. In autoimmune disorders such as systemic lupus erythrematosus (SLE) and rheumatoid arthritis (RA), chronic inflammation may persist for years, with symptoms becoming progressively worse over time. Other chronic disorders such as seasonal allergy arise at predictable times during each year, and inflammation may produce only minor, annoying symptoms.

PharmFacts

INFLAMMATORY DISORDERS

- Arthritis, the most common inflammatory disorder, is the leading cause of disability in the United States.
- Approximately 1–2 million Americans have inflammatory bowel disease. Most commonly the disease is first diagnosed between the ages of 15–40.
- In the United States, more than 98 million nonsteroidal anti-inflammatory drug (NSAID) prescriptions are written each year.
- It is estimated that NSAIDs cause more than 16,000 deaths annually, largely as a result of gastrointestinal (GI) complications. This is more mortality than is caused from gastric cancer.
- As many as 20% of pediatric fevers occur without any apparent cause.

33.2 The Role of Chemical Mediators in Inflammation

Whether the injury is due to pathogens, chemicals, or physical trauma, the damaged tissue releases a number of chemical mediators that act as "alarms" to notify the surrounding area of the injury. Chemical mediators of inflammation include histamine, leukotrienes, bradykinin, complement, and prostaglandins. Some of these inflammatory mediators are important targets for anti-inflammatory drugs. For example, aspirin and ibuprofen are prostaglandin inhibitors that are effective at treating fever, pain, and inflammation. Table 33.1 describes the sources and actions of these mediators.

Histamine is a key chemical mediator of inflammation. It is stored primarily within **mast cells** located in tissue spaces under epithelial membranes such as the skin, bronchial tree, digestive tract, and along blood vessels.

Table 33.1 Chemical Mediators of Inflammation

Mediator	Description
Bradykinin	Present in an inactive form in plasma and mast cells; vasodilator that causes pain; effects are similar to those of histamine; broken down by angiotensin-converting enzyme (ACE)
Complement	Series of at least 20 proteins that combine in a cascade fashion to neutralize or destroy an antigen; stimulates histamine release by mast cells
C-Reactive protein	Protein found in the plasma that is an early marker of inflammation.
Cytokines	Proteins produced by macrophages, leukocytes, and dendritic cells that mediate and regulate immune and inflammatory reactions
Histamine	Stored and released by mast cells; causes vasodilation, smooth-muscle constriction, tissue swelling, and itching
Leukotrienes	Stored and released by mast cells; effects are similar to those of histamine; contribute to symptoms of asthma and allergies
Prostaglandins	Present in most tissues and stored and released by mast cells; increase capillary permeability, attract white blood cells to the site of inflammation, cause pain, and induce fever

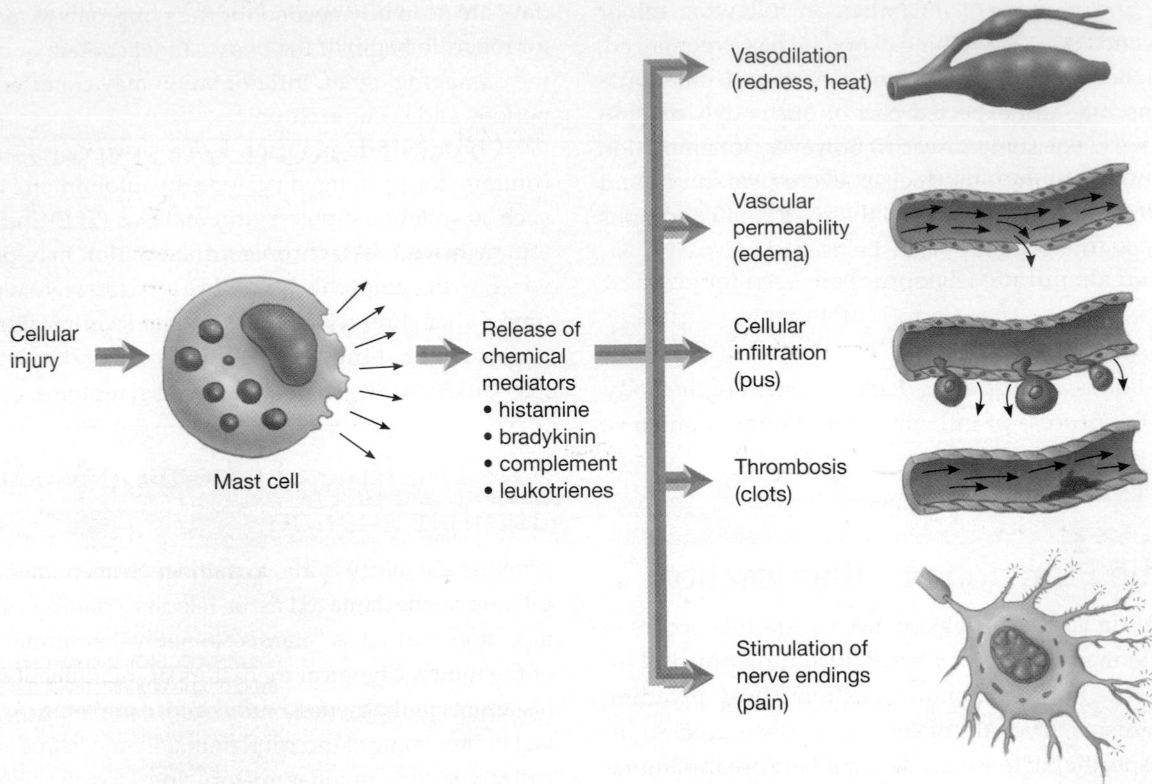

FIGURE 33.1 Steps in acute inflammation

Mast cells detect foreign agents or injury and respond by releasing histamine, which initiates the inflammatory response within seconds. Drugs that act as antagonists at histamine receptors are in widespread therapeutic use for the treatment of allergic rhinitis (see chapter 39).

When released at an injury site, histamine dilates nearby blood vessels, causing capillaries to become more permeable. Plasma, complement proteins, and phagocytes can then enter the area to neutralize foreign agents. The affected area may become congested with blood, which can lead to significant swelling and pain. Figure 33.1 illustrates the fundamental steps in acute inflammation.

The rapid release of the inflammatory mediators on a large scale throughout the body is responsible for **anaphylaxis,** a life-threatening allergic response that may result in shock and death. A number of chemicals, insect stings, foods, and some therapeutic drugs can cause this widespread release of histamine from mast cells if the person has an allergy to these substances. The pharmacotherapy of anaphylaxis is presented in chapter 29.

33.3 General Strategies for Treating Inflammation

Because inflammation is a nonspecific process and may be caused by a variety of physical and infectious etiologies, it may occur in virtually any tissue or organ system. When treating inflammation, the following general principles apply:

- Inflammation is not a disease, but a symptom of an underlying disorder. Whenever possible, the *cause* of the inflammation is identified and treated or removed.
- Inflammation is a natural process for ridding the body of antigens, and it is usually self-limiting. For mild symptoms, nonpharmacologic treatments such as ice packs and rest should be used whenever applicable.
- Topical anti-inflammatory agents should be used when applicable because they cause few adverse effects. Inflammation of the skin and mucous membranes of the mouth, nose, rectum, and vagina are best treated with topical drugs. These include anti-inflammatory creams, ointments, patches, suppositories, and intranasal sprays. Many of these products are available over the counter (OTC).

The goal of pharmacotherapy with anti-inflammatory drugs is to prevent or decrease the intensity of the inflammatory response and reduce fever, if present. Most anti-inflammatory medications are nonspecific; the drug will exhibit the same inhibitory actions regardless of the cause of the inflammation. Common diseases that benefit from anti-inflammatory therapy include allergic rhinitis, anaphylaxis, ankylosing spondylitis, contact dermatitis, Crohn's disease, glomerulonephritis, Hashimoto's thyroiditis, peptic ulcer disease, RA, SLE, and ulcerative colitis.

The two primary drug classes used for nonspecific inflammation are the NSAIDs and the corticosteroids. For mild to moderate pain, inflammation, and fever, NSAIDs are the preferred class of drugs. Should inflammation become severe or disabling, corticosteroid therapy is begun. Due to their serious long-term adverse effects, corticosteroids are usually used for short-term control of acute inflammation. The patient is then switched to NSAIDs.

A few anti-inflammatory drug classes are specific for certain disorders. For example, sulfasalazine (Azulfidine) is specific to treating inflammatory bowel disease, and colchicine and allopurinol (Zyloprim) are used for gouty arthritis. These more specific anti-inflammatory drugs are less widely prescribed because they exhibit more serious adverse effects than the NSAIDs. In addition, some of the newer biologic therapies are very expensive.

NONSTEROIDAL ANTI-INFLAMMATORY DRUGS

NSAIDs such as aspirin and ibuprofen have analgesic, antipyretic, and anti-inflammatory properties. They are widely prescribed for mild to moderate inflammation. Doses for these drugs are listed in Table 33.2.

Table 33.2 Selected Nonsteroidal Anti-Inflammatory Drugs

Drug	Route and Adult Dose (max dose where indicated)	Adverse Effects
aspirin (ASA and others) (see page 252 for the Prototype Drug box)	PO: 350–650 mg every 4 h (max: 4 g/day) for pain or fever PO: 3.6–5.4 g/day in four to six divided doses for arthritic conditions	*Stomach pain, heartburn, nausea, vomiting, tinnitus, prolonged bleeding time* Severe GI bleeding, bronchospasm, anaphylaxis, hemolytic anemia, Reye's syndrome in children, metabolic acidosis
SELECTIVE COX-2 INHIBITOR		
celecoxib (Celebrex)	PO: 100–400 mg bid (max: 800 mg/day)	*Back pain, peripheral edema, abdominal pain, dyspepsia, flatulence, dizziness, headache, insomnia, hypertension (HTN)* Increased risk of cardiovascular events, acute renal failure
IBUPROFEN AND SIMILAR DRUGS		
diclofenac (Cataflam, Voltaren, others)	PO: 150–200 mg in 3–4 divided doses (immediate release) or 75–100 mg daily (extended release);	*Dyspepsia, dizziness, headache, drowsiness, tinnitus, rash, pruritus, increased liver enzymes, prolonged bleeding time, edema, nausea, vomiting, occult blood loss* Peptic ulcer, GI bleeding, anaphylactic reactions with bronchospasm, blood dyscrasias, renal impairment, myocardial infarction (MI), heart failure (HF), hepatotoxicity
diflunisal	PO: 250–500 mg bid (max: 1,500 mg/day)	
etodolac	PO: 200–1200 mg in divided doses (max: 1,200 mg/day)	
fenoprofen (Nalfon)	PO: 200–600 mg tid–qid (max: 3,200 mg/day)	
flurbiprofen (Ansaid)	PO: 50–300 mg/day q6–12h (max: 300 mg/day)	
ibuprofen (Advil, Motrin, others)	PO: 400–800 mg tid–qid (max: 3,200 mg/day)	
indomethacin (Indocin, Tivorbex)	PO: 25–50 mg bid or tid (immediate release) or 75–100 mg one to two times/day (extended release)	
ketoprofen	PO: 25–75 mg tid (immediate release) or 200 mg/day (extended release)	
ketorolac (Sprix, Toradol)	IV/IM: 30–60 mg q6h (max: 120 mg/day) PO: 10–20 mg q6h (max: 40 mg/day) Intranasal: one spray (15.75 mg) in each nostril every 4–6 h (max: 126 mg/day). Maximum of 5 days for all dosage forms	
meclofenamate	PO: 200–400 mg/day in 3–4 divided doses (max: 400 mg)	
mefenamic acid (Ponstel)	PO: 500 mg initial dose then 250 mg q6h not to exceed 7 days	
meloxicam (Mobic)	PO: 7.5–15 mg once daily	
nabumetone	PO: 1,000 mg/day (max: 2,000 mg/day)	
naproxen (Aleve, Anaprox, Naprosyn, others)	PO: 250–500 mg bid (max: 1,000 mg/day)	
oxaprozin (Daypro)	PO: 600–1,200 mg/day (max: 1,800 mg/day)	
piroxicam (Feldene)	PO: 10–20 mg one to two times/day (max: 20 mg/day)	
sulindac (Clinoril)	PO: 150–200 mg bid (max: 400 mg/day)	
tolmetin (Tolectin)	PO: 400 mg tid (max: 1,800 mg/day)	

Note: *Italics* indicate common adverse effects; underlining indicates serious adverse effects.

33.4 Treating Inflammation With NSAIDS

Because of their relatively high safety margin and availability as OTC drugs, the NSAIDs are drugs of choice for the treatment of mild to moderate inflammation. The NSAID class includes some of the most frequently used drugs in medicine, including aspirin and ibuprofen. All NSAIDs have approximately the same efficacy, although the adverse-effect profiles vary among the different drugs. NSAIDs also exhibit analgesic and antipyretic actions. Although acetaminophen shares the analgesic and antipyretic properties of these other drugs, it has no anti-inflammatory action and is not classified as an NSAID.

NSAIDs act by inhibiting the synthesis of prostaglandins. **Prostaglandins** are lipids found in all tissues that have potent physiological effects, in addition to promoting inflammation, depending on the tissue in which they are found. NSAIDs block inflammation by inhibiting **cyclooxygenase (COX),** the key enzyme in the biosynthesis of prostaglandins. This inhibition is illustrated in Figure 33.2.

There are two forms of COX, cyclooxygenase-1 (COX-1) and cyclooxygenase-2 (COX-2). COX-1 is present in all tissues and serves *protective* functions such as reducing gastric acid secretion, promoting renal blood flow, and regulating smooth muscle tone in blood vessels and the bronchial tree. COX-2, on the other hand, is formed only after tissue injury and serves to promote inflammation. Thus, two nearly identical enzymes serve very different functions. First-generation NSAIDs such as aspirin and ibuprofen block both COX-1 and COX-2. Although this inhibition reduces inflammation, the inhibition of COX-1 results in *undesirable* effects such as bleeding, gastric upset, and reduced kidney function. Most of the adverse effects of aspirin and ibuprofen are due to inhibition of COX-1, the protective form of the enzyme.

Salicylates

Aspirin belongs to the chemical family known as the **salicylates.** Since the discovery of salicylates in 1828, aspirin has become one of the most highly used drugs in the world. Aspirin binds to both COX-1 and COX-2 enzymes, changing their structures and preventing them from forming

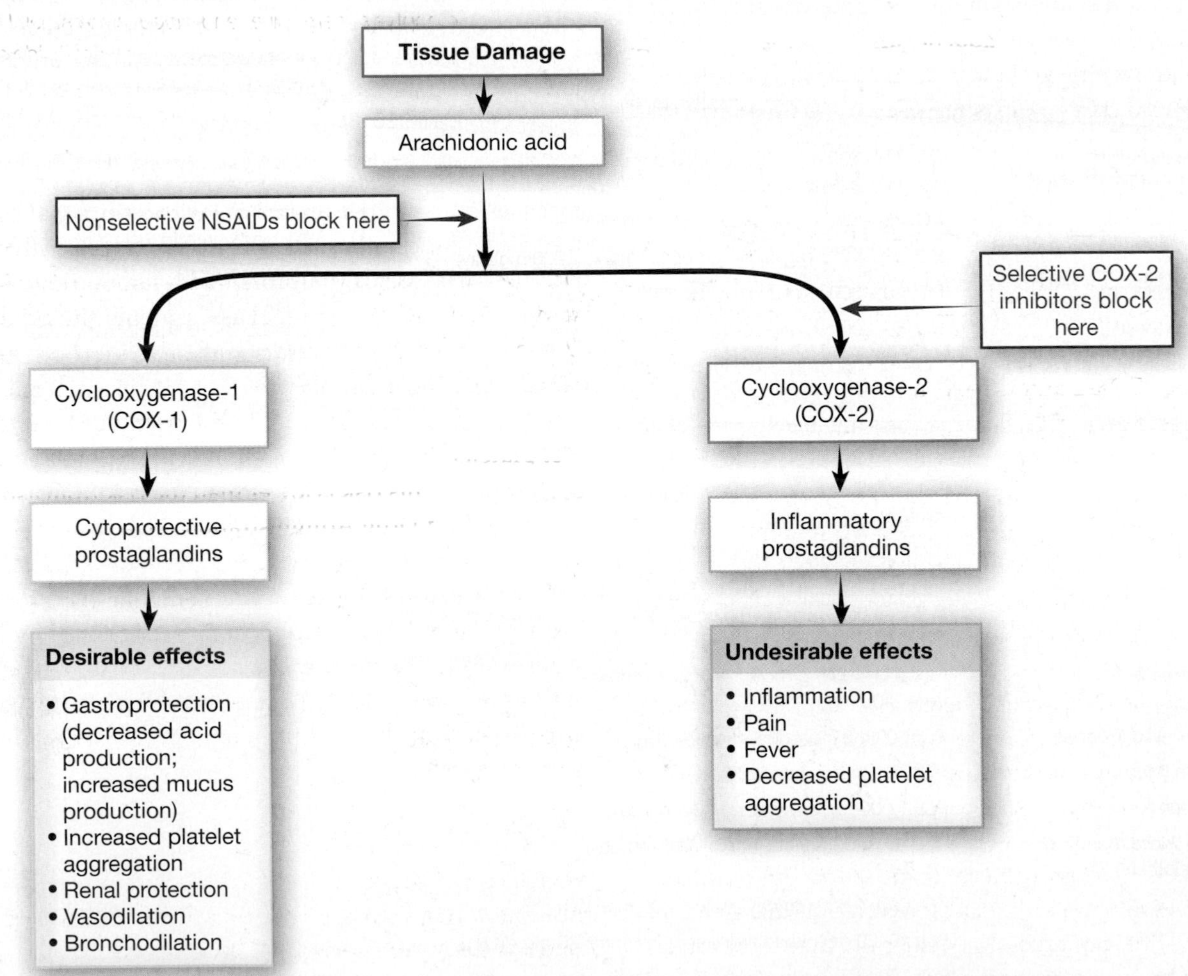

FIGURE 33.2 Inhibition of cyclooxygenase 1 and 2. Nonselective NSAIDs block the cytoprotective effects as well as inflammation. Selective COX-2 inhibitors block only the inflammation effects

NSAIDs = Long term tx

inflammatory prostaglandins. This inhibition of COX is particularly prolonged in platelets; a single dose of aspirin may cause total inhibition for the entire 8- to 11-day life span of a platelet. Because it is readily available, inexpensive, and effective, aspirin is often used for treating mild pain and inflammation. Aspirin has a protective effect on the cardiovascular system and is taken daily in small doses to prevent abnormal clot formation, MIs, and strokes. The fundamental pharmacology and a drug prototype for aspirin are presented in chapter 18.

Unfortunately, the large doses of aspirin that are needed to suppress severe inflammation may result in a high incidence of adverse effects, especially on the digestive system. By increasing gastric acid secretion and irritating the stomach lining, aspirin can cause epigastric pain, heartburn, and even bleeding due to ulceration. Some aspirin formulations are buffered or given an enteric coating to minimize adverse GI effects. In some patients, however, even small doses may cause GI bleeding. Risk factors for aspirin-induced GI bleeding include history of peptic ulcers, age greater than 60, use of anticoagulants or corticosteroids, *Helicobacter pylori* infection, smoking, and use of alcohol. Because aspirin also has a potent antiplatelet effect, the potential for bleeding must be carefully monitored. High doses may produce **salicylism,** a syndrome that includes symptoms such as tinnitus (ringing in the ears), dizziness, headache, and excessive sweating. Children under age 19 should never be administered products that contain aspirin when they have flu symptoms, fever, or chickenpox due to the risk of Reye's syndrome, a potentially fatal disease.

Complementary and Alternative Therapies

FISH OILS FOR INFLAMMATION

Fish oils, also known as marine oils, are lipids found primarily in cold water fish. These oils are rich sources of long-chain polyunsaturated fatty acids of the omega-3 type. The two most studied fatty acids found in fish oils are eicosapentaenoic acid (EPA) and docosahexaenoic acid (DHA). These fatty acids are known for their triglyceride-lowering activity. Several mechanisms are believed to account for the anti-inflammatory activity of EPA and DHA. The two competitively inhibit the conversion of arachidonic acid to the proinflammatory prostaglandins, thus reducing their synthesis.

An analysis of the literature concluded that diets high in fish oil may have beneficial effects on inflammatory conditions such as RA and possibly asthma. However, there is insufficient evidence as to their cardiovascular effects, or as to their beneficial effects in inflammatory bowel diseases such as Crohn's disease (Yates, Calder, & Rainger, 2014). One of the current areas of research is the type of omega-3 fatty acids. Laidlaw, Cockerline, and Rowe (2014) found that concentrated fish oil resulted in higher levels of EPA and DHA than other fish oils, but the clinical significance of the differences in levels have not been studied.

Interactions may occur between fish oil supplements and aspirin, other NSAIDs, and anticoagulants. Although rare, such interactions might be manifested by increased susceptibility to bruising, nosebleeds, hemoptysis, hematuria, and blood in the stool. In general, fish oils are well-tolerated and usually have minor GI side effects such as gas or diarrhea (National Center for Complementary and Integrative Health, 2013).

Ibuprofen and Ibuprofen-Like NSAIDs

Ibuprofen (Motrin, Advil) and a large number of ibuprofen-like drugs are NSAIDs that were developed as alternatives to aspirin. Like aspirin, they exhibit their effects through inhibition of both COX-1 and COX-2, although the inhibition by these drugs is reversible. Sharing the same mechanism of action, all drugs in this class have similar efficacy for treating pain, fever, and inflammation. For some patients, the choice of NSAID is based on cost and availability: aspirin, ibuprofen, and naproxen (Aleve) are inexpensive NSAIDs sold OTC in generic forms. NSAIDs differ in their duration of action, which may be important when patients are taking these drugs on an ongoing basis. Although drugs in this class have similar overall effectiveness, there is variability in response to NSAIDs, with some patients responding better to a particular drug. The choice of prescription NSAID is often based on the clinical experiences and preference of the prescriber.

Most ibuprofen-like NSAIDs share a low incidence of adverse effects when used intermittently. The most common side effects are nausea and vomiting. These medications have the potential to cause gastric ulceration and bleeding; however, the incidence is less than that of aspirin. Adverse gastric effects are especially prominent in older patients and those with peptic ulcer disease. Some formulations combine an NSAID with a drug that protects the gastric mucosa, such as Vimovo (naproxen with esomeprazole) and Duexis (ibuprofen with famotidine). Kidney toxicity is possible, and renal assessments should be conducted periodically. Patients with significant pre-existing renal impairment usually receive acetaminophen for pain or fever, rather than an NSAID. Ibuprofen-like NSAIDs affect platelet function and increase the potential for bleeding, although this risk is lower than the risk from aspirin. A U.S. Food and Drug Administration (FDA) boxed warning states that ibuprofen and other NSAIDs are associated with an increased risk of thromboembolic events (including stroke and MI), and that the drugs may cause or worsen HTN. For the occasional user who takes the medications at recommended doses and who has no risk factors, the drugs are safe and rarely produce any significant adverse effects.

COX-2 Inhibitors

Selective inhibition of COX-2 produces analgesic, anti-inflammatory, and antipyretic effects without causing some of the serious adverse effects of the older NSAIDs. Because they do not inhibit COX-1, these drugs do not produce adverse effects on the digestive system and lack any effect on blood coagulation. Upon their approval by the

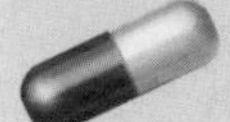

Prototype Drug | Ibuprofen *(Advil, Motrin, others)*

Therapeutic Class: Analgesic, anti-inflammatory drug, antipyretic **Pharmacologic Class:** NSAID

Actions and Uses

Ibuprofen is an older drug that is prescribed for the treatment of mild to moderate pain, fever, and inflammation. Its effectiveness is equivalent to that of aspirin and other NSAIDs. Its actions are primarily due to inhibition of prostaglandin synthesis. Common indications include pain associated with chronic musculoskeletal disorders such as RA and osteoarthritis, headache, dental pain, and dysmenorrhea. Chewable tablets, drops, and solutions are available in low doses for administration to children.

Administration Alerts

- Give the drug on an empty stomach as tolerated. If nausea, vomiting, or abdominal pain occurs, give with food.
- Be aware that patients with asthma or who have allergies to aspirin are more likely to exhibit a hypersensitivity reaction to ibuprofen.
- Pregnancy category C. Category changes to D after 30 weeks gestation.

PHARMACOKINETICS

Onset	Peak	Duration
30–60 min	1–2 h	4–6 h

Adverse Effects

When used intermittently at low to moderate doses, the adverse effects of ibuprofen are generally mild and include nausea, heartburn, epigastric pain, and dizziness. GI ulceration with occult or gross bleeding may occur, especially in patients who are taking high doses for prolonged periods. Chronic use of ibuprofen may lead to renal impairment.

Black Box Warning: NSAIDs may cause an increased risk of serious thrombotic events, MI, and stroke, which can be fatal. This risk may increase with duration of use. Patients with cardiovascular disease or risk factors for cardiovascular disease may be at greater risk. NSAIDs are contraindicated for the treatment of perioperative pain in those undergoing coronary artery bypass graft surgery. NSAIDs increase the risk of serious GI adverse events including bleeding, ulceration, and perforation of the stomach or intestines, which can be fatal. These events occur more frequently in older adults and can occur at any time during use or without warning symptoms.

Contraindications: Patients with active peptic ulcers should not take ibuprofen. This drug is also contraindicated in patients with significant renal or hepatic impairment and in those who have a syndrome of nasal polyps, angioedema, or bronchospasm due to aspirin or other NSAID use. It should be used cautiously in patients who have HF, serious HTN, or a history of stroke or MI.

Interactions

Drug–Drug: Because ibuprofen can affect platelet function, its use should be avoided when taking anticoagulants and other coagulation modifiers. Aspirin use can decrease the anti-inflammatory action of ibuprofen. The antihypertensive action of diuretics, beta blockers, and ACE inhibitors may be reduced if taken with ibuprofen. The actions of certain diuretics may be diminished when taken concurrently with ibuprofen. Use with other NSAIDs, alcohol, or corticosteroids may cause serious adverse GI events.

Lab Tests: Ibuprofen may increase bleeding time, aspartate aminotransferase (AST), and alanine aminotransferase (ALT) levels. It may decrease hemoglobin and hematocrit.

Herbal/Food: Feverfew, garlic, ginger, or ginkgo may increase the risk of bleeding.

Treatment of Overdose: There is no specific treatment for overdose. Administration of an alkaline drug may increase the urinary excretion of ibuprofen.

FDA, the COX-2 inhibitors quickly became the treatment of choice for moderate to severe inflammation.

However, in 2004, postmarketing data revealed that rofecoxib (Vioxx) doubled the risk of heart attack and stroke in patients who were taking the drug for extended periods. Based on these reports, the drug manufacturer voluntarily removed rofecoxib from the market. Shortly afterward, a second COX-2 inhibitor, valdecoxib (Bextra) was also voluntarily withdrawn, leaving celecoxib (Celebrex) the sole drug in this class. In addition to its anti-inflammatory indications, celecoxib is used to reduce the number of colorectal polyps in adults with familial adenomatous polyposis (FAP). Patients with FAP have an inherited mutation in a gene that results in hundreds of polyps and an almost 100% risk of colon cancer.

CORTICOSTEROIDS (GLUCOCORTICOIDS)

Corticosteroids have numerous therapeutic applications. One of their most useful properties is the ability to suppress severe inflammation. Because of potentially serious adverse effects, however, systemic corticosteroids are

Table 33.3 Selected Corticosteroids for Severe Inflammation

Drug	Route and Adult Dose (max dose where indicated)	Adverse Effects
betamethasone (Celestone, Diprolene)	PO: 0.6–7.2 mg/day	*Mood swings, weight gain, acne, facial flushing, nausea, insomnia, sodium and fluid retention, impaired wound healing, menstrual abnormalities, hyperglycemia, increased appetite* <u>Peptic ulcer, hypocalcemia, osteoporosis with possible bone fractures, loss of muscle mass, decreased growth in children, possible masking of infections, immunosuppression</u>
cortisone	PO/IM: 20–300 mg/day in divided doses	
dexamethasone	PO: 0.25–4 mg bid–qid	
hydrocortisone (Cortef, Solu-cortef, others) (see page 756 for the Prototype Drug box)	PO: 10–320 mg/day in three to four divided doses	
methylprednisolone (Depo-Medrol, Medrol, others)	IV/IM: 15–800 mg/day in three to four divided doses (max: 2 g/day)	
prednisolone	PO: 4–48 mg/day in divided doses	
prednisone	PO: 5–60 mg one to four times/day	
triamcinolone (Aristospan, Kenalog, others)	IM/subcutaneous: 4–48 mg/day in divided doses	

Note: *Italics* indicate common adverse effects, <u>underlining</u> indicates serious adverse effects.

reserved for the short-term treatment of severe disease. Corticosteroids are often referred to as glucocorticoids. These drugs are listed in Table 33.3.

33.5 Treating Acute or Severe Inflammation With Corticosteroids

Corticosteroids are natural hormones released by the adrenal cortex that have powerful effects on nearly every cell in the body. When corticosteroids are used as drugs to treat inflammatory disorders, the doses are many times higher than the amount naturally present in the blood. The uses of corticosteroids include the treatment of neoplasia (see chapter 38), asthma (see chapter 40), arthritis (see chapter 48), and corticosteroid deficiency (see chapter 44).

Like the NSAIDs, corticosteroids inhibit the biosynthesis of prostaglandins. Corticosteroids, however, affect inflammation by multiple mechanisms. They have the ability to suppress histamine release and can inhibit certain functions of phagocytes and lymphocytes. These multiple actions markedly reduce inflammation, making corticosteroids the most effective medications available for the treatment of severe inflammatory disorders.

When given by the oral (PO) or parenteral routes, corticosteroids have a number of serious adverse effects that limit their therapeutic utility. These include suppression of the normal functions of the adrenal gland (adrenal insufficiency), hyperglycemia, mood changes, cataracts, peptic ulcers, electrolyte imbalances, and osteoporosis. Because of their effectiveness at reducing the signs and symptoms of inflammation, corticosteroids can mask infections that may be present in a patient. This combination of masking signs of active infection and suppressing the immune response creates a potential for infections to grow rapidly and remain undetected. An active infection is usually a contraindication for corticosteroids therapy.

Because the appearance of these adverse effects is a function of the dose and duration of therapy, treatment is often limited to the short-term control of acute disease. When longer therapy is indicated, doses are kept as low as possible and alternate-day therapy is sometimes implemented; the medication is taken every other day to encourage the patient's adrenal glands to function on the days when no drug is given. During long-term therapy, nurses must be alert for signs of overtreatment with corticosteroids, a condition known as **Cushing's syndrome.** Because the body becomes accustomed to high doses of corticosteroids, patients must discontinue these drugs gradually; abrupt withdrawal can result in acute lack of adrenal function.

FEVER

Like inflammation, fever is a natural defense mechanism for neutralizing foreign organisms. Many species of bacteria are killed by high fever. Often, the health care provider must determine whether the fever needs to be dealt with aggressively or allowed to run its course. Drugs used to treat fever are called **antipyretics.**

33.6 Treating Fever With Antipyretics

In most patients, fever is more of a discomfort than a life-threatening problem. Prolonged, high fever, however, can become dangerous, especially in young children in whom fever can stimulate febrile seizures. In adults, excessively high fever can break down body tissues, reduce mental acuity, and lead to delirium or coma, particularly among older patients. In rare instances, an elevated body temperature may be fatal.

The goal of antipyretic therapy is to lower body temperature while treating the underlying cause of the fever, usually an infection. Aspirin, ibuprofen, and acetaminophen are safe, inexpensive, and effective drugs for reducing fever. Many of these antipyretics are marketed for different age groups, including special, flavored brands for infants and children. For

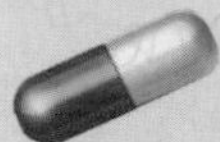

Prototype Drug | Prednisone

Therapeutic Class: Anti-inflammatory drug **Pharmacologic Class:** Corticosteroid

Actions and Uses

Prednisone is a synthetic corticosteroid. Its actions are the result of being metabolized to an active form, which is also available as a drug called prednisolone. When used for inflammation, duration of therapy is commonly limited to 4 to 10 days. For long-term therapy, alternate-day dosing is used. Prednisone is occasionally used to terminate acute bronchospasm in patients with asthma and as an antineoplastic agent for patients with certain cancers such as Hodgkin's disease, acute leukemia, and lymphomas. It is available in tablet and oral solution forms.

Administration Alerts

- Administer intramuscular (IM) injections deep into the muscle mass to avoid atrophy or abscesses.
- Do not use if signs of a systemic infection are present.
- When using the drug for more than 10 days, the dose must be slowly tapered.
- Pregnancy category C.

PHARMACOKINETICS

Onset	Peak	Duration
1–2 h	1–2 h	24–36 h

Adverse Effects

When used at low to moderate doses for short-term therapy, prednisone has few serious adverse effects. Long-term therapy may result in Cushing's syndrome, a condition that includes hyperglycemia, fat redistribution to the shoulders and face, muscle weakness, bruising, and bones that easily fracture. Because gastric ulcers may occur with long-term therapy, an antiulcer medication may be prescribed prophylactically. Use with caution in patients with peptic ulcer, ulcerative colitis, or diverticulitis.

Contraindications: Patients with active viral, bacterial, fungal, or protozoan infections should not take prednisone.

Interactions

Drug–Drug: Because barbiturates, phenytoin, and rifampin increase prednisone metabolism, increased doses may be required. Concurrent use with amphotericin B or diuretics increases potassium loss, which may be serious for patients taking digoxin. Because prednisone can raise blood glucose levels, patients with diabetes may require an adjustment in the doses of insulin or oral hypoglycemic drugs.

Lab Tests: Prednisone may inhibit antibody response to toxoids and vaccines and may increase blood glucose. Serum calcium, potassium, and thyroxine may decrease.

Herbal/Food: Herbal supplements such as aloe, buckthorn, and senna may increase potassium loss. Licorice may potentiate the effect of corticosteroids. St. John's wort may decrease prednisone levels.

Treatment of Overdose: There is no specific treatment for overdose.

fast delivery and effectiveness, drugs may come in various forms including gels, caplets, enteric-coated tablets, and suspensions. Aspirin and acetaminophen are also available as suppositories. The antipyretics come in various dosages and concentrations, including extra strength.

Although most fevers are caused by infectious processes, drugs themselves may be the cause. When the etiology of fever cannot be diagnosed, nurses should consider drugs as a possible source. In many cases, withdrawal of the agent causing the drug-induced fever will quickly return body temperature to normal. In rare cases, drug-induced fever may be lethal. It is important for nurses to recognize drugs that are most likely to cause drug-induced fever, including those in the following list:

- *Anti-infectives.* Anti-infectives, especially those derived from microorganisms such as amphotericin B or penicillin G, may be seen as foreign by the body and produce fever. When antibiotics kill microorganisms, fever-producing chemicals known as *pyrogens* may be released. Anti-infectives are the most common drugs known to induce fever.
- *Selective serotonin reuptake inhibitors (SSRIs).* Use of SSRIs such as paroxetine (Paxil) for depression or other mood disorders can result in a high fever accompanied by serious mental status and cardiovascular changes, known as serotonin syndrome (see chapter 16).
- *Conventional antipsychotic drugs.* Drugs such as chlorpromazine (Thorazine) may produce an elevated temperature with serious cardiovascular and respiratory distress, called neuroleptic malignant syndrome (see chapter 17).
- *Volatile anesthetics and depolarizing neuromuscular blockers.* Drugs such as succinylcholine can cause life-threatening malignant hyperthermia (see chapter 19).
- *Immunomodulators.* Interferons and monoclonal antibodies such as muromonab-CD3 may cause a flulike syndrome because they cause the release of fever-producing cytokines (see chapter 34).

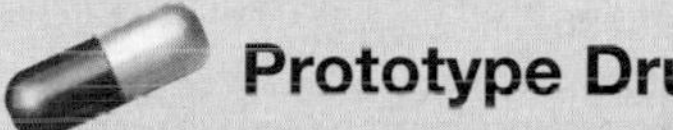

Prototype Drug | Acetaminophen *(Tylenol, others)*

Therapeutic Class: Antipyretic and analgesic **Pharmacologic Class:** Centrally acting COX inhibitor

Actions and Uses

Acetaminophen reduces fever by direct action at the level of the hypothalamus and dilation of peripheral blood vessels, which enables sweating and dissipation of heat. Acetaminophen, ibuprofen, and aspirin have equal efficacy in relieving pain and reducing fever.

Acetaminophen has no anti inflammatory properties; therefore, it is not effective in treating arthritis or pain caused by tissue swelling following injury. The primary therapeutic usefulness of acetaminophen is for the treatment of fever in children and for relief of mild to moderate pain when aspirin is contraindicated. In the treatment of severe pain, acetaminophen may be combined with opioids. This allows the dose of opioid to be reduced, thus decreasing the risk of dependence and serious opioid toxicity. It is available as tablets, caplets, solutions, and suppositories.

Acetaminophen has no effect on platelet aggregation and does not exhibit cardiotoxicity. Most importantly, it does not cause GI bleeding or ulcers, as do the NSAIDs.

Administration Alert

- Liquid forms are available in varying concentrations. Use the appropriate strength product in children to avoid toxicity.
- Never administer to patients who consume alcohol regularly due to the potential for drug-induced hepatotoxicity.
- Advise patients that acetaminophen is found in many OTC products and that extreme care must be taken to not duplicate doses by taking several of these products concurrently.
- Pregnancy category B.

PHARMACOKINETICS

Onset	Peak	Duration
30 60 min	0.5–2 h	4–6 h

Adverse Effects

Acetaminophen is generally safe, and adverse effects are uncommon at therapeutic doses. Acetaminophen causes less gastric irritation than aspirin and does not affect blood coagulation. It is not recommended in patients who are malnourished. In such cases, acute toxicity may result, leading to renal failure, which can be fatal. Other signs of acute toxicity include nausea, vomiting, chills, abdominal discomfort, and fatal hepatic necrosis.

A major concern with the use of high doses of acetaminophen is the risk for liver damage, which is especially important for patients who consume alcohol.

Black Box Warning: Acetaminophen has the potential to cause severe and even fatal liver injury and may cause serious allergic reactions with symptoms of angioedema, difficulty breathing, itching, or rash. In 2011, the FDA asked drug manufacturers to limit the strength of acetaminophen in prescription combination products to 325 mg per tablet, capsule, or dosing unit to lower the potential for acetaminophen-induced hepatotoxicity.

Contraindications: Contraindications include hypersensitivity to acetaminophen or phenacetin and chronic alcoholism.

Interactions

Drug–Drug. Acetaminophen inhibits warfarin metabolism, causing the anticoagulant to accumulate to toxic levels. High-dose or long-term acetaminophen use may result in elevated warfarin levels and bleeding. Ingestion of this drug with alcohol or other hepatotoxic drugs, such as phenytoin or barbiturates, is not recommended because of the possibility of liver failure from hepatic necrosis.

Lab Tests: Acetaminophen may increase hepatic function test values such as serum bilirubin, AST, and ALT. It may increase urinary 5-hydroxyindole acetic acid (5-HIAA) and serum uric acid.

Herbal/Food: The patient should avoid taking herbs that have the potential for liver toxicity, including comfrey, coltsfoot, and chaparral.

Treatment of Overdose: The specific treatment for overdose is the oral or intravenous (IV) administration of *N*-acetylcysteine (Acetadote) as soon as possible after the overdose. This drug protects the liver from toxic metabolites of acetaminophen.

Treating the Diverse Patient: Ethnic Differences in Acetaminophen Metabolism

Certain ethnic populations, including patients of Asian, African American, or Middle Eastern descent, may have higher rates of an enzyme deficiency that affects how they metabolize certain drugs. More than 200 million people worldwide are believed to have a hereditary deficiency of the enzyme, glucose-6-phosphate dehydrogenase (G6PD). Patients with G6PD deficiency are at risk for developing hemolysis after ingestion of certain drugs, including acetaminophen. In patients with the deficiency, therapeutic dosages of acetaminophen may cause hemolysis. Because acetaminophen is one of the most common drugs used for fever, pain control, and in many OTC cough and cold medicines, and because patients may not know that they have the deficiency, health care providers should recommend that ethnically diverse patients exercise caution when using acetaminophen and report any signs or symptoms associated with anemia. Patients with known G6PD deficiency should avoid this drug.

Community-Oriented Practice

FEVER PHOBIA AND FEVER TREATMENT

Research over the past decade as to whether single-drug or combination-drug treatment is more effective for fever management has alternated between recommendations for single and combination routines. The recent practice guideline published by the American Academy of Pediatrics has noted that either acetaminophen or ibuprofen is beneficial in the treatment of fever, and there is no evidence that one is preferable to the other. However, children who received alternating doses of acetaminophen and ibuprofen had lower temperatures after four or more hours of treatment, than when a single agent was used alone (Hoover, 2012).

There are several concerns when using antipyretics in combination. The first is that the difference in dosage may lead to an increased risk of medication errors. Another concern is that there is no consensus as to the definition of a fever, although temperatures starting at 100.4°F (38°C) are usually considered a fever (Wallenstein et al., 2012). Most providers recommend a fever greater than 38.3°C (101°F) as the threshold for treatment, and many believe there are adverse effects when a fever reaches 40°C (104°F), although there is insufficient evidence to support that claim (Hoover, 2012). A new term has begun to be discussed in research literature, "fever phobia"–the concern that a fever will continue to rise if not treated (Banks, Paul, & Wall, 2013). Wallenstein et al., (2012) reported that in a survey of caregivers, none were able to correctly identify the temperature level that would be considered a fever (38°C/100.4°F), although over 89% of caregivers would medicate the child for a fever, even if the child appeared comfortable and without distress.

For most children with fevers, treatment with either acetaminophen or ibuprofen will provide effective fever relief. However, control may be longer lasting when alternating drugs are used. Because the dosage amount of each drug may vary, nurses must ensure that parents are measuring each drug correctly and that adequate intervals are spaced between doses. This is particularly important if liquid preparations are used because these are often not measured accurately in the home setting. Instructions on avoiding concurrent use of OTC cough and cold remedies that include acetaminophen, should also be included. Most importantly, education about the temperature threshold for a fever and the potential beneficial effects of allowing a low-grade temperature to run its course unless the child's condition or provider preference necessitates treatment be given, should be part of the discussion.

- *Cytotoxic drugs.* Certain drugs used in cancer chemotherapy and to prevent transplant rejection profoundly dampen the immune response and result in fevers due to secondary infections.
- *Neutropenic drugs.* Drugs such as NSAIDs, phenothiazines, antithyroid drugs, and antipsychotic medications can cause neutropenia and a subsequent fever.

☑ Check Your Understanding 33.1

Many drug classifications may be used to reduce inflammation, including the NSAIDs, COX-2 inhibitors, and corticosteroids. Why are corticosteroids *not* routinely used for reducing inflammation? *Visit www.pearsonhighered.com/nursingresources for the answer.*

Nursing Practice Application

Pharmacotherapy With Anti-Inflammatory and Antipyretic Drugs

ASSESSMENT	POTENTIAL NURSING DIAGNOSES*
Baseline assessment prior to administration: • Obtain a complete health history including hepatic, renal, respiratory, cardiovascular or neurologic disease, pregnancy, or breast-feeding. Obtain a drug history including allergies, current prescription and OTC drugs, herbal preparations, caffeine, nicotine, and alcohol use. Be alert to possible drug interactions. • Obtain baseline vital signs and weight. • Evaluate appropriate laboratory findings (e.g., complete blood count (CBC), coagulation panels, bleeding time, electrolytes, glucose, lipid profile, hepatic or renal function studies).	• *Acute or Chronic Pain* • *Hyperthermia* • *Deficient Fluid Volume* • *Deficient Knowledge* (drug therapy) • *Risk for Injury,* related to adverse drug effects • *Risk for Infections,* related to adverse drug effects of corticosteroids • *Risk for Impaired Skin Integrity,* related to adverse drug effects of corticosteroids *NANDA I © 2014

Nursing Practice Application *continued*

ASSESSMENT	POTENTIAL NURSING DIAGNOSES*
Assessment throughout administration: • Assess for desired therapeutic effects (e.g., temperature returns to normal range, pain is decreased or absent, signs and symptoms of inflammation such as redness or swelling are decreased). • Continue periodic monitoring of CBC, coagulation studies, bleeding time, electrolytes, glucose, lipids, and hepatic and renal function studies. • Assess vital signs and weight periodically or if symptoms warrant. For patients on corticosteroids, obtain weight daily and report any weight gain over 1 kg (2 lb) in a 24-hour period or more than 2 kg (5 lb) in 1 week. • Assess for and promptly report adverse effects: symptoms of GI bleeding (dark or "tarry" stools, hematemesis or coffee-ground emesis, blood in the stool), abdominal pain, severe tinnitus, dizziness, drowsiness, confusion, agitation, euphoria or depression, palpitations, tachycardia, HTN, increased respiratory rate and depth, pulmonary congestion, or edema.	

IMPLEMENTATION

Interventions and (Rationales)	Patient-Centered Care
Ensuring therapeutic effects: • Continue assessments as described earlier for therapeutic effects. (Diminished fever, pain, or signs and symptoms of infection should begin after taking the first dose and continue to improve. The health care provider should be notified if fever remains present after 3 days or if increasing signs of infection are present.)	• Teach the patient to supplement drug therapy with nonpharmacologic measures (e.g., "RICE": **R**est, **I**ce or cool compresses, **C**ompression bandage (e.g., ACE wrap), and **E**levation of the inflamed joint or limb); increased fluid intake for fever; positioning for comfort; diversionary distractions (e.g., television or music); and rest for pain.
Minimizing adverse effects: • Continue to monitor vital signs, especially temperature if fever is present, and blood pressure and pulse for patients on corticosteroids. (Fever should begin to diminish within 1 to 3 hours after taking the drug. Corticosteroids may cause increased blood pressure, HTN, and tachycardia due to increased retention of fluids.)	• Teach the patient to report fever that does not diminish below 38°C (100.4°F), or per parameters set by the health care provider. Febrile seizures, changes in behavior or level of consciousness, tachycardia, palpitations, or increased blood pressure should be reported immediately to the health care provider. • Teach the patient on corticosteroids how to monitor pulse and blood pressure. Ensure the proper use and functioning of any home equipment obtained.
• Continue to monitor periodic laboratory work: hepatic and renal function tests, CBC, electrolytes, glucose, lipid levels, and coagulation studies or bleeding time. **Lifespan:** Monitor the older adult frequently because age-related physiological changes increase the risk of adverse renal and hepatic effects. (Aspirin and salicylates affect platelet aggregation and should be monitored if used long term or if excessive bleeding or bruising is noted. Acetaminophen can be hepatotoxic. Corticosteroids affect the CBC and a wide range of electrolytes, glucose.)	• Instruct the patient on the need to return periodically for laboratory work. • Advise the patient who is taking corticosteroids long term to carry a wallet identification card or wear medical identification jewelry indicating corticosteroid therapy. • Teach the patient to abstain from alcohol while taking acetaminophen. Men who consume more than two alcoholic beverages per day or women who consume more than one alcoholic beverage per day should not take acetaminophen.
• Monitor for abdominal pain, black or tarry stools, blood in the stool, hematemesis or coffee-ground emesis, dizziness, and hypotension, especially if associated with tachycardia. **Lifespan:** Monitor the older adult frequently for GI irritation or bleeding because age-related physiological changes increase the risk of adverse effects. (NSAIDs and corticosteroids may cause GI bleeding.)	• Instruct the patient to immediately report any signs or symptoms of GI bleeding. • Teach the patient to take the drug with food or milk to decrease GI irritation and to swallow enteric-coated tablets whole without crushing or breaking. Alcohol use should be avoided or eliminated.
• Monitor for tinnitus, difficulty hearing, light-headedness, or difficulty with balance and report promptly. (NSAIDs and salicylates may be ototoxic.)	• Instruct the patient to immediately report any signs or symptoms of ringing, humming, buzzing in ears, difficulty with balance, dizziness or vertigo, or nausea.

continued

Nursing Practice Application *continued*

IMPLEMENTATION	
Interventions and (Rationales)	**Patient-Centered Care**
• Monitor urine output and renal function studies periodically. (NSAIDs and salicylates may be renal toxic during long-term or high-dose therapy.)	• Instruct the patient on NSAIDs and salicylates to promptly report changes in quantity of urine output, darkening of urine, or edema. • Teach the patient on NSAIDs and salicylates to increase fluid intake, especially if fever is present.
• Monitor electrolyte, blood glucose, and lipid levels periodically in patients on corticosteroids. (Corticosteroids may cause hyperglycemia, hypernatremia, hyperlipidemia, and hypokalemia. Patients with diabetes may require a change in antidiabetic medication if glucose remains elevated.)	• Instruct the patient to return periodically for laboratory work as needed. • Teach the patient with diabetes to test the blood glucose more frequently and notify the health care provider if a consistent elevation is noted.
• Monitor for signs and symptoms of infection in patients on corticosteroids. (Corticosteroids suppress the body's normal immune and inflammatory response and may mask the signs and symptoms of infection.)	• Instruct the patient to immediately report any signs or symptoms of infections (e.g., increasing temperature or fever, sore throat, redness or swelling at the site of the injury, white patches in the mouth, vesicular rash).
• Monitor for osteoporosis (e.g., bone density testing) periodically in patients on corticosteroids. Encourage adequate calcium intake, weight-bearing exercise, and avoidance of carbonated sodas. (Corticosteroids affect bone metabolism and may cause osteoporosis and fractures. Weight-bearing exercise stresses bone and encourages normal bone remodeling.)	• Teach the patient to maintain adequate calcium in the diet and to do weight-bearing exercises at least three to four times per week. • Teach postmenopausal woman to consult with the health care provider about the need for additional drug therapy (e.g., bisphosphonates) for osteoporosis.
• Monitor for unusual changes in mood or affect in patients on corticosteroids. (Corticosteroids may cause mood changes, euphoria, depression, or severe mental instability.)	• Teach the patient, family, or caregiver to promptly report excessive mood swings or unusual changes in mood.
• Weigh patient on corticosteroids daily and report a weight gain of 1 kg (2 lb) or more in a 24-hour period or more than 2 kg (5 lb) per week or increasing peripheral edema. Measure intake and output in the hospitalized patient. (Daily weight is an accurate measure of fluid status and takes into account intake, output, and insensible losses. Patients on corticosteroids will experience some fluid retention.)	• Instruct the patient to weigh self daily, ideally at the same time of day. The patient should report significant weight gain or increasing peripheral edema.
• Monitor vision periodically in patients on corticosteroids. (These drugs may cause increased intraocular pressure and an increased risk of glaucoma, and may cause cataracts.)	• Teach the patient on corticosteroids to maintain eye exams twice yearly or more frequently as instructed by the health care provider. Immediately report any eye pain, rainbow halos around lights, diminished vision, or blurring and inability to focus.
• **Lifespan:** Avoid the use of aspirin or salicylates in children under 18 unless explicitly ordered by the health care provider. (Aspirin has been associated with an increased risk of Reye's syndrome in children under 18, particularly associated with the flu virus and varicella infections.)	• Instruct parents to use NSAIDs or acetaminophen in children under 18 for fever or pain control, unless otherwise ordered by the provider. • Teach parents to read labels on all OTC medications and to avoid formulations with aspirin or salicylate on the label.
• Do not stop corticosteroids abruptly. The drug must be tapered off if used longer than 1 or 2 weeks. (Adrenal insufficiency and crisis may occur with profound hypotension, tachycardia, and other adverse effects if the drug is stopped abruptly.)	• Teach the patient to not stop taking corticosteroids abruptly and to notify the health care provider if unable to take medication for more than 1 day due to illness.
Patient understanding of drug therapy: • Use opportunities during administration of medications and during assessments to provide patient education. (Using time during nursing care helps to optimize and reinforce key teaching areas.)	• The patient, family, or caregiver should be able to state the reason for the drug; appropriate dose and scheduling; what adverse effects to observe for and when to report; and the anticipated length of medication therapy.

Nursing Practice Application *continued*

IMPLEMENTATION	
Interventions and (Rationales)	**Patient-Centered Care**
Patient self-administration of drug therapy: • When administering the medication, instruct the patient, family, or caregiver in proper self-administration of the drug (e.g., with food or milk). (Proper administration will increase the effectiveness of the drug. Household measuring devices such as teaspoons differ significantly in size and amount and should not be used for pediatric or liquid doses.)	• The patient, family, or caregiver are able to discuss appropriate dosing and administration needs, including: • Corticosteroids should be taken in the morning at the same time each day. • NSAIDs and corticosteroids should be taken with food or milk to decrease GI upset. • Liquid doses of acetaminophen or NSAIDs should be measured with the enclosed dosage cup, dropper, or spoon. If that measuring device is no longer available, do NOT use a household spoon but obtain another calibrated measuring cup or dropper.

See Table 33.2 and 33.3 for a list of the drugs to which these nursing actions apply. Acetaminophen is also covered in this Nursing Process Application.

Chapter Review

KEY Concepts

The numbered key concepts provide a succinct summary of the important points from the corresponding numbered section within the chapter. If any of these points are not clear, refer to the numbered section within the chapter for review.

33.1 Inflammation is a natural, nonspecific body defense that limits the spread of invading microorganisms or injury. Acute inflammation occurs over several days, whereas chronic inflammation may continue for months or years.

33.2 Pathogens, chemicals, and physical trauma cause the release of chemical mediators that trigger the inflammatory response. Histamine is one of the key chemical mediators in inflammation. Release of histamine produces vasodilation, allowing capillaries to become leaky, thus causing tissue swelling. Rapid and large-scale release of mediators may lead to shock and death.

33.3 Inflammation may be treated with nonpharmacologic and pharmacologic therapies. When possible, topical drugs are used because they produce fewer adverse effects than oral or parenteral drugs. The two primary drug classes used for inflammation are the nonsteroidal anti-inflammatory drugs (NSAIDs) and corticosteroids.

33.4 NSAIDs are the primary medications for the treatment of mild to moderate inflammation. All drugs in this class have similar effectiveness in treating inflammation. The selective COX-2 inhibitors cause less GI distress but have significant cardiovascular side effects.

33.5 Systemic corticosteroids are effective in treating acute or severe inflammation. Overtreatment with these drugs can cause a serious condition called Cushing's syndrome; thus, therapy for inflammation is generally short term.

33.6 Acetaminophen and NSAIDs are the primary drugs used to treat fever. Certain medications may cause drug-induced fever, which may range from mild to life-threatening.

REVIEW Questions

1. A patient with a history of hypertension is to start drug therapy for rheumatoid arthritis. Which of the following drugs would be contraindicated, or used cautiously, for this patient? (Select all that apply.)
   1. Aspirin
   2. Ibuprofen (Advil, Motrin)
   3. Acetaminophen (Tylenol)
   4. Naproxen (Aleve)
   5. Methylprednisolone (Medrol)

2. The patient has been taking aspirin for several days for headache. During the assessment, the nurse discovers that the patient is experiencing ringing in the ears and dizziness. What is the most appropriate action by the nurse?
   1. Question the patient about history of sinus infections.
   2. Determine whether the patient has mixed the aspirin with other medications.
   3. Tell the patient not to take any more aspirin.
   4. Tell the patient to take the aspirin with food or milk.

3. While educating the patient about hydrocortisone (Cortef), the nurse would instruct the patient to contact the health care provider immediately if which of the following occurs?
   1. There is a decrease of 1 kg (2 lb) in weight.
   2. There is an increase in appetite.
   3. There is tearing of the eyes.
   4. There is any difficulty breathing.

4. The nurse is admitting a patient with rheumatoid arthritis. The patient has been taking prednisone (Orasone) for an extended time. During the assessment, the nurse observes that the patient has a very round moon-shaped face, bruising, and an abnormal contour of the shoulders. What does the nurse conclude based on these findings?
   1. These are normal reactions with the illness.
   2. These are probably birth defects.
   3. These are symptoms of myasthenia gravis.
   4. These are symptoms of adverse drug effects from the prednisone.

5. A 24-year-old patient reports taking acetaminophen (Tylenol) fairly regularly for headaches. The nurse knows that a patient who consumes excessive acetaminophen per day or regularly consumes alcoholic beverages should be observed for what adverse effect?
   1. Hepatic toxicity
   2. Renal damage
   3. Thrombotic effects
   4. Pulmonary damage

6. The nurse is counseling a mother regarding antipyretic choices for her 8-year-old daughter. When asked why aspirin is not a good drug to use, what should the nurse tell the mother?
   1. It is not as good an antipyretic as is acetaminophen.
   2. It may increase fever in children under age 10.
   3. It may produce nausea and vomiting.
   4. It increases the risk of Reye's syndrome in children under 19 with viral infections.

PATIENT-FOCUSED Case Study

As the nurse in the neighborhood, your neighbors turn to you for medication advice. Carlos Alvera, your new next-door neighbor, is requesting advice for medication to take for occasional headache pain. He asks you about acetaminophen (Tylenol) because he knows that the drug is available OTC.

1. What advice will you provide Mr. Alvera about his choice of acetaminophen?
2. What additional information will you gather from Mr. Alvera that will be important to cover when teaching him about acetaminophen?

CRITICAL THINKING Questions

1. A 64-year-old patient with diabetes is on prednisone for rheumatoid arthritis. The patient has recently been admitted to the hospital for stabilization of hyperglycemia. What are the nurse's primary concerns when caring for this patient?

2. The mother of a 7-year-old child calls the health care provider's office stating that her daughter has a temperature of 38.3°C (101°F). She states the child is also complaining of being tired and "achy" all over. The mother asks how much aspirin she can give her daughter for her temperature. How should the nurse respond?

Visit www.pearsonhighered.com/nursingresources for answers and rationales for all activities.

REFERENCES

Banks, T., Paul, S. P., & Wall, M. (2013). Managing fevers in children with a single antipyretic. *Nursing Times, 109*(7), 24–25.

Herdman, T. H., & Kamitsuru, S. (2014). *NANDA International nursing diagnoses: Definitions and classification, 2015–2017*. Oxford, United Kingdom: Wiley-Blackwell.

Hoover, L. (2012). AAP reports on the use of antipyretics for fever in children. *American Family Physician, 85*, 518–519.

Laidlaw, M., Cockerline, C. A., & Rowe, W. J. (2014). A randomized clinical trial to determine the efficacy of manufacturers' recommended doses of omega-3 fatty acids from different sources in facilitating cardiovascular disease risk reduction. *Lipids in Health and Disease, 13*, 99. doi:10.1186/1476-511X-13-99

National Center for Complementary and Integrative Health, (2013). *Omega-3 supplements: An introduction*. Retrieved from http://nccam.nih.gov/health/omega3/introduction.htm#moreinfo

Wallenstein, M. B., Schroeder, A. R., Hole, M. K., Ryan, C., Fijalkowski, N., Alvarez, E., & Carmichael, S. L. (2013). Fever literacy and fever phobia. *Clinical Pediatrics, 52*, 254–259. doi:10.1177/0009922812472252

Yates, C. M., Calder, P. C., & Rainger, E. G. (2014). Pharmacology and therapeutics of omega-3 polyunsaturated fatty acids in chronic inflammatory disease. *Pharmacology & Therapeutics, 141*, 272–282. doi:10.1016/j.pharmthera.2013.10.010

SELECTED BIBLIOGRAPHY

Atkinson, T. J., Fudin, J., Jahn, H. L., Kubotera, N., Rennick, A. L., & Rhorer, M. (2013). What's new in NSAID pharmacotherapy: Oral agents to injectables. *Pain Medicine, 14*(Suppl. 1), S11–S17. doi:10.1111/pme.12278

Conaghan, P. G. (2012). A turbulent decade for NSAIDs: Update on current concepts of classification, epidemiology, comparative efficacy, and toxicity. *Rheumatology International, 32*, 1491–1502. doi:10.1007/s00296-011-2263-6

Consumer Reports Best Buy Drugs (2013). *The nonsteroidal anti-inflammatory drugs: Treating osteoarthritis and pain*. Retrieved from http://www.consumerreports.org/health/resources/pdf/best-buy-drugs/Nsaids2.pdf

Farrell, S. E. (2014). *Acetaminophen toxicity*. Retrieved from http://emedicine.medscape.com/article/820200-overview#aw2aab6b2b4

Hymes, S. R. (2014). *Fever without a focus*. Retrieved from http://emedicine.medscape.com/article/970788-overview

Kumar, P., & Banik, S. (2013). Pharmacotherapy options in rheumatoid arthritis. *Clinical Medicine Insights: Arthritis and Musculoskeletal Disorders, 6*, 35. doi:10.4137/CMAMD.S5558

Niven, D. J., Stelfox, H. T., & Laupland, K. B. (2013). Antipyretic therapy in febrile critically ill adults: A systematic review and meta-analysis. *Journal of Critical Care, 28*, 303–310. doi:10.1016/j.jcrc.2012.09.009

Rowe, W.A. (2015). *Inflammatory bowel disease*. Retrieved from http://emedicine.medscape.com/article/179037-overview#aw2aab6b2b4

Shah, S., & Mehta, V. (2012). Controversies and advances in non-steroidal anti-inflammatory drug (NSAID) analgesia in chronic pain management. *Postgraduate Medical Journal, 88*, 73–78. doi:10.1136/postgradmedj-2011-130291

Chapter 34

Drugs for Immune System Modulation

Drugs at a Glance

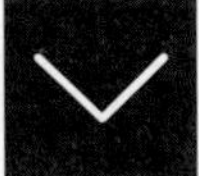

Learning Outcomes

After reading this chapter, the student should be able to:

1. Compare and contrast innate and adaptive body defenses.
2. Compare and contrast the humoral and cell-mediated immune responses.
3. For each of the major vaccines, list the recommended dosage schedule.
4. Distinguish between active immunity and passive immunity.
5. Identify indications for pharmacotherapy with biologic response modifiers.
6. Explain the need for immunosuppressant medications following organ and tissue transplants.
7. Identify the classes of medications used as immunosuppressants.
8. Describe the nurse's role in the pharmacologic management of immune disorders.
9. For each of the drug classes listed in Drugs at a Glance, know representative drugs, and explain their mechanism of drug action, primary actions related to the immune system, and important adverse effects.
10. Use the nursing process to care for patients receiving pharmacotherapy for immune conditions.

indicates a prototype drug, each of which is featured in a Prototype Drug box.

The human body is under continuous attack from a host of foreign invaders that include viruses, bacteria, fungi, protozoa, and even multicellular animals such as lice. Some of these pathogens intentionally seek out humans because the body is an essential part of their life cycle, whereas others become opportunistic when a cut or scrape allows entrance into the body. Our extensive body defenses are capable of mounting a rapid and effective response against many of these pathogens.

Immunomodulator is a general term referring to any drug or therapy that affects body defenses. In some patients, immunomodulators are used to *stimulate* body defenses so that microbes or cancer cells can be more effectively attacked. On other occasions, it is desirable to *suppress* body defenses to prevent a transplanted organ from being rejected by the immune system. The purpose of this chapter is to examine the pharmacotherapy of drugs that are used to modulate the body's response to disease.

PharmFacts

VACCINES

- Vaccines have eradicated smallpox from the world and the poliovirus from the Western Hemisphere.
- Vaccines lowered the number of diphtheria cases in the United States from 175,000 in 1922 to zero cases since 1980.
- Vaccines have lowered the number of measles cases in the United States to about 08 cases annually. Measles cases in the United States are usually due to lack of vaccine compliance and importation from other countries.
- Of the vaccine-preventable diseases, pneumococcal pneumonia is the most lethal, with about 4,250 deaths occurring annually in the United States. The Centers for Disease Control and Prevention (CDC, 2015) recommends 1 or 2 doses of the pneumococcal vaccine for adults age 19 and older.

34.1 Innate (Nonspecific) Body Defenses and the Immune Response

The lymphatic system provides the body with the ability to resist injury and protects the body from pathogens. This system consists of lymphoid cells, tissues, and organs such as the spleen, thymus, tonsils, and lymph nodes. The different components of the lymphatic system are in continuous communication and work together as a single unit to accomplish effective immune surveillance.

The first line of protection from pathogens consists of the **innate (nonspecific) body defenses,** which serve as general barriers to microbes or environmental hazards. The innate defenses are unable to distinguish one type of threat from another; the response or protection is the same regardless of the pathogen. The innate defenses, also called nonspecific defenses, include physical barriers, such as the epithelial lining of the skin, and the respiratory and gastrointestinal mucous membranes, which are potential entry points for pathogens. Other innate defenses are phagocytes, natural killer (NK) cells, the complement system, fever, and interferons. From a pharmacologic perspective, one of the most important of the innate defenses is inflammation. Because of its significance, inflammation is discussed separately, in chapter 33.

The body also has the ability to mount a *second* line of defense that is specific to particular threats. For example, a specific defense may act against only a single species of bacteria and be ineffective against all others. These are known as **adaptive (specific) body defenses,** or more commonly, the **immune response.** The primary cell of the immune response is the lymphocyte.

Microbes and foreign substances that elicit an immune response are called **antigens.** Foreign proteins, such as those present on the surfaces of pollen grains, bacteria, nonhuman cells, and viruses, are the strongest antigens. It is estimated that the immune system has the ability to recognize and react to over a billion different antigens.

The immune response is extremely complex. Basic steps involve recognition of the antigen, communication and coordination with other defense cells, and destruction or suppression of the antigen. A large number of chemical messengers and interactions are involved in the immune response, many of which have yet to be discovered. The two primary divisions of the immune response are antibody-mediated (humoral) immunity and cell-mediated immunity. These are shown in Figure 34.1.

34.2 Humoral Immune Response and Antibodies

The **humoral immune response** is initiated when an antigen encounters a type of lymphocyte known as a **B cell.** The B cell becomes activated and divides rapidly to form millions of copies, or clones, of itself. Most cells in this clone are called **plasma cells** whose primary function is to secrete antibodies specific to the antigen that initiated the challenge. Circulating through the body are **antibodies,** also known as immunoglobulins (Ig), which physically interact with the antigens to neutralize or mark them for destruction by other cells of the immune response. Peak production of antibodies occurs about 10 days after an initial antigen challenge. The important functions of antibodies are illustrated in Figure 34.2.

After the antigen challenge, memory B cells are formed that will remember the specific antigen–antibody interaction. Should the body be exposed to the same antigen in the future, the body will be able to manufacture even higher levels of antibodies in a shorter period, approximately 2 to 3 days. For some antigens, such as those for measles, mumps, or chickenpox, memory may be retained for an entire lifetime. Vaccines are sometimes administered to produce these memory cells in advance of

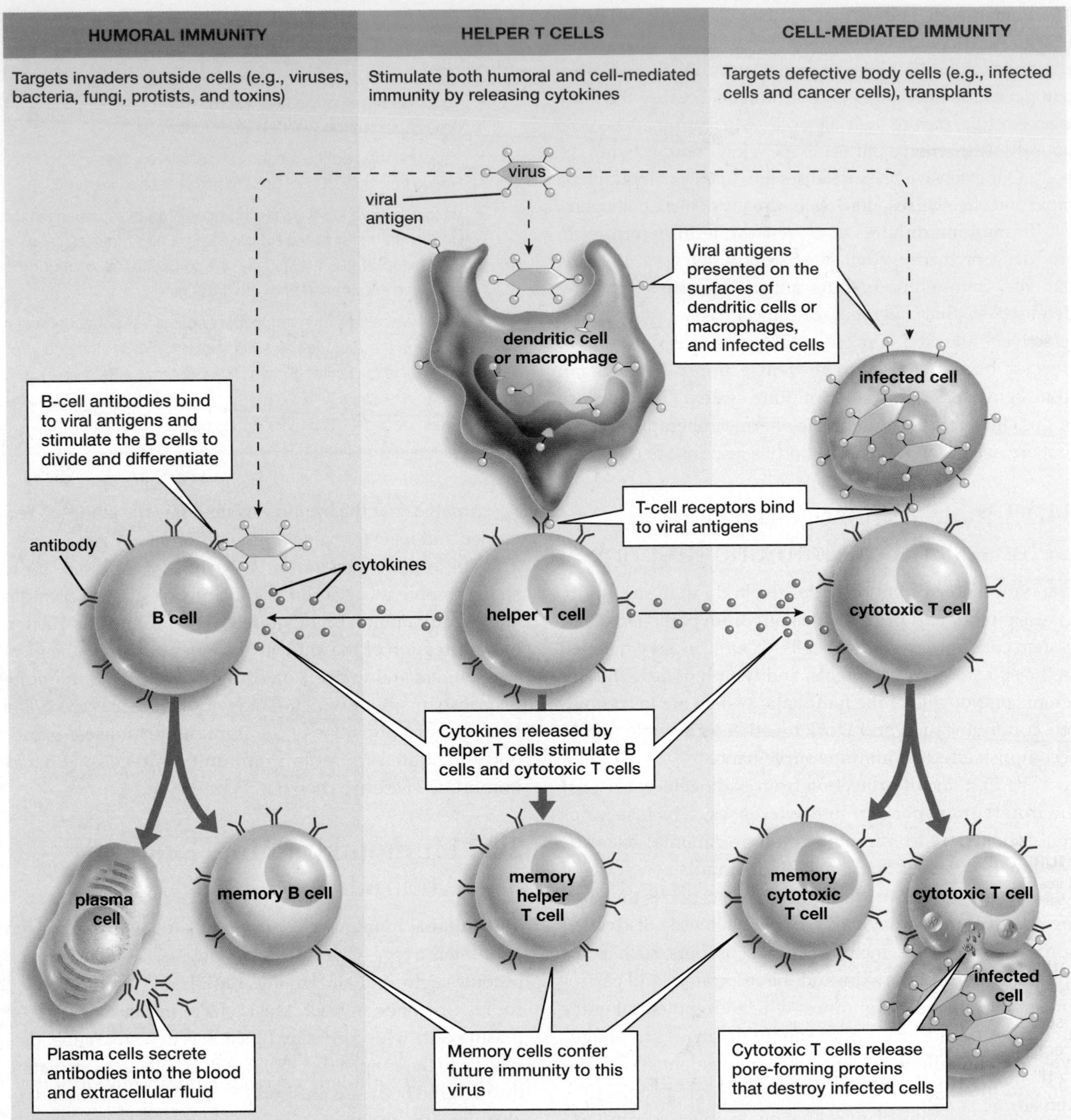

FIGURE 34.1 Steps in the humoral and cell-mediated immune response
Source: *Life on Earth With Physiology, 9th ed.*, by G. Audesirk, T. Audesirk, and B. E. Byers, 2011. Reprinted by permission of Pearson Education, Inc., Upper Saddle River, NJ.

exposure to the antigen, so that when the body is exposed to the actual organism it can mount a fast, effective response to prevent disease.

IMMUNIZATION AGENTS

Vaccines are biologic agents used to stimulate the immune system. Vaccinations are one of the most important medical interventions for the prevention of serious infectious disease.

34.3 Administration of Vaccines

Vaccination, or **immunization,** is the process of introducing foreign proteins or inactive cells (vaccines) into the body to trigger immune activation *before* the patient is exposed to the real pathogen. As a result of the vaccination, memory B cells are formed. When later exposed to the actual infectious organism, these cells will react by rapidly producing large quantities of antibodies that help to

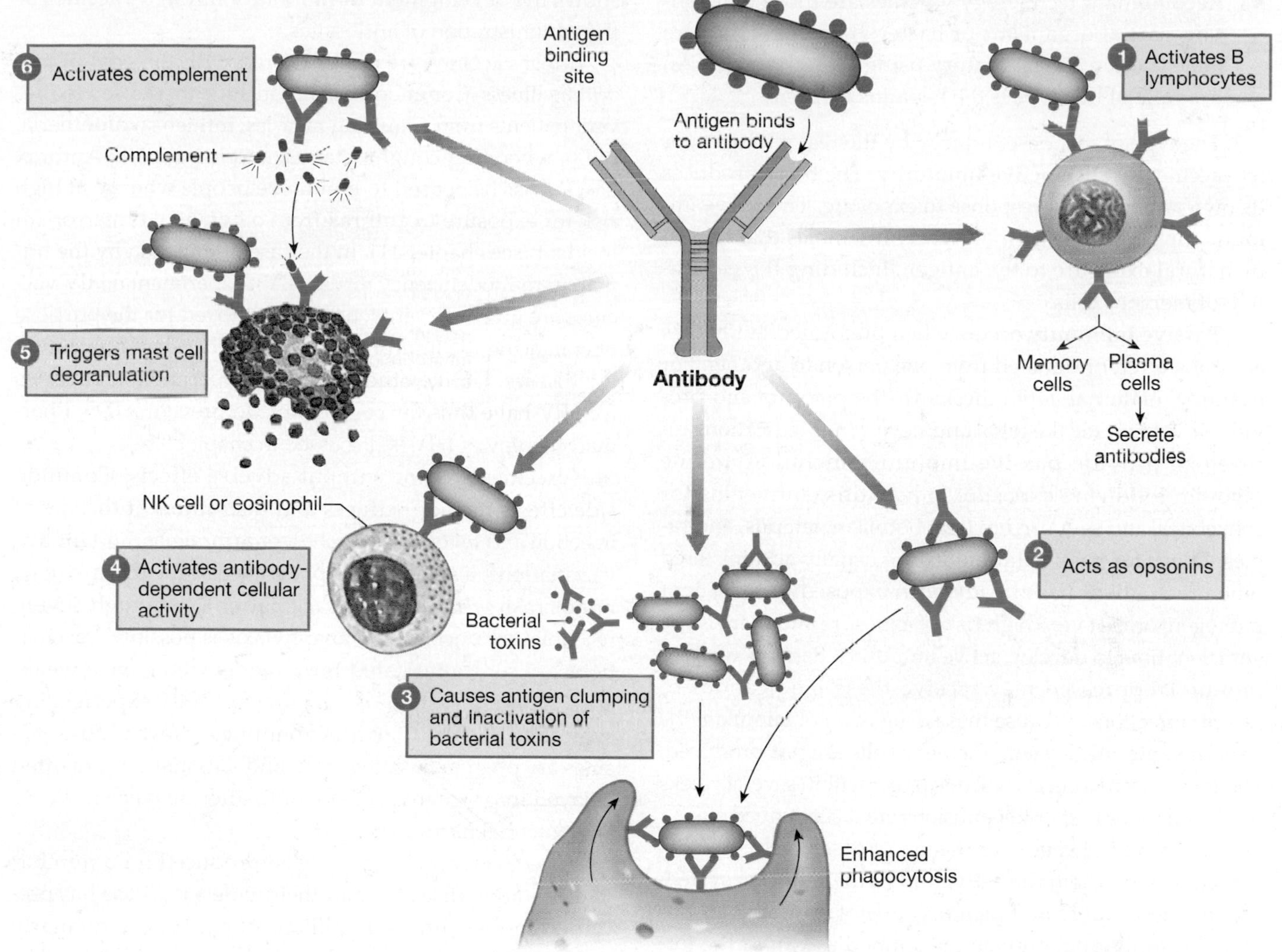

FIGURE 34.2 Functions of antibodies.
Source: *Human Physiology: An Integrated Approach*, 5th ed., by D. U. Silverthorn, 2010. Reprinted and electronically reproduced by Pearson Education, Inc., Upper Saddle River, NJ.

neutralize or destroy the pathogen. Whereas some immunizations are needed only once, most require follow-up doses, called *boosters,* to provide sustained protection. The effectiveness of most vaccines can be assessed by measuring the amount of antibody produced after the vaccine has been administered, a quantity called **titer.** If the titer falls below a specified protective level over time, a booster, or revaccination, is indicated.

The goal of vaccine administration is to induce long-lasting immunity to a pathogen *without* producing an illness in an otherwise healthy person. Therefore, the microorganisms and other substances used as vaccines must be able to strongly activate the immune system but be modified to pose no significant risk of disease development. The four methods of producing safe and effective vaccines are the following:

- Attenuated (live) vaccines contain microbes that are alive but weakened (attenuated) so they are unable to produce disease unless the patient is immunocompromised. Some attenuated vaccines cause a mild or subclinical case of the disease. An example of a live attenuated vaccine is the measles, mumps, and rubella (MMR) vaccine.
- Inactivated (killed) vaccines contain microbes that have been inactivated by heat or chemicals and are unable to replicate or cause disease. In some cases, inactivated vaccines contain only a subunit of the microbe, such as pieces of the foreign plasma membrane or modified microbial proteins. Boosters may be necessary to prolong immunity. Examples of inactivated vaccines include the influenza, human papillomavirus, and hepatitis A vaccines.
- Toxoid vaccines contain bacterial toxins that have been chemically modified to be incapable of causing disease. When injected, toxoid vaccines induce the formation of antibodies that are capable of neutralizing the real toxins. Examples include diphtheria and tetanus toxoids.

- Recombinant technology vaccines are those that contain partial organisms or bacterial proteins that are generated in the laboratory using biotechnology. An example of this type is the hepatitis B vaccine.

The type of response induced by the real pathogen, or its vaccine, is called **active immunity:** The body produces its own antibodies in response to exposure. The active immunity induced by vaccines closely resembles that caused by natural exposure to the antigen, including the generation of memory cells.

Passive immunity occurs when preformed antibodies are transferred or donated from one person to another. For example, maternal antibodies cross the placenta and provide protection for the fetus and newborn. Medications infused to provide passive immunity include immune globulin following exposure to hepatitis, antivenins for snakebites, and sera used to treat botulism, tetanus, and rabies. Drugs for passive immunity are usually administered when the patient has already been exposed to a virulent pathogen, or is at very high risk of exposure and there is not sufficient time to develop active immunity. Patients who are immunosuppressed may receive these medications to *prevent* infections. Because these drugs do not stimulate the patient's immune system, memory cells are not produced, and the protective effects will disappear within several weeks to several months after the infusions are discontinued.

A second indication for the use of passive immunity is for situations where the activation of the immune system and the development of memory are not desirable. In this case, the individual is given the antibodies *against* the foreign agent and the immune system does not mount a response. The administration of RhoGAM is an example of this type of indication. Table 34.1 lists selected immune globulin preparations. Pharmacotherapy Illustrated 34.1 shows the development of immunity through vaccines or the administration of antibodies.

Most vaccines are administered with the goal of *preventing* illness. Common vaccines include those used to prevent patients from acquiring measles, influenza, diphtheria, polio, whooping cough, tetanus, and hepatitis B. Anthrax vaccine has been used to immunize people who are at high risk for exposure to anthrax from a potential bioterrorism incident (see chapter 11). In the case of infection by the human immunodeficiency virus (HIV), experimental HIV vaccines are given *after* infection has occurred for the purpose of enhancing the immune response, rather than preventing the disease. Unlike other vaccines, experimental vaccines for HIV have thus far been unable to prevent AIDS. Pharmacotherapy of HIV is discussed in chapter 37.

Vaccines are not without adverse effects. Common side effects include redness and discomfort at the site of injection and fever, minor aches, or arthralgias; and for live vaccinations, a subclinical appearance of the disease (e.g., minor rash with measles vaccination). Although severe reactions are uncommon, anaphylaxis is possible. Vaccinations are contraindicated for patients who have a weakened immune system or who are currently experiencing symptoms such as diarrhea, vomiting, or fever. Most vaccines are pregnancy category C and vaccinations are often delayed in pregnant patients until after delivery to avoid any potential harm to the fetus.

Effective vaccines have been produced for a number of debilitating diseases, and their widespread use has prevented serious illness in millions of patients, particularly children. One disease, smallpox, has been completely eliminated from the planet through immunization, and others such as polio have diminished to extremely low levels. Nurses play a key role in encouraging patients to be

Table 34.1 Immune Globulin Preparations

Drug	Route and Adult Dose (max dose where indicated)	Adverse Effects
cytomegalovirus immune globulin (CytoGam)	IV (for prophylaxis): 150 mg/kg within 72 h of transplantation; then 100 mg/kg for 2, 4, 6, and 8 wk post-transplant; then 50 mg/kg for 12 and 16 wk post-transplant	*Local reactions at injection site (pain, erythema, myalgia), flu-like symptoms (malaise, fever, chills), headache* <u>Anaphylaxis, renal toxicity, thrombosis</u>
hepatitis B immune globulin (HBIG)	IM: 0.06 mL/kg as soon as possible after exposure, preferably within 24 h, but no later than 7 days; repeat 28–30 days after exposure	
immune globulin intravenous (Carimune, Gammagard, HyQvia, IGIV, Octagam)	IV: 100–400 mg/kg q3–4wk IM: 1.2 mL/kg followed by 0.6 mL/kg q2–4wk	
rabies immune globulin (BayRab, Imogam Rabies-HT, HyperRAB)	IM (for postexposure prophylaxis): 20 international units/kg as a single dose with rabies vaccine	
Rh_0(D) immune globulin (RhoGAM)	IM/IV: one vial or 300 mcg at approximately 28 wk; followed by one vial of minidose or 120 mcg within 72 h of delivery if infant is Rh-positive	
tetanus immune globulin (BayTet, HyperTet, HyperTet S/D)	IM (for prophylaxis): 250 units as single dose	
varicella zoster immune globulin (Varizig)	IM: 625 international units within 10 days after exposure	

Note: *Italics* indicate common adverse effects; <u>underlining</u> indicates serious adverse effects.

Pharmacotherapy Illustrated

34.1 | Mechanisms of Active and Passive Immunity

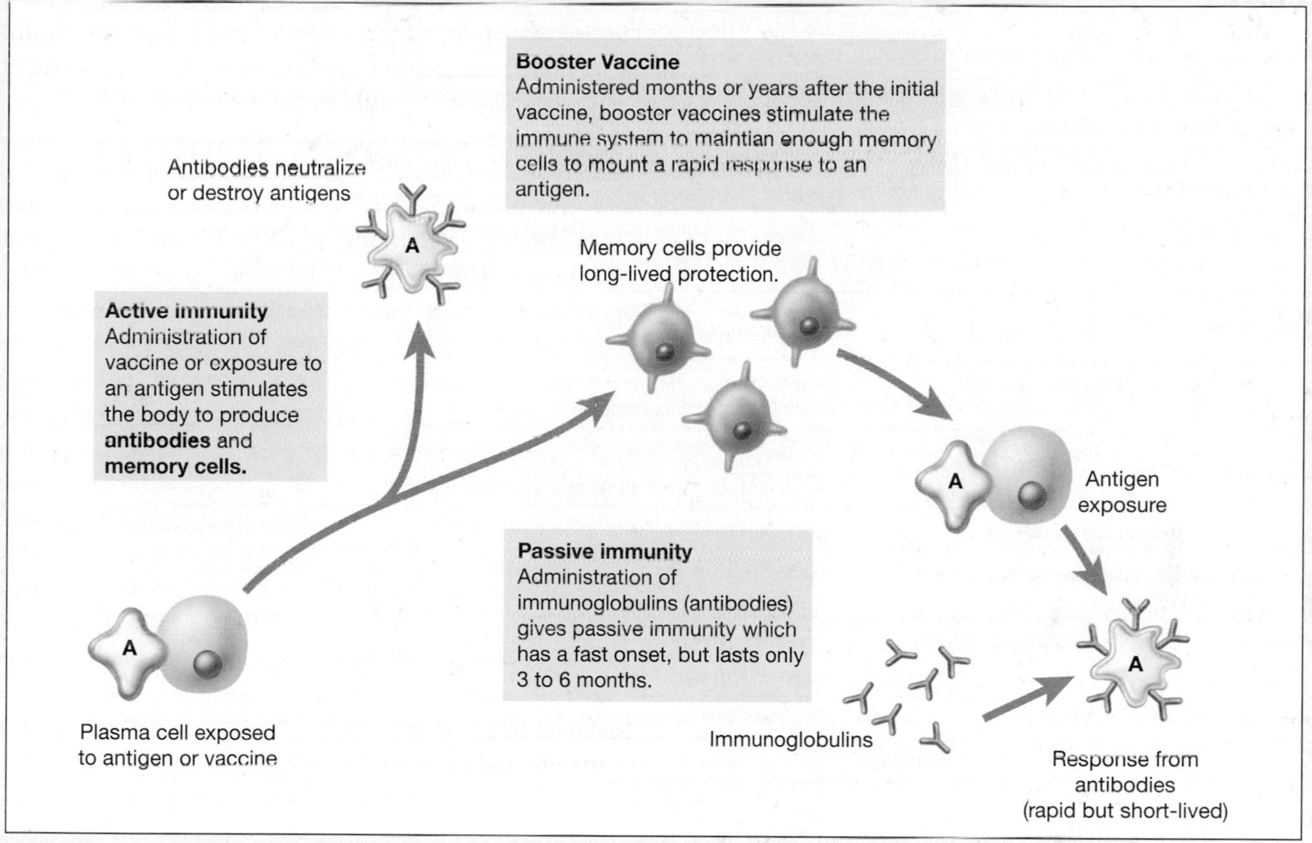
Booster Vaccine
Administered months or years after the initial vaccine, booster vaccines stimulate the immune system to maintian enough memory cells to mount a rapid response to an antigen.
Antibodies neutralize or destroy antigens
A
Memory cells provide long-lived protection.
Active immunity
Administration of vaccine or exposure to an antigen stimulates the body to produce **antibodies** and **memory cells.**
A
Antigen exposure
Passive immunity
Administration of immunoglobulins (antibodies) gives passive immunity which has a fast onset, but lasts only 3 to 6 months.
A
A
Plasma cell exposed to antigen or vaccine
Immunoglobulins
Response from antibodies (rapid but short-lived)

vaccinated according to established guidelines. Table 34.2 lists selected vaccines and their recommended schedules.

Although vaccinations have proved to be a resounding success in children, many adults die of diseases that could be prevented by vaccination. Most mortality from vaccine-preventable disease in adults is from influenza and pneumococcal disease. The CDC publishes an adult immunization schedule that contains both age-based and risk-based recommendations. Risk-based considerations include pregnancy, diabetes, heart disease, renal failure, and various other serious and debilitating conditions.

34.4 Cell-Mediated Immunity and Cytokines

A second branch of the immune response involves T-lymphocytes, or **T cells.** Two major types of T cells are called helper T cells and cytotoxic T cells. These cells are sometimes named after a protein receptor on their plasma membrane; the helper T cells have a CD4 receptor, and the cytotoxic T cells have a CD8 receptor. The helper T cells are particularly important because they are responsible for activating most other immune cells, including B cells. Cytotoxic T cells travel throughout the body, directly killing certain bacteria, parasites, virus-infected cells, and cancer cells.

T cells rapidly form clones after they are activated or sensitized by an encounter with their specific antigen. Unlike B cells, however, T cells do not produce antibodies. Instead, activated T cells produce huge amounts of **cytokines,** which are hormone-like proteins that regulate the intensity and duration of the immune response and mediate cell-to-cell communication. Some cytokines kill foreign organisms directly, whereas others induce inflammation or enhance the killing power of macrophages. Specific cytokines released by activated T cells include interleukins, gamma interferon, and tumor necrosis factor. Some cytokines are used therapeutically to stimulate the immune system, as discussed in section 34.5. Small amounts of cytokines are also secreted by macrophages, B cells, mast cells, endothelial cells, and cells of the spleen, thymus, and bone marrow.

Like B cells, some sensitized T cells become memory cells. If the person then encounters the same antigen in the future, the memory T cells assist in mounting a more rapid immune response.

Table 34.2 Selected Vaccines and Their Schedules*

Vaccine	Schedule and Age
Adacel and Boostrix (combinations of tetanus toxoid and DTaP)	IM: single dose as an active booster after age 10 (Boostrix) or between age 11 and 64 (Adacil)
Comvax (combination of haemophilus and hepatitis B vaccines)	IM: ages 2 months, 4 months, and 12–15 months
diphtheria, tetanus, and pertussis (Daptacel, DTaP, Infanrix, Tripedia)	IM: ages 2 months, 4 months, 6 months, 15–18 months, and 4–6 years
haemophilus influenza type B conjugate (ActHIB, Hiberix, PedvaxHIB)	IM: ages 2 months, 4 months, 6 months, and 12–15 months
hepatitis A (Havrix, VAQTA)	Children: IM: age 12 months, followed by a booster 6 months to 12 months later Adults: IM: 1 mL followed by a booster 6 months to 12 months later
hepatitis B (Engerix-B, Recombivax HB)	Children: IM: three doses, with the second dose 1 month after the first, and the third dose 6 months after the first
human papillomavirus (Cervarix, Gardasil)	Age 9–26 years: IM: three doses, with the second dose 2 months after the first, and the third dose 6 months after the first
influenza vaccine (Afluria, Fluarix, FluLaval, FluMist, Fluvirin, Fluzone)	Children: IM: two doses 1 month apart; then annual dose Adults: IM: single annual dose or intranasal (FluMist)
measles, mumps, and rubella (MMR II)	Subcutaneous: single dose at age 12–15 months; second dose at age 4–6 years
meningococcal conjugate vaccine (Menactra, Menomune, Menveo)	IM: first dose at age 11–12 years and second dose at age 16 years
pneumococcal, polyvalent (Pneumovax 23), or 7-valent (Prevnar)	Adults (Pneumovax 23 or Pnu-Immune 23): subcutaneous or IM; single dose Children (Prenvar): IM: four doses at ages 2 months, 4 months, 6 months, and 12–15 months
poliovirus, inactivated (IPOL, poliovax)	Children: subcutaneous: at ages 2 months, 4 months, 6–18 months, and 4–6 years
Proquad (combination of MMR and varicella vaccines)	Subcutaneous: first dose usually at age 12–15 months; second dose (if needed) at age 4–6 years
rotavirus (Rotarix, RotaTeq)	PO: three doses at ages 2 months, 4 months, and 6 months (Rotarix does not require a dose at 6 months)
tetanus toxoid	IM: (primary immunization, age 7 or older): three doses; the second dose is given 4–8 wk after the first dose; the third dose is given 6–12 months after the second dose
Twinrix (combination of hepatitis A and hepatitis B vaccines)	Over age 18: IM: three doses, with the second dose 1 month after the first, and the third dose 6 months after the first
varicella (Varivax, Zostavax)	Subcutaneous (Varivax): at ages 12–15 months and 4–6 years Subcutaneous (Zostavax): single dose at age 50 or older

*Vaccine schedules change often and the nurse should frequently check the most recent professional guidelines for updates.

Check Your Understanding 34.1

What are the four different types of vaccination? Name an example of each. *Visit www.pearsonhighered.com/nursingresources for the answer.*

IMMUNOSTIMULANTS

Despite attempts over many decades to develop effective drugs that stimulate the immune system to fight disease, only a few such medications are available. These medications include interferons and interleukins produced by recombinant DNA technology. Immunostimulants are listed in Table 34.3.

34.5 Pharmacotherapy With Biologic Response Modifiers

When challenged by specific antigens, certain cells in the immune system secrete cytokines that help defend against the invading organisms. These natural cytokines have been identified, and through recombinant DNA technology, sufficient quantities have been produced to treat certain disorders. Sometimes called **biologic response modifiers,** some of these drugs boost specific functions of the immune system. Biologic response modifiers that enhance hematopoiesis, such as colony-stimulating factors, epoetin alfa, and oprelvekin (Neumega), are presented in chapter 32.

Interferons (IFNs) are cytokines secreted by lymphocytes and macrophages that have been infected with a virus. IFNs are unable to protect the infected cell, but they warn surrounding cells that a viral infection has occurred. IFNs attach to nearby uninfected cells, inducing the production of protective antiviral proteins. When the virus attempts to attack the protected cell, the pathogen is inactivated. IFNs have antiviral, anticancer, and anti-inflammatory properties. The actions of IFNs include modulation of immune functions such as increasing phagocytosis and enhancing the cytotoxic activity of T cells.

Prototype Drug | Hepatitis B Vaccine *(Engerix-B, Recombivax HB)*

Therapeutic Class: Vaccine **Pharmacologic Class:** Vaccine

Actions and Uses

Hepatitis B vaccine is used to provide active immunity in individuals who are at risk for exposure to hepatitis B virus (HBV). It is indicated for infants born to mothers who are HBV-positive and those at high risk for exposure to HBV-infected blood, including nurses, health care providers, dentists, dental hygienists, morticians, and paramedics. Because HBV infection is extremely difficult to treat, it is prudent for all health care workers to receive the HBV vaccine before beginning their clinical education, if not already vaccinated, unless contraindicated. The vaccine is also indicated for all persons who engage in high-risk sexual practices such as heterosexual activity with multiple partners, prostitution, or homosexual or bisexual activities, and for persons who repeatedly contract sexually transmitted infections. Other recommended groups include sexually active adolescents, dialysis patients, prisoners in correctional facilities, anyone living or traveling for more than 6 months where HBV is common, and subpopulations with known high rates of infection such as Alaskan natives, Pacific Islanders, and refugees from areas where the infection is endemic. HBV vaccine does *not* provide protection against exposure to other (non-B) hepatitis viruses. HBV vaccine is produced through recombinant DNA technology using yeast cells. It is not prepared from human blood.

HBV vaccination requires three intramuscular (IM) injections; the second dose is given 1 month after the first, and the third dose 6 months after the first dose. The drug is over 90% effective in providing immunity to HBV. The effectiveness of the vaccine in producing immunity in adults declines with age.

Administration Alerts

- In adults, use the deltoid muscle for the injection site, unless contraindicated.
- Because none of the formulas of *Recombivax HB* contain a preservative, once the single-dose vial has been penetrated, the withdrawn vaccine should be used promptly, and the vial discarded.
- Epinephrine (1:1,000) should be immediately available to treat a possible anaphylactic reaction.
- Pregnancy category C.

PHARMACOKINETICS

Onset	Peak	Duration
Antibodies appear in 2 wk	6 months	Immunity lasts 5 to 7 years

Adverse Effects

The most common adverse effects from HBV vaccination are pain at the injection site and mild to moderate fever and chills. Approximately 15% of patients will experience minor symptoms such as fatigue, dizziness, fever, and headache. Hypersensitivity reactions such as urticaria or anaphylaxis are possible.

Contraindications: This vaccine is contraindicated in patients with hypersensitivity to yeast or HBV vaccine. Patients who demonstrated severe hypersensitivity to the first dose of the vaccine should not receive subsequent doses. The drug should be administered with caution in patients with fever or active infections, or those with compromised cardiopulmonary status. The vaccine should be given to pregnant or lactating women only if clearly needed to protect the health of the mother or child.

Interactions

Drug–Drug: Immunosuppressants will decrease the effectiveness of the HBV vaccine.

Lab Tests: Unknown.

Herbal/Food: Unknown.

Treatment of Overdose: Overdoses have not been recorded.

Lifespan Considerations: Geriatric

The Shingles Vaccination

Whereas most vaccinations are given in childhood, vaccination against varicella-zoster virus (VZV), the virus that causes shingles (also known as herpes zoster), is recommended for adults age 60 or older. Like Varivax, which is given in childhood to prevent varicella (chickenpox), Zostavax is given to boost immunity against shingles. Worldwide, the incidence of herpes zoster is as high as five out of 1,000 people and as many as 30% of those with herpes zoster will develop post-herpetic neuropathy (Kawai, Gebremeskel, & Acosta, 2014). The rash that develops in shingles is extremely painful and significantly impacts the patient's ability to work or carry on normal daily activities. In addition, the blisters that appear with the rash represent an exposure risk to other people in the patient's environment, including pregnant women, people without immunity to varicella, and patients who are immunocompromised. Post-herpetic neuralgia may develop, causing months or years of acute pain even after the shingles rash has resolved. Antiviral drugs such as acyclovir (Zovirax) may be used to reduce the overall period of active shingles but they do not cure the disease, and relapses may occur. Nurses working with the older adult population should review the patients' vaccination history and suggest booster vaccinations when needed. The VZV vaccine Zostavax should also be recommended for healthy older adults over the age of 60 (CDC, 2015).

Table 34.3 Immunostimulants

Drug	Route and Adult Dose (max dose where indicated)	Adverse Effects
aldesleukin (Proleukin): interleukin-2	IV: 600,000 units/kg (0.037 mg/kg) q8h by a 15-min IV infusion for a total of 14 doses	*Flulike symptoms (fever, chills, malaise), rash, anemia, nausea, vomiting, diarrhea, confusion, agitation, dyspnea, lethargy* Cardiac arrest, hypotension, tachycardia, thrombocytopenia, oliguria, anuria, pulmonary edema, capillary leak syndrome, sepsis
Bacillus Calmette-Guérin (BCG) vaccine (TheraCys, Tice)	Intradermal (Tice): 0.2–0.3 mL as vaccine Intravesical (TheraCys): bladder instillation for bladder carcinoma	*Flulike symptoms, dysuria, hematuria, anemia,* Thrombocytopenia, cystitis, urinary tract infection (UTI), disseminated mycobacteria
INTERFERONS		
interferon alfa-2b (Intron-A)	IM/subcutaneous: hairy cell leukemia: 2 million units/m² three times/wk Kaposi's sarcoma: 30 million units/m² three times/wk Chronic hepatitis: 3–5 million units/m² three times/wk for 18–24 months	*Flulike symptoms, myalgia, fatigue, headache, anorexia, diarrhea, nausea, vomiting, dyspnea, cough, alopecia, pharyngitis, injection site reactions (IFN beta)* Myelosuppression, thrombocytopenia, leukopenia, anemia, suicide ideation, severe depression, seizures (IFN beta), myasthenia gravis (IFN beta), myocardial infarction (MI), anaphylaxis, hepatotoxicity
interferon alfacon-1 (Infergen)	Subcutaneous: 9 mcg three times/wk	
interferon alfa-n3 (Alferon N)	Intralesion: 0.05 mL (250,000 international units) per wart twice/wk for up to 8 wk	
interferon beta-1a (Avonex, Rebif)	IM (Avonex): 30 mcg/wk Subcutaneous (Rebif); 44 mcg three times/wk	
interferon beta-1b (Betaseron, Extavia)	Subcutaneous: 0.25 mg (8 million units) every other day	
peginterferon alfa-2a (Pegasys)	Subcutaneous: 180 mcg/wk for 48 wk	
peginterferon alfa-2b (PegIntron, Sylatron)	Subcutaneous: PegIntron: 1.5 mcg/kg/wk Sylatron: 6 mcg/kg/wk for eight doses followed by 3 mcg/kg/wk for up to 5 years	
interferon gamma-1b (Actimmune)	Subcutaneous: 50 mcg/m² three times/wk	

Note: *Italics* indicate common adverse effects; underlining indicates serious adverse effects.

The class of IFNs having the greatest clinical utility is the alpha interferons, for which six different formulations are available. These are IFN alfa-2b, IFN alfacon-1, IFN alfa-n3, pegIFN alfa-2a, and pegIFN alfa-2b (note that when used as medications, the spelling is changed from alpha to alfa). In the two peg formulations the inert molecule polyethylene glycol (PEG) is attached to the IFN. This addition of PEG extends the half-life of the drug to allow for once-weekly dosing. Indications for IFN alfa therapy include hairy cell leukemia, AIDS-related Kaposi's sarcoma, non-Hodgkin's lymphoma, malignant melanoma, and chronic hepatitis virus B or C infections. The use of IFN alfa in the pharmacotherapy of hepatitis is presented in chapter 37.

Interferon beta consists of two different formulations, beta-1a and beta-1b, which are primarily reserved for the treatment of severe multiple sclerosis (see chapter 21). A third drug in this class, IFN gamma-1b, has limited clinical application in the treatment of chronic granulomatous disease and severe osteoporosis.

Interleukins (ILs) are another class of cytokines that are synthesized primarily by lymphocytes, monocytes, and macrophages that enhance the capabilities of the immune system. The ILs have widespread effects on immune function including stimulation of cytotoxic T-cell activity against tumor cells, increased B-cell and plasma cell production, and promotion of inflammation. At least 30 different ILs have been identified, though only a few are available as medications. Interleukin-2, derived from T helper lymphocytes, promotes the proliferation of both T lymphocytes and activated B lymphocytes. It is available as aldesleukin (Proleukin), which is approved for the treatment of metastatic renal carcinoma and metastatic melanoma. Aldesleukin therapy is sometimes limited by capillary leak syndrome, a serious condition in which plasma proteins and other substances leave the blood and enter the interstitial spaces because of "leaky" capillaries. Interleukin-11, which is derived from bone marrow cells, is a growth factor with multiple hematopoietic effects. It is marketed as oprelvekin (Neumega) for its ability to stimulate platelet production in immunosuppressed patients (see chapter 32).

Prototype Drug | Interferon alfa-2b *(Intron-A)*

Therapeutic Class: Immunostimulant **Pharmacologic Class:** Interferon, biologic response modifier

Actions and Uses

Interferon alfa-2b is a biologic response modifier prepared by recombinant DNA technology that is approved to treat cancers (hairy cell leukemia, malignant melanoma, non-Hodgkin's lymphoma, AIDS-related Kaposi's sarcoma) as well as viral infections (human papillomavirus, chronic hepatitis virus B and C). Off-label indications may include chronic myelogenous leukemia, bladder cancer, herpes simplex virus, renal cell cancer, varicella-zoster virus, and West Nile virus. It is available for IV, IM, and subcutaneous administration. For treating condylomata acuminata (genital warts) the drug is injected directly into the lesion 3 times a week for 3 weeks.

Peginterferon alfa-2b (PegIntron) has a molecule of PEG attached to the interferon molecule, which gives the drug an extended half-life. Peginterferon alfa-2b (PegIntron) is approved in combination with ribavirin to treat chronic hepatitis C virus infections. In 2011, peginterferon alfa-2b (Sylatron) was approved to treat melanoma.

Administration Alerts

- The drug should be administered under the careful guidance of a health care provider experienced with its use.
- Subcutaneous administration is recommended for patients at risk for bleeding (platelet count less than 50,000/mm^3).
- Pregnancy category C.

PHARMACOKINETICS

Onset	Peak	Duration
3 h (IM); immediate (IV)	3–12 h (IM); end of infusion (IV)	2–3 h

Adverse Effects

A flulike syndrome of fever, chills, dizziness, and fatigue occurs in 50% of patients, although this usually diminishes as therapy progresses. Headache, nausea, vomiting, diarrhea, and anorexia are relatively common. Depression and suicidal ideation have been reported and may be severe enough to require discontinuation of the drug. With prolonged therapy, serious toxicity such as immunosuppression, hepatotoxicity, and neurotoxicity may be observed.

Black Box Warning: IFNs may cause or aggravate fatal or life-threatening neuropsychiatric, autoimmune, ischemic, or infectious disorders.

Contraindications: Contraindications include hypersensitivity to IFNs, autoimmune hepatitis, and hepatic decompensation. Neonates and infants should not receive this drug because it contains benzyl alcohol, which is associated with an increased incidence of neurologic and other serious complications in these age groups.

Interactions

Drug–Drug: Use with ethanol may cause excessive drowsiness and dehydration. There is additive myelosuppression with antineoplastics. Zidovudine may increase hematologic toxicity.

Lab Tests: Large declines in hematocrit, leukocyte counts, and platelet counts may occur after 3–5 days of therapy. Hepatic enzymes may become elevated during IFN therapy and may require discontinuation of the drug. Interferon alfa-2b may elevate triglyceride levels.

Herbal/Food: Unknown.

Treatment of Overdose: Overdose may cause lethargy and coma. Treatment is by general supportive measures.

Complementary and Alternative Therapies

ECHINACEA FOR BOOSTING THE IMMUNE SYSTEM

Echinacea purpurea, or purple coneflower, is a popular botanical that is native to the midwestern United States and central Canada. The flowers, leaves, and stems of this plant are harvested and dried. Preparations include dried powder, tincture, fluid extracts, and teas. No single ingredient seems to be responsible for the herb's activity; a large number of potentially active chemicals have been identified from the extracts.

Echinacea was used by Native Americans to treat various wounds and injuries. It is believed to boost the immune system by increasing phagocytosis and inhibiting the bacterial enzyme hyaluronidase. Some substances in echinacea appear to have antiviral activity; thus, the herb is sometimes taken to treat the common cold and influenza—an indication for which it has received official approval in Germany. Clinical evidence for the effects of echinacea on upper respiratory tract infections is mixed, with some studies showing no effect and others showing a beneficial effect (National Center of Complementary and Integrative Health [NCCIH], 2012). An analysis of 24 controlled clinical trials concluded that Echinacea products may be more effective than a placebo at shortening the duration of cold symptoms, although the treatment effects are weak and not statistically significant (Karsch et al., 2014). Side effects are rare; however, echinacea may interfere with drugs that have immunosuppressant effects.

Nursing Practice Application *continued*

IMPLEMENTATION	
Interventions and (Rationales)	**Patient-Centered Care**
• Assess the patient's diet and consumption of grapefruit juice. (Grapefruit juice significantly increases cyclosporine levels and should be avoided while on immunosuppressant therapy.)	• Teach the patient to avoid or eliminate grapefruit and grapefruit juice while on the drug. Flavored beverages without juice are permissible.
• **Lifespan:** Assess for pregnancy. (Pregnancy should be avoided for up to 4 months after discontinuing immunosuppressive therapy. Women who become pregnant while on the drug should consult their health care provider.)	• Discuss pregnancy and family planning with women of childbearing age. Explain the effect of medications on pregnancy and breast-feeding and the need to discuss any pregnancy plans with the health care provider. Discuss the need for additional forms of contraception, including barrier methods, with patients taking immunosuppressants.
• Assess for the development of hirsutism or alopecia. (Hirsutism is reversible when the drug is discontinued. Alopecia may indicate significant immunosuppression.)	• Advise the patient to notify the provider of changes to hair growth or texture.
Patient understanding of drug therapy: • Use opportunities during administration of medications and during assessments to provide patient education. (Using time during nursing care helps to optimize and reinforce key teaching areas.)	• The patient, family, or caregiver should be able to state the reason for the drug; appropriate dose and scheduling; what adverse effects to observe for and when to report; and the anticipated length of medication therapy.
Patient self-administration of drug therapy: • When administering medications, instruct the patient, family, or caregiver in proper self-administration techniques followed by teach-back. (Proper administration will increase the effectiveness of the drug.)	• Teach the patient to take the medication as follows: • Use enclosed equipment to measure or mix the drug. • Use glass and not paper or plastic cups unless package directions indicate they are to be used. • Mix the drug with milk, chocolate milk, or orange juice, stirring well. After taking the drug, rinse the cup with additional liquid to ensure that the entire dose is taken.

See Table 34.4 for a list of drugs to which these nursing actions apply.

Chapter Review

KEY Concepts

The numbered key concepts provide a succinct summary of the important points from the corresponding numbered section within each chapter. If any of these points are not clear, refer to the numbered section within the chapter for review.

34.1 Innate defenses deny entrance of pathogens to the body by providing general responses that are not specific to a particular threat. Adaptive body defenses are activated by specific antigens, and each is effective against one particular microbe species.

34.2 Antibody-mediated, or humoral, immunity involves the production of antibodies by plasma cells, which neutralize the foreign agent or mark it for destruction by other defense cells.

34.3 Vaccines are biologic agents used to prevent illness by boosting antibody production and producing active immunity. Passive immunity is obtained through the administration of antibodies.

34.4 Cell-mediated immunity involves the activation of specific T cells and the secretion of cytokines such as interleukins and interferons that enhance the immune response and rid the body of the foreign agent.

34.5 Immunostimulants are biologic response modifiers, including interferons and interleukins, that boost the patient's immune system. They are used to treat certain viral infections, immunodeficiencies, and specific cancers.

34.6 Immunosuppressants inhibit the patient's immune system and are used to treat severe autoimmune disease and to prevent tissue rejection following organ transplantation.

REVIEW Questions

1. A 55-year-old female patient is receiving cyclosporine (Neoral, Sandimmune) after a heart transplant. The patient exhibits a white blood cell count of 12,000 cells/mm^3, a sore throat, fatigue, and a low-grade fever. The nurse suspects which of the following conditions?
   1. Transplant rejection
   2. Heart failure
   3. Dehydration
   4. Infection
2. Which of the following statements by a patient who is taking cyclosporine (Neoral, Sandimmune) would indicate the need for more teaching by the nurse?
   1. "I will report any reduction in urine output to my health care provider."
   2. "I will wash my hands frequently."
   3. "I will take my blood pressure at home every day."
   4. "I will take my cyclosporine at breakfast with a glass of grapefruit juice."
3. The nurse is evaluating drug effects in a patient who has been given interferon alfa-2b (Intron-A) for hepatitis B and C. Which of the following is a common adverse effect?
   1. Depression and thoughts of suicide
   2. Flulike symptoms of fever, chills, or fatigue
   3. Edema, hypotension, and tachycardia
   4. Hypertension, renal or hepatic insufficiency
4. The nurse would question an order for peginterferon alfa-2a (Pegasys) if the patient had which of the following conditions? (Select all that apply.)
   1. Pregnancy
   2. Renal disease
   3. Hepatitis
   4. Liver disease
   5. Malignant melanoma
5. A nurse is preparing to administer a hepatitis B vaccination to a patient. Which of the following would cause the nurse to withhold the vaccination and check with the health care provider?
   1. The patient smokes cigarettes, one pack per day.
   2. The patient is frightened by needles and injections.
   3. The patient is allergic to yeast and yeast products.
   4. The patient has hypertension.
6. A 5-year-old child is due for prekindergarten immunizations. After interviewing her mother, which of the following responses may indicate a possible contraindication for giving this preschooler a live vaccine (e.g., measles, mumps, and rubella [MMR]) at this visit and would require further exploration by the nurse?
   1. Her cousin has the flu.
   2. The mother has just finished her series of hepatitis B vaccines.
   3. Her arm became very sore after her last tetanus shot.
   4. They are caring for her grandmother who has just finished her second chemotherapy treatment for breast cancer.

PATIENT-FOCUSED Case Study

Genoa Brown, 43-years-old, experienced chronic kidney disease secondary to polycystic kidney disease and underwent a renal transplant 6 months ago. She has been taking cyclosporine (Neoral, Sandimmune) daily.

1. What is the purpose of the cyclosporine?
2. As the nurse, what three precautions will you review with Genoa concerning her cyclosporine treatment?

CRITICAL THINKING Questions

1. A patient is taking sirolimus (Rapamune) following a liver transplant. On the most recent CBC, the nurse notes a marked 50% decrease in platelets and leukocytes. During the physical assessment, what signs and symptoms should the nurse look for? What are appropriate nursing interventions?

2. A patient has been exposed to hepatitis A and has been referred for an injection of gamma globulin. The patient is hesitant to get a "shot" and says that his immune system is fine. How should the nurse respond?

Visit www.pearsonhighered.com/nursingresources for answers and rationales for all activities.

REFERENCES

Centers for Disease Control and Prevention (2015). *2015 recommended immunizations for adults: By age.* Retrieved from http://www.cdc.gov/vaccines/schedules/downloads/adult/adult-schedule-easy-read.pdf

Herdman, T. H., & Kamitsuru, S. (2014). *NANDA International nursing diagnoses: Definitions and classification, 2015–2017*. Oxford, United Kingdom: Wiley-Blackwell.

Karsch-Völk, M., Barrett, B., Kiefer, D., Bauer, R., Ardjomand-Woelkart, K., & Linde K. (2014). Echinacea for preventing and treating the common cold. *Cochrane Database of Systematic Reviews*, 2, Art. No.: CD000530. doi:10.1002/14651858.CD000530.pub3

Kawai, K., Gebremeskel, B. G., & Acosta, C. J. (2014). Systematic review of incidence and complications of herpes zoster: Towards a global perspective. *BMJ Open, 4*, e004833. doi:10.1136/bmjopen-2014-004833

National Center of Complementary and Integrative Health. (2012). *Echinacea: At a glance.* Retrieved from https://nccih.nih.gov/health/echinacea/ataglance.htm

SELECTED BIBLIOGRAPHY

Centers for Disease Control and Prevention. (2014). *Parent's guide to childhood immunizations.* Retrieved from http://www.cdc.gov/vaccines/pubs/parents-guide/downloads/parents-guide-508.pdf

Centers for Disease Control and Prevention. (2014). *Vaccines and immunizations: HPV vaccination.* Retrieved from http://www.cdc.gov/vaccines/vpd-vac/hpv/default.htm

Centers for Disease Control and Prevention. (2014). *Vaccine recommendations of the ACIP.* Retrieved from http://www.cdc.gov/vaccines/hcp/acip-recs/index.html

DiPiro, J. T., Talbert, R. L., Yee, G. C., Matzke, G. R., Wells, B. G., & Posey, L. M. (Eds.). (2012). *Pharmacotherapy: A pathophysiologic approach* (7th ed.). New York, NY: McGraw-Hill.

Immunization Action Coalition. (2014). *Ask the experts: Diseases and vaccines: Measles, mumps, and rubella.* Retrieved from http://www.immunize.org/askexperts/experts_mmr.asp

Janniger, C. K. (2014). *Herpes zoster.* Retrieved from http://emedicine.medscape.com/article/1132465-overview

Kaufman, C. (2011). The secret life of lymphocytes. *Nursing, 41*(6), 50–54. doi:10.1097/01.NURSE.0000396267.88998.f9

Krensky, A. M., Bennett, W. M., & Vincenti, E. (2012). Immunosuppressants, tolerogens, and immunostimulants. In L. L. Brunton, B. A. Chabner, & B. C. Knollman (Eds.), *Goodman and Gilman's the pharmacological basis of therapeutics* (12th ed., pp. 1005–1030). New York, NY: McGraw-Hill.

Krogh, D. (2011). *Biology: A guide to the natural world* (5th ed.). San Francisco, CA: Benjamin Cummings.

Macartney, K. K., Chiu, C., Georgousakis, M., & Brotherton, J. M. (2013). Safety of human papillomavirus vaccines: A review. *Drug Safety, 36*, 393–412. doi:10.1007/s40264-013-0039-5

Madigan, M. T., Martinko, J. M., Stahl, D. A., & Clark, D. P. (2012). *Brock biology of microorganisms* (13th ed.). Upper Saddle River, NJ: Pearson.

Marin, M., Güris, D., Chaves, S. S., Schmid, S., & Seward, J. F. (2007). Prevention of varicella: Recommendations of the Advisory Committee on Immunization Practices (ACIP). *Morbidity and Mortality Weekly Report, 56*(RR04), 1–40.

Markowitz, L. E., Dunne, E. F., Saraiya, M., Chesson, H. W., Curtis, C. R., Gee, J., . . . Unger, E. R. (2014). Human papillomavirus vaccination: Recommendations of the Advisory Committee on Immunization Practices (ACIP). *Morbidity and Mortality Weekly Report, 63*(RR05), 1–30.

Pelligrino, B. (2013). *Immunosuppression.* Retrieved from http://emedicine.medscape.com/article/432316-overview

Silverthorn, D. U. (2013). *Human physiology: An integrated approach* (6th ed.). Upper Saddle River, NJ: Pearson Education.

Chapter 35

Drugs for Bacterial Infections

Drugs at a Glance

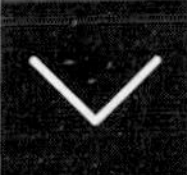

Learning Outcomes

After reading this chapter, the student should be able to:

1. Distinguish between the terms pathogenicity and virulence.
2. Explain how bacteria are described and classified.
3. Compare and contrast the terms bacteriostatic and bactericidal.
4. Using a specific example, explain how resistance can develop to an anti-infective drug.
5. Identify the role of culture and sensitivity testing in the selection of an effective antibiotic.
6. Explain how host factors can affect the success of anti-infective chemotherapy.
7. For each of the drug classes listed in Drugs at a Glance, know representative drug examples, and explain their mechanism of action, primary actions, and important adverse effects.
8. Explain how the pharmacotherapy of tuberculosis differs from that of other infections.
9. Use the nursing process to care for patients who are receiving pharmacotherapy for bacterial infections.

Indicates a prototype drug, each of which is featured in a Prototype Drug box.

The human body has adapted quite well to living in a world teeming with microorganisms (microbes). Present in the air, water, food, and soil, microbes are an essential component of life on earth. In some cases, such as with microorganisms in the colon, microbes play a beneficial role in human health. When in an unnatural environment or when present in unusually high numbers, however, microorganisms can cause a variety of ailments ranging from mildly annoying to fatal. The development of the first anti-infective drugs in the mid-1900s was a milestone in the field of medicine. In the last 50 years, pharmacologists have attempted to keep pace with microbes that rapidly become resistant to therapeutic agents. This chapter examines two groups of anti-infectives, the antibacterial medications and the specialized drugs used to treat tuberculosis.

35.1 Pathogenicity and Virulence

Microbes that are capable of causing disease are called **pathogens.** Human pathogens include viruses, bacteria, fungi, unicellular organisms (protozoans), and multicellular animals (fleas, mites, and worms). To infect humans, pathogens must bypass a number of elaborate body defenses, such as those described in chapters 33 and 34. Pathogens may enter through broken skin, or by ingestion, inhalation, or contact with a mucous membrane such as the nasal, urinary, or vaginal mucosa.

Some pathogens are extremely infectious and life threatening to humans, whereas others simply cause annoying symptoms or none at all. The ability of an organism to cause infection, or **pathogenicity,** depends on the organism's ability to evade or overcome body defenses. Fortunately, of the millions of species of microbes, only a relative few are harmful to human health. Another common word used to describe a pathogen is **virulence.** A highly virulent microbe is one that can produce disease when present in minute numbers.

After gaining entry, pathogens generally cause disease by one of two basic mechanisms: invasiveness or toxin production. **Invasiveness** is the ability of a pathogen to grow extremely rapidly and cause direct damage to surrounding tissues by their sheer numbers. Because a week or more may be needed to mount an immune response against the organism, this rapid growth can easily overwhelm body defenses. A second mechanism is the production of toxins. Even very small amounts of some bacterial toxins may disrupt normal cellular activity and, in extreme cases, cause death.

35.2 Describing and Classifying Bacteria

Because of the enormous number of different bacterial species, several descriptive systems have been developed to simplify their study. It is important for nurses to learn these classification schemes, because drugs that are effective against one organism in a class are likely to be effective against other pathogens in the same class. Common bacterial pathogens and the types of diseases that they cause are listed in Table 35.1.

One of the simplest methods of classifying bacteria is to examine them microscopically after a crystal violet Gram stain is applied. Some bacteria contain a thick cell wall and retain a purple color after staining. These are called **gram-positive bacteria** and include staphylococci, streptococci, and enterococci. Bacteria that have thinner cell walls will lose the violet stain and are called **gram-negative bacteria.** Examples of gram-negative bacteria include bacteroides, *Escherichia coli*, klebsiella, pseudomonas, and salmonella. The distinction between gram-positive and gram-negative bacteria is a profound one that reflects important biochemical and physiological differences between the two groups. Some antibacterial medications are effective only against gram-positive bacteria, whereas others are used to treat gram-negative bacteria.

A second descriptive method is based on cellular shape. Bacteria assume several basic shapes that can be readily determined microscopically. Rod shapes are called *bacilli*, spherical shapes are called *cocci*, and spirals are called *spirilla*.

A third factor used to classify bacteria is based on their ability to use oxygen. Those that thrive in an oxygen-rich environment are called **aerobic;** those that grow best without oxygen are called **anaerobic.** Some organisms have the

PharmFacts

BACTERIAL INFECTIONS

- The most frequent infectious causes of death in the United States are influenza and pneumonia.
- Food-borne illness is responsible for 48 million illnesses, 128,000 hospitalizations, and 3,000 deaths each year. *Salmonella* is the most common infection.
- Infections are a major cause of hospitalization and death in long-term care facilities. Approximately 380,000 patients die of infections in these facilities each year.
- The most common bacteria responsible for health care acquired infections (HAIs) are coagulase-negative staphylococci, *Staphylococcus aureus*, and *Enterococcus* species.
- Nearly all strains of *S. aureus* in the United States are resistant to penicillin.
- Since 2005, the rates of invasive (life-threatening) methicillin-resistant *Staphylococcus aureus* (MRSA) infections in health care settings have declined about 58%.
- Approximately 110 million sexually transmitted infections occur annually in the United States, with over half the new infections occurring in people ages 15–24.

Table 35.1 Common Bacterial Pathogens and Disorders

Name of Organism	Disease(s)	Description
Bacillus anthracis	Anthrax	Appears in cutaneous and respiratory forms
Borrelia burgdorferi	Lyme disease	Acquired from tick bites
Chlamydia trachomatis	Venereal disease, eye infection	Most common cause of sexually transmitted disease in the United States
Enterococci	Wounds, urinary tract infection (UTI), endocarditis, bacteremia	Part of host flora of the genitourinary and intestinal tracts; common opportunistic pathogen
Escherichia coli	Traveler's diarrhea, UTI, bacteremia, meningitis in children	Part of host flora of the intestinal tract
Haemophilus	Pneumonia, meningitis in children, bacteremia, otitis media, sinusitis	Some species are part of the normal host flora of the upper respiratory tract
Klebsiella	Pneumonia, UTI	Common opportunistic pathogen
Mycobacterium tuberculosis	Tuberculosis	Very high incidence in patients infected with HIV
Mycoplasma pneumoniae	Pneumonia	Most common cause of pneumonia in patients ages 5–35
Neisseria gonorrhoeae	Gonorrhea and other sexually transmitted diseases, endometriosis, neonatal eye infection	Some species are part of the normal host flora
Neisseria meningitidis	Meningitis in children	Some species are part of the normal host flora
Pneumococci	Pneumonia, otitis media, meningitis, bacteremia, endocarditis	Part of normal host flora in the upper respiratory tract
Proteus mirabilis	UTI, skin infections	Part of normal host flora in the gastrointestinal (GI) tract
Pseudomonas aeruginosa	UTI, skin infections, septicemia	Common opportunistic microbe
Rickettsia rickettsii	Rocky Mountain spotted fever	Acquired from tick bites
Salmonella enteritidis	Food poisoning	Acquired from infected animal products; raw eggs, undercooked meat or chicken
Staphylococcus aureus	Pneumonia, food poisoning, impetigo, wounds, bacteremia, endocarditis, toxic shock syndrome, osteomyelitis, UTI	Some species are part of the normal host flora on the skin and mucous membranes
Streptococcus	Pharyngitis, pneumonia, skin infections, septicemia, endocarditis, otitis media	Some species are part of the normal host flora of the respiratory, genital, and intestinal tracts

ability to change their metabolism and survive in *either* aerobic or anaerobic conditions, depending on their external environment. Antibacterial drugs differ in their effectiveness in treating aerobic versus anaerobic bacteria.

35.3 Classification of Anti-Infective Drugs

Anti-infective is a general term that applies to any drug that is effective against pathogens. In its broadest sense, an anti-infective drug may be used to treat bacterial, fungal, viral, or parasitic infections. The most frequent term used to describe an anti-infective drug is *antibiotic*. Technically, **antibiotic** refers to a natural substance produced by bacteria that can kill other bacteria. In clinical practice, however, the terms antibacterial, anti-infective, antimicrobial, and antibiotic are often used interchangeably.

With more than 300 anti-infective drugs available, it is helpful to group these drugs into classes that have similar properties. Two means of grouping are widely used: chemical classes and pharmacologic classes.

Class names such as aminoglycosides, fluoroquinolones, and sulfonamides refer to the fundamental *chemical* structure of the anti-infectives. Anti-infectives belonging to the same chemical class usually share similar antibacterial properties and adverse effects. Although chemical names are often long and difficult to pronounce, placing drugs into chemical classes will assist the student in mentally organizing these drugs into distinct therapeutic groups.

Pharmacologic classes are used to group anti-infectives by their *mechanism of action*. Examples include cell wall inhibitors, protein synthesis inhibitors, folic acid inhibitors, and reverse transcriptase inhibitors. Like chemical classes, placing an antibiotic into a pharmacologic class allows nurses to develop a mental framework on which to organize these medications and to predict similar actions and adverse effects.

Systemic sulfonamides, such as sulfisoxazole (Gantrisin) and TMP-SMZ, are readily absorbed when given PO and excreted rapidly by the kidneys. Silver sulfadiazine (Silvadene) is a topical cream used to prevent infections in patients with serious burns. The topical sulfonamides are not preferred drugs because many patients are allergic to substances containing sulfur. One combination, sulfadoxine–pyrimethamine (Fansidar), has an exceptionally long half-life and is occasionally prescribed for malarial prophylaxis.

In general, the sulfonamides are safe drugs; however, some adverse effects may be serious. Adverse effects include the formation of crystals in the urine, hypersensitivity reactions, nausea, and vomiting. Although not common, potentially fatal blood abnormalities, such as aplastic anemia (loss of bone marrow function), acute hemolytic anemia, and agranulocytosis (a severe reduction in leukocytes), can occur.

Urinary antiseptics are drugs given PO for their antibacterial action in the urinary tract. The kidney concentrates the drugs; thus, their actions are specific to the urinary system. Urinary antiseptics reach therapeutic levels in the kidney tubules, and their anti-infective action continues as they travel to the urinary bladder. The urinary antiseptics are listed in Table 35.8.

The advantage of the urinary antiseptics is that they are able to treat local infections in the urinary tract without reaching high levels in the blood that might produce systemic toxicity. Although not considered first-line drugs for UTI, they serve important roles as secondary medications, especially in patients who present with infections resistant to TMP-SMZ or the fluoroquinolones.

OTHER ANTIBACTERIAL DRUGS

35.15 Carbapenems and Miscellaneous Antibacterials

Some anti-infectives cannot be grouped into classes, or the class is too small to warrant separate discussion. That is not to diminish their importance in medicine, because some of the miscellaneous anti-infectives are critical drugs for specific infections. The miscellaneous antibiotics are listed in Table 35.9.

Imipenem (Primaxin), ertapenem (Invanz), doripenem (Doribax), and meropenem (Merrem IV) belong to a relatively new class of antibiotics called carbapenems. These drugs are bactericidal and have some of the broadest antimicrobial spectrums of any class of antibiotics. They contain a beta-lactam ring and kill bacteria by inhibiting construction of the cell wall. The ring in carbapenems is very resistant to destruction by beta-lactamase. Of the three carbapenems, imipenem has the broadest antimicrobial spectrum and is the most widely prescribed drug in this small class. Imipenem is always administered in a fixed-dose combination with cilastatin, which increases the serum levels of the antibiotic. Meropenem is approved only for peritonitis and bacterial meningitis. Ertapenem has a narrower spectrum but longer half-life than the other carbapenems. It is approved for the treatment of serious abdominopelvic and skin infections, community-acquired pneumonia, and complicated UTI. A disadvantage of the carbapenems is that they can only be given parenterally. Diarrhea, nausea, rashes, and thrombophlebitis at injection sites are the most common adverse effects.

Clindamycin (Cleocin, others) is effective against both gram-positive and gram-negative bacteria and is considered to be appropriate treatment when less toxic alternatives are not effective options. Susceptible bacteria include *Fusobacterium* and *Clostridium perfringens*. Clindamycin is sometimes the drug of choice for abdominal infections caused by *bacteroides*. It is contraindicated in patients with a history of hypersensitivity to clindamycin or lincomycin, regional enteritis, or ulcerative colitis. Indications for clindamycin are limited because some patients develop PMC, the most severe adverse effect of this drug. Serious adverse effects such as diarrhea, rashes, difficulty breathing, itching, or difficulty swallowing should be reported to the health care provider immediately.

Metronidazole (Flagyl) is another older anti-infective that is effective against anaerobes that are common causes of abscesses, gangrene, diabetic skin ulcers, and deep-wound infections. A relatively new use is for the treatment of *H. pylori* infections of the stomach associated with peptic ulcer disease (see chapter 41). Metronidazole is one of only a few drugs that have dual activity against both bacteria and multicellular parasites; it is a prototype for the antiprotozoan medications discussed in chapter 36. When metronidazole is given PO, adverse effects are generally minor, the most common being nausea, dry mouth, and headache. High doses can produce neurotoxicity.

Quinupristin/dalfopristin (Synercid) is a combination drug that belongs to a class of antibiotics called *streptogramins*. This drug is primarily indicated for treatment of vancomycin-resistant *Enterococcus faecium* infections. It is contraindicated in patients with hypersensitivity to the drug and should be used cautiously in patients with renal or hepatic dysfunction. Hepatotoxicity is the most serious adverse effect of this drug. The patient should be advised to report significant adverse effects immediately, including irritation, pain, or burning at the IV infusion site, joint and muscle pain, rash, diarrhea, or vomiting.

Linezolid (Zyvox) is one of two drugs in a class of antibiotics called the oxazolidinones. Linezolid is an alternative to vancomycin for treating MRSA infections. It also is approved

Table 35.9 Carbapenems and Miscellaneous Antibacterials

Drug	Route and Adult Dose (max dose where indicated)	Adverse Effects
CARBAPENEMS		
doripenem (Doribax)	IV: 500 mg q8h for 5–14 days	*Nausea, diarrhea, headache*
ertapenem (Invanz)	IV/IM: 1 g/day	Anaphylaxis, superinfection, PMC, confusion, seizures
imipenem-cilastatin (Primaxin)	IV: 250–500 mg tid–qid (max: 4 g/day)	
meropenem (Merrem)	IV: 1–2 g tid	
MISCELLANEOUS ANTIBACTERIALS		
aztreonam (Azactam, Cayston)	IV/IM: 0.5–2 g bid–qid (max: 8 g/day)	*Nausea, vomiting, diarrhea, rash, fever, insomnia, cough* Anaphylaxis, superinfections
chloramphenicol	PO: 50 mg/kg qid	*Nausea, vomiting, diarrhea* Anaphylaxis, superinfections, pancytopenia, bone marrow suppression, aplastic anemia
clindamycin (Cleocin, others)	PO: 150–450 mg qid IV: 600–1,200 mg/day in divided doses	*Nausea, vomiting, diarrhea, rash* Anaphylaxis, superinfections, cardiac arrest, PMC, blood dyscrasias
dalbavancin (Dalvance)	IV: 1,000 mg followed I week later by 500 mg	*Nausea, headache, vomiting, diarrhea, rash* Hypersensitivity, CDAD
daptomycin (Cubicin)	IV: 4 mg/kg once q24h for 7–14 days	*Nausea, diarrhea, constipation, headache* Anaphylaxis, superinfections, myopathy, PMC
lincomycin (Lincocin)	PO: 500 mg tid–qid (max: 8 g/day)	*Nausea, vomiting, diarrhea* Anaphylaxis, superinfections, cardiac arrest, PMC, blood dyscrasias
linezolid (Zyvox)	IM: 600 mg q12h (max: 8 g/day) PO/IV: 600 mg bid (max: 1,200 mg/day)	*Nausea, diarrhea, headache* Anaphylaxis, myelosuppression, thrombocytopenia
metronidazole (Flagyl) (see page 580 for the Prototype Drug box)	PO: 7.5 mg/kg q6h (max: 4 g/day) IV loading dose: 15 mg/kg IV maintenance dose: 7.5 mg/kg q6h (max: 4 g/day)	*Dizziness, headache, anorexia, abdominal pain, metallic taste and nausea, Candida infections* Seizures, peripheral neuropathy, leukopenia
oritavancin (Orbactiv)	IV: one 1,200 mg dose infused over 3 h	*Headache, nausea, vomiting, interference with coagulation test results, infusion-related reactions* Hypersensitivity
quinupristin–dalfopristin (Synercid)	IV: 7.5 mg/kg infused over 60 min q8h	*Pain and inflammation at the injection site, myalgia, arthralgia, diarrhea* Superinfections, PMC
tedizolid (Sivextro)	PO/IV: 200 mg once daily for 6 days	*Nausea, headache diarrhea* Thrombocytopenia, anemia
telavancin (Vibativ)	IV: 10 mg administered over 60 min, once daily for 7–10 days	*Nausea, vomiting, and foamy urine* Nephrotoxicity, QT interval prolongation, infusion-related reactions, birth defects
telithromycin (Ketek)	PO: 800 mg once daily	*Nausea, vomiting, diarrhea* Visual disturbances, hepatotoxicity, dysrhythmias
vancomycin (Vancocin)	IV: 500 mg qid or 1 g bid PO: 500 mg – 2g in three to four divided doses for 7–10 days	*Nausea, vomiting* Anaphylaxis, superinfections, nephrotoxicity, ototoxicity, red-man syndrome

Note: *Italics* indicate common adverse effects; underlining indicates serious adverse effects.

to treat VRE infections. The drug is administered IV or PO. Most patients can be converted from IV to PO in about 5 days. Linezolid is contraindicated in patients with hypersensitivity to the drug and in pregnancy and should be used with caution in patients who have hypertension. Cautious use is also necessary in patients who are taking serotonin reuptake inhibitors because the drugs can interact, causing a hypertensive crisis (serotonin syndrome). Linezolid can cause thrombocytopenia. Patients should be advised to report serious adverse effects such as bleeding, diarrhea, headache, nausea, vomiting, rash, dizziness, or fever to the health care provider immediately. Tedizolid (Sivextro) is a second drug in the oxazolidinone class that was approved in 2014 to treat skin and skin structure infections. It has the advantage of once daily dosing and may be given for 6 days, rather than the 10 days recommended for linezolid.

Vancomycin (Vancocin) is an antibiotic usually reserved for severe infections from gram-positive organisms such as *S. aureus* and *Streptococcus pneumoniae*. It is often used after bacteria have become resistant to other, safer antibiotics. Vancomycin is the most effective drug for treating MRSA infections. Because of the drug's ototoxicity, hearing must be evaluated frequently throughout the course of therapy. Vancomycin can also cause nephrotoxicity, leading to uremia. Peak and trough levels are drawn after three doses have been administered. A reaction that can occur with rapid IV administration is known as **red man syndrome** and results as large amounts of histamine are released in the body. Symptoms include hypotension with flushing and a red rash most often of the face, neck, trunk, or upper body. Other significant side effects include superinfections, generalized tingling after IV administration, chills, fever, skin rash, hives, hearing loss, and nausea. Similar in chemical structure to vancomycin, oritavancin (Orbactiv) was approved in 2014 to treat skin and skin structure infections. Oritavancin appears to have fewer serious adverse effects than vancomycin and has a long half-life that permits it to be given as a one-time, single infusion.

Daptomycin (Cubicin) is the first in a class of antibiotics called the cyclic lipopeptides. It is approved for the treatment of serious skin and skin-structure infections such as major abscesses, postsurgical skin-wound infections, and infected ulcers caused by *S. aureus*, *Streptococcus pyogenes*, *Streptococcus agalactiae*, and *E. faecalis*. The most frequent adverse effects are GI distress, injection site reactions, fever, headache, dizziness, insomnia, and rash.

Telithromycin (Ketek) is the first in a class of antibiotics known as the *ketolides* that is prescribed for respiratory infections. Its indications include acute bacterial exacerbation of chronic bronchitis, acute bacterial sinusitis, and community-acquired pneumonia due to *S. pneumoniae*. Telithromycin is an oral drug, and its most common adverse effects are diarrhea, nausea, and headache.

TUBERCULOSIS

Tuberculosis (TB) is a highly contagious infection caused by the organism *Mycobacterium tuberculosis*. The incidence is staggering: More than 1.8 billion people, or 32% of the world population, are believed to be infected. It is treated with multiple anti-infectives for a prolonged period. The antitubercular drugs are listed in Table 35.10.

35.16 Pharmacotherapy of Tuberculosis

Although *M. tuberculosis* typically invades the lung, it may travel to other body systems, particularly bone, via the blood or lymphatic system. *M. tuberculosis* activates the body's immune defenses, which attempt to isolate the pathogens by creating a wall around them. The slow-growing mycobacteria usually become dormant, existing inside cavities called **tubercles.** They may remain dormant during an entire lifetime or become reactivated if the patient's immune response becomes suppressed. Because of the immune suppression characteristic of AIDS, the incidence of TB greatly increased from 1985 to 1992; as many as 20% of all patients with AIDS develop active TB infections. Although the overall incidence of TB has been declining in the United States since 1992, the disease is still significant in regions of high immigration from countries where TB is endemic.

Drug therapy of TB differs from that of most other infections. Mycobacteria have a cell wall that is resistant to penetration by anti-infective drugs. For medications to reach the microorganisms isolated in the tubercles, therapy must continue for 6 to 12 months. Although the patient may not be infectious this entire time and may have no symptoms, it is critical that therapy continue for the entire period. Some patients develop multidrug-resistant infections and require therapy for as long as 24 months.

A second distinguishing feature of pharmacotherapy for TB is that at least two, and sometimes four or more, antibiotics are administered concurrently. During the 6- to 24-month treatment period, different combinations of drugs may be used. Multiple drug therapy is necessary because the mycobacteria grow slowly, and resistance is common. Using multiple drugs in different combinations during the long treatment period lowers the potential for resistance and increases therapeutic success. Although many different drug combinations are used, a typical regimen for patients with no complicating factors includes the following:

- *Initial phase.* 2 months of daily therapy with isoniazid, rifampin (Rifadin, Rimactane), pyrazinamide (PZA), and ethambutol (Myambutol). If C&S testing reveals that the strain is sensitive to the first three drugs, ethambutol is dropped from the regimen.
- *Continuation phase.* 4 months of therapy with isoniazid and rifampin, two to three times per week.

There are two broad categories of antitubercular drugs. One category consists of primary, first-line drugs, which are generally the most effective and best tolerated by patients. Secondary (second-line) drugs, more toxic and less effective than the first-line agents, are used when resistance develops. Infections due to multidrug-resistant *M. tuberculosis* can be rapidly fatal and can cause serious public health problems in some communities.

Table 35.10 Antituberculosis Drugs

Drug	Route and Adult Dose (max dose where indicated)	Adverse Effects
FIRST-LINE AGENTS		
ethambutol (Myambutol)	PO: 15–25 mg/kg/day (max: 1,600 mg for daily therapy)	*Nausea, vomiting, headache, dizziness* Anaphylaxis, optic neuritis
isoniazid (INH)	**Latent TB** PO: 300 mg/day or 900 mg twice weekly for 6–9 months **Active TB** PO: daily therapy 5 mg/kg/day or 300 mg/day; if given by DOT, 15 mg/kg or 900 mg twice weekly	*Nausea, vomiting, diarrhea, epigastric pain* Anaphylaxis, peripheral neuropathy, optic neuritis, hepatotoxicity, blood dyscrasias
pyrazinamide (PZA)	PO: 5–15 mg/kg tid–qid (max: 2 g/day)	*Gouty arthritis, increase in serum uric acid, rash* Anaphylaxis, hepatotoxicity, fatal hemoptysis, hemolytic anemia
rifabutin (Mycobutin)	PO: 300 mg once daily (for prophylaxis) or 5 mg/kg/day (for active TB) (max: 300 mg/day)	*Nausea, vomiting, heartburn, epigastric pain, anorexia, flatulence, diarrhea, cramping, orange discoloration of urine, sweat, tears*
rifampin (Rifadin, Rimactane)	PO/IV: 600 mg/day as a single dose or 900 mg twice weekly for 4 months	PMC, acute renal failure, hepatotoxicity, hyperuricemia, blood dycrasias
ritapentine (Priftin)	PO: 600 mg twice a week for 2 months; then once a week for 4 months	
Rifater: combination of pyrazinamide with isoniazid and rifampin	PO: 6 tablets/day (for patients weighing 121 lb or more)	(See individual drugs)
SECOND-LINE AGENTS		
amikacin (Amikin)	IV/IM: 5–7.5 mg/kg as a loading dose; then 7.5 mg/kg bid	(See Table 35.6)
aminosalicylic acid (Paser)	PO: 150 mg/kg/day in 3–4 equally divided doses	*GI intolerance, anorexia, diarrhea, fever* Hypersensitivity, inhibition of vitamin B_{12} absorption, hepatotoxicity
bedaquiline (Sirturo)	PO: 400 mg for 2 weeks, then 200 mg 3 times/week for 22 weeks	*Nausea, arthralgia, headache* Prolongation of QT interval, hepatotoxicity
capreomycin (Capastat)	IM: 1 g/day (not to exceed 20 mg/kg/day) for 60–120 days, then 1 g two to three times/wk	*Rash, pain, and inflammation at the injection site* Blood dyscrasias, nephrotoxicity, ototoxicity
ciprofloxacin (Cipro)	PO/IV: 250–750 mg bid	(See Table 35.7)
cycloserine (Seromycin)	PO: 250 mg q12h for 2 wk; may increase to 500 mg q12h (max 1 g/day)	*Drowsiness, headache, lethargy* Convulsions, psychosis, confusion
ethionamide (Trecator-SC)	PO: 0.5–1 g/day divided q8–12h (max: 1 g given in three to four divided doses)	*Nausea, vomiting, epigastric pain, diarrhea* Convulsions, hallucinations, mental depression
kanamycin (Kantrex)	IM: 5–7.5 mg/kg bid–tid	(See Table 35.6)
ofloxacin (Floxin)	PO: 200–400 mg bid	(See Table 35.7)
streptomycin	IM: 15 mg/kg up to 1 g/day as a single dose	*Nausea, vomiting, pain at the injection site, drowsiness, headache* Anaphylaxis, ototoxicity, profound CNS depression in infants, respiratory depression, exfoliative dermatitis, nephrotoxicity

Note: *Italics* indicate common adverse effects; underlining indicates serious adverse effects.

A third feature of antitubercular therapy is that drugs are extensively used for *preventing* the disease in addition to treating it. Chemoprophylaxis is initiated for close contacts of patients recently infected with TB or for those who are susceptible to infections because they are immunosuppressed. Therapy usually begins immediately after a patient is diagnosed with the infection. Patients with immunosuppression, such as those with AIDS or those who are receiving immunosuppressant drugs, may receive chemoprophylaxis with antituberculosis drugs. Nine months of therapy with isoniazid is the most effective prevention. A short-term therapy of 2 months,

Prototype Drug | Isoniazid (*INH*)

Therapeutic Class: Antituberculosis drug **Pharmacologic Class:** Mycolic acid inhibitor

Actions and Uses

Isoniazid is a first-line drug for the treatment of *M. tuberculosis*. This is because decades of experience have shown it to have a superior safety profile and to be the most effective, single drug for the infection. Isoniazid acts by inhibiting the synthesis of mycolic acids, which are essential components of mycobacterial cell walls. It is bactericidal for actively growing organisms but bacteriostatic for dormant mycobacteria. It is selective for *M. tuberculosis*. INH may be used alone for chemoprophylaxis, or in combination with other antituberculosis drugs for treating active disease. Approximately 10% of patients will develop resistance to INH during long-term therapy.

Administration Alerts

- Give on an empty stomach, 1 hour after or 2 hours before meals.
- For IM administration, inject deep IM, and rotate sites.
- Pregnancy category C.

PHARMACOKINETICS

Onset	Peak	Duration
30 min	1–2 h	6–8 h

Adverse Effects

The most common adverse effects of INH are numbness of the hands and feet, rash, and fever. Neurotoxicity is a concern during therapy, and patients may exhibit paresthesia of the feet and hands, convulsions, optic neuritis, dizziness, coma, memory loss, and various psychoses.

Black Box Warning: Although rare, hepatotoxicity is a serious and sometimes fatal adverse effect; thus, the patient should be monitored carefully for jaundice, fatigue, elevated hepatic enzymes, or loss of appetite. Liver enzyme tests are usually performed monthly during therapy to identify early hepatotoxicity. Hepatotoxicity usually appears in the first 1 to 3 months of therapy but may occur at any time during treatment. Older adults and those with daily alcohol consumption are at greater risk of developing hepatotoxicity.

Contraindications: Isoniazid is contraindicated in patients with hypersensitivity to the drug and in patients with severe hepatic impairment.

Interactions

Drug–Drug: Aluminum-containing antacids should not be administered concurrently because they can decrease the absorption of INH. When disulfiram is taken with INH, lack of coordination or psychotic reactions may result. Drinking alcohol with INH increases the risk of hepatotoxicity. INH may increase serum levels of phenytoin and carbamazepine.

Lab Tests: INH may increase values of AST and ALT.

Herbal/Food: Food interferes with the absorption of INH. Foods containing tyramine may increase INH toxicity.

Treatment of Overdose: INH overdose may be fatal. Treatment is mostly symptomatic. Pyridoxine (vitamin B_6) may be infused in a dose equal to that of the INH overdose to prevent seizures and to correct metabolic acidosis. The dose may be repeated several times until the patient regains consciousness.

consisting of a combination treatment with isoniazid (INH) and pyrazinamide (PZA), is approved for TB prophylaxis in patients who may not adhere to a longer term treatment.

Two other types of mycobacteria infect humans. *Mycobacterium leprae* is responsible for leprosy, a disease rarely seen in the United States. *M. leprae* is treated with multiple drugs, usually beginning with dapsone (DDS). *Mycobacterium avium complex* (MAC) causes an infection of the lungs most commonly observed in patients with AIDS. The most effective drugs against MAC are the macrolides azithromycin (Zithromax) and clarithromycin (Biaxin).

Complementary and Alternative Therapies

ANTIBACTERIAL PROPERTIES OF GOLDENSEAL

Goldenseal (*Hydrastis canadensis*) was once a common plant found in the woods in the eastern and midwestern United States. Native Americans used the root for a variety of medicinal applications, including skin diseases, ulcers, and gonorrhea. Recent uses include the treatment of colds and other respiratory tract infections, infectious diarrhea, eye infections, vaginitis, wounds, canker sores, and cancer (National Center for Complementary and Integrative Health, 2012). Goldenseal was once reported to mask the appearance of drugs in the urine of patients wanting to hide drug abuse, but this claim has since been proved false.

The roots and leaves of goldenseal are dried and are available as capsules, tablets, salves, and tinctures. Two of the active ingredients in goldenseal are berberine and hydrastine, which are reported to have antibacterial properties. When used topically or locally, goldenseal is claimed to be of value in treating bacterial and fungal skin infections and oral conditions such as gingivitis and thrush. As an eyewash, it can soothe inflamed eyes. Considered safe for most people, it is contraindicated in pregnancy and hypertension.

Nursing Practice Application

Pharmacotherapy With Antibacterial Drugs

ASSESSMENT	POTENTIAL NURSING DIAGNOSES*
Baseline assessment prior to administration: • Obtain a complete health history including neurologic, cardiovascular, respiratory, hepatic, or renal disease, and the possibility of pregnancy. Obtain a drug history including allergies, including specific reactions to drugs; current prescription and over-the-counter (OTC) drugs; herbal preparations; and alcohol use. Be alert to possible drug interactions. • Assess signs and symptoms of current infection noting location, characteristics; presence or absence of drainage and character of drainage; duration, and presence or absence of fever or pain. • Evaluate appropriate laboratory findings (e.g., CBC, C&S, hepatic and renal function studies).	• *Infection* • *Acute Pain* • *Hyperthermia* • *Deficient Knowledge* (drug therapy) • *Risk for Injury,* related to adverse drug effects • *Risk for Deficient Fluid Volume,* related to fever, diarrhea caused by adverse drug effects *NANDA I © 2014
Assessment throughout administration: • Assess for desired therapeutic effects (e.g., diminished signs and symptoms of infection and fever). • Continue periodic monitoring of CBC, hepatic and renal function, urinalysis, C&S, peak and trough drug levels. • Assess for adverse effects: nausea, vomiting, abdominal cramping, diarrhea, drowsiness, dizziness, and photosensitivity. Severe diarrhea, especially containing mucus, blood, or pus; yellowing of sclera or skin; and decreased urine output or darkened urine should be reported immediately.	

IMPLEMENTATION

Interventions and (Rationales)	Patient-Centered Care
Ensuring therapeutic effects: • Continue assessments as described earlier for therapeutic effects. (Diminished fever, pain, or signs and symptoms of infection should begin after taking the first dose and continue to improve. The health care provider should be notified if fever and signs of infection remain after 3 days or if the entire course of the drug has been taken and signs of infection are still present.)	• Teach the patient to report a fever that does not diminish below 37.8°C (100°F) within 3 days; increasing signs and symptoms of infection; or symptoms that remain present after taking the entire course of the drug. • Teach the patient to take the entire course of the antibacterial; not to share doses with other family members with similar symptoms; and to return to the health care provider if symptoms have not resolved after the entire course of therapy.
Minimizing adverse effects: • Continue to monitor vital signs. Immediately report undiminished fever, changes in level of consciousness (LOC), or febrile seizures to the health care provider. (A continued or increasing fever after 3 days of antibiotic use may be a sign of worsening infection, adverse drug effects, or antibiotic resistance.)	• Teach the patient to report fever that does not diminish below 37.8°C (100°F) or per parameters set by the health care provider within 3 days, increasing signs and symptoms of infection, or symptoms that remain after taking the entire course of antibacterial therapy. Immediately report febrile seizures and changes in behavior or LOC to the health care provider.
• Continue to monitor periodic laboratory work: hepatic and renal function tests, CBC, urinalysis, C&S, and peak and trough drug levels. (Many antibacterials are hepatic and/or renal toxic. Periodic C&S tests may be ordered if infections are severe or are slow to resolve to confirm appropriate therapy. Drug levels will be monitored for drugs with known severe adverse effects.)	• Instruct the patient on the need for periodic laboratory work.
• Monitor for hypersensitivity and allergic reactions, especially with the first dose of any antibacterial. Continue to monitor for up to 2 weeks after completing antibacterial therapy. (Anaphylactic reactions are possible, particularly with the first dose of an antibacterial. Post-use residual drug levels, depending on length of half-life, may cause delayed reactions.)	Teach the patient to immediately report any itching; rashes; swelling, particularly of face, tongue, or lips; urticaria; flushing; dizziness; syncope; wheezing; throat tightness; or difficulty breathing. **Safety:** Instruct the patient with known antibacterial allergies to carry a wallet identification card or wear medical identification jewelry indicating allergy.

continued

Nursing Practice Application *continued*

IMPLEMENTATION	
Interventions and (Rationales)	**Patient-Centered Care**
• Continue to monitor for hepatic, renal, and ototoxicity. (Antibacterials that are hepatic, renal, or ototoxic require frequent monitoring to prevent adverse effects. Increasing fluid intake will prevent drug accumulation in the kidneys. **Lifespan:** Age-related physiological differences may place the young child or older adult at greater risk for renal toxicity.)	• Teach the patient to immediately report any nausea; vomiting; yellowing of skin or sclera; abdominal pain; light or clay-colored stools; diminished urine output or darkening of urine; ringing, humming, or buzzing in the ears; and dizziness or vertigo. • Advise the patient to increase fluid intake to 2 to 3 L per day.
• Continue to monitor for dermatologic effects including red or purplish skin rash, blisters, and sunburning. Immediately report severe rashes, especially associated with blistering. (Tetracyclines, sulfonamides, and fluoroquinolones may cause significant dermatologic effects including Stevens–Johnson syndrome. Sunscreens and protective clothing should be used for antibacterials that cause photosensitivity.)	• Teach the patient to wear sunscreens and protective clothing for sun exposure and to avoid tanning beds, and to immediately report any severe sunburn or rashes.
• Monitor for development of superinfections (e.g., CDAD, PMC, fungal or yeast infections). (Superinfections with opportunistic organisms may occur when normal host flora are diminished or killed by the antibacterial. Severe diarrhea may indicate the presence of CDAD or PMC, superinfections caused by *C. difficile.*)	• Instruct the patient to report any diarrhea that increases in frequency or amount, or contains mucus, blood, or pus. • Instruct the patient to consult the health care provider before taking any antidiarrheal drugs because they cause the retention of harmful bacteria. • Teach the patient to observe for white patches in the mouth, whitish thick vaginal discharge, itching in the urogenital area, or blistering itchy rash. • Teach the patient infection control measures such as frequent hand washing, allowing for adequate drying after bathing, and increasing intake of live-culture–rich dairy foods.
• Monitor for significant GI effects, including nausea, vomiting, and abdominal pain or cramping. Give the drug with food or milk to decrease adverse GI effects. (Many antibiotics are associated with significant GI effects. Food or milk may impair absorption of some antibiotics such as macrolides, but if patient compliance with the drug regimen can be ensured with lessened GI effects, give with a snack and continue to monitor for therapeutic effects.)	• Teach the patient to take the drug with food or milk but to avoid acidic foods and beverages or carbonated drinks. • Teach the patient to observe for continuing signs of improvement in infection.
• Monitor for signs and symptoms of neurotoxicity (e.g., dizziness, drowsiness, severe headache, changes in LOC, and seizures). (Penicillins, cephalosporins, sulfonamides, aminoglycosides, and fluoroquinolones have an increased risk of neurotoxicity. Previous seizure disorders or head injuries may increase this risk. **Lifespan:** Be particularly cautious with the older adult who is at greater risk for falls.)	• Instruct the patient to immediately report increasing headache, dizziness, drowsiness, changes in behavior or LOC, or seizures. • Caution the patient that drowsiness may occur and to be cautious with driving or other activities requiring mental alertness until the effects of the drug are known. If dizziness occurs, the patient should sit or lie down and not attempt to stand or walk, until the sensation passes.
• Monitor for signs and symptoms of blood dyscrasias (e.g., low-grade fevers, bleeding, bruising, and significant fatigue). (Penicillins, aminoglycosides, and fluoroquinolones may cause blood dyscrasias with resulting decreases in RBCs, WBCs, and/or platelets. Periodic monitoring of CBC may be required.)	• Teach the patient to report any low-grade fever, sore throat, rashes, bruising or increased bleeding, and unusual fatigue or shortness of breath, especially after taking an antibiotic for a prolonged period.
• Monitor for development of red man syndrome in patients receiving vancomycin. Report any significantly large area of reddening such as the trunk, head or neck, limbs, or gluteal area, especially if associated with decreased blood pressure or tachycardia. (Vancomycin hypersensitivity may cause the release of large amounts of histamine, which may result in vasodilation with hypotension and reflex tachycardia. Prevancomycin antihistamines, e.g., diphenhydramine, may be ordered. IV infusions should be given slowly and monitored closely.)	• Instruct the patient to immediately report unusual flushing, especially involving a large body area; dizziness; dyspnea; or palpitations.

Nursing Practice Application *continued*

IMPLEMENTATION	
Interventions and (Rationales)	**Patient-Centered Care**
• Monitor electrolytes, pulse, and ECG if indicated in patients on penicillins. (Some preparations of penicillin may be based in sodium or potassium salts and may cause hypernatremia and hyperkalemia.)	• Teach the patient to promptly report any palpitations or dizziness.
• Monitor patients on fluoroquinolones for leg or heel pain, or difficulty walking. (Fluoroquinolones have been associated with tendinitis and tendon rupture, especially of the Achilles tendon.)	• Instruct the patient to immediately report any significant or increasing heel, lower leg, or calf pain, or difficulty walking to the provider.
• Assess for the possibility of pregnancy or breast-feeding in patients prescribed tetracycline antibiotics. (Tetracyclines affect fetal bone growth and teeth development, causing permanent yellowish-brown staining of teeth.) • **Lifespan:** Women of child bearing age who are taking penicillin antibiotics should use an alternative form of birth control to prevent pregnancy. (Penicillins may reduce the effectiveness of oral contraceptives.)	• Advise women who are pregnant, breast-feeding, or attempting to become pregnant to advise their health care provider before receiving any tetracycline antibiotic. • Teach women of child-bearing age on oral contraceptives to consult their health care provider about birth control alternatives if penicillin antibiotics are used.
Patient understanding of drug therapy: • Use opportunities during administration of medications and during assessments to provide patient education. (Using time during nursing care helps to optimize and reinforce key teaching areas.)	• The patient, family, or caregiver should be able to state the reason for the drug; appropriate dose and scheduling; what adverse effects to observe for and when to report; and the anticipated length of medication therapy.
Patient self-administration of drug therapy: • When administering medications, instruct the patient, family, or caregiver in proper self-administration techniques followed by teach-back. (Proper administration increases the effectiveness of the drug.)	• Teach the patient to take the medication as follows: • Complete the entire course of therapy unless otherwise instructed. • Avoid or eliminate alcohol. Some antibiotics (e.g., cephalosporins) cause significant reactions when taken with alcohol and alcohol increases adverse GI effects of the antibacterial. • Take the drug with food or milk but avoid acidic beverages. If instructed to take the drug on an empty stomach, take with a full glass of water. • Take the medication as evenly spaced throughout each day as feasible. • Do not take tetracycline with milk products, with iron-containing preparations such as multivitamins, or with antacids. • Increase overall fluid intake while taking the antibacterial drug. • Discard outdated medications or those that are no longer in use. Review the medicine cabinet twice a year for old medications.

See Tables 35.2 through 35.9 for lists of drugs to which these nursing actions apply.

CRITICAL THINKING Questions

1. An 18-year-old woman comes to a clinic for prenatal care. She is 8 weeks pregnant. She is healthy and takes no other medication other than low-dose tetracycline for acne. What is a priority of care for this patient?
2. A 32-year-old patient has a diagnosis of otitis externa, and the health care provider has ordered erythromycin PO. This patient has a history of hepatitis B, allergies to sulfa and penicillin, and mild hypertension. Should the nurse give the erythromycin?

Visit www.pearsonhighered.com/nursingresources for answers and rationales for all activities.

REFERENCES

Herdman, T. H., & Kamitsuru, S. (2014). *NANDA International nursing diagnoses: Definitions and classification, 2015–2017*. Oxford, United Kingdom: Wiley-Blackwell.

National Center for Complementary and Integrative Health. (2012). *Herbs at a glance: Goldenseal*. Retrieved from https://nccih.nih.gov/health/goldenseal

SELECTED BIBLIOGRAPHY

Anderson, R. J., Groundwater, P. W., Todd, A., & Worsley, A. J. (2012). Macrolide antibiotics, in *Antibacterial agents: Chemistry, mode of action, mechanisms of resistance and clinical applications* (pp. 173–196). Chichester, United Kingdom: John Wiley & Sons, Ltd. doi:10.1002/9781118325421.ch8

Barnes, B. E., & Sampson, D. A. (2011). A literature review on community-acquired methicillin-resistant *Staphylococcus aureus* in the United States: Clinical information for primary care nurse practitioners. *Journal of the American Academy of Nurse Practitioners, 23*, 23–32. doi:10.1111/j.1745-7599.2010.00571.x

Centers for Disease Control and Prevention. (2013). *CDC fact sheet: Incidence, prevalence and cost of sexually transmitted infections in the United States*. Retrieved from http://www.cdc.gov/std/stats/sti-estimates-fact-sheet-feb-2013.pdf

Centers for Disease Control and Prevention. (2013). *Get smart: Know when antibiotics work. Antibiotic resistance questions and answers*. Retrieved from http://www.cdc.gov/getsmart/antibiotic-use/antibiotic-resistance-faqs.html

Centers for Disease Control and Prevention. (2013). *Tuberculosis (TB)*. Retrieved from http://www.cdc.gov/tb/?404; http://www.cdc.gov:80/tb/pubs/mmwr/maj_guide.htm

Centers for Disease Control and Prevention. (2014). *Antibiotic resistance threats in the United States, 2013*. Retrieved from http://www.cdc.gov/drugresistance/threat-report-2013/

Centers for Disease Control and Prevention. (2014). *Estimates of foodborne illness in the United States*. Retrieved from http://www.cdc.gov/foodborneburden/

Centers for Disease Control and Prevention. (2014). *General information about MRSA in healthcare settings*. Retrieved from http://www.cdc.gov/mrsa/healthcare/index.html

Centers for Disease Control and Prevention. (2015). *Deaths and mortality*. Retrieved from http://www.cdc.gov/nchs/fastats/deaths.htm

Centers for Disease Control and Prevention. (2015). *Nursing homes and assisted living (long-term care facilities)*. Retrieved from http://www.cdc.gov/longtermcare/

Chang, C., Mahmood, M. M., Teuber, S. S., & Gershwin, M. E. (2012). Overview of penicillin allergy. *Clinical Reviews in Allergy & Immunology, 43*(1–2), 84–97. doi:10.1007/s12016-011-8279-6

Custodio, H. T. (2014). *Hospital-acquired infections*. Retrieved from http://emedicine.medscape.com/article/967022-overview#aw2aab6b2b5aa

Gumbo, T. (2011). General principles of antimicrobial therapy. In L. L. Brunton, B. A. Chabner, & B. C. Knollman (Eds.), *Goodman and Gilman's the pharmacological basis of therapeutics* (12th ed., pp. 1365–1382). New York, NY: McGraw-Hill.

Gurusamy, K. S., Koti, R., Toon, C. D., Wilson, P., & Davidson, B. R. (2013). Antibiotic therapy for the treatment of methicillin-resistant Staphylococcus aureus (MRSA) infections in surgical wounds. *Cochrane Database of Systematic Reviews, 8*, Art. No.: CD009726. doi:10.1002/14651858.CD009726

Madigan, M. T., Martinko, J. M., Stahl, A. A., & Clark, D. P. (2012). *Brock biology of microorganisms* (13th ed.). San Francisco, CA: Benjamin Cummings.

Spellberg, B., Bartlett, J. G., & Gilbert, D. N. (2013). The future of antibiotics and resistance. *The New England Journal of Medicine, 368*, 299–302. doi:10.1056/NEJMp1215093

Tortora, G. J., Funke, B. R., & Case, C. L. (2012). *Microbiology: An introduction* (11th ed.). San Francisco, CA: Benjamin Cummings.

Chapter 36

Drugs for Fungal, Protozoan, and Helminthic Infections

Drugs at a Glance

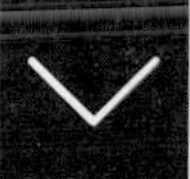

Learning Outcomes

After reading this chapter, the student should be able to:

1. Compare and contrast the pharmacotherapy of superficial and systemic fungal infections.
2. Identify the types of patients who are at greatest risk for acquiring serious fungal infections.
3. Identify protozoan and helminthic infections that may benefit from pharmacotherapy.
4. Explain how an understanding of the *Plasmodium* life cycle is important to the effective pharmacotherapy of malaria.
5. Describe the nurse's role in the pharmacologic management of fungal, protozoan, and helminthic infections.
6. For each of the classes shown in Drugs at a Glance, know representative examples, and explain their mechanism of drug action, primary actions, and important adverse effects.
7. Use the nursing process to care for patients receiving pharmacotherapy for fungal, protozoan, and helminthic infections.

Indicates a prototype drug, each of which is featured in a Prototype Drug box.

Fungi, protozoa, and multicellular parasites are more complex than bacteria. Because of structural and functional differences, most antibacterial drugs are ineffective against these organisms. Although there are fewer medications to treat these types of infections, the available medications are usually effective.

FUNGAL INFECTIONS

36.1 Characteristics of Fungi

Fungi are single-celled or multicellular organisms whose primary role on the planet is to serve as decomposers of dead plants and animals, returning their elements to the soil for recycling. Fungi include mushrooms, yeasts, and molds. Although 1.5 million species exist in soil, air, and water, only about 50 are associated with significant disease in humans. A few species of fungi grow as part of the normal host flora on the skin, mouth, and urogenital tract. **Yeasts,** which include the common pathogen *Candida albicans,* are unicellular fungi.

Most exposure to pathogenic fungi occurs through inhalation of fungal spores or by handling contaminated soil. Thus, many fungal infections involve the respiratory tract, the skin, hair, and nails. In addition, the lungs serve as a route for *invasive* fungi to enter the body and infect internal organs. An additional common source of fungal infections, especially of the mouth or vagina, is overgrowth of normal flora.

Unlike bacteria, which grow rapidly to overwhelm hosts' defenses, fungi grow slowly, and infections may progress for many months before symptoms develop. Fungi cause disease by replication; only a few secrete toxins like some bacterial species. With a few exceptions (such as athlete's foot), fungal infections are not readily transmitted through casual contact. In addition to causing infections, fungal spores may trigger a hypersensitivity response in susceptible patients, resulting in allergies to mold or mildew.

The human body is remarkably resistant to infection by these organisms, and patients with healthy immune systems experience few serious fungal diseases. Patients who have a suppressed immune system, however, such as those infected with HIV, may experience frequent fungal infections, some of which may require aggressive pharmacotherapy.

The species of pathogenic fungi that attack a person with a healthy immune system are often distinct from those that infect patients who are immunocompromised. Patients with intact immune defenses are afflicted with community-acquired infections such as sporotrichosis, blastomycosis, histoplasmosis, and coccidioidomycosis. Opportunistic fungal infections acquired in a nosocomial setting are more likely to be candidiasis, aspergillosis, cryptococcosis, and mucormycosis. Table 36.1 lists the most common fungi that cause disease in humans.

36.2 Classification of Mycoses

Fungal infections are called **mycoses.** A simple and useful method of classifying mycoses is to consider them as either systemic or superficial.

Table 36.1 Fungal Pathogens

Name of Fungus	Disease and Primary Organ System Affected
SYSTEMIC	
Aspergillus fumigatus and other species	Aspergillosis: opportunistic; most commonly affects the lung but can spread to other organs
Blastomyces dermatitidis	Blastomycosis: begins in the lungs and spreads to other organs
Candida albicans and other species	Candidiasis: most common opportunistic fungal infection; may affect nearly any organ
Coccidioides immitis	Coccidioidomycosis: begins in the lungs and spreads to other organs
Cryptococcus neoformans	Cryptococcosis: opportunistic; begins in the lungs but is the most common cause of meningitis in patients with AIDS
Histoplasma capsulatum	Histoplasmosis: begins in the lungs and spreads to other organs
Pneumocystis jiroveci	Pneumocystis pneumonia: opportunistic; primarily causes pneumonia of the lung but can spread to other organs
SUPERFICIAL	
Candida albicans and other species	Candidiasis: affects the skin, nails, oral cavity (thrush), vagina
Epidermophyton floccosum	Athlete's foot (tinea pedis), jock itch (tinea cruris), and other skin disorders
Microsporum species	Ringworm of the scalp (tinea capitis)
Sporothrix schenckii	Sporotrichosis: primarily affects the skin and superficial lymph nodes
Trichophyton species	Affects the scalp, skin, and nails

PharmFacts

FUNGAL, PROTOZOAN, AND HELMINTHIC DISEASES

- Ninety percent of human fungal infections are caused by just a few dozen species.
- Of all human fungal infections, 86% are caused by *Candida albicans*. The second most common (1.3%) is caused by the species of *Aspergillus*.
- Giardiasis is a protozoan disease that affects 6–8% of children in developed countries and about 33% of all people in underdeveloped countries.
- Over 200 million cases of malaria occur worldwide each year, with an estimated 660,000 deaths due to the disease.
- Fungal infections of the eye are rare, although they may be serious. The most common source is from an eye injury caused by plant matter such as a stick or thorn.
- *Ascaris lumbricoides* is the most common intestinal helminth infection, affecting 1 billion people worldwide.

Superficial mycoses affect the scalp, skin, nails, and mucous membranes such as the oral cavity and vagina. In most cases, the fungus invades only the surface layers of these regions. Mycoses of this type are often treated with topical drugs because the incidence of adverse effects is much lower using this route of administration. Fungi may invade the deeper layers of the skin or mucous membranes. Because topical antifungal preparations may not penetrate deep enough to reach the pathogen, infections in the cutaneous and subcutaneous layers may require oral (PO) antifungal therapy.

Systemic mycoses are those affecting internal organs, typically the lungs, brain, and digestive organs. Although much less common than superficial mycoses, systemic fungal infections affect multiple body systems and are sometimes fatal to patients with suppressed immune systems. Mycoses of this type require aggressive oral or parenteral medications that produce more adverse effects than the topical agents.

Historically, the antifungal drugs used for superficial infections were clearly distinct from those prescribed for systemic infections. In recent years, this distinction has blurred, because some of the newer antifungal medications may be used for either superficial or systemic infections. Furthermore, some superficial infections may be treated with oral, rather than topical, drugs. For example, nail infections are superficial but are often treated with oral antifungal drugs. This therapeutic division between superficial and systemic mycoses is still useful, however, because it separates the pharmacotherapy of relatively benign infections (superficial) from those that may be life threatening (systemic).

36.3 Mechanism of Action of Antifungal Drugs

Biologically, fungi are classified as eukaryotes; their cellular structure and metabolic pathways are more similar to those of humans than to bacteria. Anti-infectives that are efficacious against bacteria are ineffective in treating mycoses because of these differences in physiology. Thus, an entirely different set of drugs is needed to eliminate fungal infections.

One important difference between fungal cells and human cells is the steroid used in constructing plasma membranes. Whereas cholesterol is essential for animal cell membranes, **ergosterol** is present in fungi. The largest class of antifungal drugs, the azoles, inhibits ergosterol biosynthesis, causing the fungal plasma membrane to become porous or leaky. Amphotericin B (Fungizone), terbinafine (Lamisil), and nystatin (Mycostatin) also act by this mechanism.

Some antifungals take advantage of enzymatic differences between fungi and humans. For example, in fungi, flucytosine (Ancobon) is converted to the toxic antimetabolite 5-fluorouracil, which inhibits both DNA and RNA synthesis in the pathogen. Humans do not have the enzyme necessary for this conversion. Indeed, 5-fluorouracil itself is a common antineoplastic drug (see chapter 38).

ANTIFUNGAL DRUGS

Drugs for Systemic Fungal Infections

Systemic or invasive fungal disease may require intensive pharmacotherapy for extended periods. Amphotericin B (Fungizone) and fluconazole (Diflucan) are preferred drugs for these serious infections. Selected systemic antifungal drugs are listed in Table 36.2.

36.4 Pharmacotherapy of Systemic Fungal Diseases

Because human immune defenses provide a formidable barrier to fungi, serious fungal infections are rarely encountered in persons with healthy body defenses. The AIDS epidemic, however, has resulted in the frequent clinical occurrence of previously rare mycoses, such as cryptococcosis and coccidioidomycosis. Opportunistic fungal disease in patients with AIDS spurred the development of several new drugs for systemic fungal infections over the past 20 years. Others who may experience systemic mycoses include those patients who are receiving prolonged therapy with corticosteroids, experiencing extensive burns, receiving antineoplastic drugs, having indwelling vascular catheters, or having recently received organ transplants. Systemic antifungal drugs have little or no antibacterial activity, and pharmacotherapy is sometimes continued for several months.

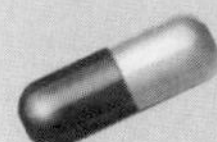

Prototype Drug | Amphotericin B *(Fungizone)*

Therapeutic Class: Antifungal (systemic type) **Pharmacologic Class:** Polyene

Actions and Uses

Amphotericin B has a broad spectrum of activity and is effective against most of the fungi pathogenic to humans; thus, it is a preferred drug for many systemic mycoses. It may also be indicated as prophylactic antifungal therapy for patients with severe immunosuppression. It acts by binding to ergosterol in fungal cell membranes, causing them to become permeable or leaky. Because amphotericin B is not absorbed from the gastrointestinal (GI) tract, it is usually given by intravenous (IV) infusion, although topical preparations are available for superficial mycoses. Several months of pharmacotherapy may be required for a complete cure. Resistance to amphotericin B is not common.

To reduce the toxicity of amphotericin B, the original drug molecule has been formulated with several lipid molecules:

- Liposomal amphotericin B (AmBisome): consists of closed spherical vesicles. Amphotericin B is integrated into the lipid membrane.
- Amphotericin B lipid complex (Abelcet): contains amphotericin B complexed with two phospholipids in a 1:1 ratio.
- Amphotericin B cholesteryl sulfate complex (Amphotec): consists of a colloidal suspension of amphotericin B in a 1:1 ratio with the lipid cholesteryl sulfate in microscopic disk-shaped particles.

The principal advantage of the lipid formulations is reduced nephrotoxicity and less infusion-related fever and chills. The reduced toxicity is believed to be due to the decreased plasma levels of the drug. Because of their expense, the lipid preparations are generally used only after therapy with other antifungals has failed.

Administration Alerts

- Infuse slowly because cardiovascular collapse may result if the medication is infused too rapidly.
- Administer premedication, such as acetaminophen, antihistamines, and corticosteroids, to decrease the risk of hypersensitivity reactions.
- Withhold the drug if the blood urea nitrogen (BUN) exceeds 40 mg/dL or serum creatinine rises above 3 mg/dL.
- Pregnancy category B.

PHARMACOKINETICS (IV)

Onset	Peak	Duration
Immediate IV	1–2 h	20 h

Adverse Effects

Amphotericin B can produce frequent and sometimes serious adverse effects. Many patients develop fever and chills, vomiting, and headache at the beginning of therapy, which subside as treatment continues. Phlebitis is common during IV therapy. Some degree of nephrotoxicity is observed in 80% of the patients taking this drug and electrolyte imbalances such as hypokalemia frequently occur. Cardiac arrest, hypotension, and dysrhythmias are possible. Because amphotericin B can cause ototoxicity, nurses should assess for hearing loss, vertigo, unsteady gait, or tinnitus.

Contraindications: The only contraindication is hypersensitivity to the drug. Caution must be observed when using amphotericin B in patients with renal impairment.

Interactions

Drug–Drug: Amphotericin B interacts with many drugs. Concurrent therapy with drugs that reduce renal function, such as aminoglycosides, vancomycin, or carboplatin is not recommended. Use with corticosteroids, skeletal muscle relaxants, and thiazole may potentiate hypokalemia. Use with digoxin increases the risk of digoxin toxicity in patients with pre-existing hypokalemia.

Lab Tests: Amphotericin B may increase values of the following: serum creatinine, alkaline phosphatase, BUN, aspartate aminotransferase (AST), and alanine aminotransferase (ALT); may decrease values for serum potassium, calcium, and magnesium.

Herbal/Food: Unknown.

Treatment for Overdose: Overdose may result in cardiorespiratory arrest. No specific therapy is available; patients are treated symptomatically.

There are relatively few drugs available for treating systemic mycoses. Amphotericin B has been the preferred drug for systemic fungal infections since the 1960s; however, this medication can cause a number of serious side effects. The newer azole drugs such as itraconazole are considerably safer and have become preferred drugs for less severe infections. Flucytosine (Ancobon) is sometimes combined with amphotericin B to treat septicemia or pulmonary and urinary tract infections due to *Candida* and *Cryptococcus* species. Flucytosine can cause immunosuppression, renal impairment, and liver toxicity.

Table 36.2 Drugs for Systemic Mycoses*

Drug	Route and Adult Dose (max dose where indicated)	Adverse Effects
amphotericin B (Abelcet, AmBisome, Amphotec, Fungizone)	IV: 0.25–1.5 mg/kg/day, infused over 2–4 h (max 1.5 mg/kg/day)	*Hypokalemia, hypomagnesemia, rash, fever and chills, nausea and vomiting, anorexia, headache* Nephrotoxicity, liver failure, anaphylaxis, cardiac arrest, thrombocytopenia, leukopenia, agranulocytosis, anemia
anidulafungin (Eraxis)	IV: loading dose 100–200 mg on day 1 followed by 50–100 mg/day	*Minor allergic reactions such as rash, urticaria, flushing, diarrhea, hypokalemia* Anaphylaxis
caspofungin (Cancidas)	IV: 70 mg on day 1, followed by 50 mg once daily	*Diarrhea, pyrexia, hypokalemia, increased alkaline phosphatase* Anaphylaxis, hepatic impairment
flucytosine (Ancobon)	PO: 50–150 mg/kg/day divided q6h	*Nausea, vomiting, headache* Blood dyscrasias, cardiac toxicity, renal failure, psychosis
micafungin (Mycamine)	IV: 150 mg/day for active *Candida* infection, 50 mg/day for *Candida* prophylaxis	*Headache, nausea, rash, phlebitis* Leukopenia, serious allergic reactions, delirium

*Azole antifungal drugs for systemic infections are included in Table 36.3.
Note: *Italics* indicate common adverse effects; underlining indicates serious adverse effects.

A newer class of antifungals called β-glucan synthesis inhibitors has been added to the treatment options for systemic mycoses. Caspofungin (Cancidas), anidulafungin (Eraxis), and micafungin (Mycamine) are important alternatives to amphotericin B in the treatment of invasive candidiasis. These drugs are expensive and usually prescribed after other antifungal therapy has been unsuccessful. Adverse effects include phlebitis, headaches, and possible renal or hepatic impairment.

Azoles

The **azole** drugs consist of two different chemical classes, the imidazoles and the triazoles. Azole antifungal drugs interfere with the biosynthesis of ergosterol, which is essential for fungal cell membranes. Depleting fungal cells of ergosterol impairs their growth. The azole drugs are listed in Table 36.3.

36.5 Pharmacotherapy With the Azole Antifungals

The azole class is the largest and most versatile group of antifungals. These drugs have a broad spectrum and are used to treat nearly any systemic or superficial fungal infection. Fluconazole (Diflucan), itraconazole (Sporanox), ketoconazole (Nizoral), and voriconazole (Vfend) are used for both systemic and topical infections. The remainder of the azoles are prescribed for superficial infections.

Systemic Azoles

The systemic azole drugs have a spectrum of antifungal activity similar to that of amphotericin B, are considerably less toxic, and have the major advantage that they can be administered PO. Because of these characteristics, azoles have replaced amphotericin B in the pharmacotherapy of less serious systemic fungal infections.

The most common adverse effects of the systemic azoles are nausea and vomiting. Severe nausea may require dose reduction or the concurrent administration of an antiemetic. Anaphylaxis and rash have been reported. Fatal drug-induced hepatitis has occurred with ketoconazole, although the incidence is rare and has not been reported with the other systemic azoles. Itraconazole has begun to replace ketoconazole in the therapy of systemic mycoses because it is less hepatotoxic and may be given either PO or IV. It also has a broader spectrum of activity than the other systemic azoles. Posaconazole (Noxafil) and isavuconazonium (Cresemba) are newer azoles used to prevent invasive *Aspergillus* infections in immunosuppressed patients. Azoles may affect glycemic control in patients with diabetes. Various reproductive abnormalities have been reported with systemic azoles, including menstrual irregularities, gynecomastia in men, and a decline in testosterone levels. Decreased libido and temporary sterility in men are other potential side effects. The azoles should be used with caution in pregnant patients.

Check Your Understanding 36.1

Why would a patient with neutropenia be more susceptible to fungal infections? *Visit www.pearsonhighered.com/nursingresources for the answer.*

Topical Azoles

Ten topical formulations are available for superficial mycoses. Clotrimazole (Mycelex, others) is a preferred drug for superficial fungal infections of the skin, vagina, and mouth. Fluconazole and itraconazole are additional options for oral candidiasis. Several of the azoles are available to treat vulvovaginal candidiasis, including tioconazole, butoconazole, and miconazole. Transient burning and irritation at the application sites are the most common adverse effects of the superficial azoles.

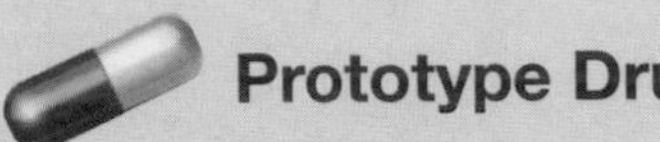

Prototype Drug | Fluconazole *(Diflucan)*

Therapeutic Class: Antifungal **Pharmacologic Class:** Inhibitor of fungal cell membrane synthesis; azole

Actions and Uses

Like other azoles, fluconazole acts by interfering with the synthesis of ergosterol. Fluconazole, however, offers several advantages over other systemic antifungals. It is rapidly and completely absorbed when given PO, and it is particularly effective against *Candida albicans*. Unlike itraconazole and ketoconazole, fluconazole is able to penetrate most body membranes to reach infections in the central nervous system (CNS), bone, eye, urinary tract, and respiratory tract.

A major disadvantage of fluconazole is its relatively narrow spectrum of activity. Although it is effective against *Candida albicans,* it is not as effective against non–*albicans Candida* species, which account for a significant percentage of opportunistic fungal infections. The drug is approved for prophylaxis of fungal infections in patients with AIDS, those undergoing bone marrow transplants, and those receiving antineoplastic drugs.

Administration Alerts

- Do not mix IV fluconazole with other drugs.
- Pregnancy category C.

PHARMACOKINETICS

Onset	Peak	Duration
Rapid IV; unknown PO	1 h IV; 1–2 h PO	2–4 days

Adverse Effects

Fluconazole is well tolerated by most patients. Nausea, vomiting, and diarrhea are reported at high doses. Unlike ketoconazole, hepatotoxicity is rare with fluconazole, although patients with hepatic impairment should be monitored carefully. Stevens–Johnson syndrome has been reported in patients with immunosuppression.

Contraindications: Fluconazole is contraindicated in patients with hypersensitivity to the drug. Because most of the drug is excreted by the kidneys, it should be used cautiously in patients with pre-existing kidney disease.

Interactions

Drug–Drug: Fluconazole is a strong inhibitor of hepatic CYP enzymes and has the potential to interact with many drugs. Use of fluconazole with warfarin may cause increased risk for bleeding. Hypoglycemia may result if fluconazole is administered concurrently with certain oral hypoglycemics, including glyburide. Fluconazole levels may be decreased with concurrent rifampin or cimetidine use. The effects of fentanyl, alfentanil, or methadone may be prolonged with concurrent administration of fluconazole.

Lab Tests: Values for AST, ALT, and alkaline phosphatase may be increased.

Herbal/Food: Unknown.

Treatment of Overdose: There is no specific treatment for overdose. Dialysis can be used to lower the serum drug level.

Drugs for Superficial Fungal Infections

Superficial mycoses are generally not severe, and patients are often treated with topical medications. Selected agents used to treat superficial mycoses are listed in Table 36.4.

36.6 Pharmacotherapy of Superficial Fungal Infections

Superficial fungal infections of the hair, scalp, nails, and the mucous membranes of the mouth and vagina are rarely medical emergencies. Infections of the nails and skin, for example, may be ongoing for months or even years before a patient seeks treatment. Unlike systemic fungal infections, superficial infections may occur in any patient, not just those who have suppressed immune systems. For example, about 75% of all adult women experience vulvovaginal candidiasis at least once in their lifetime. Athlete's foot (tinea pedis) and jock itch (tinea cruris) are two commonly experienced skin mycoses.

Antifungal drugs applied topically are much safer than their systemic counterparts because penetration into the deeper layers of the skin or mucous membranes is poor, and only small amounts are absorbed into the circulation. Adverse effects are generally minor and limited to the region being treated. Burning or stinging at the site of application, drying of the skin, rash, or contact dermatitis are the most frequent side effects from the topical agents.

Many medications for superficial mycoses are available as over-the-counter (OTC) creams, gels, powders, and ointments. If the infection has grown into the deeper skin layers, oral antifungal drug therapy may be indicated. Extensive superficial mycoses may be treated with both oral and topical antifungal medications to ensure that the infection is eliminated from deeper skin or mucous membrane layers.

Selection of a particular antifungal drug is based on the location of the infection and characteristics of the lesion. Griseofulvin (Fulvicin) is an inexpensive, older medication given PO that is indicated for mycoses of the hair, skin, and nails

Table 36.3 Azole Antifungals

Drug	Route and Adult Dose (max dose where indicated)	Adverse Effects
butoconazole (Femstat, Gynazole)	Intravaginal: Femstat: 1 applicator for 3 days. Gynazole: 1 applicator as a single dose	**Oral and parenteral routes:** *Fever, chills, rash, dizziness, drowsiness, nausea, vomiting, diarrhea* Hepatotoxicity, anaphylaxis, blood dyscrasias, QT interval prolongation **Topical route:** *Drying of skin, stinging sensation at the application site, pruritus, urticaria, contact dermatitis* No serious adverse effects
clotrimazole (FemCare, Lotrimin AF, Mycelex, others)	Topical: apply 1% cream bid for 4 weeks Intravaginal: 1 applicator for 7 days; one 100-mg tablet vaginally for 7 days or one 500-mg tablet once Troche: dissolve one in the mouth over 15–30 min	
econazole (Spectazole)	Topical: apply bid for 4 wk	
fluconazole (Diflucan)	PO/IV: 100–400 mg PO (vaginal candidiasis): 150 mg single dose	
isavuconazonium (Cresemba)	PO/IV: 372 mg daily	
itraconazole (Sporanox)	PO: 200 mg/day (max: 400 mg/day)	
ketoconazole (Nizoral)	PO: 200–400 mg/day Topical: apply once or twice daily to the affected area	
luliconazole (Luzu)	Topical: apply 1% cream to affected area once daily for 2 weeks	
miconazole (Micatin, Monistat-3, Oravig)	Topical (Micatin): apply bid for 2–4 wk Intravaginal (Monistat-3): insert one suppository daily for 3 days Buccal (Oravig): apply one tablet to the gum region daily for 2 wk	
oxiconazole (Oxistat)	Topical: apply daily in the evening for 2 months	
posaconazole (Noxafil)	PO (delayed release tablet): 100–300 mg/day (max: 400 mg/day)	
sertaconazole (Ertaczo)	Topical: 2% cream bid for 4 wk	
sulconazole (Exelderm)	Topical: apply once or twice daily for 2–6 wk	
terconazole (Terazol)	Intravaginal: 1 applicator for 3–7 days	
tioconazole (Vagistat)	Intravaginal: 1 applicator as single dose	
voriconazole (Vfend)	IV: (Vfend): 3–6 mg/kg q12h PO (maintenance dose): 200 mg q12h	

Note: *Italics* indicate common adverse effects; underlining indicates serious adverse effects.

Table 36.4 Selected Drugs for Superficial Mycoses*

Drug	Route and Adult Dose (max dose where indicated)	Adverse Effects
butenafine (Mentax)	Topical: apply daily for 4 wk for tineas	*Drying of skin, stinging sensation at the application site, pruritus, urticaria, contact dermatitis* Granulocytopenia (griseofulvin), cholestatic hepatitis (oral terbinafine), neutropenia (oral terbinafine)
ciclopirox cream, gel, shampoo (Loprox) or nail lacquer (Penlac)	Topical: apply cream bid for 4 wk for tineas Topical: apply lacquer to the nail for 48 wk for onychomycoses	
griseofulvin (Fulvicin)	PO: 500 mg microsize or 330–375 mg ultramicrosize daily for tineas and onychomycoses	
naftifine (Naftin)	Topical: apply cream daily or gel bid for 4 wk for tineas	
natamycin (Natacyn)	Ophthalmic solution: 1 drop q2h	
nystatin: topical powder (Mycostatin, Nystop); oral suspension (Nilstat); capsule (Bio-Statin); cream, ointment (Mycostatin, Nystex)	PO: 500,000–1,000,000 units tid Topical: apply two to three times/day to the affected area Capsule: PO: 500,000 to 1 million units q6h Intravaginal: 1–2 tablets daily for 2 wk	
tavaborole (Kerydin)	Topical: apply 5% solution once daily for 45 wk	
terbinafine (Lamisil)	Topical: apply once daily or bid for 7 wk for tineas PO: 250 mg daily for 6–12 wk for onychomycoses	
tolnaftate (Aftate, Tinactin)	Topical: apply bid for 2–4 wk	
undecylenic acid (Fungi-Nail, Gordochom, others)	Topical: apply once or twice daily	

*Azole antifungal drugs for superficial infections are included in Table 36.3.
Note: *Italics* indicate common adverse effects; underlining indicates serious adverse effects.

Prototype Drug | Nystatin *(Mycostatin, Nystop, others)*

Therapeutic Class: Superficial antifungal **Pharmacologic Class:** Polyene

Actions and Uses

Nystatin binds to sterols in the fungal cell membrane, causing leakage of intracellular contents as the membrane becomes weakened. Although it belongs to the same chemical class as amphotericin B, the **polyenes,** nystatin is available in a wider variety of formulations, including cream, ointment, powder, tablet, and lozenge. Too toxic for parenteral administration, nystatin is primarily used topically for *Candida* infections of the vagina, skin, and mouth. It may also be administered PO to treat candidiasis of the intestine, because it travels through the GI tract without being absorbed. Some formulations, such as Mytrex and Mycolog II cream, combine nystatin with triamcinolone (a corticosteroid) for treating inflamed subcutaneous lesions.

Administration Alerts

- For oral candidiasis, apply with a swab to the affected area in infants and children because swishing is difficult or impossible.
- For adults with oral candidiasis, the drug should be swished in the mouth for at least 2 minutes.
- Pregnancy category C (oral preparations) or A (topical preparations).

PHARMACOKINETICS

Onset	Peak	Duration
Rapid	Unknown	6–12 h

Adverse Effects

When given topically, nystatin produces few adverse effects other than minor skin irritation. There is a high incidence of contact dermatitis, related to the preservatives found in some of the formulations. When given PO, it may cause diarrhea, nausea, and vomiting.

Contraindications: The only contraindication is hypersensitivity to the drug.

Interactions

Drug–Drug: Unknown.

Lab Tests: Unknown.

Herbal/Food: Unknown.

Treatment of Overdose: There is no specific treatment for overdose.

Nursing Practice Application
Pharmacotherapy With Antifungal Drugs

ASSESSMENT

Baseline assessment prior to administration:

- Obtain a complete health history including neurologic, cardiovascular, respiratory, hepatic, or renal disease, and the possibility of pregnancy. Obtain a drug history including allergies, including specific reactions to drugs, current prescription and OTC drugs, herbal preparations, and alcohol use. Be alert to possible drug interactions.
- Assess signs and symptoms of current infection, noting location, characteristics, presence or absence of drainage and character of drainage, duration, and presence or absence of fever or pain.
- Evaluate appropriate laboratory findings (e.g., complete blood count [CBC], electrolytes, urinalysis, culture and sensitivity [C&S], hepatic and renal function studies).
- Obtain baseline weight and vital signs, especially blood pressure and pulse.

Assessment throughout administration:

- Assess for desired therapeutic effects (e.g., diminished signs and symptoms of infection and fever).
- Continue periodic monitoring of CBC, electrolytes, hepatic and renal function, and C&S.
- Continue to monitor vital signs, especially blood pressure and pulse, in patients on IV antifungals.
- Assess for adverse effects: nausea, vomiting, abdominal cramping, diarrhea, malaise, muscle cramping or pain, chills, drowsiness, dizziness, headache, tinnitus, vertigo, flushing, skin rash, urticaria, seizures, hypotension, and electrolyte imbalances (e.g., hypokalemia, hypomagnesemia). Immediately report hypotension, tachycardia, dysrhythmias, change in level of consciousness (LOC), diminished urine output, or seizures.

POTENTIAL NURSING DIAGNOSES*

- *Infection*
- *Acute Pain*
- *Hyperthermia*
- *Deficient Knowledge* (drug therapy)
- *Risk for Injury,* related to adverse drug effects
- *Risk for Deficient Fluid Volume,* related to adverse drug effects
- *Risk for Decreased Cardiac Output,* related to adverse drug effects

*NANDA I © 2014

Nursing Practice Application *continued*

IMPLEMENTATION	
Interventions and (Rationales)	**Patient-Centered Care**
Ensuring therapeutic effects: • Continue assessments as described earlier for therapeutic effects. (Diminished fever, pain, or signs and symptoms of infection should be noted.)	• Teach the patient taking oral antifungals that several months of treatment may be required. The entire course of therapy should be completed and the patient should return to the provider if symptoms have not resolved.
Minimizing adverse effects: • Continue frequent monitoring of vital signs, especially blood pressure and pulse, and respiratory rate and depth in patients on IV antifungals. Immediately report dysrhythmias, increasing pulmonary congestion, hypotension, or tachycardia. (Hypotension, tachycardia, dysrhythmias, cardiac collapse, and cardiac arrest are possible adverse effects of IV antifungal drugs. **Lifespan:** Be particularly cautious with older adults who are at increased risk for hypotension and falls.)	• Instruct the patient on the need for frequent monitoring. Explain the rationale for all monitoring equipment used. • Teach the patient to rise from lying to sitting or standing slowly to avoid dizziness or falls if hypotension is noted. If dizziness occurs, the patient should sit or lie down and not attempt to stand or walk, until the sensation passes.
• Continue to monitor periodic laboratory work: hepatic and renal function tests, CBC, urinalysis, C&S, and electrolyte levels. (Antifungals are hepatic and renal toxic and laboratory findings should be monitored frequently. **Lifespan:** Age-related physiological differences may place the older adult at greater risk for renal toxicity. Antifungals, particularly when given IV, may cause electrolyte imbalances, especially hypokalemia and hypomagnesemia, and electrolyte replacement may be needed.)	• Teach the patient about the need for frequent laboratory testing. If prescribed oral antifungals for home use, instruct the patient on the need to return for laboratory work, depending on the type of drug and the length of therapy.
• Ensure adequate hydration in patients on oral or IV antifungal drugs. Weigh the patient daily and report a weight gain of 1 kg (2 lb) or more in a 24-hour period. Measure intake and output in the hospitalized patient. (Systemic antifungal drugs may be renal toxic. Adequate hydration helps to prevent adverse renal effects. Daily weight is an accurate measure of fluid status and takes into account intake, output, and insensible losses. Excessive weight gain or edema may indicate renal dysfunction.)	• Have the patient who is taking oral antifungal drugs at home weigh self daily, ideally at the same time of day, and record weight along with blood pressure and pulse measurements. Have the patient report a weight gain of more than 1 kg (2 lb) in a 24-h period.
• Monitor for hypersensitivity and allergic reactions, especially with the first dose of IV antifungal. Continue to monitor the patient throughout therapy. (Anaphylactic reactions are possible and most common with the first IV infusion. Chills, fever, vomiting, and headache are common reactions. A test-dose of a small amount administered slowly may be given before main infusion. Premedication may include antipyretics, antihistamines, antiemetics, and corticosteroids to prevent reactions.)	• Instruct the patient to promptly report any chills, nausea, tremors, or headache.
• Ensure adequate hydration in patients on oral or IV antifungals. (Antifungal drugs are renal toxic and adequate hydration helps to prevent adverse renal effects.)	• Teach the patient to increase fluid intake to 2 L per day if on oral antifungals. Explain the rationale for increased IV fluid hydration in patients on IV antifungals.
• Continue to monitor for signs of ototoxicity. (Antifungals may cause ototoxicity and require frequent monitoring to prevent adverse effects.)	• Teach the patient to immediately report any ringing, humming, or buzzing in the ears, and dizziness or vertigo.
• Continue to monitor for hepatic toxicity (e.g., jaundice, right upper quadrant (RUQ) pain, darkened urine, diminished urine output, tinnitus, vertigo) in patients on systemic antifungal therapy. (Antifungals may cause hepatic toxicity. **Diverse Patients:** Because fluconazole is metabolized through the P450 system pathways, monitor ethnically diverse patients frequently to ensure optimal therapeutic effects and minimize adverse effects.)	• Teach the patient to immediately report any nausea, vomiting, yellowing of the skin or sclera, abdominal pain, light or clay-colored stools, or darkening of urine.
• Monitor the IV site frequently for any signs of extravasation or thrombophlebitis. (IV antifungal medication is irritating to veins and the IV site should be monitored frequently. A central line may be used when possible.)	• Instruct the patient to immediately report any pain, burning, or redness at the site of the peripheral IV. Explain the rationale for all equipment used.

continued

Nursing Practice Application *continued*

IMPLEMENTATION	
Interventions and (Rationales)	**Patient-Centered Care**
• Monitor blood glucose in patients who are taking ketoconazole. (Ketoconazole may increase glucose levels. Patients with diabetes may require a change in their antidiabetic drug routine.)	• Teach the patient with diabetes to test glucose more frequently, reporting any consistent elevations to the health care provider.
• Monitor for significant GI effects, including nausea, vomiting, and abdominal pain or cramping. Give the drug with food or milk to decrease adverse GI effects. (Food or milk may decrease GI effects but an antiemetic may also be required if nausea is severe.)	• Teach the patient to take the drug with food or milk but to avoid acidic foods and beverages or carbonated drinks.
Patient understanding of drug therapy: • Use opportunities during administration of medications and during assessments to provide patient education. (Using time during nursing care helps to optimize and reinforce key teaching areas.)	• The patient, family, or caregiver should be able to state the reason for the drug; appropriate dose and scheduling; what adverse effects to observe for and when to report; and the anticipated length of medication therapy.
Patient self-administration of drug therapy: • When administering medications, instruct the patient, family, or caregiver in proper self-administration techniques. (Proper administration will increase the effectiveness of the drug.)	• Teach the patient to take oral or topical antifungal medications as follows: • Complete the entire course of therapy unless otherwise instructed. Several months of oral therapy may be required to adequately treat the infection. • Avoid or eliminate alcohol while on oral antifungals to avoid hepatic complications. • Dissolve oral antifungal lozenges (troches) in the mouth or rinse with liquids after meals and at bedtime. If dentures are worn, remove them before using the drug and leave out overnight. Swish the liquid drug around the mouth and hold in the mouth at least 2 minutes before expectorating. Do not swallow unless instructed to do so by the provider and do not rinse the mouth with water afterwards. • Do not use occlusive dressings when topical antifungals are used. Apply a thin, even layer to the affected area. • Allow affected skin areas to air dry and wear loose-fitting and breathable fabric clothes to allow adequate ventilation. Gently cleanse areas with mild soap and water and avoid vigorous scrubbing.

See Tables 36.2, 36.3, and 36.4 for a list of drugs to which these nursing actions apply.

that have not responded to conventional topical preparations. Itraconazole (Sporanox) and terbinafine (Lamisil) are oral preparations that have the advantage of accumulating in nail beds, allowing them to remain active many months after therapy is discontinued. Miconazole and clotrimazole are frequently used OTC drugs for vulvovaginal *Candida* infections, although several other medications are equally effective. Some of the therapies for vulvovaginal candidiasis require only a single dose. Tolnaftate and undecylenic acid are frequently used to treat athlete's foot and jock itch.

PROTOZOAN INFECTIONS

Protozoa are single-celled organisms that inhabit water, soil, and animal hosts. Although only a few of the more than 20,000 species cause disease in humans, they cause significant morbidity and mortality in Africa, South America, Central America, and Asia. Travelers to these continents may acquire these infections overseas and bring them back to the United States and Canada. These parasites often thrive in conditions where sanitation and personal hygiene are poor and population density is high. In addition, protozoan infections often occur in patients who are immunosuppressed, such as those with AIDS or who are receiving antineoplastic drugs. Drugs for malarial infections are listed in Table 36.5.

ANTIPROTOZOAN DRUGS

36.7 Pharmacotherapy of Malaria

Drug therapy of protozoan infections is difficult because of the parasites' complicated life cycles, during which they

Table 36.5 Selected Drugs for Malaria

Drug	Route and Adult Dose (max dose where indicated)	Adverse Effects
artemether and lumefantrine (Coartem)	For acute infections: PO: 4 tablets as an initial dose followed by 4 tablets 8 h later, then 4 tablets bid for the following 3 days	*Headache, dizziness, anorexia, fever, arthralgia, myalgia, nausea* Hypersensitivity, QT prolongation
atovaquone and proguanil (Malarone)	For acute infections: PO: 4 tablets/day for 3 days For prophylaxis: PO: 1 tablet/day starting 1–2 days before travel, and continuing until 7 days after return	*Nausea, vomiting, abdominal pain, diarrhea, headache, myalgia* Neutropenia, hypotension
chloroquine (Aralen)	For acute infections: PO: 620 mg initial dose, then 310 mg at 6, 18, and 28 h	*Nausea, vomiting and diarrhea; visual changes, including blurred vision, photophobia, and difficulty focusing*
hydroxychloroquine (Plaquenil) (see page 838 for the Prototype Drug box)	For prophylaxis: PO: 310 mg starting 2 wk before travel and continuing 4–6 wk following return	Hemolytic anemia in patients with G6PD deficiency; irreversible retinal damage
mefloquine	For acute infections: 1,250 mg as a single dose For prophylaxis: PO: 250 mg once a week for 4 wk before travel, then 250 mg every other week during travel and 2 doses following return	*Vomiting, nausea, diarrhea, myalgia, dizziness, anorexia, abdominal pain* AV block, bradycardia, tachycardia, psychosis
primaquine	For acute infections: PO: 15 mg/day for 2 wk For prophylaxis: PO; 15 mg/day following return for 14 days	*Vomiting, nausea, diarrhea, myalgia, headache, anorexia, abdominal pain* Hemolytic anemia in patients with G6PD deficiency
quinine (Qualaquin)	For acute infections: PO: 650 mg tid for 3 days	*Vomiting, nausea, diarrhea* Cinchonism (tinnitus, ototoxicity, vertigo, fever, visual impairment), hypothermia, coma, cardiovascular collapse, agranulocytosis

Note: *Italics* indicate common adverse effects; underlining indicates serious adverse effects.

may change form and travel to infect distant organs. When faced with adverse conditions, protozoans can form cysts that allow the pathogen to survive in harsh environments and infect other hosts. When cysts occur inside the host, the parasite is often resistant to pharmacotherapy. With few exceptions, antibiotic, antifungal, and antiviral drugs are ineffective against protozoans.

Malaria is caused by four species of the protozoan *Plasmodium*. Although rare in the United States and Canada, malaria is the second most common fatal infectious disease in the world, with 300 to 500 million cases occurring annually.

Malaria begins with a bite from an infected female *Anopheles* mosquito, which is the *carrier* for the parasite. Once inside the human host, *Plasmodium* multiplies in the liver and transforms into progeny called **merozoites.** About 14 to 25 days after the initial infection, the merozoites are released into the blood. The merozoites infect red blood cells, which eventually rupture, releasing more merozoites, and causing severe fever and chills. This phase is called the **erythrocytic stage** of the infection. *Plasmodium* can remain in a latent state in body tissues for extended periods. Relapses may occur months, or even years, after the initial infection. The life cycle of *Plasmodium* is shown in Figure 36.1.

Pharmacotherapy of malaria attempts to interrupt the complex life cycle of *Plasmodium*. Although successful early in the course of the disease, therapy becomes increasingly difficult as the parasite enters different stages of its life cycle. Goals of antimalarial therapy include the following:

- *Prevention of the disease.* Prevention of malaria is the best therapeutic option, because the disease is very difficult to treat after it has been acquired. Travelers to infested areas should receive prophylactic antimalarial drugs prior to and during their visit, and for at least 1 week after leaving. Chloroquine (Aralen) is the traditional drug of choice, unless travel is to a region known to have a high incidence of chloroquine-resistant strains of *Plasmodium*. Other options include the combination drugs atovaquone-proguanil (Malarone), doxycycline, mefloquine, or primaquine.
- *Treatment of acute attacks.* After an infection is confirmed, drug therapy should begin immediately. Drugs are used to interrupt the erythrocytic stage and eliminate the merozoites from red blood cells. Chloroquine is the traditional antimalarial for treating the acute stage, although other medications are prescribed in regions of the world where chloroquine resistance is prevalent.
- *Prevention of relapse.* Patients who acquire an acute infection will always experience relapses. Drugs are given to eliminate the dormant forms of *Plasmodium* residing in the liver. Primaquine is one of the few drugs able to eliminate hepatic cysts and achieve a total cure (Table 36.5).

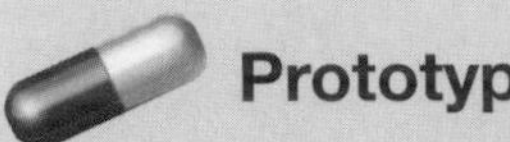

Prototype Drug | Chloroquine *(Aralen)*

Therapeutic Class: Antimalarial drug **Pharmacologic Class:** Heme complexing agent

Actions and Uses

Developed to counter the high incidence of malaria among American soldiers in the Pacific Islands during World War II, chloroquine has been the prototype medication for the prophylaxis and treatment of malaria for more than 60 years. It is effective in treating the erythrocytic stage but has no activity against latent *Plasmodium*. Both chloroquine and the closely related hydroxychloroquine (Plaquenil) are also used off-label for the treatment of rheumatic and inflammatory disorders, including lupus erythematosus and rheumatoid arthritis.

Chloroquine concentrates in the food vacuoles of *Plasmodium* residing in red blood cells. Once in the vacuoles, it is believed to prevent the metabolism of heme, which then builds to toxic levels within the parasite.

Chloroquine can reduce the high fever of patients in the acute stage in less than 48 hours. It also is used to *prevent* malaria by being administered 2 weeks before the patient enters an endemic area and continuing 4 to 6 weeks after the patient leaves. Although chloroquine is a drug of choice, many other drugs are available because resistance to chloroquine is common.

Administration Alerts

- Pediatric dosage should be monitored closely, because children are susceptible to overdose.
- If administering intramuscularly (IM), inject into a deep muscle and aspirate prior to injecting the medication because of its irritating effects to the tissues.
- Pregnancy category C.

PHARMACOKINETICS

Onset	Peak	Duration
8–10 h	3–4 h	Variable (several days to weeks)

Adverse Effects

Chloroquine exhibits few serious adverse effects at low to moderate doses. Nausea and diarrhea may occur. At higher doses, CNS and cardiovascular toxicity may be observed. Symptoms include confusion, convulsions, reduced reflexes, hypotension, and dysrhythmias. Chloroquine can cause retinal toxicity, including blurred vision, photophobia, and difficulty focusing.

Contraindications: Because chloroquine can cause retinal toxicity, it is contraindicated in patients with pre-existing retinal or visual field changes. It is also contraindicated in patients with renal impairment and in those with hypersensitivity to the drug.

Interactions

Drug–Drug: Antacids and laxatives containing aluminum and magnesium can decrease chloroquine absorption and must not be given within 4 hours of each other. Chloroquine may also interfere with the response to rabies vaccine.

Lab Tests: Unknown.

Herbal/Food: Unknown.

Treatment of Overdose: Overdose may be fatal. Symptomatic treatment may include anticonvulsants and vasopressors for shock. Ammonium chloride may be used to acidify the urine to hasten excretion of chloroquine.

Lifespan Considerations: Pediatric Treating Oropharyngeal Candidiasis in Infants

Oropharyngeal candidiasis (thrush) is a common infection in infants that may be alarming to parents. If severe, the infant may refuse to suck or feed because of mouth irritation. Transmission of this infection often occurs during a vaginal birth when the infant comes into contact with the mother's natural flora, or during feedings, including breast-feeding. Most often, the infection is self-limiting and resolves spontaneously. If the infection is severe or lasts over two months, treatment with antifungal drugs may be needed to prevent adverse feeding effects or the spread of the infection to the infant's GI or respiratory tracts.

Fluconazole (Diflucan) or nystatin (Mycostatin) are often the drugs chosen to treat infant candidasis. The antifungal liquid should be administered to the infant after feedings. Small sips of water may be given immediately before the medication to rinse away milk sugars and proteins from the mouth. A cotton swab is used to administer the medication around the infant's mouth or for the young child. The mother may also require treatment to prevent retransmission.

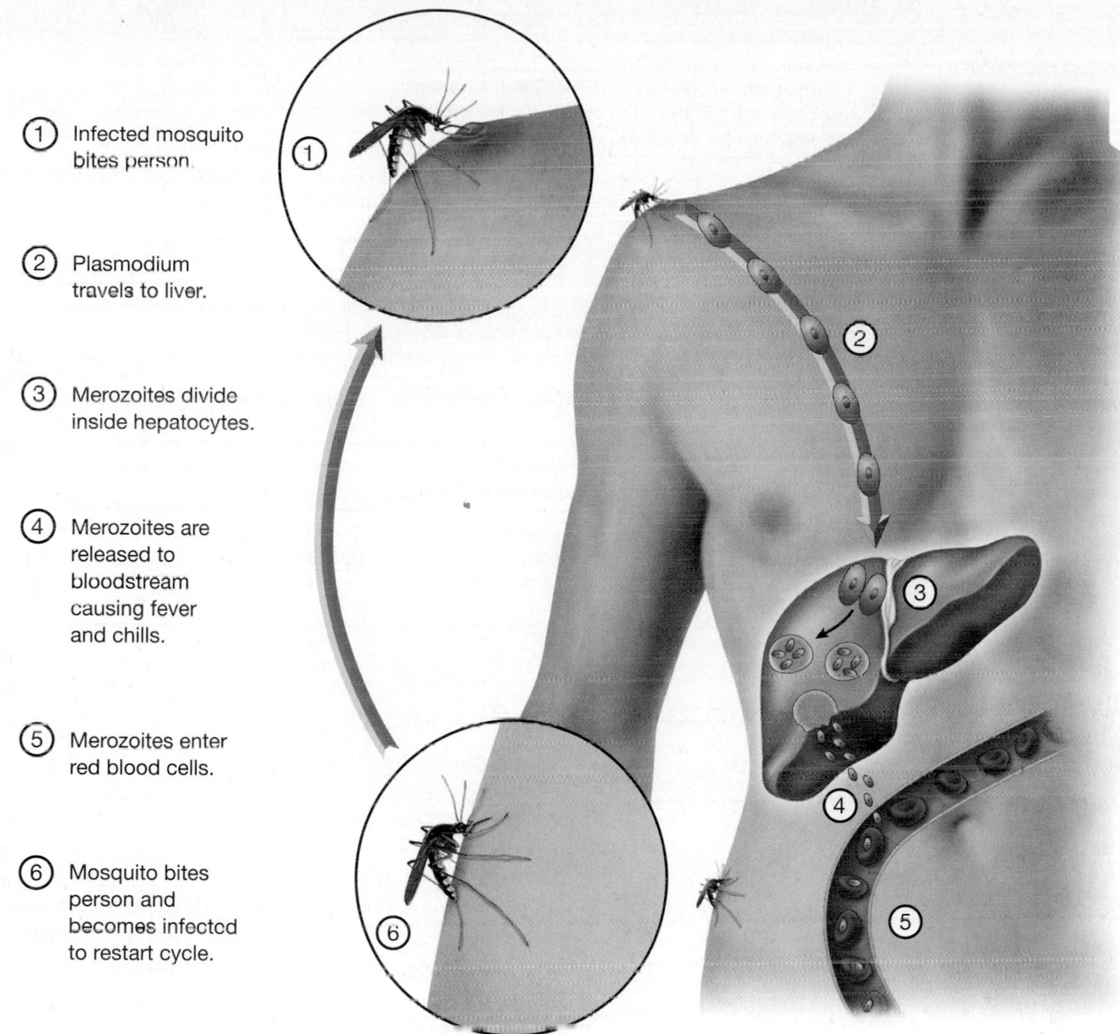

1 Infected mosquito bites person.
2 Plasmodium travels to liver.
3 Merozoites divide inside hepatocytes.
4 Merozoites are released to bloodstream causing fever and chills.
5 Merozoites enter red blood cells.
6 Mosquito bites person and becomes infected to restart cycle.

FIGURE 36.1 Life cycle of *Plasmodium*

36.8 Pharmacotherapy of Nonmalarial Protozoan Infections

Although infection by *Plasmodium* is the most significant protozoan disease worldwide, infections caused by other protozoans affect significant numbers of people in endemic areas. These infections include amebiasis, toxoplasmosis, giardiasis, cryptosporidiosis, trichomoniasis, trypanosomiasis, and leishmaniasis. Protozoans can invade nearly any tissue in the body. For example, *Plasmodia* prefer erythrocytes, *Giardia* the colon, and *Entamoeba* travels to the liver.

Like *Plasmodium* infections, the nonmalarial protozoan infections occur more frequently in regions where public sanitation is poor and population density is high. Drinking water may not be disinfected before consumption and may be contaminated with pathogens from human waste. In such regions, parasitic infections are endemic and contribute significantly to mortality, especially in children, who are often more susceptible to the pathogens. Several of these infections occur in severely immunocompromised patients. Each of the organisms has unique differences in its distribution pattern and physiology. Descriptions of common nonmalarial protozoan infections are given in Table 36.6.

One such protozoan infection, amebiasis, affects more than 50 million people and causes 100,000 deaths worldwide. Caused by the protozoan *Entamoeba histolytica*, amebiasis is common in Africa, Latin America, and Asia. Although primarily a disease of the large intestine, where it causes ulcers, *E. histolytica* can invade the liver and create abscesses. The primary symptom of amebiasis is amebic **dysentery,** a severe form of diarrhea. Drugs used to treat amebiasis include those that act directly on amoebas in the intestine and those that are administered for their systemic effects on the liver and other organs. Drugs for amebiasis and other nonmalarial protozoan infections are listed in Table 36.7.

Although several treatment options are available, metronidazole (Flagyl) has been the traditional drug of choice for nonmalarial protozoan infections. Tinidazole (Tindamax) is an alternative treatment for trichomoniasis, giardiasis, and amebiasis. This drug is very similar to metronidazole but has a longer duration of action that allows for less frequent dosing.

Table 36.6 Selected Protozoan Infections

Name of Disease and Protozoan Specie(s)	Description	Source of Infection
Amebiasis/*Entamoeba histolytica*	Primarily infects the large intestine, causing severe diarrhea; commonly travels to the liver to form liver abscesses; rarely travels to other organs such as the brain, lungs, or kidney	Fecal-contaminated water
Cryptosporidiosis/*Cryptosporidium parvum*	Infects the intestines, causing diarrhea; often seen in immunocompromised patients	Fecal-contaminated water; humans and other animals
Giardiasis/*Giardia lamblia* and other species	Infects the intestines, causing malabsorption, fatigue, and abdominal pain	Fecal-contaminated water
Malaria/*Plasmodium* (various species)	Infects red blood cells to cause fever, chills, and fatigue; some *Plasmodia* invade the liver and other tissues	Bite of female *Anopheles* mosquito
Toxoplasmosis/*Toxoplasma gondii*	Can invade any organ; causes a fatal encephalitis in immunocompromised patients	Congenital transmission; cat feces
Trichomoniasis/*Trichomonas vaginalis*	Common sexually transmitted infection (STI) that causes vaginitis in females and urethritis in males	Transmission through sexual contact with infected fluids
Trypanosomiasis/*Trypanosoma cruzi* (American)/*Trypanosoma brucei* (African)	The American form (Chagas' disease) invades cardiac tissue and autonomic ganglia; the African form (sleeping sickness) causes fatigue and CNS depression	Bite of kissing bug (American) or tsetse fly (African)

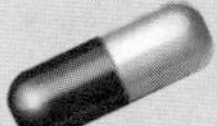

Prototype Drug | Metronidazole *(Flagyl)*

Therapeutic Class: Anti-infective, antiprotozoan **Pharmacologic Class:** Drug that disrupts nucleic acid synthesis

Actions and Uses

Metronidazole is the prototype drug for most forms of amebiasis, being effective against both the intestinal and hepatic stages of the disease. Resistant forms of *E. histolytica* have not yet emerged as a clinical problem with metronidazole therapy. Metronidazole is also a preferred drug for giardiasis and trichomoniasis.

Metronidazole is unique among antiprotozoan drugs in that it also has antibiotic activity against anaerobic bacteria and thus is used to treat a number of respiratory, bone, skin, and CNS infections. Topical forms of metronidazole (MetroGel, MetroCream, MetroLotion) are used to treat rosacea, a disease characterized by skin reddening and hyperplasia of the sebaceous glands, particularly around the nose and face. Helidac is a combination drug containing metronidazole, bismuth, and tetracycline that is used to eradicate *H. pylori* infection associated with peptic ulcer disease. Off-label uses include the pharmacotherapy of pseudomembranous colitis and Crohn's disease.

Administration Alerts

- The extended-release form must be swallowed whole and taken on an empty stomach.
- Metronidazole is contraindicated during the first trimester of pregnancy.
- Pregnancy category B.

PHARMACOKINETICS (PO)

Onset	Peak	Duration
Rapid	1–3 h	6–8 h

Adverse Effects

Although adverse effects occur relatively frequently, most are not serious enough to cause discontinuation of therapy. The most common adverse effects of metronidazole are anorexia, nausea, diarrhea, dizziness, and headache. Dryness of the mouth and an unpleasant metallic taste may be experienced. Although rare, metronidazole can cause bone marrow suppression.

Black Box Warning: Metronidazole (oral and injection) is carcinogenic in laboratory animals and should be used only for approved indications.

Contraindications: Metronidazole is contraindicated in patients with trichomoniasis during the first trimester of pregnancy and those with hypersensitivity to the drug. Metronidazole can cause bone marrow suppression; thus, it is contraindicated for patients with blood dyscrasias.

Interactions

Drug–Drug: Metronidazole interacts with oral anticoagulants to potentiate hypoprothrombinemia. In combination with alcohol, or other medications that may contain alcohol, metronidazole may elicit a disulfiram reaction. In patients who are taking lithium, the drug may elevate lithium levels.

Lab Tests: Metronidazole may decrease values for AST and ALT.

Herbal/Food: Unknown.

Treatment of Overdose: There is no specific treatment for overdose.

Table 36.7 Selected Drugs for Nonmalarial Protozoan Infections

Drug	Infection	Route and Adult Dose (max dose where indicated)	Adverse Effects
iodoquinol (Yodoxin)	Intestinal amebiasis	PO: 630–650 mg tid for 20 days (max: 2 g/day)	*Nausea, vomiting, headache, dizziness* Loss of vision, agranulocytosis, peripheral neuropathy
metronidazole (Flagyl)	Trichomoniasis, giardiasis, gardnerella	PO: 500–750 mg bid or tid	*Dizziness, headache, anorexia, abdominal pain, metallic taste, nausea* Seizures, peripheral neuropathy, transient leukopenia
miltefosine (Impavido)	Leishmaniasis	PO: 100–150 mg daily for 28 days	*Skin rash, elevated hepatic enzyme levels, reduced sperm counts* Stevens–Johnson syndrome, melena, thrombocytopenia, embryo and fetal toxicity
nifurtimox (Lampit)	American trypanosomiasis	PO: 8–10 mg/kg three to four times/day for 90–120 days	*Rash, dizziness, headache, nausea/vomiting* Seizures, paresthesia with myalgia, pneumonia
nitazoxanide (Alinia)	Diarrhea caused by cryptosporidiosis or giardiasis in children	PO: 100–200 mg q12h for 3 days	*Abdominal pain, diarrhea, nausea, vomiting, headache* No serious adverse effects
paromomycin (Humatin)	Intestinal amebiasis	PO: 25–35 mg/kg in three divided doses for 5–10 days	*Nausea, vomiting, headache, diarrhea, abdominal cramps* Ototoxicity, nephrotoxicity
pentamidine (NebuPent, Pentam)	*Pneumocystis* pneumonia, trypanosomiasis, leishmaniasis	IV/IM: 4 mg/kg/day for 14–21 days; infuse over 60 min	*Cough, bronchospasm, nausea, anorexia* Leukopenia, hypoglycemia, abscess or pain at the injection site, hypotension, nephrotoxicity
tinidazole (Tindamax)	Amebiasis, giardiasis, trichomoniasis, bacterial vaginosis	PO: giardiasis: 50 mg/kg in single dose (max: 2 g); amebiasis: 2 g/day for 3–5 days	*Anorexia, metallic taste, and nausea* Seizures, peripheral neuropathy, transient leukopenia

Note: *Italics* indicate common adverse effects; underlining indicates serious adverse effects.

HELMINTHIC INFECTIONS

Helminths consist of various species of parasitic worms, which have more complex anatomy, physiology, and life cycles than the protozoans. Diseases due to these pathogens affect more than 2 billion people worldwide and are common in areas lacking high standards of sanitation. Helminthic infections in the United States and Canada are neither common nor fatal, although drug therapy may be indicated.

ANTIHELMINTHIC DRUGS

Drugs used to treat these infections, the antihelminthics, are listed in Table 36.8.

36.9 Pharmacotherapy of Helminthic Infections

Helminths are classified as roundworms (nematodes), flukes (trematodes), or tapeworms (cestodes). The most common helminth disease worldwide is ascariasis, which is caused by the roundworm *Ascaris lumbricoides.* In the United States, this worm is most common in the Southeast, and primarily infects children aged 3 to 8 years, because this group is most likely to be exposed to contaminated soil without proper hand washing. Enteriobiasis, an infection by the pinworm *Enterobius vermicularis,* is the most common helminth infection in the United States. For ascariasis, oral mebendazole (Vermox) for 3 days is the standard treatment. Pharmacotherapy of enterobiasis includes a single dose of mebendazole, albendazole (Albenza) or pyrantel (Antiminth, Ascarel, Pin-X, Pinworm Caplets).

Like protozoa, helminths have several stages in their life cycle, which include immature and mature forms. Typically, the immature forms of helminths enter the body through the skin or the digestive tract. Most attach to the human intestinal tract, although some species form cysts in skeletal muscle or in organs such as the liver.

Not all helminthic infections require pharmacotherapy, because the adult parasites often die without reinfecting the host. When the infestation is severe or complications occur, pharmacotherapy is initiated. Complications caused by extensive infestations may include physical obstruction in the intestine, malabsorption, increased risk for secondary bacterial infections, and severe fatigue. Pharmacotherapy is targeted at killing the parasites locally in the intestine and systemically in the tissues and organs they have invaded. Some antihelminthics have a broad spectrum and are effective against multiple organisms, whereas others are specific for a certain species. Resistance has not yet become a clinical problem with antihelminthics.

Table 36.8 Selected Drugs for Helminthic Infections

Drug	Route and Adult Dose (max dose where indicated)	Adverse Effects
albendazole (Albenza)	PO: 400 mg bid with meals (max: 800 mg/day)	*Abnormal liver function tests, abdominal pain, nausea, vomiting* Agranulocytosis, leukopenia
ivermectin (Stromectol)	PO: 150–200 mcg/kg as a single dose	*Fever, pruritus, dizziness, arthralgia, lymphadenopathy* Acute allergic or inflammatory response
mebendazole (Vermox)	PO: 100 mg as a single dose, or 100 mg bid for 3 days	*Abdominal pain, diarrhea, rash* Angioedema, convulsions
praziquantel (Biltricide)	PO: 5 mg/kg as a single dose, or 25 mg/kg tid	*Headache, dizziness, malaise, fever, abdominal pain* cerebrospinal fluid reaction syndrome
pyrantel (Antiminth, Ascarel, Pin-X, Pinworm Caplets)	PO: 11 mg/kg as a single dose (max: 1 g per dose)	*Nausea, tenesmus, anorexia, diarrhea, fever* No serious adverse effects

Note: *Italics* indicate common adverse effects; underlining indicates serious adverse effects.

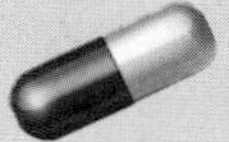

Prototype Drug | Mebendazole *(Vermox)*

Therapeutic Class: Drug for worm infections **Pharmacologic Class:** Antihelminthic

Actions and Uses

Mebendazole is the most widely prescribed antihelminthic in the United States. It is used in the treatment of a wide range of helminth infections, including those caused by roundworm (*Ascaris*) and pinworm (*Enterobiasis*). As a broad-spectrum drug, it is particularly valuable in mixed helminth infections, which are common in regions with poor sanitation. It is effective against both the adult and larval stages of these parasites. Because very little of mebendazole is absorbed systemically, it retains high concentrations in the intestine where it kills the pathogens. For pinworm infections, a single dose is usually sufficient; other infections require 3 consecutive days of therapy.

Administration Alerts

- The drug is most effective when chewed and taken with a fatty meal.
- Pregnancy category C.

PHARMACOKINETICS

Onset	Peak	Duration
2–4 h	1–7 h	3–9 h

Adverse Effects

Because so little of the drug is absorbed, mebendazole does not generally cause serious systemic side effects. As the worms die, some abdominal pain, distention, and diarrhea may be experienced.

Contraindications: The only contraindication is hypersensitivity to the drug.

Interactions

Drug–Drug: Carbamazepine and phenytoin can increase the metabolism of mebendazole.

Lab Tests: Unknown.

Herbal/Food: High-fat foods may increase the absorption of the drug.

Treatment of Overdose: There is no specific treatment for overdose.

Nursing Practice Application

Pharmacotherapy With Antiprotozoan or Antihelminthic Drugs

ASSESSMENT	POTENTIAL NURSING DIAGNOSES*
Baseline assessment prior to administration: • Obtain a complete health history including neurologic, cardiovascular, respiratory, hepatic, or renal disease, and the possibility of pregnancy. Obtain a drug history including allergies, including specific reactions to drugs, current prescription and OTC drugs, herbal preparations, and alcohol use. Be alert to possible drug interactions. • Assess signs and symptoms of current infection and assess family members or others living in the home. • Obtain a travel history, noting dates of travel and note when current symptoms started in relation to travel (i.e., before, during, or after travel). • Evaluate appropriate laboratory and diagnostic test findings (e.g., CBC, C&S, fecal ova and parasites, hepatic and renal function studies, ECG as appropriate).	• *Diarrhea* • *Nausea* • *Deficient Fluid Volume* • *Fatigue* • *Imbalanced Nutrition, Less than Body Requirements* • *Acute Pain* • *Impaired Skin Integrity* • *Deficient Knowledge* (drug therapy) *NANDA I © 2014
Assessment throughout administration: • Assess for desired therapeutic effects (e.g., diminished diarrhea, chills, fever, muscle pain). • Continue periodic monitoring of CBC, hepatic and renal function, C&S, fecal ova and parasites, and ECG as appropriate. • Assess for adverse effects: nausea, vomiting, abdominal cramping, increasing diarrhea, drowsiness, dizziness, paresthesias, metallic taste, darkened urine, dysrhythmias, and palpitations. Immediately report severe diarrhea, especially containing mucus, blood, or pus; yellowing of sclera or skin; decreased urine output; numbness of extremities; seizures; dysrhythmias; hypotension; and tachycardia.	

IMPLEMENTATION

Interventions and (Rationales)	Patient-Centered Care
Ensuring therapeutic effects: • Continue assessments as described earlier for therapeutic effects. (Diminished fever, pain, diarrhea, or signs of infection should begin soon after taking the first dose and continue to improve. The health care provider should be notified if signs of infection remain after 3 days or if the entire course of treatment has been taken and signs of infection are still present.)	• Teach the patient to report a fever that does not diminish below 37.8°C (100°F) within 3 days, increasing signs and symptoms of infection, or symptoms that remain present after taking the entire course of the drug. • Teach the patient to complete the entire course of the antibacterial; not to share doses with other family members with similar symptoms; and to return to the provider if symptoms have not resolved after the entire course of therapy.
Minimizing adverse effects: • Continue to monitor vital signs, especially temperature if fever is present. Report undiminished fever or changes in LOC to the health care provider immediately. (Fever should begin to diminish within 1 to 3 days after starting the drug. Continued fever may be a sign of worsening infection, adverse drug effects, or antibiotic resistance.)	• Teach the patient to immediately report a fever that does not diminish below 37.8°C (100°F) or per parameters, or changes in behavior or LOC to the health care provider.
• Continue to monitor periodic laboratory work: hepatic and renal function tests, CBC, ECG, C&S, and fecal ova and parasites. (Hepatic and renal panels, particularly with IV therapy, should be monitored. Periodic C&S tests or fecal ova and parasites tests may be ordered if infections are severe or are slow to resolve to confirm appropriate therapy. Periodic vision and retinal screening will be required with chloroquine therapy because the drug can cause irreversible damage to the retina. ECG monitoring may be required with some antimalarial drugs.)	• Instruct the patient on the need for periodic laboratory work. Provide a kit and instructions for home use if fecal specimens are required. • Cultures are collected *before* drug therapy is started or if started in an emergency (e.g., overwhelming infection with significant body-wide symptoms), as soon as feasibly possible, and thereafter as ordered by the health care provider. • Instruct the patient to immediately contact the provider if vision symptoms of blurring, difficulty focusing, or photophobia occur.

continued

Nursing Practice Application *continued*

IMPLEMENTATION	
Interventions and (Rationales)	**Patient-Centered Care**
• Monitor for hypersensitivity and allergic reactions, especially with the first few doses of any drug treatment. (Anaphylactic reactions are possible, particularly with the first dose. As parasites die, increasing diarrhea, abdominal pain, or chills may occur.)	• Teach the patient to immediately report any itching; rashes; swelling, particularly of tongue or face; urticaria; flushing; dizziness; syncope; wheezing; throat tightness; or difficulty breathing. Report significant increases in abdominal pain, diarrhea, chills, or fever to the health care provider.
• Continue to monitor for hepatic or renal toxicity. (Increasing fluid intake will prevent drug accumulation in the kidneys. **Lifespan:** Age-related physiological differences may place the older adult at greater risk for hepatic or renal toxicity.)	• Teach the patient to immediately report any nausea, vomiting, yellowing of the skin or sclera, abdominal pain, light or clay-colored stools, diminished urine output, or darkening of urine. • Advise the patient to increase fluid intake to 2 to 3 L per day. Alcohol use should be avoided or eliminated.
• Monitor for significant GI effects, including nausea, vomiting, and abdominal pain or cramping. Give the drug with food or milk to decrease adverse GI effects. (An antiemetic may be considered if nausea is severe. Alcohol use, especially in patients on metronidazole, may cause a disulfiram-like reaction with excessive nausea, vomiting, and possible hypotension.)	• Teach the patient to take the drug with food or milk but to avoid acidic foods and beverages, carbonated drinks, and alcohol, especially in patients on metronidazole.
• Monitor for signs and symptoms of neurologic effects (e.g., dizziness, drowsiness, and headache) and ensure patient safety. **Lifespan:** Be particularly cautious with the older adult who may be at increased risk for dizziness and falls. (Dizziness and drowsiness increase the risk for falls.)	• Teach the patient to rise from lying or sitting to standing slowly to avoid dizziness or falls and to avoid driving or other activities requiring mental alertness or physical coordination until the effects of the drug are known. If dizziness occurs, the patient should sit or lie down and not attempt to stand or walk until the sensation passes. • Instruct the hospitalized patient to call for assistance prior to getting out of bed or attempting to walk alone.
• Monitor pulse and ECG as indicated in patients on antimalarial treatment. (Some antimalarials may cause dysrhythmias and hypotension.)	• Teach the patient to promptly report any palpitations, lightheadedness, or dizziness.
• Monitor for signs and symptoms of bone marrow suppression and blood dyscrasias (e.g., low-grade fevers, bleeding, bruising, or significant fatigue). (Bone marrow suppression may cause blood dyscrasias with resulting decreases in RBCs, WBCs, and/or platelets. Periodic monitoring of CBC may be required.)	• Teach the patient to report any low-grade fevers, sore throat, rashes, bruising or increased bleeding, unusual fatigue, or shortness of breath, especially after taking drug therapy for a prolonged period.
• Assess the patient's sexual partners for infection and treat current partners to avoid reinfection. (The infection may be reintroduced by the nontreated sexual partner.)	• Have the patient notify sexual partners for assessment and treatment.
• Teach general hygiene measures to prevent reinfestation with parasites. (Families with young children should practice thorough hand washing, proper disposal of diapers, and to notify day care or child care providers of the infection. Assess for family pets that may carry infection and also require treatment. International travelers should practice scrupulous hygiene, especially in developing countries.)	• Teach the patient and family or caregiver hygiene measures, and encourage veterinary assessment of family pets, even if asymptomatic. • Encourage international travelers to consult the Centers for Disease Control and Prevention's website on "Travelers' Health" to learn the latest information about potential disease risk, preventive and treatment measures, and other valuable travel-related health information before embarking on their trip.
Patient understanding of drug therapy: Use opportunities during administration of medications and during assessments to provide patient education. (Using time during nursing care helps to optimize and reinforce key teaching areas.)	• The patient, family, or caregiver should be able to state the reason for the drug; appropriate dose and scheduling; what adverse effects to observe for and when to report; and the anticipated length of medication therapy.

Nursing Practice Application *continued*

IMPLEMENTATION

Interventions and (Rationales)	Patient-Centered Care
Patient self-administration of drug therapy: • When administering medications, instruct the patient, family, or caregiver in proper self-administration techniques followed by teach-back. (Proper administration increases the effectiveness of the drug.)	• Teach the patient to take the medication as follows: • Complete the entire course of therapy unless otherwise instructed. • Avoid or eliminate alcohol. Some medications (e.g., metronidazole) cause significant reactions when taken with alcohol, and alcohol increases adverse GI effects of many drugs. • Take the drug with food or milk and avoid acidic beverages. If instructed to take the drug on an empty stomach, take with a full glass of water. • Take the medication as evenly spaced throughout each day as feasible. • Increase overall fluid intake while taking the antibacterial drug. • Discard outdated medications or those that are no longer in use. Review the medicine cabinet twice a year for old medications.

See Tables 36.5, 36.7, and 36.8 for a list of drugs to which these nursing actions apply.

Chapter Review

KEY Concepts

The numbered key concepts provide a succinct summary of the important points from the corresponding numbered section within the chapter. If any of these points are not clear, refer to the numbered section within the chapter for review.

36.1 Most serious fungal infections occur in patients with suppressed immune defenses. The species of pathogenic fungi that attack a person with a healthy immune system are often distinct from those that infect patients who are immunocompromised.

36.2 Fungal infections are classified as systemic (affecting internal organs) or superficial (affecting hair, skin, nails, and mucous membranes).

36.3 Antibacterial medications are not effective in treating mycoses because of the physiologic differences in these organisms. Antifungal drugs target pathways that are specific to fungi.

36.4 There are relatively few drugs available for treating systemic mycoses. Systemic antifungal drugs have little or no antibacterial activity, and pharmacotherapy is sometimes continued for several months. Amphotericin B (Fungizone) is the traditional drug of choice for serious fungal infections.

36.5 The azole class is the largest and most versatile group of antifungals. These drugs have a broad spectrum and are used to treat nearly any systemic or superficial fungal infection.

36.6 Antifungal drugs to treat superficial mycoses may be given topically or orally. They exhibit few serious side effects and are effective in treating infections of the skin, nails, and mucous membranes.

36.7 Malaria is the most common protozoan disease and requires multidrug therapy owing to the complicated life cycle of the parasite. Drugs may be administered for prophylaxis, acute attacks, and prevention of relapses.

36.8 Treatment of non-*Plasmodium* protozoan disease requires a different set of medications from those used for malaria. Other protozoan diseases that may be indications for pharmacotherapy include amebiasis, toxoplasmosis, giardiasis, cryptosporidiosis, trichomoniasis, trypanosomiasis, and leishmaniasis.

36.9 Helminths are parasitic worms that cause significant disease in certain regions of the world. The goals of pharmacotherapy are to kill the parasites locally in the intestine and to disrupt their life cycle systemically in the tissues and organs they have invaded.

REVIEW Questions

1. A patient has been diagnosed with a fungal nail infection. The health care provider has prescribed griseofulvin (Fulvicin). The nurse will include which of the following in her teaching to the patient?
   1. Drug therapy will be for a very short time, probably 2 to 4 weeks.
   2. Carefully inspect all intramuscular injection sites for bruising.
   3. Notify the provider if symptoms of infection worsen.
   4. Limit fluid intake to approximately 1,000 mL/day.

2. A patient with type 2 diabetes treated with oral antidiabetic medication is receiving oral fluconazole (Diflucan) for treatment of chronic tinea cruris (jock itch). The nurse instructs the patient to monitor blood glucose levels more frequently because of what potential drug effect?
   1. Fluconazole (Diflucan) antagonizes the effects of many antidiabetic medications, causing hyperglycemia.
   2. Fluconazole (Diflucan) interacts with certain antidiabetic drugs, causing hypoglycemia.
   3. Fluconazole (Diflucan) causes hyperglycemia.
   4. Fluconazole (Diflucan) causes hypoglycemia.

3. A patient with a severe systemic fungal infection is to be given amphotericin B (Fungizone). Before starting the amphotericin infusion, the nurse premedicates the patient with acetaminophen (Tylenol), diphenhydramine (Benadryl), and prednisone (Deltasone). What is the purpose of premedicating the patient prior to the amphotericin?
   1. It delays the development of resistant fungal infections.
   2. It decreases the risk of hypersensitivity reactions to the amphotericin.
   3. It prevents hyperthermia reactions from the amphotericin.
   4. It works synergistically with the amphotericin so a lower dose may be given.

4. A patient was prescribed chloroquine (Aralen) prior to a trip to an area where malaria is known to be endemic. The nurse will instruct the patient to remain on the drug for up to 6 weeks after returning, and the patient asks why this is necessary. What is the nurse's best response?
   1. "You may be carrying microscopic malaria parasites back with you on clothes or other personal articles."
   2. "It helps prevent transmission to any of your family members."
   3. "It will prevent any mosquito that bites you from picking up the malaria infection."
   4. "It continues to kill any remaining malarial parasites that may have been acquired during the trip that are in your red blood cells."

5. A 32-year-old female patient is started on metronidazole (Flagyl) for treatment of a trichomonas vaginal infection. What must the patient eliminate from her diet for the duration she is on this medication?
   1. Caffeine
   2. Acidic juices
   3. Antacids
   4. Alcohol

6. Metronidazole (Flagyl) is being used to treat a patient's *Giardia lamblia* infection, a protozoan infection of the intestines. Which of the following are appropriate to teach this patient? (Select all that apply.)
   1. Metronidazole may leave a metallic taste in the mouth.
   2. The urine may turn dark amber brown while on the medication.
   3. The metronidazole may be discontinued once the diarrhea subsides to minimize adverse effects.
   4. Taking the metronidazole with food reduces GI upset.
   5. Current sexual partners do not require treatment for this infection.

PATIENT-FOCUSED Case Study

Jessica Treadway is a 23-year-old patient, recently diagnosed with type-1 diabetes for which she has been prescribed insulin. She developed a vaginal discharge and made an appointment with her provider. She was diagnosed with a vaginal yeast infection with *Candida albicans* and prescribed fluconazole (Diflucan) topically for the infection.

1. Why do you think that Jessica is at risk for this type of infection?
2. What patient teaching will she need regarding this treatment?

CRITICAL THINKING Questions

1. A nurse is caring for a severely immunosuppressed patient who is on IV amphotericin B (Fungizone). The nurse understands that this medication is highly toxic to the patient. What are three priority nursing assessment areas for patients on this medication?
2. A patient is traveling to Africa for 3 months and is requesting a prescription for Malarone to prevent malaria. What premedication assessment must be done for this patient?

Visit www.pearsonhighered.com/nursingresources for answers and rationales for all activities.

REFERENCE

Herdman, T. H., & Kamitsuru, S. (2014). *NANDA International nursing diagnoses: Definitions and classification, 2015–2017*. Oxford, United Kingdom: Wiley-Blackwell.

SELECTED BIBLIOGRAPHY

Bennet, J. E. (2011). Antifungal agents. In L. L. Brunton, B. A. Chabner, & B. C. Knollman (Eds.), *Goodman and Gilman's the pharmacological basis of therapeutics* (12th ed., pp. 1571–1592). New York, NY: McGraw-Hill.

Brown, T., & Dresser, L. (2014). Superficial fungal infections. In J. T. De Piro (Ed.), *Pharmacotherapy: A pathophysiologic approach* (9th ed., pp. 1911–1930). New York, NY: McGraw-Hill.

Carver, P. L. (2014). Invasive fungal infections. In J. T. De Piro (Ed.), *Pharmacotherapy: A pathophysiologic approach* (9th ed., pp. 1931–1962). New York, NY: McGraw-Hill.

Cecinati, V., Guastadisegni, C., Russo, F. G., & Brescia, L. P. (2013). Antifungal therapy in children: An update. *European Journal of Pediatrics, 172*, 437–446. doi:10.1007/s00431-012-1758-9

Centers for Disease Control and Prevention. (n.d.). *Travelers' Health*. Retrieved from http://wwwnc.cdc.gov/travel

Centers for Disease Control and Prevention. (2015). *Parasites: Giardia*. Retrieved from http://www.cdc.gov/parasites/giardia/infection-sources.html

Centers for Disease Control and Prevention. (2014). *Sources of fungal eye infections*. Retrieved from http://www.cdc.gov/fungal/diseases/fungal-eye-infections/sources.html

Centers for Disease Control and Prevention. (2015). *Malaria*. Retrieved from http://www.cdc.gov/malaria/

de Sa., D. C., Lamas, A. P., & Tosti, A. (2014). Oral therapy for onychomycosis: An evidence-based review. *American Journal of Clinical Dermatology, 15*, 17–36. doi:10.1007/s40257-013-0056-2

Dhawan, V. K. (2015). *Amebiasis*. Retrieved from http://emedicine.medscape.com/article/212029-overview

Gupta, A. K., & Simpson, F. C. (2014). New pharmacotherapy for the treatment of onychomycosis: An update. *Expert Opinion on Pharmacotherapy, 16*, 227–236. doi:10.1517/14656566.2015 993380

Hidalgo, J. A. (2014). *Candidiasis*. Retrieved from http://emedicine.medscape.com/article/213853-overview

Nilles, E. J., & Arguin, P. M. (2012). Imported malaria: An update. *American Journal of Emergency Medicine, 30*, 972–980. doi:10.1016/j.ajem.2011.06.016

Phillips, M. A., & Stanley, S. L. (2011). Chemotherapy of protozoal infections: Amebiasis, giardiasis, trichomoniasis, trypanosomiasis, leishmaniasis and other protozoal infections. In L. L. Brunton, B. A. Chabner, & B. C. Knollman (Eds.), *Goodman and Gilman's the pharmacological basis of therapeutics* (12th ed., pp. 1419–1442). New York, NY: McGraw-Hill.

Scheinfeld, N. S. (2015). *Cutaneous candidiasis*. Retrieved from http://emedicine.medscape.com/article/1090632-overview#a0101

Tosti, A. (2015). *Onychomycosis*. Retrieved from http://emedicine.medscape.com/article/1105828-overview

Tragiannidis, A., Tsoulas, C., Kerl, K., & Groll, A. H. (2013). Invasive candidiasis: Update on current pharmacotherapy options and future perspectives. *Expert Opinion on Pharmacotherapy, 14*(11), 1515–1528. doi:10.1517/14656566.2013.805204

Vinetz, J. M., Clain, J., Bounkeua, V., Eastman, R. T., & Fidock, D. T. (2011). Chemotherapy of malaria. In L. L. Brunton, B. A. Chabner, & B. C. Knollman (Eds.), *Goodman and Gilman's the pharmacological basis of therapeutics* (12th ed., pp. 1383–1418). New York, NY: McGraw-Hill.

World Health Organization. (2014). *Malaria*. Retrieved from http://www.who.int/mediacentre/factsheets/fs094/en/

Chapter 37

Drugs for Viral Infections

Drugs at a Glance

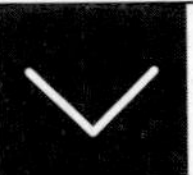

Learning Outcomes

After reading this chapter, the student should be able to:

1. Describe the major characteristics of viruses.
2. Identify viral infections that benefit from pharmacotherapy.
3. Explain the purpose and expected outcomes of HIV pharmacotherapy.
4. Explain the advantages of highly active antiretroviral therapy (HAART) in the pharmacotherapy of HIV infection.
5. Describe the nurse's role in the pharmacologic management of patients receiving medications for HIV, herpesviruses, influenza viruses, and hepatitis viruses.
6. For each of the classes listed in Drugs at a Glance, know representative drugs, and explain the mechanism of drug action, primary actions, and important adverse effects.
7. Use the nursing process to care for patients receiving pharmacotherapy for viral infections.

(pill icon) indicates a prototype drug, each of which is featured in a Prototype Drug box.

VIRUSES

Viruses are tiny infectious agents capable of causing disease in humans and other organisms. After infecting an organism, viruses use host enzymes and cellular structures to replicate. Although the number of antiviral drugs has increased dramatically because of research into the AIDS epidemic, antivirals remain the least effective of all the anti-infective drug classes.

37.1 Characteristics of Viruses

Viruses are nonliving agents that infect bacteria, plants, and animals. Viruses contain none of the cellular organelles necessary for self-survival that are present in living organisms. In fact, the structure of viruses is quite primitive compared with that of even the simplest cell. Surrounded by a protective protein coat, or **capsid,** a virus possesses only a few dozen genes, either in the form of ribonucleic acid (RNA) or deoxyribonucleic acid (DNA), that contain the necessary information needed for viral replication. Some viruses also have a lipid envelope that surrounds the capsid. The viral envelope contains glycoprotein and protein "spikes" that are recognized as foreign by the host's immune system and trigger body defenses to remove the invader. A mature infective particle is called a **virion.** Figure 37.1 shows the basic structure of the human immunodeficiency virus (HIV).

Although nonliving and structurally simple, viruses are capable of remarkable feats. They infect their host by locating and entering a target cell and then using the machinery inside that cell to replicate. Thus, viruses are **intracellular parasites:** They must be inside a host cell to cause infection. Virions do, however, bring along a few enzymes that assist the pathogen in duplicating its genetic material, inserting its genes into the host's chromosome, and assembling newly

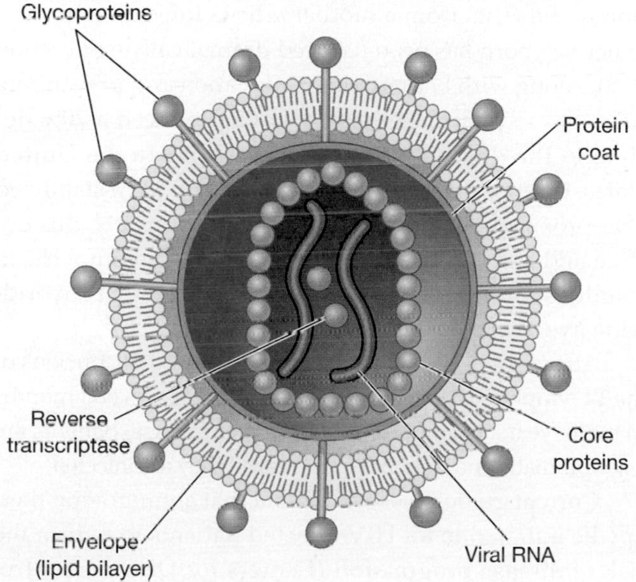

FIGURE 37.1 Structure of HIV

PharmFacts

VIRAL INFECTIONS

- Of the 1.2 million Americans living with HIV infection, almost 1 in 7 are unaware they are infected.
- About 16% of the U.S. population is infected with genital herpes: the infection is twice as common in women than in men.
- Approximately 800,000 to 1.4 million individuals in the United States are living with chronic hepatitis B infection. About 2,000 to 4,000 deaths are attributed to this disease annually.
- Chronic hepatitis C infection is the leading cause of liver transplantation.
- Although men who have sex with men comprise only about 4% of the male population in the United States, about 63% of all new genital herpes infections occur in this group.
- Since the beginning of AIDS, more than 600,000 Americans have died of this disease.

formed virions. These unique viral enzymes sometimes serve as important targets for antiviral drug action.

The host organism and cell are often very specific; it may be a single species of plant, bacteria, or animal, or even a single type of cell within that species. Most often viruses infect only one species, although cases have been documented in which viruses mutated and crossed species, as is likely the case for HIV.

Many viral infections, such as the rhinoviruses that cause the common cold, are self-limiting and require no medical intervention. Although symptoms may be annoying, they resolve in 7 to 10 days, and the virus causes no permanent effects if the patient is otherwise healthy. Some viral infections, however, require drug therapy to prevent the infection or to alleviate symptoms. For example, HIV is uniformly fatal if left untreated. The hepatitis B virus can cause permanent liver damage and increase a patient's risk of hepatocellular carcinoma. Although not life threatening in most patients, herpesviruses can cause significant pain and, in the case of ocular herpes, permanent disability.

Antiviral pharmacotherapy can be extremely challenging because of the rapid mutation rate of viruses, which can quickly render drugs ineffective. Also complicating therapy is the intracellular nature of the virus, which makes it difficult to eliminate the pathogen without giving excessively high doses of drugs that injure normal cells. Antiviral drugs have narrow spectrums of activity, usually limited to one specific virus. The three basic strategies used for antiviral pharmacotherapy are as follows:

- Prevent viral infections through the administration of vaccines (see chapter 34).
- Treat active infections with drugs such as acyclovir (Zovirax) that interrupt an aspect of the virus's replication cycle.

- For prophylaxis, use drugs that boost the patient's immune response (immunostimulants) so that the virus remains in latency with the patient symptom free.

HIV-AIDS

Acquired immune deficiency syndrome (AIDS) is characterized by profound immunosuppression that leads to opportunistic infections and malignancies not commonly found in patients with healthy immune defenses. Antiretroviral drugs slow the growth of the causative agent for AIDS, the **human immunodeficiency virus (HIV),** by several mechanisms. Resistance to these drugs is a major clinical problem, and a pharmacologic cure for **HIV-AIDS** is not yet achievable.

37.2 Replication of HIV

Infection with HIV occurs by exposure to contaminated body fluids, most commonly blood or semen. Transmission may occur through sexual activity (oral, anal, or vaginal) or through contact of infected fluids with broken skin, mucous membranes, or needlesticks. Newborns can receive the virus during birth or from breast-feeding.

Shortly after entry into the body, the virus attaches to its preferred target—the **CD4 receptor** on T4 (helper) lymphocytes. During this early stage, structural proteins on the surface of HIV fuse with the CD4 receptor. Coreceptors known as CCR5 and CXCR4 have been discovered that assist HIV in binding to the T4 lymphocyte.

The virus uncoats and the genetic material of HIV, single-stranded RNA, enters the host cell. HIV converts its RNA strands to double-stranded DNA, using the viral enzyme **reverse transcriptase.** The viral DNA eventually enters the nucleus of the T4 lymphocyte where it becomes incorporated into the host's chromosomes. This action is performed by HIV **integrase,** another enzyme unique to HIV. It may remain in the host DNA for many years before it becomes activated to begin producing more viral particles. The new virions eventually bud from the host cell and enter the bloodstream. The new virions, however, are not yet infectious. As a final step, the viral enzyme **protease** cleaves some of the proteins associated with the HIV DNA, enabling the virion to infect other T4 lymphocytes. Once budding occurs, the immune system recognizes that the cell is infected and kills the T4 lymphocyte. Unfortunately, it is too late; a patient who is infected with HIV may produce as many as 10 billion new virions every day, and the patient's devastated immune system is unable to remove them. Knowledge of the replication cycle of HIV is critical to understanding the pharmacotherapy of HIV-AIDS, as shown in Pharmacotherapy Illustrated 37.1.

Only a few viruses such as HIV are able to use reverse transcriptase to construct DNA from RNA; no bacteria, plants, or animals are able to perform this unique metabolic function. All living organisms make RNA from DNA. Because of their "backward" or reverse synthesis, these viruses are called retroviruses, and drugs used to treat HIV infections are called **antiretrovirals.** Progression of HIV to AIDS is characterized by gradual destruction of the immune system, as measured by the decline in the number of CD4 T-lymphocytes. Unfortunately, the CD4 T-lymphocyte is the primary cell coordinating the immune response. When the CD4 T-cell count falls below a certain level, the patient begins to experience opportunistic bacterial, fungal, and viral infections and certain malignancies. A point is reached at which the patient is unable to mount any immune defenses, and death ensues.

37.3 General Principles of HIV Pharmacotherapy

The widespread appearance of HIV infection in 1981 created enormous challenges for public health and an unprecedented need for the development of new antiviral drugs. HIV-AIDS is unlike any other infectious disease because it is most often sexually transmitted, is uniformly fatal, and demands a continuous supply of new drugs for patient survival. The challenges of HIV-AIDS have resulted in the development of over 20 new antiretroviral drugs. Unfortunately, the initial hopes of curing HIV-AIDS through antiretroviral therapy or vaccines have not been realized; none of these drugs produces a cure for this disease. Stopping antiretroviral therapy almost always results in a rapid rebound in HIV replication. HIV mutates extremely rapidly, and resistant strains develop so quickly that the creation of novel approaches to antiretroviral drug therapy must remain an ongoing process.

Although pharmacotherapy for HIV-AIDS has not produced a cure, it has resulted in a number of therapeutic successes. For example, many patients with HIV infection are able to live symptom free with the disease for a longer time because of medications. Furthermore, the transmission of the virus from a mother who is infected with HIV to her newborn has been reduced dramatically (see section 37.8). Along with better patient education and prevention, successes in pharmacotherapy have produced a 70% decline in the death rate due to HIV-AIDS in the United States. Overall deaths due to the infection have stabilized at approximately 50,000 annually. Unfortunately, this decline and stabilization has not been observed in African countries: About 70% of people infected with HIV worldwide live in sub-Saharan Africa.

After HIV incorporates its viral DNA into the nucleus of the T4 lymphocyte, it may remain dormant for several months to many years. During this chronic **latent phase,** patients are asymptomatic and may not even realize they are infected.

Current guidelines recommend that antiretroviral therapy be initiated in all HIV-infected patients to reduce the risk of disease progression (Centers for Disease Control and Prevention (CDC), 2014). Starting therapy immediately

Pharmacotherapy Illustrated

37.1 | Replication of HIV

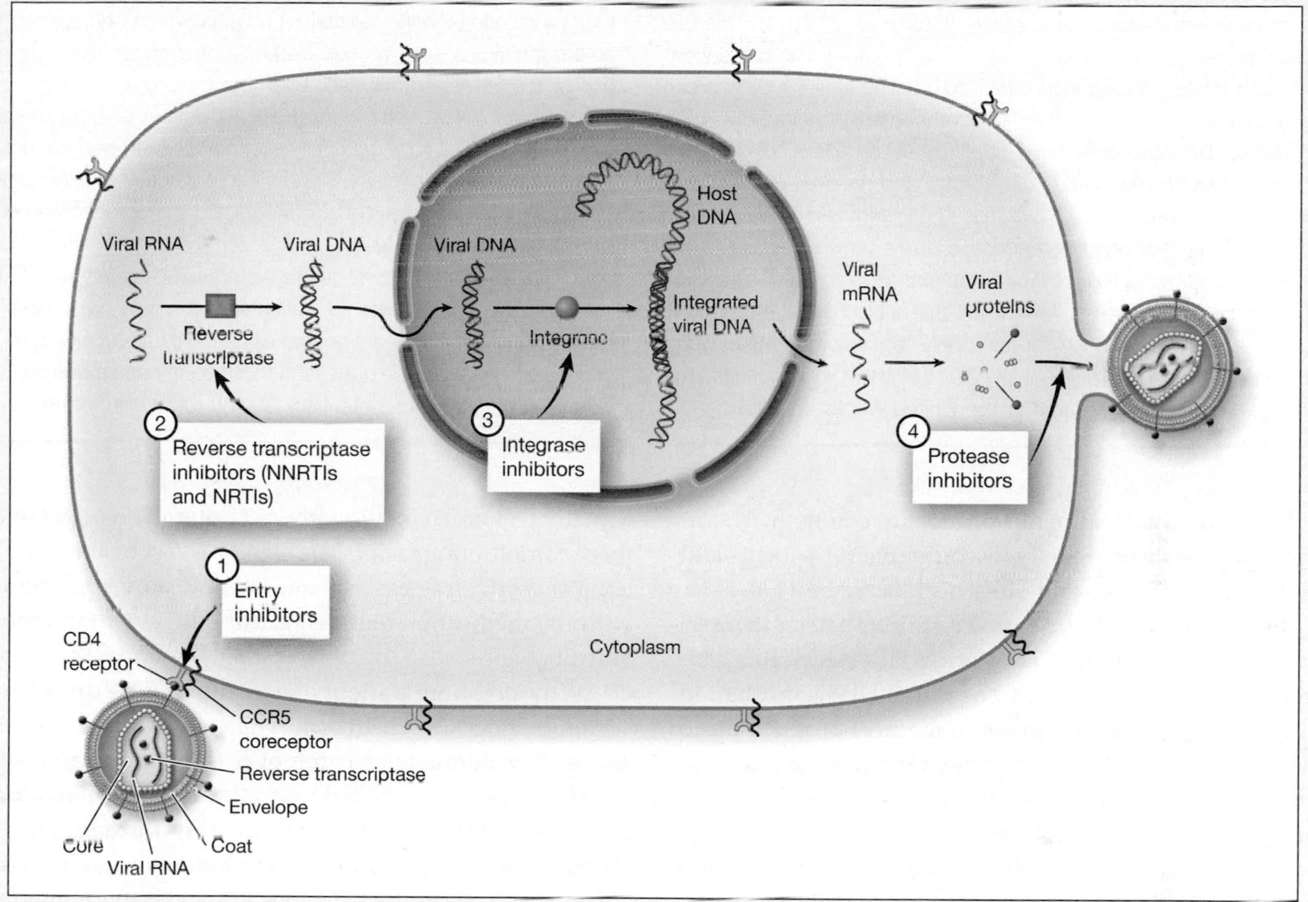

after diagnosis can reduce the number of virions in the blood and thus delay the onset of acute symptoms and the progression to AIDS.

The decision to begin treatment immediately after diagnosis has certain negative consequences. Drugs for HIV-AIDS are expensive; treatment with some of the newer agents costs as much as $60,000 per year. These drugs produce a number of uncomfortable and potentially serious adverse effects that lower the quality of life for the patient. Continuous pharmacotherapy over many years promotes viral resistance.

The therapeutic goals for the pharmacotherapy of HIV-AIDS include the following:

- Reduce HIV-related morbidity and prolong the duration and quality of survival
- Restore and preserve immunologic function
- Promote maximum suppression of plasma HIV viral load
- Prevent HIV transmission.

Two laboratory tests used to monitor the progress of pharmacotherapy of HIV are absolute CD4 T-cell count and measurement of HIV RNA in the plasma. The number of CD4 T-cells is an important indicator of immune function and predicts the likelihood of opportunistic disease and the need for prophylactic antibiotic therapy; however, it does not indicate how rapidly HIV is replicating. CD4 counts are performed every 3 to 6 months to assess the degree of effectiveness of antiretroviral therapy.

Viral load is determined by measuring the amount of HIV RNA in the blood. Viral load is the most important indicator of how the virus is responding to antiretroviral therapy. After the initial measurement, viral load is determined regularly to determine the effectiveness of pharmacotherapy, especially if a treatment regimen is modified or if treatment failure occurs. The goal of antiretroviral therapy is to reduce plasma HIV RNA to less than 75 copies/mL. For most patients, 12 to 24 weeks of HIV pharmacotherapy is required to achieve this level.

Antiretroviral therapy does not totally eliminate the virus from the body, and treatment must continue for the lifetime of the HIV-infected patient. Given the high mutation rate of the virus and decades of therapy, it is easy to

Treating the Diverse Patient: Test-and-Treat Strategies for HIV Prevention

In the HIV Prevention Trials Network (HPTN) 052 study in 2011, early antiretroviral therapy after diagnosis of HIV was shown to decrease HIV viral load and significantly lessen the chance for transmission of the virus to others (Cohen et al., 2011). This has subsequently come to be known as a "treatment as prevention" (TasP) strategy (Nachenga et al., 2014). The earlier a patient can be identified as having HIV infection, the earlier treatment can be started. Because early signs of HIV infection often include flulike symptoms of fever, chills, sore throat, and malaise, patients may not seek treatment until the disease has progressed.

Despite demonstrated success, there remain barriers to the TasP strategy to reduce HIV infections and thus, transmission (Kulkami, Shah, Sarma, & Mahajan, 2013; Nachenga et al., 2014). Patients who feel healthy or have only vague symptoms may not seek treatment or may not believe treatment is needed at this time. Health care systems in the United States and throughout the world may not be equipped for large-scale testing and the follow-through necessary to ensure that each positive individual receives the appropriate drug therapy. Patients may stop taking their medications, especially when adverse effects occur. Vulnerable populations such as sex workers, intravenous (IV) drug users, or the homeless may lack even basic access to health care to seek and obtain testing. In addition the cost of drug therapy may be prohibitive for a patient or even for a health department or international health ministry. Nurses can advocate for HIV testing for all patients, regardless of risk factors, to help increase the number of patients having testing and lessen the stigma. Nurses can also advocate for improved health systems and "safety nets," i.e., settings that provide care for patients who would not otherwise have access to health care so that all patients can receive testing. Nurses can also provide education to increase patient compliance with drug therapy, thus potentially altering the course of HIV.

understand why treatment failures are common. Therapeutic failures are extremely discouraging for patients and challenging for nurses and other health care providers.

Drug resistance has become a serious barrier to pharmacotherapeutic success in treating HIV-AIDS. It is estimated that 6% to 16% of all transmitted HIV is resistant to at least one class of antiretroviral medications, and up to 8% of transmitted HIV has resistance to more than one drug class (Panel on Antiretroviral Guidelines for Adults and Adolescents, 2015). HIV drug resistance testing is now recommended when first diagnosed with HIV infection and when viral load measurements suggest that pharmacotherapy is becoming less effective. When standard therapies fail, viral resistance must always be considered as a potential source of the failure. Genotypic drug testing identifies specific mutations in viral genes that are associated with drug resistance for the different classes of HIV medications. This gentotypic testing assists in determining which drugs(s) would be most effective for each patient. If a strain of HIV in a patient is determined to have a mutation that makes it resistant to one class of antiviral medications, another class is substituted.

Antiretroviral drugs may cause many adverse effects, including nausea, diarrhea, rash, lipid abnormalities, hepatotoxicity, neuropathy, and increased risk of cardiovascular events. Patients always take at least two of these drugs (and usually more), which often interact with other medications to cause additional adverse effects. Serious adverse effects often require an immediate change in pharmacotherapy.

To be successful, antiretroviral therapy requires strict patient compliance with a complex regimen. Unfortunately, many factors deter patients from compliance. Some antiretroviral drugs have inconvenient schedules and must be taken three to four times per day or be given parenterally. Others make the patient feel quite ill; patients may actually feel much better without taking the drugs. Given these complicating factors, and the prospect of a lifetime of drug therapy, it is easy to understand why compliance with the medication regimen is difficult, even for a motivated patient.

Why do some patients succumb to HIV infections within months after diagnosis, while others survive for decades? Considerable research over three decades has focused on genetic factors that have allowed some individuals to live with HIV for a long time without progressing to AIDS. These patients are known as long-term nonprogressors (LTNPs). Scientists have looked for specific antibodies, cytokines, and protective immune responses in these patients with the hope of developing therapies to help other infected patients. While some progress has been made in this area, researchers are far from understanding the protective genetic makeup of these LTNPs. Until knowledge advances, HIV infection will continue to be potentially fatal in every patient who acquires the infection.

DRUGS FOR TREATING HIV-AIDS

37.4 Classification of Drugs for HIV-AIDS

Antiretroviral drugs target specific phases of the HIV replication cycle. The standard pharmacotherapy for HIV-AIDS includes aggressive treatment with multiple drugs concurrently, a regimen called **highly active antiretroviral therapy (HAART).** The goal of HAART is to reduce the plasma HIV RNA to its lowest possible level. It must be understood, however, that HIV is harbored in locations other than the blood, such as lymph nodes; therefore,

Table 37.1 Antiretroviral Drugs for HIV-AIDS

Drug	Route and Adult Dose (max dose where indicated)	Adverse Effects
NONNUCLEOSIDE REVERSE TRANSCRIPTASE INHIBITORS		
delavirdine (Rescriptor)	PO: 400 mg tid (max: 1,200 mg/day)	*Rash, fever, nausea, diarrhea, headache, stomatitis*
efavirenz (Sustiva)	PO: 600 mg/day (max: 600 mg/day)	
etravirine (Intelence)	PO: 200 mg bid (max: 400 mg/day)	Paresthesia, hepatotoxicity, Stevens–Johnson syndrome, central nervous system (CNS) toxicity (efavirenz), increased rsik for depressive disorders (rilpivirine)
nevirapine (Viramune)	PO: 200 mg once daily for 14 days; then increase to bid	
rilpivirine (Edurant)	PO: 25 mg once daily	
NUCLEOSIDE AND NUCLEOTIDE REVERSE TRANSCRIPTASE INHIBITORS		
abacavir (Ziagen)	PO: 300 mg bid (max: 600 mg/day)	*Fatigue, generalized weakness, myalgia, nausea, headache, abdominal pain, vomiting, anorexia, rash*
didanosine (ddI, Videx)	PO: 125–300 mg bid	
emtricitabine (Emtriva, FTC)	PO: 200 mg/day (max: 200 mg/day)	
lamivudine (Epivir, 3TC)	PO: 150 mg bid (max: 300 mg/day)	Bone marrow suppression, neutropenia, anemia, granulocytopenia, lactic acidosis with steatorrhea, peripheral neuropathy (stavudine), pancreatitis (lamivudine), hypersensitivity reactions (abacavir), Fanconi syndrome (tenofovir)
stavudine (d4T, Zerit)	PO: 40 mg bid (max: 80 mg/day)	
tenofovir (TDF, Viread)	PO: 300 mg/day	
zidovudine (AZT, Retrovir)	PO: 300 mg bid or 200 mg tid	
	IV: 1–2 mg/kg q4h (1,200 mg/day)	
PROTEASE INHIBITORS		
atazanavir (Reyataz)	PO: 400 mg/day; 300 mg/day with 100 mg/day ritonavir; 300 mg/day with 150 mg cobicstat (Evotaz)	*Nausea, vomiting, diarrhea, abdominal pain, headache*
darunavir (Prezista)	PO: 800 mg with 100 mg bid ritonavir; 800 mg/day with 150 mg/day cobicstat (Prezcobix)	Anemia, leukopenia, deep venous thrombosis, pancreatitis, lymphadenopathy, hemorrhagic colitis, nephrolithiasis (indinavir), increased bilirubin and serum cholesterol (atazanavir), thrombocytopenia (saquinavir), pancytopenia (saquinavir), Stevens–Johnson syndrome (darunavir), hepatotoxicity (darunavir, ritonavir, tipranavir); new onset diabetes (fosamprenavir), intracranial hemorrhage (tipranavir)
fosamprenavir (Lexiva)	PO: 700–1,400 mg bid; 700–1,400 mg daily with 100–200 mg ritonavir daily	
indinavir (Crixivan)	PO: 800 mg tid	
lopinavir/ritonavir (Kaletra)	PO: 400/100 mg bid; increase dose to 500/125 mg bid, with concurrent efavirenz, fosamprenavir, nelfinavir, or nevirapine	
nelfinavir (Viracept)	PO: 750 mg tid	
ritonavir (Norvir)	PO: 600 mg bid (max: 12,000 mg/day)	
saquinavir (Invirase)	PO: 1000 mg bid taken with 100 mg ritonavir bid	
tipranavir (Aptivus)	PO: 500 mg/day taken with 200 mg of ritonavir bid	
FUSION AND INTEGRASE INHIBITORS		
dolutegravir (DTG, Tivicay)	PO: 50 mg once daily	*Pain and inflammation at the injection site (enfuvirtide), nausea, diarrhea, fatigue, abdominal pain, cough, dizziness, musculoskeletal symptoms, pyrexia, rash, upper respiratory tract infections*
elvitegravir (Vitekta): only administered concurrently with cobicistat, tenofovir, and emtricitabine	PO: 85–150 mg/day	
enfuvirtide (Fuzeon)	Subcutaneous: 90 mg bid	Hepatotoxicity, myocardial infarction, hypersensitivity, neutropenia, thrombocytopenia, nephrotoxicity (enfuvirtide), myopathy (raltegravir), Fanconi syndrome (elvitegravir)
maraviroc (Selzentry)	PO: 150–600 mg bid (max: 1,200 mg/day)	
raltegravir (Isentress)	PO: 400 mg bid (max: 800 mg/day)	

Note: *Italics* indicate common adverse effects; underlining indicates serious adverse effects.

elimination of the virus from the blood is not a cure. The simultaneous use of drugs from several classes reduces the probability that HIV will become resistant to treatment. These drugs are listed in Table 37.1.

HIV-AIDS antiretrovirals are classified into the following groups, based on their mechanisms of action:

- Nucleoside/nucleotide reverse transcriptase inhibitors (NRTIs/NtRTIs)
- Nonnucleoside reverse transcriptase inhibitors (NNRTIs)
- Protease inhibitors (PIs)
- Entry inhibitors (includes fusion inhibitors and CCR5 antagonists)
- Integrase inhibitors and other miscellaneous antivirals.

Throughout the AIDS epidemic, pharmacotherapeutic regimens for treating the infection have continuously evolved.

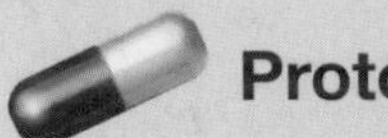

Prototype Drug | Zidovudine *(Retrovir, AZT)*

Therapeutic Class: Antiretroviral **Pharmacologic Class:** Nucleoside reverse transcriptase inhibitor (NRTI)

Actions and Uses

Zidovudine was first discovered in the 1960s, and its antiviral activity was demonstrated prior to the AIDS epidemic. Structurally, it resembles thymidine, one of the four nucleoside building blocks of DNA. As the reverse transcriptase enzyme begins to synthesize viral DNA, it mistakenly uses zidovudine as one of the nucleosides, thus creating a defective DNA strand. Zidovudine is used in combination with other antiretrovirals for symptomatic and asymptomatic patients who are infected with HIV. This combination is also used for postexposure prophylaxis in health care workers who have been exposed to HIV (see section 37.9). An important indication is reduction of the risk of transmission rate of HIV from a mother who is HIV positive to her fetus.

Because of the drugs' widespread use since the beginning of the AIDS epidemic, resistant HIV strains have become common. Most treatment guidelines do not include zidovudine as a drug of first choice due to the potential for resistance. Combination products containing zidovudine include Combivir (zidovudine and lamivudine) and Trizivir (zidovudine, lamivudine, and abacavir).

Administration Alerts

- Administer on an empty stomach with a full glass of water.
- Avoid administering with fruit juice.
- Pregnancy category C.

PHARMACOKINETICS

Onset	Peak	Duration
1–2 h	1–2 h	Unknown

Adverse Effects

Many patients experience fatigue and generalized weakness, anorexia, nausea, and diarrhea. Headache will occur in the majority of patients who are taking zidovudine, and more serious CNS effects have been reported.

Black Box Warning: Rare cases of fatal lactic acidosis with hepatomegaly and steatosis have been reported with zidovudine use. Bone marrow suppression may result in neutropenia or severe anemia. Myopathy may occur with long-term use.

Contraindications: Hypersensitivity to the drug is the only contraindication. Because the drug can suppress bone marrow function, it should be used with caution in patients with pre-existing anemia or neutropenia. Blood counts and other laboratory blood tests should be monitored frequently during therapy to prevent hematologic toxicity. Patients with significant renal or hepatic impairment require a reduction in dosage, because zidovudine may accumulate to toxic levels in these patients.

Interactions

Drug-Drug: Zidovudine interacts with many drugs. Concurrent administration with other drugs that depress bone marrow function, such as ganciclovir, interferon alfa, dapsone, flucytosine, or vincristine should be avoided due to cumulative immunosuppression. The following drugs may increase the risk of AZT toxicity: atovaquone, amphotericin B, aspirin, doxorubicin, fluconazole, methadone, and valproic acid. Use with other antiretroviral agents may cause lactic acidosis and severe hepatomegaly with steatosis.

Lab Tests: Mean corpuscular volume may be increased during zidovudine therapy. White blood cell (WBC) and hemoglobin (Hgb) may decrease due to neutropenia and anemia, respectively.

Herbal/Food: Use with caution with herbal supplements, such as St. John's wort, which may cause a decrease in antiretroviral activity.

Treatment of Overdose: There is no specific treatment for overdose.

The regimens are often different for patients who are receiving these drugs for the first time (treatment *naïve*) versus patients who have been taking antiretrovirals for months or years (treatment *experienced*). In current clinical practice, the most successful regimens consist of three medications given concurrently: two NRTIs (one of which is emtricitabine or lamivudine) plus one NNRTI, enhanced PI, or integrase inhibitor. The following are currently recommended regimens (Panel on Antiretroviral Guidelines for Adults and Adolescents, 2015):

- Integrase inhibitor-based regimens
  - dolutegravir + abacavir + lamivudine
  - dolutegravir + tenofovir + emtricitabine
  - elvitegravir (with cobicistat) + tenofovir + emtricitabine
  - raltegravir + tenofovir + emtricitabine
- PI-based regimen
  - darunavir (ritonavir-boosted) + tenofovir + emtricitabine

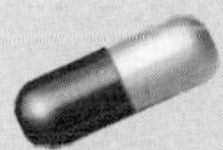

Prototype Drug | Efavirenz *(Sustiva)*

Therapeutic Class: Antiretroviral **Pharmacologic Class:** Nonnucleoside reverse transcriptase inhibitor (NNRTI)

Actions and Uses

Efavirenz is given orally (PO) in combination with other antiretrovirals in the treatment of HIV infection. The drug acts by inhibiting reverse transcriptase. It has the advantage of once-daily dosing and penetration into cerebrospinal fluid. Efavirenz is a preferred drug for the initial therapy of HIV infection.

Resistance to NNRTIs can develop rapidly, and cross resistance among drugs in this class can occur. High-fat meals increase the absorption by as much as 50% and may cause toxicity. Atripla is a fixed-dose combination of three antiretroviral drugs: efavirenz, emtricitabine, and tenofovir.

Administration Alerts

- Administer on an empty stomach.
- Administer at bedtime to limit adverse CNS effects.
- Pregnancy category C.

PHARMACOKINETICS

Onset	Peak	Duration
Rapid	3–5 h	24 h

Adverse Effects

CNS adverse effects are observed in at least 50% of the patients when first initiating therapy, including sleep disorders, nightmares, dizziness, reduced ability to concentrate, and delusions. These symptoms gradually diminish after 3–4 weeks of therapy. Like other drugs in this class, rash is common and must be monitored carefully to prevent the development of severe blistering or desquamation.

Contraindications: Efavirenz is a known teratogen in laboratory animals, causing neural tube defects and must not be given to patients who may become pregnant. If a patient taking efavirenz presents for prenatal care after the first 4-6 weeks of pregnancy, efavirenz may be continued. Patients in their child-bearing years should be advised to use reliable methods of birth control to avoid pregnancy.

Interactions

Drug–Drug: Patients who are receiving antiepileptic medications metabolized by the liver—such as carbamazepine, phenytoin, and phenobarbital—may require periodic monitoring of plasma levels because efavirenz may increase the incidence of seizures. Efavirenz can decrease serum levels of the following: statins, methadone, sertraline, and calcium channel blockers. The CNS adverse effects of efavirenz are worsened if the patient takes psychotropic drugs or consumes alcohol. Levels of warfarin may either increase or decrease.

Lab Tests: Efavirenz may give false-positive results for the presence of marijuana. It may increase serum lipid values.

Herbal/Food: St. John's wort may cause a decrease in antiretroviral activity.

Treatment of Overdose: There is no specific treatment for overdose.

Clearly, the pharmacotherapy of HIV-AIDS is rapidly evolving. Many of the initial clinical trials for these medications included very small numbers of patients, and health care providers are still learning which drug combinations are most effective. Nurses should always review the latest medical literature before treating patients with HIV-AIDS.

Drug manufacturers have responded to the need for simpler treatment regimens by combining several medications into a single capsule or tablet. Combinations include Atripla (efavirenz + emtricitabine + tenofovir), Combivir (lamivudine + zidovudine), Complera (emtricitabine + rilpivirene + tenofovir), Epzicom (abacavir + lamivudine), Stribild (emtricitabine + tenofovir + elvitegravir + cobicistat), Trizivir (abacavir + lamivudine + zidovudine), Triumeq (abacavir + dolutgravir + lamivudine) and Truvada (emtricitabine + tenofovir). These once- or twice-daily tablets lower the pill burden and likely improve patient compliance with complicated regimens.

Although no drug or drug combination has yet been found to cure HIV-AIDS, some progress has been made on its prevention. Truvada (emtricitabine + tenofovir) has been found to reduce the risk of acquiring HIV infection and may be recommended for people at very high risk for the disease. It is important for patients to be taught, however, that this drug is not 100% effective, and that it should not replace established methods for HIV prevention such as abstinence, the use of condoms, or other safe sex measures.

Reverse Transcriptase Inhibitors

Reverse transcriptase inhibitors are drugs that are structurally similar to nucleosides, the building blocks of DNA. There are three types of reverse transcriptase inhibitors: nucleoside reverse transcriptors (NRTIs), nonnucleoside

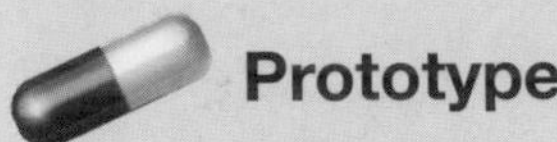

Prototype Drug | Lopinavir With Ritonavir *(Kaletra)*

Therapeutic Class: Antiretroviral **Pharmacologic Class:** Protease inhibitor

Actions and Uses

Kaletra is a combination drug containing the PIs lopinavir and ritonavir. Lopinavir is the active component of the combination. The small amount of ritonavir inhibits the hepatic breakdown of lopinavir, thus permitting serum levels of lopinavir to increase by more than 100-fold. Kaletra has an extended half-life that allows for once- or twice-daily dosing.

Resistance to lopinavir/ritonavir has been reported in patients treated with other PIs prior to Kaletra therapy. Kaletra is a preferred drug for the initial therapy of HIV infection.

Administration Alerts

- The oral solution form should be taken with food to enhance absorption. Tablets may be taken with or without food.
- Pregnancy category C.

PHARMACOKINETICS

Onset	Peak	Duration
Rapid	3–4 h	12 h

Adverse Effects

Kaletra is well tolerated, with the most frequently reported problem being diarrhea. Headache and GI-related effects are common, including nausea, vomiting, dyspepsia, and abdominal pain. Hyperglycemia has been reported, and Kaletra may cause or worsen symptoms of diabetes mellitus. Lipodystrophy syndrome occurs in many patients receiving long-term therapy with PIs. Large increases in total cholesterol and triglycerides may occur during therapy. Pancreatitis is a rare, though potentially fatal, adverse event.

Contraindications: Patients with liver impairment, especially those with pre-existing viral hepatitis, should be carefully monitored. Hepatic enzyme levels should be regularly evaluated in these patients to prevent hepatic failure. Patients with diabetes should be monitored regularly because Kaletra may exacerbate this condition. Kaletra should be used with caution in patients with cardiac disease because the drug can prolong the PR interval and cause third-degree heart block. Breast-feeding is contraindicated due to the potential risk of transmitting HIV to the newborn.

Interactions

Drug–Drug: Lopinavir is extensively metabolized by hepatic enzymes, and drugs that undergo hepatic metabolism may interact with Kaletra. Drugs that may *reduce* the effectiveness of the antiretroviral include nevirapine, efavirenz, barbiturates, rifampin, phenytoin, and carbamazepine. Drugs that may *increase* levels of lopinavir include aldesleukin, ketoconazole, delavirdine, indinavir, and ritonavir. Statins should not be administered with Kaletra due to an increased risk for myopathy. Concurrent use of rifampin may lower the effectiveness of Kaletra. Potentially life-threatening dysrhythmias may occur if Kaletra is used concurrently with terfenadine, cisapride, pimozide, and many antidysrhythmic agents. Kaletra may increase adverse effects associated with selective serotonin reuptake inhibitors, tricyclic antidepressants, and phenothiazines.

Lab Tests: Total cholesterol and triglycerides may increase.

Herbal/Food: St. John's wort may cause a decrease in antiretroviral activity and is contraindicated.

Treatment of Overdose: There is no specific treatment for overdose.

reverse transcriptase inhibitors (NNRTIs) and nucleotide reverse transcriptase inhibitors (NtRTIs).

37.5 Pharmacotherapy With Reverse Transcriptase Inhibitors

Following penetration into a T4 lymphocyte, the single-stranded viral RNA is used as a template to synthesize double-stranded viral DNA. HIV virions come "prepackaged" with reverse transcriptase, the enzyme necessary to perform this critical step. Because reverse transcriptase is a viral enzyme not found in human cells, it has been possible to design drugs capable of selectively inhibiting viral replication.

Viral DNA synthesis requires building blocks called *nucleosides and nucleotides,* which form the backbone of the DNA molecule. Nucleoside and nucleotide reverse transcriptase inhibitors (NRTIs and NtRTIs) chemically resemble the natural building blocks of DNA. In essence, reverse transcriptase is fooled by these drugs and inserts them into the proviral DNA strand. As the "false" nucleosides and nucleotides are used to build DNA, however, the proviral DNA chain is prevented from lengthening.

A second mechanism for inhibiting reverse transcriptase targets the enzyme's function. NNRTIs act by binding near the active site, causing a structural change in the enzyme molecule. The enzyme can no longer bind nucleosides and is unable to construct viral DNA.

Three NRTI's, abacavir, tenofovir, and lamivudine, have emerged as first-line drugs in the initial pharmacotherapy of HIV infection. Because some of the NRTIs, such as zidovudine (Retrovir, AZT), have been used consistently for more than 30 years, the potential for resistance must be considered when selecting the specific agent. There is a high degree of cross-resistance among NRTIs. The NRTIs and NNRTIs are always used in multidrug combinations in HAART. All fixed dose combination products for antiretroviral therapy contain one or more NRTIs.

The NRTIs are generally well tolerated, although nausea, vomiting, diarrhea, headache, and fatigue are common during the first few weeks of therapy. After prolonged therapy with NRTIs, inhibition of mitochondrial function can cause various organ abnormalities, blood disorders, lactic acidosis, and lipodystrophy, a disorder in which fat is redistributed to specific areas in the body. Areas such as the face, arms, and legs tend to lose fat, whereas the abdomen, breasts, and base of the neck (buffalo hump) accumulate excessive fat deposits. Tesamorelin (Egrifta) was approved in 2010 as an option to reduce excessive abdominal fat caused by NRTI-induced lipodystrophy. Patients receiving a regimen containing abacavir (Ziagen) should receive a laboratory test called HLA-B*5701, due to a very serious hypersensitivity reaction that can occur within the first six weeks of treatment with this drug. Patients reporting positive for HLA-B*5701 should not receive abacavir.

The NNRTIs are also generally well tolerated and exhibit few serious adverse effects. The adverse effects from these drugs, however, are different from those of the NRTIs. Rash is common, and liver toxicity is possible, increasing the risk of drug–drug interactions. Efavirenz (Sustiva) exhibits a high incidence of CNS effects such as dizziness, sleep disorders, and fatigue. However, these symptoms are rare in patients taking nevirapine (Viramune). Unlike some other antiretrovirals that negatively affect lipid metabolism, nevirapine actually improves the lipid profiles of many patients by increasing HDL levels. Rilpivirine (Edurant), a newer drug in this class, offers the convenience of once daily dosing but may increase the risk for depressive disorders.

Protease Inhibitors

Drugs in the PI class block the viral enzyme protease, which is responsible for the final assembly of the HIV virions. They have become key drugs in the pharmacotherapy of HIV infection.

37.6 Pharmacotherapy With Protease Inhibitors

Near the end of its replication cycle, HIV has assembled all the necessary components to create new virions. HIV RNA has been synthesized using the metabolic machinery of the host cell, and the structural and regulatory proteins of HIV are ready to be packaged into a new virion. As the newly formed virions bud from the host cell and are released into the surrounding extracellular fluid, one final step remains before the HIV is mature: A long polypeptide chain must be cleaved by the enzyme protease to produce the final HIV proteins. The enzyme performing this step is HIV protease.

The PIs attach to the active site of HIV protease, thus preventing the final maturation of the virions. The virions are noninfectious without this final step. When combined with other antiretroviral drug classes, the PIs are capable of lowering plasma levels of HIV RNA to an undetectable range. Since their development in 1995, the PIs have become essential drugs in the treatment of HIV-AIDS.

The PIs are metabolized in the liver and have the potential to interact with many different drugs. In general, they are well tolerated, with gastrointestinal (GI) complaints being the most common side effects. Various lipid abnormalities have been reported, including elevated cholesterol and triglyceride levels and abdominal obesity. Some of the PIs are associated with hyperglycemia and can cause diabetes or worsen existing diabetes. Cross resistance among the various PIs has been reported.

Darunavir is a recommended drug for the initial treatment of HIV, although others in this class will be frequently encountered in clinical practice. The tolerability and effectiveness of the PIs has been enhanced by combining them with other medications in a practice called **pharmacokinetic boosting.** Addition of small amounts of the "booster" drug allows less frequent dosing intervals and increases the plasma concentration of the PI. The two drugs used as boosters include:

- Ritonovir. This was the first booster discovered, and it remains the most frequently used. Ritonovir exhibits some antiretroviral activity, but it is used for its effect on pharmacokinetics. Ritonavir raises the serum levels of the primary PI by inhibiting the enzyme that metabolizes the drug. Although ritonavir may be prescribed at high doses as an antiretroviral, it is nearly always used at low doses as a booster.
- Cobicistat. This is a newer booster that exhibits no antiretroviral activity of its own. Cobicistat was initially developed to boost the activity of elvitegravir (an integrase inhibitor) and it is likely to be used in future fixed-dose combinations of PIs. The enzyme inhibition is more selective than that of ritonavir and fewer drug interactions have been reported.

Entry Inhibitors and Integrase Inhibitors

Because HIV develops resistance to most of the frequently prescribed antiretrovirals, scientists have been looking intensively for unique mechanisms of drug action. In recent years, entry inhibitors and integrase inhibitors have been discovered.

37.7 Pharmacotherapy With Entry Inhibitors and Integrase Inhibitors

Entry inhibitors prevent the entry of the viral nucleic acid into the T4 lymphocyte. The two drugs in this class block the entry of HIV by different mechanisms. Enfuvirtide (Fuzeon) blocks the fusion of the viral membrane with the bilipid layer of the host's plasma membrane, a step required for entry of the virus. Because this mechanism is so different from other antiretrovirals, many patients who are resistant to other drug classes are still sensitive to the effects of enfuvirtide. However, the use of enfuvirtide is limited because it is expensive to manufacture and it is given by subcutaneous injection twice daily. Its current use is for treating HIV infections in treatment-experienced patients with strains resistant to other antiretrovirals. Almost every patient taking enfuvirtide will experience an injection-site reaction, which involves severe pain, pruritus, erythema, cysts, abscesses, and cellulitis. Nausea, diarrhea, and fatigue are other common adverse effects.

The second entry inhibitor, maraviroc (Selzentry), was developed after scientists discovered that HIV needs coreceptors (in addition to the CD4 receptor) to enter into human cells. CCR5 is the name of one of the coreceptors required for entry. Maraviroc blocks CCR5 and has the ability to significantly reduce viral load and increase T-cell production. Maraviroc is approved for combination therapy with other antiretrovirals in treatment-naïve patients. The drug is well tolerated with the most frequently reported adverse effects being upper respiratory tract infections, cough, pyrexia, rash, and dizziness. Caution should be used when administering this drug to patients with preexisting hepatic or cardiac disease.

The integrase inhibitors are one of the newest classes for treating HIV infection. HIV requires the integrase enzyme to insert its viral DNA strand into the human chromosome. Like entry inhibitors, the integrase inhibitors offer a new mechanism for managing patients with HIV infections who have developed resistance to older antiretrovirals. The three drugs in this class include dolutegravir (Tivicay), elvitegravir (Vitekta) and raltegravir (Isentress). The integrase inhibitors are indicated for combination therapy with other antiretroviral agents for the treatment of HIV infection in adult patients. Insomnia, fatigue, headache, and GI-related symptoms such as diarrhea and nausea are the most frequently reported adverse effects. Caution should be used when administering raltegravir to patients with myopathy or rhabdomyolysis because it may worsen these conditions.

Nursing Practice Application

Pharmacotherapy for HIV-AIDS

ASSESSMENT	POTENTIAL NURSING DIAGNOSES*
Baseline assessment prior to administration: • Obtain a complete health history including neurologic, cardiovascular, respiratory, hepatic, or renal disease, and the possibility of pregnancy. Obtain a drug history including allergies, including specific reactions to drugs, current prescription and over-the-counter (OTC) drugs, herbal preparations, and alcohol use. Be alert to possible drug interactions. • Assess signs and symptoms of current infection, noting onset, duration, characteristics, and presence or absence of fever or pain. • Evaluate appropriate laboratory findings (e.g., complete blood count [CBC], CD4 count, HIV viral load, culture and sensitivity [C&S] for any concurrent infections, hepatic and renal function studies, lipid levels, serum amylase, and glucose).	• *Infection* • *Activity Intolerance* • *Fatigue* • *Anxiety* • *Imbalanced Nutrition, Less Than Body Requirements* • *Deficient Fluid Volume* • *Diarrhea* • *Impaired Oral Mucous Membranes* • *Impaired Skin Integrity* • *Insomnia* • *Social Isolation* • *Confusion (Acute or Chronic)* • *Ineffective Therapeutic Regimen Management* • *Hopelessness* • *Spiritual Distress* • *Deficient Knowledge* (drug therapy) • *Risk for Injury,* related to adverse drug effects • *Risk for Falls,* related to adverse drug effects • *Risk for Caregiver Role Strain* *NANDA I © 2014

Nursing Practice Application *continued*

ASSESSMENT	POTENTIAL NURSING DIAGNOSES*
Assessment throughout administration: • Assess for desired therapeutic effects (e.g., CD4 counts and HIV viral load remain within acceptable limits, able to attend to normal activities of daily living [ADLs], absence of signs and symptoms of concurrent infections). • Continue periodic monitoring of CBC, hepatic and renal function, CD4 and HIV viral load, lipid levels, serum amylase, and glucose. • Assess for adverse effects: nausea, vomiting, anorexia, abdominal cramping, diarrhea, fatigue, drowsiness, dizziness, mental changes, insomnia, delusions, fever, muscle or joint pain, paresthesias, hypotension, syncope, and hyperglycemia. Immediately report severe diarrhea, jaundice, decreased urine output or darkened urine, purplish-red blistering rash on the body or oral mucous membranes, acute abdominal pain, and increasing mental or behavioral changes or decreased level of consciousness (LOC).	

IMPLEMENTATION

Interventions and (Rationales)	Patient-Centered Care
Ensuring therapeutic effects: • Continue assessments as described earlier for therapeutic effects: maintenance of normal or increasing appetite, increasing energy level and ability to maintain ADLs, CD4 counts and HIV viral load within acceptable limits and stabilized, and maintaining therapeutic regimen. (Drugs will be required long term and have many potential adverse effects, making compliance with the medication regimen difficult. The health care provider should be notified if fever and signs and symptoms of concurrent infections increase, excessive fatigue is present, or adverse effects place compliance with drug therapy at risk.)	• Teach the patient to continue to take the course of medications; to not share doses with others; and to return to the provider if adverse effects make compliance with the regimen difficult to continue.
Minimizing adverse effects: • Continue to monitor vital signs, especially temperature if fever is present. Immediately report increasing fever, diarrhea or vomiting, dyspnea, tachycardia, dizziness, syncope, changes in behavior, lethargy, or LOC to the health care provider. (Increasing fever, especially when accompanied by worsening symptoms, may be a sign of worsening infection, adverse drug effects, or drug resistance.)	• Teach the patient, family, or caregiver to immediately report fever that exceeds 38.3°C (101°F), or per parameters; changes in behavior or LOC; shortness of breath; inability to maintain hydration or nutrition; or dizziness and fainting to the health care provider.
• Continue to monitor periodic laboratory work: hepatic and renal function tests, CBC, CD4 counts, HIV viral load, lipid levels, serum amylase, C&S if concurrent infections are present, and glucose. (Drugs used for the treatment of HIV are hepatic and renal toxic. Bone marrow suppression and resulting blood dyscrasias, particularly anemia and leukopenia, are also adverse effects and will be monitored by CBC. Lipid levels and serum amylase will be monitored to assess for pancreatitis and glucose levels checked for hyperglycemia.)	• Instruct the patient on the need for periodic laboratory work, correlating any symptoms with the need for possible laboratory tests (e.g., serum amylase if the patient is having upper abdominal pain). Advise laboratory personnel of the patient's HIV status.
• Monitor for hypersensitivity and allergic reactions, especially with the first dose of any antiretroviral or protease inhibitor. Continue to monitor the patient as needed based on the drug used or the patient's condition. (Anaphylactic reactions are possible. Because reactions may not always be predictable, caution and frequent monitoring are essential to ensure prompt treatment.)	• Teach the patient to immediately report any itching; rashes; swelling, particularly of face, tongue, or lips; urticaria; flushing; dizziness; syncope; wheezing; throat tightness; or difficulty breathing.

continued

Nursing Practice Application *continued*

IMPLEMENTATION	
Interventions and (Rationales)	**Patient-Centered Care**
• Continue to monitor for hepatic and renal toxicities. (Antiretrovirals and PIs may be hepatic and renal toxic and require frequent monitoring to prevent adverse effects. **Lifespan:** Age-related physiological changes may place the older adult at greater risk for hepatic or renal toxicity. **Diverse Patients:** Because zidovudine is metabolized through the P450 system pathways, monitor ethnically diverse patients frequently to ensure optimal therapeutic effects and minimize adverse effects. Increasing fluid intake will prevent drug accumulation in the kidneys.)	• Teach the patient to immediately report any nausea, vomiting, yellowing of the skin or sclera, abdominal pain, light or clay-colored stools, and diminished urine output or darkening of urine. • Advise the patient to increase fluid intake to 2 to 3 L per day.
• Continue to monitor for dermatologic effects such as red or purplish skin rash, blisters, or peeling skin, including oral mucous membranes. Assess oral mucous membranes for signs of stomatitis, because drug effects or immunosuppression may result in the overgrowth of oral flora. Immediately report severe rashes, especially those associated with blistering. (These drugs may cause significant dermatologic effects including stomatitis, as well as Stevens–Johnson syndrome, a potentially fatal condition.)	• Teach the patient to inspect the oral cavity at least once a day and maintain regular dental exams; to maintain good oral hygiene and rinse the mouth with plain water or solution as prescribed by the health care provider after eating; and to use protective clothing for sun exposure and immediately report any significant rashes or sunburned appearance.
• Monitor for signs and symptoms of neurotoxicity (e.g., drowsiness, dizziness, mental changes, insomnia, delusions, paresthesias, headache, changes in LOC, and seizures). (Many HIV-AIDS drugs cause peripheral neuropathy and have neurologic adverse effects.)	• Instruct the patient or caregiver to immediately report increasing headache; dizziness; drowsiness; worsening insomnia; numbness of the hands, feet, or extremities; and changes in behavior or LOC. • **Safety:** Caution the patient that drowsiness may occur and to be cautious with driving or other activities requiring mental alertness until effects of the drug are known. • Caution the patient to be careful when in contact with heat or cold because numbness from peripheral neuropathy may make sensing accurate temperature more difficult. • Encourage sleep hygiene measures (e.g., restful routines before bed and avoiding large meals within 1 or 2 hours of sleep). Have the patient consult with the health care provider if insomnia causes daytime sleepiness or continues.
• Monitor for signs and symptoms of blood dyscrasias (e.g., low-grade fevers, bleeding, bruising, and significant fatigue). (Bone marrow suppression may occur and may cause blood dyscrasias with resulting decreases in red blood cells [RBCs], WBCs, and/or platelets. Periodic monitoring of complete blood count [CBC] will be required.)	• Teach the patient to report any low-grade fevers, sore throat, rashes, bruising or increased bleeding, and unusual fatigue or shortness of breath, especially after taking the drug for a prolonged period.
• Monitor for significant GI effects, including nausea, vomiting, abdominal pain or cramping, and diarrhea. Administer the drugs as per guidelines. Additional pharmacologic treatment may be necessary to limit adverse GI effects. Ensure adequate nutrition and caloric intake. (Adverse GI effects are common to most antiretrovirals and protease inhibitors. Always check administration guidelines before administering with or without food or milk.)	• Teach the patient to take the drug with food or milk if appropriate or to take the drug on an empty stomach with a full glass of water. Avoid acidic foods and beverages or carbonated drinks, which may cause stomach upset. • **Collaboration:** Assist the patient in obtaining a dietary consultation as needed if nausea or diarrhea makes maintaining intake difficult.
• Monitor for symptoms of pancreatitis including severe abdominal pain, nausea, vomiting, and abdominal distention. (Some antiretroviral drugs may cause pancreatitis. Serum amylase and lipid levels should be monitored periodically.)	• Instruct the patient to immediately report fever, severe abdominal pain, nausea, vomiting, and abdominal distention.
• Monitor blood glucose in patients who are taking antiretrovirals. (These drugs may cause hyperglycemia. Patients with diabetes may require a change in their antidiabetic drug routine.)	• Teach the patient with diabetes to test for glucose more frequently, reporting any consistent elevations to the health care provider.
• Encourage infection control and good hygiene measures based on the extent of disease condition, and follow established protocol in hospitalized patients. (These drugs decrease the level of HIV infection but do not cure the disease. Excellent hygiene measures will limit the chance for secondary infections in the immunocompromised patient.)	• Teach the patient adequate infection control and hygiene measures such as frequent hand washing, avoiding crowded indoor places, and adequate nutrition and rest, especially if currently immunocompromised. • Practice abstinence or always use barrier protection during sexual activity. • Do not share needles with others and do not donate blood.

Nursing Practice Application *continued*

IMPLEMENTATION

Interventions and (Rationales)	Patient-Centered Care
• Provide resources for medical and emotional support. (Treatment requires a multidisciplinary approach.)	• **Collaboration:** Advise the patient about community resources and support groups. Assist the caregiver with respite care as needed.
Patient understanding of drug therapy: • Use opportunities during administration of medications and during assessments to provide patient education. (Using time during nursing care helps to optimize and reinforce key teaching areas.)	• The patient, family, or caregiver should be able to state the reason for the drug; appropriate dose and scheduling; what adverse effects to observe for and when to report; and the anticipated length of medication therapy.
Patient self-administration of drug therapy: • When administering medications, instruct the patient, family, or caregiver in proper self-administration techniques followed by teach-back. (Proper administration increases the effectiveness of the drug.)	• Teach the patient to take the medication as follows: • Complete the entire course of therapy unless otherwise instructed. The duration of the required therapy may be quite lengthy but it is necessary to prevent active infection. Do not stop the medication when starting to feel better. • Eliminate alcohol while on these medications. These drugs cause significant reactions when taken with alcohol. • Take the drug with food or milk but avoid acidic beverages. If instructed to take the drug on an empty stomach, take with a full glass of water. • Take the medication as evenly spaced throughout each day as feasible. • Increase overall fluid intake while taking these drugs.

See Table 37.1 for a list of drugs to which these nursing actions apply.

37.8 Prevention of Perinatal Transmission of HIV

One of the most tragic aspects of the AIDS epidemic is transmission of the virus from a mother to her child during pregnancy, delivery, or breast-feeding. Newborns with HIV may succumb to the infection within weeks, or symptoms may be delayed for months or years. The prognosis for these children is generally poor; thus, the best approach to dealing with HIV infections in neonates is prevention.

Clinical trials have confirmed that perinatal transmission of HIV can be markedly reduced through pharmacotherapy. In pregnant women with HIV, antiretroviral therapy is recommended regardless of the viral load or CD4 count. To determine the most effective regimen, genotypic drug resistance testing is recommended for all treatment-naïve pregnant women prior to the initiation of antiretroviral therapy (Panel on Antiretroviral Guidelines for Adults and Adolescents, 2015).The risk of transmission may be reduced approximately 70% using the following regimen:

- Oral administration of zidovudine to the mother, beginning at week 14 of gestation and continuing to week 34 of gestation.
- IV administration of zidovudine to the mother during labor.
- Oral administration of zidovudine to the newborn to begin immediately after delivery and continuing for 6 weeks following delivery. (HIV infection is established in infants by age 1 to 2 weeks; starting antiretroviral therapy more than 48 hours after birth is ineffective in preventing the infection.)

The specific drugs chosen depend on whether the mother is treatment experienced prior to the pregnancy and on the results of resistance studies. Treatment with at least three drugs is recommended: usually two NRTIs combined with either a NNRTI or a boosted PI. Although zidovudine was the NRTI included in the early research studies, more resent research suggests that combinations with tenofovir, emtricitabine, abacavir, or lamivudine can also be considered preferred treatment (Panel on Treatment of HIV-Infected Pregnant Women and Prevention of Perinatal Transmission, 2015).

Virologic tests for HIV can be conducted at birth for babies born to HIV-infected mothers who did not receive prenatal antiretroviral therapy. However, sensitivity of the test increases rapidly by about 2 weeks after birth. Antiretroviral therapy may be discontinued if the neonate has two consecutive negative HIV virologic tests (one at 2 weeks, the other at one month). Infants may be retested at ages 6 and 12 months to confirm the negative diagnosis. In addition to antiretrovirals, infants born to women with HIV infection usually receive trimethoprim-sulfamethoxazole to prevent *Pneumocystis jiroveci* pneumonia at 4 to 6 weeks of age.

37.9 Postexposure Prophylaxis of HIV Infection Following Occupational Exposure

Since the start of the AIDS epidemic, nurses and other health care workers have been concerned about acquiring the infection from their patients with HIV-AIDS. Fortunately, if proper precautions are observed, the disease is rarely transmitted from patient to caregiver. Accidents have occurred, however, in which health care workers have acquired the infection by exposure to the blood or body fluids of a patient infected with HIV. Although the risk is very small, the question remains: Can HIV transmission be prevented *after* accidental occupational exposure to HIV? The answer is a qualified yes.

The success of postexposure prophylaxis (PEP) therapy following HIV exposure is difficult to assess because of the lack of controlled studies and the small number of cases. Enough data have been accumulated, however, to demonstrate that PEP is successful in certain circumstances. For prevention to be most successful, PEP should be started as quickly as possible or within 24 to 36 hours after exposure to a patient who is *known* to be HIV positive. The longer the time between suspected exposure and initiation of treatment, the less successful will be the PEP. The exposed health care professional should receive a baseline HIV RNA level test as soon as possible after exposure and subsequent follow-up testing at 6 weeks, 12 weeks, and 6 months postexposure. PEP is continued for about 4 months.

If the HIV status of the patient is *unknown*, PEP is decided case by case, based on the type of exposure and the likelihood that the blood or body fluid contained HIV. In some cases, PEP is initiated for a few days until the patient can be tested. PEP should be initiated only if the exposure was sufficiently severe and the source fluid is known, or strongly suspected, to contain HIV. Using PEP outside established guidelines is both expensive and dangerous; the antiretrovirals used for PEP therapy produce adverse effects in more than half the patients. The preferred PEP treatment includes a three drug regimen that includes raltegravir (Isentris) plus Truvada (tenofovir plus emtricitabine) (Kuhar et al., 2013).

HERPESVIRUSES

Herpes simplex viruses (HSVs) are a family of DNA viruses that cause repeated blister-like lesions on the skin, genitals, and other mucosal surfaces. Antiviral drugs can lower the frequency of acute herpes episodes and diminish the intensity of acute disease. These drugs are listed in Table 37.2.

37.10 Pharmacotherapy of Herpesvirus Infections

Herpesviruses are usually acquired through direct physical contact with an infected person, but they may also be transmitted from infected mothers to their newborns, sometimes resulting in severe CNS disease. The herpesvirus family includes the following:

- *HSV-1.* Primarily infections of the eye, mouth, and lips, although the incidence of genital infections is increasing
- *HSV-2.* Primarily genital infections
- *Cytomegalovirus (CMV).* Affects multiple body systems in immunosuppressed patients

Table 37.2 Drugs for Herpesviruses

Drug	Route and Adult Dose (max dose where indicated)	Adverse Effects
acyclovir (Zovirax)	PO: 400 mg tid IV: 5–10 mg/kg q8h for 7–14 days	Systemic Agents *Nausea, vomiting, diarrhea, headache, pain and inflammation at the injection sites (parenteral drugs)* Thrombocytopenic purpura/hemolytic uremic syndrome, nephrotoxicity, seizures (foscarnet), electrolyte imbalances (foscarnet), hematologic toxicity/bone marrow suppression (ganciclovir) Topical Agents *Burning, irritation, or stinging at the site of application, headache* Photophobia, keratopathy, and edema of eyelids (ocular drugs)
cidofovir (Vistide)	IV: 5 mg/kg once weekly for 2 consecutive wk	
docosanol (Abreva)	Topical: 10% cream applied to the cold sore up to five times/day for 10 days	
famciclovir (Famvir)	PO: 500 mg tid for 7 days (max: 1,500 mg/day)	
foscarnet (Foscavir)	IV: 40–60 mg/kg infused over 1–2 h tid (max: 180 mg/kg/day)	
ganciclovir (Cytovene, Zirgan)	PO: 1 g tid IV: 5 mg/kg infused over 1 h bid Topical (Zirgan): 1 drop in affected eye five times/day	
idoxuridine (Dendrid, Herplex)	Topical: 1 drop in each eye qh during waking hours and q2h during the night	
penciclovir (Denavir)	Topical: apply q2h while awake for 4 days	
trifluridine (Viroptic)	Topical: 1 drop in each eye q2h during waking hours (max: 9 drops/day)	
valacyclovir (Valtrex)	PO: 500 mg–2.0 g daily (max: 3 g/day)	

Note: *Italics* indicate common adverse effects; underlining indicates serious adverse effects.

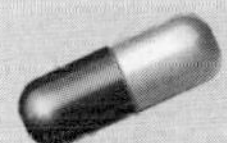

Prototype Drug | Acyclovir *(Zovirax)*

Therapeutic Class: Antiviral for herpesviruses **Pharmacologic Class:** Nucleoside analog

Actions and Uses

Approved by the U.S. Food and Drug Administration (FDA) in 1982 as one of the first antiviral drugs, acyclovir is limited to pharmacotherapy for herpesviruses, for which it is a drug of choice. It is most effective against HSV-1 and HSV-2, and it is effective only at high doses against CMV and varicella zoster. By preventing viral DNA synthesis, acyclovir decreases the duration and severity of acute herpes episodes. When given for prophylaxis, it may decrease the frequency of herpes appearance, but it does not cure the patient. It is available as a 5% ointment for application to active lesions, in oral form for prophylaxis, and as an IV for severe episodes. Because of its short half-life, acyclovir is sometimes administered PO up to five times a day.

Administration Alerts

- When given IV, the drug may cause painful inflammation of vessels at the site of infusion.
- Administer around the clock, even if sleep is interrupted.
- Administer with food.
- Pregnancy category C.

PHARMACOKINETICS (PO)

Onset	Peak	Duration
1–2 h	1.5–2 h	4–8 h

Adverse Effects

There are few adverse effects from acyclovir when it is administered topically or PO. Nephrotoxicity and neurotoxicity are possible when the medication is given IV. Resistance has developed to the drug, particularly in patients with HIV-AIDS.

Contraindications: Acyclovir is contraindicated in patients with hypersensitivity to drugs in this class.

Interactions

Drug–Drug: Concurrent use of acyclovir with nephrotoxic agents should be avoided. Probenecid decreases acyclovir elimination, and zidovudine may cause increased drowsiness and lethargy.

Lab Tests: Values for kidney function tests such as blood urea nitrogen (BUN) and serum creatinine may increase.

Herbal/Food: Unknown.

Treatment of Overdose: There is no specific treatment for overdose.

- *Varicella-zoster virus (VZV).* Shingles (zoster) and chickenpox (varicella)
- *Epstein–Barr virus (EBV).* Infectious mononucleosis and a form of cancer called Burkitt's lymphoma
- *Herpesvirus-type 6.* Roseola in children and hepatitis or encephalitis in immunosuppressed patients.

Following its initial entrance into the patient, HSV may remain in a latent, asymptomatic state in nerve ganglia for many years. Immunosuppression, physical challenges, or emotional stress can promote active replication of the virus and the appearance of the characteristic lesions. Complications include secondary infections of nongenital tissues.

The pharmacologic goals for the management of herpes infections are twofold: to *relieve acute symptoms* and to *prevent recurrences*. It is important to understand that the antiviral drugs used to treat herpesviruses do not cure patients; the virus remains in patients for the rest of their lives.

Initial, acute HSV-1 and HSV-2 infections are usually treated with oral antiviral therapy for 5 to 10 days. Commonly prescribed antivirals for HSV and VZV include acyclovir (Zovirax), famciclovir (Famvir), and valacyclovir (Valtrex). Topical forms of several antivirals are available for application to herpes lesions, although they are not as effective as the oral forms. In immunocompromised patients, IV acyclovir may be indicated.

Recurrent herpes lesions are usually mild and often require no drug treatment. If drug therapy is initiated within 24 hours after recurrent symptoms first appear, the length of the acute episode may be shortened. Patients who experience particularly severe or frequent recurrences (more than six episodes per year) may benefit from low doses of prophylactic antiviral therapy. Prophylactic therapy may also be of benefit to immunocompromised patients, such as those receiving antineoplastic therapy or those with AIDS.

Herpes of the eye is the most common infectious cause of corneal blindness in the United States. Ocular herpes causes a painful, inflamed lesion on the eyelid or surface of the eye. Prompt treatment with antiviral drugs prevents permanent tissue destruction. As with genital herpes, once patients acquire ocular herpes, they often experience recurrences, which may occur years after the initial symptoms. Ocular herpes is treated with local application of drops or ointment. Trifluridine (Viroptic) and idoxuridine

(Dendrid, Herplex) are available in ophthalmic formulations. Oral acyclovir is used when topical drops or ointments are contraindicated. Uncomplicated ocular herpes usually resolves after 1 to 2 weeks of pharmacotherapy.

INFLUENZA

Influenza is a viral infection characterized by acute symptoms that include sore throat, sneezing, coughing, fever, and chills. The infectious viral particles are easily spread via airborne droplets. In immunosuppressed patients, an influenza infection may be fatal. In 1918–1919, a worldwide outbreak of influenza killed an estimated 20 million people. Influenza viruses are designated with the letters A, B, or C. Type A is the most common and has been responsible for several serious pandemics throughout history. The RNA-containing influenza viruses should not be confused with *Haemophilus influenzae*, which is a bacterium that causes respiratory disease.

Lifespan Considerations: Geriatric
Increasing Influenza Vaccination Participation in Older Adults

Despite frequent media campaigns about influenza vaccination, many people continue to avoid the getting vaccinated. As recent years have shown, influenza continues to have a deadly outcome for even healthy members of the population. Older adults are especially at risk for infection and potentially greater morbidity. McIntyre, Zecevic, and Diachun (2014) explored factors that influenced older adults to avoid or obtain the influenza vaccine. Among reasons for avoidance: belief that they were not at risk, accessibility (e.g., cost, transportation), general lack of knowledge about the vaccination, and fear of adverse reactions. Trust in the health care provider's recommendation was the main reason participants in the study received the vaccine, followed by knowing others who had received it. This highlights the crucial role nurses play in educating their patients about the need for vaccinations.

37.11 Pharmacotherapy of Influenza

The best approach to influenza infection is *prevention* through annual vaccination. Past recommendations specified certain groups be vaccinated, such as residents of long-term care facilities, healthy adults age 65 and older, and health care workers who are involved in the direct care of patients at high risk for acquiring influenza. The Advisory Committee on Immunization Practices now recommends that everyone over the age of 6 months be vaccinated annually against influenza (CDC, 2015). Additional details on the influenza vaccine are presented in chapter 34.

Antivirals may be used to prevent influenza or decrease the severity of acute symptoms. Amantadine (Symmetrel) and rimantadine (Flumadine) have been available to prevent and treat influenza for many years, but are no longer recommended due to widespread resistance. Antivirals for influenza are listed in Table 37.3.

The neuroaminidase inhibitors were introduced in 1999 to treat *active* influenza infections. If given within 48 hours of the onset of symptoms, oseltamivir (Tamiflu) and zanamivir (Relenza) are reported to shorten the normal 7-day duration of influenza symptoms to 5 days. Oseltamivir is given PO, whereas zanamivir is inhaled. A newer drug in this class is peramivir (Rapivab) which was approved in 2014 by the IV route for the treatment of acute, uncomplicated influenza. Because these agents are expensive and produce only modest results, prevention through vaccination remains the best alternative.

It is important to understand that these antivirals are not effective against the common cold virus. About 200 different viruses, including rhinoviruses, cause symptoms identified with the common cold. Despite considerable attempts to develop drugs to prevent this annoying infection, success has not yet been achieved. There are drugs, however, that may relieve symptoms of the common cold, and these are presented in chapter 39.

☑ Check Your Understanding 37.1

Viral infections are very often more difficult to treat than bacterial infections. What are several reasons for this? *Visit www.pearsonhighered.com/nursingresources for the answer.*

Table 37.3 Drugs for Influenza

Drug	Route and Adult Dose (max dose where indicated)	Adverse Effects
INFLUENZA PROPHYLAXIS		
amantadine (Symmetrel)	PO: 100 mg bid (max: 400 mg/day)	*Nausea, dizziness, nervousness, difficulty concentrating, insomnia*
rimantadine (Flumadine)	PO: 100 mg bid (max: 200 mg/day)	Leukopenia, hallucinations, orthostatic hypotension, urinary retention
INFLUENZA TREATMENT: NEUROAMINIDASE INHIBITORS		
oseltamivir (Tamiflu)	PO: 75 mg bid for 5 days	*Nausea, vomiting, diarrhea, dizziness*
peramivir (Rapimab)	IV: 600 mg once	Bronchitis, bronchospasm, skin hypersensitivity reactions, neuropsychiatric events and abnormal behavior (peramivir), Steven's–Johnson syndrome (peramivir)
zanamivir (Relenza)	Inhalation: 2 inhalations/bid for 5 days	

Note: *Italics* indicate common adverse effects; underlining indicates serious adverse effects.

VIRAL HEPATITIS

Viral **hepatitis** is a common infection caused by a number of different viruses. The three primary types of viral hepatitis are hepatitis A, hepatitis B, and hepatitis C. Although each has its own unique clinical features, all hepatitis viruses cause inflammation and necrosis of liver cells and produce similar symptoms. Acute symptoms include fever, chills, fatigue, anorexia, nausea, and vomiting. Chronic hepatitis may result in prolonged fatigue, jaundice, liver cirrhosis, and ultimately hepatic failure.

37.12 Pharmacotherapy of Viral Hepatitis

Hepatitis A

Hepatitis A virus (HAV) is spread by the oral–fecal route and causes epidemics in regions of the world having poor sanitation. Outbreaks in the United States are most often sporadic events caused by the consumption of contaminated food. HAV is the most common cause of acute hepatitis in the United States.

Although approximately 20% of patients infected with HAV require some hospitalization for symptoms related to the infection, most recover without pharmacotherapy and develop lifelong immunity to the virus. Fatalities due to chronic disease are rare, and only a small number of patients develop severe liver failure. Thus, HAV is normally considered an acute disease, having no significant chronic form. This makes HAV very different from hepatitis B or C.

Like all forms of hepatitis, the best treatment for HAV is prevention. HAV vaccine (Havrix, VAQTA) is indicated for all children ages 2 to 18, travelers to countries with high HAV infection rates, men who have sex with men, and illegal drug users. When a booster is given 6 to 12 months after the initial dose, close to 100% immunity is obtained. The average length of protection is approximately 5 to 8 years, although protection may last 20 years or longer in some patients. The availability of the HAV vaccine has led to a dramatic drop in the rate of this infection in the United States.

Prophylaxis or postexposure treatment for a patient recently exposed to HAV includes hepatitis A immunoglobulins (HAIg), a concentrated solution of antibodies. HAIg is administered as prophylaxis for patients traveling to endemic areas and to close personal contacts of infected patients to prevent transmission of the virus. A single intramuscular (IM) dose of HAIg can provide passive protection and prophylaxis for about 3 months. It is estimated that the immunoglobulins are 85% effective at preventing HAV in patients exposed to the virus.

Therapy for acute HAV infection is symptomatic. No specific drugs are indicated; in otherwise healthy adults, the infection is self-limiting.

Hepatitis B

Hepatitis B virus (HBV) in the United States is transmitted primarily through exposure to contaminated blood and body fluids. Major risk factors for HBV infection include injected drug abuse, sex with an HBV-infected partner, and sex between men. Health care workers are at risk because of accidental exposure to HBV-contaminated needles or body fluids. In many regions of the world, the primary mode of transmission of HBV is by the perinatal route and from child to child.

Treatment of acute HBV infection is symptomatic, because no specific therapy is available. Ninety percent of acute HBV infections resolve with complete recovery and do not progress to chronic disease. Lifelong immunity to HBV is usually acquired following resolution of the infection.

Symptoms of chronic HBV may develop as long as 10 years following exposure. HBV has a much greater probability of progression to chronic hepatitis and a greater mortality rate than does HAV. The final stage of the infection is hepatic cirrhosis. In addition, chronic HBV infections are associated with an increased risk of hepatocellular carcinoma.

As with HAV, the best treatment for HBV infection is *prevention* through immunization. HBV vaccine (Engerix-B, Recombivax HB) is indicated for health care workers and others who are routinely exposed to blood and body fluids, men who have sex with men, and people who inject street drugs, have more than one sex partner, are under age 60 with diabetes, have HIV infection, have chronic kidney disease, or travel to countries where HBV is common. Universal vaccination of all children is now recommended, with three doses starting at birth to 18 months of age. Three doses of the vaccine provide up to 90% of patients with protection against HBV following exposure to the virus. Combination vaccines that contain HBV vaccine include Comvax (hepatitis B-*Haemophilus influenzae* type b conjugate vaccine), Pediatrix (hepatitis B, diphtheria, tetanus, acellular pertussis [DTaP], and inactivated poliovirus vaccine), and Twinrix (HAV and HBV vaccine).

For someone who has been recently exposed to HBV, therapy with hepatitis B immunoglobulins (HBIg) may be initiated. Indications for HBIg therapy include probable exposure to HBV through the perinatal, sexual, or parenteral routes, or exposure of an infant to a caregiver with HBV. HBIg is administered as soon as possible after suspected exposure to HBV.

Once chronic hepatitis becomes symptomatic, pharmacotherapy with antivirals is indicated to stop viral replication, or to administer immunomodulators that boost body defenses. Three different therapies are approved for chronic HBV pharmacotherapy:

- *Interferon alfa or PEG interferon.* Between 30% to 40% of patients respond to 4 months of therapy.
- *Tenofovir disoproxil (Viread).* Following 48 weeks of therapy, about 78% of patients respond to tenofovir. Long-term studies show that resistance to tenofovir is very low.

Table 37.4 Drugs for Hepatitis

Drug	Route and Adult Dose (max dose where indicated)	Adverse Effects
INTERFERONS		
interferon alfa-2b (Intron A) (see page 525 for the Prototype Drug box)	Subcutaneous/IM: 3 million units/m^2 three times/wk	*Flulike symptoms, myalgia, fatigue, headache, anorexia, diarrhea*
interferon alfacon-1 (Infergen)	Subcutaneous: 9 mcg three times/wk for 24 wk As combination therapy: 15 mcg daily with ribavirin for up to 48 wk	Myelosuppression, thrombocytopenia, suicide ideation, anaphylaxis, hepatotoxicity
peginterferon alfa-2a (Pegasys)	Subcutaneous: 180 mcg once per wk for 48 wk	
peginterferon alfa-2b (PEG-Intron)	Subcutaneous: 1 mcg/kg/wk for 48 wk	
ANTIVIRALS		
adefovir dipivoxil (Hepsera)	PO: 10 mg once daily	*Asthenia, headache, nausea, dizziness, fatigue, nasal disturbances (lamivudine), rash with photosensitivity (simeprivir), hyperbilirubinemia (simeprivir)*
boceprevir (Victrelis)	PO: 800 mg tid	
daclatasvir (Daklinza)	PO: 60 mg once daily in combination with sofosbuvir	
entecavir (Baraclude)	PO: 0.5–1 mg once daily	Nephrotoxicity and lactic acidosis (adefovir, telbivudine), pancreatitis (lamivudine), hepatomegaly with steatorrhea (lamivudine, entecavir), cardiac arrest (ribavirin), hemolytic anemia (ribavirin), apnea (ribavirin), myopathy (telbivudine), peripheral neuropathy (telbivudine)
lamivudine (Epivir)	PO: 100 mg once daily	
ribavirin (Copegus, Rebetrol, others)	PO: 600 mg bid	
simeprevir (Olysio)	PO: 150 mg once daily	
sofosbuvir (Sovaldi)	PO: 400 mg once daily	
telaprevir (Incivek)	PO: 750 mg tid	
telbivudine (Tyzeka)	PO: 600 mg once daily	
tenofovir (Viread)	PO: 300 mg once daily	

Note: *Italics* indicate common adverse effects; underlining indicates serious adverse effects.

- *Entecavir (Baraclude).* About 70% of patients respond after 48 weeks of therapy. Long-term studies show that resistance to entecavir is very low.

The remaining medications for HBV infection are considered second-line agents because they exhibit lower effectiveness, increased adverse effects, or greater resistance than the first-line agents. The second-line drugs such as lamivudine (Epivir) and adefovir (Hepsera) may be useful when resistance develops, or when used in combination with first-line agents. Clinical guidelines for the treatment of chronic HBV infection continue to evolve as long-term research becomes available.

Hepatitis C and Other Hepatitis Viruses

The hepatitis C, D, E, and G viruses are sometimes referred to as non A–non B viruses. Of the non A–non B viruses, hepatitis C has the greatest clinical importance.

Transmitted primarily through exposure to infected blood or body fluids, hepatitis C virus (HCV) is more common than HBV. Approximately half of all patients with HIV-AIDS are coinfected with HCV. About 70% of patients infected with HCV proceed to chronic hepatitis, and up to 30% may develop end-stage cirrhosis. HCV is the most common cause of liver transplants.

Unlike with HAV and HBV, no vaccine is available to prevent hepatitis C. In addition, postexposure prophylaxis of HCV with immunoglobulins is not recommended because its effectiveness has not been demonstrated. Drugs for treating HCV are shown in Table 37.4.

Current pharmacotherapy for chronic HCV infection includes several types of interferon (IFN) and the antiviral ribavirin. Combination therapy has been found to produce a more sustained viral suppression than monotherapy with either agent. Commercially available interferons for hepatitis include both the regular and pegylated formulations. **Pegylation** is a process that attaches polyethylene glycol (PEG) to an interferon to extend its duration of action, thus allowing it to be administered less frequently. Whereas standard interferon formulations must be administered three times per week, pegylated versions require only one dose per week. The PEG molecule is inert and does not influence antiviral activity. Additional information on interferons used for other indications may be found in chapter 34.

Boceprivir (Victelis) and telaprivir (Incivek) have emerged as important drugs in the pharmacotherapy of chronic HCV infections. These drugs inhibit HCV protease, an enzyme that is essential to viral replication in infected host cells. Addition of a PI to the PEG-IFN–ribavirin regimen is becoming the standard of care for treating this infection. The three-drug combination produces a more sustained viral inhibition, especially in patients with cirrhosis.

In 2013 two drugs were approved by the FDA that represent a new generation of medications for treating HCV. Research discovered that several proteins (NS3, NS4, NS5A, NS5B) are necessary for HCV to replicate.

Nursing Practice Application

Pharmacotherapy for Non-HIV Viral Infections

ASSESSMENT	POTENTIAL NURSING DIAGNOSES*
Baseline assessment prior to administration: • Obtain a complete health history including immunizations; respiratory, neurologic, hepatic, or renal disease; and the possibility of pregnancy. Obtain a drug history including allergies, including specific reactions to drugs, current prescription and OTC drugs, herbal preparations, and alcohol use. Be alert to possible drug interactions. • Assess signs and symptoms of current infection, noting onset, duration, characteristics, and presence or absence of fever or pain. • Evaluate appropriate laboratory findings (e.g., CBC, hepatic and renal function studies, viral cultures).	• *Infection* • *Impaired Oral Mucous Membranes* • *Impaired Skin Integrity* • *Fatigue* • *Activity Intolerance* • *Social Isolation* • *Deficient Knowledge* (drug therapy) • *Risk for Deficient Fluid Volume,* related to adverse drug effects • *Risk for Imbalanced Nutrition, Less Than Body Requirements,* related to adverse drug effects *NANDA I © 2014
Assessment throughout administration: • Assess for desired therapeutic effects (e.g., diminished or absence of signs and symptoms of herpesvirus infection and without symptoms of concurrent infections). • Continue periodic monitoring of CBC and hepatic and renal function. • Assess for adverse effects: nausea, vomiting, diarrhea, anorexia, fatigue, drowsiness, dizziness, and headache. Decreased urine output or darkened urine, increased bruising or bleeding, and increasing fever or symptoms of infections should be reported immediately.	

IMPLEMENTATION

Interventions and (Rationales)	Patient-Centered Care
Ensuring therapeutic effects: • Continue assessments as described earlier for therapeutic effects: diminishing signs of original infection, maintenance of normal appetite and fluid intake, and increasing energy level. (Drug effects may not be immediately observable. Gradual improvement should be noted, and the patient should be encouraged to continue taking medication.)	• Teach the patient to continue to take the course of medications; to not share doses with others; and to return to the provider if adverse effects make compliance with the regimen difficult. • Encourage adequate nutrition, rest, and activity levels as improvement is noted.
Minimizing adverse effects: • Continue to monitor vital signs. Immediately report increasing fever, dizziness, headache, or diminished urine output to the health care provider. (Increasing fever, especially when accompanied by worsening symptoms, may be a sign of worsening infection or adverse drug effects.)	• Teach the patient, family, or caregiver to promptly report fever that exceeds 38.3°C (101°F) or per parameters set by the health care provider; inability to maintain hydration or nutrition; or dizziness to the health care provider.
• Continue to monitor periodic laboratory work: CBC, hepatic and renal function tests, and viral cultures. (Antiviral drugs may be toxic to the liver and kidneys. Blood dyscrasias due to bone marrow suppression, particularly thrombocytopenia, are adverse effects and are monitored by CBC.)	• Instruct the patient on the need for periodic laboratory work, correlating any symptoms with the need for possible laboratory tests (e.g., increased bruising or bleeding).
• Continue to monitor for hepatic and renal toxicities. (Hepatic and renal toxicities may occur. **Lifespan:** Age-related physiological differences may place older adult at greater risk for hepatic or renal toxicity. Increasing fluid intake may prevent drug accumulation in the kidneys.)	• Teach the patient to immediately report any nausea, vomiting, yellowing of the skin or sclera, abdominal pain, light or clay-colored stools, or diminished urine output or darkening of urine. • Advise the patient to maintain fluid intake at 2 to 3 L per day.
• Monitor for signs and symptoms of neurotoxicity, particularly in patients on IV acyclovir (e.g., drowsiness, dizziness, tremors, headache, confusion, changes in LOC, and seizures). Ensure patient safety, and have the patient rise slowly from lying or sitting to standing. (Acyclovir, especially when given IV, may be neurotoxic. **Lifespan:** The older adult patient should be monitored closely to prevent falls.)	• Instruct the patient, family, or caregiver to immediately report increasing headache, dizziness, drowsiness, tremors, confusion, or changes in LOC. If dizziness occurs, the patient should sit or lie down and not attempt to stand or walk, until the sensation passes. • **Safety:** Caution the patient that drowsiness may occur and to be cautious with driving or other hazardous activities until the effects of the drug are known. • If dizziness occurs, rise from a lying or sitting position to standing slowly.

continued

Nursing Practice Application *continued*

IMPLEMENTATION	
Interventions and (Rationales)	**Patient-Centered Care**
• Monitor patients on amantadine for changes in behavior, psychiatric symptoms, or suicidal thoughts. (An increased risk of CNS or psychiatric symptoms, or suicidal thoughts has been known to occur with amantadine, especially in patients with preexisting CNS or psychiatric disorders.)	• Have the patient, family, or caregiver immediately report any changes in behavior, confusion, delusion, or expressed thoughts of suicide.
• Monitor for signs and symptoms of blood dyscrasias (e.g., bleeding, bruising, significant fatigue, and increasing signs of infection). (Bone marrow suppression may occur and cause decreases in RBCs, WBCs, or platelets. Periodic monitoring of CBC will be required.)	• Instruct the patient to report any low-grade fevers, sore throat, rashes, bruising or increased bleeding, or unusual fatigue or shortness of breath, especially if on drug therapy for a prolonged period.
• Monitor for significant GI effects, including nausea, vomiting, and diarrhea. Ensure adequate nutrition and caloric intake. (Adverse GI effects are common and the patient may also have disease-related effects, e.g., mouth sores. Maintaining adequate nutrition and fluids is essential to healing.)	• Teach the patient to avoid acidic foods and beverages, carbonated drinks, or excessively hot or cold foods and beverages, which may cause mouth irritation. • Encourage the patient to try small, frequent meals, which may be better tolerated than fewer, larger meals. High-caloric foods and supplemental beverages may help add additional calories and supply additional fluids. Assist the patient in obtaining a dietary consultation as needed if nausea or diarrhea makes maintaining intake difficult.
• Encourage infection control and good hygiene measures based on disease condition, and follow the established protocol in hospitalized patients. (Antiviral drugs decrease the level of infection but do not cure the disease. Excellent hygiene measures will limit the chance for secondary infections in the immunocompromised patient. Infection control measures prevent disease transmission.)	• Teach the patient adequate infection control and hygiene measures such as frequent hand washing, appropriate disposal of dressing material, and adequate nutrition and rest, especially if currently immunocompromised. • The patient may need to be isolated in the hospital or remain at home during peak transmission periods, leading to social isolation. **Collaboration:** Ascertain if the patient has assistance available if a prolonged period of homebound status is anticipated. • Teach the patient to practice abstinence or to use barrier protection during sexual activity even if genital lesions are not present. Genital HSV infections may be transmitted even in the asymptomatic period. Have the patient consult with the health care provider about suppressive therapy.
Patient understanding of drug therapy: • Use opportunities during administration of medications and during assessments to provide patient education. (Using time during nursing care helps to optimize and reinforce key teaching areas.)	• The patient, family, or caregiver should be able to state the reason for the drug; appropriate dose and scheduling; what adverse effects to observe for and when to report; and the anticipated length of medication therapy.

Patient self-administration of drug therapy:
• When administering medications, instruct the patient, family, or caregiver in the proper self-administration techniques followed by teach-back. (Proper administration will improve the effectiveness of the drug.)
	• Teach the patient to:
	  • Complete the entire course of therapy unless otherwise instructed.
	  • Take the medication as evenly spaced throughout each day as feasible.
	  • Increase overall fluid intake.
	  • If using ointments or creams, wash hands well before applying and again after application. If family or caregivers administer the medicine, gloves should be worn.

See Table 37.2 for a list of drugs to which these nursing actions apply.

Simeprevir (Olysia) inhibits the viral proteins NS3 and NS4; sofosbuvir (Sovaldi) inhibits NS5B. Both are recommended as combination therapy with PEG-IFN and ribavirin. Both are administered PO once daily and exhibit few serious adverse effects. Sofosbuvir may be used with ribavirin alone (without PEG-IFN).

In 2014 sofosbuvir was combined with ledipasvir, a new NS5A inhibitor, in a fixed dose combination (Harvoni). Harvoni is taken once daily, with fatigue and headache being the two most common adverse effects. Viekira Pak was also approved in 2014. Viekira Pak is a four drug combination containing ombitasvir (NS5A inhibitor), paritaprevir (NS3A/4A inhibitor), dasabuvir (NS5B inhibitor), and ritonavir. Ombitasvir, paritaprevir, and ritonavir are in a single tablet given once daily. Dasabuvir is in a separate tablet taken twice daily. The most frequent adverse effects from Viekira Pak include fatigue, nausea, pruritus, skin reactions, insomnia, and asthenia.

Chapter Review

KEY Concepts

The numbered key concepts provide a succinct summary of the important points from the corresponding numbered section within the chapter. If any of these points are not clear, refer to the numbered section within the chapter for review.

37.1 Viruses are nonliving intracellular parasites that require host organelles to replicate. Some viral infections are self-limiting, whereas others benefit from pharmacotherapy.

37.2 HIV targets the T4 lymphocyte, using reverse transcriptase to make viral DNA. The result is gradual destruction of the immune system.

37.3 Antiretroviral drugs used in the treatment of HIV-AIDS do not cure the disease, but they do help many patients live longer. Pharmacotherapy may be initiated in the acute (symptomatic) or chronic (asymptomatic) phase of HIV infection.

37.4 Drugs from five drug classes are used in various combinations in the pharmacotherapy of HIV-AIDS. The specific combinations of drugs that are most effective against HIV is continually evolving, based on ongoing clinical research.

37.5 The reverse transcriptase inhibitors block HIV replication at the level of the reverse transcriptase enzyme. These include the NRTIs, NNRTIs, and the NtRTIs.

37.6 The protease inhibitors inhibit the final assembly of the HIV virion. When combined with other antiretroviral drug classes, the PIs are capable of lowering plasma HIV RNA to undetectable levels.

37.7 Entry inhibitors prevent the entry of the viral nucleic acid into the T4 lymphocyte. HIV integrase inhibitors prevent integrase enzyme from inserting its viral DNA strand into the human chromosome.

37.8 The risk of perinatal transmission of HIV can be markedly reduced by implementing drug therapy in the mother during pregnancy and the newborn following birth.

37.9 Postexposure prophylaxis of HIV infection is designed to prevent the accidental transmission of the virus to health care workers.

37.10 Pharmacotherapy can lessen the severity of acute herpes simplex infections and prolong the latent period of the disease.

37.11 Drugs are available to prevent and to treat influenza infections. Vaccination is the best choice, because drugs are relatively ineffective once influenza symptoms appear.

37.12 Hepatitis A and B are best treated through immunization. Newer drugs for HBV and HCV have led to therapies for chronic hepatitis.

REVIEW Questions

1. A patient is started on efavirenz (Sustiva) for HIV. What should the nurse teach the patient about this drug?
   1. Efavirenz (Sustiva) will cure the disease over time.
   2. Efavirenz (Sustiva) will not cure the disease but may significantly extend the life expectancy.
   3. Efavirenz (Sustiva) will be used prior to vaccines.
   4. Efavirenz (Sustiva) will prevent the transmission of the disease.
2. A patient with HIV has been taking lopinavir with ritonavir (Kaletra) for the past 8 years and has noticed a redistribution of body fat in the arms, legs, and abdomen (lipodystrophy). The nurse will evaluate this patient for what other additional adverse effects associated with this drug? (Select all that apply.)
   1. Renal failure
   2. Hyperglycemia
   3. Pancreatitis
   4. Bone marrow suppression
   5. Hepatic failure
3. Which of the following findings would suggest that myelosuppression is occurring in a patient who is taking zidovudine (Retrovir)?
   1. Increase in serum blood urea nitrogen (BUN) levels
   2. Increase in white blood cell (WBC) count
   3. Decrease in platelet count
   4. Decrease in blood pressure
4. A patient has received a prescription for zanamivir (Relenza) for flulike symptoms. The patient states, "I think I'll hold off on starting this. I don't feel that bad yet." What is the nurse's best response?
   1. "The drug has a stable shelf life so you can save it for later infections."
   2. "It can be saved for later but you will also require an antibiotic to treat your symptoms if you wait."
   3. "It can be started within two weeks after the onset of symptoms."
   4. "To be effective, it must be started within 48 hours after the onset of symptoms."
5. The nurse is teaching a community health class to a group of young adults who have recently immigrated to the United States about preventing hepatitis B. What is the most effective method of preventing a hepatitis B infection?
   1. Peginterferon alfa-2a (Pegasys)
   2. Hepatitis B vaccine (Engerix-B)
   3. Adefovir dipivoxil (Hepsera)
   4. Entecavir (Baraclude)
6. A patient has been diagnosed with genital herpes and has been started on oral acyclovir (Zovirax). What should be included in the teaching instructions for this patient? (Select all that apply.)
   1. Increase fluid intake up to 2 L per day.
   2. Report any dizziness, tremors, or confusion.
   3. Decrease the amount of fluids taken so that the drug can be more concentrated.
   4. Take the drug only when having the most itching or pain from the outbreak.
   5. Use barrier methods such as condoms for sexual activity.

PATIENT-FOCUSED Case Study

Nathan Whitcomb is a 23-year-old college student seeking treatment in the student health clinic for recurrent cold sores (herpes simplex virus [HSV]). Like many college students, he eats on the run and seldom sleeps more than 4 to 5 hours per night. His weekends are even more hectic with his job, school, and social activities. Nathan requests something to help rid him of his existing cold sore immediately. Topical acyclovir (Zovirax) is prescribed.

1. As the nurse, how would you explain the mode of transmission and onset of symptoms for HSV to Nathan?
2. How would you respond when Nathan asked, "Is there any medication that I can take to prevent the cold sores from returning?"
3. Topical acyclovir is prescribed for this patient. What patient education would you provide?

CRITICAL THINKING Questions

1. A 72-year-old woman who lives in an assisted living community is talking with the nurse about her health. The nurse advises the patient of the importance of receiving a seasonal influenza vaccination. What is the rationale supporting this recommendation? If the patient does become infected with the flu, what options are available?

2. A newly diagnosed HIV-positive patient has been started on antiretroviral therapy with efavirenz (Sustiva), tenofovir (Viread), and emtricitabine (Emtriva). What should the nurse teach this patient about taking the drugs? What other factors should the nurse consider when talking with this patient? Identify priorities of nursing care for this patient.

Visit www.pearsonhighered.com/nursingresources for answers and rationales for all activities.

REFERENCES

Centers for Disease Control and Prevention. (2014). *Recommendations for HIV prevention with adults and adolescents with HIV in the United States, 2014*. Retrieved from http://stacks.cdc.gov/view/cdc/26062

Centers for Disease Control and Prevention. (2015). *Advisory Committee on Immunization Practices (ACIP) reaffirms recommendation for annual influenza vaccination*. Retrieved from http://www.cdc.gov/media/releases/2015/s0226-acip.html

Cohen, M. S., Chen, Y. Q., McCauley, M., Gamble, T., Hosseinipour, M. C., Kumarasamy, N., . . . Fleming, T. R. (2011). Prevention of HIV-1 infection with early antiretroviral therapy. *New England Journal of Medicine, 365*, 493–505. doi:10.1056/NEMoa1105243

Herdman, T. H., & Kamitsuru, S. (2014). *NANDA International nursing diagnoses: Definitions and classification, 2015–2017*. Oxford, United Kingdom: Wiley-Blackwell.

Kuhar, D. T., Henderson, D. K., Struble, K. A., Heneine, W., Thomas, V., Cheever, L. W., . . . US Public Health Service Working Group. (2013). Updated US Public Health Service guidelines for the management of occupational exposures to human immunodeficiency virus and recommendations for postexposure prophylaxis. *Infection Control and Hospital Epidemiology, 34*, 875–892. doi:10.1086/672271

Kulkarni, S. P., Shah, K. R., Sarma, K. V., & Mahajan, A. P. (2013). Clinical uncertainties, health service challenges and ethical complexities of HIV "test-and-treat": A systematic review. *American Journal of Public Health, 103*(6), e14–23. doi:10.2105/AJPH.2013.301273

McIntyre, A., Zecevic, A., Diachun, L. (2014). Influenza vaccination: Older adults' decision-making process. *Canadian Journal on Aging, 33*, 92–98. doi:10.1017/S0714980813000640

Nachenga, J. B., Uthman, O. A., del Rio, C., Mugaverno, M. J., Rees, H., & Mills, E. J. (2014). Addressing the Achilles' heel in the HIV care continuum for the success of a test-and-treat strategy to achieve an AIDS-free generation. *Clinical Infectious Diseases, 59*, S21–27. doi:10.1093/cid/ciu299

Panel on Antiretroviral Guidelines for Adults and Adolescents. (2015). *Guidelines for the use of antiretroviral agents in HIV-1-infected adults and adolescents*. Department of Health and Human Services. Retrieved from http://www.aidsinfo.nih.gov/ContentFiles/AdultandAdolescentGL.pdf

Panel on Treatment of HIV-Infected Pregnant Women and Prevention of Perinatal Transmission. (2015). *Recommendations for use of antiretroviral drugs in pregnant HIV-1-infected women for maternal health and interventions to reduce perinatal HIV transmission in the United States*. Retrieved from http://aidsinfo.nih.gov/contentfiles/PerinatalGL.pdf

SELECTED BIBLIOGRAPHY

AIDS.gov. (2014). *HIV in the United States: At a glance*. Retrieved from https://www.aids.gov/hiv-aids-basics/hiv-aids-101/statistics/

Ambrosioni, J., Nicolas, D., Sued, O., Agüero, F., Manzardo, C., & Miro, J. M. (2014). Update on antiretroviral treatment during primary HIV infection. *Expert Review of Anti-Infective Therapy, 12*, 793–807. doi:10.1586/14787210.2014.913981

Buggs, A. M. (2014). *Viral hepatitis*. Retrieved from http://emedicine.medscape.com/article/775507-overview

Chou, R., Hartung, D., Rahman, B., Wasson, N., Cottrell, E. B., & Fu, R. (2013). Comparative effectiveness of antiviral treatment for hepatitis C virus infection in adults: A systematic review. *Annals of Internal Medicine, 158*, 114–123. doi:10.7326/0003-4819-158-2-201301150-00576

Centers for Disease Control and Prevention. (2014). *CDC says "take 3" actions to fight the flu*. Retrieved from http://www.cdc.gov/flu/protect/preventing.htm

Centers for Disease Control and Prevention. (2014). *Genital herpes-CDC fact sheet*. Retrieved from http://www.cdc.gov/std/herpes/stdfact-herpes-detailed.htm

Centers for Disease Control and Prevention. (2014). *Hepatitis B FAQs for health professionals*. Retrieved from http://www.cdc.gov/hepatitis/HBV/HBVfaq.htm#overview

Centers for Disease Control and Prevention. (2015). *Hepatitis C FAQs for health professionals*. Retrieved from http://www.cdc.gov/hepatitis/HCV/HCVfaq.htm#section1

Derlet, R. W. (2015). *Influenza*. Retrieved from http://emedicine.medscape.com/article/219557-overview

Kim, S. R., Khan, F., & Tyring, S. K. (2014). Varicella zoster: An update on current treatment options and future perspectives. *Expert Opinion on Pharmacotherapy, 15*, 61–71. doi:10.1517/14656566.2014.860443

Kiser, J. J., & Flexner, C. (2013). Direct-acting antiviral agents for hepatitis C virus infection. *Annual Review of Pharmacology and Toxicology, 53*, 427–449. doi:10.1146/annurev-pharmtox-011112-140254

Macías, J., Neukam, K., Merchante, N., & Pineda, J. A. (2014). Latest pharmacotherapy options for treating hepatitis C in HIV-infected patients. *Expert Opinion on Pharmacotherapy, 15*, 1837–1848. doi:10.1517/14656566.2014.934810

Muir, P. (2014). Management of herpes simplex and varicella-zoster infections. *Prescriber, 25*(3), 14–23. doi:10.1002/psb.1156

Pyrsopoulos, N. T. (2015). *Hepatitis B*. Retrieved from http://emedicine.medscape.com/article/177632-overview

Rakhmanina, N., & Phelps, B. R. (2012). Pharmacotherapy of pediatric HIV infection. *Pediatric Clinics of North America, 59*, 1093–1115. doi:10.1016/j.pcl.2012.07.009

Chapter 38

Drugs for Neoplasia

Drugs at a Glance

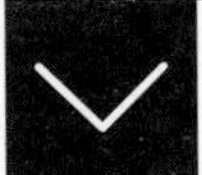

Learning Outcomes

After reading this chapter, the student should be able to:

1. Explain differences between normal cells and cancer cells.
2. Identify factors associated with an increased risk of cancer.
3. Describe lifestyle factors associated with a reduced risk of acquiring cancer.
4. Identify the three primary therapies for cancer.
5. Explain the significance of growth fraction and the cell cycle to the success of chemotherapy.
6. Describe the nurse's role in the pharmacologic management of cancer.
7. Explain how combination therapy and special dosing protocols increase the effectiveness of chemotherapy.
8. Describe the general adverse effects of chemotherapeutic drugs.
9. For each of the drug classes listed in Drugs at a Glance, know representative drugs, and explain their mechanism of drug action, primary actions, and important adverse effects.
10. Categorize anticancer drugs based on their classification and mechanism of action.
11. Use the nursing process to care for patients receiving pharmacotherapy for cancer.

indicates a prototype drug, each of which is featured in a Prototype Drug box.

Cancer is one of the most feared diseases in society for a number of valid reasons. It is often silent, producing no symptoms until it reaches an advanced stage. It sometimes requires painful and disfiguring treatments. It may strike at an early age, even during childhood, to deprive people of a normal life span. Perhaps worst of all, the medical treatment of cancer often cannot offer a cure, and progression to death is sometimes slow, painful, and psychologically difficult for patients and their loved ones.

Despite its feared status, many successes have been made in the diagnosis, understanding, and treatment of cancer. Modern treatment methods result in a cure for nearly two of every three people and the 5-year survival rate has steadily increased for many types of cancer. This chapter examines the role of drugs in the treatment of cancer. Medications used to treat this disease are called anticancer drugs, antineoplastics, or cancer chemotherapeutic agents.

CANCER

38.1 Characteristics of Cancer

Cancer, or carcinoma, is a disease characterized by abnormal, uncontrolled cell division. Cell division is a normal process occurring extensively in most body tissues from conception to late childhood. At some point in time, however, suppressor genes responsible for cell growth stop this rapid division. This may result in a total lack of replication, as in the case of muscle cells and perhaps brain cells. In other cells, genes controlling replication can be turned on when it becomes necessary to replace worn-out cells, as in the case of blood cells and the mucosa of the digestive tract.

Cancer is thought to result from damage to the genes controlling cell growth. Once damaged, the cell is no longer responsive to normal chemical signals checking its growth. The cancer cells lose their normal functions, divide rapidly, and invade surrounding cells. The abnormal cells often travel to distant sites where they populate new tumors, a process called **metastasis.** Figure 38.1 illustrates some characteristics of cancer cells.

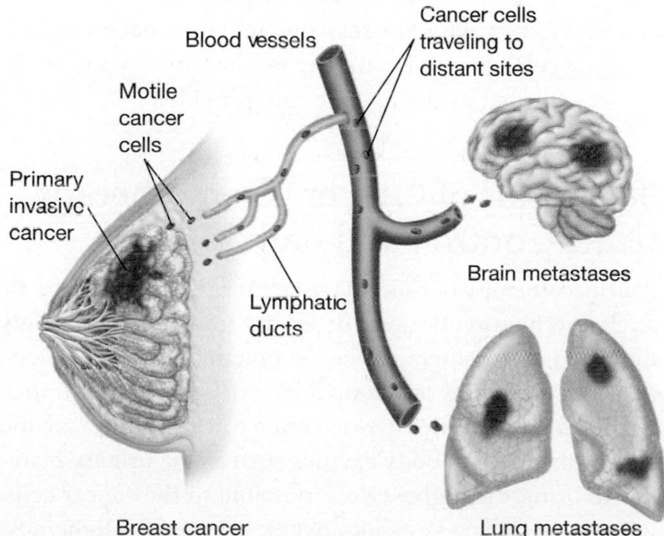

FIGURE 38.1 Invasion and metastasis by cancer cells

Tumor is defined as a swelling, abnormal enlargement, or mass. The word **neoplasm** is often used interchangeably with tumor. Tumors may be solid masses, such as lung or breast cancer, or they may be widely disseminated in the blood, such as leukemia. Tumors are named according to their tissue of origin, generally with the suffix *-oma*. Table 38.1 describes common types of tumors.

38.2 Causes of Cancer

Numerous factors have been found to cause cancer or to be associated with a higher risk for acquiring the disease. These factors are known as *carcinogens*.

Many chemical carcinogens have been identified. For example, chemicals in tobacco smoke are responsible for about one third of all cancers in the United States. Alcohol ingestion has also been linked to certain cancers, including esophageal, oral, breast, and liver cancers. Some chemicals, such as asbestos and benzene, have been associated with a higher incidence of cancer in the workplace. In some cases,

PharmFacts

CANCER

- It is estimated that more than 1,658,000 new cancer cases occur each year, with more than 589,000 deaths (more than 1,620 people each day). Overall, cancer-related deaths have decreased 22% from a high in 1991.
- 78% of cancer diagnoses occur in adults over the age of 55.
- Cancer is the second most common cause of death, and the most common cause of death by disease in children younger than age 14.
- Leukemia is the most common childhood cancer (30%), followed by brain and nervous system tumors (26%).
- Lung cancer has the highest mortality rate: It is responsible for 28% of all cancer deaths.
- Prostate cancer is the second leading cause of cancer death in men.
- The highest 5-year survival rates are for cancers of the prostate, testis, and thyroid. The lowest survival rates are for pancreatic, liver, and lung cancers.
- African Americans are more likely to develop and die from cancer than any other ethnic group.
- Although breast cancer is predominant in women (second in cancer deaths), about 2,300 men are diagnosed with the disease each year.

Data from *Cancer Facts and Figures, American Cancer Society, 2015,* http://www.cancer.org/acs/groups/content/@editorial/documents/document/acspc-044552.pdf

Table 38.1 Classification and Naming of Tumors

Name	Description	Examples
Benign tumor	Slow growing; does not metastasize and rarely requires drug treatment	Adenoma, papilloma and lipoma, osteoma, meningioma
Carcinoma	Cancer of epithelial tissue; most common type of malignant neoplasm; grows rapidly and metastasizes	Malignant melanoma, squamous cell carcinoma, renal cell carcinoma, adenocarcinoma, hepatocellular carcinoma
Glioma	Cancer of glial (interstitial) cells in the brain, spinal cord, pineal gland, posterior pituitary gland, or retina	Telangiectatic glioma, brainstem glioma
Leukemia	Cancer of the blood-forming cells in bone marrow; may be acute or chronic	Myelocytic leukemia, lymphocytic leukemia
Lymphoma	Cancer of lymphoid tissue	Hodgkin's disease, lymphoblastic lymphoma
Malignant tumor	Grows rapidly, becomes resistant to treatment and results in death if untreated	Malignant melanoma
Sarcoma	Cancer of connective tissue; grows extremely rapidly and metastasizes early in the progression of the disease	Osteogenic sarcoma, fibrosarcoma, Kaposi's sarcoma, angiosarcoma

the site of the cancer may be distant from the entry location, as with bladder cancer caused by the inhalation of certain industrial chemicals. A number of physical factors are also associated with cancer. For example, exposure to large amounts of x-rays is associated with a higher risk of leukemia. Ultraviolet light from the sun is a known cause of skin cancer.

It is estimated that viruses are associated with about 15% of all human cancers. Examples include herpes simplex types I and II, Epstein-Barr, human papillomavirus (HPV), cytomegalovirus, and human T-lymphotrophic viruses. Factors that suppress the immune system, such as HIV or drugs given after transplant surgery, may encourage the growth of cancer cells.

Some cancers have a strong genetic component. The fact that close relatives may acquire the same type of cancer suggests that certain genes may predispose close relatives to the condition. These abnormal genes interact with chemical, physical, and biologic agents to promote cancer formation. Other genes, called *tumor suppressor genes,* may inhibit the formation of tumors. If these suppressor genes are damaged, cancer may result. Damage to the suppressor gene p53 is associated with cancers of the breast, lung, brain, colon, and bone.

Although the development of cancer has a genetic component, it is also greatly influenced by factors in the environment. Maintaining or adopting healthy lifestyle habits can reduce the risk of acquiring cancer. Following proper nutrition, avoiding chemical and physical risks, and maintaining a regular schedule of health checkups can help prevent cancer from developing into a fatal disease. The following are lifestyle factors regarding cancer prevention or diagnosis that should be used by nurses when teaching patients about cancer prevention:

- Eliminate tobacco use and exposure to secondhand smoke.
- Limit or eliminate alcoholic beverage use.
- Maintain a healthy diet low in fat and high in fresh vegetables and fruit.
- Choose most foods from plant sources; increase fiber in the diet.
- Exercise regularly and maintain body weight within recommended guidelines.
- Self-examine your body monthly for abnormal lumps and skin lesions.
- Avoid chronic or prolonged exposure to direct sunlight and/or wear protective clothing or sunscreen.
- Have periodic diagnostic testing performed at recommended intervals:
    - Women should have periodic mammograms, according to the schedule recommended by their health care provider.
    - Men should receive prostate screening, as recommended by their health care provider.
    - Both men and women should receive a screening colonoscopy, according to the schedule recommended by their health care provider.
    - Women who are sexually active or have reached age 21 should have a Pap test every 3–5 years, or as directed by their health care provider.

38.3 Goals of Cancer Chemotherapy: Cure, Control, and Palliation

Pharmacotherapy of cancer is sometimes simply referred to as **chemotherapy.** Because drugs are transported through the blood, chemotherapy has the potential to reach cancer cells in virtually any location. Certain drugs are able to cross the blood-brain barrier to reach brain tumors. Others are instilled directly into body cavities such as the urinary bladder to bring the highest dose possible to the cancer cells without producing systemic adverse effects. Chemotherapy has three general goals: cure, control, and palliation.

Complementary and Alternative Therapies

ACUPUNCTURE

Acupuncture is a practice that involves stimulating specific points on the body through fine, metal needles or by electrical stimulation (National Center for Complementary and Integrative Health, 2014). Acupuncture has been used as a component of traditional Chinese medicine for thousands of years but only recently has it gained more acceptance as a valid treatment in Western medicine. Research has focused on its effectiveness when used to treat pain, including cancer and neuropathic pain, hiccups, dyspnea, hot flashes, dry mouth (xerostomia), and many other conditions, including psychological symptoms.

Research and large clinical trials have supported acupuncture as a valid treatment for cancer pain and symptoms related to chemotherapy and radiation such as nausea; for pain from arthritis; for joint and low back pain; and for reduction in the frequency of migraines (Haddad & Palesh, 2014; Rithirangsriroj, Manchana, & Akkayagorn, 2015). Acupuncture did not prevent the progression of the disease, but provided relief from symptoms related to the disease. And in most studies, manual acupuncture, rather than the use of electrically stimulated acupuncture, was the most successful. There is not yet enough clinical evidence to support the use of acupuncture in the treatment of xerostomia, depression, anxiety, sleep disturbances, or other conditions.

When diagnosed with cancer, the primary goal desired by most patients is to achieve a complete cure; that is, permanent removal of all cancer cells from the body. The possibility for cure is much greater if a cancer is identified and treated in its early stages, when the tumor is small and localized to a well-defined region. Indeed, the 5-year survival rates for nearly all types of cancer have increased in the past several decades due to improved detection and more effective therapies. Examples in which chemotherapy has been used successfully as curative treatments include Hodgkin's lymphoma, certain leukemias, and choriocarcinoma.

When cancer has progressed and cure is not possible, a second goal of chemotherapy is to control or manage the disease. Although the cancer is not eliminated, preventing the growth and spread of the tumor may extend the patient's life. Essentially, the cancer is managed as a chronic disease, such as hypertension or diabetes.

In its advanced stages, cure or control of the cancer may not be achievable. For these patients, chemotherapy is used as **palliation.** Chemotherapy drugs are administered to reduce the size of the tumor, easing the severity of pain and other tumor symptoms, thus improving the quality of life. Examples of advanced cancers for which palliation is frequently used include osteosarcoma, pancreatic cancer, and Kaposi's sarcoma.

Chemotherapy may be used alone or in combination with other treatment modalities such as surgery or radiation therapy. Surgery is especially useful for removing solid tumors that are localized. Surgery lowers the number of cancer cells in the body so that radiation therapy and pharmacotherapy can be more successful. Surgery is not an option for tumors of blood cells or when it would not be expected to extend a patient's life span or to improve the quality of life.

Approximately 50% of patients with cancer receive radiation therapy as part of their treatment. Radiation therapy is most successful and produces the fewest adverse effects for cancers that are localized, when high doses of ionizing radiation can be aimed directly at the tumor and be confined to a small area. Radiation treatments are frequently prescribed postoperatively to kill cancer cells that may remain following an operation. Radiation is sometimes given as palliation for inoperable cancers to shrink the size of a tumor that may be pressing on vital organs, and to relieve pain, difficulty breathing, or difficulty swallowing.

Adjuvant chemotherapy is the administration of antineoplastic drugs *after* surgery or radiation therapy. The purpose of adjuvant chemotherapy is to rid the body of any cancerous cells that could not be removed during surgery or to treat any microscopic metastases that may be developing. In a few cases, drugs are given as *chemoprophylaxis* with the goal of preventing cancer from occurring in patients at high risk for developing tumors. For example, some patients who have had a primary breast cancer removed may receive tamoxifen, even if there is no evidence of metastases, because there is a high likelihood that the disease will recur. Chemoprophylaxis of cancer is uncommon, because most of these drugs have potentially serious adverse effects.

38.4 Growth Fraction and Success of Chemotherapy

Although cancers grow rapidly, not all cells in a tumor are replicating at any given time. Because antineoplastic drugs are generally more effective against cells that are replicating, the percentage of tumor cells dividing at the time of chemotherapy is critical.

Both normal and cancerous cells go through a sequence of events known as the cell cycle, illustrated in Figure 38.2. Cells spend most of their lifetime in the G_0 phase. Although sometimes called the resting stage, the G_0 is the phase during which cells conduct their everyday activities such as metabolism, impulse conduction,

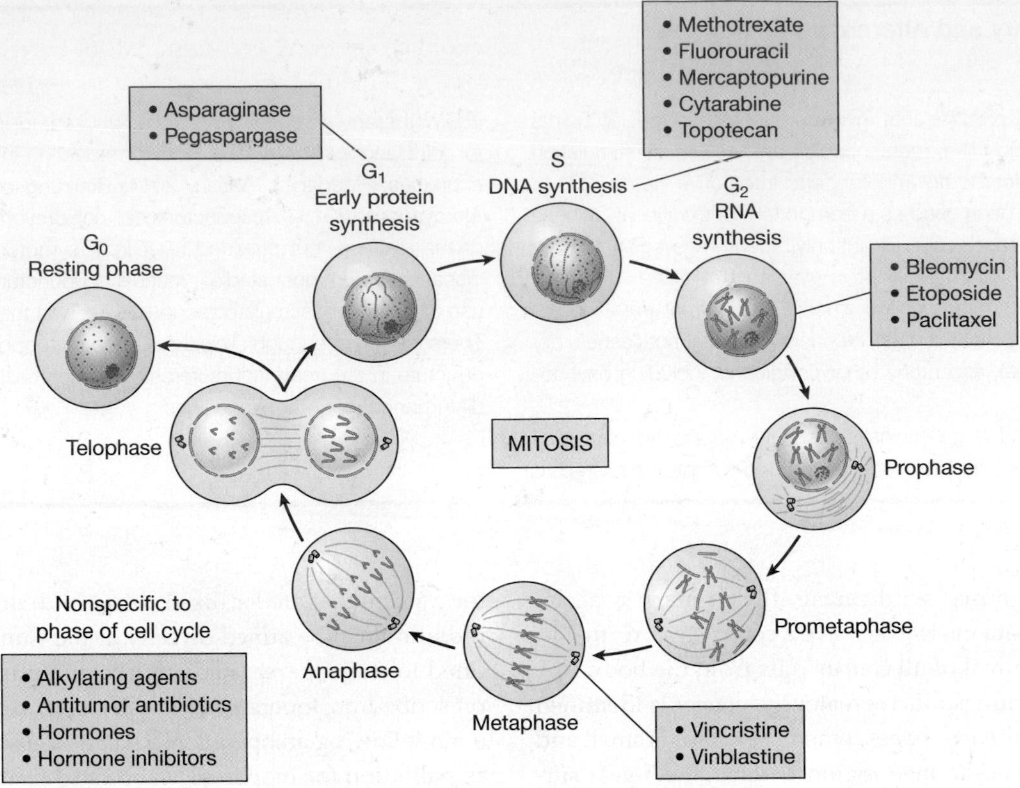

FIGURE 38.2 Antineoplastic agents and the cell cycle

contraction, or secretion. If the cell receives a signal to divide, it leaves G_0 and enters the G_1 phase, during which it synthesizes the RNA, proteins, and other components needed to duplicate its DNA during the S phase. Following duplication of its DNA, the cell enters the premitotic phase, or G_2. Following mitosis in the M phase, the cell re-enters its resting G_0 phase, where it may remain for extended periods, depending on the specific tissue and surrounding cellular signals.

The actions of many of the antineoplastic drugs are specific to certain phases of the cell cycle, whereas others are mostly independent of the cell cycle. For example, mitotic inhibitors such as vincristine (Oncovin) affect the M phase, which includes prophase, metaphase, anaphase, and telophase. Antimetabolites such as fluorouracil (5-FU, Adrucil, Carac, Efudex) are most effective during the S phase. The effects of alkylating agents such as cyclophosphamide (Cytoxan) are generally independent of the phases of the cell cycle. Some of these drugs are shown in Figure 38.2.

The **growth fraction** is a measure of the number of cells undergoing mitosis in a tissue. It is a ratio of the number of *replicating* cells to the number of *resting* cells. Antineoplastic drugs are much more toxic to tissues and tumors with high growth fractions. For example, solid tumors such as breast and lung cancer generally have a *low* growth fraction; thus, they are less sensitive to antineoplastic drugs. Certain leukemias and lymphomas have a *high* growth fraction and therefore have a greater antineoplastic success rate. Because certain normal tissues, such as hair follicles, bone marrow, and the gastrointestinal (GI) epithelium, also have a high growth fraction, they are sensitive to the effects of the antineoplastics.

38.5 Achieving a Total Cancer Cure

To cure a patient, it is believed that every single cancer cell in a tumor must be eliminated from the body. Leaving even a single malignant cell could result in regrowth of the tumor. Eliminating every cancer cell, however, is a very difficult task.

As an example, consider that a small, 1-cm breast tumor may already contain 1 billion cancer cells before it can be detected on a manual examination. A drug that could kill 99% of these cells would be considered a very effective drug indeed. Yet even with this fantastic achievement, 10 million cancer cells would remain, any one of which could potentially cause the tumor to return and kill the patient. The relationship between cell kill and chemotherapy is shown in Figure 38.3.

It is likely that no antineoplastic drug (or combination of drugs) will kill 100% of the tumor cells. The large burden of cancer cells, however, may be lowered sufficiently to permit the patient's immune system to control or

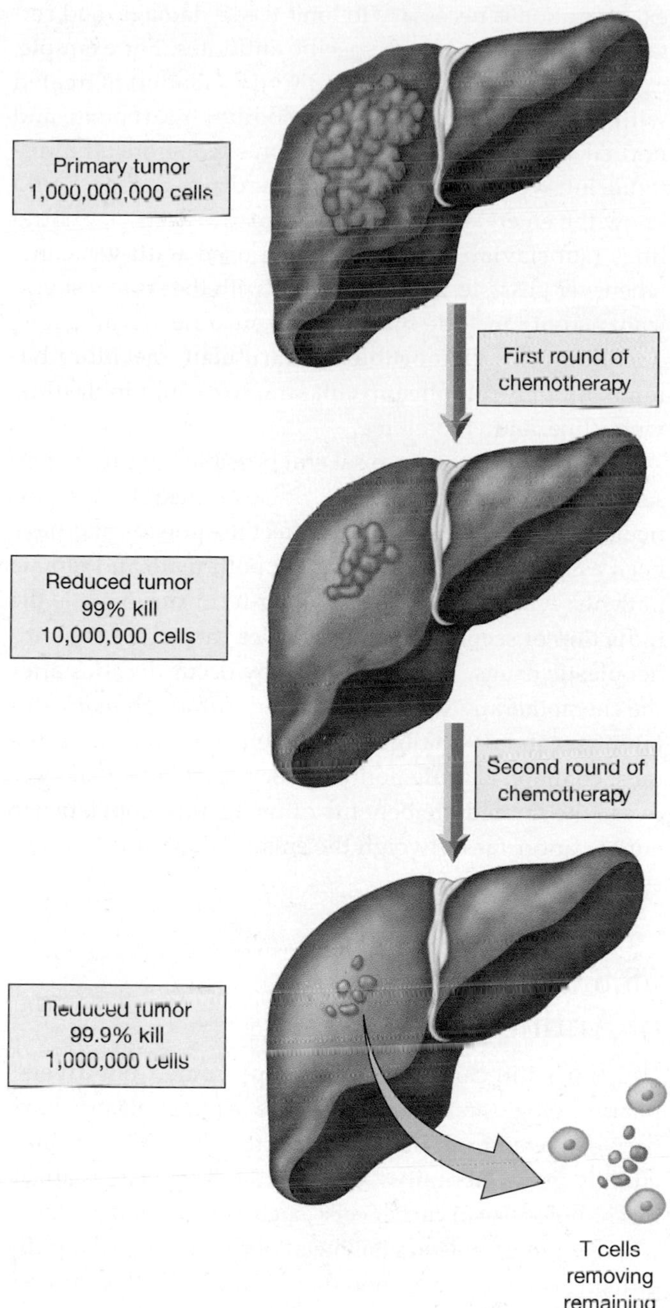

FIGURE 38.3 Cell kill and chemotherapy

eliminate the remaining cancer cells. Because the immune system is able to eliminate only a relatively small number of cancer cells, it is imperative that as many cancerous cells as possible be eliminated during treatment. This example reinforces the need to diagnose and treat tumors at an *early* stage when the number of cancer cells is smaller.

38.6 Special Chemotherapy Protocols and Strategies

Tumor cells exhibit a high mutation rate that continually changes their genetic structure, resulting in a more heterogenous mass as the tumor grows. Essentially, the tumor becomes a mass of hundreds of different types of cancer cells with different growth rates and physiological properties. An antineoplastic drug may kill only a small portion of the tumor, leaving some clones unaffected. Complicating the chances for a cure is that cancer cells often develop resistance to antineoplastic drugs. Thus, a therapy that was very successful in reducing the tumor mass at the start of chemotherapy may become less effective over time. The tumor becomes "refractory" to treatment. A number of treatment strategies have been found to increase the effectiveness of chemotherapy.

Combination Chemotherapy

In most cases, multiple drugs from different antineoplastic classes are given during a course of chemotherapy. The use of multiple drugs affects different stages of the cancer cell's life cycle and attacks the various clones within the tumor via several mechanisms of action, thus increasing the percentage of cell kill. Combination chemotherapy also allows lower dosages of each individual drug, thus reducing toxicity and slowing the development of resistance. Examples of combination therapies include cyclophosphamide-methotrexate-fluorouracil for breast cancer and cyclophosphamide-doxorubicin-vincristine for lung cancer. Each type of cancer has its own individual protocol, which is continually being refined and revised based on current research.

Dosing Schedules

Specific dosing schedules, or protocols, have been found to increase the effectiveness of the antineoplastic drugs. For example, some of the anticancer drugs are given as a single dose or perhaps several doses over a few days. A few weeks may pass before the next series of doses begins. This gives normal cells time to recover from the adverse effects of the drugs and allows tumor cells that may not have been replicating at the time of the first dose to begin dividing and become more sensitive to the next round of chemotherapy. Sometimes the optimal dosing schedule must be delayed until the patient sufficiently recovers from the drug toxicities, especially bone marrow suppression. The specific dosing schedule depends on the type of tumor, stage of the disease, and the patient's overall condition.

38.7 Toxicity of Antineoplastic Drugs

Although cancer cells are clearly abnormal in structure and function, much of their physiology is identical to that of normal cells. Because it is difficult to kill cancer cells *selectively* without profoundly affecting normal cells, all anticancer drugs have the potential to cause serious toxicity. These drugs are often pushed to their maximum possible dosages, so that the greatest tumor kill can be obtained.

Such high dosages always result in adverse effects in the patient. Normal cells that are replicating are most susceptible to adverse effects. Hair follicles are damaged, resulting in hair loss or **alopecia.** The epithelial lining of the digestive tract commonly becomes inflamed, a condition known as **mucositis.** Consequences of mucositis include painful ulcerations, difficulty eating or swallowing, GI bleeding, intestinal infections, or severe diarrhea. The vomiting center in the medulla is triggered by many antineoplastics, resulting in significant nausea and vomiting. Because of this effect, antineoplastics are sometimes classified by their **emetogenic potential.** Before starting therapy with the highest emetic potential medications, patients may be pretreated with antiemetic drugs such as ondansetron (Zofran), prochlorperazine (Compazine), metoclopramide (Reglan, others), or lorazepam (Ativan) (see chapter 42).

Stem cells in the bone marrow may be destroyed by antineoplastics, causing anemia, leukopenia, and thrombocytopenia. These adverse effects are dose limiting and the ones that most often cause discontinuation or delays of chemotherapy. Severe bone marrow suppression is a contraindication to therapy with most antineoplastics.

Each antineoplastic drug has a documented **nadir,** the lowest point to which the erythrocyte, neutrophil, or platelet count is depressed by the drug. Although chemotherapy decreases all types of white blood cells (WBCs), neutrophils are the type most affected. A patient is diagnosed with neutropenia when the neutrophil count is less than 1,500 cells/mL. Patients are very susceptible to infections while they are neutropenic. Many times patients who are neutropenic are placed in reverse isolation to protect them from exposure to any infections from family members or health care providers. Even an infection from a mild cold could be fatal to patients with extremely low neutrophil counts. If a patient with neutropenia develops a fever, antibiotics are indicated.

Efforts to minimize bone marrow toxicity may include bone marrow transplantation, platelet infusions, or therapy with growth factors such as epoetin alfa (Epogen, Procrit), filgrastim (Neupogen), or oprelvekin (Neumega) (see chapter 32). The administration of filgrastim often prevents or shortens the time period of neutropenia, thus lowering the risk of opportunistic infections and allowing the patient to maintain an optimal dosing schedule.

When possible, antineoplastics are given locally by topical application or through direct instillation into a tumor site to minimize systemic toxicity. Most antineoplastics, however, must be administered intravenously. Many antineoplastics are classified as **vesicants,** agents that can cause serious tissue injury if they escape from an artery or vein during an infusion or injection. Extravasation from an injection site can produce severe tissue and nerve damage, local infection, and even loss of a limb. Rapid treatment of extravasation is necessary to limit tissue damage, and certain antineoplastics have specific antidotes. For example, extravasation of carmustine (BiCNU, Gliadel) is treated with injections of equal parts of sodium bicarbonate and normal saline into the extravasation site. Before administering intravenous (IV) antineoplastic drugs, nurses should know the emergency treatment for extravasation. Central lines (subclavian vein) should be used with vesicants whenever possible. Antineoplastics with the strongest vesicant activity include busulfan, carmustine, dacarbazine, dactinomycin, daunorubicin, idarubicin, mechlorethamine, mitomycin, plicamycin, streptozocin, vinblastine, vincristine, and vinorelbine.

Cancer survivors face several possible long-term consequences from chemotherapy. Some antineoplastics, particularly the alkylating agents, affect the gonads and have been associated with infertility in both male and female patients. A second concern for long-term survivors is the induction of secondary malignancies caused by the antineoplastic drugs. These tumors may occur decades after the chemotherapy was administered. Although many different secondary malignancies have been reported, the most common is acute nonlymphocytic leukemia. In most cases, the immediate benefits of using antineoplastics to cure a cancer far outweigh the small risk of developing a secondary malignancy.

38.8 Classification of Antineoplastic Drugs

Drugs used in cancer chemotherapy come from diverse pharmacologic and chemical classes. Antineoplastics have been extracted from plants and bacteria as well as created entirely in the laboratory. Some of the drug classes attack macromolecules in cancer cells, such as DNA and proteins, whereas others poison vital metabolic pathways of rapidly growing cells. The common theme among all the antineoplastic medications is that they kill or at least stop the growth of cancer cells.

Classification of the various antineoplastics is quite variable because some of these drugs kill cancer cells by different mechanisms and have characteristics from more than one class. Furthermore, the mechanisms by which some antineoplastics act are not completely understood. A simple method of classifying this complex group of drugs includes the following categories:

- Alkylating agents
- Antimetabolites
- Antitumor antibiotics
- Natural products
- Hormones and hormone antagonists
- Biologic response modifiers and targeted therapies
- Miscellaneous antineoplastic drugs.

ALKYLATING AGENTS

The first alkylating agents, the nitrogen mustards, were developed in secrecy as chemical warfare agents during World War II. Although the drugs in this class have different chemical structures, all share the common characteristic of forming bonds or linkages with DNA, a process called **alkylation.** Figure 38.4 illustrates the process of alkylation.

38.9 Pharmacotherapy With Alkylating Agents

Alkylation changes the shape of the DNA double helix and prevents the nucleic acid from completing normal cell division. Each alkylating agent attaches to DNA in a different manner; however, collectively the alkylating agents have the effect of inducing cell death, or at least slowing the replication of tumor cells. Although the process of alkylation occurs independently of the cell cycle, the killing action does not occur until the affected cell attempts to divide. The alkylating agents have a broad spectrum and are used against many types of malignancies. They are some of the most widely prescribed antineoplastic drugs. These drugs are listed in Table 38.2.

Because blood cells are particularly sensitive to alkylating agents, bone marrow suppression is the primary dose-limiting toxicity of drugs in this class. Within days after administration, the numbers of erythrocytes, leukocytes, and platelets begin to decline, reaching a nadir at

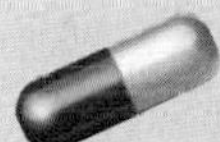

Prototype Drug | Cyclophosphamide *(Cytoxan)*

Therapeutic Class: Antineoplastic **Pharmacologic Class:** Alkylating agent; nitrogen mustard

Actions and Uses

Cyclophosphamide is a commonly prescribed nitrogen mustard. It is used alone, or in combination with other drugs, against a wide variety of cancers, including Hodgkin's disease, lymphoma, multiple myeloma, breast cancer, and ovarian cancer. Cyclophosphamide acts by attaching to DNA and disrupting replication, particularly in rapidly dividing cells. It is one of only a few anticancer drugs that are well absorbed when given orally (PO).

Cyclophosphamide is a powerful immunosuppressant. While this is considered an adverse effect during cancer chemotherapy, the drug is used to *intentionally* cause immunosuppression for the prophylaxis of organ transplant rejection and to treat severe rheumatoid arthritis and systemic lupus erythematosus (SLE).

Administration Alerts

- Dilute prior to IV administration.
- Monitor platelet count prior to IM administration; if low, hold dose.
- To avoid GI upset, take with meals or divide doses.
- Pregnancy category C.

PHARMACOKINETICS (PO)

Onset	Peak	Duration
1–2 h	1–2 h	Unknown

Adverse Effects

Bone marrow suppression is a potentially life-threatening adverse reaction that occurs during days 9–14 of therapy; the patient is at dangerous risk for severe infection and sepsis during this period. Thrombocytopenia is common, though less severe than with many other alkylating agents. Nausea, vomiting, anorexia, and diarrhea are frequently experienced. Cyclophosphamide causes reversible alopecia, although the hair may regrow with a different color or texture. Several metabolites of cyclophosphamide may cause hemorrhagic cystitis if the urine becomes concentrated; patients should be advised to maintain high fluid intake during therapy. The drug may cause permanent sterility in some patients. Unlike other nitrogen mustards, cyclophosphamide exhibits little neurotoxicity.

Contraindications: Cyclophosphamide is contraindicated in patients with hypersensitivity to the drug and for those who have active infections or severely suppressed bone marrow.

Interactions

Drug–Drug: Immunosuppressant drugs used concurrently with cyclophosphamide will increase the risk of infections and further development of neoplasms. There is an increased chance of bone marrow toxicity if cyclophosphamide is used concurrently with allopurinol. There is an increased risk of bleeding if given with anticoagulants.

If used concurrently with digoxin, decreased serum levels of digoxin occur. Use with insulin may lead to hypoglycemia. Phenobarbital, phenytoin, or glucocorticoids used concurrently may lead to an increased rate of cyclophosphamide metabolism by the liver. Thiazide diuretics increase the possibility of leukopenia.

Lab Tests: Serum uric acid levels may increase. Blood cell counts will diminish due to bone marrow suppression. Positive reactions to Candida, mumps, and tuberculin skin tests are suppressed. Pap smears may give false positives.

Herbal/Food: St. John's wort may increase the toxic effects of cyclophosphamide.

Treatment of Overdose: There is no specific treatment for overdose.

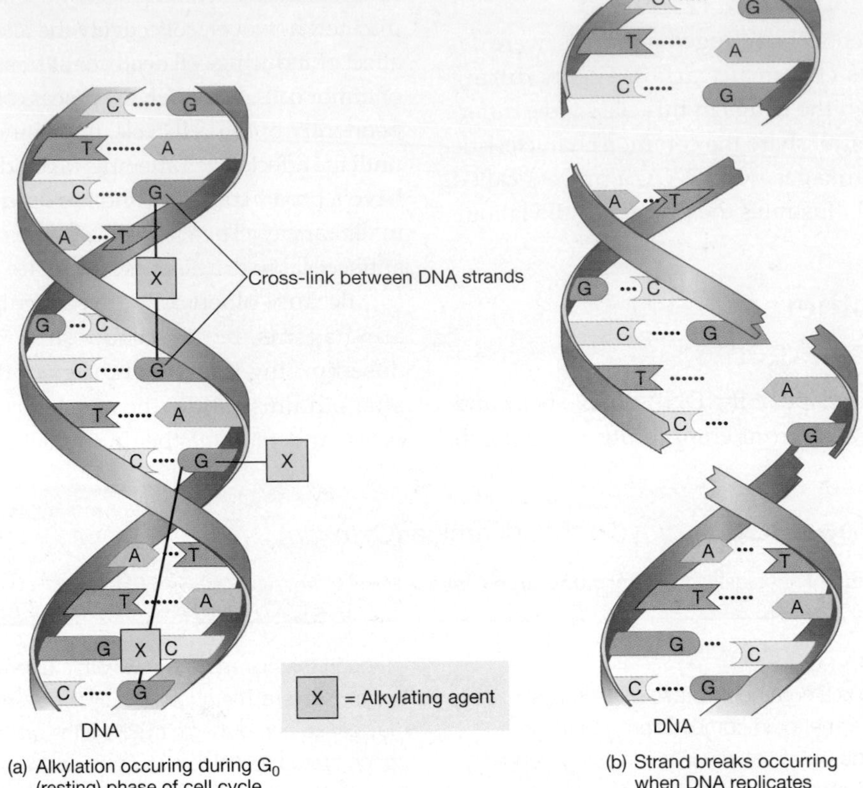
Cross-link between DNA strands
X = Alkylating agent
DNA
(a) Alkylation occuring during G_0 (resting) phase of cell cycle
DNA
(b) Strand breaks occurring when DNA replicates during S phase of cell cycle

FIGURE 38.4 Mechanism of action of the alkylating agents

Table 38.2 Alkylating Agents

Drug	Route and Adult Dose (max dose where indicated)	Adverse Effects
NITROGEN MUSTARDS		
bendamustine (Treanda)	IV: 90–120 mg/m² on days 1 and 2 of a 28-day cycle	*Nausea, vomiting, stomatitis, anorexia, rash, headache, alopecia, fluid retention* Bone marrow suppression (neutropenia, anemia, thrombocytopenia), severe nausea and vomiting, diarrhea, Stevens–Johnson syndrome (SJS), hemorrhagic cystitis, pulmonary toxicity, neurotoxicity (carboplatin, cisplatin, oxaliplatin), ototoxicity (cisplatin), hypersensitivity reactions (including anaphylaxis), nephrotoxicity, fetal toxicity
chlorambucil (Leukeran)	PO: Initial dose: 0.1–0.2 mg/kg/day for 3–6 wk	
cyclophosphamide (Cytoxan)	PO: Initial dose: 1–5 mg/kg/day; Maintenance dose: 1–5 mg/kg every 7–10 days	
estramustine (Emcyt)	PO: 14 mg/kg/day	
ifosfamide (Ifex)	IV: 1.2 g/m²/day for 5 consecutive days	
mechlorethamine (Mustargen)	IV: 0.4 mg/kg as a single or divided dose	
melphalan (Alkeran)	PO: 6 mg/day for 2–3 wk	
NITROSOUREAS		
carmustine (BiCNU, Gliadel)	IV: 200 mg/m² once every 6 wk	
lomustine (CeeNU, CCNU)	PO: 130 mg/m² as a single dose once every 6 wk	
streptozocin (Zanosar)	IV: 500 mg/m² for 5 consecutive days, every 6 wk	
OTHER ALKYLATING AGENTS		
busulfan (Myleran)	PO: 4–8 mg/day	
carboplatin (Paraplatin)	IV: 0.8 mg/kg qid for 4 days	
cisplatin (Platinol)	IV: 360 mg/m² once every 4 wk	
dacarbazine (DTIC-Dome)	IV: 20 mg/m²/day for 5 days	
oxaliplatin (Eloxatin)	IV: 2–4.5 mg/kg/day for 10 days, repeated every 4 wk	
procarbazine (Matulane)	IV: 85 mg/m² for 2 h	
temozolomide (Temodar)	PO: 2–4 mg/kg/day for 1 wk	
thiotepa	PO: 150 mg/m²/day for 5 consecutive days IV: 0.3–0.4 mg/kg every 1–4 wks	

Note: *Italics* indicate common adverse effects; underlining indicates serious adverse effects.

9 to 14 days (depending upon the specific drug used). Epithelial cells lining the GI tract are also damaged, resulting in nausea, vomiting, and diarrhea. Alopecia is expected from most of the alkylating agents. The nitrosoureas and mechlorethamine are strong vesicants. A small percentage of the patients treated with alkylating agents develop acute nonlymphocytic leukemia 4 years or more after chemotherapy has been completed.

ANTIMETABOLITES

Antimetabolites are antineoplastic drugs that chemically resemble essential building blocks of cells. These drugs interfere with aspects of the nutrient or nucleic acid metabolism of rapidly growing tumor cells.

38.10 Pharmacotherapy With Antimetabolites

Rapidly growing cancer cells require large quantities of nutrients to construct cellular proteins and nucleic acids. Antimetabolite drugs are structurally similar to these nutrients, but they do not perform the same functions as their natural counterparts. When cancer cells attempt to synthesize proteins, RNA, or DNA using the antimetabolites, metabolic pathways are disrupted and the cancer cells die or their growth is slowed. The three classes of antimetabolites include the folic acid analogs, the purine analogs, and the pyrimidine analogs. Bone marrow toxicity is the principal dose-limiting adverse effect of many drugs in this class. Some also cause serious GI toxicity, including ulcerations of the mucosa. Mercaptopurine and thioguanine can cause hepatotoxicity, including cholestatic jaundice. These medications are prescribed for leukemias and solid tumors and are listed in Table 38.3. Figure 38.5 illustrates the structural similarities of some of these antimetabolites to their natural counterparts.

Folic Acid Analogs

Folic acid, or folate, is vitamin B_9, which is essential for the growth and maintenance of cells. Lack of this vitamin during pregnancy can cause neural tube defects in the fetus. Three folic acid analogs are used as antineoplastic drugs. Methotrexate, the oldest, is prescribed for several autoimmune disorders in addition to cancer. Pemetrexed (Alimta) and pralatrexate (Folotyn) have very limited therapeutic applications. As antineoplastics, folic acid analogs are given at high doses, which can be toxic to normal cells as well as cancer cells. To "rescue" normal cells, the drug

Table 38.3 Antimetabolites

Drug	Route and Adult Dose (max dose where indicated)	Adverse Effects
FOLIC ACID ANALOGS		
methotrexate (Rheumatrex, Trexall)	PO: 10–30 mg/day for 5 days	*Nausea, vomiting, stomatitis, anorexia, rash, headache, alopecia* <u>Bone marrow suppression (neutropenia, anemia, thrombocytopenia), severe nausea, vomiting and diarrhea, hepatotoxicity, mucositis, pulmonary toxicity, hypersensitivity reactions (including anaphylaxis), neurotoxicity (cytarabine, fluorouracil, fludarabine, cladribine)</u>
pemetrexed (Alimta)	IV: 500 mg/m² on day 1 of each 21-day cycle	
pralatrexate (Folotyn)	IV: 30 mg/m² administered over 3–5 minutes	
PYRIMIDINE ANALOGS		
capecitabine (Xeloda)	PO: 2,500 mg/m²/day for 2 wk	
cytarabine (Cytosar, Depot-Cyt)	IV: 200 mg/m² as a continuous infusion over 24 h	
floxuridine (FUDR)	Intra-arterial: 0.1–0.6 mg/kg/day as a continuous infusion	
fluorouracil (5-FU, Adrucil, Carac, Efudox)	IV: 12 mg/kg/day for 4 consecutive days	
gemcitabine (Gemzar)	IV: 1,000 mg/m² once every wk for 7 wk	
PURINE ANALOGS		
cladribine (Leustatin)	IV: 0.09 mg/m²/day as a continuous infusion	
clofarabine (Clolar)	IV: 52 mg/m²/day over 2 h for 5 days	
fludarabine (Fludara)	IV: 25 mg/m²/day for 5 consecutive days	
mercaptopurine (Purinethol)	PO: 2.5 mg/kg/day	
nelarabine (Arranon)	IV: 1,500 mg/m² on days 1, 3, and 5, repeated every 21 days	
pentostatin (Nipent)	IV: 4 mg/m² bolus or infusion every 2 wk	
thioguanine (Tabloid)	PO: 2 mg/kg/day	

Note: *Italics* indicate common adverse effects; <u>underlining</u> indicates serious adverse effects.

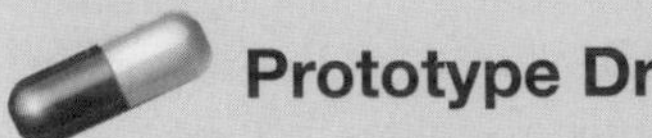

Prototype Drug | Methotrexate *(Rheumatrex, Trexall)*

Therapeutic Class: Antineoplastic **Pharmacologic Class:** Antimetabolite, folic acid analog

Actions and Uses

Methotrexate is an antimetabolite available by the oral, parenteral, and intrathecal routes. By blocking the synthesis of folic acid (vitamin B_9), methotrexate inhibits replication, particularly in rapidly dividing cells. It is prescribed alone or in combination with other drugs for choriocarcinoma, osteogenic sarcoma, leukemias, head and neck cancers, breast carcinoma, and lung carcinoma. Its primary use as an antineoplastic agent is in combination therapy to maintain induced remissions in those persons who have had surgical resection or amputation for a primary tumor.

In addition to its role as an antimetabolite, methotrexate has powerful immunosuppressant properties. While immunosuppression is considered an adverse effect in patients with cancer, this action of methotrexate can be used to advantage in treating patients with severe rheumatoid arthritis, ulcerative colitis, SLE, and psoriasis.

Administration Alerts

- Avoid skin exposure to the drug.
- Avoid inhaling drug particles.
- Dilute prior to IV administration.
- Pregnancy category X.

PHARMACOKINETICS

Onset	Peak	Duration
1–4 h PO; 0.5–2 h IM/IV	1–2 h	Unknown

Adverse Effects

Methotrexate has many adverse effects, some of which can be life threatening. Nausea and vomiting are severe at high doses.

Black Box Warning: Methotrexate carries multiple black box warnings. Methotrexate combined with nonsteroidal anti-inflammatory drugs (NSAIDs) may cause severe and sometimes fatal myelosuppression, which is the primary dose-limiting toxicity of this drug. The drug is hepatotoxic and may cause liver cirrhosis with prolonged use. Ulcerative stomatitis and diarrhea require suspension of therapy because they may lead to hemorrhagic enteritis and death from intestinal perforation. Potentially fatal opportunistic infections, including *Pneumocystis* pneumonia, may occur during therapy. Pulmonary toxicity may result in acute or chronic interstitial pneumonitis at any dose level. Severe, sometimes fatal, dermatologic reactions such as toxic epidermal necrolysis and Stevens–Johnson syndrome (SJS) have been reported. Low doses of methotrexate have been associated with the development of malignant lymphomas. High doses can result in renal failure.

Contraindications: The use of methotrexate as an antineoplastic is contraindicated in thrombocytopenia, anemia, leukopenia, concurrent administration of hepatotoxic drugs and hematopoietic suppressants, alcoholism, or lactation. Methotrexate is teratogenic and is contraindicated in pregnant patients. Patients with alcoholism or other chronic liver disease should not receive methotrexate. Immunosuppressed patients or those with blood dyscrasias should not receive methotrexate.

Interactions

Drug–Drug: Bone marrow suppressants such as chemotherapy agents or radiation therapy may cause increased effects; the patient will require a lower dose of methotrexate. Concurrent use with NSAIDs may lead to severe methotrexate toxicity. Aspirin may interfere with excretion of methotrexate, leading to increased serum levels and toxicity. Concurrent administration with live oral vaccines may result in decreased antibody response and increased adverse reactions to the vaccine.

Lab Tests: Serum uric acid levels may increase. Blood cell counts will diminish due to bone marrow suppression.

Herbal/Food: Food delays the oral absorption of methotrexate. Echinacea may increase the risk of hepatotoxicity. More than 180 mg per day of caffeine (3 to 4 cups of coffee) may decrease the effectiveness of methotrexate when taken for arthritis.

Treatment of Overdose: Leucovorin (folinic acid), a reduced form of folic acid, is sometimes administered with methotrexate to "rescue" normal cells or to protect against severe bone marrow damage. It is most effective if administered as soon as possible after the overdose is discovered. In addition, the urine may be alkalinized to protect the kidneys from methotrexate toxicity.

leucovorin is administered following chemotherapy with methotrexate. Leucovorin, or folinic acid, is a reduced form of folic acid that is able to enter normal cells but not cancer cells. When used with fluorouracil (5-FU) in the treatment of colorectal cancer, leucovorin has been found to enhance cell killing.

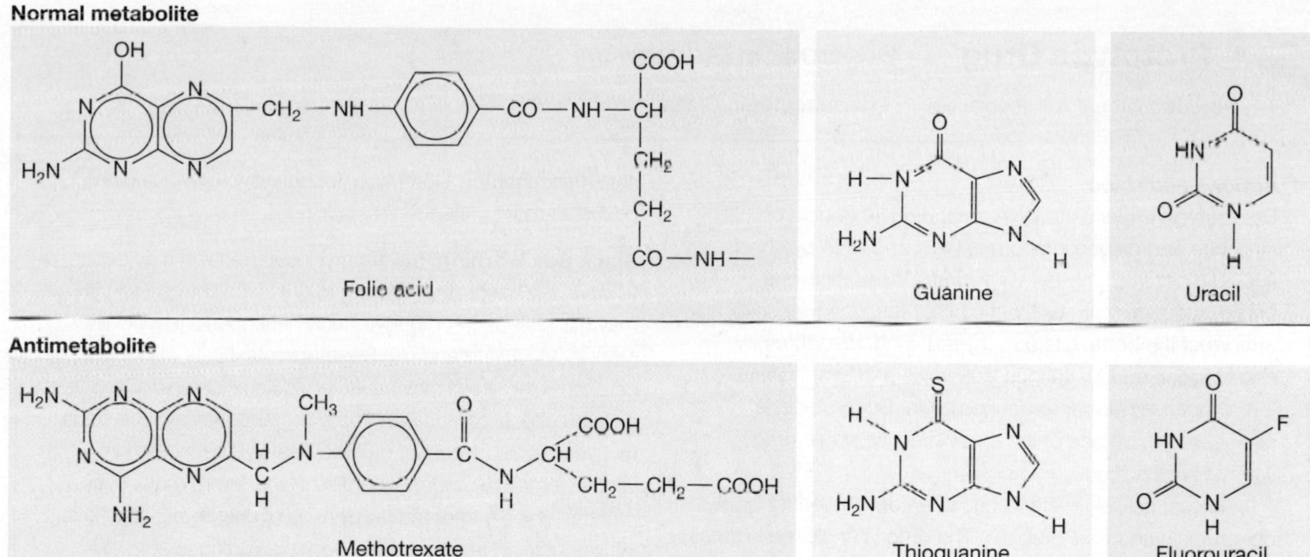

FIGURE 38.5 Structural similarities between antimetabolites and their natural counterparts

Purine and Pyrimidine Analogs

Purines and pyrimidines are bases used in the biosynthesis of DNA and RNA. The purine and pyrimidine analogs are drugs structurally similar to their naturally occurring counterparts that can act in several ways. They can inhibit the synthesis of the natural purine or pyrimidine bases, thus limiting the precursors needed for DNA and RNA biosynthesis. The analogs themselves can also become incorporated into the structures of DNA and RNA, resulting in a disruption of nucleic acid function.

ANTITUMOR ANTIBIOTICS

Antitumor antibiotics are drugs obtained from bacteria that have the ability to kill cancer cells. Although not widely used, they are very effective against certain tumors. The antitumor antibiotics are listed in Table 38.4.

38.11 Pharmacotherapy With Antitumor Antibiotics

A number of substances isolated from microorganisms have been found to possess antitumor properties. These chemicals are more cytotoxic than traditional antibiotics and, with the exception of doxorubicin, their use is limited to treating a few specific types of cancer. For example, the only indication for idarubicin (Idamycin) is acute myelogenous leukemia. Breast carcinoma is the only approved use for epirubicin (Ellence).

The antitumor antibiotics bind to DNA and affect its function by a mechanism similar to that of the alkylating agents. Thus, their general actions and side effects are similar to those of the alkylating agents. Unlike the alkylating agents, however, all the antitumor antibiotics must be administered IV or through direct instillation via a catheter into a body

Table 38.4 Antitumor Antibiotics

Drug	Route and Adult Dose (max dose where indicated)	Adverse Effects
bleomycin (Blenoxane)	IV: 0.25–0.5 unit/kg every 4–7 days	*Nausea, vomiting, stomatitis, anorexia, rash, headache, alopecia* Bone marrow suppression, severe nausea, vomiting, diarrhea, cardiotoxicity, tissue necrosis due to extravasation, mucositis, pulmonary toxicity, hypersensitivity reactions (including anaphylaxis)
dactinomycin (Actinomycin-D, Cosmegen)	IV: 500 mcg/day for a maximum of 5 days	
daunorubicin (Cerubidine)	IV: 30–60 mg/m²/day for 3–5 days	
daunorubicin liposomal (DaunoXome)	IV: 40 mg/m² every 2 wk	
doxorubicin (Adriamycin)	IV: 60–75 mg/m² as a single dose at 21-day intervals, or 30 mg/m² on each of 3 consecutive days (max: total cumulative dose 550 mg/m²)	
doxorubicin liposomal (Doxil, Evacet)	IV: 20 mg/m² every 3 wk	
epirubicin (Ellence)	IV: 100–120 mg/m² as a single dose	
idarubicin (Idamycin)	IV: 8–12 mg/m² /day for 3 days	
mitomycin (Mutamycin)	IV: 2 mg/m² as a single dose	
mitoxantrone (Novantrone)	IV: 12 mg/m²/day for 3 days	

Note: *Italics* indicate common adverse effects; underlining indicates serious adverse effects.

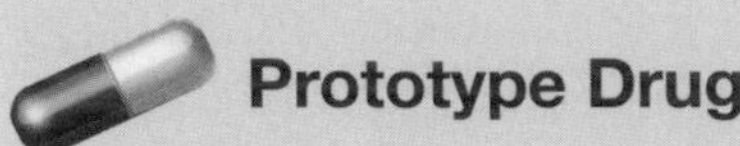

Prototype Drug | Doxorubicin *(Adriamycin)*

Therapeutic Class: Antineoplastic **Pharmacologic Class:** Antitumor antibiotic

Actions and Uses

Doxorubicin attaches to DNA, distorting its double helical structure and preventing normal DNA and RNA synthesis. It is administered only by IV infusion. Doxorubicin is a broad-spectrum cytotoxic antibiotic, prescribed for solid tumors of the bone, GI tract, thyroid, lung, breast, ovary, and bladder, and for various leukemias and lymphomas. It is structurally similar to daunorubicin. Doxorubicin is considered to be one of the most effective single drugs against solid tumors.

A novel delivery method has been developed for both doxorubicin and daunorubicin. The drug is enclosed in small lipid sacs, or vesicles, called *liposomes.* The liposomal vesicle is designed to open and release the antitumor antibiotic when it reaches a cancer cell. The goal is to deliver a higher concentration of drug to the cancer cells, thus sparing normal cells. An additional advantage is that doxorubicin liposomal has a half-life of 50 to 60 hours, which is about twice that of regular doxorubicin. Doxorubicin liposomal is approved for use in patients with Kaposi's sarcoma, refractory ovarian tumors, and relapsed multiple myeloma.

Administration Alerts

- Extravasation can cause severe pain and extensive tissue damage. Skin contact or extravasation should be treated immediately with local ice packs to reduce absorption of the drug.
- For infants and children, verify concentration and rate of IV infusion with the health care provider.
- Avoid skin contact with the drug. If exposure occurs, wash thoroughly with soap and water.
- Pregnancy category D.

PHARMACOKINETICS

Onset	Peak	Duration
Rapid	30 min–2 h	Up to 30–40 h

Adverse Effects

Doxorubicin has many adverse effects, some of which are serious. The most serious dose-limiting adverse effect of doxorubicin is cardiotoxicity. Like many anticancer drugs, doxorubicin may profoundly lower blood cell counts. Acute nausea and vomiting are common and often require antiemetic therapy. Complete, though reversible, hair loss occurs in most patients.

Black Box Warning: Severe myelosuppression may occur, which is the major dose-limiting toxicity with doxorubicin. It may manifest as thrombocytopenia, leukopenia (especially granulocytes), and anemia. Doxorubicin exhibits significant cardiotoxicity, which may be either acute or chronic. Cardiac adverse effects can be life threatening and may include sinus tachycardia, bradycardia, delayed heart failure, acute left ventricular failure, and myocarditis. Heart failure may occur months or years after the termination of chemotherapy. Acute, infusion-related reactions may occur, including anaphylaxis. Severe local necrosis may result if extravasation occurs. Secondary malignancies, especially acute myelogenous leukemia, may occur 1 to 3 years following therapy.

Contraindications: Contraindications include pregnancy, lactation, myelosuppression, thrombocytopenia, pre-existing cardiac disease, obstructive jaundice, lactation, or previous treatment with complete cumulative doses of doxorubicin or daunorubicin.

Interactions

Drug–Drug: If digoxin is taken concurrently, patient serum digoxin levels will decrease. Use with phenobarbital may lead to increased plasma clearance of doxorubicin and decreased effectiveness. Use with phenytoin may lead to decreased phenytoin level and possible seizure activity. Hepatotoxicity may occur if mercaptopurine is taken concurrently. Use with verapamil may increase serum doxorubicin levels, leading to doxorubicin toxicity.

Lab Tests: Serum uric acid and aspartate aminotransferase (AST) levels may increase. Blood cell counts will diminish due to bone marrow suppression.

Herbal/Food: Green tea may enhance the antitumor activity of doxorubicin. St. John's wort may decrease the effectiveness of doxorubicin.

Treatment of Overdose: The primary result of doxorubicin overdosage is immunosuppression. Treatment includes prophylactic antimicrobials, platelet transfusions, symptomatic treatment of mucositis, and possibly hemopoietic growth factor (G-CSF, GM-CSF).

cavity. These drugs can cause major damage to the skin, subcutaneous tissue, and nerves should extravasation occur.

As with many other antineoplastics, bone marrow suppression is a major dose-limiting adverse effect of drugs in this class. Doxorubicin, daunorubicin, epirubicin, and idarubicin are all closely related in structure, and cardiac toxicity is a major limiting adverse effect. Cardiotoxicity may occur within minutes of administration or be delayed for months or years after chemotherapy has been completed.

NATURAL PRODUCTS (PLANT EXTRACTS AND ALKALOIDS)

Plants have been a valuable source for antineoplastic drugs. These natural products act by preventing the division of cancer cells.

38.12 Pharmacotherapy With Natural Products

Substances with antineoplastic activity have been isolated from a number of plants, including the common periwinkle (*Vinca rosea*), Pacific yew (*Taxus baccata*), mandrake (May apple), and the shrub *Camptotheca acuminata*. Although structurally very different, medications in this class have the common ability to affect cell division; thus, some of them are called *mitotic inhibitors*. The plant extracts, or natural products, are listed in Table 38.5. There are three primary subdivisions of natural products used as antineoplastics:

- Vinca alkaloids
- Taxanes
- Topoisomerase inhibitors.

The **vinca alkaloids,** vincristine (Oncovin) and vinblastine (Velban), are two older drugs derived from more than 100 alkaloids isolated from the periwinkle plant. The medicinal properties of this plant were described in folklore in several regions of the world long before their antineoplastic properties were discovered. Despite being derived from the same plant, vincristine, vinblastine, and the semisynthetic vinorelbine (Navelbine) exhibit different effects and toxicity profiles. Vincristine is a common component of regimens for treating pediatric leukemias, lymphomas, and solid tumors. Vinblastine has traditionally been used to treat Hodgkin's disease and testicular tumors.

The **taxanes,** which include cabazitaxel (Jevtana), paclitaxel (Taxol), and docetaxel (Taxotere), were originally isolated from the bark of the Pacific yew, an evergreen found in forests throughout the western United States. Like the vinca alkaloids, the taxanes are mitotic inhibitors. Paclitaxel is approved for metastatic ovarian and breast cancer and for Kaposi's sarcoma; however, off-label uses include many other cancers. A newer form of paclitaxel (Abraxane), was approved in 2012. It is bound to albumin and delivers a higher dose of the drug directly to the cancer cells with fewer side effects. Docetaxel is approved to treat solid tumors, and cabazitaxel, a newer taxane, is indicated for hormone refractory metastatic prostate cancer. Bone marrow toxicity is usually the dose-limiting factor for the taxanes.

American Indians described uses of the May apple or wild mandrake (*Podophyllum peltatum*) long before pharmacologists isolated podophyllotoxin, the primary active

Table 38.5 Natural Products With Antineoplastic Activity

Drug	Route and Adult Dose (max dose where indicated)	Adverse Effects
VINCA ALKALOIDS		
vinblastine (Velban)	IV: 3.7–18.5 mg/m² every 7–10 days	*Nausea, vomiting, asthenia, stomatitis, anorexia, rash, alopecia*
vincristine (Oncovin)	IV: 1.4 mg/m² once every wk (max: 2 mg/m²)	Bone marrow suppression (neutropenia, anemia, thrombocytopenia), severe nausea and vomiting, diarrhea, cardiotoxicity, mucositis, pulmonary toxicity, hypersensitivity reactions (including anaphylaxis), neurotoxicity (docetaxel, vincristine), nephrotoxicity (vincristine), hemorrhage (omacetaxine)
vincristine liposome (Marqibo)	IV: 2.25 mg/m² once every wk	
vinorelbine (Navelbine)	IV: 30 mg/m² once every wk	
TAXANES		
cabazitaxel (Jevtana)	IV: 25 mg/m² once every 3 wk	
docetaxel (Taxotere)	IV: 60–100 mg/m² once every 3 wk	
paclitaxel (Abraxane, Taxol)	IV: 135–175 mg/m² once every 3 wk	
TOPOISOMERASE INHIBITORS		
etoposide (VePesid)	IV: 50–100 mg/m²/day for 5 days	
irinotecan (Camptosar)	IV: 125 mg/m² once every wk for 4 wk	
teniposide (Vumon)	IV: 165 mg/m² every 3–4 days for 4 wk	
topotecan (Hycamtin)	IV: 1.5 mg/m²/day for 5 days	
MISCELLANEOUS NATURAL PRODUCTS		
eribulin (Halaven)	IV: 1.4 mg/m² on days 1 and 8 of a 21-day cycle	
omacetaxine (Synribo)	Subcutaneous: 1.25 mg/m² for 14 consecutive days	

Note: *Italics* indicate common adverse effects; underlining indicates serious adverse effects.

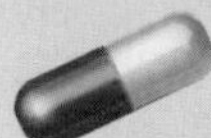

Prototype Drug | Vincristine *(Oncovin)*

Therapeutic Class: Antineoplastic **Pharmacologic Class:** Vinca alkaloid, mitotic inhibitor, natural product

Actions and Uses

Vincristine is specific for the M-phase of the cell cycle where it kills cancer cells by preventing their ability to complete mitosis. It exerts this action by inhibiting microtubule formation in the mitotic spindle. Although vincristine must be given IV, its major advantage is that it causes minimal immunosuppression. It has a wider spectrum of clinical activity than vinblastine and is usually prescribed in combination with other antineoplastics for the treatment of Hodgkin's and non-Hodgkin's lymphomas, leukemias, Kaposi's sarcoma, Wilms' tumor, bladder carcinoma, and breast carcinoma.

Administration Alerts

- Extravasation may result in serious tissue damage. Stop the injection immediately if extravasation occurs, apply local heat, and inject hyaluronidase as ordered. Observe the site for sloughing.
- Avoid eye contact, which can cause severe irritation and corneal changes.
- Pregnancy category D.

PHARMACOKINETICS

Onset	Peak	Duration
15–20 min	Unknown	7 days

Adverse Effects

The most serious dose-limiting adverse effects of vincristine relate to nervous system toxicity. Children are particularly susceptible. Symptoms include numbness and tingling in the limbs, muscular weakness, loss of neural reflexes, and pain. Severe constipation is common and paralytic ileus may occur in young children. Reversible alopecia occurs in most patients.

Black Box Warning: Myelosuppression may be severe and predispose to opportunistic infections. Extravasation can cause intense pain, inflammation, and tissue necrosis. If extravasation occurs, treatment with warm compresses and hyaluronidase is recommended; cold compresses will significantly increase the toxicity of vinca alkaloids.

Contraindications: Contraindications to the use of vincristine include obstructive jaundice, men and women of child-bearing age, active infection, adynamic ileus, radiation of the liver, infants, pregnancy, and lactation.

Interactions

Drug–Drug: Asparaginase used concurrently with or before vincristine may cause increased neurotoxicity secondary to decreased hepatic clearance of vincristine. Doxorubicin or prednisone may increase bone marrow toxicity. Calcium channel blockers may increase vincristine accumulation in cells. Concurrent use with digoxin may decrease digoxin levels. When vincristine is given with methotrexate, the patient may need lower doses of methotrexate. Vincristine may decrease serum phenytoin levels, leading to increased seizure activity.

Lab Tests: Serum uric acid levels may increase.

Herbal/Food: Unknown.

Treatment of Overdose: Overdose with vincristine may cause life-threatening symptoms or death. Symptoms are extensions of the drug's adverse effects. Supportive treatment may include administration of leucovorin (folinic acid).

ingredient in the plant. As a botanical, podophyllum has been used as an antidote for snakebites, as a cathartic, and as a topical treatment for warts. Teniposide (Vumon) and etoposide (VePesid) are semisynthetic products of podophyllotoxin. These drugs, known as **topoisomerase I inhibitors,** act by inhibiting **topoisomerase I,** an enzyme that helps repair DNA damage. By binding in a complex with topoisomerase and DNA, these antineoplastics cause strand breaks that accumulate and permanently damage the tumor DNA. Etoposide is approved for refractory testicular carcinoma, small-cell carcinoma of the lung, and choriocarcinoma. Teniposide is approved only for refractory acute lymphoblastic leukemia in children, topotecan is approved for small-cell lung cancer, and irinotecan is indicated for metastatic colorectal cancer. Bone marrow toxicity is the primary dose-limiting adverse effect of drugs in this class.

HORMONES AND HORMONE ANTAGONISTS

Use of hormones or their antagonists as antineoplastic agents is a strategy for slowing the growth of hormone-dependent tumors. Hormonal therapy is limited to treating hormone-sensitive tumors of the breast or prostate.

38.13 Pharmacotherapy With Hormones and Hormone Antagonists

A number of hormones are used in cancer chemotherapy, including corticosteroids, progestins, estrogens, and androgens. In addition, several hormone antagonists have been found to exhibit antitumor activity. The mechanism of hormone antineoplastic activity is largely unknown. It is likely, however, that these antitumor properties are independent of their normal hormone mechanisms because the doses used in cancer chemotherapy are magnitudes larger than the amount normally present in the body. Only the antitumor properties of these drugs are discussed in this section; for other indications and actions, the student should refer to other chapters in this text. The antitumor hormones and hormone antagonists are listed in Table 38.6.

The hormones and hormone antagonists are believed to act by blocking substances essential for tumor growth. Because hormonal drugs are not cytotoxic, they produce few of the debilitating adverse effects seen with other antineoplastics. They can, however, produce significant adverse effects when given at high doses for prolonged periods. Because they rarely produce cancer cures when used singly, these medications are normally given for palliation. These agents may be classified into four general groups:

- Corticosteroids
- Gonadal hormones
- Estrogen antagonists
- Androgen antagonists.

Table 38.6 Hormone and Hormone Antagonists Used for Neoplasia

Drug	Route and Adult Dose (max dose where indicated)	Adverse Effects
HORMONES		
dexamethasone (Decadron, others)	PO: 0.25 bid–qid	*Weight gain, insomnia, abdominal distension, sweating, flushing, diarrhea, nervousness, gynecomastia, hirsutism (testosterone, testolactone)* Thrombophlebitis, muscle wasting (prednisone, dexamethasone), osteoporosis, hepatotoxicity (testosterone, testolactone)
diethylstilbestrol (DES, Stilbestrol)	PO: for treatment of prostate cancer, 500 mg tid; for palliation 1–15 mg/day	
ethinyl estradiol (Estinyl, others)	PO: for treatment of breast cancer, 1 mg tid for 2–3 months; for palliation of prostate cancer, 0.15–3 mg/day	
fluoxymesterone (Halotestin)	PO: 10 mg tid	
medroxyprogesterone (Provera, Depo-Provera) (see page 795 for the Prototype Drug box)	IM: 400–1,000 mg once every wk	
megestrol (Megace)	PO: 40–160 mg bid–qid	
prednisone (Deltasone, others) (see page 508 for the Prototype Drug box)	PO: 20–100 mg/day	
testosterone enanthate (Delatestryl) (see page 809 for the Prototype Drug box)	IM: 200–400 mg every 2–4 wk	
HORMONE ANTAGONISTS		
abiraterone (Zytiga)	PO: 1 g once daily in combination with prednisone	*Hot flashes, insomnia, breast enlargement/pain, headache, diarrhea, asthenia, nausea* Hypersensitivity reactions (including anaphylaxis), thrombophlebitis, heart failure (bicalutamide, goserelin), hepatotoxicity (abiraterone, flutamide), sexual dysfunction (goserelin, nilutamide, tamoxifen), ocular toxicity (toremifene), adrenocortical deficiency (abiraterone)
anastrozole (Arimidex)	PO: 1 mg/day	
bicalutamide (Casodex)	PO: 50 mg/day	
degarelix (Firmagon)	Subcutaneous: 240 mg loading dose followed by 80 mg every 28 days	
exemestane (Aromasin)	PO: 25 mg/day after a meal	
flutamide (Eulexin)	PO: 250 mg tid	
fulvestrant (Faslodex)	IM: 500 mg on days 1, 15, 29, then once a month thereafter	
goserelin (Zoladex)	Subcutaneous: 3.6 mg every 28 days	
histrelin (Supprelin LA, Vantas)	Subcutaneous implant: 1 implant every 12 months (50 mg)	
letrozole (Femara)	PO: 2.5 mg/day	
leuprolide (Eligard, Lupron, Viadur)	Subcutaneous: 1 mg/day IM depot (Lupron); 11.25 mg every 3 months Subcutaneous (Eligard): 7.5–45 mg every 1–6 months Subcutaneous implant (Viadur); 1 implant every 12 months (65 mg)	
nilutamide (Nilandron)	PO: 300 mg/day for 30 days; then 150 mg/day	
raloxifene (Evista) (see page 831 for the Prototype Drug box)	PO: 60 mg once daily	
tamoxifen	PO: 20 mg daily in two divided doses	
toremifene (Fareston)	PO: 60 mg/day	
triptorelin (Trelstar)	IM: 3.75 mg every 4 wk, 11.25 mg every 12 wk, or 22.5 mg every 24 wk.	

Note: *Italics* indicate common adverse effects; underlining indicates serious adverse effects.

Chapter Review

KEY Concepts

The numbered key concepts provide a succinct summary of the important points from the corresponding numbered section within the chapter. If any of these points are not clear, refer to the numbered section within the chapter for review.

38.1 Cancer is characterized by rapid, uncontrolled growth of cells that eventually invade normal tissues and metastasize.

38.2 The causes of cancer may be chemical, physical, or biologic. Many environmental and lifestyle factors are associated with a higher risk of cancer.

38.3 Cancer may be treated using surgery, radiation therapy, and drugs. Chemotherapy may be used for cure, control, or palliation of cancer.

38.4 The growth fraction, the percentage of cancer cells undergoing mitosis at any given time, is a major factor determining success of chemotherapy. Antineoplastics are more effective against cells that are rapidly dividing.

38.5 To achieve a total cure, every malignant cell must be removed or killed through surgery, radiation, or drugs, or by the patient's immune system.

38.6 Use of multiple drugs and special dosing protocols are strategies that allow for lower doses, fewer side effects, and greater success of chemotherapy.

38.7 Serious toxicity, including bone marrow suppression, severe nausea, vomiting, and diarrhea, limits therapy with most antineoplastic drugs. Long-term consequences of chemotherapy include possible infertility and an increased risk for secondary tumors.

38.8 Classes of antineoplastic drugs include alkylating agents, antimetabolites, antitumor antibiotics, natural products, hormones and hormone antagonists, biologic response modifiers and monoclonal antibodies, and miscellaneous antineoplastics.

38.9 Alkylating agents have a broad spectrum of activity and act by changing the structure of DNA in cancer cells. Their use is limited because they can cause significant bone marrow suppression.

38.10 Antimetabolites act by disrupting critical pathways in cancer cells, such as folate metabolism or DNA synthesis. The three types of antimetabolites are folic acid analogs, purine analogs, and pyrimidine analogs.

38.11 Due to their cytotoxicity, a few antibiotics are used to treat cancer by inhibiting cell growth. They have a narrow spectrum of clinical activity.

38.12 Some plant extracts have been isolated that kill cancer cells by preventing cell division. These include the vinca alkaloids, taxanes, and topoisomerase inhibitors.

38.13 Some hormones and hormone antagonists are antineoplastic agents that are effective against tumors of the breast or prostate. They are less cytotoxic than other antineoplastics.

38.14 Biologic response modifiers have been found to be effective against tumors by stimulating or assisting the patient's immune system. These include interferons, interleukins, and targeted therapies.

38.15 A large number of miscellaneous antineoplastics act by mechanisms other than those given in prior sections.

REVIEW Questions

1. A patient who is undergoing cancer chemotherapy asks the nurse why she is taking three different chemotherapy drugs. What is the nurse's best response?
   1. "Your cancer was very advanced and therefore requires more medications."
   2. "Each drug attacks the cancer cells in a different way, increasing the effectiveness of the therapy."
   3. "Several drugs are prescribed to find the right drug for your cancer."
   4. "One drug will cancel out the side effects of the other."
2. What is the most effective treatment method for the nausea and vomiting that accompanies many forms of chemotherapy?
   1. Administer an oral antiemetic when the patient complains of nausea and vomiting.

2. Administer an antiemetic by intramuscular injection when the patient complains of nausea and vomiting.
3. Administer an antiemetic prior to the antineoplastic medication.
4. Encourage additional fluids prior to administering the antineoplastic medication.

3. Which of the following statements by a patient who is undergoing antineoplastic therapy would be of concern to the nurse? (Select all that apply.)
   1. "I have attended a meeting of a cancer support group."
   2. "My husband and I are planning a short trip next week."
   3. "I am eating six small meals plus two protein shakes a day."
   4. "I am taking my 15-month-old granddaughter to the pediatrician next week for her baby shots."
   5. "I am going to go shopping at the mall next week."

4. A patient on chemotherapy has a complete blood count (CBC) drawn and the nurse calculates the absolute neutrophil count (ANC). The white blood cell (WBC) count is 2,500 mm^3 with 0.22 segmented neutrophils (segs) and 0.06 banded neutrophils (bands). What is the ANC?
   1. 18.93
   2. 89
   3. 700
   4. 2500.28

5. A 2-year-old patient is receiving vincristine (Oncovin) for Wilms' tumor. Which of the following findings will the nurse monitor to prevent or limit the main adverse effect for this patient? (Select all that apply.)
   1. Numbness of the hands or feet
   2. Angina or dysrhythmias
   3. Constipation
   4. Diminished reflexes
   5. Dyspnea and pleuritis

6. The nurse notes that the patient has reached his nadir. What does this finding signify?
   1. The patient is receiving the highest dose possible of the chemotherapy.
   2. The patient is experiencing bone marrow suppression and his blood counts are at their lowest point.
   3. The patient has peaked on his chemotherapy level and should be going home in a few days.
   4. The patient is experiencing extreme depression and will be having a psychiatric consult.

PATIENT-FOCUSED Case Study

Ramon de la Cruz is a 27-year-old financial analyst who has recently begun chemotherapy for treatment of Hodgkin's lymphoma. He has tolerated the chemotherapy fairly well but has experienced mild, daily nausea with occasional vomiting, usually controlled by granisetron (Kytril). His main concern is the fatigue he experiences and the impact it has on his work. He also admits that he has been experiencing anorexia and "just doesn't feel like eating much," something which may be contributing to his fatigue. He has lost 2 kg (more than 4 lb) since his last clinic visit 2 weeks ago.

1. As Ramon's nurse, how might you manage his chemotherapy-related nausea and anorexia?
2. What suggestions might assist Ramon in managing his fatigue?

CRITICAL THINKING Questions

1. Chemotherapy medications often cause neutropenia in patients with cancer. What would be a priority for the nurse to teach a patient who is receiving chemotherapy at home?
2. A nurse is taking chemotherapy IV medication to a patient's room and the IV bag suddenly leaks solution (approximately 50 mL) on the floor. What action should the nurse take?

Visit www.pearsonhighered.com/nursingresources for answers and rationales for all activities.

REFERENCES

American Cancer Society. (2015). *Cancer facts and figures, 2015.* Retrieved from http://www.cancer.org/acs/groups/content/@editorial/documents/document/acspc-044552.pdf

Haddad, N. E., & Palesh, O. (2014). Acupuncture in the treatment of cancer-related psychological symptoms. *Integrative Cancer Therapies, 13,* 371–385. doi:10.1177/1534735413520181

Herdman, T. H., & Kamitsuru, S. (2014). *NANDA International nursing diagnoses: Definitions and classification, 2015–2017.* Oxford, United Kingdom: Wiley-Blackwell.

National Center for Complementary and Integrative Health. (2014). *Acupuncture: What you need to know.* Retrieved from https://nccih.nih.gov/health/acupuncture/introduction

Rithirangsriroj, K., Manchana, T., & Akkayagorn, L. (2015). Efficacy of acupuncture in prevention of delayed chemotherapy induced nausea and vomiting in gynecologic cancer patients. *Gynecologic Oncology, 136,* 82–86. doi:10.1016/j.ygyno.2014.10.025

SELECTED BIBLIOGRAPHY

American Cancer Society. (2014). *What are the key statistics about breast cancer?* Retrieved from http://www.cancer.org/cancer/breastcancer/detailedguide/breast-cancer-key-statistics

Bruce, S. D. (2013). Before you press that button: A look at chemotherapy errors. *Clinical Journal of Oncology Nursing, 17*(1), 31–32. doi:10.1188/13.CJON.31-32

Chabner, B. A., Barnes, J., Neal, J., Olson, E., Mujagic, H., Sequist, L., . . . Richardson, P. (2011). Targeted therapies: Tyrosine kinase inhibitors, monoclonal antibodies and cytokines. In L. L. Brunton, B. A. Chabner, & B. C. Knollman (Eds.), *Goodman and Gilman's the pharmacological basis of therapeutics* (12th ed., pp. 1731–1754). New York, NY: McGraw-Hill.

Chabner, B. A., Bertino, J., Cleary, J., Ortiz, T., Lane, A., Supko, J. G., & Ryan, D. (2011). Cytotoxic agents. In L. L. Brunton, B. A. Chabner, & B. C. Knollman (Eds.), *Goodman and Gilman's the pharmacological basis of therapeutics* (12th ed., pp. 1677–1730). New York, NY: McGraw-Hill.

Cho, W. C. (2012). Targeting the signaling pathways in cancer therapy. *Expert Opinion on Therapeutic Targets, 16,* 1–3. doi:10.1517/14728222.2011.648618

Khatcheressian, J. L., Hurley, P., Bantug, E., Esserman, L. J., Grunfeld, E., Halberg, F., . . . Davidson, N. E. (2013). Breast cancer follow-up and management after primary treatment: American Society of Clinical Oncology clinical practice guideline update. *Journal of Clinical Oncology, 31,* 961–965. doi:10.1200/JCO.2012.45.9859

Lizée, G., Overwijk, W. W., Radvanyi, L., Gao, J., Sharma, P., & Hwu, P. (2013). Harnessing the power of the immune system to target cancer. *Annual Review of Medicine, 64,* 71–90. doi:10.1146/annurev-med-112311-083918

Mendelsohn, J. (2013). Personalizing oncology: Perspectives and prospects. *Journal of Clinical Oncology, 31,* 1904–1911. doi:10.1200/JCO.2012.45.3605

Unit 6

The Respiratory System

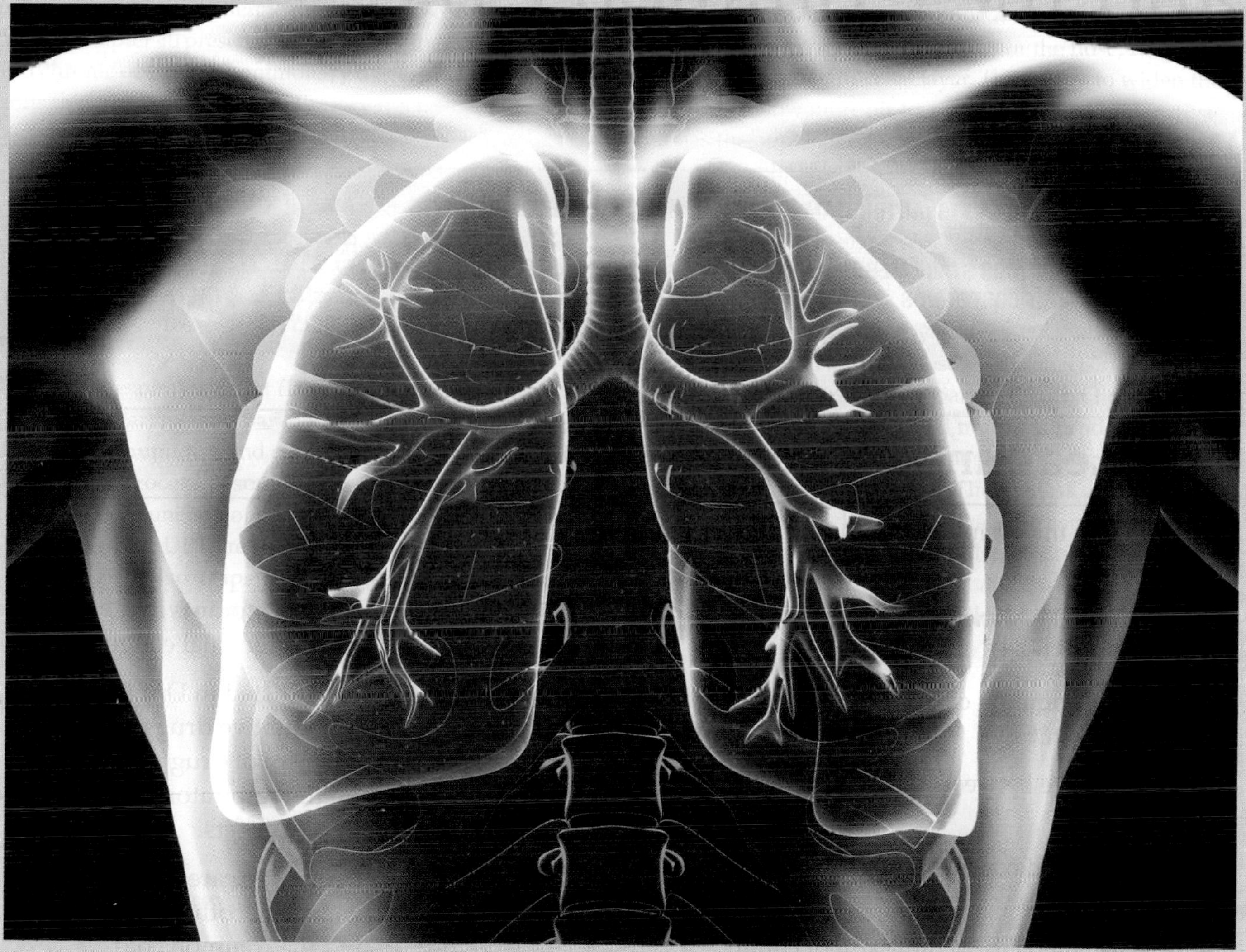

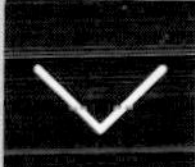

The Respiratory System

ALLERGIC RHINITIS

Allergic rhinitis, or hay fever, is inflammation of the nasal mucosa due to exposure to allergens. Although not life threatening, allergic rhinitis is a condition affecting millions of patients, and pharmacotherapy is frequently necessary to control symptoms and to prevent secondary complications.

39.2 Pharmacotherapy of Allergic Rhinitis

Symptoms of allergic rhinitis resemble those of the common cold: tearing eyes, sneezing, nasal congestion, postnasal drip, and itching of the throat. In addition to the acute symptoms, potential complications of allergic rhinitis include loss of taste or smell, sinusitis, chronic cough, hoarseness, and middle ear infections in children.

As with other allergies, the cause of allergic rhinitis is exposure to an antigen. An antigen, or **allergen,** is anything that is recognized as foreign and provokes a response from the body's defense system. The specific allergen responsible for a patient's allergic rhinitis is often difficult to pinpoint; however, the most common agents are pollens from weeds, grasses, and trees; mold spores; dust mites; certain foods; and animal dander. Chemical fumes, tobacco smoke, or air pollutants such as ozone are nonallergenic factors that may worsen symptoms. In addition, there is a strong genetic predisposition to allergic rhinitis.

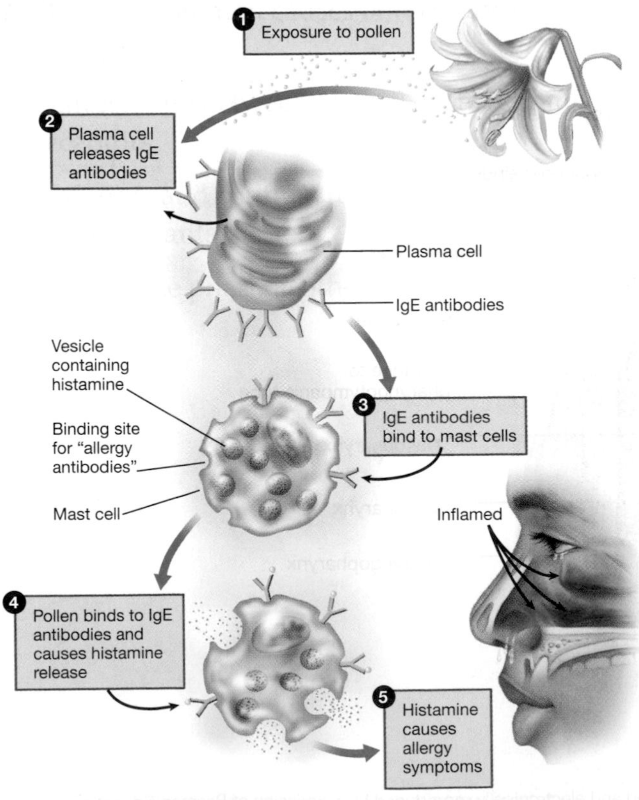

FIGURE 39.2 Allergic rhinitis

Some patients experience symptoms of allergic rhinitis only at specific times of the year, when pollen levels are at high levels in the environment. These periods are typically in the spring and fall when plants and trees are blooming, thus the name *seasonal* allergic rhinitis. Obviously, the blooming season changes with the geographic location and with each species of plant. These patients may need symptom relief for only a few months during the year. Other patients, however, are afflicted with allergic rhinitis throughout the year because they are continuously exposed to indoor allergens, such as dust mites, animal dander, or mold. This variation is called *perennial* allergic rhinitis. These patients may require continuous pharmacotherapy.

It is often not clear whether a person is experiencing seasonal or perennial allergic rhinitis. Patients with seasonal allergies may also be sensitive to some of the perennial allergens. It is also common for one allergen to sensitize the patient to another. For example, during ragweed season, a patient may become hyper-responsive to other allergens such as mold spores or animal dander. The body's response and the symptoms of allergic rhinitis are the same, however, regardless of the specific allergens. Allergy testing can help to identify the specific allergens producing the symptoms.

The fundamental pathophysiology responsible for allergic rhinitis is inflammation of the mucous membranes in the nose, throat, and airways. The nasal mucosa is rich with mast cells (a type of connective tissue cell) and basophils (a type of leukocyte), which recognize antigens as they enter the body. Patients with allergic rhinitis contain greater numbers of mast cells. An *immediate* hypersensitivity response releases histamine and other inflammatory mediators from the mast cells and basophils, producing sneezing, itchy nasal membranes, and watery eyes. A *delayed* hypersensitivity reaction also occurs 4 to 8 hours after the initial exposure, causing continuous inflammation of the mucosa and adding to the chronic nasal congestion experienced by these patients. Because histamine is released during an allergic response, many signs and symptoms of allergy are similar to those of inflammation (see chapter 33). The pathophysiology of allergic rhinitis is illustrated in Figure 39.2.

The therapeutic goals of treating allergic rhinitis are to prevent its occurrence and to relieve symptoms. Thus, drugs used to treat allergic rhinitis may be grouped into two simple categories:

- *Preventers* are used for prophylaxis and include antihistamines, intranasal corticosteroids, and mast cell stabilizers.
- *Relievers* are used to provide immediate, though temporary, relief for acute allergy symptoms once they have occurred. Relievers include the oral and intranasal decongestants, usually drugs from the sympathomimetic class.

In addition to treating allergic rhinitis with medications, nurses should help patients identify sources of the allergies and recommend appropriate interventions. These may include removing pets from the home environment, cleaning moldy surfaces, using microfilters on air conditioning units, and cleaning dust mites out of bedding, carpet, or couches.

H_1-RECEPTOR ANTAGONISTS (ANTIHISTAMINES) AND MAST CELL STABILIZERS

Antihistamines block the actions of histamine at the H_1 receptor. They are widely used as over-the-counter (OTC) remedies for relief of allergy symptoms, motion sickness, and insomnia. These medications are listed in Table 39.1.

39.3 Pharmacology of Allergic Rhinitis With H_1-Receptor Antagonists and Mast Cell Stabilizers

Histamine is a chemical mediator of inflammation that is responsible for many of the symptoms of allergic rhinitis. When released from mast cells and basophils, histamine reaches its receptors to cause itching, increased mucus secretion, and nasal congestion. In more severe allergic states, histamine release may cause bronchoconstriction, edema, hypotension, and other symptoms of anaphylaxis. The histamine receptors responsible for allergic symptoms are called **H_1 receptors.** The other major histamine receptor, H_2, is found in the gastric mucosa and is responsible for peptic ulcers (see chapter 41).

Antihistamines are drugs that selectively block histamine from reaching its H_1 receptors, thereby alleviating allergic symptoms. Because the term *antihistamine* is nonspecific and does not indicate which of the two histamine receptors are affected, H_1-receptor antagonist is a more accurate name. In clinical practice, as well as in this text, the two terms are used interchangeably.

The most frequent therapeutic use of antihistamines is for the treatment of allergies. These medications provide symptomatic relief from the characteristic sneezing, runny nose, and itching of the eyes, nose, and throat of allergic rhinitis. Antihistamines are often combined with decongestants and antitussives in OTC cold and sinus medicines. Common OTC antihistamine combinations used to treat allergies are listed in Table 39.2. Antihistamines are most effective when taken prophylactically to *prevent*

Table 39.1 H_1-Receptor Antagonists

Drug	Route and Adult Dose (max dose where indicated)	Adverse Effects
FIRST-GENERATION DRUGS		
brompheniramine (Dimetapp, others)	PO: 4–8 mg tid–qid (max: 40 mg/day)	*Dry mouth, headache, dizziness, urinary retention, thickening of bronchial secretions, nausea, vomiting* Paradoxical excitation, sedation, hypersensitivity reactions, hypotension, extrapyramidal symptoms (promethazine), agranulocytosis (brompheniramine, promethazine), respiratory depression
chlorpheniramine (Chlor-Trimeton, others)	PO: 2–4 mg tid–qid (max: 24 mg/day)	
clemastine (Tavist)	PO: 1.34–2.68 mg bid (max: 8.04 mg/day)	
cyproheptadine	PO: 4–20 mg tid or qid (max: 0.5 mg/kg/day)	
dexchlorpheniramine (Dexchlor, Poladex, Polaramine)	PO: 2 mg q4–6h (max: 12 mg/day)	
dimenhydrinate (Dramamine)	PO: 50–100 mg q4–6h	
diphenhydramine (Benadryl, others)	PO: 25–50 mg tid to qid (max: 300 mg/day)	
promethazine (Phenergan)	PO: 6.25–25 mg q8h	
triprolidine	PO: 2.5 mg bid or tid (max: 10 mg/day)	
SECOND-GENERATION DRUGS		
acrivastine with pseudoephedrine (Semprex-D)	PO: One capsule daily (8 mg acrivastine/60 mg pseudoephedrine)	*Dry mouth, headache, dizziness, drowsiness, bitter taste (olopatadine), nausea* Paradoxical excitation, hypersensitivity reactions, hypotension
azelastine (Astelin, Astepro, Optivar)	Intranasal: 1–2 sprays per nostril once daily or bid Ophthalmic (Optivar): 1 drop in each affected eye bid	
cetirizine (Zyrtec)	PO: 5–10 mg/day (max: 10 mg/day)	
desloratadine (Clarinex)	PO: 5 mg/day (max: 5 mg/day)	
fexofenadine (Allegra)	PO: 60 mg bid or 180 mg once daily	
levocetirizine (Xyzal)	PO: 5 mg (1 tablet or 2 teaspoons) once daily	
loratadine (Claritin)	PO: 10 mg/day	
olopatadine (Patanase, Patanol)	Intranasal (Patanase): 2 sprays per nostril bid Ophthalmic (Patanol): 1 drop in each affected eye bid	

Note: *Italics* indicate common adverse effects; underlining indicates serious adverse effects.

Table 39.2 Selected OTC Antihistamine Combinations

Brand Name	Antihistamine	Decongestant	Analgesic
Actifed Cold and Allergy tablets	chlorpheniramine	phenylephrine	—
Actifed Plus tablets	triprolidine	pseudoephedrine	acetaminophen
Benadryl Allergy/Cold tablets	diphenhydramine	phenylephrine	acetaminophen
Chlor-Trimeton Allergy/Decongestant tablets	chlorpheniramine	pseudoephedrine	—
Dimetapp Children's Cold and Allergy elixir	brompheniramine	phenylephrine	—
Sudafed PE Severe Cold tablets	diphenhydramine	phenylephrine	acetaminophen
Sudafed PE Sinus and Allergy tablets	chlorpheniramine	phenylephrine	—
Tavist Allergy tablets	clemastine	—	—
Triaminic Cold/Allergy	chlorpheniramine	phenylephrine	—
Tylenol Allergy Multisystem Gels	chlorpheniramine	phenylephrine	acetaminophen
Tylenol PM Gelcaps	diphenhydramine	—	acetaminophen

allergic symptoms; their effectiveness in *reversing* allergic symptoms is limited. Their effectiveness may diminish with long-term use.

In addition to producing their antihistamine effects, these drugs cause typical anticholinergic effects, such as increased heart rate, urinary retention, constipation, and blurred vision. Anticholinergic effects are responsible for certain beneficial effects of the antihistamines, such as drying of mucous membranes, which results in less nasal congestion and tearing eyes.

A large number of H_1-receptor antagonists are available as medications. They all have the same basic mechanism of action and are equally effective in treating allergic rhinitis and other mild allergies. Adverse effects are similar but differ in intensity among the various antihistamines. The older, first-generation drugs have the potential to cause significant drowsiness, which can be a limiting adverse effect in some patients. After a few doses, tolerance generally develops to this sedative action. The newer, second-generation drugs have less tendency to cause sedation. Alcohol and other central nervous system (CNS) depressants should be used with caution when taking antihistamines, because their sedating effects may be additive, even for the second-generation drugs. Some patients exhibit CNS *stimulation,* which can cause insomnia, nervousness, and tremors.

Anticholinergic adverse effects are also common in some patients. These include excessive drying of mucous membranes, which can lead to dry mouth, and urinary hesitancy, an effect that is troublesome for patients with BPH. Some antihistamines produce more pronounced anticholinergic effects than others. Diphenhydramine and clemastine produce the greatest incidence of anticholinergic side effects, whereas the second-generation drugs—loratadine, desloratadine, and fexofenadine—produce the least.

Although most antihistamines are given via the oral route (PO), azelastine (Astelin, Astepro) and olopatadine (Patanase) are available by the intranasal route. These medications are as effective as the PO antihistamines, but because they are applied locally to the nasal mucosa, limited systemic absorption occurs. Both these drugs are also available as ophthalmic drops for the treatment of allergic conjunctivitis.

In addition to allergic rhinitis, antihistamines have been used to treat a number of other disorders, including the following:

- *Vertigo and motion sickness.* Nausea resulting from vertigo or motion sickness responds well to antihistamines. These drugs act by suppressing the vomiting center in the medulla and depressing neurons of the vestibular apparatus of the inner ear. To be effective, they must be taken prior to the onset of symptoms. Meclizine (Antivert) and dimenhydrinate (Dramamine) are two common antihistamines used for this purpose. The pharmacotherapy of nausea is discussed in chapter 42.
- *Parkinson's disease.* Drugs with significant anticholinergic actions are used to treat mild forms of Parkinson's disease. They are also used to treat the tremor and certain other adverse effects of conventional antipsychotic drugs. Because diphenhydramine exhibits greater anticholinergic action, it is sometimes used to treat these conditions. The pharmacotherapy of Parkinson's disease is discussed in chapter 20.
- *Insomnia.* Many patients become drowsy after taking first-generation antihistamines. OTC products promoted as sleep aids usually include antihistamines such as diphenhydramine and doxylamine. After a few days, patients will become tolerant to the drowsiness produced by these drugs; thus, they should be used for 2 weeks or less.
- *Urticaria and other skin rashes.* Urticaria, or hives, is often caused by the release of histamine; thus, the

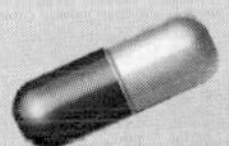

Prototype Drug | Diphenhydramine *(Benadryl, others)*

Therapeutic Class: Drug to treat allergies **Pharmacologic Class:** H_1-receptor antagonist; antihistamine

Actions and Uses

Diphenhydramine is a first-generation H_1-receptor antagonist whose primary use is to treat minor symptoms of allergy and the common cold such as sneezing, runny nose, and tearing of the eyes. Diphenhydramine is often combined with an analgesic, decongestant, or expectorant in OTC cold and flu products. Diphenhydramine is also administered topically to treat rashes, and intramuscular (IM) and intravenous (IV) forms are available for severe allergic reactions. Other indications for diphenhydramine include Parkinson's disease, motion sickness, and insomnia.

Administration Alerts

- There is an increased risk of anaphylactic shock when this drug is administered parenterally.
- When administering IV, inject at a rate of 25 mg/min to reduce the risk of shock.
- When administering IM, inject deep into a large muscle to minimize tissue irritation.
- Pregnancy category C.

PHARMACOKINETICS (PO)

Onset	Peak	Duration
15–30 min	1–4 h	4–7 h

Adverse Effects

First-generation H_1-receptor antagonists such as diphenhydramine cause significant drowsiness, although this usually diminishes with long-term use. Occasionally, paradoxical CNS stimulation and excitability will be observed, rather than drowsiness. Excitation is more frequent in children than adults. Anticholinergic effects such as dry mouth, tachycardia, and mild hypotension occur in some patients. Diphenhydramine may cause photosensitivity.

Contraindications: Hypersensitivity to the drug, benign prostatic hypertrophy (BPH), narrow-angle glaucoma, and gastrointestinal (GI) obstruction are contraindications of use. The drug should be used cautiously in patients with asthma or hyperthyroidism.

Interactions

Drug–Drug: Use with CNS depressants such as alcohol or opioids will cause increased sedation. Other OTC cold preparations may increase anticholinergic side effects. Monoamine oxidase inhibitors (MAOIs) may cause a hypertensive crisis.

Lab Tests: Drug should be discontinued at least 4 days prior to skin allergy tests; otherwise, false-negative tests may result.

Herbal/Food: Henbane may cause increased anticholinergic effects.

Treatment of Overdose: Overdose may cause either CNS depression or excitation. There is no specific treatment for overdose.

condition responds well to H_1-receptor antagonists. Symptomatic treatment may include any of the first- or second-generation drugs, either using oral drugs, topical creams, or lotions.

☑ Check Your Understanding 39.1

Alcohol use should be avoided by a patient who is taking antihistamines. Does this hold true for the second-generation antihistamines, or does it just apply to the first-generation drugs? *Visit www.pearsonhighered.com/nursingresources for the answer.*

INTRANASAL CORTICOSTEROIDS

Corticosteroids, also known as glucocorticoids, are applied directly to the nasal mucosa to prevent symptoms of allergic rhinitis. They have largely replaced antihistamines as preferred drugs for the treatment of perennial allergic rhinitis. These drugs are listed in Table 39.3.

39.4 Pharmacotherapy of Allergic Rhinitis With Intranasal Corticosteroids

The importance of the corticosteroids in treating severe inflammation is presented in chapter 33. Although corticosteroids are very effective, their use as *systemic* therapy is limited by potentially serious adverse effects. *Intranasal* corticosteroids, however, produce virtually no serious adverse effects. Because of their effectiveness and safety, the intranasal corticosteroids are often first-line drugs in the treatment of allergic rhinitis. Some of the corticosteroids are also administered by inhaler for the treatment of asthma (see chapter 40).

When sprayed onto the nasal mucosa, corticosteroids decrease the secretion of inflammatory mediators, reduce tissue edema, and cause a mild vasoconstriction. They are administered with a metered-spray device that delivers a consistent dose of drug per spray. All have equal

Table 39.3 Intranasal Corticosteroids and Miscellaneous Drugs for Allergic Rhinitis

Drug	Route and Adult Dose (max dose where indicated)	Adverse Effects
INTRANASAL CORTICOSTEROIDS		
beclomethasone (Beconase AQ, Qnasl, Qvar) (see page 665 for the Prototype Drug box)	Intranasal: 1–2 sprays in each nostril one to four times daily	*Transient nasal irritation, burning, sneezing, or dryness, nasopharyngitis*
budesonide (Rhinocort Aqua)	Intranasal: 2 sprays in each nostril bid	Hypercorticism (only if large amounts are swallowed)
ciclesonide (Omnaris)	Intranasal: 2 sprays once daily (max 200 mcg/day)	
flunisolide	Intranasal: 2 sprays in each nostril bid; may increase to tid if needed	
fluticasone (Flonase, Veramyst, others)	Intranasal: 1 spray in each nostril once (Veramyst) or twice (Flonase) daily	
mometasone (Nasonex)	Intranasal: 2 sprays in each nostril/day	
triamcinolone (Nasacort AQ)	Intranasal: 2 sprays in each nostril daily	
MISCELLANEOUS DRUGS		
cromolyn (NasalCrom)	Intranasal: 1 spray tid–qid	*Nasal burning and irritation* Anaphylaxis
ipratropium (Atrovent) (see page 663 for the Prototype Drug box)	Intranasal: 2 sprays tid to qid up to 4 days	*Transient nasal irritation, burning, sneezing, or dryness, cough, headache* Urinary retention, worsening of narrow-angle glaucoma
montelukast (Singulair)	PO: 10 mg/day	*Headache, nausea, diarrhea* No serious adverse effects

Note: *Italics* indicate common adverse effects; underlining indicates serious adverse effects.

effectiveness. Unlike the sympathomimetics, however, intranasal corticosteroids do not have immediate benefits. One to three weeks may be required to achieve peak response, especially when treating perennial rhinitis. Because of this delayed effect, intranasal corticosteroids are most effective when taken in advance of expected allergen exposure. Two of the drugs in this class, triamcinolone (Nasacort Allergy 24 HR) and fluticasone (Flonase Allergy Relief) have recently been approved for OTC use.

When corticosteroids are administered correctly, their action is limited to the nasal passages. The most frequently reported adverse effect is an intense burning sensation in the nose that occurs immediately after spraying. Excessive drying of the nasal mucosa may occur, leading to epistaxis.

There are several alternatives for patients who do not respond to intranasal corticosteroids. Intranasal cromolyn (NasalCrom) is approved as an OTC drug for the treatment of allergy and cold symptoms. Because it inhibits the release of histamine from mast cells, cromolyn is called a mast cell stabilizer. Most effective when given prior to allergen exposure, cromolyn has few adverse effects. Other alternatives to the intranasal corticosteroids in treating allergies include montelukast (Singulair) and ipratropium (Atrovent). Further information on cromolyn, montelukast, and ipratropium is presented in chapter 40, because asthma is a second indication for these drugs.

DECONGESTANTS

Decongestants are drugs that relieve nasal congestion. They are administered by either the oral or intranasal routes and are often combined with antihistamines in the pharmacotherapy of allergies or the common cold. Doses for the nasal decongestants are listed in Table 39.4.

39.5 Pharmacotherapy of Nasal Congestion With Decongestants

Most decongestants are sympathomimetics: drugs that activate the sympathetic nervous system. Sympathomimetics with alpha-adrenergic activity are effective at relieving the nasal congestion associated with the common cold or allergic rhinitis when given by either the oral or intranasal route. The intranasal preparations such as oxymetazoline (Afrin, others) are available OTC as sprays or drops and produce an effective response within minutes.

Intranasal sympathomimetics produce few systemic effects because almost none of the drug is absorbed into the circulation. The most serious, limiting side effect of the intranasal preparations is **rebound congestion,** a condition characterized by hypersecretion of mucus and worsening nasal congestion once the drug effects wear off. This can lead to a cycle of increased drug use as the condition worsens. Because of this rebound congestion, intranasal sympathomimetics should be used for no longer than 3 to 5 days. Patients with allergic

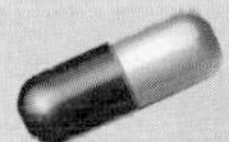

Prototype Drug | Fluticasone *(Flonase, Veramyst, others)*

Therapeutic Class: Drug for allergic rhinitis **Pharmacologic Class:** Intranasal corticosteroid

Actions and Uses

Fluticasone is typical of the intranasal corticosteroids used to treat seasonal allergic rhinitis. Therapy usually begins with two sprays in each nostril, twice daily, and decreases to one dose per day. Fluticasone acts to decrease local inflammation in the nasal passages, thus reducing nasal stuffiness.

In 2007 fluticasone (Veramyst) was approved for the treatment of both seasonal and perennial allergic rhinitis. Veramyst offers the advantage of once daily dosing along with improvement of both nasal and ocular symptoms associated with allergies. In 2012, Dymista was approved which combines fluticasone with azelastine, an H_2-receptor antagonist. Fluticasone is also available in oral inhalation and topical formulations. Flovent is administered by oral inhalation to reduce bronchial inflammation for the therapy of asthma and COPD (see chapter 50). In 2014, a second oral inhalation formulation of fluticasone (Arnuity Ellipta) was approved for the maintenance therapy of asthma. Topical fluticasone ointments and creams are applied to the skin for various inflammatory conditions, including atopic dermatitis, eczema, psoriasis, and contact dermatitis.

Administration Alerts

- Instruct the patient to carefully follow the directions for use provided by the manufacturer.
- Pregnancy category C.

PHARMACOKINETICS

Onset	Peak	Duration
12 h to several days	Unknown	Several days

Adverse Effects

When administered intranasally, adverse effects of fluticasone are rare. Swallowing large amounts increases the potential for systemic corticosteroid adverse effects. Nasal irritation and epistaxis occur in a small number of patients. When inhaled to treat asthma or COPD, the most frequent side effects are headache and nasopharyngitis.

Contraindications: The only contraindication to fluticasone is prior hypersensitivity to the drug. Because corticosteroids can mask signs of infection, patients with known bacterial, viral, fungal, or parasitic infections (especially of the respiratory tract) should not receive intranasal corticosteroids.

Interactions

Drug–Drug: Concomitant use of an intranasal decongestant increases the risk of nasal irritation or bleeding. Use with ritonavir should be avoided, because this drug significantly increases plasma fluticasone levels.

Lab Tests: Unknown.

Herbal/Food: Use with caution with licorice, which may potentiate the effects of corticosteroids.

Treatment of Overdose: There is no specific treatment for overdose.

Table 39.4 Nasal Decongestants

Drug	Route and Adult Dose (max dose where indicated)	Adverse Effects
naphazoline (Privine)	Intranasal: 2 drops q3–6h	*Intranasal: transient nasal irritation, burning, sneezing, or dryness, headache*
oxymetazoline (Afrin 12 Hour, Neo-Synephrine 12 Hour, others)	Intranasal (0.05%): 2–3 sprays bid for up to 3–5 days	*PO: nervousness, insomnia, headache, dry mouth* Intranasal: rebound congestion CNS excitation, tremors, dysrhythmias, tachycardia, difficulty in voiding, severe vasoconstriction
phenylephrine (Afrin 4–6 Hour, Neo-Synephrine 4–6 Hour, others)	Intranasal (0.1%): 2–3 drops or sprays every 3–4 h, as needed	
pseudoephedrine (Sudafed)	PO: 30–60 mg q4–6h (max: 240 mg/day) Sustained release: 120 mg q12h	
tetrahydrozoline (Tyzine)	Intranasal: 2–4 drops or sprays q3h	
xylometazoline	Intranasal (0.1%): 1–2 sprays bid (max: three doses/day)	

Note: *Italics* indicate common adverse effects; underlining indicates serious adverse effects.

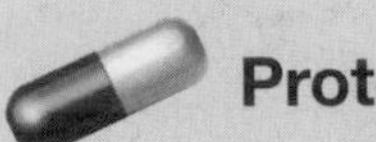

Prototype Drug | Oxymetazoline *(Afrin, others)*

Therapeutic Class: Nasal decongestant **Pharmacologic Class:** Sympathomimetic

Actions and Uses

Oxymetazoline activates alpha-adrenergic receptors in the sympathetic nervous system. This causes arterioles in the nasal passages to constrict, thus drying the mucous membranes. Relief from nasal congestion occurs within minutes and lasts for 10 or more hours. Oxymetazoline is administered with a metered spray device or by nasal drops.

Oxymetazoline (Visine LR) is also available as eyedrops. It causes vasoconstriction of vessels in the eye and is used to relieve redness and provide relief from dryness and minor eye irritations.

Administration Alerts

- Wash hands carefully after administration to prevent anisocoria (blurred vision and inequality of pupil size).
- Pregnancy category C.

PHARMACOKINETICS

Onset	Peak	Duration
5–10 min	Unknown	6–10 h

Adverse Effects

Rebound congestion is common when oxymetazoline is used for longer than 3 to 5 days. Minor stinging and dryness in the nasal mucosa may be experienced. Systemic adverse effects are unlikely, unless a large amount of the medicine is swallowed.

Contraindications: Patients with thyroid disorders, hypertension, diabetes, or heart disease should use sympathomimetics only on the direction of their health care provider.

Interactions

Drug–Drug: No clinically important interactions occur, because absorption of oxymetazoline is limited.

Lab Tests: Unknown.

Herbal/Food: Use with caution with herbal supplements such as St. John's wort that have properties of MAOIs.

Treatment of Overdose: There is no specific treatment for overdose.

rhinitis who develop tolerance to the effects of decongestants should be gradually switched to intranasal corticosteroids because they do not cause rebound congestion.

When administered *orally*, sympathomimetics do not produce rebound congestion. Their onset of action by this route, however, is much slower than when administered intranasally, and they are less effective at relieving severe congestion. The possibility of systemic adverse effects is also greater with the oral drugs. Potential adverse effects include hypertension and CNS stimulation that may lead to insomnia and anxiety.

Prior to 2000, pseudoephedrine was the most common decongestant included in oral OTC cold and allergy medicines. Pseudoephedrine, however, is the starting chemical for the illegal synthesis of methamphetamine by drug traffickers. Although pseudoephedrine is still available OTC, pharmacists are required to monitor its distribution by keeping a log of patient names and addresses, checking the photo identification of the buyers, and limiting the quantities of the drug that are sold at one time. It should be noted that these precautions are being taken not because pseudoephedrine itself is a dangerous drug, but to limit the availability of the drug to illicit makers of methamphetamine. Manufacturers have reformulated their OTC cold medicines to contain phenylephrine rather than pseudoephedrine. A drug prototype feature for phenylephrine is included in chapter 13.

Because the sympathomimetics relieve only nasal congestion, they are often combined with antihistamines to control sneezing and tearing eyes. It is interesting to note that some OTC drugs having the same basic name (Neo-Synephrine, Afrin, and Vicks) may contain different sympathomimetics. For example, Neo-Synephrine decongestants with 12-hour duration contain the drug oxymetazoline; Neo-Synephrine preparations that last 4 to 6 hours contain phenylephrine.

COMMON COLD

The common cold is a viral infection of the URT that produces a characteristic array of annoying symptoms. It is fortunate that the disorder is self-limiting, because there is no cure or effective prevention for colds. Therapies used to relieve symptoms include some of the same drug classes used for allergic rhinitis, including antihistamines and decongestants. A few additional drugs, such as those that suppress cough and loosen bronchial secretions, are used for symptomatic treatment.

ANTITUSSIVES

Antitussives are drugs used to dampen the cough reflex. They are of value in treating coughs due to allergies or the common cold.

Table 39.5 Selected Antitussives, Expectorants, and Mucolytics

Drug	Route and Adult Dose (max dose where indicated)	Adverse Effects
ANTITUSSIVES: OPIOIDS		
codeine	PO: 10–20 mg q4–6h prn (max: 120 mg/24 h)	*Nausea, vomiting, constipation, confusion, dizziness, sedation*
hydrocodone combined with homatropine (Hycodan, others)	PO: 1 tablet or 5 mL q4–6h as needed (max: 30 mL/day or 6 tablets/day)	<u>Hypotension, seizures, bradycardia, respiratory depression, severe somnolence</u>
ANTITUSSIVES: NONOPIOIDS		
benzonatate (Tessalon)	PO: 100 mg tid prn (max: 600 mg/day)	*Drowsiness, constipation, GI upset* <u>Paradoxical excitation, tremors, euphoria, insomnia</u>
dextromethorphan (Delsym, Robitussin DM, others)	PO: 10–20 mg q4h or 30 mg q6–8h (max: 120 mg/day)	*Drowsiness, headache, GI upset* <u>CNS depression, paradoxical excitation, respiratory depression</u>
EXPECTORANT		
guaifenesin (Mucinex)	PO: 200–400 mg q4h (max: 2.4 g/day) Extended release PO: 600–1,200 mg q12h (max: 2,400 mg/day)	*Drowsiness, headache, GI upset* <u>No serious adverse effects</u>
MUCOLYTIC		
acetylcysteine (Mucomyst)	Inhalation: 1–10 mL of 20% solution q4–6h or 2–20 mL of 10% solution q4–6h	*Unpleasant odor, nausea* <u>Severe nausea and vomiting, bronchospasm</u>

Note: *Italics* indicate common adverse effects; <u>underlining</u> indicates serious adverse effects.

39.6 Pharmacotherapy With Antitussives

Cough is a natural reflex mechanism that serves to forcibly remove excess secretions and foreign material from the respiratory system. In diseases such as emphysema and bronchitis, or when liquids have been aspirated into the bronchi, it is not desirable to suppress the normal cough reflex. Dry, hacking, nonproductive cough, however, can be irritating to the membranes of the throat and can deprive a patient of much-needed rest. It is these types of conditions in which therapy with medications that control cough, known as **antitussives,** may be warranted. Antitussives are classified as opioid or nonopioid and are listed in Table 39.5.

Opioids, the most effective antitussives, act by raising the cough threshold in the CNS. Codeine and hydrocodone are the most frequently used opioid antitussives. Doses needed to suppress the cough reflex are very low; thus, there is minimal potential for dependence. Most opioid cough mixtures are classified as Schedule III, IV, or V drugs and are reserved for serious cough conditions. Though not common, overdose from opioid cough remedies may cause significant respiratory depression. Care must be taken when using these medications in patients with asthma, because bronchoconstriction may occur. Opioids may be combined with other drugs such as antihistamines, decongestants, and nonopioid antitussives in the therapy of severe cold or flu symptoms. Some of these combinations are listed in Table 39.6.

The most frequently used nonopioid antitussive for a mild cough is dextromethorphan, which is available in OTC cold and flu medications. Dextromethorphan is chemically similar to the opioids and also acts on the CNS to raise the cough threshold. Although it does not have the same level of abuse potential as the opioids, large amounts of dextromethorphan produce symptoms that include hallucinations, slurred speech, dizziness, drowsiness, euphoria, and lack of motor coordination. Nurses should be aware of the potential for abuse of this drug, especially among teens, and should counsel patients to not exceed the recommended dose.

Table 39.6 Selected Opioid Combination Drugs for Severe Cold Symptoms

Trade Name	Opioid	Nonopioid Active Ingredients
Cheratussin AC	codeine	guaifenesin
Codimal DH	hydrocodone	phenylephrine, pyrilamine
Novahistine DH	codeine	phenylephrine, chlorpheniramine
Obredon	hydrocodone	guaifenesin
Phenergan with Codeine	codeine	promethazine
Tussigon	hydrocodone	homatropine
Tussionex	hydrocodone	chlorpheniramine
Zutipro	hydrocodone	pseudoephedrine, chlorpheniramine

Evidence-Based Practice: Combination Antihistamine, Decongestant, and Analgesic Drugs for the Common Cold

Clinical Question: How effective are combination remedies for treating the common cold?

Evidence: In a review of randomized controlled trials (RCTs) conducted on combinations of antihistamines, decongestants, and analgesics, De Sutter, van Driel, Kumar, Lessar, and Skrt (2012) sought to determine if combination remedies were effective treatments for the common cold. All combinations were shown to have some overall benefits in shortening the duration of the cold in older children and adults but had no benefit in young children. The combination of an antihistamine, decongestant, and analgesic had more adverse effects than other combinations or with placebo use, but the difference was not statistically significant. Without significant findings, the authors caution that combination remedies should be used after weighing the risk of adverse effects against the benefits of treatment.

Nursing Implications: Nurses are often asked by patients, family members, friends, or neighbors for recommendations about treatments for the common cold. Although the use of antihistamines, decongestants, and analgesics will provide some benefit, even OTC drugs are not without potential adverse effects, and these effects should be weighed against the benefit in treating the symptoms. When possible, a single-remedy drug should be used to treat specific symptoms. Whereas these combinations in general may be beneficial to older children and adults, their use is not recommended for young children.

Benzonatate (Tessalon) is a nonopioid antitussive that acts by a different mechanism. Chemically related to the local anesthetic tetracaine (Pontocaine), benzonatate suppresses the cough reflex by anesthetizing stretch receptors in the lungs. If chewed, the drug can cause the side effect of numbing the mouth and pharynx. Adverse effects are uncommon but may include sedation, nausea, headache, and dizziness.

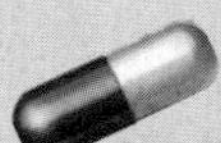

Prototype Drug | Dextromethorphan *(Delsym, Robitussin DM, others)*

Therapeutic Class: Cough suppressant **Pharmacologic Class:** Drug for increasing cough threshold

Actions and Uses

Dextromethorphan is a nonopioid drug that is a component in many OTC severe cold and flu preparations. It is available in a large variety of formulations, including tablets, liquid-filled capsules, lozenges, and liquids. It has a rapid onset of action, usually within 15 to 30 minutes. Like codeine, it acts in the medulla, although it lacks the analgesic and euphoric effects of the opioids and does not produce dependence. Patients whose cough is not relieved by dextromethorphan after several days of therapy should notify their health care provider.

Administration Alerts

- Avoid pulmonary irritants, such as smoking or other fumes, because these agents may decrease drug effectiveness.
- Pregnancy category C.

PHARMACOKINETICS

Onset	Peak	Duration
15–30 min	Unknown	3–8 h

Adverse Effects

At therapeutic doses, adverse effects due to dextromethorphan are rare. Dizziness, drowsiness, and GI upset occur in some patients. In abuse situations, the drug can cause CNS toxicity with a wide variety of symptoms, including slurred speech, ataxia, hyperexcitability, stupor, respiratory depression, seizures, coma, and toxic psychosis.

Contraindications: Dextromethorphan is contraindicated in the treatment of chronic cough due to excessive bronchial secretions, such as in asthma, smoking, and emphysema. Suppressing the cough reflex is not desirable in these patients. The U.S. Food and Drug Administration (FDA) has issued advisories that nonprescription cough and cold products (including those containing dextromethorphan) not be used in children under 6 years of age and that they be used with extreme caution in all children.

Interactions

Drug–Drug: Drug interactions with dextromethorphan include excitation, hypotension, and hyperpyrexia when used concurrently with MAOIs. Use with alcohol, opioids, or other CNS depressants may result in sedation.

Lab Tests: Unknown.

Herbal/Food: Grapefruit juice can raise serum levels of dextromethorphan and cause toxicity.

Treatment of Overdose: There is no specific treatment for overdose.

EXPECTORANTS AND MUCOLYTICS

Several drugs are available to control excess mucus production. Expectorants increase bronchial secretions, and mucolytics help loosen thick bronchial secretions. These drugs are listed in Table 39.5.

39.7 Pharmacotherapy With Expectorants and Mucolytics

Expectorants are drugs that reduce the thickness or viscosity of bronchial secretions, thus increasing mucus flow that can then be removed more easily by coughing. The most effective OTC expectorant is guaifenesin (Mucinex). Like dextromethorphan, guaifenesin produces few adverse effects and is a common ingredient in many OTC multi-symptom cold and flu preparations. It is most effective in treating dry, nonproductive cough, but it may also be of benefit for patients with productive cough. Research has questioned the effectiveness of guaifenesin in reducing acute cold symptoms. The dosage range used in cold remedies is usually too low to have much positive benefit for patients. Nonprescription cough and cold products (including those containing guaifenesin) should not be used in children under 6 years of age.

Acetylcysteine (Mucomyst) is one of the few drugs available to *directly* loosen thick, viscous bronchial secretions. Drugs of this type, which are called **mucolytics,** break down the chemical structure of mucus molecules. The mucus becomes thinner and can be removed more easily by coughing. Acetylcysteine is delivered by the inhalation route and is not available OTC. It is used in patients who have cystic fibrosis, chronic bronchitis, or other diseases that produce large amounts of thick bronchial secretions. Mucomyst can trigger bronchospasm and has an offensive odor resembling rotten eggs. Acetylcysteine (Acetadote) is also administered by the IV route as an antidote for patients who have received an overdose of acetaminophen. Its use in the pharmacotherapy of acetaminophen toxicity is presented in chapter 33.

A second mucolytic, dornase alfa (Pulmozyme), is approved for maintenance therapy in the management of thick bronchial secretions. Dornase alfa breaks down DNA molecules in the mucus, causing it to become less viscous.

Nursing Practice Application

Pharmacotherapy for Symptomatic Cold Relief

ASSESSMENT	POTENTIAL NURSING DIAGNOSES*
Baseline assessment prior to administration: • Obtain a complete health history including previous history and length of symptoms; existing cardiovascular, respiratory, hepatic, or renal disease; presence of fever; pregnancy or breast-feeding; alcohol use; or smoking. Obtain a drug history, including allergies, current prescription and OTC drugs, herbal preparations, caffeine, nicotine, and alcohol use. Be alert to possible drug interactions. • Obtain baseline vital signs. • Evaluate appropriate laboratory findings (e.g., complete blood count [CBC], hepatic and renal laboratory values).	• *Ineffective Airway Clearance* • *Ineffective Breathing Pattern* • *Disturbed Sleep Pattern*, related to adverse drug effects • *Deficient Knowledge* (drug therapy) • *Risk for Injury*, related to adverse drug effects • *Risk for Falls*, related to adverse drug effects *NANDA I © 2014
Assessment throughout administration: • Assess for desired therapeutic effects (e.g., decreased nasal congestion, tearing or itching eyes, cough, increased ease in expectorating mucus, clearer nasal passages). • Assess vital signs, especially pulse rate and rhythm, in patients with existing cardiac disease. • Assess for adverse effects: dizziness, drowsiness, blurred vision, headache, and epistaxis. Report immediately any increasing fever, tachycardia, palpitations, syncope, dyspnea, pulmonary congestion, or confusion.	

IMPLEMENTATION	
Interventions and (Rationales)	**Patient-Centered Care**
Ensuring therapeutic effects: • Continue assessments as described earlier for therapeutic effects. (Improvement in signs and symptoms of allergies or the common cold should begin after taking the first dose. The health care provider should be notified if symptoms increase, especially if respiratory involvement worsens or if fever is present.)	• Teach the patient to supplement drug therapy with nonpharmacologic measures such as increased fluid intake to liquefy and mobilize mucus and moisten the respiratory tract. • Instruct the patient to contact the health care provider if symptoms worsen or if fever is present or increasing.

continued

Nursing Practice Application *continued*

IMPLEMENTATION	
Interventions and (Rationales)	**Patient-Centered Care**
• For treatment of seasonal allergies, drug therapy should be started before the beginning of the allergy season and appearance of symptoms. (Beginning drug therapy before the circulating histamine increases will result in greater therapeutic effects. Starting drug therapy after allergy symptoms are severe will require several doses before marked improvement of symptoms is noted.)	• Teach the patient to begin taking the drug before allergy season begins or at the earliest possible appearance of symptoms for best results, and to maintain consistent dosing. • **Lifespan:** Teach parents or caregivers that antihistamines are not recommended for use in children under 6 unless recommended by the health care provider.
Minimizing adverse effects: • Observe for drowsiness or dizziness. (**Lifespan:** Drowsiness or dizziness may occur, increasing the risk of falls, especially in older adults.)	• **Safety:** Instruct the patient to call for assistance prior to getting out of bed or attempting to walk alone, and to avoid driving or other activities requiring mental alertness or physical coordination until the effects of the drug are known. If dizziness occurs, the patient should sit or lie down and not attempt to stand or walk until the sensation passes.
• Continue to monitor vital signs, especially pulse rate and rhythm for patients taking decongestants, including nasal decongestants. (Sympathomimetic decongestants may cause tachycardia and dysrhythmias in patients with a history of cardiac disease. **Lifespan:** Undetected cardiac disease may place the older adult at greater risk for cardiovascular adverse effects.)	• Instruct the patient to immediately report dizziness, palpitations, or syncope. • Teach the patient, family, or caregiver how to monitor pulse and blood pressure as appropriate. Ensure the proper use and functioning of any home equipment obtained.
• Monitor for persistent dry cough, increasing cough severity, increasing congestion, or dyspnea. (Some of these drugs are used with caution or are contraindicated in patients with existing respiratory disease, including COPD. A change in the severity of the cough may indicate worsening disease process or a more serious respiratory infection and should be reported immediately.)	• Instruct the patient to report promptly any change in the severity or frequency of cough. Any cough accompanied by shortness of breath, increasing congestion, fever, or chest pain should be reported immediately. • Encourage the patient to increase fluid intake to liquefy mucous secretions and moisten the upper respiratory tract.
• Assess the color and consistency of any expectorated sputum. (Increasing thickness, color, hemoptysis, or quantity of sputum may indicate a serious respiratory infection and should be reported immediately.)	• Instruct the patient to report any significant change in the color, consistency, or quantity of expectorated mucus to the health care provider.
• Assess for CNS effects including restlessness, nervousness, insomnia, headache, tremors, fatigue, or weakness. Report severe symptoms or any disorientation or confusion immediately. (CNS depressant effects such as drowsiness, fatigue, or mild weakness are common. Paradoxical excitement such as restlessness, nervousness, or insomnia may occur, especially in children. Alcohol consumption increases the CNS depressant effects and should be avoided.)	• Instruct the patient, family, or caregiver to report increasing lethargy, disorientation, confusion, changes in behavior or mood, agitation or aggression, slurred speech, or ataxia immediately. • Instruct the patient to avoid or eliminate alcohol consumption.
• If used for sleep, ensure patient safety on awakening. Avoid using antihistamines for sleep for more than 2 weeks and consult the health care provider if insomnia continues. (Morning or daytime drowsiness, a "hangover" effect, may occur in some patients taking antihistamines for sleep and may impair normal activities. Patients may become tolerant to drowsiness-inducing effects within 2 weeks.)	• **Safety:** Caution the patient about possible morning or daytime sleepiness and to exercise caution with activities requiring mental alertness or physical coordination until daytime effects of the drug are known. Do not keep the medication at the bedside to prevent overdosage from occurring if additional doses are taken when drowsy. Do not take the medication concurrently with alcohol.
• Assess for changes in visual acuity, blurred vision, loss of peripheral vision, seeing rainbow halos around lights, acute eye pain, or any of these symptoms accompanied by nausea and vomiting, and report immediately. (Increased intraocular pressure in patients with narrow-angle glaucoma may occur with antihistamines.)	• Instruct the patient to immediately report any visual changes or eye pain.
• Monitor for anticholinergic-related adverse effects including dry mouth, thickened mucus, nasal dryness, slightly blurred vision, and headache. (Mild anticholinergic effects are common and are treated symptomatically. Significant symptoms as listed previously are reported immediately. **Lifespan:** Be aware that the older adult male with an enlarged prostate is at higher risk for mechanical obstruction.)	• Instruct the patient to immediately report the inability to void and increasing bladder pressure or pain.

Nursing Practice Application *continued*

IMPLEMENTATION	
Interventions and (Rationales)	**Patient-Centered Care**
• Have the patient use appropriate administration techniques to self-administer the drug. (Clearing the nasal passages before administering the nasal spray and allowing the first of two sprays' time to constrict local vessels and mucosa will allow the spray to reach higher into passages. Swallowing additional drug may increase the risk of systemic adverse effects.)	• Teach the patient to clear nasal passages, and then administer the decongestant spray. After a waiting period of 5 to 10 minutes, follow with additional nasal sprays as ordered. Any excess that drains into the mouth should be spit out and not swallowed. • Teach the patient to limit use of decongestant nasal sprays to 3 to 5 days, unless otherwise ordered by the provider, to avoid rebound congestion.
• Encourage the use of single-symptom drug preparations when possible. (Multisystem formulations increase the risk of adverse effects. Additional drugs not needed in multiuse preparations should be avoided.)	• Teach the patient to consider symptoms when selecting OTC cold remedies and choose preparations based on current symptoms. • Instruct the patient that multiuse cold remedies containing acetaminophen must be taken in prescribed doses to avoid acetaminophen overdose and potential liver damage.
Patient understanding of drug therapy: • Use opportunities during administration of medications and during assessments to provide patient education. (Using time during nursing care helps to optimize and reinforce key teaching areas.)	• The patient should be able to state the reason for the drug, appropriate dose and scheduling, and what adverse effects to observe for and when to report them.
Patient self-administration of drug therapy: • When administering the medication, instruct the patient, family, or caregiver in the proper self-administration of the drug (e.g., take the drug before allergy season or before symptoms are severe). (Proper administration will increase the effectiveness of the drug.)	• The patient and family or caregiver are able to discuss appropriate dosing and administration needs, including: • Antihistamines: Begin taking the drug before allergy season begins or at the earliest possible appearance of symptoms for best results. • Cough suppressants: Cough syrups should be swallowed without water and allowed to coat the throat for soothing effects, followed by increased fluid intake 30 to 60 minutes later. • Expectorants: Syrups should be taken with a full glass of liquid and increased fluid intake throughout the day to assist in thinning mucus for ease of expectoration. • Nasal decongestants: Nasal passages should be cleared by blowing, followed by the nasal spray.

See Tables 39.1, 39.3, 39.4, 39.5, and 39.6 for a list of drugs to which these nursing actions apply.

Chapter Review

KEY Concepts

The numbered key concepts provide a succinct summary of the important points from the corresponding numbered section within the chapter. If any of these points are not clear, refer to the numbered section within the chapter for review.

39.1 The upper respiratory tract humidifies and cleans incoming air. The nasal mucosa is richly supplied with vascular tissue and is the first line of immuno logic defense.

39.2 Allergic rhinitis is a disorder characterized by tearing eyes, sneezing, and nasal congestion. Pharmacotherapy is targeted at preventing the disorder or relieving its symptoms.

39.3 Antihistamines, or H_1-receptor antagonists, can provide relief from the symptoms of allergic rhinitis. Major side effects include drowsiness and anticholinergic effects such as dry mouth. Newer drugs in this class are nonsedating.

39.4 Intranasal corticosteroids have become first-line drugs for treating allergic rhinitis due to their high efficacy and safety. For maximum effectiveness, they must be administered 2 to 3 weeks prior to allergen exposure.

39.5 The most commonly used decongestants are oral and intranasal sympathomimetics that alleviate the nasal congestion associated with allergic rhinitis and the common cold. Intranasal drugs are more efficacious but should be used for only 3 to 5 days due to rebound congestion.

39.6 Antitussives are effective at relieving cough caused by the common cold. Opioids are used for severe cough. Nonopioids such as dextromethorphan are used for mild or moderate cough.

39.7 Expectorants promote mucus secretion, making it thinner and easier to remove by coughing. Mucolytics directly break down mucus molecules.

REVIEW Questions

1. The patient has been prescribed oxymetazoline (Afrin) nasal spray for seasonal rhinitis. The nurse will provide which of the following instructions?
   1. Limit use of this spray to 5 days or less.
   2. The drug may be sedating so be cautious with activities requiring alertness.
   3. This drug should not be used in conjunction with antihistamines.
   4. This is an over-the-counter drug and may be used as needed for congestion.

2. A patient has a prescription for fluticasone (Flonase). Place the following instructions in the order in which the nurse will instruct the patient to use the drug.
   1. Instill one spray directed high into the nasal cavity.
   2. Clear the nose by blowing.
   3. Prime the inhaler prior to first use.
   4. Spit out any excess liquid that drains into the mouth.

3. A male, age 67, reports taking diphenhydramine (Benadryl) for hay fever. Considering this patient's age, the nurse assesses for which of the following findings?
   1. A history of prostatic or urinary conditions
   2. Any recent weight gain
   3. A history of allergic reactions
   4. A history of peptic ulcer disease

4. The nurse is teaching a patient about the use of dextromethorphan with guaifenesin (Robitussin-DM) syrup for a cough accompanied by thick mucus. Which instruction should be included in the patient's teaching?
   1. Lie supine for 30 minutes after taking the liquid.
   2. Drink minimal fluids to avoid stimulating the cough reflex.
   3. Take the drug with food for best results.
   4. Avoid drinking fluids immediately after the syrup but increase overall fluid intake throughout the day.

5. A patient has been prescribed fluticasone (Flonase) to use with oxymetazoline (Afrin). How should the patient be taught to use these drugs?
   1. Use the fluticasone first, then the oxymetazoline after waiting 5 minutes.
   2. Use the oxymetazoline first, then the fluticasone after waiting 5 minutes.
   3. The drugs may be used in either order.
   4. The fluticasone should be used only if the oxymetazoline fails to relieve the nasal congestion.

6. Which of the following is the best advice that the nurse can give a patient with viral rhinitis who intends to purchase an over-the-counter combination cold remedy?
   1. Dosages in these remedies provide precise dosing for each symptom that you are experiencing.
   2. These drugs are best used in conjunction with an antibiotic.
   3. It is safer to use a single-drug preparation if you are experiencing only one symptom.
   4. Since these drugs are available over the counter, it is safe to use any of them as long as needed.

PATIENT-FOCUSED Case Study

George Orlanski, who is 60-years-old, has had bronchitis with coughing for several days. He has been losing sleep because of the severity of the cough, and it is starting to affect his work. He finally goes to the local urgent care clinic for treatment. He is diagnosed with acute viral bronchitis and is given a prescription for an antitussive.

1. As the nurse, of the two antitussive medications, dextromethorphan and codeine, which is the drug of choice for this patient? Why?
2. George asks why the provider did not give him an antibiotic prescription. What is the best answer to his question?
3. What additional measures can George try to relieve his cough and what additional information does he need?

CRITICAL THINKING Questions

1. A 74-year-old male patient informs the nurse that he is taking diphendydramine (Benadryl) to reduce seasonal allergy symptoms. This patient has a history of BPH and mild glaucoma (controlled by medication). What is the nurse's response?
2. A 67-year-old patient has allergic rhinitis and always carries a handkerchief in his pocket because he has nasal discharge nearly every day. Sometimes his nose is stuffy and dry. The health care provider prescribes fluticasone (Flonase). He is to take one spray intranasally at bedtime. The patient starts to take fluticasone and a week later calls the provider's office and talks to the nurse. He says, "This Flonase is not helping me." What is the nurse's best response?

Visit www.pearsonhighered.com/nursingresources for answers and rationales for all activities.

REFERENCES

De Sutter, A. I., van Driel, M. L., Kumar, A. A., Lessar, O., & Skrt, A. (2012). Oral antihistamine-decongestant-analgesic combinations for the common cold. *Cochrane Database of Systematic Reviews Online, 2*, Art. No.: CD004976. doi:10.1002/14651858.CD004976.pub3

Herdman, T. H., & Kamitsuru, S. (2014). *NANDA International nursing diagnoses: Definitions and classification, 2015–2017*. Oxford, United Kingdom: Wiley-Blackwell.

SELECTED BIBLIOGRAPHY

American Lung Association. (n.d.). *Facts about the common cold*. Retrieved from http://www.lung.org/lung-disease/influenza/in-depth-resources/facts-about-the-common-cold.html

Hoyte, F. C., Meltzer, E. O., Ostrom, N. K., Nelson, H. S., Bensch, G. W., Spangler, D. L., . . . Katial, R. K. (2014). Recommendations for the pharmacologic management of allergic rhinitis. *Allergy and Asthma Proceedings, 35*(Suppl. 1), S20–S27. doi:10.2500/aap.2014.35.3761

Isbister, G. K., Prior, F., & Kilham, H. A. (2012). Restricting cough and cold medicines in children. *Journal of Paediatrics and Child Health, 48*, 91–98. doi:10.1111/j.1440-1754.2010.01780.x

Paul, I. M. (2012). Therapeutic options for acute cough due to upper respiratory infections in children. *Lung, 190*, 41–44. doi:10.1007/s00408-011-9319-y

Ridolo, E., Montagni, M., Melli, V., Braido, F., Incorvaia, C., & Canonica, G. W. (2014). Pharmacotherapy of allergic rhinitis: Current options and future perspectives. *Expert Opinion on Pharmacotherapy, 15*, 73–83. doi:10.1517/14656566.2014.860445

Ryan, N. M., & Gibson, P. G. (2014). Recent additions in the treatment of cough. *Journal of Thoracic Disease, 6*(Suppl. 7), S739–S747. doi:10.3978/j.issn.2072-1439.2014.03.13

Smith, S. M., Schroeder, K., & Fahey, T. (2012). Over-the-counter (OTC) medications for acute cough in children and adults in ambulatory settings. *Cochrane Database of Systematic Reviews, 8*, Art. No.: CD001831. doi:10.1002/14651858.CD001831.pub4

Tharpe, C. A., & Kemp, S. F. (2015). Pediatric allergic rhinitis. *Immunology and Allergy Clinics of North America, 35*, 185–198. doi:10.1016/j.iac.2014.09.003

Turner, P. J., & Kemp, A. S. (2012). Allergic rhinitis in children. *Journal of Paediatrics and Child Health, 48*, 302–310. doi:10.1111/j.1440-1754.2010.01779.x

U.S. Food and Drug Administration. (2011). *Unapproved cough, cold and allergy products: FDA prompts removal from the market*. Retrieved from http://www.fda.gov/Safety/MedWatch/SafetyInformation/SafetyAlertsforHumanMedicalProducts/ucm245279.htm

U.S. Government Accountability Office. (2013). *Drug control: State approaches taken to control access to key methamphetamine ingredient show varied impact on domestic drug labs*. Retrieved from http://www.gao.gov/products/GAO-13-204

Yanai, K., Rogala, B., Chugh, K., Paraskakis, E., Pampura, A. N., & Boev, R. (2012). Safety considerations in the management of allergic diseases: Focus on antihistamines. *Current Medical Research & Opinion, 28*, 623–642. doi:10.1185/03007995.2012.672405

Chapter 40

Drugs for Asthma and Other Pulmonary Disorders

Drugs at a Glance

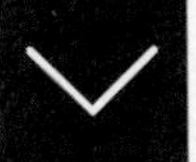

Learning Outcomes

After reading this chapter, the student should be able to:

1. Identify anatomic structures associated with the lower respiratory tract and their functions.
2. Explain how the autonomic nervous system regulates airflow in the lower respiratory tract, and how this process can be modified with drugs.
3. Compare the advantages and disadvantages of using the inhalation route of administration for pulmonary drugs.
4. Describe the types of devices used to deliver aerosol therapies via the inhalation route.
5. Compare and contrast the pharmacotherapy of acute and chronic asthma.
6. Describe the nurse's role in the pharmacologic treatment of lower respiratory tract disorders.
7. For each of the classes listed in Drugs at a Glance, know representative drugs, and explain their mechanism of drug action, primary actions on the respiratory system, and important adverse effects.
8. Use the nursing process to care for patients who are receiving pharmacotherapy for lower respiratory tract disorders.

indicates a prototype drug, each of which is featured in a Prototype Drug box.

The flow of oxygen, carbon dioxide, and other gases into and out of the human body is dynamic and in constant flux. Continuous control of the airways is necessary to bring an abundant supply of essential gases to the pulmonary capillaries and to rid the body of waste products. Any restriction in this dynamic flow, even for brief periods, may result in serious consequences. This chapter examines drugs used in the pharmacotherapy of two primary pulmonary disorders—asthma and chronic obstructive pulmonary disease (COPD).

THE LOWER RESPIRATORY SYSTEM

40.1 Physiology of the Lower Respiratory Tract

The primary function of the respiratory system is to bring oxygen into the body and to remove carbon dioxide. The process by which gases are exchanged is called respiration. The basic structures of the lower respiratory tract are shown in Figure 40.1.

Ventilation is the process of moving air into and out of the lungs. As the diaphragm contracts and lowers in position, it creates a negative pressure that draws air into the lungs, and inspiration occurs. During expiration, the diaphragm relaxes and air leaves the lungs passively with no energy expenditure required. Ventilation is a purely mechanical process that occurs approximately 12 to 18 times per minute in adults, a rate determined by neurons in the brainstem. This rate may be modified by a number of factors, including emotions, fever, stress, the pH of the blood, and certain medications.

The respiratory tree ends in dilated sacs called alveoli, which have no smooth muscle but are abundantly rich in capillaries. An extremely thin membrane in the alveoli separates the airway from the pulmonary capillaries, allowing gases to readily move between the internal environment of the blood and the inspired air. As oxygen crosses this membrane, it is exchanged for carbon dioxide, a cellular waste product that travels from the blood to the air. The lung is richly supplied with blood. Blood flow through the lungs is called **perfusion**. The process of gas exchange is shown in Figure 40.1.

40.2 Bronchiolar Smooth Muscle

Bronchioles are muscular, elastic structures whose diameter, or lumen, varies with the contraction or relaxation of smooth muscle. Bronchodilation opens the lumen, allowing air to enter the lungs more freely, thus increasing the supply of oxygen to the body's tissues. Bronchoconstriction closes the lumen, resulting in less airflow. Bronchodilation and bronchoconstriction are largely regulated by the two branches of the autonomic nervous system.

- The sympathetic branch activates beta$_2$-adrenergic receptors, which causes bronchiolar smooth muscle to relax, the airway diameter to increase, and bronchodilation to occur.
- The parasympathetic branch causes bronchiolar smooth muscle to contract, the airway diameter to narrow, and bronchoconstriction to occur.

Drugs that enhance bronchodilation will enable the patient to breathe easier. Drugs that stimulate beta$_2$-adrenergic receptors, commonly called bronchodilators, are some of the most frequently prescribed drugs for

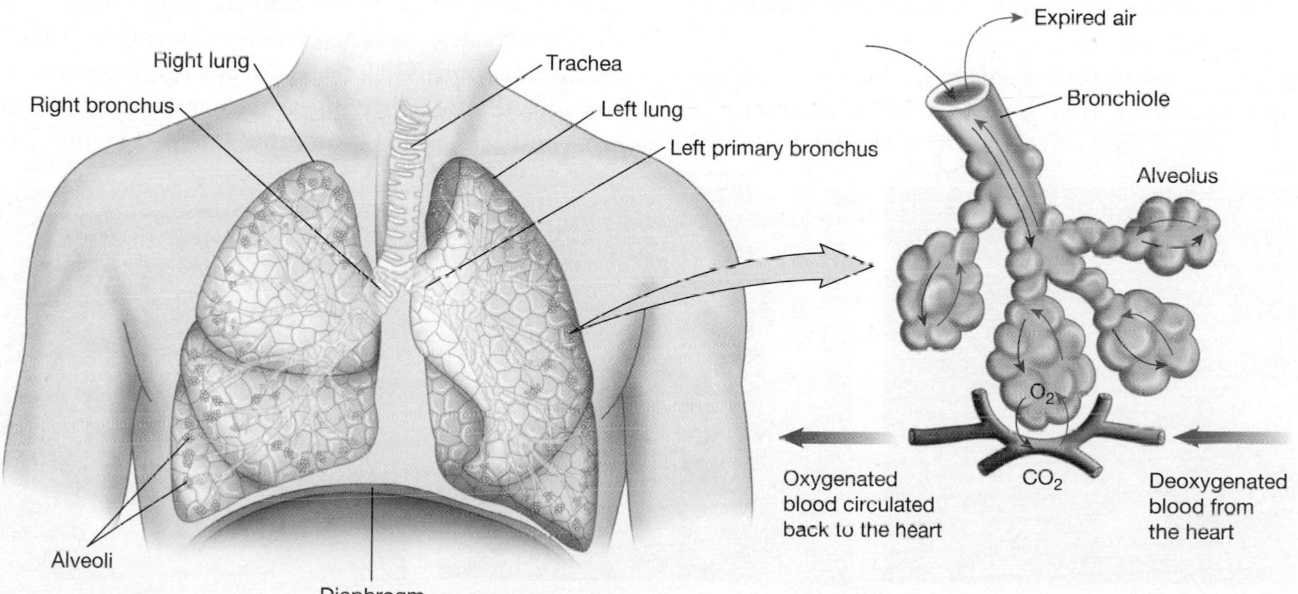

FIGURE 40.1 The lower respiratory tract and the process of gas exchange

treating pulmonary disorders. On the other hand, drugs that cause bronchoconstriction may cause breathing to become labored and the patient to become short of breath.

40.3 Administration of Pulmonary Drugs Via Inhalation

The respiratory system offers a rapid and efficient mechanism for delivering drugs. The enormous surface area of the bronchioles and alveoli, and the rich blood supply to these areas, results in an almost instantaneous onset of action for inhaled substances.

Medications are delivered to the respiratory system by aerosol therapy. An **aerosol** is a suspension of minute liquid droplets or fine solid particles suspended in a gas. The major advantage of aerosol therapy is that it delivers pulmonary drugs to their immediate site of action, thus reducing systemic side effects. To produce an equivalent therapeutic action, an oral drug would have to be given at higher doses and be distributed to all body tissues. Aerosol therapy can give immediate relief for **bronchospasm,** an acute condition during which the bronchiolar smooth muscle rapidly contracts, leaving the patient gasping for breath. Drugs may also be given to loosen viscous mucus in the bronchial tree.

It should be clearly understood that drugs delivered by inhalation have the potential to produce *systemic* effects because there is always some degree of drug absorption across the pulmonary capillaries. For example, anesthetics such as nitrous oxide and isoflurane (Forane) are delivered via the inhalation route and are rapidly distributed to cause central nervous system (CNS) depression (see chapter 19). Solvents such as paint thinners and glues are sometimes intentionally inhaled and can cause serious adverse effects on the nervous system and even death. In general, however, drugs administered by the inhalation route for respiratory conditions produce minimal systemic toxicity when administered correctly.

Several devices are used to deliver drugs via the inhalation route. A **nebulizer** is a small machine that vaporizes a liquid medication into a fine mist that is inhaled, using a face mask or handheld device. If the drug is a solid, it may be administered using a **dry powder inhaler (DPI).** A DPI is a small device that is activated during inhalation to deliver a fine powder directly to the bronchial tree. Turbuhaler and Flexhaler are types of DPIs. A **metered-dose inhaler (MDI)** is the most common type of device used to deliver respiratory drugs. MDIs consist of a propellant inside a canister filled with medication. The patient depresses the canister while inhaling a slow, deep breath. This helps to deliver a measured dose of medication to the lungs during each breath.

There are disadvantages to administering aerosol therapy. The precise dose received by the patient is difficult to measure because it depends on the patient's breathing pattern and the correct use of the inhaler device. Even under optimal conditions, only 10% to 50% of the drug actually reaches the lower respiratory tract. Accurate hand-breath coordination is essential to receiving the correct dose. Therefore, patients must be carefully instructed on the correct use of these devices.

Swallowing medication that has been deposited in the oral cavity may cause systemic adverse effects if the drug is absorbed in the gastrointestinal (GI) tract. In addition, patients should rinse their mouth thoroughly following drug use to reduce the potential for absorption of the drug across the oral mucosa. Three devices used to deliver respiratory drugs are shown in Figure 40.2.

ASTHMA

Asthma is a chronic pulmonary disease with inflammatory and bronchospasm components. Drugs may be given to decrease the frequency of asthmatic attacks or to terminate attacks in progress.

40.4 Pathophysiology of Asthma

Asthma is one of the most common chronic conditions in the United States, affecting 20 million Americans. Although the disorder can affect a person of any age, asthma is often considered a pediatric disease. Characterized by acute bronchospasm, asthma can cause intense breathlessness,

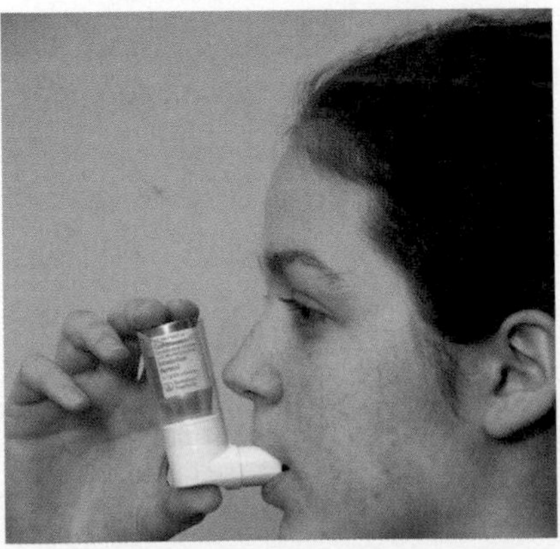

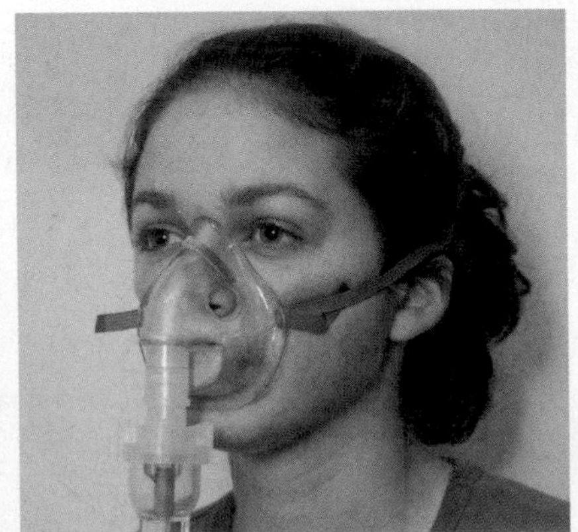

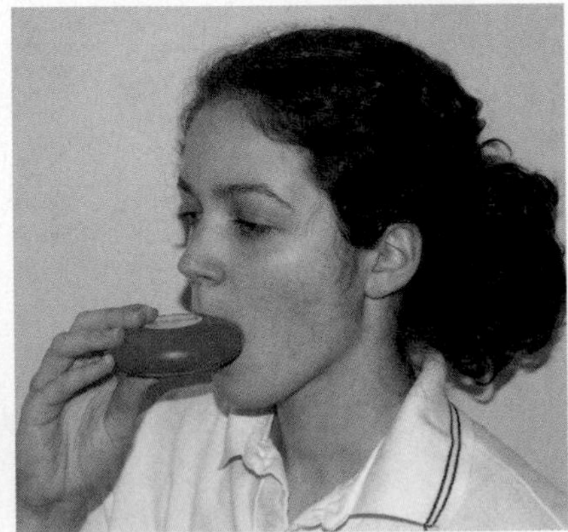

FIGURE 40.2 Devices used to deliver respiratory drugs: (a) metered-dose inhaler; (b) nebulizer with face mask; (c) dry powder inhaler
Ph College/Pearson Education, Inc.

PharmFacts

ASTHMA

- Approximately 8% of adults and 9.3% of children in the United States have asthma.
- Asthma is responsible for about 1.8 million emergency department visits and more than 400,000 hospitalizations each year.
- More than 3,000 people die of asthma each year.
- Non-Hispanic black children were more likely to have ever been diagnosed with asthma (22%) and to still have asthma (16%) than Hispanic (14% and 9%) or non-Hispanic white (12% and 8%) children.
- Asthma is the most common chronic disease of childhood, affecting more than 1 child in 20.

coughing, and gasping for air. Along with bronchoconstriction, an acute inflammatory response stimulates the secretion of histamine and other inflammatory mediators, which increases mucus and edema in the airways. As in allergic rhinitis, the airway becomes hyper-responsive to allergens. Both bronchospasm and inflammation contribute to airway obstruction, as illustrated in Figure 40.3.

The patient with asthma can present with acute or chronic symptoms. Intervals between symptoms may vary from days to weeks to months. Some patients experience asthma when exposed to specific triggers, such as those listed in Table 40.1. Others experience the disorder on exertion, a condition called *exercise-induced asthma.* **Status asthmaticus** is a severe, prolonged form of asthma unresponsive to drug treatment that may lead to respiratory failure.

Table 40.1 Common Triggers of Asthma

Cause	Sources
Air pollutants	Tobacco smoke
	Ozone
	Nitrous and sulfur oxides
	Fumes from cleaning fluids or solvents
	Burning leaves
Allergens	Pollen from trees, grasses, and weeds
	Animal dander
	Household dust
	Mold
Chemicals and food	Drugs, including aspirin, ibuprofen, and beta blockers
	Sulfite preservatives
	Food and condiments, including nuts, monosodium glutamate (MSG), shellfish, and dairy products
Respiratory infections	Bacterial, fungal, and viral
Stress	Emotional stress/anxiety
	Exercise in dry, cold climates

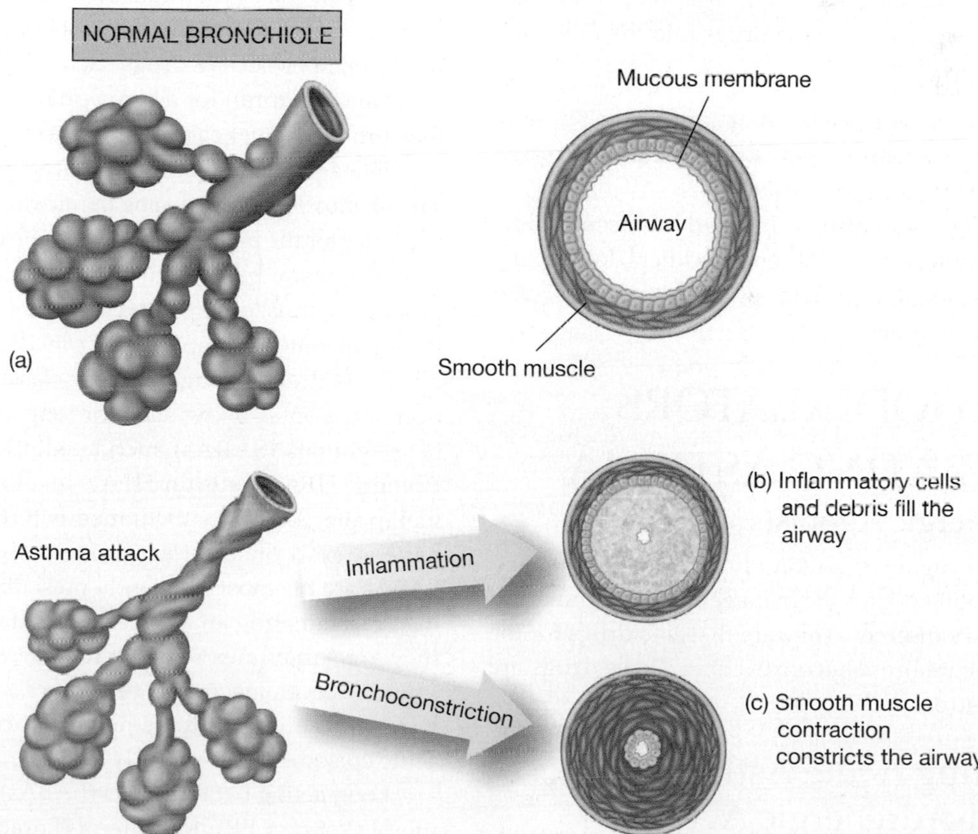

FIGURE 40.3 Changes in the bronchioles during an asthma attack: (a) normal bronchiole; (b) the inflammatory component plugs the airway; (c) bronchoconstriction narrows the airway

Table 40.2 Overview of Drug Classes for Asthma Management

Class	Mechanism	Use
QUICK-RELIEF MEDICATIONS		
Short-acting $beta_2$-adrenergic agonists (SABAs)	Bronchodilation	Preferred drugs for relief of acute symptoms.
Anticholinergics	Bronchodilation	Alternate drugs for those who cannot tolerate SABAs.
Corticosteroids: systemic	Anti-inflammatory	Although not rapid acting, these oral drugs are used for short periods to reduce the frequency of acute exacerbations.
LONG-ACTING MEDICATIONS		
Corticosteroids: inhaled	Anti-inflammatory	Preferred drugs for long-term asthma management. Oral doses may be required for severe, persistent asthma.
Mast cell stabilizers	Anti-inflammatory	Alternative drugs to control mild, persistent asthma or exercise-induced asthma.
Leukotriene modifiers	Anti-inflammatory	Alternative drugs to control mild, persistent asthma or as adjunctive therapy with inhaled corticosteroids.
Long-acting $beta_2$-adrenergic agonists (LABAs)	Bronchodilation	Used in combination with inhaled corticosteroids for prophylaxis of moderate to severe persistent asthma.
Methylxanthines	Bronchodilation	Used in combination with inhaled corticosteroids for prophylaxis of mild to moderate persistent asthma.
Immunomodulators	Monoclonal antibody	Used as adjunctive therapy for patients who have allergies and severe, persistent asthma.

Data from *Expert Panel Report 3: Guidelines for the Diagnosis and Management of Asthma,* by the National Heart, Blood, and Lung Institute, National Asthma Education and Prevention, 2007.

Because asthma has both a bronchoconstriction component and an inflammation component, pharmacotherapy of the disease focuses on one or both of these mechanisms. The goals of drug therapy are twofold: to *terminate* acute bronchospasms in progress and to *reduce the frequency* of asthma attacks. Different medications are needed to achieve each of these goals. The National Asthma Education and Prevention Program categorizes asthma drugs into the following two simple classes (Table 40.2):

- Quick-relief medications. Short and intermediate-acting $beta_2$-adrenergic agonists, anticholinergics and systemic corticosteroids.
- Long-acting medications. Inhaled corticosteroids, mast cell stabilizers, leukotriene modifiers, long-acting $beta_2$-adrenergic agonists, methylxanthines, and immunomodulators.

BRONCHODIALATORS FOR TREATING ASTHMA

Beta-Adrenergic Agonists

$Beta_2$-adrenergic agonists (or simply beta agonists) are effective bronchodilators for the management of asthma and other pulmonary diseases. They are first-line drugs for the treatment of acute bronchoconstriction. These drugs are listed in Table 40.3.

40.5 Treating Acute Asthma With Beta-Adrenergic Agonists

Beta-adrenergic agonists are drugs that activate the sympathetic nervous system, which relaxes bronchial smooth muscle resulting in bronchodilation. Beta-agonist medications may act either on $beta_1$ receptors, which are located in the heart, or on $beta_2$ receptors, which are found in the smooth muscle of the lung, uterus, and other organs. Beta agonists that activate both $beta_1$ and $beta_2$ receptors are called *nonselective* bronchodilators. Beta agonists that activate only the $beta_2$ receptors are called *selective* drugs. The selective $beta_2$-adrenergic agonists have largely replaced the older, nonselective drugs such as epinephrine and isoproterenol (Isuprel) for asthma pharmacotherapy because they produce fewer cardiac side effects.

Beta agonists are bronchodilators that relax bronchial smooth muscle, thus widening the airway and making breathing easier for the patient. Although quite effective at relieving bronchospasm, beta agonists have no anti-inflammatory properties; thus, other drug classes are required to control the inflammatory component of *chronic* asthma.

Beta-adrenergic agonists are classified by their duration of action as being short or long acting. Short-acting beta agonists (SABAs) such as albuterol (ProAir HFA, Prventil HFA, Ventolin HFA), levalbuterol (Xonopex), metaprotereol, and subcutaneous terbutaline (Brethine) have a rapid onset of action, usually several minutes. SABAs are the most frequently prescribed drugs for aborting or terminating an acute asthma attack. For this reason, they are sometimes referred to as *rescue drugs*. Their effects, however, last only 2 to 6 hours, so the use of SABAs is generally limited to as-needed (prn) management of acute episodes.

Long-acting beta agonists (LABAs) which include albuterol (VoSpire ER), formoterol (Foradil), and salmeterol (Serevent Diskus), have therapeutic effects that last up to 12 hours. The LABAs carry a black box warning that their use

Table 40.3 Bronchodilators

Drug	Route and Adult Dose (max dose where indicated)	Adverse Effects
BETA-ADRENERGIC AGONISTS		
albuterol (ProAir HFA, Proventi, HFAI, Ventolin HFA, VoSpire ER)	MDI: 2 inhalations q4–6h as needed (max: 12 inhalations/day) Nebulizer: 1.25–5 mg q4–8h as needed PO (VoSpire ER): 4–8 mg q12h (max: 32 mg/day divided)	*Headache, dizziness, tremor, nervousness, throat irritation, drug tolerance* Tachycardia, dysrhythmias, hypokalemia, hyperglycemia, paradoxical bronchoconstriction, increased risk for asthma-related death (LABAs)
arformoterol (Brovana)	Nebulizer (for COPD): 15 mcg bid (max: 30 mcg/day)	
formoterol (Foradil, Perforomist)	DPI (Foradil for asthma and COPD): 12 mcg inhalation capsule q12h (max: 24 mcg/day) Nebulizer (Performist for COPD): 20 mcg bid (max: 40 mcg/day)	
indacaterol (Arcapta neohaler)	Inhalation (for COPD): one 75 mcg capsule/day using the Neohaler	
levalbuterol (Xopenex)	Nebulizer: 0.63 mg tid–qid MDI: 2 inhalations q4–6h Inhalation: 2–3 inhalations (max: 12 inhalations/day) PO: 20 mg tid–qid	
metaproterenol	Nebulizer: 5–10 inhalations	
olodaterol (Stiverdi Respimat)	Inhalation (for COPD): 2 inhalations daily	
salmeterol (Serevent Diskus)	DPI (for asthma and COPD): 1 inhalation bid	
terbutaline (Brethine)	PO: 2.5–5 mg tid (max: 15 mg/day) Subcutaneous: 250 mcg (may be repeated in 15 min)	
ANTICHOLINERGICS		
aclidinium (Tudorza Pressair)	DPI (for COPD): 1 inhalation (400 mcg) bid	*Headache, cough, dry mouth, bad taste, paradoxical bronchospasm* Pharyngitis, paradoxical bronchospasm, worsening of urinary retention
ipratropium (Atrovent HFA)	MDI (for COPD): 2 inhalations qid (max: 12 inhalations/day) Nebulizer: 500 mcg q6–8h	
tiotropium (Spiriva Handihaler, Spiriva Respimat)	DPI (for COPD): 2 inhalations of 1 capsule (18 mcg)/day for Spiriva Handihaler or 2 inhalations (5 mcg)/day for Spiriva Respimat)	
umeclidinium (Incruse Ellipta)	DPI: 1 inhalation (62.5 mcg) daily.	
METHYLXANTHINES		
aminophylline	IV: 0.1–0.5 mg/kg/h (rate dependent on patient parameters)	*Nervousness, tremors, dizziness, headache, nausea, vomiting, anorexia* Tachycardia, dysrhythmias, hypotension, seizures, circulatory failure, respiratory arrest
theophylline	PO: 300–600 mg/day in divided doses (max: 900 mg/day)	

Note: *Italics* indicate common adverse effects; underlining indicates serious adverse effects.

is associated with an increased risk in asthma-related deaths. These medications have a relatively slow onset of action and will not abort an acute bronchospasm. Because some LABAs are delivered via handheld inhalers, patients may assume they have the same rapid actions as the short-acting drugs. Therefore, patients must be alerted to the dangers of taking LABAs during an acute episode. Although the risk of asthma-related death is small, LABAs should be used only as adjunctive therapy for patients who cannot be adequately controlled with other medications, such as inhaled corticosteroids, or for patients with severe asthma who require two medications for disease management. They are contraindicated as monotherapy for this disease. A newer LABA, olodaterol (Striverdi Respimat), was approved in 2014 for the maintenance therapy of COPD.

Beta-adrenergic agonists are available in oral (PO), inhaled, and parenteral formulations. When taken for respiratory conditions, inhalation is the most common route. Inhaled beta agonists exhibit minimal systemic toxicity when used appropriately because only small amounts of the drugs are absorbed. When given PO, a longer duration of action is achieved, but systemic adverse effects are more frequently experienced. Systemic effects may include some activation of beta$_1$ receptors in the heart, which could cause an angina attack or a dysrhythmia in patients with cardiac impairment. With chronic use, tolerance may develop to the bronchodilation effect and the duration of action will become shorter. Should this occur, the dose of beta$_2$ agonist may need to be increased, or a second drug may be added to the therapeutic regimen. Increased use of a beta agonist over a period of hours or days is an indication that the patient's condition is rapidly deteriorating, and medical attention should be sought immediately.

Refer to the Nursing Practice Application: Pharmacotherapy With Adrenergic Drugs, in chapter 13, for patients receiving these drugs.

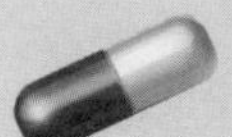

Prototype Drug | Albuterol *(ProAir HFA, Proventil, HFA, Ventolin HFA, VoSpire ER)*

Therapeutic Class: Bronchodilator **Pharmacologic Class:** Beta$_2$-adrenergic agonist

Actions and Uses

Albuterol is a SABA that is used to relieve the bronchospasm of asthma. Its rapid onset and excellent safety profile have made inhaled albuterol a preferred drug for the termination of acute bronchospasm. In addition to relieving bronchospasm, the drug facilitates mucus drainage and can inhibit the release of inflammatory chemicals from mast cells. When inhaled 15 to 30 minutes prior to physical activity, it can prevent exercise-induced bronchospasm. Short-acting beta$_2$ agonists such as albuterol are not recommended for asthma prophylaxis.

Oral forms of albuterol include immediate-release and extended-release tablets (VoSpire) and an oral solution. The oral forms have a longer onset of action and are not suitable for terminating acute asthma attacks.

Administration Alerts

- The proper use of the inhaler is important to the effective delivery of the drug; use only the actuator that comes with the canister. Observe and instruct the patient in proper use.
- Pregnancy category C.

PHARMACOKINETICS

Onset	Peak	Duration
5–15 min inhalation; 30 min PO	0.5–2 h	2–6 h inhalation; 8–12 h PO, sustained release.

Adverse Effects

Serious adverse effects from inhaled albuterol are uncommon. Some patients experience palpitations, headaches, throat irritation, tremor, nervousness, restlessness, and tachycardia. Less common adverse reactions include insomnia and dry mouth. Uncommon adverse effects include chest pain, paradoxical bronchospasm, and allergic reactions.

Contraindications: Use is contraindicated in patients with hypersensitivity to the drug. Because albuterol may exhibit cardiovascular effects in some patients, caution is required when administering these drugs to persons with a history of cardiac disease or hypertension (HTN).

Interactions

Drug–Drug: Concurrent use with beta blockers will inhibit the bronchodilation effect of albuterol. Patients should also avoid monoamine oxidase inhibitors (MAOIs) within 14 days of beginning therapy.

Lab Tests: May cause hypokalemia at high doses.

Herbal/Food: Products containing caffeine may cause nervousness, tremor, or palpitations.

Treatment of Overdose: Overdose results in an exaggerated sympathetic activation, causing dysrhythmias, hypokalemia, and hyperglycemia. In severe cases, administration of a cardioselective beta-adrenergic antagonist may be necessary.

☑ Check Your Understanding 40.1

Beta-adrenergic drugs used in the treatment of asthma include short and long-acting drugs. For the treatment of an acute asthma attack, which form of the drug should be used? Why? *Visit www.pearsonhighered.com/nursingresources for the answer.*

Anticholinergics

Although beta agonists are preferred drugs for treating acute asthma, anticholinergics are alternative bronchodilators.

Community-Oriented Practice

THE ROLE OF THE SCHOOL NURSE IN ASTHMA MANAGEMENT

Children are in school up to one-third of their waking hours during the academic year. It is estimated that over 7 million children have asthma, and asthma is the largest cause of school absenteeism (National Association of School Nurses [NASN], 2015). The costs of asthma are many and include loss of learning time due to emergency department visits and absenteeism; lower grades due to the lost learning time; lost wages for families due to absenteeism; ever-increasing costs for treatment; and long-term health effects for the child (Rodriguez et al., 2013).

The school nurse may be the most important person in assisting teachers and parents to proactively manage childhood asthma rather than reactively seeking assistance when an attack occurs. Working as a team, the school nurse can help teachers and parents become more knowledgeable about asthma triggers, symptoms, and treatment, and more skilled in symptom recognition and prevention measures. NASN has developed evidence-based practice guidelines for the prevention and treatment of asthma, and maintains a tool kit for use by nurses and teachers (Maughan & Schantz, 2014; NASN, 2015). Working as partners to lobby for school policies that aim for "asthma-free" school conditions and placing a registered nurse in every school, developing care guidelines, and establishing outcome measures that can help the team prioritize goals and interventions, may decrease the incidence and impact of childhood asthma (Engelke, Swanson, & Guttu, 2014).

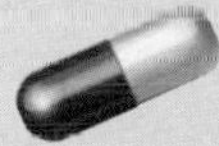

Prototype Drug | Ipratropium *(Atrovent)*

Therapeutic Class: Bronchodilator **Pharmacologic Class:** Anticholinergic

Actions and Uses

Ipratropium is an anticholinergic drug that is delivered by the inhalation and intranasal routes. The inhalation form is approved to relieve and prevent the bronchospasm that is characteristic of asthma and COPD. When combined with albuterol (Combivent Respimat), it is a first-line drug for treating bronchospasms due to COPD, including bronchitis and emphysema. Although it has not received U.S Food and Drug Administration (FDA) approval for the treatment of asthma, it is prescribed off-label for the disorder. The primary role of ipratropium is as an alternative to SABAs and for patients experiencing severe asthma exacerbations. It is sometimes combined with beta agonists or corticosteroids to provide additive bronchodilation.

The nasal spray formulation of ipratropium is approved for the symptomatic relief of runny nose associated with the common cold and allergic rhinitis. The drug inhibits nasal secretions but does not have decongestant action. Treatment is limited to 3 weeks.

Administration Alerts

- The proper use of the MDI is important to the effective delivery of drug. Observe and instruct the patient in proper use.
- Wait 2–3 minutes between dosages.
- Avoid contact with eyes; otherwise, blurred vision may occur.
- Pregnancy category B.

PHARMACOKINETICS

Onset	Peak	Duration
5–15 min	1.5–2 h	3–6 h

Adverse Effects

Because very little is absorbed by the lungs, ipratropium produces few systemic adverse effects. Irritation of the upper respiratory tract may result in cough, drying of the nasal mucosa, or hoarseness. It produces a bitter taste, which may be relieved by rinsing the mouth after use. Intranasal administration may cause epistaxis and excessive drying of the nasal mucosa.

Contraindications: Ipratropium is contraindicated in patients with hypersensitivity to soya lecithin or related food products such as soybean and peanut. Soya lecithin is used as a propellant in the inhaler.

Interactions

Drug–Drug: Use with other drugs in this class such as atropine may lead to additive anticholinergic side effects. Ipratropium should not be used concurrently with the antidiabetic drug pramlintide because both slow peristalsis and can cause serious or life-threatening GI symptoms.

Lab Tests: Unknown.

Herbal/Food: Unknown.

Treatment of Overdose: Overdose with ipratropium does not occur because very little of the drug is absorbed when given by aerosol.

Only three anticholinergics are used for pulmonary disease, and these drugs are listed in Table 40.3.

40.6 Treating Chronic Asthma With Anticholinergics

Anticholinergics (also called cholinergic blockers or antagonists) are alternative bronchodilators for patients with pulmonary disease. Anticholinergics block the parasympathetic nervous system. Because the parasympathetic response is largely the opposite of the sympathetic response, blocking the parasympathetic nervous system results in actions similar to those of stimulating the sympathetic nervous system (see chapter 12). It is predictable, then, that anticholinergic drugs would cause bronchodilation and have potential applications in the pharmacotherapy of pulmonary disease.

Although anticholinergics such as atropine have been available for many decades, drugs in this class exhibit many adverse effects when administered by the PO or parenteral routes. However, the discovery of anticholinergics that can be delivered by inhalation led to the approval of several important drugs in this class for pulmonary disease.

Ipratropium (Atrovent) is the most common anticholinergic prescribed for the pharmacotherapy of pulmonary disease. It has a slower onset of action than most beta agonists and produces a less intense bronchodilation. However, combining ipratropium with a beta agonist produces a greater and more prolonged bronchodilation than using either drug separately. Taking advantage of this increased effect, Combivent Respimat is a mixture of ipratropium and albuterol in a single MDI canister. Tiotropium (Spiriva Handihaler, Spiriva Respimat) has a longer duration of action than ipratropium and is indicated for the long-term maintenance treatment and prophylaxis of bronchospasm in patients with COPD, including chronic bronchitis and emphysema.

Two newer anticholinergics include aclidinium (Tudorza Pressair) and umeclidinium (Incruse Ellipta). Both of these medications are used for the long-term maintenance treatment of bronchospasm associated with COPD. Umeclidinium is combined with other pulmonary medications in the treatment of COPD (see section 40.12).

The inhaled anticholinergics are relatively safe medications and systemic anticholinergic adverse effects are uncommon. Dry mouth, headache, cough, GI distress, headache, and anxiety are the most common patient complaints.

Refer to the Nursing Practice Application: Pharmacotherapy With Anticholinergic Drugs in chapter 12 for patients receiving these drugs.

Methylxanthines

The methylxanthines were considered drugs of choice for treating asthma 30 years ago. Now they are primarily reserved for the long-term management of persistent asthma that is unresponsive to beta agonists or inhaled corticosteroids. These drugs are shown in Table 40.3.

40.7 Treating Chronic Asthma With Methylxanthines

The **methylxanthines,** theophylline and aminophylline, are bronchodilators chemically related to caffeine. The methylxanthines are infrequently prescribed because they have a narrow safety margin, especially with prolonged use. Adverse effects such as nausea, vomiting, and CNS stimulation occur frequently, and dysrhythmias may be observed at high doses. Like caffeine, methylxanthines can cause nervousness and insomnia. These drugs also have significant interactions with numerous other drugs.

Methylxanthines are administered by the PO or intravenous (IV) routes, rather than by inhalation. Having been largely replaced by safer and more effective drugs, theophylline is currently used primarily for the long-term oral prophylaxis of asthma that is unresponsive to beta agonists or inhaled corticosteroids.

ANTI-INFLAMMATORY DRUGS FOR TREATING ASTHMA

Corticosteroids

Inhaled corticosteroids (ICS) are used for the long-term prevention of asthmatic attacks. Oral corticosteroids may be used for the short-term management of acute severe asthma. These drugs are listed in Table 40.4.

Table 40.4 Anti-Inflammatory Drugs for Asthma

Drug	Route and Adult Dose (max dose where indicated)	Adverse Effects
INHALED CORTICOSTEROIDS*		
beclomethasone (Qvar)	MDI: 1–2 inhalations (40–160 mcg) bid (max: 320 mcg bid)	*Hoarseness, dry mouth, cough, sore throat*
budesonide (Pulmicort Flexhaler, Pulmicort Respules)	DPI (Pulmicort Flexhaler): 1–2 inhalations (360 mcg) bid (max: 720 mcg bid)	<u>Oropharyngeal candidiasis, hypercorticism, hypersensitivity reactions</u>
	Nebulizer (Pulmicort Respules): 0.5 mg/day either once daily or divided into 2 doses (max: 0.5–1 mg/day)	
ciclesonide (Alvesco)	MDI: 1–2 inhalations (80–320 mcg) bid	
flunisolide (AeroSpan)	MDI: 2–3 inhalations (160 mcg) bid (max: 320 mcg bid)	
fluticasone (Flovent Diskus, Flovent HFA) (see page 647 for the Prototype Drug box)	DPI (Flovent Diskus): 100–500 mcg bid (max: 1,000 mcg bid)	
	MDI (Flovent HFA): 88–220 mcg bid (max: 880 mcg bid)	
mometasone (Asmanex HFA)	MDI: 2 inhalations (100–200 mcg) bid (max: 200 mcg bid)	
MAST CELL STABILIZERS		
cromolyn (Intal)	MDI: 1 inhalation qid	*Nausea, sneezing, nasal stinging, throat irritation, unpleasant taste*
nedocromil (Tilade)	MDI: 2 inhalations qid	<u>Anaphylaxis, angioedema, bronchospasm</u>
LEUKOTRIENE MODIFIERS AND MISCELLANEOUS DRUGS		
montelukast (Singulair)	PO: 10 mg/day in evening	*Headache, nausea, diarrhea, throat pain, weight loss (romflumilast)*
roflumilast (Daliresp)	PO (for COPD): 500 mcg once daily	
zafirlukast (Accolate)	PO: 20 mg bid 1 h before or 2 h after meals	<u>Liver toxicity (zileuton), increased AST, psychiatric events including suicidality (romflumilast)</u>
zileuton (Zyflo CR)	PO: 1,200 mg bid	

Note: *For doses of systemic corticosteroids, refer to chapter 44.
Note: *Italics* indicate common adverse effects; <u>underlining</u> indicates serious adverse effects.

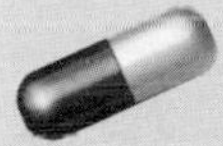

Prototype Drug | Beclomethasone *(Qvar)*

Therapeutic Class: Anti-inflammatory drug for asthma and allergic rhinitis **Pharmacologic Class:** Inhaled corticosteroid

Actions and Uses

Beclomethasone is a corticosteroid available through aerosol inhalation for asthma (Qvar) or as a nasal spray (Beconase AQ, Qnasl) for allergic rhinitis. Beclomethasone and other drugs in this class are preferred drugs for the long-term management of persistent asthma in both children and adults. Three or four weeks of therapy may be necessary before optimal benefits are obtained. Beclomethasone acts by reducing inflammation, thus decreasing the frequency of asthma attacks. It is not a bronchodilator and should not be used to terminate asthma attacks in progress.

Intranasal beclomethasone is effective at reducing the symptoms of allergic rhinitis. Beconase AQ is also approved to prevent recurrence of nasal polyps following surgical removal.

Administration Alerts

- Do not use if the patient is experiencing an acute asthma attack.
- Oral inhalation products and nasal spray products are not to be used interchangeably.
- Pregnancy category C.

PHARMACOKINETICS

Onset	Peak	Duration
1–4 wk	30–70 min	Unknown

Adverse Effects

Inhaled beclomethasone produces few systemic adverse effects. Because small amounts may be swallowed with each dose, the patient should be observed for signs of corticosteroid toxicity. Local effects may include hoarseness, dry mouth, and changes in taste. Inhaled corticosteroid use has been associated with the development of cataracts in adults. Long-term intranasal or inhaled corticosteroids may cause growth inhibition in children.

As with all corticosteroids, the anti-inflammatory properties of beclomethasone can mask signs of infections, and the drug is contraindicated if an active infection is present. A significant percentage of patients who take beclomethasone on a long-term basis will develop oropharyngeal candidiasis, a fungal infection in the throat, due to the constant deposits of drug in the oral cavity.

Contraindications: Beclomethasone is contraindicated in those with hypersensitivity to the drug. The growth of pediatric patients should be monitored carefully, because inhaled corticosteroids may reduce growth velocity in some children.

Interactions

Drug–Drug: Unknown.

Lab Tests: Unknown.

Herbal/Food: Unknown.

Treatment of Overdose: Overdose does not occur when the drug is given by the inhalation route.

40.8 Prophylaxis of Asthma With Corticosteroids

Corticosteroids, also known as glucocorticoids, are the most potent natural anti-inflammatory substances known. Because asthma has a major inflammatory component, it should not be surprising that drugs in this class play a major role in the management of this disorder. Corticosteroids dampen the activation of inflammatory cells and increase the production of anti-inflammatory mediators. Mucus production and edema is diminished, thus reducing airway obstruction. Although corticosteroids are not bronchodilators, they sensitize the bronchial smooth muscle to be more responsive to beta-agonist stimulation. In addition, they reduce the bronchial hyper-responsiveness to allergens that is responsible for triggering some asthma attacks. In the pharmacotherapy of asthma, corticosteroids may be given systemically or by inhalation.

Inhaled corticosteroids are the preferred therapy for *preventing* asthma attacks. When inhaled on a daily schedule, corticosteroids suppress inflammation without producing major adverse effects. Although symptoms will improve in the first 1 to 2 weeks of therapy, 4 to 8 weeks may be required for maximum benefit. For patients with persistent asthma, a LABA may be prescribed along with the inhaled corticosteroid to obtain an additive effect. Inhaled corticosteroids must be taken daily to produce their therapeutic effect, and these drugs are not effective at terminating acute asthmatic episodes in progress. Most patients with asthma carry an inhaler containing a rapid-acting beta agonist to terminate acute attacks if they occur.

For severe, unstable asthma that is unresponsive to other treatments, systemic corticosteroids such as oral prednisone may be prescribed. Treatment time is limited to the shortest length possible, usually 5 to 7 days. At the end

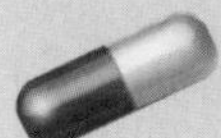

Prototype Drug | Montelukast *(Singulair)*

Therapeutic Class: Anti-inflammatory drug for asthma prophylaxis **Pharmacologic Class:** Leukotriene modifier

Actions and Uses

Montelukast is used for the prophylaxis of persistent, chronic asthma, exercise-induced bronchospasm, and allergic rhinitis. It prevents airway edema and inflammation by blocking leukotriene receptors in the airways. The drug is given PO and acts rapidly, although it is not recommended for termination of acute bronchospasm. It is the only agent in this class that is approved for pediatric use. To aid in administration, montelukast is available in chewable tablets and as granules that are recommended by the manufacturer to be mixed with applesauce, mashed carrots, or ice cream.

Administration Alerts

- Do not use to terminate acute asthma attacks.
- If preventing exercise-induced bronchospasm, take drug at least 2 hours before the activity.
- Pregnancy category B.

PHARMACOKINETICS

Onset	Peak	Duration
Rapid	3–4 h	Unknown

Adverse Effects

Montelukast produces few serious adverse effects. Headache is the most common complaint, and nausea and diarrhea are reported by some patients. Although rare, some patients have experienced serious neuropsychiatric events, including suicidal ideation, hallucinations, aggressiveness, or depression.

Contraindications: The only contraindication is hypersensitivity to the drug. Because a few rare cases of hepatic failure have been reported in patients who are taking montelukast, those with pre-existing hepatic impairment should be treated with caution.

Interactions

Drug–Drug: Montelukast exhibits fewer drug-drug interactions than other medications in this class.

Lab Tests: Montelukast may increase serum alanine aminotransferase (ALT) values.

Herbal/Food: None known

Treatment of Overdose: There is no specific treatment for overdose.

of the brief treatment period, patients are switched to inhaled corticosteroids for long-term management.

Inhaled corticosteroids are absorbed into the circulation so slowly that systemic adverse effects are rarely observed. Local side effects include hoarseness and oropharyngeal candidiasis. If taken for longer than 10 days, *systemic* corticosteroids can produce significant adverse effects, including adrenal gland atrophy, peptic ulcers, and hyperglycemia. Growth retardation is a concern with the use of these drugs in children. Because these adverse effects are all dose and time dependent, they can be avoided by limiting systemic therapy to less than 10 days. When taken long term, both PO and inhaled formulations of corticosteroids have the potential to affect bone physiology in adults and children. Adults who are at risk for osteoporosis should receive periodic bone mineral density tests. When taken for longer than 14 days, corticosteroids should be discontinued slowly, by gradually reducing the dose. Other uses and adverse effects of corticosteroids are presented in chapters 33 and 44.

Refer to the Nursing Practice Application: Pharmacotherapy With Systemic Corticosteroids, in chapter 44, for patients receiving these drugs.

Leukotriene Modifiers

The leukotriene modifiers are second choice drugs used to reduce inflammation and ease bronchoconstriction. Leukotriene modifiers are used as alternative drugs in the management of asthma symptoms. These drugs are listed in Table 40.4.

40.9 Prophylaxis of Asthma With Leukotriene Modifiers

Leukotrienes are mediators of the immune response that are involved in allergic and asthmatic reactions. Although the prefix *leuko-* implies white blood cells, these inflammatory mediators are synthesized by mast cells as well as neutrophils, basophils, and eosinophils. When released in the airway, leukotrienes promote edema, inflammation, and bronchoconstriction.

There are currently three drugs that modify leukotriene function. Zileuton (Zyflo CR) acts by blocking lipoxygenase, the enzyme used to synthesize leukotrienes. The remaining two drugs in this class, zafirlukast (Accolate) and montelukast (Singulair), act by blocking leukotriene receptors. All three reduce inflammation. They are not considered bronchodilators like the $beta_2$ agonists, although they do reduce bronchoconstriction indirectly.

The leukotriene modifiers are oral medications approved for the prophylaxis of chronic asthma. Zileuton has a more rapid onset of action (2 hours) than the other two leukotriene modifiers, which take as long as 1 week to produce optimal therapeutic benefit. Because of their delayed onset, leukotriene modifiers are ineffective in terminating acute asthma attacks. The current role of leukotriene modifiers in the management of asthma is for persistent asthma that cannot be controlled with inhaled corticosteroids or SABAs.

Few serious adverse effects are associated with the leukotriene modifiers. Headache, cough, nasal congestion, or GI upset may occur. Patients who are older than age 65 have been found to experience an increased frequency of infections when taking leukotriene modifiers. These drugs may be contraindicated in patients with significant hepatic dysfunction or in chronic alcohol users, because they are extensively metabolized by the liver.

Mast Cell Stabilizers

Two mast cell stabilizers serve limited, though important, roles in the prophylaxis of asthma. These drugs act by inhibiting the release of histamine from mast cells, and their doses are listed in Table 40.4.

40.10 Prophylaxis of Asthma With Mast Cell Stabilizers

Cromolyn (Intal) and nedocromil (Tilade) are classified as mast cell stabilizers because their action serves to inhibit mast cells from releasing histamine and other chemical mediators of inflammation. By reducing inflammation, they are able to prevent asthma attacks. Like the corticosteroids, these drugs should be taken on a daily basis because they are not effective for terminating acute attacks. Maximum therapeutic benefit may take several weeks. Both cromolyn and nedocromil are pregnancy category B and exhibit no serious toxicity. The mast cell stabilizers are less effective in preventing chronic asthma than the inhaled corticosteroids.

Cromolyn (Intal), the first mast stabilizer discovered, is administered by several routes for different indications. Via an MDI or a nebulizer, cromolyn is indicated for asthma prophylaxis. An intranasal form (Nasalcrom) is used in the treatment of seasonal allergic rhinitis (see chapter 39). An ophthalmic solution (Crolom) is used to treat various allergic disorders of the conjunctiva. Gastrocrom is a PO dosage form of cromolyn that is the only FDA-approved drug to treat systemic mastocytosis, a rare condition in which the patient has an excessive number of mast cells. Gastrocrom is also used off-label to treat ulcerative colitis and to prevent symptoms associated with food allergies.

Adverse effects of cromolyn include stinging or burning of the nasal mucosa, irritation of the throat, and nasal congestion. Although not common, bronchospasm and anaphylaxis have been reported. Because of its short half-life, cromolyn must be inhaled four to six times per day.

Nedocromil (Tilade) has actions and uses similar to those of cromolyn. Administered with an MDI, the drug produces adverse effects similar to those of cromolyn, although the longer half-life of nedocromil allows less-frequent dosing. Patients often experience a bitter, unpleasant taste, which is a common cause for discontinuation of therapy. An ophthalmic form (Alocril) is available to treat allergic conjunctivitis.

Monoclonal Antibodies

40.11 Monoclonal Antibodies for Asthma Prophylaxis

Omalizumab (Xolair) is a monoclonal antibody that was the first biologic therapy approved to treat asthma, offering a novel approach to the management of the disease. Monoclonal antibodies are designed to attach to a specific receptor on a target cell or molecule. Although most monoclonal antibodies are designed to attack cancer cells, omalizumab is designed to attach to a receptor on immunoglobulin E (IgE). The normal function of IgE is to react to antigens and cause the release of inflammatory chemical mediators. By binding to IgE, omalizumab prevents inflammation and dampens the body's response to allergens that trigger asthma. The student should refer to chapter 38 for a complete discussion of monoclonal antibodies.

Lifespan Considerations: Geriatric
Proper Inhaler Use by Older Adults With COPD

Inhaler use in the treatment of COPD is common, and correct use of the inhaler is necessary for adequate therapeutic outcomes and compliance with the treatment regimen. Proper inhaler use can be a challenge for all patients but the older adult is more likely to have one or more factors that impede appropriate use than does a younger patient (Lareau & Hodder, 2012). These factors include patient issues (e.g., cognitive ability, dexterity, presence of tremors, visual or hearing impairments), disease-based issues (e.g., ability to inhale adequately, decreased inspiratory volume), device issues (e.g., devices with differing instructions, use of multiple devices), and cost. Nurses who work with patients with respiratory disease should be familiar with the use and functioning of all types of inhalers and provide detailed instructions for appropriate use. Recognizing additional barriers that older adults might experience will help nurses to plan teaching strategies to improve inhaler use for these patients, thus resulting in improved therapeutic outcomes.

Omalizumab is approved for treating allergic rhinitis and moderate to severe, persistent asthma in patients at least 12 years of age who cannot be controlled satisfactorily with inhaled corticosteroids. Although it is only available by the subcutaneous route, injections are scheduled every 2 to 4 weeks, depending on the patient's response to therapy. Adverse effects may be serious and include anaphylaxis, bleeding-related events, or severe dysmenorrhea. Less serious adverse effects include rash, headache, and viral infections. Omalizumab is reserved for patients with persistent asthma because of its expense, potential adverse effects, and the need for regular parenteral injections.

CHRONIC OBSTRUCTIVE PULMONARY DISEASE

Chronic obstructive pulmonary disease (COPD) is a progressive pulmonary disorder characterized by chronic and recurrent obstruction of airflow. The two most common examples of conditions causing chronic pulmonary obstruction are chronic bronchitis and emphysema.

40.12 Pharmacotherapy of COPD

COPD is a major cause of death and disability. The two primary COPD conditions are chronic bronchitis and emphysema. Chronic bronchitis and emphysema are strongly associated with smoking tobacco products (cigarette smoking accounts for 85% to 90% of all cases of nonasthmatic COPD) and, secondarily, breathing air pollutants. In **chronic bronchitis,** excess mucus is produced in the lower respiratory tract due to the inflammation and irritation from cigarette smoke or pollutants. The airway becomes partially obstructed with mucus, thus resulting in the classic signs of dyspnea and coughing. An early sign of bronchitis is often a productive cough on awakening. Gas exchange may be impaired; thus, wheezing and decreased exercise tolerance are additional clinical signs. Microbes thrive in the mucus-rich environment, and pulmonary infections are common. Because most patients with COPD are lifelong tobacco users, they often have serious comorbid cardiovascular conditions such as heart failure and HTN.

COPD is progressive, with the terminal stage being **emphysema.** After years of chronic inflammation, the bronchioles lose their elasticity, and the alveoli dilate to maximum size to allow more air into the lungs. The patient suffers extreme dyspnea from even the slightest physical activity. The clinical distinction between chronic bronchitis and emphysema is sometimes unclear, because patients may exhibit symptoms of both conditions concurrently.

The goals of pharmacotherapy of COPD are to relieve symptoms and avoid complications of the condition. Various classes of drugs are used to treat infections, control cough, and relieve bronchospasm. Most patients receive the same classes of bronchodilators and anti-inflammatory agents that are used for asthma. Both short-acting and long-acting bronchodilators are prescribed. Mucolytics and expectorants (see chapter 39) are sometimes used to reduce the viscosity of the bronchial mucus and to aid in its removal. Long-term oxygen therapy assists breathing and has been shown to decrease mortality in patients with advanced COPD. Antibiotics may be prescribed for patients who experience multiple bouts of pulmonary infections.

Some newer agents and drug combinations have been approved specifically for the maintenance treatment of COPD. These include the following:

- Roflumilast (Daliresp) exhibits anti-inflammatory effects on the airways by inhibiting the enzyme phosphodiesterase-4. It is an oral tablet that is administered once daily.
- Incruse ellipta, approved in 2013, contains the anticholinergic drug umeclidinium that relaxes bronchial smooth muscle to cause bronchodilation. It is administered once daily by oral inhalation.
- Anoro ellipta, approved in 2013, contains umeclidinium and vilanterol (a LABA). It is given once daily by oral inhalation.
- Breo ellipta, approved in 2013, is a fixed dose combination of vilanterol and fluticasone (a corticosteroid). Like anora ellipto, it is given once daily by oral inhalation.
- Stiolto Respimat, approved in 2015, combines tiotropium with olodaterol, a newer LABA. Given once daily, it is indicated for the long-term maintenance of COPD.

Patients with COPD should not receive drugs that have beta-adrenergic antagonist activity or otherwise cause bronchoconstriction. Respiratory depressants such as opioids and barbiturates should be avoided. It is important to note that none of the pharmacotherapies offer a cure for COPD; they only treat the symptoms of a progressively worsening disease. The most important teaching point for the nurse is to strongly encourage smoking cessation in these patients. Smoking cessation has been shown to slow the progression of COPD and to result in fewer respiratory symptoms.

Nursing Practice Application

Pharmacotherapy for Asthma and COPD

ASSESSMENT	POTENTIAL NURSING DIAGNOSES*
Baseline assessment prior to administration: • Obtain a complete health history including previous history of symptoms and association to seasons, foods, or environmental exposures; existing cardiovascular, respiratory, hepatic, renal, or neurologic disease; glaucoma; prostatic hypertrophy or difficulty with urination; presence of fever or active infections; pregnancy or breast-feeding; alcohol use; or smoking. Obtain a drug history, noting the type of adverse reaction experienced to any medications. • If asthma symptoms are of new onset, assess for any recent changes in diet, soaps including laundry detergent or softener, cosmetics, lotions, environment, or recent carpet cleaning (particularly in young children) that may correlate with onset of symptoms. • Obtain baseline vital signs, noting respiratory rate and depth. • Assess pulmonary function with pulse oximeter, peak expiratory flow meter, and/or arterial blood gases to establish baseline levels. • Evaluate appropriate laboratory findings (e.g., complete blood count [CBC], hepatic and renal laboratory tests). • Assess symptom-related effects on eating, sleep, and activity level.	• *Impaired Gas Exchange* • *Ineffective Tissue Perfusion* • *Anxiety* • *Disturbed Sleep Pattern*, related to adverse drug effects • *Activity Intolerance* • *Deficient Knowledge* (drug therapy) *NANDA I © 2014
Assessment throughout administration: • Assess for desired therapeutic effects (e.g., increased ease of breathing, improvement in pulmonary function studies, improved signs of peripheral oxygenation, increased activity levels, and maintenance of normal eating and sleep periods). • Continue periodic monitoring of pulmonary function with pulse oximeter, peak expiratory flowmeter, and/or arterial blood gases as appropriate. • Assess vital signs, especially respiratory rate and depth. Assess breath sounds, noting presence of adventitious sounds, and any mucus production. Assess for the frequency of inhaler use because too-frequent use may indicate poor control of the condition. • Assess for adverse effects: dizziness, tachycardia, palpitations, blurred vision, or headache. Report immediately any fever, confusion, tachycardia, palpitations, hypotension, syncope, dyspnea, or increasing pulmonary congestion.	

IMPLEMENTATION

Interventions and (Rationales)	Patient-Centered Care
Ensuring therapeutic effects: • Continue assessments as described earlier for therapeutic effects. (Increased ease of breathing; lessened adventitious breath sounds; improved signs of tissue oxygenation; and normal appetite, eating, and sleep patterns should occur. The health care provider should be notified if symptoms worsen, especially if respiratory involvement increases or fever is present.)	• Teach the patient to supplement drug therapy with nonpharmacologic measures such as increased fluid intake to liquefy and mobilize mucus and to reduce exposure to allergens where possible. • **Safety:** Advise the patient to carry a wallet identification card or wear medical identification jewelry indicating the presence of asthma or respiratory condition, any significant allergies or anaphylaxis, and use of inhaler therapy.
• Monitor pulmonary function periodically with pulse oximeter, peak expiratory flow meter, and/or arterial blood gases. (Periodic monitoring is necessary to assess drug effectiveness.)	• Teach the patient the use of the peak expiratory flowmeter or other equipment ordered to monitor pulmonary function. • Instruct the patient to immediately report symptoms of deteriorating respiratory status such as increased dyspnea, breathlessness with speech, increased anxiety, or orthopnea.

continued

Nursing Practice Application *continued*

IMPLEMENTATION

Interventions and (Rationales)	Patient-Centered Care
• To abort an acute asthmatic attack, inhaler therapy should be started at the first sign of respiratory difficulty. For preventive therapy, long-term bronchodilation by inhaler or PO will be used. *LABAs and long-acting bronchodilators are not to be used to abort an acute attack.* (Acute asthmatic attacks are managed with quick-acting bronchodilation such as $beta_2$ agonists. For preventing attacks, LABAs, anticholinergics, mast cell stabilizers, and corticosteroid therapy may be used. It is crucial to know and recognize the difference in quick-acting and long-acting inhalers.)	• Provide explicit instructions on the use of quick-acting versus long-acting inhalers. Teach the patient to use quick-acting inhalers at the earliest possible appearance of symptoms. Long-acting inhalers or oral therapy may be used to maintain bronchodilation, but do not discard quick-acting inhalers if on long-term maintenance therapy. They may still be needed for periodic acute attacks.
Minimizing adverse effects: • Continue to monitor respirations, rate, depth, breath sounds, mucus production, increasing dyspnea, adventitious breath sounds, signs of tissue hypoxia, anxiety, confusion, and decreasing pulmonary functions studies. (Increasing dyspnea, adventitious breath sounds, diminished oxygenation, or increasing anxiety or confusion may indicate inadequate drug therapy, worsening disease process, or respiratory infection and should be reported immediately. **Diverse Patients:** Because some drugs such as theophylline metabolize through the P450 system pathways, monitor ethnically diverse patients to ensure optimal therapeutic effects and to minimize adverse effects.)	• Instruct the patient to immediately report symptoms of deteriorating respiratory status such as increased dyspnea, breathlessness with speech, increased anxiety, or orthopnea.
• Monitor eating and sleep patterns and the ability to maintain functional activities of daily living (ADLs). Provide for calorie-rich, nutrient-dense foods; frequent rest periods between eating or activity; and a cool room for sleeping. (Respiratory difficulty and fatigue are associated with hypoxia, and the work of breathing may affect appetite and the ability to maintain required ADLs. Maintaining adequate nutrition, fluids, rest, and sleep are essential to support optimal health.)	• Teach the patient to supplement drug therapy with nonpharmacologic measures including: • Increase fluid intake to liquefy and mobilize mucus. • Consume small, frequent meals of calorie- and nutrient-dense foods to prevent fatigue and maintain normal nutrition. • Get adequate rest periods between eating and activities. • Decrease room temperature for ease of breathing during sleep. • Reduce exposure to allergens where possible. • Instruct the patient to report any significant change in appetite, an inability to maintain normal intake, inadequate sleep periods, or an inability to carry out required ADLs.
• Maintain consistent dosing of long-acting bronchodilators. (Regular, consistent dosing with LABAs, anticholinergics, mast-cell stabilizers, and corticosteroids is used to prevent or limit acute bronchoconstrictive attacks.)	• Teach the patient the importance of consistent administration of bronchodilation therapy to prevent acute attacks.
• Use an appropriate spacer between the inhaler and the mouth as appropriate and rinse the mouth after using the inhaler, especially after corticosteroids. (Spacers between MDIs assist in the coordination and timing of inhalation and prevent medication from being delivered to the back of the pharynx. Rinsing the mouth after the use of corticosteroid inhalers prevents systemic absorption or localized reactions to the drug such as ulceration or thrush infections from *Candida*.)	• Instruct the patient in the proper use of spacers if ordered, followed by teach-back. • Teach the patient to rinse the mouth after each use of the inhaler and to spit out after rinsing if a corticosteroid inhaler is used.
• Continue to monitor cardiac status, hepatic function, and ophthalmology exam findings. (Beta-adrenergic drugs given for asthma and COPD may cause cardiac adverse effects. Corticosteroids may increase the risk of cataract formation. **Lifespan:** Monitor the older adult frequently because age-related physiological changes increase the risk of adverse effects.)	• Teach the patient about any follow-up laboratory or other testing needed, such as annual eye exams.

Nursing Practice Application *continued*

IMPLEMENTATION	
Interventions and (Rationales)	**Patient-Centered Care**
• Monitor for anticholinergic adverse effects in patients taking ipratropium (Atrovent) and other anticholinergic drugs. (**Lifespan:** Be aware that the male older adult with an enlarged prostate is at higher risk for mechanical obstruction. The older adult is also at increased risk of constipation due to slowed peristalsis.)	• Teach the patient about the importance of drinking extra fluids and increasing fiber intake. Instruct the patient to notify the health care provider if difficulty with urination occurs or if constipation is severe.
Patient understanding of drug therapy: • Use opportunities during the administration of medications and during assessments to provide patient education. (Using time during nursing care helps to optimize and reinforce key teaching areas.)	• The patient should be able to state the reason for the drug, appropriate dose and scheduling, and what adverse effects to observe for and when to report them.
Patient self-administration of drug therapy: • When administering the medication, instruct the patient, family, or caregiver in the proper self-administration of the drug (e.g., take the drug at the first appearance of symptoms before symptoms are severe). (Proper administration increases the effectiveness of the drugs.)	• The patient recognizes the difference between quick-acting and long-acting inhalers and knows when each is to be used. • Instruct the patient in proper administration techniques for inhalers, followed by teach-back, including: • Use a spacer if instructed between the MDI and the mouth. • Shake the inhaler or load the inhaler with the tablet or powder as instructed. • If using bronchodilator and corticosteroid inhalers, use the bronchodilator first, wait 5–10 minutes, then use the corticosteroid to ensure that the drug reaches deeper into the bronchi. • Rinse the mouth after using any inhaler. • Rinse the inhaler and spacer with water at least daily and allow to air-dry. • **Lifespan:** Supervise inhaler use in children under the age of 5 to ensure proper use.

See Tables 40.3 and 40.4 for a list of drugs to which these nursing actions apply.

Chapter Review

KEY Concepts

The numbered key concepts provide a succinct summary of the important points from the corresponding numbered section within the chapter. If any of these points are not clear, refer to the numbered section within the chapter for review.

40.1 The physiology of the respiratory system involves two main processes. Ventilation moves air into and out of the lungs, and perfusion allows for gas exchange across capillaries.

40.2 Bronchioles are lined with smooth muscle that controls the amount of air entering the lungs. Dilation and constriction of the airways are controlled by the autonomic nervous system.

40.3 Inhalation is a common route of administration for pulmonary drugs because it delivers drugs directly to the sites of action. Nebulizers, DPIs, and MDIs are devices used for aerosol therapies.

40.4 Asthma is a chronic disease that has both inflammatory and bronchoconstriction components. Drugs are used to prevent asthmatic attacks and to terminate an attack in progress.

40.5 Beta-adrenergic agonists are the most effective drugs for relieving acute bronchospasm. These drugs act by activating $beta_2$ receptors in bronchial smooth muscle to cause bronchodilation.

40.6 The anticholinergic ipratropium is a bronchodilator occasionally used as an alternative to the beta agonists in asthma therapy.

40.7 Methylxanthines such as theophylline are less effective and produce more side effects than the beta agonists.

40.8 Inhaled corticosteroids are often preferred drugs for the long-term prophylaxis of asthma. Oral corticosteroids are used for the short-term therapy of severe, unstable asthma.

40.9 The leukotriene modifiers, primarily used for asthma prophylaxis, act by reducing the inflammatory component of asthma.

40.10 Mast cell stabilizers are safe drugs for the prophylaxis of asthma. They are less effective than the inhaled corticosteroids and are ineffective at relieving acute bronchospasm.

40.11 Monoclonal antibodies offer a novel approach for the prevention of asthma symptoms. These drugs are only used for persistent cases of the disease when other therapies have been unsuccessful.

40.12 Chronic obstructive pulmonary disease (COPD) is a progressive disorder treated with multiple pulmonary drugs. Bronchodilators, mucolytics, expectorants, oxygen, and antibiotics may offer symptomatic relief.

REVIEW Questions

1. A patient is receiving treatment for asthma with albuterol (Proventil). The nurse teaches the patient that while serious adverse effects are uncommon, the following may occur. (Select all that apply.)
   1. Tachycardia
   2. Sedation
   3. Temporary dyspnea
   4. Nervousness
   5. Headache

2. A patient with asthma has a prescription for two inhalers, albuterol (Proventil) and beclomethasone (Qvar). How should the nurse instruct this patient on the proper use of the inhalers?
   1. Use the albuterol inhaler, and use the beclomethasone only if symptoms are not relieved.
   2. Use the beclomethasone inhaler, and use the albuterol only if symptoms are not relieved.
   3. Use the albuterol inhaler, wait 5–10 minutes, then use the beclomethasone inhaler.
   4. Use the beclomethasone inhaler, wait 5–10 minutes, then use the albuterol inhaler.

3. A patient has been using a fluticasone (Flovent) inhaler as a component of his asthma therapy. He returns to his health care provider's office complaining of a sore mouth. On inspection, the nurse notices white patches in the patient's mouth. What is a possible explanation for these findings?
   1. The patient has been consuming hot beverages after the use of the inhaler.
   2. The patient has limited his fluid intake, resulting in dry mouth.
   3. The residue of the inhaler propellant is coating the inside of the mouth.
   4. The patient has developed thrush as a result of the fluticasone.

4. A 65-year-old patient is prescribed ipratropium (Atrovent) for the treatment of asthma. Which of the following conditions should be reported to the health care provider before giving this patient the ipratropium?
   1. A reported allergy to peanuts
   2. A history of intolerance to albuterol (Proventil)
   3. A history of bronchospasms
   4. A reported allergy to chocolate

5. A patient who received a prescription for montelukast (Singulair) returns to his provider's office after three days, complaining that "the drug is not working." She reports mild but continued dyspnea and has had to maintain consistent use of her bronchodilator inhaler, albuterol (Proventil). What does the nurse suspect is the cause of the failure of the montelukast?
   1. The patient is not taking the drug correctly.
   2. The patient is not responding to the drug and will need to be switched to another formulation.
   3. The drug has not had sufficient time of use to have full effects.
   4. The albuterol inhaler is interacting with the montelukast.

6. Which of the following drugs is most immediately helpful in treating a severe acute asthma attack?
   1. Beclomethasone (Qvar)
   2. Zileuton (Zyflo CR)
   3. Albuterol (Proventil, Ventolin)
   4. Salmeterol (Serevent Diskus)

PATIENT-FOCUSED Case Study

Caleb Saldano, 9-years-old, has a history of asthma. He goes to the health room at his elementary school and states that he has increased shortness of breath and chest tightness. On assessment, you, the school nurse, note scattered expiratory wheezes throughout his upper and middle lung fields and a decreased peak meter flow. The current therapeutic regimen for this child includes salmeterol (Serevent Diskus) two puffs every 12 h, montelukast (Singulair) 5 mg/day PO in the evening, flunisolide (AeroSpan) two puffs tid, and albuterol (Proventil) two puffs every 4 h prn.

1. What are the drug classifications and use of the medications that Caleb is taking?
2. After observing the child's technique in using the MDI, you wish to reinforce the child's education as it relates to the administration technique of his inhalants. What areas should be emphasized?

CRITICAL THINKING Questions

1. A 72-year-old male patient has recently been started on an ipratropium (Atrovent) inhaler. What teaching is important for the nurse to provide?
2. A 45-year-old patient with chronic asthma is on beclomethasone (Qvar). What must the nurse monitor when caring for this patient?

Visit www.pearsonhighered.com/nursingresources for answers and rationales for all activities.

REFERENCES

Engelke, M. K., Swanson, M., & Guttu, M. (2014). Process and outcomes of school nurse case management for students with asthma. *Journal of School Nursing, 30,* 196–205. doi:10.1177/1059840513507084

Herdman, T. H., & Kamitsuru, S. (2014). *NANDA International nursing diagnoses: Definitions and classification, 2015–2017.* Oxford, United Kingdom: Wiley-Blackwell.

Lareau, S. C., & Hodder, R. (2012). Teaching inhaler use in chronic obstructive pulmonary disease patients. *Journal of the American Academy of Nurse Practitioners, 24,* 113–120. doi:10.1111/j.1745-7599.2011.00681.x

Maughan, E. D., & Schantz, S. (2014). NASN's first evidence-based clinical guidelines: Asthma. *NASN School Nurse, 29,* 221–223. doi:10.1177/1942602X14545227

National Association of School Nurses (2015). *Asthma online tool kit.* Retrieved from http://www.nasn.org/ToolsResources/Asthma

National Heart, Blood, and Lung Institute, National Asthma Education and Prevention Program. (2007). *Expert panel report 3: Guidelines for the diagnosis and management of asthma.* Retrieved from http://www.nhlbi.nih.gov/guidelines/asthma/asthgdln.htm

Rodriguez, E., Rivera, D. A., Perlroth, D., Becker, E., Wang, N. E., & Landau, M. (2013). School nurses' role in asthma management, school absenteeism, and cost savings: A demonstration project. *Journal of School Health, 83,* 842–850. doi:10.1111/josh.12102

SELECTED BIBLIOGRAPHY

Albertson, T. E., Schivo, M., Gidwani, N., Kenyon, N. J., Sutter, M. E., Chan, A. L., & Louie, S. (2013). Pharmacotherapy of critical asthma syndrome: Current and emerging therapies. *Clinical Reviews in Allergy & Immunology, 48*, 7–30. doi:10.1007/s12016-013-8393-8

American Academy of Allergy, Asthma and Immunology. (n.d.). *Asthma statistics*. Retrieved from http://www.aaaai.org/about-the-aaaai/newsroom/asthma-statistics.aspx

Antus, B. (2013). Pharmacotherapy of chronic obstructive pulmonary disease: A clinical review. *ISRN Pulmonology, 2013*, Article ID 582807, 11 pp. doi:10.1155/2013/582807

Bjerg, A., Lundbäck, B., & Lötvall, J. (2012). The future of combining inhaled drugs for COPD. *Current Opinion in Pharmacology, 12*, 252–255. doi:10.1016/j.coph.2012.03.004

Centers for Disease Control and Prevention. (2015). *Asthma*. Retrieved from http://www.cdc.gov/nchs/fastats/asthma.htm

Colbert, B. J., Gonzales, L. S., & Kennedy, B. J. (2012). *Integrated cardiopulmonary pharmacology* (3rd ed.). Upper Saddle River, NJ: Pearson Education.

Ferry-Rooney, R. (2013). Asthma in primary care: A case-based review of pharmacotherapy. *Nursing Clinics of North America, 48*, 25–34. doi:10.1016/j.cnur.2012.12.005

Garvey, C., Hanania, N. A., & Altman, P. (2014). Optimizing care of your patients with COPD. *Nursing: Research & Reviews, 2014*(4), 7–18. doi:10.2147/NRR.S54396

National Center for Health Statistics. (2012). *Summary health statistics for U.S. children: National health interview survey, 2012*. Retrieved from http://www.cdc.gov/nchs/data/series/sr_10/sr10_258.pdf

Slejko, J. F., Ghushchyan, V. H., Sucher, B., Globe, D. R., Lin, S. L., Globe, G., & Sullivan, P. W. (2014). Asthma control in the United States, 2008–2010: Indicators of poor asthma control. *Journal of Allergy and Clinical Immunology, 133*, 1579–1587. doi.org/10.1016/j.jaci.2013.10.028

Taylor-Fishwick, J. C., Okafor, M., & Fletcher, M. (2015). Effectiveness of asthma principles and practice course in increasing nurse practitioner knowledge and confidence in the use of asthma clinical guidelines. *Journal of the American Association of Nurse Practitioners, 27*, 197–204. doi:10.1002/2327-6924.12147

Unit 7

The Gastrointestinal System

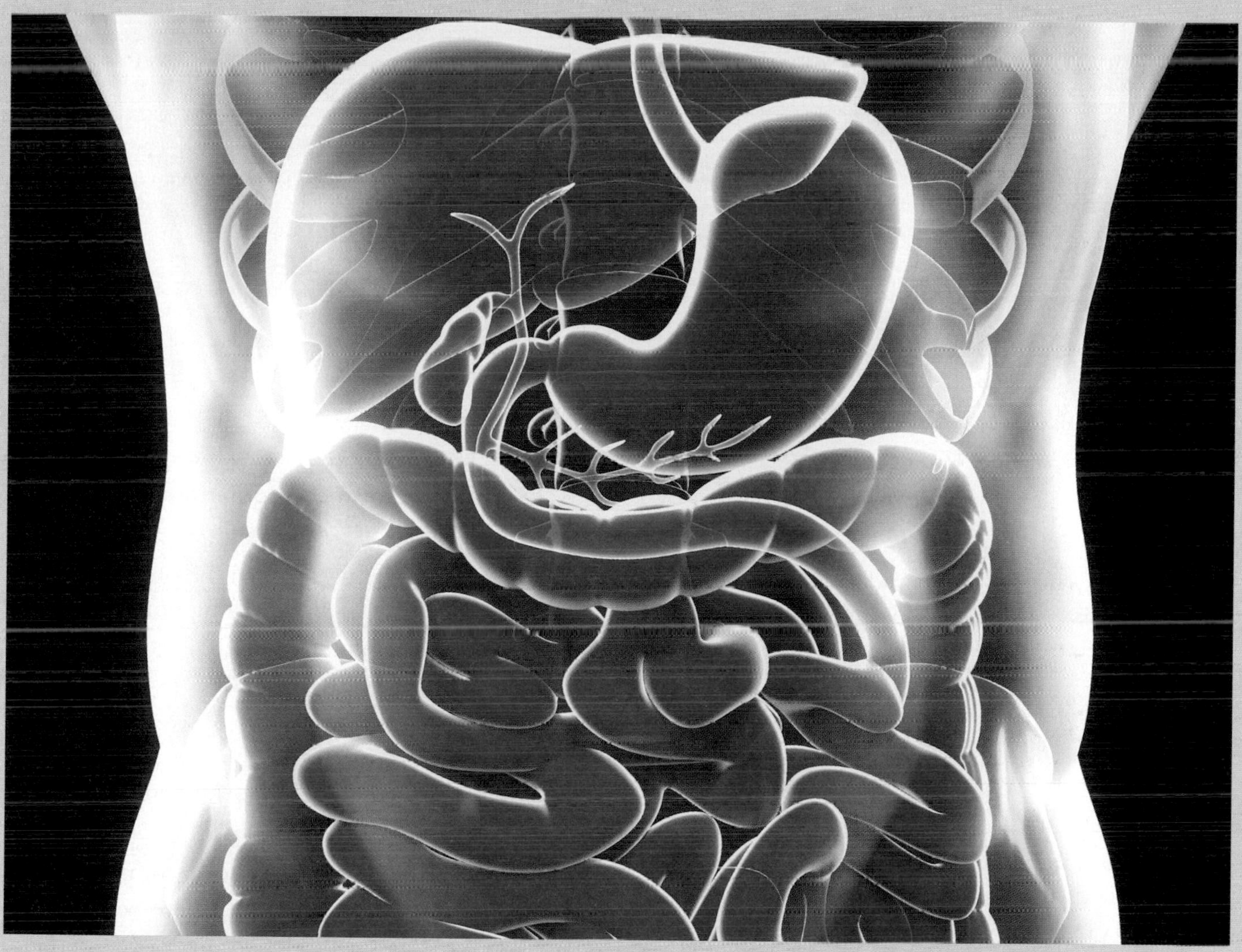

The Gastrointestinal System

Chapter 41

Drugs for Peptic Ulcer Disease

Drugs at a Glance

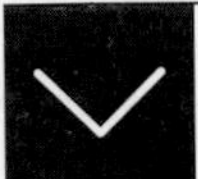

Learning Outcomes

After reading this chapter, the student should be able to:

1. Describe the major anatomic structures of the upper gastrointestinal tract.
2. Identify causes, signs, and symptoms of peptic ulcer disease and gastroesophageal reflux disease.
3. Compare and contrast duodenal ulcers and gastric ulcers.
4. Describe treatment goals for the pharmacotherapy of gastroesophageal reflux disease.
5. Identify the classification of drugs used to treat peptic ulcer disease and gastroesophageal reflux disease.
6. Explain the pharmacologic strategies for eradicating *Helicobacter pylori.*
7. Describe the nurse's role in the pharmacologic management of patients with peptic ulcer disease.
8. For each of the classes listed in Drugs at a Glance, know representative drugs, and explain their mechanism of drug action, primary actions, and important adverse effects.
9. Use the nursing process to care for patients who are receiving pharmacotherapy for peptic ulcer and gastroesophageal reflux diseases.

(pill icon) indicates a prototype drug, each of which is featured in a Prototype Drug box.

Very little of the food we eat is directly available to body cells. Food must be broken down, absorbed, and chemically modified before it is in a useful form. The digestive system performs these functions and more. Some disorders of the digestive system are mechanical in nature, providing for the transit of substances through the gastrointestinal (GI) tract. Others are metabolic, involving the secretion of digestive enzymes and fluids or the absorption of essential nutrients. Many signs and symptoms of digestive disorders are nonspecific and may be caused by a number of different pathologies. This chapter examines the pharmacotherapy of two common disorders of the upper digestive system: peptic ulcer disease (PUD) and gastroesophageal reflux disease (GERD).

PharmFacts

UPPER GASTROINTESTINAL TRACT DISORDERS

- Approximately 4.5 million Americans are affected by peptic ulcers annually.
- Approximately 10% of Americans will experience a peptic ulcer in their lifetime.
- At one time the incidence of PUD was higher in men; however, now the incidence is nearly equal in men and women.
- Seven to ten percent of Americans suffer from daily symptoms of GERD; 25%–45% will experience symptoms of GERD at some point during their lifetime.

THE DIGESTIVE SYSTEM

41.1 Normal Digestive Processes

The digestive system consists of two basic anatomic divisions: the alimentary canal and the accessory organs. The alimentary canal, or GI tract, is a long, continuous, hollow tube that extends from the mouth to the anus. The accessory organs of digestion include the salivary glands, liver, gallbladder, and pancreas. Major structures of the digestive system are illustrated in Figure 41.1.

The inner lining of the alimentary canal is the mucosa layer, which provides a surface area for the various acids, bases, mucus, and enzymes to break down food. In many parts of the alimentary canal, the mucosa is folded and contains deep grooves and pits. The small intestine is lined with tiny projections called *villi* and *microvilli*, which provide a huge surface area for the absorption of food and medications.

Substances are propelled along the GI tract by **peristalsis,** which is a series of rhythmic contractions of layers of smooth muscle. The speed at which substances move through the GI tract is critical to the absorption of nutrients and water and for the removal of wastes. If peristalsis is too fast, nutrients and drugs will not have sufficient contact with the mucosa to be absorbed. In addition, the large intestine will not have enough time to absorb water, and diarrhea may result. Abnormally slow transit may result in constipation or even obstructions in the small or large intestine. Disorders of the lower digestive tract are discussed in chapter 42.

To chemically break down ingested food, a large number of enzymes and other substances are required. Digestive enzymes are secreted by the salivary glands, stomach, small intestine, and pancreas. The liver makes bile, which is stored in the gallbladder until needed for lipid digestion. Because these digestive substances are not common targets for drug therapy, their discussion in this chapter is limited, and the student should refer to anatomy and physiology texts for additional information.

41.2 Acid Production by the Stomach

Food passes from the esophagus to the stomach by traveling through the lower esophageal (cardiac) sphincter. This ring of smooth muscle usually prevents the stomach contents from moving backward, a condition known as **esophageal reflux.** A second ring of smooth muscle, the pyloric sphincter, is located at the entrance to the small intestine. This sphincter regulates the flow of substances leaving the stomach.

The stomach thoroughly mixes ingested food and secretes substances that promote the processes of chemical digestion. Gastric glands extending deep into the mucosa of the stomach contain several cell types critical to digestion and important to the pharmacotherapy of digestive disorders. **Chief cells** secrete pepsinogen, an inactive form of the enzyme pepsin that chemically breaks down proteins. **Parietal cells** secrete 1 to 3 L of hydrochloric acid each day. This strong acid helps break down food, activates pepsinogen, and kills microbes that may have been ingested. Parietal cells also secrete **intrinsic factor,** which is essential for the absorption of vitamin B_{12} (see chapter 43). Parietal cells are targets for the classes of antiulcer drugs that limit acid secretion.

The combined secretion of the chief and parietal cells, gastric juice, is the most acidic fluid in the body, having a pH of 1.5 to 3.5. A number of natural defenses protect the stomach mucosa from this extremely acidic fluid. Certain cells that line the surface of the stomach secrete a thick mucus layer and bicarbonate ions to neutralize the acid. These form such an effective protective layer that the pH at the mucosal surface is nearly neutral. Once they reach the duodenum, the stomach contents are further neutralized by bicarbonate from pancreatic and biliary secretions. These natural defenses are shown in Figure 41.2.

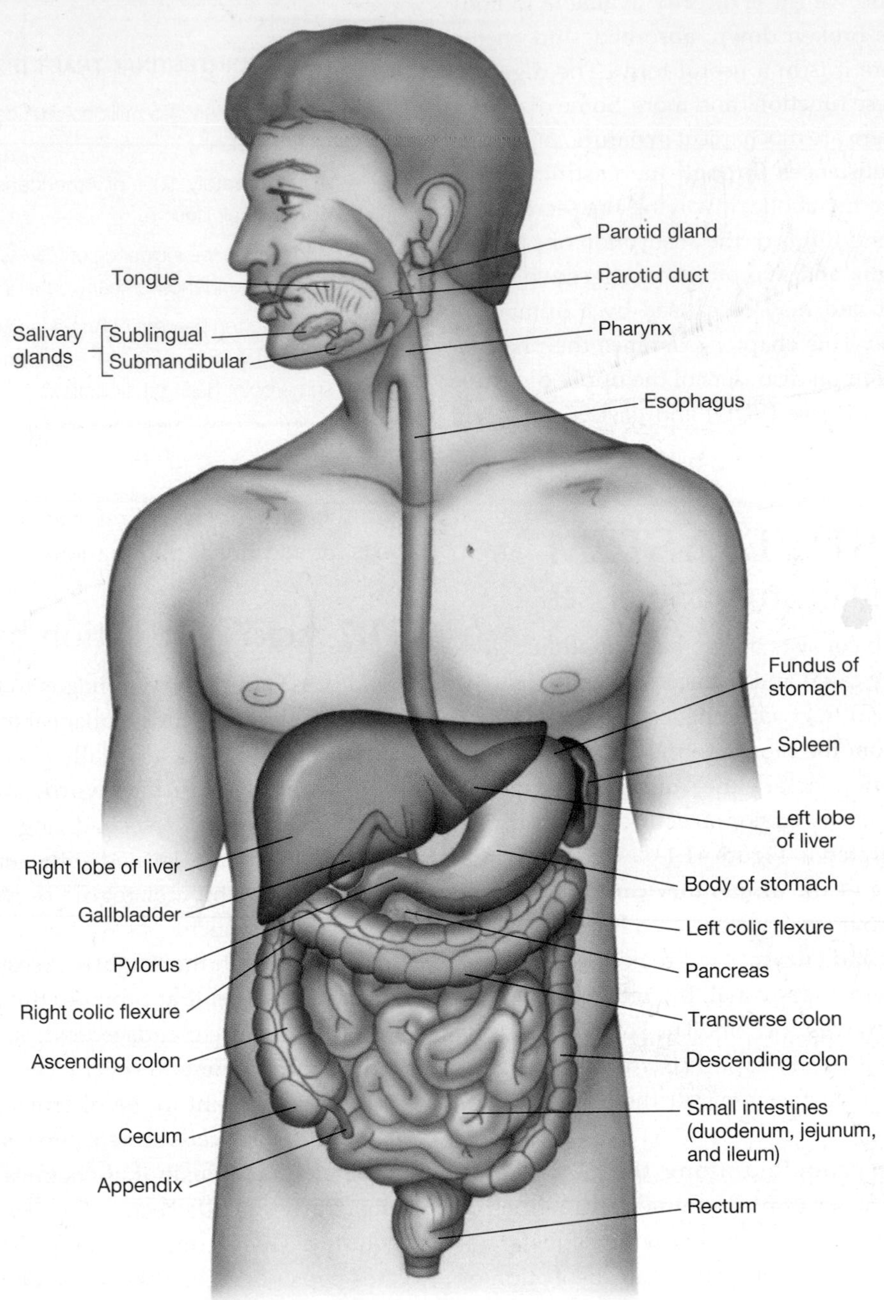

FIGURE 41.1 The digestive system

Source: *Human Diseases: A Systemic Approach,* by M. L. Mulvihill, M. Zelman, P. Holdaway, E. Tompary, and J. Raymond, 2006. Reprinted and electronically reproduced by permission of Pearson Education, Inc., Upper Saddle River, NJ.

PEPTIC ULCER DISEASE AND GASTROESOPHAGEAL REFLUX DISEASE

41.3 Pathogenesis of Peptic Ulcer Disease

An *ulcer* is an erosion of the mucosal layer of the GI tract, usually associated with acute inflammation. Although ulcers may occur in any portion of the alimentary canal, the duodenum is the most common site. The term **peptic ulcer** refers to a lesion located in either the stomach (gastric) or small intestine (duodenal). Peptic ulcer disease is associated with the following risk factors:

- Close family history of PUD
- Blood group O
- Smoking tobacco (increases gastric acid secretion)
- Consumption of beverages and food that contain caffeine

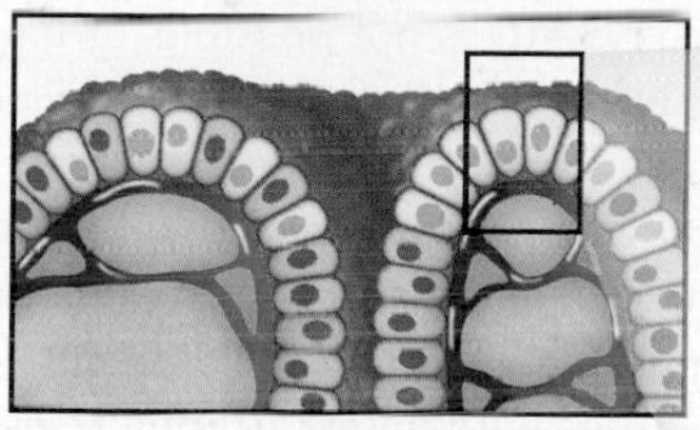
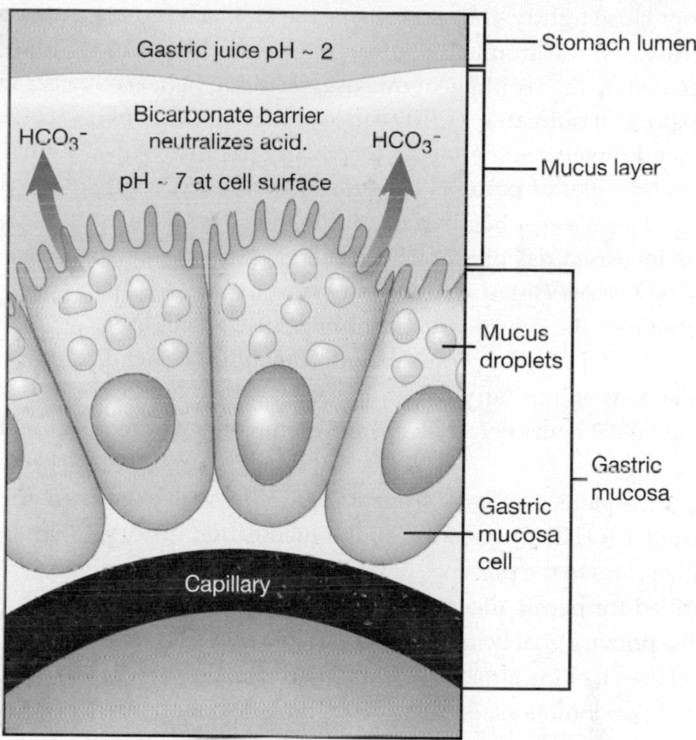

FIGURE 41.2 Natural defenses against stomach acid

- Drugs, particularly corticosteroids, nonsteroidal anti-inflammatory drugs (NSAIDs), and platelet inhibitors such as aspirin and clopidogrel
- Excessive psychological stress
- Infection with *Helicobacter pylori*.

The primary cause of PUD is infection by the gram-negative bacterium ***Helicobacter pylori.*** Approximately 50% of the population has *H. pylori* present in their stomach and proximal small intestine (see section 41.9). In *non-infected* patients, the most common cause of PUD is drug therapy with NSAIDs, including aspirin. NSAIDs cause direct cellular damage to GI mucosal cells and decrease the secretion of protective mucus and bicarbonate ion. NSAIDs and *H. pylori* infection act synergistically to promote ulcers. The combination poses a 3.5-fold greater risk of ulcers than either factor alone.

The characteristic symptom of *duodenal* ulcer is a gnawing or burning upper abdominal pain that occurs 1 to 3 hours after a meal. The pain is worse when the stomach is empty and often disappears on ingestion of food. Nighttime pain, nausea, and vomiting are uncommon. If the erosion progresses deeper into the mucosa, bleeding occurs, which may be evident as either bright red blood in vomit or black, tarry stools. Many duodenal ulcers heal spontaneously, although they frequently recur after months of remission. Long-term medical follow-up is usually not necessary.

Gastric ulcers are less common than the duodenal type and have different symptoms. Although relieved by food, pain may continue even after a meal. Loss of appetite, known as anorexia, as well as weight loss and vomiting are more common. Remissions may be infrequent or absent. Medical follow-up of gastric ulcers should continue for several years, because a small percentage of the erosions become cancerous. The most severe ulcers may penetrate the wall of the stomach and cause death. Whereas duodenal ulcers occur most frequently in males in the 30- to 50-year age group, gastric ulcers are more common in women over age 60. NSAID-related ulcers are more likely to produce gastric ulcers, whereas *H. pylori*–associated ulcers are more likely to be duodenal.

Ulceration in the distal small intestine is known as *Crohn's disease*, and erosions in the large intestine are called *ulcerative colitis*. These diseases, together categorized as inflammatory bowel disease, are discussed in chapter 42. Together these diseases are categorized as inflammatory bowel disease.

41.4 Pathogenesis of Gastroesophageal Reflux Disease

Gastroesophageal reflux disease (GERD) is a common condition in which the acidic contents of the stomach move upward into the esophagus. This causes an intense burning (heartburn) sometimes accompanied by belching. In severe cases, untreated GERD can lead to complications such as esophagitis, or esophageal ulcers or strictures. Although most often thought a disease of people older than age 40, GERD also occurs in a significant percentage of infants.

The cause of GERD is usually a weakening of the lower esophageal sphincter (LES). When the LES sphincter does not close tightly, the contents of the stomach move upward when the stomach contracts. These acidic substances irritate the esophageal mucosa, resulting in heartburn pain. Left untreated, GERD can lead to complications such as esophagitis, esophageal ulcers, or strictures. Approximately 10% of patients diagnosed with GERD will develop Barrett's esophagus, a condition that is associated with an increased risk of esophageal cancer.

GERD is associated with obesity, and losing weight may eliminate the symptoms. Other lifestyle changes that can improve GERD symptoms include elevating the head of the bed, avoiding fatty or acidic foods, eating smaller meals at least 3 hours before sleep, and eliminating tobacco and alcohol use.

Because patients often self-treat this disorder with over-the-counter (OTC) drugs, a thorough medication history may give clues to the presence of GERD. Many of the drugs prescribed for peptic ulcers are also used to treat GERD, with the primary goal being to reduce gastric acid secretion. Drug classes include antacids, H_2-receptor antagonists, and proton pump inhibitors. Because drugs provide only symptomatic relief, surgery may become necessary to eliminate the cause of GERD in patients with persistent disease.

DRUGS FOR TREATING PEPTIC ULCER DISEASE

41.5 Pharmacotherapy of Peptic Ulcer Disease

Before initiating pharmacotherapy, patients are usually advised to change lifestyle factors contributing to the severity of PUD or GERD. For example, eliminating tobacco and alcohol use and reducing stress often allow healing of the ulcer and cause it to go into remission. Avoiding certain foods and beverages can lessen the severity of symptoms.

For patients who are taking NSAIDs, the initial approach to PUD is to switch the patient to an alternative medication, such as acetaminophen or a selective COX-2 inhibitor. This is not always possible, because NSAIDs are preferred drugs for treating chronic arthritis and other disorders associated with pain and inflammation. If discontinuation of the NSAID is not possible, or if symptoms persist after the NSAID has been withdrawn, antiulcer medications are indicated.

For patients with PUD who are infected with *H. pylori*, elimination of the bacteria using anti-infective therapy is the primary goal of pharmacotherapy. If the treatment includes only antiulcer drugs without eradicating *H. pylori*, a very high recurrence rate of PUD is observed. It has also been found that eradicating *H. pylori* infection prophylactically decreases the incidence of peptic ulcers in patients who subsequently take NSAIDs.

The goals of PUD pharmacotherapy are to provide immediate relief from symptoms, promote healing of the ulcer, and prevent future recurrence of the disease. A wide variety of both prescription and OTC drugs are available. The mechanisms of action of the primary drug classes for PUD are shown in Pharmacotherapy Illustrated 41.1:

- Proton pump inhibitors
- H_2-receptor antagonists
- Antacids
- Antibiotics
- Miscellaneous drugs.

Proton Pump Inhibitors

Proton pump inhibitors (PPIs) act by blocking the enzyme responsible for secreting hydrochloric acid in the stomach. They are drugs of choice for the short-term therapy of PUD and GERD. These medications are listed in Table 41.1.

41.6 Pharmacotherapy With Proton Pump Inhibitors

The PPIs reduce acid secretion in the stomach by binding irreversibly to **H^+, K^+-ATPase,** the enzyme that acts as a pump to release acid (also called H^+, or protons) onto the surface of the GI mucosa. They reduce acid secretion to a greater extent than the H_2-receptor antagonists and have a longer duration of action. PPIs heal more than 90% of duodenal ulcers within 4 weeks and about 90% of gastric ulcers in 6 to 8 weeks.

Several days of PPI therapy may be needed before patients gain relief from ulcer pain. Beneficial effects

Table 41.1 Proton Pump Inhibitors

Drug	Route and Adult Dose (max dose where indicated)	Adverse Effects
esomeprazole (Nexium)	PO/IV: 20–40 mg/day	*Headache, diarrhea, nausea, rash, dizziness*
lansoprazole (Prevacid)	PO/IV: 20–40 mg/day	Increased risk for osteoporosis-related fractures of the hip, wrist, or spine
omeprazole (Prilosec)	PO: 20–60 mg one to two times/day	
pantoprazole (Protonix)	PO: 40 mg/day	
rabeprazole (AcipHex)	PO: 20 mg once daily	

Note: *Italics* indicate common adverse effects; underlining indicates serious adverse effects.

Pharmacotherapy Illustrated

41.1 | Mechanisms of Action of Antiulcer Drugs

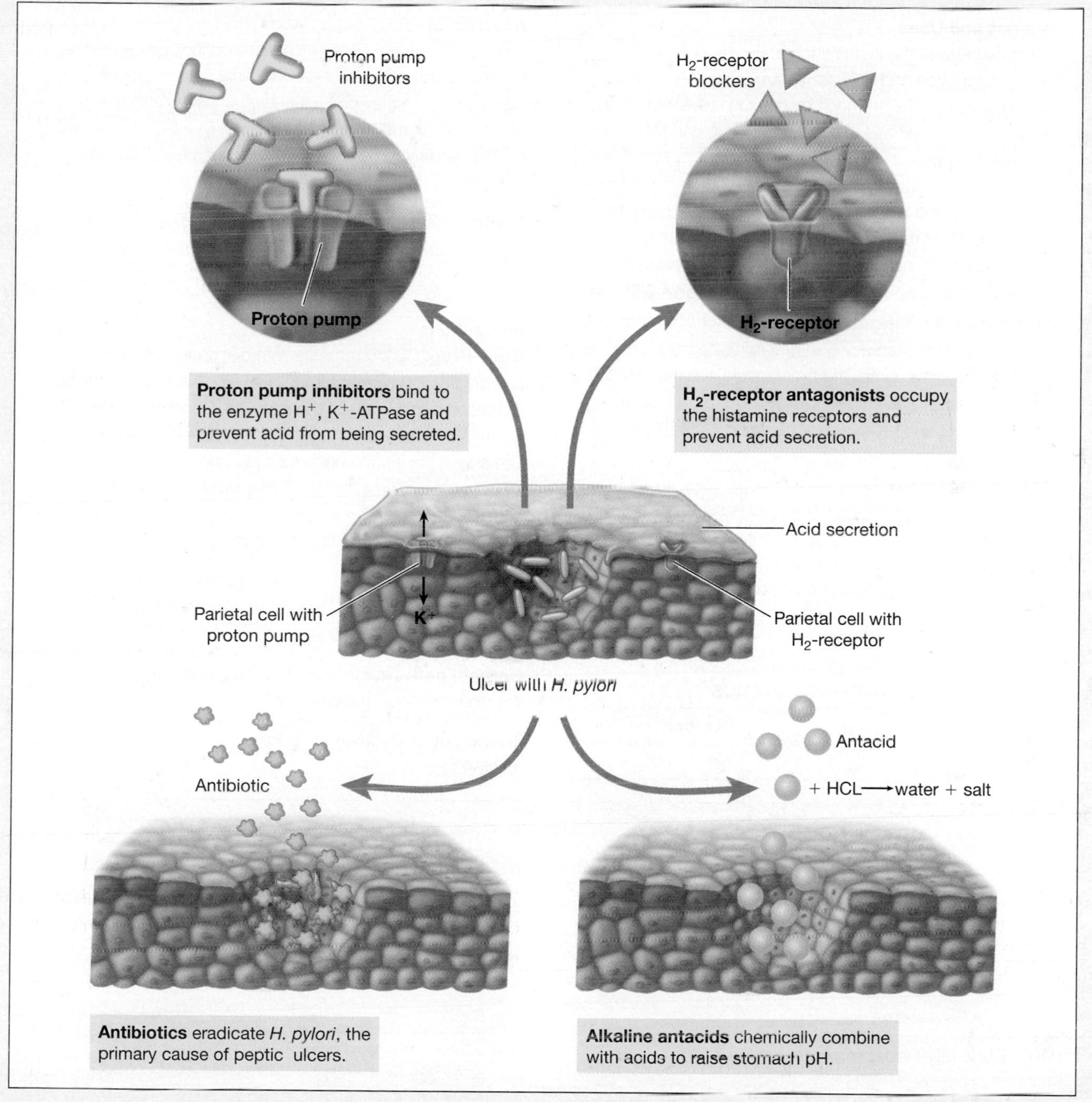
Proton pump inhibitors
Proton pump
Proton pump inhibitors bind to the enzyme H^+, K^+-ATPase and prevent acid from being secreted.
H_2-receptor blockers
H_2-receptor
H_2-receptor antagonists occupy the histamine receptors and prevent acid secretion.
Acid secretion
Parietal cell with proton pump
K^+
Parietal cell with H_2-receptor
Ulcer with H. pylori
Antibiotic
Antacid
+ HCL → water + salt
Antibiotics eradicate H. pylori, the primary cause of peptic ulcers.
Alkaline antacids chemically combine with acids to raise stomach pH.

continue for 3 to 5 days after the drugs have been stopped. These drugs are used only for the short-term control of peptic ulcers and GERD: The typical length of therapy for PUD is 4 weeks. Omeprazole and lansoprazole are used concurrently with antibiotics to eradicate *H. pylori*. Esomeprazole (Nexium) and pantoprazole (Protonix) offer the convenience of once-a-day dosing. Up to 12 weeks of therapy may be needed to reduce symptoms of GERD.

Because the proton pump is activated by food intake, the PPI should be taken 20 to 30 minutes before the first major meal of the day. All PPIs have similar efficacy and adverse effects. Headache, abdominal pain, diarrhea, nausea, and vomiting are the most frequently reported effects. Long-term therapy with PPIs increases the risk for osteoporosis-related fractures, probably because they interfere with calcium absorption. Some health care providers recommend calcium supplements during therapy to prevent these types of fractures.

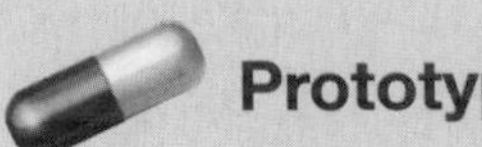

Prototype Drug | Omeprazole (*Prilosec*)

Therapeutic Class: Antiulcer drug **Pharmacologic Class:** Proton pump inhibitor

Actions and Uses

Omeprazole was the first PPI to be approved for PUD. Both prescription and OTC forms are available. It reduces acid secretion in the stomach by binding irreversibly to the enzyme H^+, K^+-ATPase. Although this drug can take 2 hours to reach therapeutic levels, its effects last up to 72 hours. It is used for the short-term, 4- to 8-week therapy of active peptic ulcers and GERD. Most patients are symptom free after 2 weeks of therapy. It is used at higher doses and for longer periods in patients who have chronic hypersecretion of gastric acid, a condition known as **Zollinger–Ellison syndrome.** It is the most effective drug for this syndrome. Omeprazole is available only in oral form. Zegerid is a combination drug containing omeprazole and the antacid sodium bicarbonate. Other indications for omeprazole include GERD and erosive esophagitis.

Administration Alerts

- If possible, administer before breakfast on an empty stomach.
- It may be administered with antacids.
- Capsules and tablets should not be chewed, divided, or crushed.
- Pregnancy category C.

PHARMACOKINETICS

Onset	Peak	Duration
1 h	2 h	72 h

Adverse Effects

Adverse effects are generally minor and include headache, nausea, diarrhea, rash, and abdominal pain. Although rare, blood disorders may occur, causing unusual fatigue and weakness. Therapy is generally limited to 2 months. Atrophic gastritis and hypomagnesemia have been reported rarely with prolonged treatment with PPIs.

Contraindications: The only contraindication is hypersensitivity to the drug. OTC use is not approved for patients under 18 years of age.

Interactions

Drug–Drug: Concurrent use with diazepam, phenytoin, and central nervous system (CNS) depressants may cause increased blood levels of these drugs. Concurrent use with warfarin may increase the likelihood of bleeding. Alcohol can aggravate the stomach mucosa and decrease the effectiveness of omeprazole. Omeprazole should not be administered concurrently with nelfinavir or rilpivirine because it lowers the serum levels of these drugs.

Lab Tests: Omeprazole may increase values for alanine aminotransferase (ALT), aspartate aminotransferase (AST), and serum alkaline phosphatase.

Herbal/Food: Ginkgo and St. John's wort may decrease the plasma concentration of omeprazole.

Treatment of Overdose: There is no specific treatment for overdose.

H_2-Receptor Antagonists

The discovery of the H_2-receptor antagonists in the 1970s marked a major breakthrough in the treatment of PUD. They have since become available OTC and are widely used in the treatment of hyperacidity disorders of the GI tract. These medications are listed in Table 41.2.

Table 41.2 H_2-Receptor Antagonists

Drug	Route and Adult Dose (max dose where indicated)	Adverse Effects
cimetidine (Tagamet)	PO (Active ulcers): 300 mg q6h or 800 mg at bedtime or 400 mg bid with food PO (GERD): 400 mg q6h or 800 mg bid for 12 wk	*Diarrhea, constipation, headache, fatigue, nausea, gynecomastia* Rare: Hepatitis, blood dyscrasias, anaphylaxis, dysrhythmias, skin reactions, galactorrhea, confusion or psychoses
famotidine (Pepcid)	PO (Active ulcers): 20 mg bid or 40 mg at bedtime for 4–8 wk PO (GERD): 20 mg bid for 6 wk	*Headache, nausea, dry mouth* Rare: Musculoskeletal pain, tachycardia, blood dyscrasia, blurred vision
nizatidine (Axid)	PO: 150–300 mg at bedtime	
ranitidine (Zantac)	PO: 100–150 mg bid or 300 mg at bedtime IV/IM: 50 mg q6–8h	

Note: *Italics* indicate common adverse effects; underlining indicates serious adverse effects.

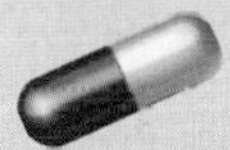

Prototype Drug | Ranitidine *(Zantac)*

Therapeutic Class: Antiulcer drug **Pharmacologic Class:** H_2-receptor antagonist

Actions and Uses

Ranitidine acts by blocking H_2 receptors in the stomach to decrease acid production. It has a higher potency than cimetidine, which allows it to be administered once daily, usually at bedtime. Adequate healing of the ulcer takes approximately 4 to 8 weeks, although those at high risk for PUD may continue on drug maintenance for prolonged periods to prevent recurrence. Gastric ulcers require longer therapy for healing to occur. Intravenous (IV) and intramuscular (IM) forms are available for the treatment of acute, stress-induced bleeding ulcers. Tritec is a combination drug with ranitidine and bismuth citrate. Ranitidine is available in a dissolving tablet form (EFFERdose) for treating GERD in children and infants older than 1 month of age. Additional indications include Zollinger-Ellison syndrome and erosive esophagitis.

Administration Alert

- Administer after meals and monitor liver and renal function.
- Pregnancy category B.

PHARMACOKINETICS

Onset	Peak	Duration
30–60 min	2–3 h	8–12 h

Adverse Effects

Adverse effects are uncommon and mild, with headache being the most common symptom. Ranitidine does not cross the blood–brain barrier to any appreciable extent, so it does not cause the confusion and CNS depression observed with cimetidine. Although rare, severe reductions in the number of red blood cells (RBCs), white blood cells (WBCs), and platelets are possible; thus, periodic blood counts may be performed. High doses may result in impotence or loss of libido in men.

Contraindications: Contraindications include hypersensitivity to H_2-receptor antagonists, acute porphyria, and OTC administration in children less than 12 years of age.

Interactions

Drug–Drug: Ranitidine has fewer drug–drug interactions than cimetidine. Ranitidine may reduce the absorption of cefpodoxime, ketoconazole, and itraconazole. Antacids should not be given within 1 hour of H_2-receptor antagonists because the effectiveness may be decreased due to reduced absorption. Smoking decreases the effectiveness of ranitidine.

Lab Tests: Ranitidine may increase the values of serum creatinine, AST, ALT, lactate dehydrogenase (LDH), alkaline phosphatase, and bilirubin. It may produce false positives for urine protein.

Herbal/Food: Absorption of vitamin B_{12} depends on an acidic environment; thus, deficiency may occur. Iron is also better absorbed in an acidic environment.

Treatment of Overdose: There is no specific treatment for overdose.

41.7 Pharmacotherapy With H_2-Receptor Antagonists

Histamine has two types of receptors: H_1 and H_2. Activation of H_1 receptors produces the classic symptoms of inflammation and allergy, whereas the H_2 receptors are responsible for increasing acid secretion in the stomach. The **H_2-receptor antagonists** are effective at suppressing the volume and acidity of parietal cell secretions. Duodenal ulcers usually heal in 6 to 8 weeks, and gastric ulcers may require up to 12 weeks of therapy. All of the H_2-receptor antagonists are available OTC for the short-term (2 weeks) treatment of GERD.

All H_2-receptor antagonists have similar safety profiles: Adverse effects are minor and rarely cause discontinuation of therapy. Patients who are taking high doses, or those with renal or hepatic disease, may experience confusion, restlessness, hallucinations, or depression. The first drug in this class, cimetidine (Tagamet), is used less frequently than other H_2-receptor antagonists because of numerous drug–drug interactions (it inhibits hepatic drug-metabolizing enzymes) and because it must be taken up to four times a day. Antacids should not be taken at the same time because the absorption of the H_2-receptor antagonist will be diminished.

Antacids

Antacids are alkaline substances that have been used to neutralize stomach acid for hundreds of years. These medications, listed in Table 41.3, are readily available as OTC drugs.

41.8 Pharmacotherapy With Antacids

Prior to the development of H_2-receptor antagonists and PPIs, **antacids** were the mainstays of peptic ulcer and GERD pharmacotherapy. Indeed, many patients still use

Community-Oriented Practice

PROTON PUMP INHIBITORS AND OSTEOPOROSIS RISK

PPIs are used in many age groups, including children, to treat GERD and other hyperacidity conditions. They are available by prescription as well as in lower doses as OTC drugs, and patients may self-medicate without medical advice. Research suggests there may be a link between the use of PPIs and an increased risk for osteopenia, osteoporosis, and fractures due to malabsorption of calcium and other nutrients (Fraser, Leslie, Targownik, Papaioannou, & Adachi, 2013; Leontiadis & Moayyedi, 2014; Solomon et al., 2015). In the older adult, who is more prone to fractures related to aging, the linkage is less clear. This is because age-related changes to the GI tract could also explain some of these conditions. The research is equivocal however, and some studies suggest that combining a bisphosphonate drug such as risedronate (Actonel) to treat osteoporosis, with a PPI may reduce the risk of severe esophagitis and other GI-associated adverse effects of the bisphosphonate classification (Itoh, Sekino, Shinomiya, & Takeda, 2013). Long-term use of PPIs has also been considered a possible cause of iron and vitamin B_{12} deficiencies.

Risk reduction strategies to avoid long-term complications such as osteoporosis that may be associated with PPIs, include increasing intake of calcium and magnesium; weight-bearing exercise for a minimum of three times weekly; and increasing iron, folic acid, and vitamin B_{12}-rich foods such as fortified cereals, bread, meats, fish, and green leafy vegetables. Laboratory and radiologic studies such as a DEXA scan may indicate the need for more aggressive therapies such as the use of biphosphonates for bone building. Nurses can help patients choose appropriate foods and select age- and condition-appropriate exercise options to improve general health and reduce the risk of vitamin and mineral deficiencies. These strategies are especially important for the patient who is prescribed, or is taking OTC PPIs for gastric hyperacidity.

these inexpensive and readily available OTC drugs. Although antacids may provide temporary relief from heartburn or indigestion, they are no longer recommended as the primary drug class for PUD. This is because antacids do not promote healing of the ulcer, nor do they help to eradicate *H. pylori*.

Antacids are alkaline, inorganic compounds of aluminum, magnesium, sodium, or calcium. Combinations of aluminum hydroxide and magnesium hydroxide, the most common type, are capable of rapidly neutralizing stomach acid. Chewable tablets and liquid formulations are available. A few products combine antacids and H_2-receptor blockers into a single tablet; for example, Pepcid Complete contains calcium carbonate, magnesium hydroxide, and famotidine.

Simethicone is sometimes added to antacid preparations, because it reduces gas bubbles that cause bloating and discomfort. For example, Mylanta contains simethicone, aluminum hydroxide, and magnesium hydroxide. Simethicone is classified as an **antiflatulent,** because it reduces gas. It also is available by itself in OTC products such as Gas-X and Mylanta Gas.

Self-medication with antacids is safe when taken in doses directed on the labels. Although antacids act within 10 to 15 minutes, their duration of action is only 2 hours; thus, they must be taken often during the day. Antacids

Table 41.3 Antacids

Drug	Route and Adult Dose (max dose where indicated)	Adverse Effects
aluminum hydroxide (AlternaGEL, others)	PO: 600 mg tid–qid	*Constipation, nausea, stomach cramps* Fecal impaction, hypophosphatemia
calcium carbonate (Titralac, Tums)	PO: 1–2 g bid–tid	*Constipation, flatulence* Fecal impaction, metabolic alkalosis, hypercalcemia, renal calculi
calcium carbonate with magnesium hydroxide (Mylanta Supreme, Rolaids)	PO: 400–1,000 mg calcium/ 110–200 mg magnesium (2–4 capsules or tablets) prn (max: 12 tablets/day)	
magaldrate (Riopan)	PO: 540–1,080 mg (5–10 mL suspension or 1–2 tablets) daily	*Diarrhea, nausea, vomiting, abdominal cramping* Hypermagnesemia, dysrhythmias (when given parenterally)
magnesium hydroxide (Milk of Magnesia)	PO: 5–15 mL or 2–4 tablets as needed up to four times daily	
magnesium carbonate with aluminum hydroxide (Gaviscon)	PO: 2–4 tablets prn (max: 16 tablets/day)	
magnesium hydroxide with aluminum hydroxide and simethicone (Mylanta, Maalox Plus, others)	PO: 75–110 mg magnesium/ 31–160 mg aluminium (10–20 mL) prn (max: 120 mL/day) or 2–4 tablets prn (max: 24 tablets/day)	
sodium bicarbonate (Alka-Seltzer, baking soda) (see page 370 for the Prototype Drug box)	PO: 325 mg–2 g one to four times/day	*Abdominal distention, belching, flatulence* Metabolic alkalosis, fluid retention, edema, hypernatremia

Note: *Italics* indicate common adverse effects; underlining indicates serious adverse effects.

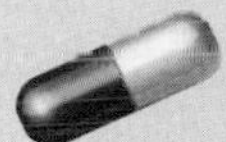

Prototype Drug | Aluminum Hydroxide *(AlternaGEL, others)*

Therapeutic Class: Antiheartburn agent **Pharmacologic Class:** Antacid

Actions and Uses

Aluminum hydroxide is an inorganic agent used alone or in combination with other antacids. Combining aluminum compounds with magnesium (Gaviscon, Maalox, Mylanta) increases their effectiveness and reduces the potential for constipation. Unlike calcium-based antacids that can be absorbed and cause systemic effects, aluminum compounds are minimally absorbed. Their primary action is to neutralize stomach acid by raising the pH of the stomach contents. Unlike H_2-receptor antagonists and PPIs, aluminum antacids do not reduce the volume of acid secretion. They are most effectively used in combination with other antiulcer drugs for the symptomatic relief of heartburn due to PUD or GERD. A second aluminum salt, aluminum carbonate (Basaljel), is also available to treat heartburn.

Administration Alerts

- Administer aluminum antacids at least 2 hours before or after other drugs because absorption could be affected.
- Pregnancy category C.

PHARMACOKINETICS

Onset	Peak	Duration
20–40 min	30 min	2–3 h

Adverse Effects

When taken regularly or in high doses, aluminum antacids cause constipation. At high doses, aluminum products bind with phosphate in the GI tract and long-term use can result in phosphate depletion. Those at risk include those who are malnourished, alcoholics, and those with renal disease.

Contraindications: This drug should not be used in patients with suspected bowel obstruction.

Interactions

Drug–Drug: Aluminum compounds should not be taken at the same time as other medications, because they may interfere with absorption. Use with sodium polystyrene sulfonate may cause systemic alkalosis.

Lab Tests: Values for serum gastrin and urinary pH may increase. Serum phosphate values may decrease.

Herbal/Food: Aluminum antacids may inhibit the absorption of dietary iron.

Treatment of Overdose: There is no specific treatment for overdose.

containing sodium, calcium, or magnesium can result in absorption of these minerals to the general circulation. Absorption of antacids is clinically unimportant unless the patient is on a sodium-restricted diet or has diminished renal function that could result in accumulation of these minerals. In fact, some manufacturers advertise their calcium-based antacid products as mineral supplements. Patients should follow the label instructions carefully and keep within the recommended dosage range.

Antacids containing calcium can cause constipation and may cause or aggravate kidney stones. Administering calcium carbonate antacids with milk or any items with vitamin D can cause **milk–alkali syndrome** to occur. Early symptoms are those of hypercalcemia and include headache, urinary frequency, anorexia, nausea, and fatigue. Milk–alkali syndrome may result in permanent renal damage if the drug is continued at high doses.

Pharmacotherapy of *H. Pylori* Infection

The gram-negative bacterium *H. pylori* is associated with 80% of patients with duodenal ulcers and 70% of those with gastric ulcers. It is also strongly associated with gastric cancer. To more rapidly and completely heal peptic ulcers, combination therapy with several antibiotics is used to eradicate this bacterium.

41.9 Pharmacotherapy With Combination Antibiotic Therapy

H. pylori has adapted well as a human pathogen by devising ways to neutralize the high acidity surrounding it and by making chemicals called *adhesins* that allow it to stick tightly to the GI mucosa. *H. pylori* infections can remain active for life if not treated appropriately. Elimination of this organism allows ulcers to heal more rapidly and remain in remission longer. Because acid-reducing drugs have little or no effect on *H. pylori*, antibiotics must be used to eliminate the bacterium.

A combination of antibiotics is used concurrently to eradicate *H. pylori*. Once eliminated from the stomach, reinfection with *H. pylori* is uncommon. Those with peptic ulcers who are not infected with *H. pylori* should not receive antibiotics because it has been shown that these patients have a worse outcome if they receive *H. pylori* treatment. Thus, patients should be tested for *H. pylori* before initiating treatment for infection. Example regimens used to eradicate *H. pylori* include the following:

- Initial regimen: Omeprazole, clarithromycin (Biaxin), and amoxicillin (Amoxil, others).
- Alternative regimens:
  - Omeprazole (or other PPI), clarithromycin (Biaxin), and metronidazole (Flagyl), or
  - Omeprazole (or other PPI), bismuth subsalicylate (Pepto-Bismol), metronidazole (Flagyl), and tetracycline.

Two or more antibiotics are given concurrently to increase the effectiveness of therapy and to lower the potential for bacterial resistance. The antibiotics are also combined with a PPI or an H_2-receptor antagonist. Bismuth compounds (Pepto-Bismol, Tritec) are sometimes added to the antibiotic regimen. Although technically not antibiotics, bismuth compounds inhibit bacterial growth and prevent *H. pylori* from adhering to the gastric mucosa. Antibiotic therapy generally continues for 7 to 14 days. Additional information on anti-infectives can be found in chapters 35 and 36.

☑ Check Your Understanding 41.1

Drug therapy for PUD and GERD may be started after other measures have not been successful. What additional nonpharmacologic measures should be tried before drug therapy is considered? *Visit www.pearsonhighered.com/nursingresources for the answer.*

Nursing Practice Application

Pharmacotherapy for Peptic Ulcer and Gastroesophageal Reflux Diseases

ASSESSMENT	POTENTIAL NURSING DIAGNOSES*
Baseline assessment prior to administration: • Obtain a complete health history including GI, hepatic, renal, respiratory, or cardiovascular disease; pregnancy; or breast-feeding. Obtain a drug history including allergies, current prescription and OTC drugs, herbal preparations, caffeine, nicotine, and alcohol use. Be alert to possible drug interactions. • Obtain a history of past and current symptoms, noting any correlations between the onset or presence of any pain related to meals, sleep, positioning, or associated with other medications. Also note what measures have been successful to relieve the pain (e.g., eating). • Obtain baseline vital signs and weight. • Evaluate appropriate laboratory findings (e.g., complete blood count [CBC], platelets, electrolytes, hepatic or renal function studies).	• *Acute Pain* • *Altered Nutrition, Less Than Body Requirements* • *Constipation or Diarrhea,* related to adverse drug effects • *Ineffective Health Management* • *Deficient Knowledge* (drug therapy) *NANDA I © 2014
Assessment throughout administration: • Assess for desired therapeutic effects (e.g., diminished gastric area pain, lessened bloating or belching). • Continue periodic monitoring of CBC, electrolytes, and hepatic and renal function laboratory tests. Testing for *H. pylori* may be needed if symptoms fail to resolve. • Assess for adverse effects: nausea, vomiting, diarrhea, headache, drowsiness, and dizziness. Severe abdominal pain, vomiting, coffee-ground or bloody vomiting, or blood in stool or tarry stools should be reported immediately.	

IMPLEMENTATION

INTERVENTIONS AND (RATIONALES)	PATIENT-CENTERED CARE
Ensuring therapeutic effects: • Follow appropriate administration guidelines. (For best results, follow administration guidelines regarding timing of the drug around meals. See "Patient Self-Administration" below.)	• Teach the patient to follow appropriate guidelines and not to crush, open, or chew tablets unless directed to do so by the health care provider or label directions.
• Encourage appropriate lifestyle changes, including an increased intake of yogurt and acidophilus-containing foods. Have the patient note correlations between discomfort or pain and meals or activities. (Smoking and alcohol use increase gastric acid and irritation and should be eliminated. Correlating symptoms with dietary habits may help to eliminate a triggering factor.)	• Encourage the patient to adopt a healthy lifestyle of low-fat food choices and increased exercise and to eliminate alcohol consumption and smoking. **Collaboration:** Provide for dietitian consultation or information on smoking cessation programs as needed. • Teach the patient to keep a food diary, noting correlations between discomfort or pain and meals or activities.

Nursing Practice Application *continued*

IMPLEMENTATION	
INTERVENTIONS AND (RATIONALES)	**PATIENT-CENTERED CARE**
Minimizing adverse effects: • Continue to monitor the presence of gastric area pain. (Continued symptoms may indicate ineffectiveness of current drug therapy or the need for testing for *H. pylori*.)	• Teach the patient that full drug effects may take several days to weeks. Consistent drug therapy will provide the best results. If gastric discomfort or pain continue or worsen after several weeks of therapy, the health care provider should be notified.
• Monitor for any severe abdominal pain, vomiting, coffee-ground or bloody vomiting, or blood in stool or tarry stools and report immediately. (The drugs used to treat PUD and GERD decrease gastric acidity, making the gastric environment less favorable for ulcer development but they do not heal existing ulcers. Severe abdominal pain or blood in emesis or stools may indicate a worsening of the disease or more serious conditions and should be reported immediately.)	• Teach the patient that severe abdominal pain or any blood in emesis or stools should be reported immediately to the health care provider.
• Continue to monitor periodic hepatic and renal function tests and CBC, platelets, and electrolyte levels. (Abnormal liver function tests may indicate drug-induced adverse hepatic effects. Long-term use of PPIs has been linked to osteopenia and osteoporosis. Calcium and magnesium supplementation or other preventive drug therapy may be required. Decreased RBC, WBC, or platelets have been noted with long-term H_2 receptor blocker therapy, and decreases should be reported to the health care provider. Excessive use of antacids may affect electrolyte levels.)	• Instruct the patient on the need to return periodically for laboratory work.
• Observe for dizziness and monitor ambulation until the effects of the drug are known. (Drowsiness or dizziness from H_2-receptor blockers may occur, which increases the risk of falls. Continued dizziness or drowsiness may require a change in drug therapy.)	• **Safety:** Instruct the patient to call for assistance prior to getting out of bed or attempting to walk alone, and to avoid driving or other activities requiring mental alertness or physical coordination until the effects of the drug are known.
• Monitor respiratory status and for fever, congestion, or adventitious breath sounds such as crackles or wheezing. (The drugs used to treat hyperacidic conditions raise the gastric pH and impact the body's normal defense mechanisms against respiratory pathogens. Antibacterial therapy may be needed if respiratory infections develop.)	• Teach the patient to report symptoms of respiratory infection and to report lung congestion or dyspnea accompanied by fever to the health care provider.
• Monitor for severe diarrhea, especially if mucus, blood, or pus is present. (The drugs used to treat hyperacidic conditions raise the gastric pH and increase the risk of *Clostridium difficile*–associated diarrhea [CDAD] or pseudomembranous colitis [PMC].)	• Instruct the patient to immediately report diarrhea that increases in frequency or amount or that contains mucus, blood, or pus. • Instruct the patient to consult the health care provider before taking any antidiarrheal drugs because they may cause the retention of harmful bacteria. • Teach the patient to increase intake of dairy products containing live active cultures, such as yogurt or kefir, to help restore normal intestinal flora.
• Continue to monitor periodic hepatic and renal function tests and CBC, platelets, and electrolyte levels. (Abnormal liver function tests may indicate drug-induced adverse hepatic effects. **Diverse Patients:** Because some drugs used in PUD therapy [e.g., omeprazole, cimetidine] are metabolized through the P450 system, monitor ethnically diverse patients frequently to ensure optimal therapeutic effects and minimize adverse effects. **Lifespan:** Age-related physiological differences may place the older adult at greater risk for hepatic or renal toxicity. Decreased RBCs, WBCs, or platelets have been noted with long-term H_2-receptor antagonist therapy, and decreases should be reported to the health care provider. Excessive use of antacids may affect electrolyte levels.)	• Instruct the patient on the need to return periodically for laboratory work.

continued

Nursing Practice Application *continued*

IMPLEMENTATION	
INTERVENTIONS AND (RATIONALES)	**PATIENT-CENTERED CARE**
• Monitor for the effectiveness of other drugs taken along with H_2-receptor antagonists or antacids. (H_2-receptor antagonists and antacids may impair the absorption or effects of other drugs.)	• Teach the patient to consult with the health care provider before taking any other drugs concurrently with these medications and to report any unusual symptoms.
Patient understanding of drug therapy:	
• Use opportunities during administration of medications and during assessments to provide patient education. (Using time during nursing care helps to optimize and reinforce key teaching areas.)	• The patient, family, or caregiver should be able to state the reason for the drug; appropriate dose and scheduling; what adverse effects to observe for and when to report; and the anticipated length of medication therapy.
Patient self-administration of drug therapy:	
• When administering the medication, instruct the patient, family, or caregiver in the proper self-administration of the drug (e.g., during evening meal). (Proper administration improves the effectiveness of the drugs.)	• Teach the patient to take the drug according to appropriate guidelines as follows: • H_2-receptor blockers: May be taken without regard to mealtimes. Do not take concurrently with antacids unless the drug is available in a combination product such as Pepcid-Complete. • PPIs: Take 30 minutes before meals. If once-a-day dosing is ordered, take the drug in the morning before breakfast. Antacids may be used concurrently. Do not continue taking the drug beyond 3 to 4 months unless directed by the health care provider. • Antacids: Take 2 hours before or after meals with a full glass of water. Do not take other medications concurrently unless available as a combination product or directed to do so by the health care provider.

See Tables 41.1, 41.2, and 41.3 for a list of drugs to which these nursing actions apply.

Lifespan Considerations: Pediatric
GERD and PUD in Children

GERD is a rare condition in children that is commonly treated with the same PPIs, H_2-receptor antagonists, and antacids that are used to treat adults. The dosage for PPIs is higher per kilogram of weight in children than in adults, but the dosages of H_2-receptor antagonists and antacids are smaller. Ideally, dietary alterations are used along with drug therapy. Thickening feedings with cereal has been shown to improve GERD symptoms in infants. Determining food intolerances such as those to soy or milk products and avoiding chocolate, tomatoes, or caffeinated beverages may also improve the conditions. As for adults, older children are encouraged to follow healthy lifestyles and exercise recommendations to decrease aggravating factors for GERD.

41.10 Miscellaneous Drugs for Peptic Ulcer Disease

Several additional drugs are beneficial in treating PUD. Sucralfate (Carafate) consists of sucrose (a sugar) plus aluminum hydroxide (an antacid). The drug produces a thick, gel-like substance that coats the ulcer, protecting it against further erosion and promoting healing. It does not affect the secretion of gastric acid. Other than constipation, adverse effects are minimal, because little of the drug is absorbed by the GI tract. A major disadvantage of sucralfate is that it must be taken four times daily.

Misoprostol (Cytotec) inhibits gastric acid secretion and stimulates the production of protective mucus. Its primary use is for the prevention of peptic ulcers in patients who are taking high doses of NSAIDs or corticosteroids. Diarrhea and abdominal cramping are relatively common adverse effects. Classified as a pregnancy category X drug, misoprostol is contraindicated during pregnancy. In fact, misoprostol may be combined with a prostaglandin to terminate pregnancies, as discussed in chapter 46.

Metoclopramide (Reglan) is occasionally used for the short-term therapy of symptomatic PUD in patients who fail to respond to first-line drugs. Available by the oral, IM, or IV routes, metoclopramide is more commonly prescribed to treat nausea and vomiting associated with surgery or cancer chemotherapy. The drug causes muscles in the upper intestine to contract, resulting in faster emptying of the stomach, and blocks food from re-entering the

Complementary and Alternative Therapies

GINGER'S TONIC EFFECTS ON THE GASTROINTESTINAL TRACT

The use of ginger (*Zingiber officinalis*) as a spice and medicinal herb dates back to antiquity in India and China. The active ingredients of ginger are located in its roots or rhizomes. The herb is sometimes standardized according to its active substances, called gingerols and shogaols. It is sold in pharmacies as dried ginger root powder, at a dose of 250 to 1,000 mg, and is readily available at most grocery stores for cooking. It has been shown to stimulate appetite, promote gastric secretions, and increase peristalsis. Its effects appear to stem from direct action on the GI tract, rather than on the CNS.

Ginger is one of the most studied herbs, and it appears to be useful for a number of digestive-related conditions. Its widest use is for treating nausea, including that caused by motion sickness, pregnancy morning sickness, and postoperative procedures. The herb is as effective as dimenhydrinate and pyridoxine in reducing the nausea that occurs during pregnancy (Maitre, Neher, & Safranek, 2011). A recent meta-analysis concluded that ginger may reduce the pain and disability associated with osteoarthritis (Bartels et al., 2015). It has no toxicity when used at recommended doses.

esophagus from the stomach, which is of benefit in patients with GERD. Adverse CNS effects such as drowsiness, fatigue, confusion, and insomnia occur in a significant number of patients. The drug carries a black box warning that it can cause tardive dyskinesia with long-term therapy. In 2009 an oral-disintegrating tablet form of this drug, Metozolv ODT, was approved for the treatment of GERD and diabetic gastroparesis.

Chapter Review

KEY Concepts

The numbered key concepts provide a succinct summary of the important points from the corresponding numbered section within the chapter. If any of these points are not clear, refer to the numbered section within the chapter for review.

41.1 The digestive system is responsible for breaking down food, absorbing nutrients, and eliminating wastes.

41.2 The stomach secretes enzymes and hydrochloric acid that accelerate the process of chemical digestion. A thick mucus layer and bicarbonate ions protect the stomach mucosa from the damaging effects of the acid.

41.3 Peptic ulcer disease (PUD) is caused by an erosion of the mucosal layer of the stomach or duodenum. Gastric ulcers are more commonly associated with cancer and require longer follow-up.

41.4 Gastroesophageal reflux disease (GERD) results when acidic stomach contents enter the esophagus. GERD and PUD are treated with similar medications.

41.5 PUD is best treated with a combination of lifestyle changes and pharmacotherapy. Treatment goals are to eliminate infection by *H. pylori*, provide relief from symptoms, promote ulcer healing, and prevent recurrence of the disease.

41.6 Proton pump inhibitors (PPIs) block the enzyme H^+, K^+-ATPase and are effective at reducing gastric acid secretion.

41.7 H_2-receptor blockers slow acid secretion by the stomach and are often drugs of choice in treating PUD and GERD.

41.8 Antacids are effective at neutralizing stomach acid and are inexpensive OTC therapy for PUD and GERD. Although they relieve symptoms, antacids do not promote ulcer healing.

41.9 Combinations of antibiotics are administered to treat *H. pylori* infections of the GI tract, the cause of many peptic ulcers. A PPI, or an H_2-receptor antagonist, and bismuth compounds are often included in the regimen.

41.10 Several miscellaneous drugs, including sucralfate, misoprostol, and metoclopramide, are also beneficial in treating PUD.

REVIEW Questions

1. A female patient reports using OTC aluminum hydroxide (AlternaGEL) for relief of gastric upset. She is on renal dialysis three times a week. What should the nurse teach this patient?
   1. Continue using the antacids but if she needs to continue them beyond a few months, she should consult the health care provider about different therapies.
   2. Take the antacid no longer than for two weeks; if it has not worked by then, it will not be effective.
   3. Consult with the health care provider about the appropriate amount and type of antacid.
   4. Continue to take the antacid; it is OTC and safe.
2. The nurse is assisting the older adult diagnosed with a gastric ulcer to schedule her medication administration. What would be the most appropriate time for this patient to take her lansoprazole (Prevacid)?
   1. About 30 minutes before her morning meal
   2. At night before bed
   3. After fasting at least 2 hours
   4. 30 minutes after each meal
3. Simethicone (Gas-X, Mylicon) may be added to some medications or given plain for what therapeutic effect?
   1. Decrease the amount of gas associated with GI disorders.
   2. Increase the acid-fighting ability of some medications.
   3. Prevent constipation associated with gastrointestinal drugs.
   4. Prevent diarrhea associated with gastrointestinal drugs.
4. The nurse is caring for a patient with gastroesophageal reflux disease and would question an order for which of the following?
   1. Amoxicillin (Amoxil)
   2. Ranitidine (Zantac)
   3. Pantoprazole (Protonix)
   4. Calcium carbonate (Tums)
5. A 35-year-old male patient has been prescribed omeprazole (Prilosec) for treatment of gastroesophageal reflux disease. Which of the following assessment findings would assist the nurse to determine whether drug therapy has been effective? (Select all that apply.)
   1. Decreased "gnawing" upper abdominal pain on an empty stomach
   2. Decreased belching
   3. Decreased appetite
   4. Decreased nausea
   5. Decreased dysphagia
6. In taking a new patient's history, the nurse notices that he has been taking omeprazole (Prilosec) consistently over the past 6 months for treatment of epigastric pain. Which recommendation would be the best for the nurse to give this patient?
   1. Try switching to a different form of the drug.
   2. Try a drug like cimetidine (Tagamet) or famotidine (Pepcid).
   3. Try taking the drug after meals instead of before meals.
   4. Check with his health care provider about his continued discomfort.

PATIENT-FOCUSED Case Study

Reginald Foxe, 68-years-old, has had chronic hyperacidity of the stomach and takes calcium carbonate (Tums) multiple times, daily. He comes to the clinic with complaints of fatigue, increasing weakness, and headaches. When taking his medication history, Mr. Foxe tells the nurse that he takes two Tums tablets (1,000 mg calcium carbonate) every four hours, and sometimes as frequently as every two hours.

1. What may be the cause of Mr. Foxe's symptoms of fatigue, weakness, and headaches?
2. As the nurse, what will you recommend to Mr. Foxe?
3. What additional teaching is necessary?

CRITICAL THINKING Questions

1. A 37-year-old male patient has been taking NSAIDs for a shoulder injury. He develops abdominal pain that is worse when his stomach is empty. After trying several OTC remedies, he schedules a visit with his health care provider. A breath test confirms the presence of *H. pylori* and a diagnosis of PUD is made. The patient is started on omeprazole (Prilosec), clarithromycin (Biaxin), and amoxicillin (Amoxil). He asks about the purpose of the drugs. How should the nurse respond?

2. A patient who is on ranitidine (Zantac) for PUD smokes and drinks alcohol daily. What education will the nurse provide to this patient?

Visit www.pearsonhighered.com/nursingresources for answers and rationales for all activities.

REFERENCES

Bartels, E. M., Folmer, V. N., Bliddal, H., Altman, R. D., Juhl, C., Tarp, S., . . . Christensen, R. (2015). Efficacy and safety of ginger in osteoarthritis patients: A meta-analysis of randomized placebo-controlled trials. *Osteoarthritis and Cartilage, 23*, 13–21. doi:10.1016/j.joca.2014.09.024

Fraser, L. A., Leslie, W. D., Targownik, L. E., Papaioannou, A., Adachi, J. D. (2013). The effect of proton pump inhibitors on fracture risk: Report from the Canadian Multicenter Osteoporosis Study. *Osteoporosis International, 24*, 1161–1168. doi:10.1007/s00198-012-2112-9

Herdman, T. H., & Kamitsuru, S. (2014). *NANDA International nursing diagnoses: Definitions and classification, 2015–2017*. Oxford, United Kingdom: Wiley-Blackwell.

Itoh, S., Sekino, Y., Shinomiya, K, & Takeda, S. (2013). The effects of risedronate administered in combination with a proton pump inhibitor for the treatment of osteoporosis. *Journal of Bone and Mineral Metabolism, 31*, 206–211. doi:10.1007/s00774-012-0406-9

Leontiadis, G. I., & Moayyedi, P. (2014). Proton pump inhibitors and risk of bone fractures. *Current Treatment Options in Gastroenterology, 12*, 414–423. doi:10.1007/s11938-014-0030-y

Maitre, S., Neher, J., & Safranek, S. (2011). Ginger for the treatment of nausea and vomiting in pregnancy. *American Family Physician, 84*(10), 1–2.

Solomon, D. H., Diem, S. J., Ruppert, K., Lian, Y. J., Liu, C. C., Wohlfart, A., . . . Finkelstein, J. S. (2015). Bone mineral density changes among women initiating proton pump inhibitors or H2 receptor antagonists: A SWAN cohort study. *Journal of Bone and Mineral Research, 30*, 232–239. doi:10.1002/jbmr.2344

SELECTED BIBLIOGRAPHY

Anand, B. S. (2015). *Peptic ulcer disease*. Retrieved from http://emedicine.medscape.com/article/181753-overview#a0101

Hsu, P.-I. (2012). New look at antiplatelet agent-related peptic ulcer: An update of prevention and treatment. *Journal of Gastroenterology and Hepatology, 27*, 654–661. doi:10.1111/j.1440-1746.2012.07085.x

Medline Plus. (2012). *Zollinger-Ellison syndrome*. Retrieved from http://www.nlm.nih.gov/medlineplus/ency/article/000325.htm

National Center for Complementary and Integrative Health. (2012). *Herbs at a glance: Ginger*. Retrieved from https://nccih.nih.gov/health/ginger

O'Keefe, S. J. D. (2010). Tube feeding, microbiota, and *Clostridium difficile* infection. *World Journal of Gastroenterology, 16*(2), 139–142. doi:10.3748/wjg.v16.i2.139

Patti, M. G. (2014). *Gastroesophageal reflux disease*. Retrieved from http://emedicine.medscape.com/article/176595-overview

Tang, R. S., & Chan, F. K. (2012). Therapeutic management of recurrent peptic ulcer disease. *Drugs, 72*, 1605–1616. doi:10.2165/11634850-000000000-00000

Chapter 42

Drugs for Bowel Disorders and Other Gastrointestinal Conditions

Drugs at a Glance

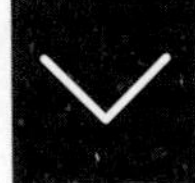

Learning Outcomes

After reading this chapter, the student should be able to:

1. Identify major anatomic structures of the lower gastrointestinal tract.
2. Explain the pathophysiology and pharmacotherapy of constipation.
3. Explain the pathophysiology and pharmacotherapy of diarrhea.
4. Compare and contrast the pharmacotherapy of inflammatory bowel disease and irritable bowel syndrome.
5. Explain the pathophysiology and pharmacotherapy of nausea and vomiting.
6. Explain the use of pancreatic enzyme replacement in the pharmacotherapy of pancreatitis.
7. Describe the nurse's role in the pharmacologic management of bowel disorders, nausea and vomiting, and other gastrointestinal conditions.
8. For each of the drug classes listed in Drugs at a Glance, know representative drugs, and explain the mechanism of drug action, primary actions, and important adverse effects.
9. Use the nursing process to care for patients who are receiving pharmacotherapy for bowel disorders, nausea and vomiting, and other gastrointestinal conditions.

(prototype drug icon) indicates a prototype drug, each of which is featured in a Prototype Drug box.

Bowel disorders, nausea, and vomiting are among the most common complaints for which patients seek medical assistance. These nonspecific symptoms may be caused by a large number of infectious, metabolic, inflammatory, neoplastic, and neuropsychological disorders. In addition, nausea, vomiting, constipation, and diarrhea are the most common adverse effects of oral medications. Although symptoms often resolve without the need for pharmacotherapy, when severe or prolonged, these conditions may lead to serious consequences unless drug therapy is initiated. This chapter examines the pharmacotherapy of these and other conditions associated with the gastrointestinal (GI) tract.

THE LOWER DIGESTIVE TRACT

42.1 Normal Function of the Lower Digestive Tract

The lower portion of the GI tract consists of the small and large intestines, as shown in Figure 42.1. The first 10 inches of the small intestine, the duodenum, is the site where partially digested food from the stomach, known as chyme, mixes with bile from the gallbladder and digestive enzymes from the pancreas. It is sometimes considered part of the upper GI tract because of its close proximity to the stomach. The most common disorder of the duodenum, peptic ulcer, is discussed in chapter 41.

The remainder of the small intestine consists of the jejunum and ileum. The jejunum is the site where most nutrient absorption occurs. The ileum empties its contents into the large intestine through the ileocecal valve. Peristalsis through the intestines is controlled by the autonomic nervous system. Activation of the parasympathetic division will increase peristalsis and speed materials through the intestine; the sympathetic division has the opposite effect. Travel time for chyme through the entire small intestine varies from 3 to 6 hours.

The large intestine, or colon, receives chyme from the ileum in a fluid state. The major functions of the colon are to reabsorb water from the waste material and to excrete the remaining fecal material from the body. The colon harbors a substantial number of bacteria and fungi, the host flora, which serve a useful purpose by synthesizing B-complex vitamins and vitamin K. Disruption of the host flora in the colon can lead to diarrhea. With few exceptions, little reabsorption of nutrients occurs during the 12- to 24-hour journey through the colon.

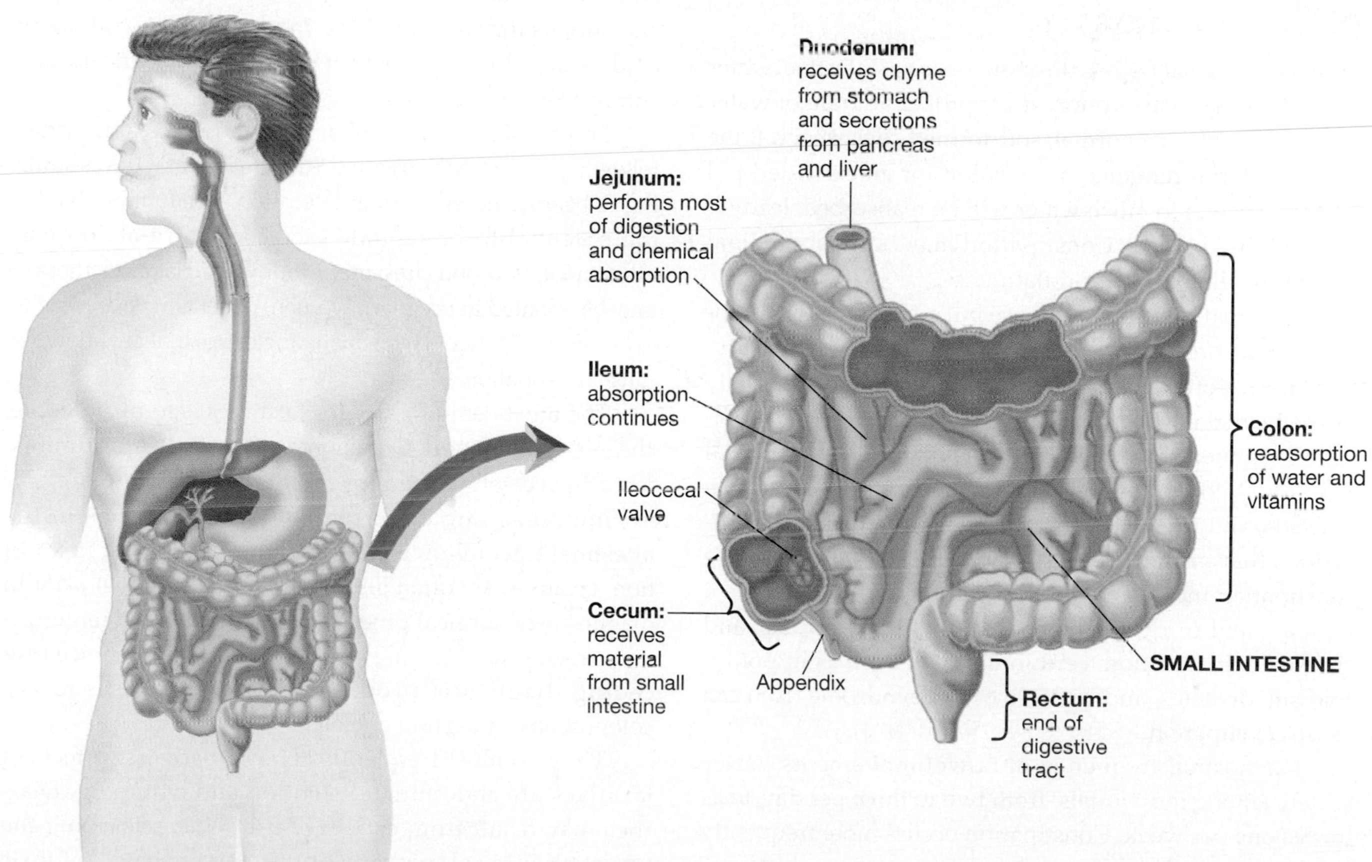

FIGURE 42.1 The digestive system: functions of the small intestine and large intestine (colon)

PharmFacts

GASTROINTESTINAL DISORDERS

- Ulcerative colitis has a peak onset from ages 15 to 40 and another smaller peak from ages 55 to 65.
- As many as 40% of those age 65 and older report recurrent constipation.
- Irritable bowel syndrome affects 10% to 20% of adults.
- The incidence of motion sickness peaks from ages 9 to 10, and then begins to decline.
- Gallstones account for most cases of acute pancreatitis, whereas chronic alcohol consumption is associated with the majority of chronic pancreatitits.
- About 70% to 80% of women experience nausea and vomiting during pregnancy, with a peak incidence of 8–12 weeks following conception.

CONSTIPATION

Constipation may be defined as a decrease in the frequency of bowel movements. Stools often become dry, hard, and difficult to evacuate from the rectum without straining.

42.2 Pathophysiology of Constipation

As waste material travels through the large intestine, water is reabsorbed. Reabsorption of the proper amount of water results in stools of a normal, soft-formed consistency. If the waste material remains in the colon for an extended period, however, too much water will be reabsorbed, leading to small, hard stools. Constipation may cause abdominal distention, discomfort, and flatulence.

Constipation is not a disease but a symptom of an underlying disorder. The etiology of constipation may be related to lack of exercise; insufficient food intake, especially insoluble dietary fiber; diminished fluid intake; or a medication regimen that includes drugs that reduce intestinal motility. Opioids, anticholinergics, antihistamines, certain antacids, and iron supplements are just some of the medications that promote constipation. Foods that can cause constipation include alcoholic beverages, products with a high content of refined white flour, dairy products, and chocolate. In addition, certain diseases such as hypothyroidism, diabetes, and irritable bowel syndrome (IBS) can cause constipation.

The normal frequency of bowel movements varies widely among individuals, from two to three per day, to as few as one per week. Constipation occurs more frequently in older adults, because fecal transit time through the colon slows with aging. This population also exercises less and has a higher frequency of chronic disorders that cause constipation. All patients should understand that variations in frequency are normal, and that a daily bowel movement is not a requirement for good health.

Occasional constipation is self-limiting and does not require drug therapy. Lifestyle modifications that incorporate increased dietary fiber, fluid intake, and physical activity should be considered before drugs are used for constipation. Chronic, infrequent, and painful bowel movements, accompanied by severe straining, may justify initiation of treatment. In its most severe form, constipation can lead to a fecal impaction and complete obstruction of the bowel.

Laxatives

Laxatives are drugs that promote bowel movements. Many are available over the counter (OTC) for the self-treatment of simple constipation. Doses of laxatives are identified in Table 42.1.

42.3 Pharmacotherapy With Laxatives

Laxatives promote the evacuation of the bowel, or defecation, and are widely used to prevent and treat constipation. **Cathartic** is a related term that implies a stronger and more complete bowel emptying. A variety of prescription and OTC products are available, including tablet, liquid, and suppository formulations. Indications for laxatives include either the *prophylaxis* of constipation or *treatment* of chronic constipation.

Prophylactic laxative pharmacotherapy is appropriate following abdominal surgeries. Such treatment reduces straining or bearing down during defecation—a situation that has the potential to precipitate increased intra-abdominal, intraocular, or blood pressure. Prophylactic laxative therapy may be initiated in pregnant women, patients who are unable to exercise, or patients who are taking drugs that are known to cause constipation.

The most common use for laxatives is to treat simple, chronic constipation. Occasionally, laxatives are administered to accelerate the movement of ingested toxins following poisoning or to remove dead parasites in the intestinal tract following antihelminthic therapy. In addition, laxatives are often given to cleanse the bowel prior to diagnostic or surgical procedures of the colon or genitourinary tract. Cathartics are usually the drugs of choice preceding diagnostic procedures of the colon, such as colonoscopy or barium enema.

The two most frequently reported adverse effects of laxatives are abdominal distention and cramping. Diarrhea may result from excessive use. When cleansing the bowel prior to colonoscopy or purging the bowel of toxic substances or parasites, forceful, frequent bowel movements are *expected* outcomes. Care must be taken to rule

Table 42.1 Laxatives and Cathartics

Drug	Route and Adult Dose (max dose where indicated)	Adverse Effects
BULK FORMING		
calcium polycarbophil (Equalactin, FiberCon, others)	PO: 1 g daily	*Abdominal fullness or cramping, fainting*
methylcellulose (Citrucel)	PO: 1 tbsp tid in 8–10 oz water	Esophageal or GI obstruction if taken with insufficient fluid
psyllium mucilloid (Metamucil)	PO: 1–2 tsp or 2–6 capsules daily in 8 oz water	
SALINE AND OSMOTIC		
lactulose (Chronulac)	PO: 15–30 mL daily	*Diarrhea, abdominal cramping*
magnesium hydroxide (Milk of Magnesia)	PO: 20–60 mL or 6–8 tablets daily	Hypermagnesemia with magnesium hydroxide (dysrhythmias, respiratory failure)
polyethylene glycol (MiraLax)	PO: 17 g daily in 8 oz of liquid	
sodium biphosphate (Fleet Phospho-Soda)	PO: 15–30 mL daily mixed in water	
STIMULANT		
bisacodyl (Correctol, Dulcolax, others)	PO: 10–15 mg daily	*Abdominal cramping, nausea, fainting, diarrhea* Fluid and electrolyte loss
STOOL SOFTENER/SURFACTANT		
docusate (Colace, Dulcolax Stool Softener)	PO: 50–500 mg/day	*Abdominal cramping, diarrhea* No serious adverse effects
HERBAL AGENTS		
castor oil (Emulsoil, Neoloid)	PO: 15–60 mL daily	*Abdominal cramping, diarrhea*
senna (Ex-Lax, Senokot, others)	PO: 8.6–17.2 mg/day	No serious adverse effects
MISCELLANEOUS DRUGS		
lubiprostone (Amitiza)	PO (idiopathic constipation): 24 mcg bid PO (IBS with constipation): 8 mcg bid	*Nausea, diarrhea, headache, abdominal pain* Allergic reactions, dyspnea
methylnaltrexone (Relistor)	Subcutaneous: 8 or 12 mg every other day	*Diarrhea, nausea, abdominal pain, flatulence, hyperhidrosis* GI perforation
mineral oil	PO: 15–30 mL bid	*Diarrhea, nausea* Nutritional deficiencies, aspiration pneumonia
naloxegol (Movantik)	PO (opioid-induced constipation): 25 mg in the morning	*Abdominal pain, nausea, vomiting, diarrhea, flatulance* GI perforation, opioid withdrawal

Note: *Italics* indicate common adverse effects; underlining indicates serious adverse effects.

out acute abdominal pathology such as bowel obstruction prior to administration because the drugs will increase colon pressure and possibly cause bowel perforation.

When taken in prescribed amounts, laxatives have few adverse effects. These drugs are often classified into five primary groups and a miscellaneous category:

- *Bulk-forming laxatives* contain fiber, a substance that absorbs water, and increases the size of the fecal mass. These are preferred drugs for the treatment and prevention of chronic constipation and may be taken on a regular basis without ill effects. Because fiber absorbs water and expands to provide bulk, these agents must be taken with plenty of water. Because of their slow onset of action, they are not used when a rapid and complete bowel evacuation is necessary.
- *Saline cathartics,* also called osmotic laxatives, are not absorbed in the intestine; they pull water into the fecal mass to create a more watery stool. These drugs can produce a bowel movement very quickly and should not be used on a regular basis because of the possibility of dehydration and fluid and electrolyte depletion. Saline laxatives are highly effective and are an important component of colonoscopy prep and for purging toxins from the body.
- *Stimulant laxatives* promote peristalsis by irritating the bowel mucosa. They are rapid acting and more likely to cause diarrhea and cramping than the bulk-forming laxatives. They should be used only occasionally because they may cause laxative dependence and depletion of fluid and electrolytes.

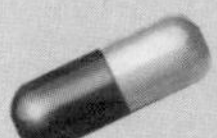

Prototype Drug | Psyllium Mucilloid *(Metamucil, others)*

Therapeutic Class: Bulk-type laxative **Pharmacologic Class:** Natural product

Actions and Uses

Psyllium is derived from a natural product, the seeds of the plantain plant. Like other bulk-forming laxatives, psyllium is an insoluble fiber that is indigestible and not absorbed from the GI tract. When taken with a sufficient quantity of water, psyllium swells and increases the size of the fecal mass, which promotes the passage of stool. Several doses of psyllium may be needed over 1 to 3 days to produce a therapeutic effect. The drug may be taken daily as a fiber supplement.

Frequent use of psyllium (7 g/day) may cause a small reduction in blood cholesterol level. Because of this effect, psyllium may be used as part of a regimen to reduce the risk of coronary heart disease.

Administration Alerts

- Mix with at least 8 oz of water, fruit juice, or milk, and administer immediately. Follow each dose with an additional 8 oz of liquid.
- Observe older adults closely for possible aspiration.
- Pregnancy category C.

PHARMACOKINETICS

Onset	Peak	Duration
12–24 h	24 h	24 h

Adverse Effects

Psyllium is a safe laxative that rarely produces adverse effects. It causes less cramping than stimulant-type laxatives and results in a more natural bowel movement. If taken with insufficient water, psyllium may swell in the esophagus and cause an obstruction.

Contraindications: Psyllium should not be administered to patients with undiagnosed abdominal pain, intestinal obstruction, or fecal impaction.

Interactions

Drug-Drug: Psyllium may decrease the absorption and effects of warfarin, digoxin, nitrofurantoin, antibiotics, tricyclic antidepressants, carbamazepine, and salicylates.

Lab Tests: Psyllium may reduce serum glucose levels in patients with type 2 diabetes.

Herbal/Food: Unknown.

Treatment of Overdose: Overdose from psyllium is unlikely.

- *Stool softeners or surfactant laxatives* cause more water and fat to be absorbed into the stools. They are most often used to *prevent* constipation, especially in patients who have undergone recent surgery.
- *Herbal agents* are natural products that are available OTC and are widely used for self-treatment of constipation. The most commonly used herbal laxative is senna, a potent herb that irritates the bowel and increases peristalsis. Other natural laxatives include castor oil, rhubarb, cascara sagrada, aloe, flaxseed, and dandelion.
- *Miscellaneous drugs* include mineral oil, which acts by lubricating the stool and the colon mucosa. The use of mineral oil should be discouraged, because it may interfere with the absorption of fat-soluble vitamins and can cause other potentially serious adverse effects. Several newer laxatives have been approved for specific types of constipation. Lubiprostone (Amitiza) is approved to treat chronic constipation as well as the constipation form of IBS in women. Methylnaltrexone (Relistor) and naloxegol (Movantik) are specifically used to treat chronic constipation in patients with advanced illness who are receiving opioids. These drugs act by an unusual mechanism: they block opioid mu receptors in the GI tract. When opioids occupy this receptor, they slow the transit of intestinal contents, causing constipation. Blocking the mu receptor occurs without affecting opioid-induced analgesia.

DIARRHEA

When the large intestine does not reabsorb enough water from the fecal mass, stools become watery. **Diarrhea** is an increase in the frequency and fluidity of bowel movements. Diarrhea is not a disease but a symptom of an underlying disorder.

42.4 Pathophysiology of Diarrhea

Like constipation, occasional diarrhea is often self-limiting and does not warrant drug therapy. Indeed, diarrhea may be considered a type of body defense, rapidly and

Complementary and Alternative Therapies

PROBIOTICS FOR DIARRHEA

Probiotics are live microorganisms that are taken in specified amounts to confer a health benefit on the host. Most commercial probiotics are bacteria from the genera *Lactobacillus* and *Bifidobacterium*. However, the yeast *Saccharomyces* is sometimes also used. Although probiotics have been used for thousands of years, only in the past 20 years has research begun to confirm their health benefits. Probiotics are claimed to improve immune function, decrease cancer risk, lower blood cholesterol, reduce blood pressure, and prevent vaginal infections. Probiotic supplements are available in certain drinks, yogurts, and tablets. Although probiotics are safe, care must be taken not to exceed recommended doses.

Most of the evidence supporting the efficacy of probiotics is related to their effects on the intestinal tract. Both *Lactobacillus* and *Bifidobacterium* are normal nonpathogenic inhabitants of a healthy digestive tract. These are considered to be protective flora, inhibiting the growth of potentially pathogenic species such as *Escherichia coli, Candida albicans, H. pylori*, and *Gardnerella vaginalis*. Probiotics restore the normal flora of the intestine following diarrhea, particularly from antibiotic therapy (Hempel et al., 2012). Some studies indicate that probiotics reduce symptoms of IBS in some patients (Whelan, 2011).

completely eliminating the body of toxins and pathogens. When prolonged or severe, especially in children, diarrhea can result in significant loss of body fluids, and pharmacotherapy is indicated. Prolonged diarrhea may lead to fluid, acid–base, or electrolyte disorders (see chapter 25).

Diarrhea may be caused by certain medications, infections of the bowel, and substances such as lactose. Inflammatory disorders such as ulcerative colitis, Crohn's disease, and IBS can cause episodes of intense diarrhea. Antibiotics often cause diarrhea by killing normal intestinal flora, thus allowing an overgrowth of opportunistic pathogenic organisms. The primary goal in treating diarrhea is to assess and treat the underlying condition causing the diarrhea. Assessing the patient's recent travels, dietary habits, immune system competence, and recent drug history may provide information about its etiology. Critically ill patients with a reduced immune response who are exposed to many antibiotics may have diarrhea related to pseudomembranous colitis (PMC), a condition that may lead to shock and death.

Antidiarrheals

For mild diarrhea, OTC products are effective at returning elimination patterns to normal. For chronic or severe cases, the opioids are the most effective of the antidiarrheal medications. The antidiarrheals are listed in Table 42.2.

42.5 Pharmacotherapy With Antidiarrheals

Pharmacotherapy related to diarrhea depends on the severity of the condition and any identifiable etiologic factors. If the cause is an infectious disease, then an antibiotic or antiparasitic drug is indicated. If the cause is inflammatory in nature, anti-inflammatory drugs are warranted. When the diarrhea appears to be an adverse effect of pharmacotherapy, the health care provider may discontinue the offending medication, lower the dose, or substitute an alternative drug.

The most effective drugs for the symptomatic treatment of diarrhea are the opioids, which can dramatically slow peristalsis in the colon. The most common opioid antidiarrheals are codeine and diphenoxylate with atropine

Table 42.2 Antidiarrheals

Drug	Route and Adult Dose (max dose where indicated)	Adverse Effects
OPIOIDS		
camphorated opium tincture (Paregoric)	PO: 5–10 mL one to four times daily	*Drowsiness, lightheadedness, nausea, dizziness, dry mouth (from atropine), constipation*
difenoxin with atropine (Motofen)	PO: 1–2 mg after each diarrhea episode (max: 8 mg/day)	Paralytic ileus with toxic megacolon, respiratory depression, central nervous system (CNS) depression
diphenoxylate with atropine (Lomotil)	PO: 5 mg qid (max: 20 mg/day)	
loperamide (Imodium)	PO: 4 mg as a single dose, then 2 mg after each diarrhea episode (max: 16 mg/day)	
MISCELLANEOUS DRUGS		
bismuth salts (Pepto-Bismol)	PO: 2 tabs or 30 mL prn	*Constipation, nausea, tinnitus* Impaction, Reye's syndrome
Lactobacillus acidophilus	PO: 1–15 billion colony forming units (CFUs) daily	*Stomach gas, diarrhea, abdominal pain* Allergic reactions
octreotide (Sandostatin)	Subcutaneous/IV: 100–600 mcg/day in two to four divided doses	*Nausea, diarrhea, abdominal pain* Changes in serum glucose, gallstones, cholestatic hepatitis

Note: *Italics* indicate common adverse effects; underlining indicates serious adverse effects.

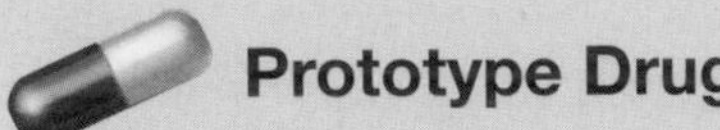

Prototype Drug | Diphenoxylate With Atropine (*Lomotil*)

Therapeutic Class: Antidiarrheal **Pharmacologic Class:** Opioid

Actions and Uses

The primary antidiarrheal ingredient in Lomotil is diphenoxylate. Like other opioids, diphenoxylate slows peristalsis, allowing time for additional water reabsorption from the colon and more solid stools. It acts within 45 to 60 minutes. It is effective for moderate to severe diarrhea but is not recommended for infants. The atropine in Lomotil is added not for any therapeutic effect, but to discourage patients from taking too much of the drug. At higher doses, the anticholinergic effects of atropine such as drowsiness, dry mouth, and tachycardia will be experienced. Diphenoxylate is discontinued as soon as the diarrhea symptoms resolve.

Administration Alerts

- If administering to young children, measure the drug accurately by using the dropper packaged with the liquid form of the drug.
- Pregnancy category C.

PHARMACOKINETICS

Onset	Peak	Duration
45–60 min	2 h	3–4 h

Adverse Effects

Unlike most opioids, diphenoxylate has no analgesic properties and has a very low potential for abuse. The drug is well tolerated at normal doses. Some patients experience dizziness or drowsiness, and they should not drive or operate machinery until the effects of the drug are known.

Contraindications: Contraindications include hypersensitivity to the drug, severe liver disease, obstructive jaundice, severe dehydration or electrolyte imbalance, narrow-angle glaucoma, and diarrhea associated with PMC.

Interactions

Drug-Drug: Diphenoxylate with atropine interacts with other CNS depressants, including alcohol, to produce additive sedation. When taken with monoamine oxidase inhibitors (MAOIs), diphenoxylate may cause hypertensive crisis.

Lab Tests: Diphenoxylate with atropine may increase serum amylase.

Herbal/Food: Unknown.

Treatment of Overdose: Overdose with Lomotil may be serious. Narcotic antagonists such as naloxone may be administered parenterally to reverse respiratory depression within minutes.

(Lomotil). Diphenoxylate is a Schedule V controlled drug that acts directly on the intestine to slow peristalsis, thereby allowing more fluid and electrolyte absorption in the large intestine. The opioids cause CNS depression at high doses and are generally reserved for the short-term therapy of acute diarrhea because of the potential for dependence. Details on indications and adverse effects of opioids may be found in chapter 18.

OTC drugs for diarrhea act by a number of different mechanisms. Loperamide (Imodium) is similar to meperidine but it has no narcotic effects and is not classified as a controlled substance. Low-dose loperamide is available OTC; higher doses are available by prescription. Other OTC treatments include bismuth subsalicylate (Pepto-Bismol), which acts by binding and absorbing toxins. Psyllium preparations may also slow diarrhea because they absorb large amounts of fluid, which helps form bulkier stools. Probiotic supplements containing *Lactobacillus*, a normal inhabitant of the human gut and vagina, are sometimes taken to correct the altered GI flora following a serious diarrhea episode.

Antidiarrheal medications should never be used to treat diarrhea caused by poisoning or infection by toxin-producing organisms. For these patients, it is important that the toxic substances and organisms be expelled from the body. Use of antidiarrheals in these circumstances will retain these harmful substances in the body. Antidiarrheal use is contraindicated in cases of diarrhea caused by PMC that is caused by *Clostridium difficile*. This infection can cause fatal toxic megacolon.

☑ Check Your Understanding 42.1

What drug(s) may cause constipation or diarrhea? *Visit www.pearsonhighered.com/nursingresources for the answer.*

IRRITABLE BOWEL SYNDROME

Irritable bowel syndrome (IBS), also known as spastic colon or mucous colitis, is a common disorder of the lower GI tract. Symptoms include abdominal pain, bloating, excessive gas, and colicky cramping. Bowel habits are altered, with diarrhea

Evidence-Based Practice: Fecal Microbiota Transplant

Clinical Question: Can healthy intestinal flora be used to combat *Clostridium difficile* infection?

Evidence: The role that normal intestinal flora, or "intestinal microbiota," plays in maintaining body health and immunity is becoming more apparent and appreciated. Multiple organisms populate the intestinal tract. It has been found that the functions of these microorganisms include boosting immune protection against toxins produced by some pathogenic bacteria and guarding against septic shock. In addition, they may play a role in the prevention of obesity (Brandt, 2013). When normal intestinal flora is disrupted, such as by antibiotic therapy which kills beneficial organisms along with pathogenic, the pathogenic bacteria may overgrow and cause serious infection. *Clostridium difficile*, or "*C. dif.*," as it is commonly called, is a serious bowel infection that results from antibiotic therapy. It results in watery diarrhea that contains blood and pus. Dehydration may result quickly from fluid loss.

The standard treatment for *C. dif.* has included fluid replacement and the use of the antibiotic, vancomycin. Recently, research has explored the use of transplanting small amounts of healthy intestinal flora from a donor into a recipient with *C. dif.* associated diarrhea (CDAD), and the results are promising.

Fecal microbiota transplant (FMT) is accomplished by instilling small amounts of stool from a donor who has been prescreened for serious viral diseases (e.g., HIV, hepatitis), syphilis, ova and parasites, and colon cancer (Brandt, 2013). Instillation is accomplished by suspending the donor stool in liquid, then instilling it into the patient by enema, colonoscopy, or nasogastric tube (Brandt, 2013; Youngster et al., 2014). In recent studies, significant improvement was noted with resolution of the CDAD in 90 to 98% of patients (Baron & Kozarek, 2013; Brandt, 2013; Patel, Griesbach, DiBaise, & Orenstein, 2013; Youngster et al., 2014). It was also shown to be effective in cases of relapsing CDAD, and a second transplant proved successful in all but one patient (Pathak, Enuh, Patel, & Wickremesinghe, 2013). After analyzing the cost of FMT versus the traditional use of antibiotics, Konijeti, Sauk, Shrime, Gupta, and Ananthakrishnan (2014) found that the transplant was the most cost-efficient treatment.

Because the U.S. Food and Drug Administration (FDA) considers a drug to be a substance that produces a biologic response in the body and is used to diagnose, treat, cure, or prevent a disease or condition, FMT is currently considered a drug therapy. Because standardization of the administration exists, efforts are underway to reclassify FMT as a tissue transplant, which would allow health care providers more flexibility and timeliness for treating patients (Vyas, Aekka, & Vyas, 2015).

Nursing Implications: Patients with CDAD are often seriously ill and as FMT becomes more common and discussed in the media, some patients may turn to friends or family members for a "do it yourself" FMT (Brandt, 2013). It is essential that nurses help patients and their families to understand the importance of seeking treatment from a qualified health care provider, such as a gastroenterologist.

alternating with constipation, and there may be mucus in the stool. IBS is considered a functional bowel disorder, meaning that the normal operation of the digestive tract is impaired without the presence of detectable organic disease.

The diagnosis of IBS is sometimes one of exclusion, ruling out other diseases such as colon cancer, ulcerative colitis, intestinal infections, Crohn's disease, and diverticulitis. A diagnosis of IBS requires that the patient has experienced recurrent abdominal pain or discomfort for at least 3 days per month during the previous 3 months that is associated with two or more of the following:

- Relieved by defecation
- Onset associated with a change in stool frequency
- Onset associated with a change in stool form or appearance.

42.6 Pharmacotherapy of Irritable Bowel Syndrome

Because constipation and diarrhea often alternate in patients with IBS, pharmacotherapy can be challenging. Indeed, drugs used to treat IBS do not alter the course of the illness, and, in some cases, they may actually worsen patient symptoms. Research has not demonstrated that drugs are any more effective than nonpharmacologic treatments such as IBS support groups, relaxation therapy, or dietary changes. Most patients keep a diary to record "triggers" that induce IBS symptoms. Some triggers include caffeine, wheat products, lactose-based products, and foods that cause bloating such as beans or cabbage. Fiber supplements ease symptoms in some patients, and worsen symptoms in others. There is no prototype drug for this condition. Drug therapy of IBS is targeted at symptomatic treatment, depending on whether constipation or diarrhea is the predominant symptom. Table 42.3 lists drugs that are used to treat IBS.

Drugs that provide symptomatic relief for some patients with IBS include anticholinergics such as dicyclomine (Bentyl) and hyoscyamine (Anaspaz, Gastrosed), which act as antispasmodics to slow GI motility. Lubiprostone (Amitiza) is indicated for treating constipation-predominant IBS in women over age 18. Alosetron (Lotronex) is available for treating severe diarrhea in women over age 18 but only under a limited distribution program due to the potential for serious GI adverse effects.

A newer drug for IBS is linaclotide, which was approved in 2012 for the treatment of constipation-dominant IBS. Linaclotide accelerates fecal transport by drawing more water into the intestine. Linaclotide is contraindicated in children age 6 and younger.

Table 42.3 Selected Drugs for Inflammatory Bowel Disease and Irritable Bowel Syndrome

Drug	Route and Adult Dose (maximum dose where indicated)	Adverse Effects
FIRST-LINE DRUGS FOR INFLAMMATORY BOWEL DISEASE		
balsalazide (Colazal)	PO: 2.25 g tid for 8–12 wk (max: 6.75 g/day)	*Headache, abdominal pain, diarrhea, nausea, vomiting, rash, flulike illness, allergic reactions*
mesalamine (Apriso, Asacol, Canasa, Lialda, others)	PO (delayed-release tablets): 800 mg tid for 6 wk PO (delayed-release capsules): 1 g qid for 8 wk	Hepatotoxicity, blood dyscrasias, renal impairment, salicylate hypersensitivity, crystalluria (sulfasalazine)
olsalazine (Dipentum)	PO: 500 mg bid (max: 3 g/day)	
sulfasalazine (Azulfidine)	PO: 1–2 g/day in four divided doses (max: 8 g/day)	
DRUGS FOR IRRITABLE BOWEL SYNDROME		
alosetron (Lotronex)	PO: Begin with 1 mg daily for 4 wk; may increase to 1 mg bid (max: 2 mg/day)	*Constipation, abdominal discomfort, nausea, and rash* Ischemic colitis, ileus
dicyclomine (Bentyl)	PO: 20–40 mg qid (max: 160 mg/day IM: 80 mg/day	*Dry mouth, blurred vision, drowsiness, constipation, urinary hesitancy, and tachycardia* Confusion, paralytic ileus
hyoscyamine (Anaspaz, Gastrosed, Levsin)	PO: 0.15–0.3 mg one to four times/day	
eluxadoline (Viberzi)	PO: 100 mg bid	*Constipation, nausea, abdominal pain* Pancreatitis
linaclotide (Linzess)	PO: 145–290 mcg once daily	*Abdominal pain and distention, flatulence* Severe diarrhea
lubiprostone (Amitiza)	Chronic idiopathic constipation: PO: 24 mcg bid IBS with constipation: PO: 8 mcg bid (max: 48 mcg/day)	*Nausea, diarrhea, headache, dyspnea* Allergic reactions
rifaximin (Xifaxan)	PO: 550 mg tid	*Flatulence, headache, nausea, increase in alanine aminotransferase* Hypersensitivity

Note: Italics indicate common adverse effects; underlining indicates serious adverse effects.

For patients with diarrhea-predominant IBS, two new drugs were approved in 2015. Eluxadoline (Viberzi) acts on opioid receptors in the nervous system to lessen bowel contractions. The most common side effects of eluxadoline are constipation, nausea, and abdominal pain. Also approved in 2015, rifaximin (Xifaxan) is an antibiotic closely resembling rifampin, which was previously approved for traveler's diarrhea. It is believed that rifaximin changes the bacterial composition of the GI tract and reduces gas. The most common adverse effects are flatulence, headache, and abdominal pain.

INFLAMMATORY BOWEL DISEASE

Inflammatory bowel disease (IBD) is characterized by the presence of ulcers in the distal (terminal) portion of the small intestine (**Crohn's disease**) or mucosal erosions in the large intestine (**ulcerative colitis**). Over 1 million Americans are estimated to have IBD.

The etiology of IBD remains largely unknown. Several genes involved with immune responses have been identified as being associated with the disorder. It is believed that these defective genes cause hyperactivity of immune responses that result in chronic intestinal inflammation. In addition to genetic susceptibility, certain environmental triggers such as smoking, the use of nonsteroidal anti-inflammatory drugs (NSAIDs), and high levels of stress worsen symptoms of IBD.

Symptoms of IBD range from mild to acute, and the condition is often characterized by alternating periods of remission and exacerbation. The most common clinical presentation of ulcerative colitis is abdominal cramping with frequent bowel movements. Severe disease may result in weight loss, bloody diarrhea, high fever, and dehydration. The patient with Crohn's disease also presents with abdominal pain, cramping, and diarrhea, which may have been present for years before the patient sought treatment. Symptoms of Crohn's disease are sometimes similar to those of ulcerative colitis.

42.7 Pharmacotherapy of Inflammatory Bowel Disease

Multiple medications are used to treat IBD, and pharmacotherapy is conducted in a stepwise manner, starting with the safest and best established medications for the disorder. The expected outcomes for the pharmacotherapy of IBD are as follow:

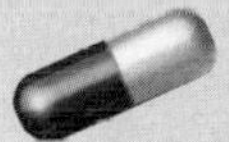

Prototype Drug | Sulfasalazine *(Azulfidine)*

Therapeutic Class: Drug for inflammatory bowel disease **Pharmacologic Class:** 5-aminosalicylate, sulfonamide

Actions and Uses

Sulfasalazine is an oral drug with anti-inflammatory properties that is approved to treat mild to moderate symptoms of ulcerative colitis for those age 6 and older. Sulfasalazine is used off-label to treat Crohn's disease. It is approved as an alternate drug in the pharmacotherapy of rheumatoid arthritis and is classified as a disease-modifying antirheumatic drug (DMARD) (see chapter 48).

Sulfasalazine inhibits mediators of inflammation in the colon such as prostaglandins and leukotrienes. Colon bacteria metabolize sulfasalazine to active metabolites. One of these metabolites, mesalamine, is available as an IBD drug.

Administration Alerts

- Do not administer this drug to patients who have allergies to sulfonamide antibiotics or furosemide (Lasix).
- This drug is not approved for children under age 2.
- Do not crush or chew extended-release tablets.
- Pregnancy category B.

PHARMACOKINETICS

Onset	Peak	Duration
Unknown	1.5–6 h	5–10 h

Adverse Effects

The most frequent adverse effects of sulfasalazine are GI related: nausea, vomiting, diarrhea, dyspepsia, and abdominal pain. Dividing the total daily dose evenly throughout the day and using the enteric-coated tablets may improve adherence. Headache is common. Blood dyscrasias occur infrequently during therapy. Skin rashes are relatively common and may be a sign of a more serious adverse effect such as Stevens–Johnson syndrome. The drug may impair male fertility, which reverses when the drug is discontinued. Sulfasalazine can cause photosensitivity.

Contraindications: Sulfasalazine is contraindicated in patients with sulfonamide or salicylate (aspirin or 5-ASA) hypersensitivity. Patients with pre-existing anemia, folate disorders, or other hematologic disorders should use the drug with caution because it may worsen blood dyscrasias. Sulfasalazine should be used with caution in patients with hepatic impairment because the drug can cause hepatotoxicity. The drug is contraindicated in patients with urinary obstruction and should be used with caution in dehydrated patients because it may cause crystalluria. Patients with diabetes or hypoglycemia should use sulfasalazine with caution because the drug can increase insulin secretion and worsen hypoglycemia.

Interactions

Drug–Drug: Sulfasalazine may worsen bone marrow suppression caused by methotrexate and also result in additive hepatotoxicity. Absorption of digoxin may be decreased. Sulfasalazine can displace warfarin from its protein binding sites, causing increased anticoagulant effects.

Lab Tests: Unknown.

Herbal/Food: Sulfasalazine may decrease the absorption of iron and folic acid.

Treatment of Overdose: Overdose will cause abdominal pain, anuria, drowsiness, gastric distress, nausea, seizures, and vomiting. Treatment is supportive.

- Reduce the acute symptoms of active disease by induction therapy, and place the disease in remission.
- Keep the disease in remission with maintenance therapy.
- Change the natural course or progression of the disease.

The first step of IBD treatment is usually with 5-aminosalicylic acid (5-ASA) medications. These include the sulfonamide sulfasalazine (Azulfidine), olsalazine (Dipentum), balsalazide (Colazal), and mesalamine (Asacol, Canasa, Lialda, others). For many patients, these drugs provide the most rapid symptom relief.

If the 5-ASA drugs fail to provide symptomatic relief, oral corticosteroids such as prednisone, methylprednisolone, or hydrocortisone are used. Budesonide (Entocort-EC, Uceris) is a corticosteroid with interesting properties that allow it to be used as a first-line therapy for IBD. Entocort EC is encapsulated to prevent significant absorption in the stomach or duodenum. The drug is released slowly and reaches a high concentration in the terminal ileum and proximal colon, the two most frequently affected sites for IBD. Thus, the drug is in direct contact with the GI mucosa and, in effect, it produces a *topical* anti-inflammatory effect. This drug shows few of the adverse effects seen with the long-term use of other corticosteroids. It is approved for mild to moderate Crohn's disease (Entocort-EC) and ulcerative colitis (Uceris).

If corticosteroid therapy fails to resolve symptoms, step 3 of IBD therapy includes immunosuppressant drugs such as azathioprine (Imuran) or methotrexate (MTX, Rheumatrex, Trexall). These drugs are not used for initial therapy because they have a 3-month onset of action; however, they are effective at extending the time between relapses.

Biologic therapies have given clinicians another valuable tool in the pharmacotherapy of IBD. Biologic therapies are currently recommended only when corticosteroid therapy is unable to control symptoms. Examples include the tumor necrosis factor (TNF) inhibitor infliximab (Remicade), which has been shown to effectively reduce acute symptoms and provide maintenance therapy for both Crohn's disease and ulcerative colitis. A second anti-TNF drug, adalimumab (Humira), is approved for Crohn's disease. A newer pegylated TNF inhibitor, certolizumab pegol (Cimzia), offers dosing at 2- to 4-week intervals. Natalizumab (Tysabri), a drug previously approved for multiple sclerosis, is now approved for treating Crohn's disease but it has potentially serious side effects. Similar in action to natalizumab but with fewer serious adverse effects, vedolizumab (Entyvio) was approved in 2014 to treat IBD. Vedolizumab is given intravenously (IV) for both the induction and remission phases of IBD. The biologic therapies are expensive and patients experience a much higher rate of serious infections due to their immunosuppressive actions.

Nursing Practice Application

Pharmacotherapy for Bowel Disorders

ASSESSMENT	POTENTIAL NURSING DIAGNOSES*
Baseline assessment prior to administration: • Obtain a complete health history including GI, cardiovascular, hepatic, or renal disease; pregnancy; or breast-feeding. Obtain a drug history including allergies, current prescription and OTC drugs, herbal preparations, caffeine, nicotine, and alcohol use. Be alert to possible drug interactions. • Obtain a history of past and current symptoms, noting what measures have been successful at relieving the symptoms (e.g., increased fluids, fiber, dietary changes). • Obtain baseline weight and vital signs. • Evaluate appropriate laboratory findings (e.g., complete blood count [CBC], electrolytes, hepatic or renal function studies). • Obtain an abdominal assessment (e.g., bowel sounds, firmness, distention, presence of tenderness).	• *Constipation* • *Diarrhea* • *Deficient Knowledge* (drug therapy) • *Risk for Deficient Fluid Volume* *NANDA I © 2014
Assessment throughout administration: • Assess for desired therapeutic effects (e.g., adequate pattern of elimination, normal stool consistency and volume). • Continue periodic monitoring of abdominal assessment findings, especially bowel sounds. • Continue periodic monitoring of CBC, electrolytes, and hepatic and renal function laboratory tests as appropriate. • Assess for adverse effects: nausea, vomiting, diarrhea, constipation, headache, drowsiness, and dizziness. Severe abdominal pain, coffee-ground or bloody vomiting, blood in stool, or tarry stools should be reported immediately.	

IMPLEMENTATION

Interventions and (Rationales)	Patient-Centered Care
Ensuring therapeutic effects: • Treat the cause if a definitive cause for the current symptoms can be identified (e.g., infection, food poisoning, inadequate fluid intake); correct the cause where possible. (Constipation and diarrhea are usually symptoms of other underlying conditions such as infections, inadequate fluid or fiber intake, stress, or sedentary lifestyle.)	• For recurrent constipation or diarrhea, encourage the patient to maintain a diary of correlations between symptoms and foods, beverages, stress, or medications to help identify causative factors.
• Encourage appropriate lifestyle changes. Have the patient keep a diary, noting correlations between symptoms and foods, beverages, stress, or medications. (Ensuring adequate amounts of daily fluids and dietary fiber, and increasing activity levels, assists in encouraging normal peristaltic activity. Correlating symptoms with medications or stress may help to identify a triggering factor.)	• Encourage the patient to adopt a healthy lifestyle of increased dietary fiber and fluid intake, increased intake of yogurt and probiotic-containing foods, stress management techniques, increased exercise, and limited or eliminated alcohol consumption and smoking. **Collaboration:** Provide for dietitian consultation or information on smoking cessation programs as needed. • Encourage the patient to keep a diary noting correlations between symptoms and foods, beverages, stress, or medications.

Nursing Practice Application *continued*

IMPLEMENTATION	
Interventions and (Rationales)	**Patient-Centered Care**
• Follow appropriate administration guidelines. Do not administer laxatives if bowel obstruction is possible. Do not administer antidiarrheal drugs if infection is possible. (Bowel obstruction must be ruled out in the presence of hypoactive or absent bowel sounds. If infection is suspected, giving antidiarrheal drugs may decrease peristalsis giving the infection an opportunity to increase and spread.)	• Teach the patient to take the drug following appropriate guidelines or label directions, particularly for any additional fluid intake required, for best results. • Instruct the patient that diarrhea or constipation associated with increasing nausea or vomiting, especially if accompanied by abdominal pain, should be reported to the health care provider before taking the drug.
Minimizing adverse effects:	
• Continue to monitor abdominal assessment findings. (Any significant change in bowel sound activity or increased discomfort or pain may signal the development of worsening bowel disease or of adverse drug effects.)	• Teach the patient that some easing of discomfort related to constipation or diarrhea may be noticed soon after beginning drug therapy but the full effects may take several days or longer. If gastric discomfort or pain continue or worsen, the health care provider should be notified.
• Monitor for any severe abdominal pain, vomiting, coffee-ground or bloody emesis, blood in stool, or tarry stools. (Severe abdominal pain or blood in emesis or stools may indicate a worsening of disease or more serious conditions and should be reported immediately.)	• Teach the patient that severe abdominal pain or any blood in emesis or stools should be reported immediately to the health care provider.
• Observe for dizziness, and monitor ambulation until the effects of the drug are known. Obtain electrolyte levels if dizziness continues. (Drowsiness or dizziness from opioid-based or related antidiarrheals may occur. **Lifespan:** The older adult is at increased risk of falls. Continued dizziness may indicate electrolyte imbalance.)	• **Safety:** Instruct the patient to call for assistance prior to getting out of bed or attempting to walk alone if dizziness or drowsiness occurs. Provide a commode or bedpan nearby. For home use, instruct the patient to avoid driving or other activities requiring mental alertness or physical coordination until the effects of the drug are known.
• Continue to monitor periodic hepatic and renal function tests and electrolyte levels as needed. (Abnormal liver function tests may indicate drug-induced adverse hepatic effects. Excessive use of laxatives or continued diarrhea may affect electrolyte levels.)	• Instruct the patient on the need to return periodically for laboratory work.
• Monitor vital signs, particularly respiratory rate and depth, on patients who are taking opioid or opioid-related drugs. (Opioids may decrease respiratory rate and depth. Intervention with narcotic antagonists may be needed if overdose occurs.)	• Teach the patient to take the drug as ordered and not to increase the dose or frequency unless instructed to do so by the health care provider. Any drowsiness, dizziness, or disorientation should be promptly reported to the provider.
Patient understanding of drug therapy:	
• Use opportunities during administration of medications and during assessments to provide patient education. (Using time during nursing care helps to optimize and reinforce key teaching areas.)	• The patient, family, or caregiver should be able to state the reason for the drug; appropriate dose and scheduling; what adverse effects to observe for and when to report; and the anticipated length of medication therapy.
Patient self-administration of drug therapy:	
• When administering the medication, instruct the patient, family, or caregiver in the proper self-administration of the drug (e.g., taken with additional fluids). (Proper administration increases the effectiveness of the drug.)	• Teach the patient on laxatives to take the drug according to appropriate guidelines, as follows: • *All laxative drugs:* Take the drug with additional fluids and increase fluid intake throughout the day. Increase the intake of dietary fiber. Exceeding the recommended dose or frequent laxative use increases the risk of adverse effects and decreases normal peristalsis over time, resulting in laxative dependence. • *Bulk-forming laxatives:* Take other medications 1 hour before or 2 hours after the laxative. Powdered formulations should be mixed with a full glass of liquid and immediately taken, followed by an additional full glass of liquid. Powders should never be swallowed dry as esophageal obstruction may result.

See Tables 42.1, 42.2, and 42.3 for a list of drugs to which these nursing actions apply.

NAUSEA AND VOMITING

Nausea is an unpleasant, subjective sensation that is accompanied by weakness, diaphoresis, and hyperproduction of saliva. It is sometimes accompanied by dizziness. Intense nausea often leads to vomiting, or **emesis.**

42.8 Pathophysiology of Nausea and Vomiting

Vomiting is a defense mechanism used by the body to rid itself of toxic substances. Vomiting is a reflex primarily controlled by the vomiting center of the medulla of the brain, which receives sensory signals from the digestive tract, the inner ear, and the **chemoreceptor trigger zone (CTZ)** in the cerebral cortex. Interestingly, the CTZ is not protected by the blood–brain barrier, as is the vast majority of the brain; thus, these neurons can directly sense the presence of toxic substances in the blood. Once the vomiting reflex is triggered, wavelike contractions of the stomach quickly propel its contents upward and out of the body.

The treatment outcomes for nausea or vomiting focus on removal of the cause, whenever feasible. Nausea and vomiting are common symptoms associated with a wide variety of conditions such as GI infections, food poisoning, nervousness, emotional imbalances, motion sickness, and extreme pain. Other conditions that promote nausea and vomiting are general anesthetics, migraines, trauma to the head or abdominal organs, inner ear disorders, and diabetes. Psychological factors play a significant role, as patients often become nauseated during periods of extreme stress or when confronted with unpleasant sights, smells, or sounds.

The nausea and vomiting experienced by women during the first trimester of pregnancy is referred to as morning sickness. If this condition becomes acute, with continual vomiting, it may lead to *hyperemesis gravidarum*, a situation in which the health and safety of the mother and developing baby can become compromised. Pharmacotherapy is initiated after other antinausea measures have proved ineffective.

Nausea and vomiting are the most frequently listed adverse effects for oral medications. Nurses should remember that because the vomiting center lies in the brain, nausea and vomiting may occur with parenteral formulations as well as with oral drugs. The most extreme example of this occurs with the antineoplastic drugs, most of which cause intense nausea and vomiting regardless of the route they are administered. The capacity of a chemotherapeutic drug to cause vomiting is called its **emetogenic potential.** Nausea and vomiting is a common reason for patients' lack of compliance with the therapeutic regimen and for discontinuation of drug therapy.

When large amounts of fluids are vomited, dehydration and significant weight loss may occur. Because the contents lost from the stomach are strongly acidic, vomiting may cause a change in the pH of the blood, resulting in metabolic alkalosis. With excessive loss, severe acid–base disturbances can lead to vascular collapse, resulting in death if medical intervention is not initiated. Dehydration is especially dangerous for infants, small children, and older adults and is evidenced by dry mouth, sticky saliva, and reduced urine output that is dark yellow-orange to brown.

Antiemetics

Drugs from at least eight different classes are used to prevent nausea and vomiting. Many of these act by inhibiting dopamine or serotonin receptors in the brain. The antiemetics are listed in Table 42.4.

42.9 Pharmacotherapy With Antiemetics

A large number of **antiemetics** are available to treat nausea and vomiting. Selection of a particular agent depends on the experience of the health care provider and the cause of the nausea and vomiting. Patients seeking self-treatment can find several options available OTC. For example, simple nausea and vomiting is sometimes relieved by antacids or diphenhydramine (Benadryl). Herbal options include peppermint and ginger, the most popular herbal therapies for nausea and vomiting. Relief of serious nausea or vomiting, however, requires prescription medications. Patients who are receiving antineoplastic drugs may receive three or more antiemetics concurrently to reduce the nausea and vomiting from chemotherapy. In fact, therapy with antineoplastic drugs is one of the most common reasons for prescribing antiemetic drugs.

Serotonin (5-HT_3) Antagonists

The serotonin antagonists include dolasetron (Anzemet), granisetron (Kytril, Sancuso), ondansetron (Zofran, Zuplenz), and palonosetron (Aloxi). These are preferred drugs for the pharmacotherapy of serious nausea and vomiting caused by antineoplastic therapy, radiation therapy, or surgical procedures. They are usually given prophylactically, just prior to antineoplastic therapy. IV, oral, transdermal patches, orally-disintegrating tablets, and oral soluble film formulations are available. The few adverse effects include headache, constipation or diarrhea, and dizziness.

Antihistamines and Anticholinergics

These drugs are effective for treating simple nausea, with some being available OTC. For example, nausea due to motion sickness is effectively treated with anticholinergics or antihistamines. Motion sickness is a disorder affecting a portion of the inner ear that is associated with significant nausea. The most common drug used for motion sickness is scopolamine (Transderm Scop), which is usually administered as a transdermal patch. Antihistamines such as dimenhydrinate (Dramamine) and meclizine (Antivert) are also effective but may cause significant drowsiness in some patients. Drugs used to treat motion sickness are most effective when taken 20 to 60 minutes before travel is expected.

Table 42.4 Selected Antiemetics

Drug	Route and Adult Dose (max dose where indicated)	Adverse Effects
ANTICHOLINERGICS AND ANTIHISTAMINES		
cyclizine (Marezine)	PO: 50 mg q4–6h (max: 200 mg/day)	*Drowsiness, dry mouth, blurred vision (scopolamine)*
dimenhydrinate (Dramamine, others)	PO: 50–100 mg q4–6h (max: 400 mg/day)	Hypersensitivity reaction, sedation, tremors, seizures, hallucinations, paradoxical excitation (more common in children), hypotension
diphenhydramine (Benadryl, others) (see page 645 for the Prototype Drug box)	PO: 25–50 mg tid–qid (max: 300 mg/day)	
doxylamine with pyridoxine (Diclegis)	PO: 20–40 mg daily	
hydroxyzine (Atarax, Vistaril)	PO: 25–100 mg tid–qid	
meclizine (Antivert, Bonine, others)	PO: 25–50 mg/day, taken 1 h before travel (max: 50 mg/day)	
scopolamine (Hyoscine, Transderm-Scop)	Transdermal patch: 0.5 mg q72h	
BENZODIAZEPINE		
lorazepam (Ativan) (see page 171 for the Prototype Drug box)	IV: 1–1.5 mg prior to chemotherapy PO: 2–6 mg/day in divided doses	*Dizziness, drowsiness, ataxia, fatigue, slurred speech* Paradoxical excitation (more common in children), seizures (if abruptly discontinued), coma
CANNABINOIDS		
dronabinol (Marinol)	PO: 5 mg/m^2 1–3 h before administration of chemotherapy (max: 15 mg/m^2)	*Dizziness, drowsiness, euphoria, confusion, ataxia, asthenia, increased sensory awareness*
nabilone (Cesamet)	PO: 1–2 mg bid	Paranoia, decreased motor coordination, hypotension
CORTICOSTEROIDS		
dexamethasone (Decadron)	PO: 0.25–4 mg bid–qid	*Mood swings, weight gain, acne, facial flushing, nausea, insomnia, sodium and fluid retention, impaired wound healing, menstrual abnormalities, insomnia* Peptic ulcer, hypocalcemia, osteoporosis with possible bone fractures, loss of muscle mass, decreased growth in children, possible masking of infections
methylprednisolone (Medrol, Solu-Medrol, others)	PO: 4–48 mg/day in divided doses	
NEUROKININ RECEPTOR ANTAGONIST		
aprepitant (Emend, Fosaprepitant)	PO: 125 mg 1 h prior to chemotherapy	*Fatigue, constipation, diarrhea, anorexia, nausea, hiccups* Dehydration, peripheral neuropathy, blood dyscrasias, pneumonia
PHENOTHIAZINE AND PHENOTHIAZINE-LIKE DRUGS		
metoclopramide (Reglan)	PO: 2 mg/kg 1 h prior to chemotherapy	*Dry eyes, blurred vision, dry mouth, constipation, drowsiness, photosensitivity* Extrapyramidal symptoms (EPS), neuroleptic malignant syndrome, agranulocytosis
perphenazine (Phenazine, Trilafon)	PO: 8–16 mg bid–qid	
prochlorperazine (Compazine)	PO: 5–10 mg tid–qid	
promethazine (Phenergan, others)	PO: 12. 5–25 mg every 4 h qid	
trimethobenzamide (Tigan)	PO: 300 mg once daily IM: 200 mg tid–qid	
SEROTONIN RECEPTOR ANTAGONISTS		
dolasetron (Anzemet)	PO: 100 mg 1 h prior to chemotherapy	*Headache, drowsiness, fatigue, constipation, diarrhea* Dysrhythmias, EPS
granisetron (Kytril, Sancuso)	PO: 2 mg/day 1 h prior to chemotherapy IV: 10 mcg/kg 30 min prior to chemotherapy Transdermal patch: 1 patch 24–48 h prior to chemotherapy	
ondansetron (Zofran, Zuplenz)	PO: 4 mg tid prn IV: 32 mg single dose or three 0.15 mg/kg doses 30 min prior to chemotherapy Oral film or disintegrating tablet: three 8 mg doses 30 min prior to chemotherapy	
palonosetron (Aloxi)	PO: 0.5 mg single dose 1 h prior to chemotherapy IV: 0.25 mg 30 min prior to chemotherapy	

Note: Italics indicate common adverse effects; underlining indicates serious adverse effects.

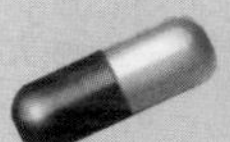

Prototype Drug | Prochlorperazine *(Compazine)*

Therapeutic Class: Antiemetic **Pharmacologic Class:** Phenothiazine antipsychotic

Actions and Uses

Prochlorperazine is a phenothiazine, a class of drugs usually prescribed for psychoses. The phenothiazines are the largest group of drugs prescribed for severe nausea and vomiting, and prochlorperazine is the most frequently prescribed antiemetic in its class. Prochlorperazine acts by blocking dopamine receptors in the brain, which inhibits signals to the vomiting center in the medulla. As an antiemetic, it is frequently given by the rectal route, where absorption is rapid. It is also available in tablet, extended-release capsule, and IM formulations.

Administration Alerts

- Administer 2 hours before or after antacids and antidiarrheals.
- Pregnancy category C.

PHARMACOKINETICS

Onset	Peak	Duration
30–40 min PO; 60 min rectal	Unknown	3–4 h PO or rectal

Adverse Effects

Prochlorperazine produces dose-related anticholinergic side effects such as dry mouth, sedation, constipation, orthostatic hypotension, and tachycardia. When used for prolonged periods at higher doses, extrapyramidal symptoms resembling those of Parkinson's disease are a serious concern, especially in older patients.

Black Box Warning (for all conventional phenothiazines)**:** Older patients with dementia who are treated with conventional phenothiazines are at an increased risk of death compared to placebo.

Contraindications: This drug should not be used in patients with hypersensitivity to phenothiazines, in comatose patients, or in the presence of profound CNS depression. It is also contraindicated in children younger than age 2 or weighing less than 20 lb. Patients with narrow-angle glaucoma, bone marrow suppression, or severe hepatic or cardiac impairment should not take this drug.

Interactions

Drug–Drug: Prochlorperazine interacts with alcohol and other CNS depressants to cause additive sedation. Antacids and antidiarrheals inhibit the absorption of prochlorperazine. When taken with phenobarbital, metabolism of prochlorperazine is increased. Use with tricyclic antidepressants may produce increased anticholinergic and hypotensive effects.

Lab Tests: Unknown.

Herbal/Food: Unknown.

Treatment of Overdose: Overdose may result in serious CNS depression and EPS. Patients may be treated with antiparkinsonism drugs (for EPS) and possibly a CNS stimulant such as dextroamphetamine.

Phenothiazine and Phenothiazine-like Drugs

The major indication for phenothiazines relates to treating psychoses, but they are also very effective antiemetics. The serious nausea and vomiting associated with antineoplastic therapy is sometimes treated with the phenothiazines. To prevent loss of the antiemetic medication due to vomiting, some of these medications are available through the intramuscular (IM), IV, and suppository routes. Nonphenothiazine antipsychotics that have high antiemetic activity include haloperidol (Haldol) and droperidol (Inapsine).

Corticosteroids

Dexamethasone (Decadron) and methylprednisolone (Solu-Medrol) are used to prevent chemotherapy-induced and postsurgical nausea and vomiting. They are reserved for the short-term therapy of acute cases because of the potential for serious long-term adverse effects.

Other Antiemetics

Aprepitant (Emend, Fosaprepitant) and netupitant belong to a class of antiemetics called neurokinin receptor antagonists, which are used to prevent nausea and vomiting following surgery or antineoplastic therapy. Netupitant with palonosetron was approved in 2014 with the trade name of (Akynzeo). The benzodiazepine lorazepam (Ativan) has the advantage of promoting relaxation along with having antiemetic properties. Cannabinoids are drugs that contain the same active ingredient as marijuana. Dronabinol (Marinol) and nabilone (Cesamet) are given orally (PO) to produce antiemetic effects and relaxation without the euphoria produced by marijuana. Dronabinol and nabilone are Schedule II controlled drugs.

Emetics

On some occasions, it is desirable to *stimulate* the vomiting reflex with drugs called **emetics.** Indications for emetics include ingestion of poisons and overdoses of oral drugs. Ipecac syrup, given orally, or apomorphine, given subcutaneously, will induce vomiting in about 15 minutes.

Nursing Practice Application

Pharmacotherapy With Antiemetic Drugs

ASSESSMENT	POTENTIAL NURSING DIAGNOSES*
Baseline assessment prior to administration: • Obtain a complete health history including GI, cardiovascular, hepatic, or renal disease; pregnancy; or breast-feeding. Obtain a drug history including allergies, current prescription and OTC drugs, herbal preparations, caffeine, nicotine, and alcohol use. Be alert to possible drug interactions. • Obtain baseline weight and vital signs, especially blood pressure and pulse. • Evaluate appropriate laboratory findings (e.g., electrolytes, glucose, CBC, hepatic or renal function studies). • Obtain an abdominal assessment (e.g., bowel sounds, firmness, distention, presence of tenderness). • Assess emesis for amount, color, and presence of blood.	• *Deficient Fluid Volume* • *Deficient Knowledge* (drug therapy) • *Risk for Falls,* related to adverse drug effects • *Risk for Injury,* related to adverse drug effects *NANDA I © 2014
Assessment throughout administration: • Assess for desired therapeutic effects (e.g., nausea is decreased, no vomiting is present, is able to tolerate fluids and increasing solids). • Continue to monitor and measure any emesis. Assess urine output and maintain intake and output measurements in the hospitalized patient. • Monitor vital signs, especially blood pressure and pulse, and report any hypotension or tachycardia to the health care provider. • Continue periodic monitoring of abdominal assessment findings, especially bowel sounds. • Continue periodic monitoring of electrolytes, glucose, CBC, and hepatic and renal function laboratory findings as appropriate. • Assess for adverse effects: headache, drowsiness, dizziness, dry mouth, blurred vision, and fatigue. Continued vomiting, severe nausea, emesis with blood present or coffee-ground appearance, hypotension, tachycardia, or confusion should be reported immediately.	

IMPLEMENTATION

Interventions and (Rationales)	Patient-Centered Care
Ensuring therapeutic effects:	
• Treat the cause if a definitive cause for the current symptoms can be identified (e.g., infection, adverse drug effects); correct the cause where possible. (Nausea and vomiting are often symptoms of other underlying conditions such as adverse drug effects or infections.)	• Review medications, foods, and the possibility of illness with the patient, family, or caregiver to help identify causative factors. • Decrease noxious stimuli (e.g., strong odors, rapid changes in position) that may increase nausea or vomiting.
• Encourage a small amount of fluids or ice chips and decrease activity level while nauseated; eliminate alcohol intake; limit or cease smoking; and increase intake of yogurt and acidophilus-containing foods after nausea has ceased. (These interventions may help ease symptoms during the acute phase. Ensuring adequate amounts of fluids, including IV fluids if necessary, will help maintain a normal fluid balance. Smoking and alcohol use cause gastric irritation.)	• Encourage the patient to limit physical movement or activity during periods of acute nausea or vomiting. Encourage increasing fluid intake gradually with ice chips or small sips of water. Ginger ale may act as a natural antinausea beverage and may be palatable for some patients.
• Administer antiemetics 30 to 60 minutes before anticipated nausea-inducing travel or drug administration (e.g., chemotherapy). Ensure adequate hydration prior to the onset of anticipated nausea. (Antiemetics are most effective when taken before nausea occurs. Ensuring adequate prehydration decreases the risk of dehydration should vomiting occur.)	• Teach the patient to take the antiemetic before travel if nausea is anticipated. Encourage the patient to consider a trial run by taking the medication in the evening before bedtime to ascertain its effects prior to taking it if driving is required. • Teach the patient on at-home chemotherapy to take antiemetics prior to chemotherapy dose or routinely as ordered by the health care provider.

continued

Nursing Practice Application *continued*

IMPLEMENTATION	
Interventions and (Rationales)	**Patient-Centered Care**
Minimizing adverse effects: • Monitor vital signs, particularly blood pressure and pulse. Take blood pressure lying, sitting, and standing to detect orthostatic hypotension. **Lifespan:** Be cautious with older adults who are at an increased risk for hypotension. Report any hypotension, especially associated with tachycardia, immediately. (Excessive vomiting may cause dehydration and decreased blood pressure or hypotension, or electrolyte imbalance. Anticholinergics, antihistamines, and phenothiazine or phenothiazine-like drugs may also decrease blood pressure.)	• **Safety:** Teach the patient to rise from lying or sitting to standing slowly to avoid dizziness or falls. If dizziness occurs, the patient should sit or lie down and not attempt to stand or walk, until the sensation passes.
• Continue to monitor abdominal assessment findings. Immediately report any significant increase or decrease in bowel sounds, distention, new onset or increase in discomfort or pain, severe abdominal pain, or vomiting that is coffee-ground in consistency or contains blood. (Increasing or severe abdominal pain or blood in emesis may indicate a worsening of the disease.)	• Teach the patient to report any increasing gastric discomfort or pain. • Instruct the patient that severe abdominal pain or any blood in emesis should be reported immediately to the health care provider.
• Continue to monitor periodic electrolyte, glucose levels, and hepatic and renal function tests as needed. (Loss of electrolytes may occur with severe vomiting. Abnormal liver function tests may indicate drug-induced adverse hepatic effects.)	• Instruct the patient on the need for laboratory work.
• Monitor intake and output in the hospitalized patient. Initiate IV fluid replacement when indicated. Hold oral fluids until acute vomiting has ceased and then gradually increase fluid intake, beginning with small sips of water or ice chips. (Continuing oral intake may worsen nausea and vomiting. Gradually resuming fluids will allow for hydration without stimulating nausea. IV fluid replacement may be required if fluid loss has been severe and dehydration is present.)	• Instruct the patient on the need to withhold fluids and food until vomiting has ceased. Initiate incremental increases in intake beginning with small sips of water and clear fluids. • Explain the rationale for any IV hydration required and any equipment used.
• **Lifespan:** If pregnancy is suspected or confirmed, hold the antiemetic until after consulting with the health care provider. (Alternative antinausea measures should be used to ease nausea when possible. The drug's pregnancy class and the pregnancy trimester will be considered by the health care provider before prescribing.)	• If the patient is pregnant, or if pregnancy is suspected, teach the patient to consult with the health care provider before taking any antiemetic drug for morning sickness. • Encourage the use of nondrug measures such as dry and unsweetened cereals or crackers taken in small amounts and avoiding noxious stimuli during periods of nausea. Ginger ale may aid in diminishing nausea.
Patient understanding of drug therapy: • Use opportunities during the administration of medications and during assessments to provide patient education. (Using time during nursing care helps to optimize and reinforce key teaching areas.)	• The patient, family, or caregiver should be able to state the reason for the drug; appropriate dose and scheduling; what adverse effects to observe for and when to report; and the anticipated length of medication therapy.
Patient self-administration of drug therapy: • When administering the medication, instruct the patient, family, or caregiver in the proper self-administration of the drug (e.g., taken with small sips of fluid). (Proper administration increases the effectiveness of the drugs.)	• The patient, family, or caregiver is able to discuss appropriate dosing and administration needs.

See Table 42.4 for a list of drugs to which these nursing actions apply.

PANCREATITIS

The pancreas secretes essential digestive enzymes: Pancreatic juice contains carboxypeptidase, chymotrypsin, and trypsin, which are converted to their active forms once they reach the small intestine. Three other pancreatic enzymes—lipase, amylase, and nuclease—are secreted in their active form but require the presence of bile for optimal activity. Because lack of secretion will result in malabsorption disorders, replacement therapy is sometimes warranted.

Pancreatitis results when digestive enzymes remain in the pancreas rather than being released into the

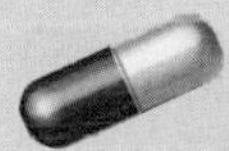

Prototype Drug | Pancrelipase (*Creon, Pancreaze, others)*

Therapeutic Class: Pancreatic enzymes **Pharmacologic Class:** None

Actions and Uses

Pancrelipase contains lipase, protease, and amylase of pork origin and is used as replacement therapy for patients with insufficient pancreatic exocrine secretions, including those with pancreatitis and cystic fibrosis. Given PO, the capsule dissolves in the alkaline environment of the duodenum and releases its enzymes. The enzymes act locally in the GI tract and are not absorbed. Pancrelipase is available in powder, tablet, and delayed-release capsule formulations.

The different trade names of pancrelipase are not interchangeable because the amounts of pancreatic enzymes in each product may vary. Dose is based on the amount of fat in the diet. Doses are taken just prior to meals or with meals.

Administration Alerts

- Do not crush or open enteric-coated tablets.
- Powder formulations may be sprinkled on food.
- Give the drug 1–2 hours before or with meals, or as directed by the health care provider.
- Pregnancy category C.

PHARMACOKINETICS

Onset	Peak	Duration
Immediate	Unknown	Unknown

Adverse Effects

Adverse effects of pancrelipase are uncommon, because the enzymes are not absorbed. The most frequent adverse effects are GI symptoms of nausea, vomiting, and diarrhea. Very high doses are associated with a risk for hyperuricemia.

Contraindications: Pancrelipase is contraindicated in patients who are allergic to the drug or to pork products. The delayed-release products should not be given to patients with acute pancreatitis.

Interactions

Drug–Drug: Pancrelipase interacts with iron, which may result in decreased absorption of iron. Antacids may decrease the effect of pancrelipase.

Lab Tests: Pancrelipase may increase serum or urinary levels of uric acid.

Herbal/Food: Unknown.

Treatment of Overdose: High levels of uric acid may occur with overdose. Patients are treated symptomatically.

duodenum. The enzymes escape into the surrounding tissue, causing inflammation in the pancreas. Pancreatitis can be either acute or chronic.

Acute pancreatitis usually occurs in middle-aged adults and is often associated with gallstones in women and alcoholism in men. Symptoms of acute pancreatitis present suddenly, often after eating a fatty meal or consuming excessive amounts of alcohol. The most common symptom is a continuous severe pain in the epigastric area that often radiates to the back. The patient usually recovers from the illness and regains normal function of the pancreas. Some patients with acute pancreatitis have recurring attacks and progress to chronic pancreatitis.

Many patients with acute pancreatitis require only bed rest and withholding food and fluids by mouth for a few days for the symptoms to subside. In more serious cases, aggressive IV fluid therapy is necessary to replace fluids lost to the intra-abdominal area. For patients with acute pain, opioid analgesics may be administered to bring effective relief. In particularly severe cases, total parenteral nutrition may be necessary. Once the acute symptoms have subsided, diagnostic tests are performed to determine the cause of the pancreatitis.

The majority of chronic pancreatitis is associated with alcoholism. Alcohol is thought to promote the formation of insoluble proteins that occlude the pancreatic duct. Pancreatic juice is prevented from flowing into the duodenum and remains in the pancreas to damage cells and cause inflammation. Symptoms include chronic epigastric or left upper quadrant pain, anorexia, nausea, vomiting, and weight loss. **Steatorrhea,** the passing of bulky, foul-smelling fatty stools, occurs late in the course of the disease. Chronic pancreatitis eventually leads to pancreatic insufficiency that may necessitate insulin therapy as well as replacement of pancreatic enzymes.

42.10 Pharmacotherapy of Pancreatitis

Drugs prescribed for the treatment of acute pancreatitis may also be used for patients with chronic pancreatitis. Opioid analgesics, IV fluids, insulin, and antiemetics may be necessary. Oral pancreatic enzyme supplementation is often used in patients with chronic pancreatitis. Pancrelipase (Creon, Pancreaze, others) is administered to help digest fats and prevent steatorrhea.

Chapter Review

KEY Concepts

The numbered key concepts provide a succinct summary of the important points from the corresponding numbered section within the chapter. If any of these points are not clear, refer to the numbered section within the chapter for review.

42.1 The small intestine is the location for most nutrient and drug absorption. The large intestine is responsible for the reabsorption of water.

42.2 Constipation, the infrequent passage of hard, small stools, is a common condition caused by insufficient dietary fiber and slow motility of waste material through the large intestine.

42.3 Laxatives and cathartics are drugs given to promote emptying of the large intestine by adding more bulk or water to the colon contents, lubricating the fecal mass, or stimulating peristalsis.

42.4 Diarrhea is an increase in the frequency and fluidity of bowel movements that occurs when the colon fails to reabsorb enough water.

42.5 For simple diarrhea, OTC medications such as loperamide or bismuth subsalicylate are effective. Opioids are the most effective drugs for controlling severe diarrhea.

42.6 Drugs for irritable bowel syndrome (IBS) are targeted at symptomatic treatment, depending on whether constipation or diarrhea is the predominant symptom.

42.7 Treatment for inflammatory bowel disease (IBD) includes 5-aminosalicylic acid (5-ASA) drugs, corticosteroids, and immunosuppressants.

42.8 Nausea and vomiting are common symptoms associated with a wide variety of conditions such as GI infections, food poisoning, nervousness, emotional imbalances, motion sickness, and extreme pain. Many oral drugs can cause nausea and vomiting as side effects.

42.9 Symptomatic treatment of nausea and vomiting includes drugs from many different classes, including serotonin receptor antagonists, antihistamines, anticholinergics, phenothiazines, corticosteroids, neurokinin receptor antagonists, benzodiazepines, and cannabinoids. Emetics are used on some occasions to stimulate the vomiting reflex.

42.10 Pancreatitis results when pancreatic enzymes remain in the pancreas rather than being released into the duodenum. Pharmacotherapy includes replacement enzymes and supportive drugs for reduction of pain and gastric acid secretion.

REVIEW Questions

1. A patient with constipation is prescribed psyllium (Metamucil) by his health care provider. What essential teaching will the nurse provide to the patient?
   1. Take the drug with meals and at bedtime.
   2. Take the drug with minimal water so that it will not be diluted in the GI tract.
   3. Avoid caffeine and chocolate while taking this drug.
   4. Mix the product in a full glass of water and drink another glassful after taking the drug.

2. A patient with severe diarrhea has an order for diphenoxylate with atropine (Lomotil). When assessing for therapeutic effects, which of the following will the nurse expect to find?
   1. Increased bowel sounds
   2. Decreased belching and flatus
   3. Decrease in loose, watery stools
   4. Decreased abdominal cramping

3. A 24-year-old patient has been taking sulfasalazine (Azulfidine) for irritable bowel syndrome and complains to the nurse that he wants to stop taking the drug because of the nausea, headaches, and abdominal pain it causes. What would the nurse's best recommendation be for this patient?
   1. The drug is absolutely necessary, even with the adverse effects.
   2. Talk to the health care provider about dividing the doses throughout the day.
   3. Stop taking the drug and see if the symptoms of the irritable bowel syndrome have resolved.
   4. Take an antidiarrheal drug such as loperamide (Imodium) along with the sulfasalazine.
4. The nurse is preparing to administer chemotherapy to an oncology patient who also has an order for ondansetron (Zofran). When should the nurse administer the odansetron?
   1. Every time the patient complains of nausea
   2. 30 to 60 minutes before starting the chemotherapy
   3. Only if the patient complains of nausea
   4. When the patient begins to experience vomiting during the chemotherapy
5. Pancrelipase (Pancreaze) granules are ordered for a patient. Which of the following will the nurse complete before administering the drug? (Select all that apply.)
   1. Sprinkle the granules on a nonacidic food.
   2. Give the granules with or just before a meal.
   3. Mix the granules with orange or grapefruit juice.
   4. Ask the patient about an allergy to pork or pork products.
   5. Administer the granules followed by an antacid.
6. The nurse has administered prochlorperazine (Compazine) to a patient for postoperative nausea. Before administering this medication, it is essential that the nurse check which of the following?
   1. Pain level
   2. Blood pressure
   3. Breath sounds
   4. Temperature

PATIENT-FOCUSED Case Study

Jerry Nobal is a 59-year old manager at a local golf center. He has been prescribed diphenoxylate with atropine (Lomotil) for continual diarrhea for the past 3 days. He has taken the drug consistently, but he returns to his provider stating that he has had diarrhea five times today.

1. What is a possible rationale for Jerry's continuing diarrhea?
2. What is the key priority for nursing care? What are additional needs that Jerry may have?

CRITICAL THINKING Questions

1. An older adult patient has been ordered prochlorperazine (Compazine) for treatment of nausea and vomiting associated with a bowel obstruction, pending planned surgery. The nurse is preparing the plan of care for this patient. What should be included in the plan?
2. A patient comes to the clinic complaining of no bowel movement for 4 days (other than small amounts of liquid stool). The patient has been taking psyllium mucilloid (Metamucil) for his constipation and wants to know why it is not working. What is the nurse's response?

Visit www.pearsonhighered.com/nursingresources for answers and rationales for all activities.

REFERENCES

Baron, T. H., & Kozarek, R. A. (2013). Fecal microbiota transplant: We know its history, but can we predict its future? *Mayo Clinic Proceedings, 88*, 782–785. doi:10.1016/j.mayocp.2013.06.007

Brandt, L. J. (2013). American Journal of Gastroenterology lecture: Intestinal microbiota and the role of fecal microbiota transplant (FMT) in treatment of *C. difficile* infection. *American Journal of Gastroenterology, 108*, 177–185. doi:10.1038/ajg.2012.450

Hempel, S., Newberry, S. J., Maher, A. R., Wang, Z., Miles, J., Shanman, R., . . . Shekelle, P. G. (2012). Probiotics for the prevention and treatment of antibiotic-associated diarrhea: A systematic review and meta-analysis. *JAMA: The Journal of the American Medical Association, 307*, 1959–1969. doi:10.1001/jama.2012.3507

Herdman, T. H., & Kamitsuru, S. (Eds.). (2014). *NANDA International nursing diagnoses: Definitions and classification, 2015–2017*. Oxford, United Kingdom: Wiley-Blackwell

Konijeti, G. G., Sauk, J., Shrime, M. G., Gupta, M., & Ananthakrishnan, A. N. (2014). Cost-effectiveness of competing strategies for management of recurrent *Clostridium difficile* infection: A decision analysis. *Clinical Infectious Diseases, 58*, 1507–1514. doi:10.1093/cid/ciu128

Patel, N. C., Griesbach, C. L., DiBaise, J. K., & Orenstein, R. (2013). Fecal microbiota transplant for recurrent *Clostridium difficile* infection: Mayo Clinic in Arizona experience. *Mayo Clinic Proceedings, 88*, 799–805. doi:10.1016/j.mayocp.2013.04.022

Pathak, R., Enuh, H. A., Patel, A., & Wickremesinghe, P. (2013). Treatment of relapsing *Clostridium difficile* infection using fecal microbiota transplantation. *Clinical and Experimental Gastroenterology, 7*, 1–6. doi:10.2147/CEG.S53410

Vyas, D., Aekka, A., & Vyas, A. (2015). Fecal transplant policy and legislation. *World Journal of Gastroenterology, 21*, 6–11. doi:10.3748/wjg.v21.i1.6

Whelan, K. (2011). Probiotics and prebiotics in the management of irritable bowel syndrome: A review of recent clinical trials and systematic reviews. *Current Opinion in Clinical Nutrition & Metabolic Care, 14*, 581–587. doi:10.1097/MCO.0b013e32834b8082

Youngster, I., Sauk, J., Pindar, C., Wilson, R. G., Kaplan, J. L., Smith, M. B., . . . Hohmann, E. L. (2014). Fecal microbiota transplant for relapsing *Clostridium difficile* infection using a frozen inoculum from unrelated donors: A randomized, open-label, controlled pilot study. *Clinical Infectious Diseases, 58*, 1515–1522. doi:10.1093/cid/ciu135

SELECTED BIBLIOGRAPHY

Basson, M.D. (2014). *Constipation*. Retrieved from http://emedicine.medscape.com/article/184704-overview

Dudley-Brown, S. (2012). The changing world of inflammatory bowel disease: Impact of generation, gender, and global trends. *Gastroenterology Nursing, 35*, 226. doi:10.1097/SGA.0b013e3182569fdc

Fukudo, S., Kaneko, H., Akiho, H., Inamori, M., Endo, Y., Okumura, T., . . . Shimosegawa, T. (2015). Evidence-based clinical practice guidelines for irritable bowel syndrome. *Journal of Gastroenterology, 50*(1), 11–30. doi:10.1007/s00535-014-1017-0

Gardner, T. B. (2014). *Acute pancreatitis*. Retrieved from http://emedicine.medscape.com/article/181364-overview

Glatter, J., Sephton, M., & Garrick, V. (2013). The revised inflammatory bowel disease (IBD) standards and the IBD nurse role. *Gastrointestinal Nursing, 11*(10), 28–34. doi:10.12968/gasn.2013.11.10.28

Hamdy, O. (2015). *Obesity*. Retrieved from http://emedicine.medscape.com/article/123702-overview

Herrstedt, J., Rapoport, B., Warr, D., Roila, F., Bria, E., Rittenberg, C., & Hesketh, P. J. (2011). Acute emesis: Moderately emetogenic chemotherapy. *Supportive Care in Cancer, 19*(Suppl. 1), 15–23. doi:10.1007/s00520-010-0951-5

Laugsand, E. A., Kaasa, S., & Klepstad, P. (2011). Management of opioid-induced nausea and vomiting in cancer patients: Systematic review and evidence-based recommendations. *Palliative Medicine, 25*, 442–453. doi:10.1177/0269216311404273

Lehrer, J. K. (2015). *Irritable bowel syndrome*. Retrieved from http://emedicine.medscape.com/article/180389-overview

Löhr, J. M., Oliver, M. R., & Frulloni, L. (2013). Synopsis of recent guidelines on pancreatic exocrine insufficiency. *United European Gastroenterology Journal, 1*, 79–83. doi:10.1177/2050640613476500

Rowe, W. A. (2015). *Inflammatory bowel disease*. Retrieved from http://emedicine.medscape.com/article/179037-overview#a0156

Saad, A. M., Kahn, S. A., Rubin, M., & Rubin, D. T. (2013). Advances in inflammatory bowel diseases 2012. *Clinical Investigation, 3*, 323–327. doi:10.4155/cli.13.11

Wallace, J. L., & Sharkey, K. A. (2011). Pharmacotherapy of inflammatory bowel disease. In L. L. Brunton, B. A. Chabner, & B. C. Knollman (Eds.), *Goodman and Gilman's the pharmacological basis of therapeutics* (12th ed., pp. 1351–1362). New York, NY: McGraw-Hill.

Wilcox, S. R. (2013). *Hyperemesis gravidarum in emergency medicine*. Retrieved from http://emedicine.medscape.com/article/796564-overview

Wood, M., Hall, L., Hockenberry, M., & Borinstein, S. (2015). Improving adherence to evidence-based guidelines for chemotherapy-induced nausea and vomiting. *Journal of Pediatric Oncology Nursing*, 1043454214563403. Advance online publication. doi:10.1177/1043454214563403

Chapter 43

Drugs for Nutritional Disorders

Drugs at a Glance

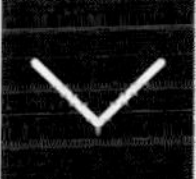

Learning Outcomes

After reading this chapter, the student should be able to:

1. Describe the role of vitamins in maintaining wellness.
2. Compare and contrast the properties of water-soluble and fat-soluble vitamins.
3. Discuss the role of the recommended dietary allowance in preventing vitamin deficiencies.
4. Identify indications for vitamin pharmacotherapy.
5. Explain how pharmacotherapy with water-soluble and fat-soluble vitamins prevents nutritional disorders.
6. Compare and contrast the properties of macrominerals and trace minerals.
7. Identify differences among oligomeric, polymeric, modular, and specialized formulations for enteral nutrition.
8. Compare and contrast enteral and parenteral methods of providing nutrition.
9. Describe the types of drugs used in the short-term management of obesity.
10. For each of the drug classes listed in Drugs at a Glance, know representative drugs, explain the mechanism of drug action, describe primary actions, and identify important adverse effects.
11. Use the nursing process to care for patients who are receiving pharmacotherapy for nutritional disorders.

(prototype drug icon) indicates a prototype drug, each of which is featured in a Prototype Drug box.

Most people are able to obtain all the necessary nutrients their body requires through a balanced diet. However, many Americans rely on nutrient-poor fast foods and processed edibles as their main diet. Although a healthy diet is the best way to maintain adequate vitamin and mineral intake, individual supplements are available as an additional way to meet the minimum daily requirements. This chapter focuses on the role of vitamins, minerals, and nutritional supplements in pharmacology.

VITAMINS

Vitamins are essential substances needed to maintain optimal wellness. Patients who have a deficient or unbalanced dietary intake, those who are pregnant, or those experiencing a chronic disease may benefit from vitamin therapy.

43.1 Role of Vitamins in Maintaining Health

Vitamins are organic compounds required by the body in small amounts for growth and for the maintenance of normal metabolic processes. Since the discovery of thiamine in 1911, more than a dozen vitamins have been identified. Because scientists did not know the chemical structures of the vitamins when they were discovered, they assigned letters and numbers such as A, B_{12}, and C. These names are still widely used today.

An important characteristic of vitamins is that, with the exception of vitamin D, human cells cannot synthesize them in adequate amounts. They, or their precursors known as **provitamins,** must be supplied in the diet. A second important characteristic is that if the vitamin is not present in adequate amounts, then the body's metabolism will be disrupted and disease will result. For most vitamin deficiencies, the symptoms of the deficiency can be reversed by administering the missing vitamin.

Vitamins serve diverse and important roles. For example, the B-complex vitamins are coenzymes essential to many metabolic pathways. Vitamin A is a precursor of retinal, a pigment needed for vision. Calcium metabolism is regulated by a hormone that is derived from vitamin D. Without vitamin K, abnormal prothrombin is produced, and blood clotting is affected.

43.2 Classification of Vitamins

A simple way to classify vitamins is by their ability to mix with water. Those that dissolve easily in water are called *water-soluble* vitamins. Examples include vitamin C and the B vitamins. Those that dissolve in lipids are called *fat-* or *lipid-soluble* and include vitamins A, D, E, and K.

This difference in solubility affects the way the vitamins are absorbed by the gastrointestinal (GI) tract and stored in the body. The water-soluble vitamins are absorbed with water in the digestive tract and readily dissolve in blood and body fluids. When excess water-soluble vitamins are absorbed, they cannot be stored for later use and are simply excreted in the urine. Because they are not stored to any significant degree, they must be ingested daily; otherwise, deficiencies will quickly develop. An exception is Vitamin B_{12}, which can be stored in the liver and recycled through enterohepatic recirculation for many years before signs of deficiency develop.

Lipid-soluble vitamins, on the other hand, cannot be absorbed in sufficient quantity in the small intestine unless they are ingested with other fats. These vitamins can be stored in large quantities in the liver and adipose tissue. Should the patient not ingest sufficient amounts, lipid-soluble vitamins are removed from storage depots in the body as needed. Unfortunately, storage may lead to dangerously high levels of these vitamins if they are taken in excessive amounts.

43.3 Recommended Dietary Allowances

Based on scientific research on humans and animals, the Food and Nutrition Board of the National Academy of Sciences has established levels for the dietary intake of vitamins and minerals called **recommended dietary allowances (RDAs).** The RDA values represent the *minimum* amount of vitamin or mineral needed daily to prevent deficiencies in nearly all (up to 98%) healthy adults. The RDAs are revised periodically to reflect the latest scientific research. Current RDAs for vitamins are listed in Table 43.1. A newer standard, the Dietary Reference Intake (DRI), is sometimes used to represent the *optimal* level of nutrient needed to ensure wellness.

PharmFacts

VITAMINS, MINERALS, AND NUTRITIONAL SUPPLEMENTS

- About 40% of Americans take vitamin supplements daily.
- There is no difference between the chemical structure of a natural vitamin and a synthetic vitamin, yet consumers pay much more for the natural type.
- Vitamin B_{12} is present only in animal products and yeast. Vegetarians may find adequate amounts in fortified cereals, nutritional supplements, or yeast.
- Administration of folic acid prior to conception and during pregnancy has been found to reduce birth defects in the nervous system of the baby.
- Patients who do not receive adequate exposure to direct sunlight often require vitamin D supplements.
- Vitamins technically cannot increase a patient's energy level. Energy can be provided only by adding calories from carbohydrates, proteins, and lipids.

Table 43.1 Vitamins

Vitamin	Function(s)	RDA (adults)		Common Cause(s) of Deficiency
		Men	Women	
A	Visual pigments, epithelial cells	900 mg RE*	700 mg RE	Prolonged dietary deprivation, particularly when rice is the main food source; pancreatic disease; cirrhosis
B complex: biotin	Coenzyme in metabolic reactions	30 mcg	30 mcg	Deficiencies are rare
cyanocobalamin (B_{12})	Coenzyme in nucleic acid metabolism	2.4 mcg	2.4 mcg	Lack of intrinsic factor, inadequate intake of foods from animal origin
folic acid/folate (B_9)	Coenzyme in amino acid and nucleic acid metabolism	400 mcg	400 mcg	Pregnancy, alcoholism, cancer, oral contraceptive use
niacin (B_3)	Coenzyme in oxidation–reduction reactions	16 mg	14 mg	Prolonged dietary deprivation, particularly when Indian corn (maize) or millet is the main food source; chronic diarrhea; liver disease; alcoholism
pantothenic acid (B_5)	Coenzyme in metabolic reactions	5 mg	5 mg	Deficiencies are rare
pyridoxine (B_6)	Coenzyme in amino acid metabolism, RBC production	1.3–1.7mg	1.3–1.5 mg	Alcoholism, oral contraceptive use, isoniazid, malabsorption diseases
riboflavin (B_2)	Coenzyme in oxidation–reduction reactions	1.3 mg	1.1 mg	Inadequate consumption of milk or animal products, chronic diarrhea, liver disease, alcoholism
thiamine (B_1)	Coenzyme in metabolic reactions, RBC formation	1.2 mg	1.1 mg	Prolonged dietary deprivation, particularly when rice is the main food source; hyperthyroidism; pregnancy; liver disease; alcoholism
C (ascorbic acid)	Coenzyme and antioxidant	90 mg	75 mg	Inadequate intake of fruits and vegetables, pregnancy, chronic inflammatory disease, burns, diarrhea, alcoholism
D	Calcium and phosphate metabolism	600 international units (15 mcg)	600 international units (15 mcg)	Low dietary intake, inadequate exposure to sunlight
E	Antioxidant	15 TE**	15 mg TE	Prematurity, malabsorption diseases
K	Cofactor in blood clotting	120 mcg	90 mcg	Some newborns, liver disease, long-term parenteral nutrition, certain drugs such as cephalosporins and salicylates

Note: *RE = retinoid equivalents; **TE = alpha-tocopherol equivalents.

Vitamin, mineral, or herbal supplements should never substitute for a balanced diet. Sufficient intake of proteins, carbohydrates, and lipids is needed for proper health. Furthermore, although the label on a vitamin supplement may indicate that it contains 100% of the RDA for a particular vitamin, the body may absorb as little as 10% to 15% of the amount ingested. With the exception of vitamins A and D, it is not harmful for most patients to consume two to three times the recommended levels of vitamins. In cases where dietary needs are increased, the RDAs will need adjustment, and supplements are indicated to achieve optimal wellness.

43.4 Indications for Vitamin Pharmacotherapy

Most people who eat a normal, balanced diet obtain all the necessary nutrients without vitamin supplementation. Indeed, megavitamin therapy is not only expensive but also harmful to health if taken for long periods. **Hypervitaminosis,** or toxic levels of vitamins, has been reported for vitamins A, C, D, E, B_6, niacin, and folic acid. In the United States, it is actually more common to observe syndromes of vitamin *excess* than of vitamin *deficiency*. Indeed, research has determined that high amounts of beta carotene supplements (usually taken to lower blood cholesterol) may increase one's risk of lung cancer, an effect seen in smokers. Most patients are unaware that taking too much of a vitamin or mineral can cause serious adverse effects.

Vitamin deficiencies follow certain patterns. The following are general characteristics of vitamin deficiency disorders:

- Patients more commonly present with *multiple* vitamin deficiencies than with a single vitamin deficiency.
- Symptoms of deficiency are *nonspecific* and often do not appear until the deficiency has been present for a long time.
- Deficiencies in the United States are most often the result of poverty, fad diets, chronic alcohol or drug abuse, or prolonged parenteral feeding.

Certain patients and conditions require higher levels of vitamins. Infancy and childhood are times of potential deficiency due to the high growth demands placed on the body. In addition, requirements for all nutrients are increased during pregnancy and lactation. With normal aging, the absorption of food diminishes and the quantity of ingested food is often reduced, leading to a higher risk of vitamin deficiencies in older adults. Men and women can have different vitamin and mineral needs as do persons who participate in vigorous exercise. Vitamin deficiencies in patients with chronic liver and kidney disease are well documented.

Certain drugs have the potential to affect vitamin metabolism. Alcohol is known for its ability to inhibit the absorption of thiamine and folic acid: Alcohol abuse is the most common cause of thiamine deficiency in the United States. Folic acid levels may be reduced in patients taking phenothiazines, oral contraceptives, phenytoin (Dilantin), or barbiturates. Vitamin D deficiency can be caused by therapy with certain anticonvulsants. Inhibition of vitamin B_{12} absorption has been reported with a number of drugs, including omeprazole (Prilosec), metformin (Glucophage), alcohol, and oral contraceptives. Nurses must be aware of these drug interactions and recommend vitamin therapy when appropriate.

Lipid-Soluble Vitamins

The lipid- or fat-soluble vitamins are abundant in both plant and animal foods and are relatively stable during cooking. Because the body stores them, it is not necessary to ingest the recommended amounts on a daily basis.

43.5 Pharmacotherapy With Lipid-Soluble Vitamins

Lipid-soluble vitamins are absorbed from the intestine with dietary lipids and are stored primarily in the liver. When consumed in high amounts, these vitamins can accumulate to toxic levels and produce hypervitaminosis. Because these are available over the counter (OTC), patients must be advised to carefully follow the instructions of the health care provider, or the label directions, for proper dosage. Medications containing lipid-soluble vitamins, and their recommended doses, are listed in Table 43.2.

One important source for vitamin A, also known as *retinol,* is foods that contain **carotenes.** Carotenes are precursors to vitamin A that are converted to retinol in the wall of the small intestine when absorbed. The most abundant and biologically active carotene is beta carotene. During metabolism, each molecule of beta carotene yields two molecules of vitamin A. Good sources of dietary vitamin A include yellow and dark leafy vegetables, butter, eggs, whole milk, and liver. Vitamin A is used as replacement therapy for conditions affecting absorption, mobilization, or storage of vitamin A, such as steatorrhea, severe biliary obstruction, liver cirrhosis, or total gastrectomy.

Vitamin D is actually a group of chemicals sharing similar activity. Vitamin D_2, also known as **ergocalciferol,** is obtained from fortified milk, margarine, and other dairy products. Vitamin D_3 is formed in the skin by a chemical reaction requiring ultraviolet radiation. Vitamin D is used to treat skeletal diseases that weaken the bones such as rickets, osteomalacia (adult rickets), osteoporosis, and hypocalcemia. Sometimes vitamin D is helpful in treating psoriasis, rheumatoid arthritis, and lupus vulgaris. The pharmacology of the D vitamins and a drug prototype for calcitriol, the active form of vitamin D, are detailed in chapter 48.

Vitamin E consists of about eight chemicals, called **tocopherols,** having similar activity. Alpha tocopherol constitutes 90% of the tocopherols and is the only one of pharmacologic importance. Dosage of vitamin E is reported as either milligrams of alpha-tocopherol or as international units (IU). Vitamin E is found in plant-seed

Table 43.2 Lipid-Soluble Vitamins for Treating Nutritional Disorders

Drug	Route and Adult Dose (max dose where indicated)	Adverse Effects
vitamin A (Aquasol A, others)	PO: 100,000 units/day for 3 days, followed by 50,000 units/day for 2 wk; then 10,000–20,000 units/day for 2 months IM: 100,000 units/day for 3 days followed by 50,000 units/day for 2 wk	*Uncommon at recommended doses* High doses: nausea, vomiting, fatigue, irritability, night sweats, alopecia, dry skin
vitamin D: calcitriol (Calcijex, Rocaltrol) (see page 828 for the Prototype Drug box)	PO: 800–1,000 units/day or 50,000 units monthly for severe deficiency PO: 0.25 mcg/day; may be increased by 0.25 mcg/day at 4–8 wk intervals for dialysis patients or at 2–4 wk intervals for hypoparathyroidism	*Uncommon at recommended doses, metallic taste* High doses: nausea, vomiting, fatigue, headache, polyuria, weight loss, hallucinations, dysrhythmias, muscle and bone pain
vitamin E (Aquasol E, Vita-Plus E, others)	PO/IM: 60–75 units/day	*Uncommon at recommended doses* High doses: nausea, vomiting, fatigue, headache, blurred vision
vitamin K (AquaMEPHYTON)	PO/IM: 2.5–10 mg for hypoprothrombinemia	*Facial flushing, pain at the injection site* IV route may result in dyspnea, hypotension, shock, cardiac arrest

Note: *Italics* indicate common adverse effects; underlining indicates serious adverse effects.

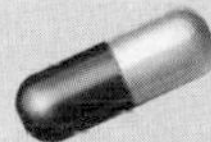

Prototype Drug | Vitamin A *(Aquasol A, others)*

Therapeutic Class: Lipid-soluble vitamin **Pharmacologic Class:** Retinoid

Actions and Uses

Vitamin A is essential for general growth and development, particularly of the bones, teeth, and epithelial membranes. It is necessary for proper wound healing, is essential for the biosynthesis of steroids, and is one of the pigments required for night vision. Vitamin A is indicated in deficiency states and during periods of increased need such as pregnancy, lactation, or undernutrition. Night blindness and slow wound healing can be effectively treated with as little as 30,000 units of vitamin A given daily over a week. It is also prescribed for GI disorders, when absorption in the small intestine is diminished or absent. Topical forms are available for acne, psoriasis, and other skin disorders. Doses of vitamin A are sometimes measured in retinoid equivalents (RE). In severe deficiency states, up to 500,000 units may be given per day for 3 days, gradually tapering off to 10,000–20,000 units/day.

Administration Alerts

- Pregnancy category A at low doses.
- Pregnancy category X at doses above the RDA.

PHARMACOKINETICS

Onset	Peak	Duration
Unknown	Unknown	Unknown

Adverse Effects

Adverse effects are not observed with normal doses of vitamin A. Acute ingestion, however, produces serious central nervous system (CNS) toxicity, including headache, irritability, drowsiness, delirium, and possible coma. Long-term ingestion of high amounts causes drying and scaling of the skin, alopecia, fatigue, anorexia, vomiting, and leukopenia. Chronic toxicity may cause liver impairment.

Contraindications: Vitamin A in excess of the RDA is contraindicated in pregnant patients or those who may become pregnant. Fetal harm may result.

Interactions

Drug–Drug: People who are taking vitamin A should avoid taking mineral oil and cholestyramine, because both may decrease the absorption of vitamin A. Concurrent use with isoretinoin may result in additive toxicity.

Lab Tests: Vitamin A may increase serum calcium, serum cholesterol, and blood urea nitrogen (BUN).

Herbal/Food: Unknown.

Treatment of Overdose: There is no specific treatment for overdose.

oils, nuts, whole-grain cereals, eggs, and certain organ meats such as the liver, pancreas, and heart. It is considered a primary antioxidant, preventing the formation of free radicals that damage plasma membranes and other cellular structures. Deficiency in adults has been observed only with severe malabsorption disorders; however,

Community-Oriented Practice

VITAMIN D AND DISEASE RISK

Vitamin D deficiency has been increasingly implicated in the development of a variety of diseases, including diabetes, cardiovascular disease, cancer, and cognitive decline (Autier, Bonjol, Pizot, & Mullie, 2014; Sun, Pan, Hu, Manson, & Rexrode, 2012; Theodoratou, Tzoulaki, Zgaga, & Ioannidid, 2014; Wang et al., 2012). However, it is difficult to prove a causal effect between low levels of vitamin D and disease risk. The U.S. Preventative Task Force found that there was insufficient evidence to recommend routine screening for vitamin D deficiency, although populations that may be at higher risk for deficiency, including people with little or no sun exposure, with low vitamin D intake, patients with obesity, or patients who by age may be at risk of fractures, may warrant such screening (LeFevre, 2015). Other factors that contribute to possible risk of deficiency include female gender, smoking, older age, sedentary lifestyle, and alcohol use (Sohl et al., 2014). There is limited evidence that vitamin D deficiency is a global health problem, although in a survey of available studies, similar risk factors were found throughout the world (Palacios & Gonzalez, 2014). In addition, there is inconclusive evidence that screening for vitamin D deficiency reduces disease risk, except in those older adults in long-term care settings and those at risk for falls (LeBlanc, Zakher, Daeges, Pappas, & Chou, 2015).

Despite inconclusive research findings, many authors suggest that because much of the world's population may have a deficiency in vitamin D, and because the vitamin is readily available, increasing vitamin D intake may improve the overall health of the population. Further research is needed, including the need to define the overall purpose for screening for deficiency, i.e., for nutrition replenishment or for disease prevention (Heaney & Armas, 2015; Schodin, 2014). Although hyper-supplementation is not recommended and may cause significant adverse effects, nurses can help to ensure that patients receive adequate intake or discuss supplementation with their health care provider to improve health and potentially decrease the development of more serious health conditions.

deficiency in premature neonates may lead to hemolytic anemia. Patients often self-administer vitamin E because it is thought to be useful in preventing heart disease and increasing sexual prowess, although research has not always supported these claims. The preferred route is oral (PO), although topical products are available to treat dry, cracked skin.

Vitamin K is also a mixture of several chemicals. Vitamin K_1 is found in plant sources, particularly green leafy vegetables, tomatoes, and cauliflower; and in egg yolks, liver, and cheeses. Vitamin K_2 is synthesized by microbial flora in the colon. Deficiency states, caused by inadequate intake or by antibiotic destruction of normal intestinal flora, may result in delayed hemostasis. The body does not have large stores of vitamin K, and a deficiency may occur in only 1 to 2 weeks. Blood clotting factors II, VII, IX, and X depend on vitamin K for their biosynthesis. Vitamin K is used as a treatment for patients with clotting disorders and is the antidote for warfarin (Coumadin) overdose. It is also given to infants at birth to promote blood clotting. Vitamin K carries a black box warning that anaphylaxis, shock, and cardiac or respiratory arrest have been reported immediately following intravenous (IV) and intramuscular (IM) administration.

Water-Soluble Vitamins

The water-soluble vitamins consist of the B-complex vitamins and vitamin C. These vitamins must be consumed on a daily basis because they are not stored in the body.

43.6 Pharmacotherapy With Water-Soluble Vitamins

The B-complex group of vitamins comprises 8 different substances that are grouped together because they were originally derived from yeast and foods that counteracted the disease beriberi. They have very different chemical structures and serve various metabolic functions. The B vitamins are known by their chemical names as well as their vitamin number. For example, vitamin B_{12} is also called *cyanocobalamin*. Medications containing water-soluble vitamins and their doses are listed in Table 43.3. Vitamins B_5 (pantothenic acid) and B_7 (biotin) are not included in the table because deficiencies in these vitamins are very rare.

Vitamin B_1, or *thiamine,* is a precursor of an enzyme responsible for several steps in the oxidation of carbohydrates. It is abundant in both plant and animal products, especially whole-grain foods, dried beans, and peanuts. Because of the vitamin's abundance, thiamine deficiency in the United States is not common, except in alcoholics and in patients with chronic liver disease. Thiamine deficiency, or **beriberi,** is characterized by neurologic signs such as paresthesia, neuralgia, and progressive loss of feeling and reflexes. With pharmacotherapy, symptoms can be completely reversed in the early stages of the disease; however, permanent disability can result in patients with prolonged deficiency.

Vitamin B_2, or *riboflavin,* is a component of coenzymes that participate in a number of different oxidation–reduction

Table 43.3 Water-Soluble Vitamins for Treating Nutritional Disorders

Drug	Route and Adult Dose (max dose where indicated)	Adverse Effects
vitamin B_1: thiamine	IV/IM: 5–30 mg tid PO: 15–30 mg/day	*Pain at the injection site* IV route may result in angioedema, cyanosis, pulmonary edema, GI bleeding, and cardiovascular collapse
vitamin B_2: riboflavin	PO: 5–10 mg/day	*Uncommon at the recommended doses*
vitamin B_3: niacin (Nicobid, Nicolar, others)	PO (for niacin deficiency): 100 mg/day PO (for hyperlipidemia): 1.5–3 g/day	*Uncommon at doses used for vitamin therapy* High doses: flushing, rash, diarrhea, hepatotoxicity
vitamin B_6: pyridoxine (Hexa-Betalin, Nestrex, others)	PO: 10–100 mg/day (max: 100 mg/day) IV: 10–20 mg/day for 3 wk	*Pain at the injection site* High doses: neuropathy, ataxia, seizures
vitamin B_9: folic acid (Folacin)	PO/IM/IV/subcutaneous: 0.4–1 mg/day	*Uncommon at the recommended doses* Parenteral routes: allergic hypersensitivity
vitamin B_{12}: cyanocobalamin (Betalin 12, Cobex, Nascobol, others) (see page 492 for the Prototype Drug box)	IM/deep subcutaneous: 30 mcg/day for 5–10 days; then 100–200 mcg/month Intranasal: 500 mcg in one nostril once weekly	*Rash, diarrhea* High doses: thrombosis, hypokalemia, pulmonary edema, heart failure
vitamin C: ascorbic acid (Ascorbicap, Cebid, Vita-C, others)	PO/IV/IM/subcutaneous: 150–500 mg/day in one to two doses	*Uncommon at the recommended doses* High doses: deep vein thrombosis (IV route), crystalluria

Note: *Italics* indicate common adverse effects; underlining indicates serious adverse effects.

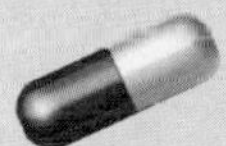

Prototype Drug | Folic Acid *(Folacin)*

Therapeutic Class: Water-soluble vitamin **Pharmacologic Class:** None

Actions and Uses

Folic acid is administered to reverse symptoms of deficiency, which most commonly occurs in patients with inadequate intake, such as with chronic alcohol abuse. Because this vitamin is destroyed at high temperatures, people who overcook their food may experience folate deficiency. Pregnancy markedly increases the need for dietary folic acid; folic acid is given during pregnancy to promote normal fetal growth and prevent neural tube defects in the fetus. Because insufficient vitamin B_{12} creates a lack of activated folic acid, deficiency symptoms resemble those of vitamin B_{12} deficiency. The megaloblastic anemia observed in folate-deficient patients, however, does not include the severe nervous system symptoms seen in patients with B_{12} deficiency. Administration of 1 mg/day of PO folic acid often reverses the deficiency symptoms within 5 to 7 days.

Administration Alerts

- Pregnancy category A (category C when taken in doses above the RDA).

PHARMACOKINETICS

Onset	Peak	Duration
Unknown	30–60 min	Unknown

Adverse Effects

Adverse effects during folic acid therapy are uncommon. Patients may feel flushed following IV injections. Allergic hypersensitivity to folic acid by the IV route is possible.

Contraindications: Folic acid is contraindicated in anemias other than those caused by folate deficiency.

Interactions

Drug–Drug: Phenytoin, trimethoprim–sulfamethoxazole, and other medications may interfere with the absorption of folic acid. Chloramphenicol may antagonize effects of folate therapy. Oral contraceptives, alcohol, barbiturates, methotrexate, and primidone may cause folate deficiency.

Lab Tests: Folic acid may decrease serum levels of vitamin B_{12}.

Herbal/Food: Unknown.

Treatment of Overdose: There is no specific treatment for overdose.

reactions. Riboflavin is abundantly found in plant and meat products, including wheat germ, eggs, cheese, fish, nuts, and leafy vegetables. As with thiamine, deficiency of riboflavin is most commonly observed in alcoholics. Signs of deficiency include corneal vascularization and anemia as well as skin abnormalities such as dermatitis and cheilosis. Most symptoms resolve by administering 25 to 100 mg/day of the vitamin until improvement is observed.

Vitamin B_3, or *niacin,* is a key component of coenzymes essential for oxidative metabolism. Niacin is synthesized from the amino acid tryptophan and is widely distributed in both animal and plant foodstuffs, including beans, wheat germ, meats, nuts, and whole-grain breads. Niacin deficiency, or **pellagra,** is most commonly seen in alcoholics and in those areas of the world where corn is the primary food source. Early symptoms include fatigue, anorexia, and drying of the skin. Advanced symptoms include three classic signs: dermatitis, diarrhea, and dementia. Deficiency is treated with niacin at dosages ranging from 10 to 25 mg/day. When used to treat hyperlipidemia, niacin doses are much higher—up to 3 g/day (see chapter 23).

Vitamin B_6, or *pyridoxine,* consists of several closely related compounds, including pyridoxine itself, pyridoxal, and pyridoxamine. Vitamin B_6 is essential for the synthesis of heme and is a primary coenzyme involved in

Complementary and Alternative Therapies

SEA VEGETABLES

Sea vegetables, or seaweeds, are a form of marine algae that grow in the upper levels of the ocean, where sunlight can penetrate. Examples of these edible seaweeds include spirulina, kelp, chlorella, arame, and nori, many of which are used in Asian cooking. Sea vegetables are found in coastal locations throughout the world. Kelp, or Laminaria, is found in the cold waters of the North Atlantic and Pacific Oceans.

Sea vegetables contain a multitude of vitamins as well as protein. Their most notable nutritional aspect, however, is their mineral content. Plants from the sea contain more minerals than most other food sources, including calcium, magnesium, phosphorous, iron, potassium, and all essential trace elements. Because they are so rich in minerals, seaweeds act as alkalizers for the blood, helping to rid the body of acidic conditions (acidosis). Spirulina, kelp, and chlorella are available in capsule or tablet form, or as part of a "greens" mix containing other nutritional ingredients.

the metabolism of amino acids. Deficiency states can result from alcoholism, uremia, hypothyroidism, or heart failure. Certain drugs can also cause vitamin B_6 deficiency, including isoniazid (INH), cycloserine (Seromycin), hydralazine (Apresoline), oral contraceptives, and pyrazinamide. Patients who are receiving these drugs may routinely receive B_6 supplements. Deficiency symptoms include skin abnormalities, cheilosis, fatigue, and irritability. Symptoms reverse after administration of about 10 to 20 mg/day for several weeks. Diclegis is a fixed dose combination of pyridoxine with the antihistamine doxylamine that is approved to treat nausea and vomiting that occurs during pregnancy.

Vitamin B_9, more commonly known as folate or folic acid, is metabolized to tetrahydrofolate, which is the activated form of the vitamin. Folic acid is essential for normal DNA synthesis and for red blood cell production. Folic acid is widely distributed in plant products, especially green leafy vegetables and citrus fruits. This vitamin is highlighted as a drug prototype in this chapter.

Vitamin B_{12}, or cyanocobalamin, is a cobalt-containing vitamin that is a required coenzyme for a number of metabolic pathways. It also has important roles in cell replication, erythrocyte maturation, and myelin synthesis. Sources include lean meat, seafood, liver, and milk. The principal disease caused by deficiency of vitamin B_{12} is **megaloblastic anemia.** When the B_{12} deficiency results from a lack of intrinsic factor, it is called **pernicious anemia.** The purified form of this vitamin (cyanocobalamin) is featured as a prototype drug in chapter 32.

Vitamin C, or *ascorbic acid,* is the most commonly purchased OTC vitamin. It is a potent antioxidant and serves many functions including collagen synthesis, tissue healing, and maintenance of bone, teeth, and epithelial tissue. Many consumers purchase the vitamin for its ability to prevent the common cold, a claim that has not been definitively proved. Deficiency of vitamin C, or **scurvy,** is caused by diets lacking fruits and vegetables. Alcoholics, cigarette smokers, patients with cancer, and those with renal failure are at highest risk for vitamin C deficiency. Symptoms include fatigue, bleeding gums and other hemorrhages, gingivitis, and poor wound healing. Symptoms can normally be reversed by the administration of 300 to 1,000 mg/day of vitamin C for several weeks.

Check Your Understanding 43.1

True vitamin deficiencies are uncommon in many parts of the world. What are some of the causes for deficiencies? *Visit www.pearsonhighered.com/nursingresources for the answer.*

MINERALS

Minerals are inorganic substances needed in small amounts to maintain homeostasis. Minerals are classified as macrominerals or microminerals; the macrominerals must be ingested in larger amounts. A normal, balanced diet will provide the proper amounts of the required minerals in most people. The primary minerals used in pharmacotherapy are listed in Table 43.4.

43.7 Indications for Mineral Pharmacotherapy

Minerals are essential substances that constitute about 4% of the body weight and serve many diverse functions. Some are essential ions or electrolytes in body fluids; others are bound to organic molecules such as hemoglobin, phospholipids, or metabolic enzymes. Those minerals that function as critical electrolytes in the body, most notably sodium and potassium, are covered in more detail in chapter 25. Sodium chloride, sodium bicarbonate, and potassium chloride are featured as drug prototypes in that chapter.

Because minerals are needed in very small amounts for human metabolism, a balanced diet will supply the necessary quantities for most patients. As with vitamins, patients should be advised not to exceed recommended doses because excess amounts of minerals can lead to toxicity. Mineral supplements are, however, indicated for certain disorders. Iron-deficiency anemia is the most common nutritional deficiency in the world and is a common indication for iron supplements. Women at high risk for osteoporosis are advised to consume extra calcium, either in their diet or as a dietary supplement.

Certain drugs affect normal mineral metabolism. For example, loop or thiazide diuretics can cause significant urinary potassium and magnesium loss. Corticosteroids and oral contraceptives are among several classes of drugs that can promote sodium retention. The uptake of iodine by the thyroid gland can be impaired by certain oral hypoglycemics and lithium carbonate (Eskalith). Oral contraceptives have been reported to lower the plasma levels of zinc and to increase those of copper. Nurses must be aware of drug-related mineral interactions and recommend changes to mineral intake when appropriate.

43.8 Pharmacotherapy With Minerals

Macrominerals

Macrominerals (major minerals) are inorganic substances that must be consumed daily in amounts of 100 mg or higher. The macrominerals include calcium, chlorine, magnesium, phosphorus, potassium, sodium, and sulfur. Approximately 75% of the total mineral content in the body consists of calcium and phosphorus salts in a bone matrix. Recommended dietary allowances have been established for each of the macrominerals except sulfur, as listed in Table 43.5.

Table 43.1 Selected Minerals for Treating Nutritional and Electrolyte Disorders

Drug	Route and Adult Dose (max dose where indicated)	Adverse Effects
potassium chloride (K-Dur, Micro-K, Klor-Con, others) (see page 366 for the Prototype Drug box)	PO: 10–100 mEq/day in divided doses IV: 10–60 mEq/h diluted to at least 10–20 mEq/100 mL of solution (max: 200–400 mEq/day)	*Nausea, vomiting, diarrhea, abdominal cramping* Hyperkalemia, hypotension, confusion, dysrhythmias
sodium bicarbonate (see page 370 for the Prototype Drug box)	PO: 0.3–2 g/day–qid or 1 tsp of powder in a glass of water	*Headache, weakness, belching, flatulence* Hypernatremia, hypertension, muscle twitching, dysrhythmias, pulmonary edema, peripheral edema
CALCIUM SALTS		
calcium acetate (PhosLo)	PO: 2–4 tablets with each meal (each tablet contains 169 mg)	*Parenteral route: flushing, nausea, vomiting, pain at the injection site* *Oral route: abdominal pain, loss of appetite, nausea, vomiting, constipation, dry mouth, increased thirst/urination* Hypercalcemia, hypotension, constipation, fatigue, anorexia, confusion, dysrhythmias
calcium carbonate (Rolaids, Tums, OsCal, others)	PO: 1–2 g bid–tid	
calcium chloride	IV: 0.5–1 g/ every 3 days	
calcium citrate (Citracal)	PO: 1–2 g bid–tid	
calcium gluconate (Kalcinate)	PO: 1–2 g bid–qid IV: 0.5–4 g by slow infusion (1 g/h)	
calcium lactate (Cal-Lac)	PO: 325 mg–1.3 g tid with meals	
calcium phosphate tribasic (Posture)	PO: 1–2 g bid–tid	
IRON SALTS		
ferrous fumarate (Feostat, others)	PO: 200 mg tid–qid	*Nausea, constipation or diarrhea, abdominal pain, leg cramps (iron sucrose)* Anaphylaxis (IV forms), hypovolemia, hematemesis, hepatotoxicity, metabolic acidosis, hypotension
ferrous gluconate (Fergon, others)	PO: 325–600 mg qid; may be gradually increased to 650 mg qid as needed and tolerated	
ferrous sulfate (Feosol, others) (see page 494 for the Prototype Drug box)	PO: 750–1,500 mg/day in single dose or two to three divided doses	
ferumoxytol (Feraheme)	IV: 510 mg single dose followed by second 510 mg dose 3–8 days later	
iron dextran (Dexferrum, others)	IM/IV: dose is individualized and determined from a table of correlations between the patient's weight and hemoglobin (max: 100 mg [2 mL] of iron dextran within 24 h)	
iron sucrose (Venofer)	IV: 100–200 mg by slow IV injection or infusion	
MAGNESIUM		
magnesium chloride (Chloromag, Slow-Mag)	PO: 270–400 mg/day	*Nausea, vomiting, diarrhea, flushing* Cardiotoxicity, respiratory failure, hypotension, deep tendon reflex reduction, facial paresthesias, weakness
magnesium hydroxide (Milk of Magnesia)	PO: 535 mg (64 mg elemental magnesium) once daily	
magnesium oxide (Mag-Ox, Uro-mag, others)	PO: 400–1,200 mg/day in divided doses	
magnesium sulfate (Epsom salts)	IV/IM: 0.5–3 g/day	
PHOSPHORUS/PHOSPHATE		
potassium/sodium phosphates (K-Phos original, K-Phos MF, K Phos neutral, Neutra-Phos-K, Uro-KP neutral)	PO: 250–1,000 mg /day	*Nausea, vomiting, diarrhea* Hyperphosphatemia, bone pain, fractures, muscle weakness, confusion
ZINC		
zinc acetate (Galzin)	PO: 50 mg tid	*Adverse effects are uncommon at the recommended doses* High doses: nausea, vomiting, fever, immunosuppression, anemia
zinc gluconate	PO: 20–100 mg (20-mg lozenges may be taken to a max of six lozenges/day)	
zinc sulfate (Orazinc, Zincate, others)	PO: 15–220 mg/day	

Note: *Italics* indicate common adverse effects; underlining indicates serious adverse effects.

Table 43.5 Recommended Dietary Allowances for Minerals

Mineral	RDA	Function
MACROMINERALS		
calcium	1.0–1.2 g	Forms bony matrix; regulates nerve conduction and muscle contraction
chloride	1.8–2.3 g	Major anion in body fluids; part of gastric acid (HCl)
magnesium	Men: 400–420 mg Women: 310–320 mg	Cofactor for many enzymes; necessary for normal nerve conduction and muscle contraction
phosphorus	700 mg	Forms bony matrix; part of ATP and nucleic acids
potassium	4.7 g	Necessary for normal nerve conduction and muscle contraction; principal cation in intracellular fluid; essential for acid–base and electrolyte balance
sodium	1.5 g	Necessary for normal nerve conduction and muscle contraction; principal cation in extracellular fluid; essential for acid–base and electrolyte balance
Sulfur	Not established	Component of proteins, B vitamins, and other critical molecules
MICROMINERALS		
chromium	25–35 mcg	Potentiates insulin and is necessary for proper glucose metabolism
cobalt	0.1 mcg	Cofactor for vitamin B_{12} and several oxidative enzymes
copper	900 mcg	Cofactor for hemoglobin synthesis
fluorine	3–4 mg	Influences tooth structure and stimulates new bone growth
iodine	150 mcg	Component of thyroid hormone
iron	Men and postmenopausal women: 8 mg Premenopausal women: 18 mg Pregnant women: 27 mg	Component of hemoglobin and some enzymes of oxidative phosphorylation
manganese	1.8–2.5 mg	Cofactor in some enzymes of lipid, carbohydrate, and protein metabolism
molybdenum	45 mcg	Cofactor for certain enzymes
selenium	55 mcg	Antioxidant cofactor for certain enzymes
zinc	Men: 11 mg Women: 8 mg	Cofactor for certain enzymes, including carbonic anhydrase; needed for proper protein structure, normal growth, and wound healing

Nursing Practice Application

Pharmacotherapy With Vitamins and Minerals

ASSESSMENT

Baseline assessment prior to administration:

- Obtain a complete health history including cardiovascular, neurologic, endocrine, hepatic, or renal disease. Obtain a drug history including allergies, current prescription and OTC drugs, and herbal preparations, alcohol use, or smoking. Be alert to possible drug interactions.
- Obtain a history of any current symptoms that may indicate vitamin deficiencies or hypervitaminosis (e.g., dry itchy skin, alopecia, sore and reddened gums or tongue, tendency to bleed easily or excessive bruising, nausea or vomiting, excessive fatigue).
- Obtain a dietary history noting adequacy of essential vitamins, minerals, and nutrients obtained through food sources.
- Note sunscreen use and the amount of sun exposure.
- Obtain baseline weight and vital signs.
- Evaluate appropriate laboratory findings (e.g., complete blood count [CBC], electrolytes, hepatic and renal function studies, ferritin and iron levels).

Assessment throughout administration:

- Assess for desired therapeutic effects depending on the reason for the drug (symptoms of deficiency are diminished or absent).
- Continue monitoring of vital signs and periodic laboratory values as appropriate.

POTENTIAL NURSING DIAGNOSES*

- *Imbalanced Nutrition: Less Than Body Requirements*
- *Impaired Health Maintenance*
- *Deficient Knowledge* (drug therapy)
- *Risk for Injury,* related to adverse drug effects

*NANDA I © 2014

Nursing Practice Application *continued*

ASSESSMENT	POTENTIAL NURSING DIAGNOSES*
• Assess for and promptly report adverse effects: nausea, vomiting, excessive fatigue, tachycardia, palpitations, hypotension, constipation, drowsiness, dizziness, disorientation, hyperreflexia, and electrolyte imbalances.	

IMPLEMENTATION

Interventions and (Rationales)	Patient-Centered Care
Ensuring therapeutic effects:	
• If a definitive cause of vitamin or mineral deficiency is identified, correct the deficiency using dietary sources of the nutrient where possible. (Natural food sources provide additional nutrients, fiber, and essential requirements not found in vitamin and mineral supplementation.)	• Review the dietary history with the patient and discuss food source options for correcting any deficiencies. Encourage the patient to adopt a healthy lifestyle of increased variety in the diet. **Collaboration:** Provide for dietitian consultation as needed. • Assist the patient and family or caregiver to become "educated consumers," aware of marketing of supplements that may not be required if the diet is adequate. Provide educational materials or Web-based references to reputable sources as needed.
Minimizing adverse effects:	
• Review the dietary and supplement history to correct any existing possibility for hypervitaminosis and adverse drug effects. (Excessive intake of vitamins A, C, D, E, B_6, niacin, and folic acid may lead to toxic effects.)	• Discuss the need for nutritional supplements if the normal diet is unable to supply these or if disease conditions (e.g., pernicious anemia) prevent absorption or use. • Discourage the overuse of supplementation, and provide information on adverse effects and symptoms related to hypervitaminosis.
• Continue to monitor periodic laboratory work as needed. (Laboratory tests appropriate to the condition [e.g., pernicious anemia and hemoglobin (Hgb) and hematocrit (Hct) levels] will help to ensure that therapeutic effects are met. With mineral replacement, electrolytes should return to normal levels.)	• Instruct the patient on the need to return periodically for laboratory work.
• Monitor the use of fat-soluble vitamins. Excessive intake may lead to toxic effects. (Fat-soluble vitamins are stored in the body and may accumulate and result in toxic levels. Monitor liver function studies and promptly report symptoms such as nausea, vomiting, headache, fatigue, dry and itchy skin, blurred vision, or palpitations.)	• Instruct the patient not to take large amounts of fat-soluble vitamins unless instructed by the health care provider. • Encourage obtaining fat-soluble vitamins from natural sources whenever possible.
• **Lifespan:** Assess for pregnancy. Assess safe storage availability for any prenatal vitamins kept in the house. (Folic acid supplementation reduces the incidence of neurologic birth defects. Excessive vitamin intake may have deleterious effects on the developing fetus and prenatal vitamin use should be monitored. Poisonings with vitamins and iron are common in children.)	• Provide education to women of child-bearing age about folic acid and its potential usefulness in preventing neurologic-related birth defects. Encourage the adequate intake of vitamin and folic acid–rich foods prior to conception. • **Safety:** Instruct the patient to keep prenatal vitamins in a secure location if young children are in the household to prevent accidental poisoning.
• Ensure adequate hydration if large doses of water-soluble vitamins are taken. (Water-soluble vitamins are not stored in the body but are excreted. Large doses of vitamin C may cause renal calculi.)	• Encourage the patient to increase fluid intake to 2 L of fluid per day, divided throughout the day.
Patient understanding of drug therapy:	
• Use opportunities during administration of medications and during assessments to provide patient education. (Using time during nursing care helps to optimize and reinforce key teaching areas.)	• The patient should be able to state the reason for the drug; appropriate dose and scheduling; what adverse effects to observe for and when to report; and the anticipated length of medication therapy.
Patient self-administration of drug therapy:	
• When administering the medication, instruct the patient, family, or caregiver in the proper self-administration of the drug (e.g., taken with additional fluids). (Proper administration will increase the effectiveness of the drug.)	• The patient is able to discuss appropriate dosing and administration needs.

See Tables 43.1, 43.2, 43.3, and 43.4 for a list of drugs to which these nursing actions apply.

Calcium is essential for nerve conduction, muscular contraction, construction of bone matrix, and hemostasis. Hypocalcemia occurs when total serum calcium falls below 8.8 mEq/L and may be caused by inadequate intake of calcium-containing foods, lack of vitamin D, chronic diarrhea, or decreased secretion of parathyroid hormone. Symptoms of hypocalcemia involve the nervous and muscular systems. The patient often becomes irritable and restless, and muscular twitches, cramps, spasms, and cardiac abnormalities are common. Prolonged hypocalcemia may lead to fractures. Pharmacotherapy includes calcium compounds, which are available in many oral salts such as calcium carbonate, calcium citrate, calcium gluconate, or calcium lactate. In severe cases, IV preparations are administered. Calcium gluconate is featured as a prototype drug for hypocalcemia and osteoporosis in chapter 48.

Phosphorus is an essential mineral, 85% of which is bound to calcium in the form of calcium phosphate in bones. In addition to playing a role in bone structure, phosphorus is a component of proteins, adenosine triphosphate (ATP), and nucleic acids. Phosphate (PO_4^{3-}) is an important buffer in the blood. Because phosphorus is a primary component of phosphate, phosphorus balance is normally considered the same as phosphate balance. Hypophosphatemia is most often observed in patients with serious medical illnesses, especially those with kidney disorders that cause excess phosphorus loss in the urine. Because of its abundance in food, the patient must be suffering from severe malnutrition or an intestinal malabsorption disorder to experience a dietary deficiency. Symptoms of hypophosphatemia include weakness, muscle tremor, anorexia, weak pulse, and bleeding abnormalities. When serum phosphorus levels fall below 3.5 mEq/L, phosphate supplements are usually administered. Sodium phosphate and potassium phosphate are available for treating phosphorus deficiencies.

Magnesium is the second most abundant intracellular cation and, like potassium, it is essential for proper neuromuscular function. Magnesium also serves a metabolic role in activating certain enzymes in the breakdown of carbohydrates and proteins. Because it produces few symptoms until serum levels fall below 1.4 mEq/L, hypomagnesemia is sometimes called the most common undiagnosed electrolyte abnormality. Patients may experience general weakness, dysrhythmias, hypertension, loss of deep tendon reflexes, and respiratory depression—signs and symptoms that are sometimes mistaken for hypokalemia. In fact, low magnesium levels and low potassium levels often occur concurrently. Pharmacotherapy with magnesium sulfate can quickly reverse the symptoms of hypomagnesemia. Magnesium sulfate is a CNS depressant and is sometimes given to prevent or terminate seizures associated with eclampsia. Magnesium salts have additional applications as cathartics or antacids (magnesium citrate, magnesium hydroxide, and magnesium oxide) and as analgesics (magnesium salicylate).

Microminerals

The nine **microminerals,** commonly called **trace minerals,** are required daily in amounts of 20 mg or less. The fact that they are needed in such small amounts does not diminish their key role in human health; deficiencies in some of the trace minerals can result in profound illness. The functions of some of the trace minerals, such as iron and iodine, are well established; the role of others is less completely understood. The RDA for each of the microminerals is listed in Table 43.5.

Iron is an essential micromineral that is most closely associated with hemoglobin. Excellent sources of dietary iron include meat, shellfish, nuts, and legumes. Excess iron in the body results in hemochromatosis, whereas lack of iron results in iron-deficiency anemia. The pharmacology of iron supplements is presented in chapter 32, where ferrous sulfate is featured as a drug prototype for anemia.

Iodine is a trace mineral needed to synthesize thyroid hormone. The most common source of dietary iodine is iodized salt. When dietary intake of iodine is low, hypothyroidism occurs and enlargement of the thyroid gland (goiter) results. At high concentrations, iodine suppresses thyroid function. *Lugol's solution*, a mixture containing 5% elemental iodine and 10% potassium iodide, is given to hyperthyroid patients prior to thyroidectomy or during a thyrotoxic crisis. Sodium iodide acts by rapidly suppressing the secretion of thyroid hormone and is indicated for patients who are having an acute thyroid crisis. Radioactive iodine (I-131) is given to destroy overactive thyroid glands. Pharmacotherapeutic uses of iodine as a drug extend beyond the treatment of thyroid disease. Iodine is an effective topical antiseptic that can be found in creams, tinctures, and solutions. Iodine salts such as iothalamate and diatrizoate are very dense and serve as diagnostic contrast agents in radiologic procedures of the urinary and cardiovascular systems. The role of potassium iodide in protecting the thyroid gland during acute radiation exposure is discussed in chapter 11.

Fluorine is a trace mineral found abundantly in nature and is best known for its beneficial effects on bones and teeth. Research has validated that adding fluoride (an anion of fluorine) to the water supply in very small amounts (1 part per billion) can reduce the incidence of dental caries. This effect is more pronounced in children,

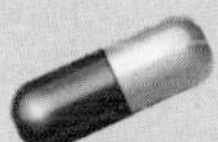

Prototype Drug | Magnesium Sulfate ($MgSO_4$)

Therapeutic Class: Magnesium supplement **Pharmacologic Class:** Electrolyte

Actions and Uses

Severe hypomagnesemia can be rapidly reversed by the administration of IM or IV magnesium sulfate. Parenteral formulations include 4%, 8%, 12.5%, and 50% solutions. Hypomagnesemia has a number of causes, including the loss of body fluids due to diarrhea, diuretic therapy, or nasogastric suctioning, and prolonged parenteral feeding with magnesium-free solutions.

After administration, magnesium sulfate is distributed throughout the body, and therapeutic effects are observed within 30–60 minutes. Oral forms of magnesium sulfate are used as cathartics when complete evacuation of the colon is desired. Its action as a CNS depressant has led to its occasional use as an anticonvulsant. It is used off-label to delay premature labor.

Administration Alerts

- Continuously monitor the patient during IV infusion for early signs of decreased cardiac function.
- Monitor serum magnesium levels every 6 hours during IV infusion.
- When giving IV infusion, give the required dose over 4 hours.
- Pregnancy category D.

PHARMACOKINETICS

Onset	Peak	Duration
1–2 h PO; 1 h IM	Unknown	3–4 h PO; 30 min IV

Adverse Effects

Patients who are receiving IV infusions of magnesium sulfate require careful observation to prevent toxicity. Early signs of magnesium overdose include flushing of the skin, sedation, confusion, intense thirst, and muscle weakness. Extreme levels cause neuromuscular blockade with resultant respiratory paralysis, heart block, and circulatory collapse. Plasma magnesium levels should be monitored frequently. Because of these potentially fatal adverse effects, the use of magnesium sulfate is restricted to severe magnesium deficiency: Mild-to-moderate hypomagnesemia is treated with oral forms of magnesium such as magnesium gluconate or magnesium hydroxide.

Contraindications: When given by the parenteral route, magnesium is contraindicated in patients with serious cardiac disease. Oral administration is contraindicated in patients with undiagnosed abdominal pain, intestinal obstruction, or fecal impaction. The drug should be used cautiously in patients with renal impairment because the drug may rapidly rise to toxic levels.

Interactions

Drug–Drug: Use with neuromuscular blockers may increase respiratory depression and apnea. Concurrent use of magnesium with alcohol or other CNS depressants may lead to increased sedation. Magnesium salts and tetracyclines should not be used concurrently because the magnesium interferes with the absorption of the antibiotic.

Lab Tests: Unknown.

Herbal/Food: Magnesium salts may decrease the absorption of certain anti-infectives such as tetracycline and fluoroquinolone antibiotics.

Treatment of Overdose: Serious respiratory and cardiac suppression may result from overdose. Calcium gluconate or gluceptate may be administered IV as an antidote.

because fluoride is incorporated into the enamel of growing teeth. Concentrated fluoride solutions can also be applied to the teeth topically by dental professionals. Sodium fluoride and stannous fluoride are components of most toothpastes and oral rinses. Because high amounts of fluoride can be quite toxic, the use of fluoride-containing products should be closely monitored in children.

Zinc is a component of at least 100 enzymes, including alcohol dehydrogenase, carbonic anhydrase, and alkaline phosphatase. This trace mineral has a regulatory function in enzymes controlling nucleic acid synthesis and is believed to have roles in wound healing, male fertility, bone formation, and cell-mediated immunity. Because symptoms of zinc deficiency are often nonspecific, diagnosis is usually confirmed by a serum zinc level of less than 70 mcg/dL. Zinc sulfate, zinc acetate, and zinc gluconate are available to prevent and treat deficiency states at doses of 60 to 120 mg/day. In addition, lozenges containing zinc are available OTC for treating sore throats and symptoms of the common cold.

NUTRITIONAL SUPPLEMENTS

Nurses will encounter many patients who are undernourished. Major goals in resolving nutritional deficiencies are to identify the specific type of deficiency and supply the missing nutrients. Nutritional supplements may be needed for short-term therapy or for the remainder of a patient's life.

43.9 Etiology of Undernutrition

Undernutrition is the ingestion or absorption of fewer nutrients than required for normal body growth and maintenance. Successful pharmacotherapy of this condition relies on the skills of nurses in identifying the symptoms and causes of patients' undernutrition.

Causes of undernutrition range from the simple to the complex and include the following:

- Advanced age
- HIV-AIDS
- Alcoholism
- Burns
- Cancer
- Chronic inflammatory bowel disease (IBD)
- Eating disorders
- GI disorders
- Chronic neurologic disease such as progressive dysphagia and multiple sclerosis
- Surgery
- Trauma.

The most obvious cause for undernutrition is low dietary intake, although reasons for the inadequate intake must be assessed. Patients may have no resources to purchase food and may be suffering from starvation. Clinical depression leads many patients to shun food. Older adult patients may have poorly fitting dentures or difficulty chewing or swallowing after a stroke. In terminal disease, patients may be comatose or otherwise unable to take food orally. Although the etiologies differ, patients with insufficient intake exhibit a similar pattern of general weakness, muscle wasting, and loss of subcutaneous fat.

When the undernutrition is caused by lack of one specific nutrient, vitamin, or mineral, the disorder is more difficult to diagnose. Patients may be on a fad diet lacking only protein or fat in their intake. Certain digestive disorders may lead to malabsorption of specific nutrients or vitamins. Patients may simply avoid certain foods such as green leafy vegetables, dairy products, or meat products, which can lead to specific nutritional deficiencies. Proper pharmacotherapy requires the expert knowledge and assessment skills of nurses, and sometimes a nutritional consult, so that the correct treatment can be administered.

43.10 Enteral Nutrition

Numerous nutritional supplements are available, and a common method of classifying these agents is by their *route of administration*. Products that are administered via the GI tract, either orally or through a feeding tube, are classified as **enteral nutrition.** Those that are administered by means of IV infusion are called **parenteral nutrition.**

When the patient's condition permits, enteral nutrition is best provided by oral consumption. Oral feeding allows natural digestive processes to occur and requires less intense nursing care. It does, however, rely on patient cooperation, because it is not feasible for the health care provider to observe the patient at every meal.

Tube feeding, or enteral tube alimentation, is necessary when the patient has difficulty swallowing or is otherwise unable to take meals orally. An advantage of tube feeding is that the amount of enteral nutrition the patient receives can be precisely measured and recorded. Various tube feeding routes are possible, including nasogastric (nose to stomach), nasoduodenal (nose to duodenum), nasojejunal (nose to jejunum), gastrostomy, or jejunostomy (tube is placed directly into the stomach or jejunum, respectively, through a surgical incision). A nasogastric tube may be inserted by a registered nurse or licensed practical nurse. The nasoduodenal and nasojejunal tubes are usually inserted by a radiologist or other health care provider. The gastrostomy and jejunostomy tubes are placed by a surgeon or a gastroenterologist. Feedings may be delivered by bolus, or by intermittent, continuous, or cyclic infusions.

The particular enteral product is chosen to address the specific nutritional needs of the patient. Because of the wide diversity in their formulas, it is difficult to categorize enteral products, and different methods are used. A simple method is to classify enteral products as oligomeric, polymeric, modular, or specialized formulations.

- *Polymeric* formulas are the most common type of enteral preparations. These products contain various mixtures of proteins, carbohydrates, and lipids. These formulas are used in patients who are generally undernourished but have a fully functioning GI tract. Polymeric formulas include blenderized diets and meal replacement formulas. Examples include Osmolite and Promote.
- *Elemental (monomeric)* formulas include products that are usually lactose free and contain only a small percentage of calories from fats. Individual amino acids are provided, which are able to be absorbed without

the aid of digestive enzymes. These formulas are used for patients who have malabsorption disorders. Examples include Criticare HN, and Vivonex TEN.

- *Semielemental (oligomeric)* formulas contain slightly larger molecules than elemental products, such as free amino acids and peptide combinations that require little or no digestion, and are easily absorbed into the body. They are usually low in fat, which allows for rapid gastric emptying, and many of these preparations are designed for administration directly into the intestines. Indications include malabsorption syndrome, partial bowel obstruction, IBD, radiation enteritis, bowel fistulas, and short-bowel syndrome. Sample products include Pepti-2000, Vital HN, Peptamen, and Subdue.
- *Modular* formulas or disease-specific supplements contain a single nutrient, protein, lipid, or carbohydrate. Although not designed to serve as a sole source of nutrition, they can be added to other products to meet a specific nutrient deficiency. For example, protein modules can be used to meet the extra nitrogen needs of patients with burns or severe trauma. Other conditions include renal failure, hepatic failure, pulmonary disease, or a specific genetic enzyme deficiency. Sample products include Casec, Polycose, Microlipid, and MCT Oil.

43.11 Parenteral Nutrition

When a patient's metabolic needs are unable to be met through enteral nutrition, parenteral nutrition (PN) is utilized. Also called **total parenteral nutrition (TPN),** or hyperalimentation, PN is administered solely by the IV route. PN is able to provide all of a patient's nutritional needs in a hypertonic solution containing amino acids, lipid emulsions, carbohydrates (as dextrose), electrolytes, vitamins, and minerals. The particular formulation may be specific to the disease state, such as renal failure or hepatic failure. TPN should be administered through an infusion pump, so that nutrition delivery can be precisely monitored. PN solutions may be modified daily based on the patient's laboratory results, the underlying disorder, the rate of metabolism, and other factors. Patients in various settings such as acute care, long-term care, and home health care often benefit from TPN therapy.

Peripheral vein PN (PPN) is used when a central venous line is not appropriate, such as patients in whom the subclavian vein is inaccessible due to scar tissue from repeated IV line punctures or in patients with extensive trauma in the region of the upper torso or chest. PPN is sometimes considered a temporary measure until a central line can be placed. The catheter site is routinely rotated to prevent infection, and the vein must be able to accommodate the larger sized venous catheter. PPN is associated with a high risk of phlebitis and is therefore reserved for patients with robust veins.

Central vein PN is the administration of the solution through a central vein such as the subclavian or the internal jugular vein. The catheter tip is positioned in the superior vena cava so that the solution can be immediately diluted to a tolerable concentration. The central vein PN solution usually consists of crystalline amino acids, dextrose, and lipid emulsions with the addition of vitamins, minerals, trace elements, essential electrolytes, and water. Central vein PN is usually considered the access of choice for long-term parenteral therapy and is always administered using an infusion pump in order to precisely monitor the amount of solution given.

OBESITY

Obesity is a growing epidemic in the United States: It is estimated that 95 million adults are overweight or obese. This represents 34% of the adult population over age 20. Obesity is closely associated with increased health risks that include premature death, hypertension, hyperlipidemia, diabetes mellitus, heart disease, sleep apnea, and osteoarthritis.

43.12 Etiology of Obesity

Obesity may be simply defined as being more than 20% above the ideal body weight. Clinically, obesity is commonly measured by the **body mass index (BMI).** BMI is determined by dividing body weight (in kilograms) by the square of height (in meters). In adults, a BMI of 25 kg/m^2 indicates the person is overweight. Obesity is defined by a BMI of 30 kg/m^2.

The etiology of obesity is a complex combination of genetic, lifestyle, and physiological factors. In a few cases, weight gain can be attributed to medical conditions, the most common being hypothyroidism. Certain rare disorders of the hypothalamus can also cause overeating. Drugs such as corticosteroids are clearly causes of weight gain.

Lifestyle choices play a key role in the development of obesity, the two most obvious factors being diet and physical activity. The fundamental shift in obesity levels in the past three decades has likely been due to high-fat, calorie-dense diets combined with less physically active lifestyles.

Despite an ongoing debate on the "best" diet, the fact remains that body weight is most likely determined by energy (calorie) balance. Simply stated, if the number of calories *consumed* equals the number of calories *expended*, body weight will be maintained (balanced) at the current level. Changes in weight are due to an energy *imbalance*. For example, an imbalance of as little as 10 surplus calories per day can lead to a 1 lb weight gain each year. While this seems insignificant, if the imbalance persists over several

Nursing Practice Application

Enteral and Parenteral Nutrition Therapy

ASSESSMENT	POTENTIAL NURSING DIAGNOSES*
Baseline assessment prior to administration: • Obtain a complete health history including cardiovascular, neurologic, endocrine, hepatic, or renal disease. Obtain a drug history including allergies, current prescription and OTC drugs, herbal preparations, alcohol use, or smoking. Be alert to possible drug interactions. • Obtain a dietary history, noting the ability to eat and take adequate fluids. • Obtain baseline height, weight, and vital signs. • Evaluate appropriate laboratory findings (e.g., CBC, electrolytes, glucose, BUN, hepatic and renal function studies, total protein, serum albumin, lipid profile, serum iron levels).	• *Imbalanced Nutrition: Less Than Body Requirements* • *Deficient Knowledge* (drug therapy) • *Risk for Imbalanced Fluid Volume* • *Risk for Infection* *NANDA I © 2014
Assessment throughout administration: • Assess for desired therapeutic effects depending on the reason for the drug (e.g., weight is maintained, electrolytes, glucose, proteins, lipid levels remain within normal limits). • Continue monitoring of vital signs and periodic laboratory values as appropriate. • Weigh daily at the same time each day and record. • Assess for and promptly report adverse effects: fever, nausea, vomiting, tachycardia, palpitations, hypotension, dyspnea, drowsiness, dizziness, disorientation, hypo- or hyperglycemia, and electrolyte imbalances.	

IMPLEMENTATION

Interventions and (Rationales)	Patient-Centered Care
Ensuring therapeutic effects: • Assess the patient's ability to take oral nutrition and encourage small oral feedings if allowed. (Supplementation with oral feedings may be allowed if enteral or parenteral nutrition will be used short term. Encouraging small amounts of oral intake will maintain normal salivation and activities of daily living [ADLs] during the time of replacement nutrition.)	• If allowed, encourage the patient to maintain small, frequent oral intake or have a caregiver assist with oral nutrition and hydration.
• Provide water between bolus feedings or each time a new enteral feeding amount is added with continuous feedings. If the patient is unable to take fluids PO, provide additional fluids through the enteral tube in addition to amounts used to flush the tube. Monitor skin turgor and mucous membranes. (Additional water will assist in maintaining dilution of concentrated feedings and replenish body water. Decreased skin turgor and dry mucous membranes may indicate dehydration and the need for additional water.)	• Encourage the patient to consume small amounts of water if allowed, assisted by the family or caregiver as needed. • Teach the patient, family, or caregiver to monitor for dry mouth or lips, dry skin, or tenting of the skin as signs that insufficient water is being given.
Minimizing adverse effects: • Monitor vital signs, particularly temperature, throughout nutrition replacement. Assess all access sites (e.g., gastric tube site, IV or port sites) frequently for redness, streaking, swelling, or drainage. Report any fever, chills, malaise, or changes in mental status immediately. (Enteral and parenteral nutritional replacement contains high glucose, protein, and lipid sources that may serve as a reservoir for infection. Tube insertion and access sites may also serve as a point-of-entry for infection.)	• Instruct the patient, family, or caregiver to immediately report any fever, chills, unusual changes to the access site, or changes in the level of consciousness to the health care provider.

Nursing Practice Application *continued*

IMPLEMENTATION	
Interventions and (Rationales)	**Patient-Centered Care**
• Use aseptic technique with all IV tubing or bag changes and enteral and IV site dressing changes. Refrigerate the TPN or enteral solutions until 30 minutes before using and store extra enteral formula in the refrigerator after opening. Follow agency guidelines on the length of time solutions and equipment are allowed to remain in use and change accordingly. (Infusion and tube insertion sites are at high risk for development of infection and must be monitored frequently. Solutions and extra formula must be refrigerated to inhibit bacterial growth.)	• Explain the rationale for all dressing and equipment monitoring and changes. • Teach appropriate technique (aseptic or clean) to the family or caregiver if nutrition is to be continued at home, followed by teach back until the family is comfortable with the routine. • Allow enteral feedings to hang no longer than 4 hours, and refrigerate unused portions of feedings. Plain water may be used to flush the enteral tube. • Provide written instructions on the frequency of bag and tubing changes and how often the solution should be changed.
• Monitor blood glucose levels. Observe for signs of hyperglycemia or hypoglycemia, and obtain capillary glucose levels as ordered. (Blood glucose levels may be affected if nutrition feeding is stopped, the rate is reduced, or is dependent on other medications the patient is taking. Supplemental insulin, subcutaneously or added to the IV solution, may be required.)	• Instruct the patient on the need for frequent glucose monitoring. Teach the patient, family, or caregiver to report signs of hyperglycemia (excessive thirst, copious urination, and insatiable hunger) or hypoglycemia (nervousness, irritability, and dizziness) promptly. • Instruct the patient, family, or caregiver in the technique to monitor capillary glucose, followed by teach-back, if the patient will be on nutrition replacement at home.
• Monitor for signs of fluid overload. (Solutions are hypertonic and may create fluid shifting with resulting changes in intravascular fluid. Monitoring for increased pulse rate and quality, increasing blood pressure, dyspnea, or edema will assist in quickly noting adverse effects.)	• Instruct the patient, family, or caregiver to immediately report shortness of breath, heart palpitations, swelling, decreased urine output, disorientation, or confusion.
• Monitor renal status. (Intake and output ratio, daily weight, and laboratory studies such as serum creatinine and BUN should be monitored.)	• Instruct the patient on home therapy to weigh self daily at the same time each day and record. An increase or loss in weight of over 1 kg (2 lb) per 24 hours should be reported to the health care provider. Report any edema or dyspnea immediately.
• Monitor for signs of venous thrombosis on the same side as the IV catheter. (Venous thrombosis may occur in or around the catheter tubing. Signs and symptoms include the inability to obtain blood on aspiration from the catheter, inability to run fluids through the catheter, neck vein distention, and facial and neck edema on the side of the catheter. The infusion should be stopped and the provider immediately contacted.	• Instruct the patient, family, or caregiver to immediately report a stoppage in the infusion, neck vein distention, or swelling of the face or neck on the side of the IV placement.
• Assess for appropriate enteral tube placement before administering any feeding. (Proper tube insertion should be confirmed radiographically before any feeding is initiated. Confirmation of placement thereafter should be completed per agency policy.) • Maintain accurate enteral feeding or TPN infusion rate with infusion pump; make rate changes gradually; and avoid abruptly discontinuing the TPN feeding. (The use of infusion pumps allows precise control over enteral feeding rate or TPN infusion.)	• Explain the rationale for checking tube placement prior to each feeding to the patient, family, or caregiver. If home enteral therapy is ordered, teach the patient, family, or caregiver the appropriate methods for checking placement prior to feeding. • Teach the patient about the rationale for all equipment used and the need for frequent monitoring. If using home equipment, ensure the proper functioning of equipment and the proper use by the patient, family, or caregiver.
• Assess lung sounds every 4 h or per agency protocol. Immediately report any dyspnea, lung congestion, or changes in sputum to the health care provider. Maintain the head of the bed at a 30-degree angle or greater per agency policy for patients on enteral feedings. (Keeping the head of the bed elevated may help to prevent regurgitation and aspiration.)	• Teach the patient, family, or caregiver to keep the patient in a semi-upright position and to immediately report dyspnea or lung congestion.
• Assess bowel sounds every 4 h, whenever a new amount of feeding is added to continuous feedings, before each bolus feeding, or per agency protocol. Assess for and report diarrhea, especially if profuse, watery, or containing blood or mucus. (Diarrhea or constipation may occur with enteral feedings. Patients on enteral feeding, particularly with elemental formulas, are at increased risk of *Clostridium difficile*–associated diarrhea [CDAD] or other pathogens.)	• Teach the patient, family, or caregiver to report diarrhea or constipation to the health care provider. Immediately report any diarrhea that is profuse, watery, or contains blood or mucus.

continued

Nursing Practice Application *continued*

IMPLEMENTATION	
Interventions and (Rationales)	**Patient-Centered Care**
• Review all oral medications the patient is to receive for appropriateness to be given via enteral tube. Contact the health care provider for alternative forms when necessary. (Oral medications may be crushed for administration via enteral tube in most cases. Enteric-coated, sustained release, gel capsules, and others may not be crushed, and an alternative form or drug may be required.)	• Instruct the patient, family, or caregiver to review any new medication ordered with the provider who has ordered the enteral feeding to ensure appropriateness for administration via the enteral tube.
Patient understanding of drug therapy:	
• Use opportunities during administration of medications and during assessments to provide patient education. (Using time during nursing care helps to optimize and reinforce key teaching areas.)	• The patient, family, or caregiver should be able to state the reason for the drug; appropriate dose and scheduling; what adverse effects to observe for and when to report; and the anticipated length of medication therapy.
Patient self-administration of drug therapy:	
• When administering the medication, instruct the patient, family, or caregiver in the proper self-administration of the drug (e.g., taken with additional fluids). (Proper administration can improve the effectiveness of the drugs.)	• The patient, family, or caregiver is able to discuss appropriate dosing and administration needs. • The patient, family, or caregiver is able to teach-back appropriate dosing and administration and care of access sites and tubes prior to home use.

decades it can lead to obesity in older adults. Of course, this calculation holds true for losing weight, but few are patient enough to wait an entire year to lose a single pound.

Therefore, to lose weight one has to expend more calories than one consumes. Although nutritionists disagree, in terms of weight loss, the *source* of the calories (carbohydrates, proteins, or lipids) probably does not matter. Of course, the source is indeed important in terms of overall health and wellness. There remains considerable debate in the medical community as to which of the energy sources (carbohydrate, protein, or lipid) contributes the most to adult obesity.

Hunger occurs when the hypothalamus recognizes the levels of certain chemicals (glucose) or hormones (insulin) in the blood. Hunger is a normal physiological response that drives people to seek nourishment. Appetite is somewhat different than hunger. Appetite is a *psychological* response that drives food intake based on associations and memory. For example, people often eat not because they are experiencing hunger but because it is a particular time of day, or because they find the act of eating pleasurable or social. This is a key concept because blocking hunger sensations with drugs does not guarantee that a person will have less appetite or consume fewer calories.

Nonpharmacologic strategies should always be attempted before initiating drug therapy for obesity. This is true for two reasons. First, drugs for treating obesity produce only modest results and should be taken for only a few months. For someone who needs to lose 25 or more pounds, nonpharmacologic strategies *must* be employed. Secondly, maintaining an optimal weight cannot be accomplished by drugs alone: Smart lifestyle choices are required. A sustainable, healthy diet and an appropriate exercise program are essential to losing weight and maintaining optimal weight.

DRUGS FOR OBESITY

Despite the public's desire for effective drugs to promote weight loss, there are few such drugs on the market. The approved drugs produce only modest results.

43.13 Pharmacotherapy of Obesity

Because of the prevalence of obesity in society and the difficulty most patients experience when following weight reduction plans for extended periods, drug manufacturers have long sought to develop safe drugs that induce rapid and sustained weight loss. In the 1970s, amphetamine and dextroamphetamine (Dexedrine) were widely prescribed to reduce appetite. However, these drugs are addictive and rarely prescribed for this purpose today. In the 1990s, the combination of fenfluramine and phentermine (fen-phen) was widely prescribed, until fenfluramine was removed from the market for causing heart valve defects. An OTC appetite suppressant, phenylpropanolamine, was removed from the market in 2000 due to an increased incidence of strokes and adverse cardiac events. Until 2004, natural alternative weight-loss products contained ephedra

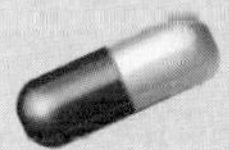

Prototype Drug | Orlistat (*Alli, Xenical)*

Therapeutic Class: Antiobesity drug **Pharmacologic Class:** Lipase inhibitor

Actions and Uses

Orlistat is prescribed for the treatment of obesity in combination with a reduced-calorie diet and exercise. Orlistat is indicated for patients with a BMI of 30 or greater, or a BMI of 27 or greater if the patient has other risk factors such as hypertension, hyperlipidemia, or diabetes. This drug produces only a modest increase in weight reduction compared to placebos.

The prescription form of orlistat (Xenical) is available at 120 mg and is given three times daily, during or just prior to a meal. An OTC dosage form (Alli) is 60 mg. The drug is only effective if taken with meals containing lipids. Orlistat is not approved for children under age 12.

Administration Alerts

- Administer the drug with or up to 1 hour before meals containing fats; if the meal does not contain fat, skip the dose.
- Keep the bottle tightly closed and at room temperature lower than 30°C (86°F). Do not use the drug past its expiration date.
- Pregnancy category B.

PHARMACOKINETICS

Onset	Peak	Duration
24–48 h	Unknown	1–2 h

Adverse Effects

The most common adverse effects of orlistat are GI related and include flatus with discharge, oily stool, fecal urgency, and abdominal pain. To avoid serious adverse GI effects, patients should restrict their fat intake. Orlistat may also decrease the absorption of other substances, including fat-soluble vitamins and warfarin (Coumadin). Rapid weight loss increases the risk for cholelithiasis. Headache is also a common adverse effect.

Contraindications: Contraindications include hypersensitivity to orlistat, malabsorption syndromes, gallbladder disease, hypothyroidism, organic causes of obesity, anorexia nervosa, and bulimia nervosa.

Interactions

Drug–Drug: The absorption of statin medications may be increased. Orlistat may decrease the absorption of fat-soluble vitamins.

Lab Tests: For patients who are taking warfarin, the prothrombin time and international normalized ratio (PT/INR) should be carefully monitored.

Herbal/Food: Unknown.

Treatment of Overdose: Tachycardia and hypertension may result from overdose. Beta-adrenergic blockers may be administered.

alkaloids, but these were removed from the market because of an increased incidence of adverse cardiovascular events.

More recent attempts to find an effective antiobesity treatment have also failed. Rimonabant (Acomplia, Zimulti) was the first of a new class of antiobesity drugs known as cannabinoid receptor (CB1) blockers. The CB1 receptors are primarily found in the brain, and their activation is responsible for the psychoactive effects of marijuana. Overeating activates CB1 receptors in the CNS; blocking them reduces appetite. Although approved in 2006, concerns about adverse effects, especially depression and suicide ideation, prevented the drug from being marketed in the United States. Approval was subsequently withdrawn.

From 2007 until 2010, sibutramine (Meridia) was approved for the adjunctive treatment of obesity. The drug was able to produce a 5% to 10% loss of body weight within 6 to 12 months of treatment. Although well tolerated by most patients, sibutramine was found to produce an unacceptable incidence of serious cardiac events and stroke and was voluntarily removed from the market.

The quest to produce a "magic pill" to lose weight has indeed been elusive. Current pharmacologic strategies for weight management focus primarily on two mechanisms: lipase inhibitors and anorexiants.

Lipase inhibitors are drugs such as orlistat (Alli, Xenical) that block the absorption of dietary fats in the small intestine. Unfortunately, lipase inhibitors may also decrease absorption of other substances, including fat-soluble vitamins and warfarin (Coumadin). To avoid having severe GI effects such as flatus with discharge, oily stool, abdominal pain, and discomfort, patients need to restrict their fat intake when taking this drug. GI effects often diminish after 4 weeks of therapy. Orlistat produces only a very small decrease in weight compared with placebos.

A second strategy to reduce weight is to block regions of the nervous system responsible for hunger with

anorexiants, also called appetite suppressants. Although several drugs in this class have been removed from the market, several newer medications are available.

Diethylpropion (Tenuate) is one of the oldest medications for weight loss that is similar to amphetamine. Given orally, its use is limited to 12 weeks of therapy because tolerance develops rapidly to the anorexiant effects of the drug. If the patient has not lost at least 2 kg (4 lb) after the first month of therapy, treatment should be discontinued. Nervous system adverse effects include confusion, agitation, nervousness, insomnia, and tremors. Diethylpropion is a Schedule IV drug and is pregnancy category B.

Phentermine, once part of the now-banned combination of fen-phen, was approved in 2012 as a fixed-dose combination with topiramate (Qysmia). Phenteramine affects the hypothalamus of the brain, causing decreased appetite. The precise mechanism of the antiobesity action of topiramate, an antiepileptic drug, is unknown. Side effects of Qysmia include paresthesia, dizziness, dysgeusia, insomnia, constipation, and dry mouth. The drug should be discontinued gradually to prevent possible seizures. Both phenteramine and topiramate are pregnancy catgory X drugs and must not be administered to pregnant patients. Phenteramine is a Schedule IV controlled substance.

Approved in 2012, locaserin (Belviq) is a newer anorexiant approved for the short-term therapy of obesity. This drug is believed to act by activating serotonin (5-HT) receptors in the hypothalamus, causing a feeling of fullness or satiety. The drug is well tolerated, with headache and upper respiratory tract infection being the most common side effects. Like other antiobesity drugs, it should be combined with a regimen of diet and exercise for optimal weight loss.

A newer anorexiant approved in 2014, Contrave is a combination of bupropion and naltrexone. Bupropion was previously approved as an atypical antidepressant and naltrexone as an opioid agonist. The combination reduces appetite by increasing dopamine activity and blocking opioid receptors in the brain. Contrave should be discontinued in four months if a weight loss of less than 5% is observed. The drug carries a black box warning that it may cause suicidal behavior. It is pregnancy category X.

Also approved in 2014, liraglutide (Saxenda) is indicated for chronic weight management, along with a calorie-restricted diet. It is only approved for obese patients with at least one comorbid condition, such as hypertension, dyslipidemia, or type 2 diabetes. The drug acts by activating receptors for glucagon-like peptide (GLP-1), which is a physiological regulator of appetite in the brain. This results in decreased calorie intake. The drug is administered daily by the subcutaneous route and carries a black box warning regarding the potential for thyroid carcinoma. It is interesting to note that liraglutide was previously approved by the trade name Tradjenta to treat type 2 diabetes. Despite being the same drug, Saxenda and Tradjenta are not considered interchangeable.

All the anorexiants have the potential to produce serious side effects; thus, their use is limited to short-term therapy. Anorexiants are prescribed for patients with a BMI of at least 30 or greater, or a BMI of 27 or greater with other risk factors for disease such as hypertension, hyperlipidemia, or diabetes.

Chapter Review

KEY Concepts

The numbered key concepts provide a succinct summary of the important points from the corresponding numbered section within the chapter. If any of these points are not clear, refer to the numbered section within the chapter for review.

43.1 Vitamins are organic substances needed in small amounts to promote growth and maintain health. Deficiency of a vitamin will result in disease.

43.2 Vitamins are classified as water-soluble (C and B complex) or lipid-soluble (A, D, E, and K). Excess quantities of lipid-soluble vitamins are stored in the liver and adipose tissue.

43.3 Failure to meet the Recommended Dietary Allowances (RDAs) for vitamins may result in deficiency disorders. The RDA is the amount of a vitamin needed to prevent symptoms of deficiency.

43.4 Vitamin therapy is indicated for conditions such as poor nutritional intake, pregnancy, and chronic disease states. Symptoms of deficiency are usually nonspecific and occur over a prolonged period.

43.5 Deficiencies of vitamins A, D, E, or K are indications for pharmacotherapy with lipid-soluble vitamins.

43.6 Deficiencies of vitamins C, thiamine, riboflavin, niacin, pyridoxine, folic acid, or cyanocobalamin are indications for pharmacotherapy with water soluble vitamins.

43.7 Minerals are essential substances needed in very small amounts to maintain normal body metabolism. Mineral deficiencies may be caused by inadequate dietary intake or by certain medications.

43.8 Pharmacotherapy with macrominerals includes medications containing calcium, phosphorus, magnesium, or potassium. Pharmacotherapy with microminerals includes agents containing iron, iodine, fluorine, or zinc.

43.9 Undernutrition may be caused by low dietary intake, fad diets, malabsorption disorders, or wasting disorders such as cancer or AIDS.

43.10 Enteral nutrition, provided orally or through a feeding tube, is a means of providing a patient's complete nutritional needs.

43.11 Parenteral nutrition, also called total parenteral nutrition (TPN) is a means of supplying nutrition to patients via a peripheral vein (short term) or central vein (long term).

43.12 Genetic, lifestyle, and physiological factors contribute to the etiology of obesity. Nonpharmacologic strategies should be attempted prior to initiating pharmacotherapy.

43.13 Lipase inhibitors cause weight loss by interfering with the absorption of fats. Anorexiants are drugs used to induce weight loss by suppressing appetite and hunger.

REVIEW Questions

1. An older adult has been diagnosed with pernicious anemia, and replacement therapy is ordered. The nurse will anticipate administering which vitamin and by what technique?
   1. B_6, orally in liquid form
   2. K, via intramuscular injection
   3. D, by light-box therapy or increased sun exposure
   4. B_{12}, by intramuscular injection

2. The nurse is preparing to administer magnesium sulfate intravenously to a patient. The nurse should assess for which of the following early signs of magnesium toxicity? (Select all that apply.)
   1. Skin flushing
   2. Anxiety or excitement
   3. Complete heart block
   4. Muscle weakness
   5. Intense thirst

3. The nurse would anticipate administering vitamin K (AquaMEPHYTON) to which of the following patients? (Select all that apply.)
   1. A newborn infant
   2. A patient with hearing impairment secondary to antibiotic use
   3. A teenager with severe acne
   4. A patient who has taken an overdose of the oral anticoagulant warfarin (Coumadin)
   5. A patient with newly diagnosed type 1 diabetes

4. The patient on home-based enteral nutrition via a gastric tube has a temperature of 38.6°C (101.5°F). After assessing the patient, the nurse uses the opportunity to talk with the family about which of the following preventive measures to decrease the risk of infection related to the enteral nutrition?
   1. Hang a feeding solution no longer than 2 hours.
   2. Refrigerate any unused portions of feeding.
   3. Use plain water to irrigate the tube between feedings.
   4. Maintain sterile technique whenever initiating a new feeding solution.

5. A patient has been discharged home on total parenteral nutrition therapy. When making a home visit, which are the most important assessments that should be monitored by the family and the home care nurse?
   1. Temperature and blood pressure
   2. Temperature and weight
   3. Pulse and blood pressure
   4. Pulse and weight

6. A patient has been prescribed orlistat (Xenical). Which of the following will the nurse teach this patient?
   1. Take the drug once in the morning.
   2. Take the drug only when feeling hungry.
   3. Take the drug before exercising daily but no more than three times per day.
   4. Take the drug with or just before a meal containing fats.

PATIENT-FOCUSED Case Study

Jackson Shoewalter is a 66-year-old man with a history of type-1 diabetes. He has been on insulin for over 20 years. During the past few months, Mr. Shoewalter has had increasing difficulty eating. At first he noticed that he felt full almost immediately and then nausea began in waves, eventually resulting in vomiting. He began to lose weight and have trouble controlling his blood glucose levels, experiencing more frequent bouts of hypoglycemia. After seeing his provider and having follow-up testing, he was diagnosed with gastroparesis diabeticorum. His provider has told him that it is most likely due to his diabetes and may be temporary. He has been started on several prokinetic drugs that encourage gastric emptying (e.g., metoclopramide/Reglan and erythromycin). A jejunostomy tube is inserted for feedings until the outcomes of drug therapy can be determined. Mr. Shoewalter has returned for his first postoperative visit to the provider's office and will need teaching about his feeding tube.

1. Mr. Shoewalter wants to know if he can still eat foods "normally." Give a rationale for your answer.
2. He does not know how to take care of his tube and wants to know if any special care is required. As the nurse, what would you teach him?
3. Create a list of potential complications to which Mr. Shoewalter and his family should be alerted.

CRITICAL THINKING Questions

1. A patient has been self-medicating with vitamin B_3 (niacin) for an elevated cholesterol level. The patient comes to the clinic with a severe case of redness and flushing and is concerned about an allergic reaction. What is the nurse's best response?
2. A patient complains of a constant headache for the past several days. The only supplements the patient has been taking are megadoses of vitamins A, C, and E. What would be a priority for the nurse with this patient?

Visit www.pearsonhighered.com/nursingresources for answers and rationales for all activities.

REFERENCES

Autier, P., Bonjol, M., Pizot, C., & Mullie, P. (2014). Vitamin D status and ill health: A systematic review. *The Lancet Diabetes & Endocrinology, 2,* 76–89. doi:10.1016/S2213-8587(13)70165-7

Heaney, R. P., & Armas, L. A. (2015). Screening for vitamin D deficiency: Is the goal disease prevention or nutrient repletion? *Annals of Internal Medicine, 162,* 144–145. doi:10.7326/M14-2573

Herdman, T. H., & Kamitsuru, S. (Eds.). (2014). *NANDA International nursing diagnoses: Definitions and classification, 2015–2017.* Oxford, United Kingdom: Wiley-Blackwell.

LeBlanc, E. S., Zakher, B., Daeges, M., Pappas, M., & Chou, R. (2015). Screening for vitamin D deficiency: A systematic review for U.S. Preventative Services Task Force. *Annals of Internal Medicine, 162,* 109–122. doi:10.7326/M14-1659

LeFevre, M. L. (2015). Screening for vitamin D deficiency in adults: U.S. Preventive Services Task Force recommendation statement. *Annals of Internal Medicine, 162,* 133–140. doi:10.7326/M14-2450

Palacios, C., & Gonzalez, L. (2014). Is vitamin D deficiency a major global public health problem? *Journal of Steroid Biochemistry and Molecular Biology, 144,* 138–145. doi:10.1016/j.jsbmb.2013.11.003

Schodin, B. A. (2014). Vitamin D testing: The controversy continues. *MLO: Medical Laboratory Observer, 46*(6), 16, 18.

Sohl, E., Heymans, M. W., de Jongh, R.T., den Jeijer, M., Visser, M., Merlijn, T., . . . van Schoor, N. M. (2014). Prediction of vitamin D deficiency by simple patient characteristics. *The American Journal of Clinical Nutrition, 99,* 1089–1095. doi:10.3945/ajcn.113.076430

Sun, Q., Pan, A., Hu, F. B., Manson, J. E., & Rexrode, K. M. (2012). 25-Hydroxyvitamin D levels and the risk of stroke: A prospective study and meta-analysis. *Stroke, 43,* 1470–1477. doi:10.1161/STROKEAHA.111.636910

Theodoratou, E., Tzoulaki, I., Zgaga, L., & Ioannidis, J. P. (2014). Vitamin D and multiple health outcomes: Umbrella review of systematic reviews and meta-analyses of observational studies and randomised trials. *BMJ, 348,* g2035. doi:10.1136/bmj.g2035

Wang, L., Song, Y., Manson, J. E., Pilz, S., März, W., Michaëlsson, K., . . . Sesso, H. D. (2012). Circulating 25-hydroxy-vitamin D and risk of cardiovascular disease: A meta-analysis of prospective studies. *Circulation: Cardiovascular Quality and Outcomes, 5,* 819–829. doi:10.1161/CIRCOUTCOMES.112.967604

SELECTED BIBLIOGRAPHY

Bistrian, B. R. (2012). The who, what, where, when, why, and how of early enteral feeding. *The American Journal of Clinical Nutrition, 95,* 1303–1304. doi:10.3945/ajcn.112.039826

Boullata, J. I. (2013). Drug and nutrition interactions: Not just food for thought. *Journal of Clinical Pharmacy and Therapeutics, 38,* 269–271. doi:10.1111/jcpt.12075

Bray, G. A. (2013). Why do we need drugs to treat the patient with obesity? *Obesity, 21,* 893–899. doi:10.1002/oby.20394

Bray, G. A., & Ryan, D. H. (2014). Update on obesity pharmacotherapy. *Annals of the New York Academy of Sciences, 1311,* 1–13. doi:10.1111/nyas.12328

Centers for Disease Control and Prevention. (2014). *Overweight and obesity: Adult obesity facts.* Retrieved from http://www.cdc.gov/obesity/data/adult.html

Dawodu, S. T. (2013). *Nutritional management in the rehabilitation setting.* Retrieved from http://emedicine.medscape.com/article/318180-overview#a1

Dibb, M., Teubner, A., Theis, V., Shaffer, J., & Lal, S. (2013). Review article: The management of long-term parenteral nutrition. *Alimentary Pharmacology and Therapeutics, 37,* 587–603. doi:10.1111/apt.12209

Hark, L., Ashton, K., & Deen, D. (Eds.). (2012). *The nurse practitioner's guide to nutrition* (2nd ed.). Oxford, United Kingdom: Wiley-Blackwell.

Hitt, E. (2011). *Updated USDA dietary guidelines released.* Retrieved from http://www.medscape.org/viewarticle/736605

Howes, R. M. (2011). Mythology of antioxidant vitamins? *Journal of Evidence-Based Complementary & Alternative Medicine, 16,* 149–159. doi:10.1177/1533210110392995

Moyer, V. A. (2014). Vitamin, mineral, and multivitamin supplements for the primary prevention of cardiovascular disease and cancer: U.S. Preventive Services Task Force recommendation statement. *Annals of Internal Medicine, 160,* 558–564. doi:10.7326/M14-0198

National Institutes of Health, Office of Dietary Supplements. (n.d.). *Nutrient recommendations: Dietary reference intakes (DRI).* Retrieved from http://ods.od.nih.gov/Health_Information/Dietary_Reference_Intakes.aspx

Rosenbloom, M. (2014). *Vitamin toxicity.* Retrieved from http://emedicine.medscape.com/article/819426-overview

Seres, D. S., Valcarcel, M., & Guillaume, A. (2013). Advantages of enteral nutrition over parenteral nutrition. *Therapeutic Advances in Gastroenterology, 6,* 157–167. doi:10.1177/1756283X12467564

Tucker, S., & Dauffenbach, V. (2011). *Nutrition and diet therapy.* Upper Saddle River, NJ: Pearson Education.

Walmsley, R. S. (2013). Refeeding syndrome: Screening, incidence, and treatment during parenteral nutrition. *Journal of Gastroenterology and Hepatology, 28*(Suppl. 4), 113–117. doi:10.1111/jgh.12345

Chapter 44

Drugs for Pituitary, Thyroid, and Adrenal Disorders

Drugs at a Glance

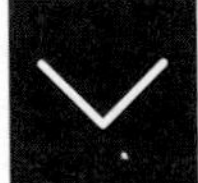

Learning Outcomes

After reading this chapter, the student should be able to:

1. Describe the general structure and functions of the endocrine system.
2. Through the use of specific examples, explain the concept of negative feedback in the endocrine system.
3. Explain the pharmacotherapy of growth hormone disorders in children and adults.
4. Explain the pharmacotherapy of antidiuretic hormone disorders.
5. Identify the signs and symptoms of hypothyroidism and hyperthyroidism.
6. Explain the pharmacotherapy of thyroid disorders.
7. Describe the signs and symptoms of Addison's disease and Cushing's syndrome.
8. Explain the pharmacotherapy of adrenal gland disorders.
9. Describe the nurse's role in the pharmacologic management of pituitary, thyroid, and adrenal disorders.
10. For each of the classes listed in Drugs at a Glance, know representative drugs, and explain the mechanisms of drug action, primary actions, and important adverse effects.
11. Use the nursing process to care for patients who are receiving pharmacotherapy for pituitary, thyroid, and adrenal disorders.

indicates a prototype drug, each of which is featured in a Prototype Drug box.

The nervous system and endocrine system are major controllers of homeostasis. Whereas nerve fibers may exert instantaneous control over a single muscle fiber or gland, hormones from the endocrine system affect thousands of cells and take as long as several days to produce an optimal response. Hormonal balance is kept within a narrow range: Too little or too much of a hormone produces profound physiological changes. This chapter examines common endocrine disorders and their pharmacotherapy. The reproductive hormones are covered in chapters 46 and 47.

THE ENDOCRINE SYSTEM

44.1 The Endocrine System and Homeostasis

The endocrine system consists of various glands that secrete **hormones,** chemical messengers released in response to a change in the body's internal environment. The role of hormones is to maintain homeostasis. For example, when the level of glucose in the blood rises above normal, the pancreas secretes insulin to return glucose levels to normal. The various endocrine glands and their hormones are illustrated in Figure 44.1.

After secretion from an endocrine gland, hormones enter the blood and are transported throughout the body. Some, such as insulin and thyroid hormone, have receptors on nearly every cell in the body; thus, these hormones have widespread effects. Others, such as parathyroid hormone (PTH) and oxytocin, have receptors on only a few specific types of cells. The cells affected by a hormone are called target cells.

Because hormones can produce profound effects on the body, their secretion and release are carefully regulated by several levels of control. The most important control mechanism is called *negative feedback*. A hormone causes an action at its target cell or tissue. As an example, a rising level of glucose in the blood serves as a stimulus and prompts the release of insulin from the pancreas, which functions as the control center. As insulin is secreted from the pancreas, glucose is removed from the bloodstream by cells in the tissues to result in a falling level of glucose. Thus, the output signal of the control center is a reversal of the initial stimulus. This is the way balance or homeostasis in the body is maintained most of the time. The fact that the feedback is "negative" means that the output signal has reversed the condition of the original stimulus.

When given as medications, hormones can affect negative feedback processes. For example, testosterone may be given as a medication to increase sperm count, or glucocorticoids may be given for a rheumatoid arthritis condition. Rising levels of steroids in the bloodstream however, will "feedback" and inhibit the release of other hormones in the brain and pituitary gland. Hormones from these areas impact secondary endocrine targets located throughout the body. Effects can be both diverse and adverse. Continued use of testosterone or glucocorticoid medications can produce serious negative feedback disruption and cause various glands in the body to atrophy or become nonfunctional. As is evident from these examples, understanding the concept of negative feedback is essential for effective hormone pharmacotherapy.

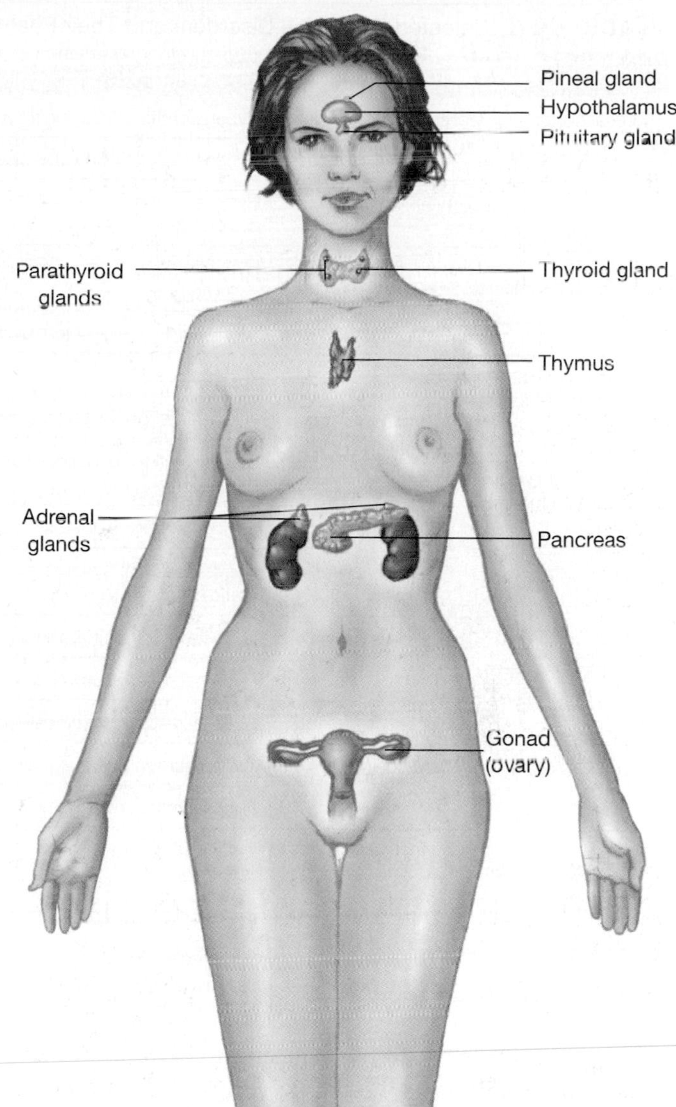

FIGURE 44.1 The endocrine system

44.2 Indications for Hormone Pharmacotherapy

The goals of hormone pharmacotherapy vary widely. In many cases, a hormone is administered as simple replacement therapy for patients who are unable to secrete sufficient quantities of their own endogenous hormones. Examples of replacement therapy include the administration of thyroid hormone after the thyroid gland has been surgically removed, or supplying insulin to patients whose pancreas is

Table 44.1 Selected Endocrine Disorders and Their Pharmacotherapy

Gland	Hormone(s)	Disorder	Drug Therapy Examples
Adrenal cortex	Corticosteroids	Hypersecretion: Cushing's syndrome	ketoconazole (Nizoral) and mitotane (Lysodren)
		Hyposecretion: Addison's disease	hydrocortisone, prednisone
Gonads	Ovaries: estrogen	Hyposecretion: menstrual and metabolic dysfunction	conjugated estrogens and estradiol
	Ovaries: progesterone	Hyposecretion: dysfunctional uterine bleeding	medroxyprogesterone (Provera, Others) and norethindrone
	Testes: testosterone	Hyposecretion: hypogonadism	testosterone
Pancreatic islets	Insulin	Hyposecretion: diabetes mellitus	insulin and oral antidiabetic drugs
Parathyroid	Parathyroid hormone	Hypersecretion: hyperparathyroidism	surgery (no drug therapy)
		Hyposecretion: hypoparathyroidism	human parathyroid hormone (Natpara), vitamin D and calcium supplements
Pituitary	Antidiuretic hormone	Hyposecretion: diabetes insipidus	desmopressin (DDAVP, Stimate) and vasopressin
		Hypersecretion: syndrome of inappropriate antidiuretic hormone (SIADH)	conivaptan (Vaprisol) and tolvaptan (Samsca)
	Growth hormone	Hyposecretion: small stature	somatropin (Genotropin, Others)
		Hypersecretion: acromegaly (adults)	octreotide (Sandostatin)
	Oxytocin	Hyposecretion: delayed delivery or lack of milk ejection	oxytocin (Pitocin)
Thyroid	Thyroid hormone (T_3 and T_4)	Hypersecretion: Graves' disease	propylthiouracil (PTU) and I-131
		Hyposecretion: myxedema (adults), cretinism (children)	thyroid hormone and levothyroxine (T4)

not functioning. Replacement therapy supplies the same physiological, low-level amounts of the hormone that would normally be present in the body. Selected endocrine disorders and their drug therapy are summarized in Table 44.1.

Some hormones are used in cancer chemotherapy to shrink the size of hormone-sensitive tumors. Examples include testosterone for breast cancer and estrogen for testicular cancer. Exactly how these hormones produce their antineoplastic action is largely unknown. When hormones are used as antineoplastics, their doses far exceed normal physiological levels. Hormones are always used in combination with other antineoplastic medications, as discussed in chapter 38.

Another goal of hormonal pharmacotherapy may be to produce an *exaggerated response* that is part of the normal action of the hormone. Administering hydrocortisone to suppress inflammation takes advantage of the normal action of the corticosteroids but to a greater extent than would normally occur in the body. Supplying estrogen or progesterone at specific times during the menstrual cycle can prevent ovulation and pregnancy. In this example, the patient is given these hormones; however, they are taken at a time when levels in the body are normally low.

Endocrine pharmacotherapy also involves the use of "antihormones." These hormone antagonists block the actions of endogenous hormones. For example, propylthiouracil (PTU) is given to block the effects of an overactive thyroid gland (see section 44.7). Tamoxifen is given to block the actions of estrogen in estrogen-dependent breast cancers (see chapter 38).

THE HYPOTHALAMUS AND PITUITARY GLAND

44.3 The Endocrine Structures of the Brain

Two endocrine structures in the brain, the hypothalamus and the pituitary gland, deserve special recognition because they control many other endocrine glands. The hypothalamus secretes **releasing hormones** that travel via blood vessels a short distance to the pituitary gland. These releasing hormones specify which hormone is to be released by the pituitary. After secretion, the pituitary hormone travels to its target tissues to cause its biologic effects. For example, the hypothalamus secretes thyrotropin-releasing hormone (TRH) that travels to the pituitary gland with the message to secrete thyroid-stimulating hormone (TSH). TSH then travels to its target organ, the thyroid gland, to stimulate the release of thyroid hormone. Although the pituitary is often called the master gland, the pituitary and hypothalamus are best visualized as an integrated unit.

The pituitary gland comprises two distinct regions. The anterior pituitary, or **adenohypophysis,** consists of *glandular tissue* and secretes adrenocorticotropic hormone

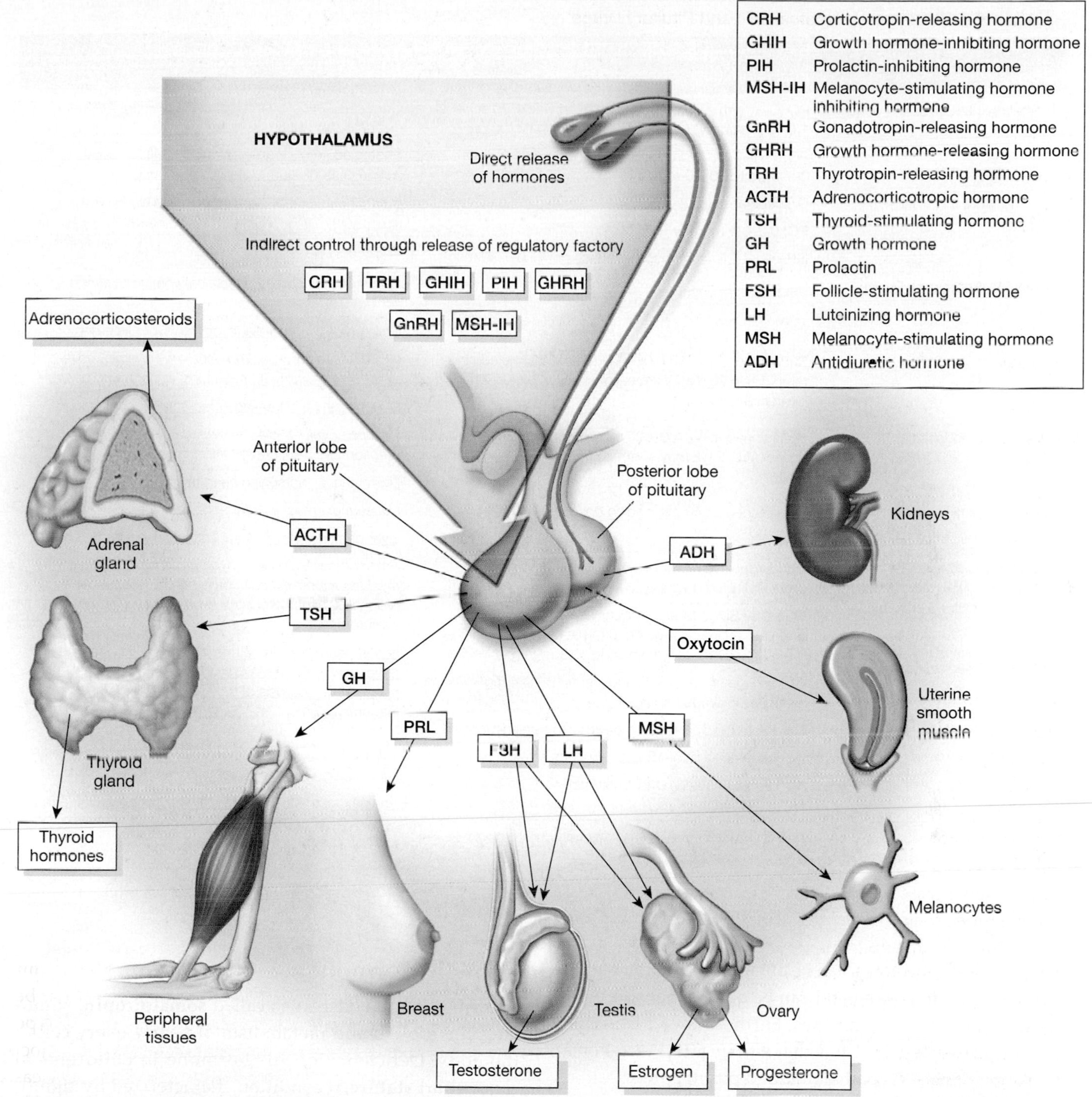

FIGURE 44.2 Hormones associated with the hypothalamus and the pituitary gland

(ACTH), TSH, growth hormone, prolactin, follicle-stimulating hormone (FSH), and luteinizing hormone (LH). The posterior pituitary, or **neurohypophysis,** contains *nervous tissue* rather than glandular tissue. Neurons in the posterior pituitary store antidiuretic hormone (ADH) and oxytocin, which are released in response to nerve impulses from the hypothalamus. Those hormones that affect the female reproductive tract are presented in chapter 46. Selected hormones associated with the hypothalamus and pituitary gland are shown in Figure 44.2.

HYPOTHALAMIC AND PITUITARY DRUGS

44.4 Pharmacotherapy With Pituitary and Hypothalamic Hormones

Of the 15 different hormones secreted by the pituitary and the hypothalamus, only a few are used in pharmacotherapy. There are valid reasons why they are not widely used.

Table 44.2 Selected Hypothalamic and Pituitary Drugs*

Drug	Route and Adult Dose (maximum dose where indicated)	Adverse Effects
bromocriptine (Cycloset, Parlodel)	PO (Cycloset): 0.8 mg daily, increased weekly to achieve 1.6–4.8 mg daily PO: 1.25–2.5 mg/day for 3 days, then increase dose every 3–7 days to 30–60 mg/day	*Orthostatic hypotension, nausea, vomiting, fatigue, dizziness, headache* Shock, acute myocardial infarction (MI), cerebral ischemia, confusion, agitation, psychosis
desmopressin (DDAVP, Stimate)	IV/subcutaneous: 2–4 mcg in two divided doses PO: 0.2–0.4 mg/day Intranasal (Stimate); 1 spray in each nostril (10–40 mcg)	*Headache, nasal congestion or irritation, nausea* Water intoxication, coma, thromboembolic disorder, hyponatremia
lanreotide (Somatuline Depot)	Subcutaneous: 60–100 mg every 4 wk	*Pain at the injection site, nausea, vomiting, diarrhea, itching* Gallstones, bradycardia, hyper- or hypoglycemia
mecasermin (Increlex)	Subcutaneous: 0.04–0.08 mg/kg bid. Must be administered within 20 min of a meal or snack (max: 0.12 mg/kg given bid)	*Injection-site reaction, iron deficiency anemia, goiter, antibody development, headache, hypertrophy of tonsils* Hypoglycemia, increased intracranial pressure
octreotide (Sandostatin)	Subcutaneous/IV: 100–600 mcg/day in two to four divided doses; after 2 wk may switch to IM depot, 20 mg every 4 wk	*Nausea, vomiting, diarrhea, headache, flushing, injection-site pain, cholelithiasis* Dysrhythmia, worsening heart failure, sinus bradycardia
pegvisomant (Somavert)	Subcutaneous: 40 mg loading dose, then 10 mg/day (max: 30 mg/day)	*Nausea, diarrhea, injection-site pain, flulike symptoms* Liver damage, elevated transaminase levels
somatotropin (Genotropin, Humatrope, Norditropin, Nutropin, Saizen, Serostim, Zorbtive)	Humatrope: Subcutaneous: 0.006 mg/kg daily (max: 0.0125 mg/kg/day) Serostim: Subcutaneous: Weight more than 55 kg: 6 mg at bedtime; 45–55 kg: 5 mg at bedtime; 35–45 kg: 4 mg at bedtime; less than 35 kg: 0.1 mg/kg at bedtime Child: Genotropin: Subcutaneous: 0.16–0.24 mg/kg/wk in six to seven divided doses Norditropin: 0.024–0.034 mg/kg six to seven times/wk	*Pain at the injection site, hyperglycemia, arthralgia, myalgia, abdominal pain, otitis media, headache, bronchitis, hypothyroidism, hypertension (HTN), flulike symptoms* Severe respiratory impairment in severely obese patients with Prader-Willi syndrome, diabetes, pancreatitis, scoliosis of the spine, papilledema, intracranial tumor
vasopressin	IM/subcutaneous: 5–10 units aqueous solution bid–qid IV: 0.2–0.4 unit/min up to 1 unit/min	*Tremor, pallor, nausea, vomiting, water retention, intoxication* Angina, acute MI, gangrene, anaphylaxis, cardiac arrest

*Hypothalamic and pituitary drugs used for conditions of the female reproductive system are presented in chapter 46.
Note: *Italics* indicate common adverse effects; underlining indicates serious adverse effects.

Some of these hormones can be obtained only from natural sources (human brains) and can be quite expensive when used in therapeutic quantities. Furthermore, it is usually more effective to give drugs that *directly* affect secretion at the target organs. Hypothalamic and pituitary medications are listed in Table 44.2.

The only hypothalamic hormone used clinically is gonadotropin-releasing hormone (GnRH). Leuprolide (Lupron), goserelin (Zoladex), and nafarelin (Synarel) are analogs of GnRH that are used to treat endometriosis, a common cause of infertility (see chapter 46). Leuprolide and goserelin are also used for the palliative treatment of advanced prostate cancer. Two pituitary hormones, prolactin and oxytocin, affect the female reproductive system and are discussed in chapter 46. Corticotropin affects the adrenal gland and is discussed later in this chapter. Of the remaining, growth hormone and antidiuretic hormone have the most clinical utility.

Growth Hormone

Growth hormone (GH), also called **somatotropin,** stimulates the growth and metabolism of nearly every cell in the body. Deficiency of this hormone in children can cause **short stature,** a condition characterized by significantly decreased physical height compared with the norm of a specific age group. Severe deficiency results in dwarfism. Short stature is caused by many conditions other than GH deficiency, and often a specific cause cannot be identified.

Prior to 1985, all GH was obtained by extracting the hormone from human pituitary glands, which severely limited the amount available for pharmacotherapy. Human GH, somatropin (Accretropin, Genotropin, others), is now available by the subcutaneous route in large quantities through recombinant DNA technology. If therapy is begun early in life, as much as 6 inches of growth may be achieved. GH therapy is contraindicated in patients after the epiphyses have closed. GH agents are usually well tolerated, although patients must undergo regular assessments of glucose tolerance and thyroid function during pharmacotherapy.

Mecasermin (Increlex) is a newer drug that has the same actions as GH. Mecasermin is indicated for the long-term treatment of growth failure in children with severe deficiency of insulin-like growth factor (IGF) or for those who have developed neutralizing antibodies to GH. It is administered once daily by the subcutaneous route. It should not be administered to adults, after the epiphyses have closed. Adverse effects include hypoglycemia, headache, dizziness, vomiting, and tonsillar hypertrophy.

Prior to 2003, GH therapy was approved only for treating short stature in children who had deficiencies in GH. GH therapy is now approved to treat children with short stature who have normal levels of GH. Therapy produces only modest improvement in height. Before proceeding, the physician and parents need to determine whether these gains are likely to be beneficial to the psychological well-being of the patient. Furthermore, the annual cost of $30,000 to $50,000 may discourage many parents from seeking this therapy for their children.

Excess secretion of GH in adults is known as **acromegaly.** Acromegaly is a rare disorder caused by a GH-secreting tumor of the pituitary gland. Because the epiphyseal plates are closed in adults, bones become deformed rather than elongated with this disorder. The onset is gradual, with enlargement of the small bones of the hands, feet, face, and skull; broad nose; protruding lower jaw; and slanting forehead.

Treatment of acromegaly consists of a combination of surgery, radiation therapy, and pharmacotherapy to suppress GH secretion or block GH receptors. Pharmacotherapy is generally attempted only in patients who are unable to undergo surgical removal of the tumor. Octreotide (Sandostatin) is a synthetic GH *antagonist* structurally related to GH–inhibiting hormone (somatostatin). In addition to inhibiting GH, octreotide promotes fluid and electrolyte reabsorption from the gastrointestinal (GI) tract and prolongs intestinal transit time. It has limited applications in treating acromegaly in adults and in treating the severe diarrhea sometimes associated with metastatic carcinoid tumors. Other choices to treat acromegaly include pegvisomant (Somavert), bromocriptine (Cycloset, Parlodel), and lanreotide (Somatuline Depot).

Antidiuretic Hormone

It is essential that the amount of fluids in the body be maintained within narrow limits. Loss of large amounts of water leads to dehydration, whereas too much body fluid leads to congestion, edema, and water intoxication. **Antidiuretic hormone (ADH)** is one of the most important means the body uses to maintain fluid homeostasis.

As its name implies, ADH conserves water in the body. ADH is secreted from the posterior pituitary gland when the hypothalamus senses that plasma volume has decreased or that the osmolality of the blood has become too high. ADH acts on the collecting ducts in the kidneys to increase water reabsorption. The increased amount of water in the body reduces serum osmolality to normal levels and ADH secretion stops. ADH is also called *vasopressin,* because it has the ability to constrict blood vessels and raise blood pressure.

A deficiency in ADH results in **diabetes insipidus (DI),** a rare condition characterized by the production of large volumes of very dilute urine, usually accompanied by increased thirst. Two ADH preparations are available for the treatment of diabetes insipidus: desmopressin (DDAVP) and vasopressin.

Desmopressin is the most common drug for treating DI. Details regarding this drug may be found in the Prototype Drug feature.

Vasopressin is a synthetic drug that has a structure identical with that of human ADH. It acts on the renal collecting tubules to increase their permeability to water, thus enhancing water reabsorption. Although it acts within minutes, vasopressin has a short half-life that requires it to be administered three to four times per day. Vasopressin tannate is formulated in peanut oil to increase its duration of action. Vasopressin is usually given by intramuscular (IM) or intravenous (IV) injection, although an intranasal form is available for mild DI.

THE THYROID GLAND

44.5 Normal Function of the Thyroid Gland

The thyroid gland secretes hormones that affect nearly every cell in the body. Thyroid hormone increases **basal metabolic rate,** which is the baseline speed at which cells perform their functions. By increasing cellular metabolism, this hormone increases body temperature. Adequate secretion of thyroid hormone is also necessary for the normal growth and development in infants and children, including mental development and attainment of sexual maturity. The thyroid strongly affects cardiovascular, respiratory, GI, and neuromuscular function.

The thyroid gland has two basic types of cells which secrete different hormones. Parafollicular cells secrete calcitonin, a hormone that is involved with calcium homeostasis (see chapter 48). **Follicular cells** in the gland secrete thyroid hormone, which actually consists of two different hormones:

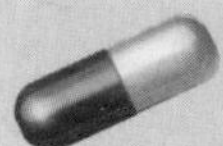

Prototype Drug | Desmopressin *(DDAVP, Stimate)*

Therapeutic Class: Antidiuretic hormone replacement **Pharmacologic Class:** Vasopressin analog

Actions and Uses

Desmopressin is a synthetic analog of human ADH that acts on the kidneys to increase the reabsorption of water. It is used to control the acute symptoms of DI in patients who have insufficient ADH secretion. The oral (PO) route is preferred, although intranasal and parenteral forms are available. It has a duration of action of up to 20 hours, whereas vasopressin has a duration of only 2–8 hours.

Desmopressin causes contraction of smooth muscle in the vascular system, uterus, and GI tract. It also produces an increase in clotting Factor VIII and von Willebrand's factor and is thus indicated for the management of bleeding in patients with hemophilia A and von Willebrand's disease (type I). When taken an hour prior to bedtime, desmopressin lowers the production of urine during the night and thus is useful in the management of nocturnal enuresis (bed-wetting).

Administration Alerts

- When administered IV for DI, desmopressin is given undiluted over 1 minute.
- Following an IV injection, fluids must be restricted and carefully monitored to prevent serious water intoxication.
- Pregnancy category B.

PHARMACOKINETICS

Onset	Peak	Duration
Immediate IV; 1 h PO	15–30 min IV; 4–7 h PO	3 h IV; 8–20 h PO

Adverse Effects

Desmopressin can cause symptoms of water intoxication: drowsiness, headache, and listlessness, progressing to convulsions and coma. Other adverse effects include transient headache, nausea, mild abdominal pain and cramping, facial flushing, HTN, pain, or swelling at the injection site. Intranasal forms can cause nasal congestion, rhinitis, and epistaxis. Tolerance develops to the effects of desmopressin when it is administered more frequently than every 48 hours or by the IV route.

Contraindications: Desmopressin is contraindicated in patients with DI that is caused by kidney disease because the drug can worsen fluid retention and overload. It is used with caution in patients with coronary artery disease and HTN and in patients at risk for hyponatremia or thrombi. Young children and older adults should be treated with caution because they are more prone to water intoxication and hyponatremia.

Interactions

Drug–Drug: Increased antidiuretic action can occur with carbamazepine, chlorpropamide, clofibrate, and nonsteroidal anti-inflammatory drugs (NSAIDs). Decreased antidiuretic action can occur with lithium, alcohol, heparin, and epinephrine.

Lab Tests: Unknown.

Herbal/Food: Unknown.

Treatment of Overdose: Overdose may cause severe water intoxication. Treatment includes water restriction and osmotic diuretics.

Nursing Practice Application

Pharmacotherapy With Hypothalamic and Pituitary Hormones

ASSESSMENT

Baseline assessment prior to administration:

- Obtain a complete health history including cardiovascular, GI, hepatic, or renal disease; pregnancy; or breast-feeding. Obtain a drug history including allergies, current prescription and over-the-counter (OTC) drugs, herbal preparations, alcohol use, or smoking. Be alert to possible drug interactions.
- Evaluate appropriate laboratory findings (e.g., urine and serum osmolality, urine specific gravity, serum protein, complete blood count [CBC], electrolytes, glucose, hepatic and renal function studies).
- Obtain baseline height, weight, and vital signs. Obtain an ECG on patients who are taking GH antagonists.

POTENTIAL NURSING DIAGNOSES*

- *Deficient Fluid Volume*
- *Diarrhea*
- *Disturbed Body Image*
- *Impaired Urinary Elimination*
- *Situational Low Self-Esteem*
- *Deficient Knowledge* (drug therapy)
- *Risk for Disproportionate Growth*
- *Risk for Delayed Development*
- *Risk for Fluid Volume Overload,* related to adverse drug effects
- *Risk for Unstable Blood Glucose Level,* related to adverse drug effects
- *Risk for Bleeding*

*NANDA I © 2014

Nursing Practice Application *continued*

ASSESSMENT	POTENTIAL NURSING DIAGNOSES*
Assessment throughout administration: • Assess for desired therapeutic effects depending on the reason the drug is being given (e.g., measurable increase in height, slowed diuresis, return to normal urine output and serum osmolality, return to normal bowel activity). • Continue periodic monitoring of urine and serum osmolality, urine specific gravity, CBC, electrolytes, glucose, and hepatic and renal function studies. • Continue monitoring vital signs, height, and weight. Monitor the ECG for patients who are taking growth hormone antagonists. • Assess for adverse effects: nausea, vomiting, diarrhea, and headache. Hypotension or HTN, tachycardia, dysrhythmias, or angina should be reported immediately.	

IMPLEMENTATION

Interventions and (Rationales)	Patient-Centered Care
Ensuring therapeutic effects:	
• *Patients who are taking GH:* Monitor height and weight at each clinical visit. Report lack of growth to the health care provider. (Lack of growth after a period of consistent growth may indicate the development of antibodies against GH.) • *Patients who are taking GH antagonists:* Monitor levels of serum GH. Monitor bowel sounds and for a decrease in diarrhea. (GH antagonists are given for acromegaly, severe diarrhea unresponsive to other drug therapy, and the treatment of portal HTN. Monitoring levels of serum GH and bowel activity will evaluate therapeutic changes.) • *Patients who are taking ADH:* For patients with DI, monitor urine output, urine and serum osmolality, and urine specific gravity for return to normal limits. If given for nocturnal enuresis, have the patient, family, or caregiver keep a diary of sleep patterns, noting any bed-wetting. (Urine output, osmolality, and specific gravity should return to normal limits. Bed-wetting has slowed or stopped.)	• Teach the patient, family, or caregiver to measure and record height and weight weekly and bring the record to each clinical visit. • Instruct the patient on the need to return periodically for laboratory work. • Instruct the patient to monitor output and to keep a record of daily weight and output and bring the record to each provider visit. Provide measuring equipment as needed. • Teach the patient, family, or caregiver to keep a diary of nighttime sleep habits and any bed-wetting. Limit oral fluids within 4 hours of bedtime. • Advise the patient of the drug's cost before beginning therapy. Explore the ability to maintain drug therapy for the duration of the treatment prescribed. **Collaboration:** Assess financial concerns and provide appropriate social service referral as needed.
Minimizing adverse effects:	
• Monitor for any complaints of muscle, joint, or bone pain, particularly in the knee or hip, or any changes in gait. (Avascular necrosis is an adverse drug effect of GH. Increasing or severe pain in joints or changes in gait should be reported promptly for follow-up evaluation.)	• Instruct the patient, family, or caregiver to report any changes in walking, discomfort or pain in the knee or hip joints, bone pain, or consistent muscle pain over joint areas to the health care provider.
• Monitor glucose levels, particularly in patients with diabetes. Report consistent elevations to the health care provider. (GH and GH antagonists may cause increases in glucose level. Patients with diabetes may need alterations in their normal medication routines if hyperglycemia occurs.)	• Instruct the patient on the need to return periodically for laboratory work. • Teach the patient with diabetes to monitor capillary glucose levels more frequently during therapy. Teach the patient to report any consistent elevations in blood glucose to the health care provider.
• Continue to monitor vital signs, especially pulse and blood pressure, especially for patients with cardiac disease. ECGs may be ordered periodically for patients with a history of dysrhythmias. Monitor daily weight, output, level of consciousness, lung sounds, and for peripheral edema. (Fluid retention secondary to ADH treatment may lead to increased intravascular volume and HTN.)	• Instruct the patient to immediately report pounding headache, dizziness, palpitations, or syncope. • Teach the patient, family, or caregiver how to monitor pulse and blood pressure as appropriate. Ensure the proper use and functioning of any home equipment obtained. • Instruct the patient to monitor output and to keep a record of daily weight and output and bring the record to each provider visit. Provide measuring equipment as needed.
• Monitor for signs of peripheral ischemia or angina and report immediately. (Vasoconstriction caused by vasopressin may cause cardiac or peripheral ischemia, angina, or infarction.)	• Instruct the patient to immediately report any chest pain, pain or numbness in toes or fingers, or cramping when walking to the health care provider.

continued

Nursing Practice Application *continued*

IMPLEMENTATION	
Interventions and (Rationales)	**Patient-Centered Care**
• For patients who are taking intranasal medications, monitor nasal passages. Report any excoriation or bleeding. (Long-term intranasal ADH therapy may cause nasal irritation and ulceration.)	• Teach the patient to report nasal congestion, irritation, increase in nasal discharge, or nasal bleeding to the health care provider.
• Continue to monitor nutritional and fluid intake. (Chronic, severe diarrhea requiring treatment with a GH antagonist may result in nutritional deficits and dehydration until the diarrhea is corrected. Dietary consultation may be required.)	• Encourage increased fluid intake, up to 2 L per day, taken in frequent small amounts. • Encourage small, high-calorie, nutrient-dense meals rather than large, infrequent meals.
Patient understanding of drug therapy: • Use opportunities during administration of medications and during assessments to provide patient education. (Using time during nursing care helps to optimize and reinforce key teaching areas.)	• The patient should be able to state the reason for the drug, appropriate dose and scheduling, and what adverse effects to observe for and when to report them.
Patient self-administration of drug therapy: • When administering the medication, instruct the patient, family, or caregiver in the proper self-administration of the drug (e.g., during evening meal.) (Proper administration will increase the effectiveness of the drug.)	• Teach the patient to take the drug according to appropriate guidelines, as follows: • Reconstitute the parenteral drug exactly per package directions and do not shake the vial but rotate gently to avoid breaking down the drug. • Direct nasal sprays high into the nasal cavity rather than back to the nasopharynx. Do not shake the nasal spray before using but rotate gently. • Store any unused reconstituted solutions in the refrigerator. Nasal sprays may be kept at room temperature but avoid excessive heat over 80°F. Discard any discolored solution or if particulate matter is present. • Administer GH drugs in the evening to mimic the body's natural rhythms. • Administer subcutaneous injections in the abdomen, buttock, or thigh areas.

See Table 44.2 for a list of drugs to which these nursing actions apply.

thyroxine (T_4) and triiodothyronine (T_3). Iodine is essential for the synthesis of these hormones and is provided through the dietary intake of common iodized salt. The names of these hormones refer to the number of bound iodine atoms in each molecule, either three (T_3) or four (T_4). Thyroxine is the major hormone secreted by the thyroid gland; however, it is converted to T_3 before it enters its target cells. T_3 is three to five times more biologically active than T_4.

As it travels through the blood, thyroid hormone is attached to a carrier protein in the plasma, **thyroxine-binding globulin (TBG),** which protects it from degradation. Any condition that causes decreased amounts of plasma proteins, such as protein malnutrition or liver impairment, can lead to a larger percentage of *free* thyroid hormone, with subsequent symptoms of hyperthyroidism.

The secretion of thyroid hormone is regulated by the hypothalamus and anterior pituitary gland by way of a negative feedback loop, as shown in Figure 44.3. When blood levels of thyroid hormone are low, the hypothalamus secretes TRH. Secretion of TRH stimulates the anterior pituitary to secrete TSH. TSH, then, stimulates the thyroid to produce and secrete T_3 and T_4. As blood levels of thyroid hormone increase, negative feedback suppresses the secretion of TSH and TRH. High levels of iodine can also cause a temporary decrease in thyroid activity that can last for several weeks. One of the strongest stimuli for increased thyroid hormone production is exposure to cold.

Disorders of the thyroid result from hypofunction or hyperfunction of the thyroid gland. Abnormal thyroid hormone levels could occur due to disease within the thyroid gland itself or be caused by abnormalities of the pituitary or hypothalamus.

THYROID DRUGS

Thyroid disorders are common and drug therapy is often indicated. The correct dose of thyroid drug is highly individualized and requires careful, periodic adjustment. The medications used to treat thyroid disease are listed in Table 44.3.

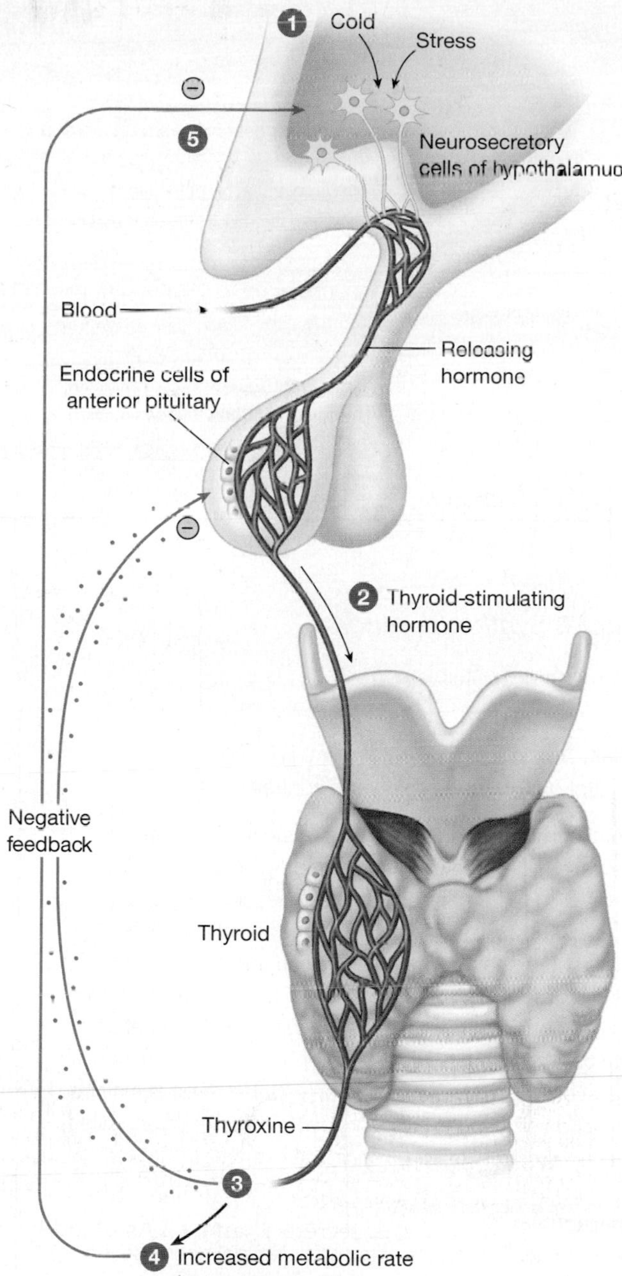

FIGURE 44.3 Feedback mechanisms of the thyroid gland: (1) stimulus; (2) release of TSH; (3) release of thyroid hormone; (4) increased BMR; (5) negative feedback

Thyroid Agents

44.6 Pharmacotherapy of Hypothyroidism

Hypothyroidism may result from either a poorly functioning thyroid gland or low secretion of TSH by the pituitary gland. The most common cause of hypothyroidism in the United States is destruction of the thyroid gland due to chronic autoimmune thyroiditis, a condition known as Hashimoto's thyroiditis. Early symptoms of hypothyroidism in adults, or **myxedema,** include general weakness, muscle cramps, and dry skin. More severe symptoms include slurred speech, bradycardia, weight gain, decreased sense of taste and smell, and intolerance to cold environments. Laboratory results generally reveal elevated TSH with diminished T_3 and T_4 levels. The etiology of myxedema may include autoimmune disease, surgical removal of the thyroid gland, or aggressive treatment with antithyroid drugs. At high doses, the antidysrhythmic drug amiodarone (Cordarone) can induce hypothyroidism in patients due to its high iodine content. Enlargement of the thyroid gland, or goiter, may be absent or present, depending on the cause of the disease.

Hypothyroidism is treated by replacement therapy with T_3 or T_4. The standard replacement regimen consists of levothyroxine (T_4), although combined therapy with levothyroxine plus liothyronine (T_3) is an option. Desiccated thyroid gland from beef, pork, or sheep sources (Thyroid USP) is an inexpensive option, although it is rarely used because of the possibility of allergic reactions to animal protein. Liothyronine sodium is a short-acting synthetic form of thyroid hormone that can be administered IV to individuals with myxedema coma. The short duration of action allows for a rapid response to critically ill patients.

Serum TSH levels are used to evaluate the progress of therapy. Because small changes in drug bioavailability can affect thyroid function, patients should avoid switching brands of medication once their condition has stabilized. When initiating therapy in older adults, the precaution is to "go low and go slow," because there is a risk for inducing acute coronary syndromes in susceptible individuals. Replacement therapy for most patients is continued lifelong.

PharmFacts

THYROID DISORDERS

- Hypothyroidism is 8 times more common in women; hyperthyroidism is 5 to 10 times more common in women.
- The two most common thyroid disorders, Graves' disease and Hashimoto's thyroiditis, are autoimmune diseases and may have a genetic link.
- One of every 4,000 babies is born without a working thyroid gland.
- One of every five women older than 75 years has Hashimoto's thyroiditis.
- Postpartum thyroiditis occurs in 5% to 9% of women and may recur in future pregnancies.
- Both hyperthyroidism and hypothyroidism can affect a woman's ability to become pregnant and can cause miscarriages.

Antithyroid Agents

Medications are often used to treat the cause of hyperthyroidism or to relieve its distressing symptoms. The goal of antithyroid therapy is to lower the activity of the thyroid gland.

Table 44.3 Thyroid and Antithyroid Drugs

Drug	Route and Adult Dose (max dose where indicated)	Adverse Effects
THYROID AGENTS		
levothyroxine (Levothroid, Synthroid, others)	PO: 100–400 mcg/day IV/IM: 50–100 mcg/day	*Weight loss, headache, tremors, nervousness, heat intolerance, insomnia, menstrual irregularities*
liothyronine (Cytomel, Triostat)	PO: 25–75 mcg/day IV: 25–100 mcg/day	Dysrhythmias, HTN, palpitations
liotrix (Thyrolar)	PO: 12.5–30 mcg/day	
thyroid, desiccated (Armour Thyroid, Thyroid USP)	PO: 60–180 mg/day	
ANTITHYROID AGENTS		
methimazole (Tapazole)	PO: 5–15 mg tid	*Nausea, rash, pruritus, weight gain, headache, fever, numbness in fingers, leukopenia, diarrhea, hypothyroidism*
potassium iodide and iodine (Lugol's Solution, Thyro-Block)	PO: 250 mg tid	
propylthiouracil (PTU)	PO: 300–450 mg tid	Agranulocytosis, bradycardia, hepatotoxicity (methimazole)
radioactive iodide (I-131)	PO: 0.8–150 mCi (a Ci or curie is a unit of radioactivity)	

Note: *Italics* indicate common adverse effects; underlining indicates serious adverse effects.

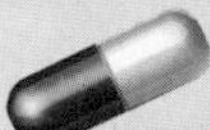

Prototype Drug | Levothyroxine *(Levothroid, Synthroid, others)*

Therapeutic Class: Thyroid hormone **Pharmacologic Class:** Thyroid hormone replacement

Actions and Uses

Levothyroxine is a synthetic form of T_4 that is a drug of choice for replacement therapy in patients with low thyroid function. Actions are those of endogenous thyroid hormone and include loss of weight, improved tolerance to environmental temperature, increased activity, and increased pulse rate.

To avoid adverse effects, doses of levothyroxine are highly individualized for each patient. When given PO, 1–3 weeks may be required to obtain full therapeutic benefits. Doses for patients with pre-existing cardiac disease are usually increased at 4- to 6-week intervals to avoid triggering dysrhythmias or angina attacks. Serum TSH levels are regularly monitored to determine whether the patient is receiving sufficient levothyroxine—high TSH levels usually indicate that the dosage of T_4 needs to be increased.

Administration Alerts

- Administer the medication at the same time every day, preferably in the morning to decrease the potential for insomnia.
- Pregnancy category A.

PHARMACOKINETICS

Onset	Peak	Duration
24 h PO, 6–8 h IV	3–4 wk	1–3 wk

Adverse Effects

At therapeutic doses, adverse effects of levothyroxine therapy are rare, although care must be taken to avoid overtreatment. Adverse effects are those of hyperthyroidism and include palpitations, dysrhythmias, anxiety, insomnia, weight loss, and heat intolerance. Menstrual irregularities may occur in females, and long-term use of levothyroxine has been associated with osteoporosis in women.

Black Box Warning: Use of thyroid hormone in the treatment of obesity or weight loss is contraindicated.

Contraindications: Levothyroxine is contraindicated if the patient is hypersensitive to the drug, is experiencing thyrotoxicosis, or has severe cardiovascular conditions or acute MI. If given to patients with adrenal insufficiency, thyroid hormone may cause a serious adrenal crisis; thus, the insufficiency should be corrected prior to administration of levothyroxine. It should be used with caution in patients with cardiac disease, HTN, and impaired kidney function, and in older adults. Symptoms of diabetes mellitus may be worsened with administration of thyroid hormone and doses of antidiabetic drugs may require adjustment.

Interactions

Drug–Drug: Cholestyramine and colestipol decrease the absorption of levothyroxine. Concurrent administration of epinephrine and norepinephrine increases the risk of cardiac insufficiency. Levothyroxine increases the effects of warfarin, resulting in an increased risk of bleeding.

Lab Tests: Unknown.

Herbal/Food: Soybean flour (infant formula), cottonseed meal, walnuts, and dietary fiber may bind and decrease the absorption of levothyroxine sodium from the GI tract. Calcium or iron supplements should be taken at least 4 hours after taking levothyroxine to prevent interference with drug absorption.

Treatment of Overdose: Overdose can cause serious thyrotoxicosis, which may not present until several days after the overdose. Treatment is symptomatic, usually targeted at preventing cardiac toxicity with beta-adrenergic antagonists such as propranolol.

Community-Oriented Practice

THE EFFECTS OF SOY INTAKE ON DRUG TREATMENT FOR HYPOTHYROIDISM

Soy and soy products are known to interact with, and inhibit absorption of thyroid replacement drugs such as levothyroxine. Fruzza, Demeterco-Berggren, and Jones (2012) reported on the impact of soy formula and soy milk on infants and toddlers who had been diagnosed with congenital hypothyroidism. Signs of clinical hypothyroidism were observed until the soy formula (infant) or soy milk (toddler) was switched to a non-soy alternative. Because the implications of hypothyroidism in infants and young children during crucial periods of brain growth are significant and may result in developmental and growth delays, parents of children with congenital hypothyroidism should be cautioned about the use of soy products, and appropriate substitutions explored. This study also has implications for adult patients on thyroid replacement therapy. Depending on the amount of soy intake, hypothyroidism may result if the intake interferes with thyroid replacement absorption. Because some patients may switch to soy as a supplement or substitute for animal proteins in the diet, nurses should include a dietary assessment for adult patients on replacement therapy, especially for those who are experiencing hypothyroidism after a period of a euthyroid state.

44.7 Pharmacotherapy of Hyperthyroidism

Hypersecretion of thyroid hormone results in symptoms that are the opposite of those caused by hypothyroidism: increased body metabolism, tachycardia, weight loss, elevated body temperature, and anxiety. The most common type of hyperthyroidism is called **Graves' disease.** Considered an autoimmune disease in which the body develops antibodies against its own thyroid gland, Graves' disease most often occurs between the ages of 30 and 40. Other causes of hyperthyroidism are adenomas of the thyroid, pituitary tumors, and pregnancy. Treatment of hyperthyroidism often requires surgical removal of all or part of the thyroid gland. In less serious cases of the disorder, pharmacotherapy can be used to diminish the secretion of thyroid hormone.

Very high levels of circulating thyroid hormone may cause **thyroid storm,** a rare, life-threatening form of hyperthyroidism. If untreated, the condition is associated with mortality rates of 80% to 90%, even with treatment. Symptoms include high fever, cardiovascular effects (tachycardia, heart failure, angina, MI), and central nervous system (CNS) effects (agitation, restlessness, delirium, progressing to coma). Thyroid storm is treated with supportive measures, efforts to reduce body temperature while trying to avoid causing shivering; fluid, glucose and electrolyte replacement; and beta-adrenergic blockers. Antithyroid drugs may be used to decrease thyroid hormone production.

The two primary drugs for hyperthyroidism are propylthiouracil (PTU) and methimazole (Tapazole). These medications act by inhibiting the incorporation of iodine atoms into T_3 and T_4. Methimazole has a much longer half-life that offers the advantage of less frequent dosing and is the preferred antithyroid drug for treating thyroid storm. Both drugs are pregnancy category D, but methimazole crosses the placenta more readily than propylthiouracil and is contraindicated in pregnant patients.

One strategy to lower thyroid hormone secretion is to destroy part of the gland (ablation) by administering radioactive iodide (I-131). Shortly after oral administration, I-131 accumulates in the thyroid gland where it destroys follicular cells. The goal of pharmacotherapy with I-131 is to destroy just enough of the thyroid gland so that levels of thyroid function return to normal. This therapy is preferred by many endocrinologists because it results in a permanent, long-term solution to hyperthyroidism. Following treatment with radioactive iodine, some patients become hypothyroid and require levothyroxine therapy.

Nonradioactive iodine is also available to treat other thyroid conditions. Lugol's solution is a mixture of 5% elemental iodine and 10% potassium iodide that is used to suppress thyroid function 10 to 14 days prior to thyroidectomy, or for the treatment of thyroid storm. Potassium iodide (Thyro-Block) is administered prior to thyroid surgery to reduce the vascularity of the gland and to protect the thyroid from radiation damage following a nuclear accident or bioterrorist act (see chapter 11).

Check Your Understanding 44.1

What are three main uses of pharmacotherapy with endocrine hormones? *Visit www.pearsonhighered.com/nursingresources for the answer.*

THE ADRENAL GLANDS

Though small, the adrenal glands secrete hormones that affect every body tissue. Adrenal disorders include those resulting from either *excess* hormone secretion or *deficient* hormone secretion. The specific pharmacotherapy depends on which portion of the adrenal gland is responsible for the abnormal secretion.

44.8 Normal Function of the Adrenal Glands

Weighing only two-tenths of an ounce, each adrenal gland is divided into two major portions: an inner medulla and an outer cortex. The adrenal medulla secretes 75% to 80% epinephrine, with the remainder of its secretion being

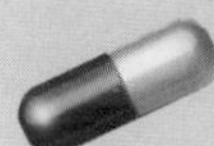

Prototype Drug | Propylthiouracil *(PTU)*

Therapeutic Class: Drug for hyperthyroidism **Pharmacologic Class:** Antithyroid drug

Actions and Uses

Propylthiouracil is administered to patients with hyperthyroidism. It acts by interfering with the synthesis of T_3 and T_4 in the thyroid gland. It also prevents the conversion of T_4 to T_3 in the target tissues. Its action may be delayed from several days to as long as 6–12 weeks. Effects include a return to normal thyroid function: weight gain, reduction in anxiety, less insomnia, and slower pulse rate. Because it has a short half-life, PTU is usually administered several times a day. Propylthiouracil is not effective in treating thyroiditis because this condition is due to overrelease, not overproduction, of thyroid hormone.

Administration Alerts

- Administer with meals to reduce GI distress.
- Pregnancy category D.

PHARMACOKINETICS

Onset	Peak	Duration
30–40 min (several weeks before effects are observed)	1–1.5 h	2–4 h

Adverse Effects

Overtreatment with PTU produces symptoms of hypothyroidism. Rash and transient leukopenia are the most frequent adverse effects. A small percentage of patients experience agranulocytosis, which is its most serious adverse effect. Periodic laboratory blood counts and TSH values are necessary to establish proper dosage.

Black Box Warning: Severe liver injury and acute hepatic failure have been reported in patients taking PTU. This drug should be reserved for those unable to tolerate methimazole and in whom radioactive iodine therapy or surgery are not appropriate treatments for hyperthyroidism.

Contraindications: PTU should not be given during pregnancy or lactation or to patients with known or suspected hypothyroidism.

Interactions

Drug–Drug: PTU increases the actions of anticoagulants, which carries an increased risk of bleeding. Iodine-containing drugs (amiodarone and potassium iodide) and thyroid hormones can antagonize the effectiveness of this drug. Cross-hypersensitivity occurs in about 50% of patients who have experienced a hypersensitivity reaction to methimazole, the other major antithyroid medication.

Lab Tests: Propylthiouracil may increase prothrombin time and increase serum levels of aspartate aminotransferase (AST), alanine aminotransferase (ALT), and alkaline phosphatase (ALP).

Herbal/Food: Unknown.

Treatment of Overdose: Overdose will cause signs of hypothyroidism. Treatment includes a thyroid agent, atropine for bradycardia, and symptomatic treatment as necessary

Nursing Practice Application

Pharmacotherapy for Thyroid Disorders

ASSESSMENT	POTENTIAL NURSING DIAGNOSES*
Baseline assessment prior to administration: • Obtain a complete health history including cardiovascular, GI, hepatic, or renal disease; pregnancy; or breast-feeding. Obtain a drug history including allergies, current prescription and OTC drugs, herbal preparations, alcohol use, or smoking. Be alert to possible drug interactions. • Evaluate appropriate laboratory findings (e.g., T_3, T_4, and TSH levels, CBC, platelets, electrolytes, glucose, and lipid levels). • Obtain baseline height, weight, and vital signs. Obtain an ECG as needed.	• *Activity Intolerance* • *Fatigue* • *Constipation* • *Deficient Knowledge* (drug therapy) • *Risk for Infection,* related to adverse drug effects • *Risk for Imbalanced Body Temperature* *NANDA I © 2014

Nursing Practice Application *continued*

ASSESSMENT	POTENTIAL NURSING DIAGNOSES*
Assessment throughout administration: • Assess for desired therapeutic effects depending on the reason the drug is being given (e.g., T_3, T_4, and TSH levels return to normal, associated symptoms of hypo- or hyperthyroidism ease). • Continue periodic monitoring of T_3, T_4, and TSH levels; CBC; platelets; and glucose. • Continue monitoring vital signs, height, and weight. Monitor the ECG as needed. • Assess for adverse effects: nausea, vomiting, diarrhea, epigastric distress, skin rash, itching, headache, tachycardia, palpitations, dysrhythmias, sweating, nervousness, paresthesias, tremors, insomnia, heat intolerance, and angina. Hypotension or HTN, tachycardia, especially associated with angina, should be reported immediately.	

IMPLEMENTATION

Interventions and (Rationales)	Patient-Centered Care
Ensuring therapeutic effects:	
• Monitor vital signs, appetite, weight, sensitivity to heat or cold, sleep patterns, and activities of daily living (ADLs) for return to normal limits. (The patient should return to more normal ADLs and feelings of wellness. Weight and pulse rate are measured to assess therapeutic response to drug therapy.)	• Advise the patient that the drug will help to stabilize thyroid hormone levels quickly, but full effects may take a week or longer to occur. • Instruct the patient to maintain consistent dosing during this initial period to allow the drug to reach therapeutic levels. • Instruct the patient to record the pulse rate and weigh self two to three times per week. Instruct the patient to bring the record of weight and pulse to each provider visit.
• Monitor diet for iodine-containing foods (e.g., iodized salt, soy sauce, tofu, yogurt, milk, strawberries, eggs). (Increasing or decreasing normal iodine intake may result in adverse drug effects.)	• Provide dietary instruction on foods to avoid. **Collaboration:** Provide dietitian consultation as needed.
• Monitor thyroid function tests. (Results help determine the effectiveness of the drug therapy and the need for dosage changes.)	• Instruct the patient on the need to return periodically for laboratory work.
Minimizing adverse effects:	
• Monitor for return of original symptoms and report consistent occurrence. (Daily fluctuations in symptoms may occur. Significant increases in original symptoms may signal suboptimal results. Dramatic "opposite" effect and hypo- or hyperthyroid symptoms may signal drug toxicity.)	• Teach the patient that small daily fluctuations may occur, especially during periods of stress or illness. Any significant or increasing changes in pulse rate, weight, nervousness or fatigue, intolerance to heat or cold, and diarrhea or constipation should be reported to the health care provider.
• Monitor for signs of infection, CBC, and platelet counts. (Antithyroid drugs may cause agranulocytosis.)	• Instruct the patient to report fever, rashes, sore throat, chills, malaise, or weakness to the health care provider.
• **Lifespan:** Monitor symptoms in older adults more frequently. (Older adults are more sensitive to thyroid replacement therapy. Minor changes in daily thyroid levels may cause a significant change in symptoms.)	• Teach the patient and family or caregiver that the lowest dose will be started and gradually increased to find the optimal level, and that any significant change in symptoms should be reported to the health care provider promptly.
• Monitor serum glucose levels, especially in patients with diabetes. Patients with diabetes should monitor capillary levels more frequently. (Thyroid and antithyroid drugs may cause changes in glucose levels.)	• Teach the patient with diabetes to monitor capillary glucose levels more frequently during therapy. Report any consistent elevations in blood glucose to the health care provider.
• Observe for dizziness and monitor ambulation until the effects of the drug are known. (Dizziness may be secondary to changes in pulse or blood pressure. **Lifespan:** The older adult is especially at risk for falls related to dizziness. Effects of thyroid hormone on bone remodeling may place the patient at risk for fractures.)	• **Safety:** Instruct the patient to call for assistance prior to getting out of bed or attempting to walk alone if dizziness occurs. If dizziness occurs, the patient should sit or lie down and not attempt to stand or walk, until the sensation passes. • Assess the safety of the home environment and discuss modifications that may be needed with the family or caregiver.

continued

Nursing Practice Application *continued*

IMPLEMENTATION	
Interventions and (Rationales)	**Patient-Centered Care**
• Ensure patient and caregiver safety if radioactive iodine is used. (Radioactive iodine provides low-dose radiation but prolonged contact by health care providers or visitors should be avoided.)	• **Safety:** Teach the patient to limit contact with family to 1 hour per day per person until the treatment period is over. Young children and pregnant women should avoid contact. • Advise the patient to increase fluid intake and to void frequently to avoid irradiation to gonads from radioactivity in the urine. • Instruct the patient not to expectorate and to cover the mouth when coughing. Any contaminated tissues should be disposed of per the protocol of the health care provider.
Patient understanding of drug therapy:	
• Use opportunities during administration of medications and during assessments to provide patient education. (Using time during nursing care helps to optimize and reinforce key teaching areas.)	• The patient should be able to state the reason for the drug, appropriate dose and scheduling, and what adverse effects to observe for and when to report them.
Patient self-administration of drug therapy:	
• When administering the medication, instruct the patient, family, or caregiver in the proper self-administration of the drug (e.g., take the drug in the morning at the same time each day). (Proper administration will increase the effectiveness of the drug.)	• Teach the patient to take the drug according to appropriate guidelines, as follows: • Take the drug at the same time each day to maintain consistent body hormone levels. • Take the drug 1 hour before or 2 hours after a meal (e.g., breakfast) consistently with respect to the chosen daily meal. • Avoid foods high in iodine unless approved by the health care provider. • To ensure a therapeutic response, take the same brand of drug and request the same manufacturer each time the drug is filled. Do not switch trade names without the approval of the health care provider.

See Table 44.3 for a list of drugs to which these nursing actions apply.

norepinephrine. Adrenal release of epinephrine is triggered by activation of the sympathetic division of the autonomic nervous system. These hormones are described in chapter 13.

The adrenal cortex secretes three classes of steroid hormones: the glucocorticoids, mineralocorticoids, and gonadocorticoids. Collectively, the glucocorticoids and mineralocorticoids are called *corticosteroids* or adrenocortical hormones. The terms *corticosteroid* and *glucocorticoid* are often used interchangeably in clinical practice. However, it should be understood that the term *corticosteroid* implies that a drug has both glucocorticoid *and* mineralocorticoid activity.

Gonadocorticoids

The gonadocorticoids secreted by the adrenal cortex are mostly androgens (male sex hormones), though small amounts of estrogen are also produced. The amounts of these adrenal sex hormones are far less than the levels secreted by the testes or ovaries. It is believed that the adrenal gonadocorticoids contribute to the onset of puberty. The adrenal glands also are the primary source of endogenous estrogen in postmenopausal women. Tumors of the adrenal cortex can cause hypersecretion of gonadocorticoids, resulting in hirsutism and masculinization, which are signs that are more noticeable in females than males. The physiological effects of androgens are detailed in chapter 47.

Mineralocorticoids

Aldosterone accounts for more than 95% of the mineralocorticoids secreted by the adrenals. The primary function of aldosterone is to regulate plasma volume by promoting sodium reabsorption and potassium excretion by the renal tubules. When plasma volume falls, the kidney secretes renin, which results in the production of angiotensin II. Angiotensin II then causes aldosterone secretion, which promotes sodium and water retention. Attempts to modify this pathway led to the development of the angiotensin-converting enzyme (ACE) inhibitor class of medications, which are often preferred drugs for treating HTN and heart failure (see chapters 26 and 27). Certain adrenal tumors cause excessive secretion of aldosterone, a condition known as *hyper-aldosteronism,* which is characterized by HTN and hypokalemia.

Glucocorticoids

More than 30 glucocorticoids are secreted from the adrenal cortex, including cortisol, corticosterone, and cortisone. Cortisol, also called *hydrocortisone,* is secreted in the highest amount and is the most important pharmacologically. Glucocorticoids affect the metabolism of nearly every cell and prepare the body for long-term stress. The effects of glucocorticoids are diverse and include the following:

- Increase the level of blood glucose (hyperglycemic effect) by inhibiting insulin secretion and promoting gluconeogenesis, the synthesis of carbohydrates from lipid and protein sources.
- Increase the breakdown of proteins and lipids and promote their utilization as energy sources.
- Suppress the inflammatory and immune responses (see chapters 33 and 34).
- Increase the sensitivity of vascular smooth muscle to norepinephrine and angiotensin II.
- Increase the breakdown of bony matrix, resulting in bone demineralization.
- Promote bronchodilation by making bronchial smooth muscle more responsive to sympathetic nervous system activation.

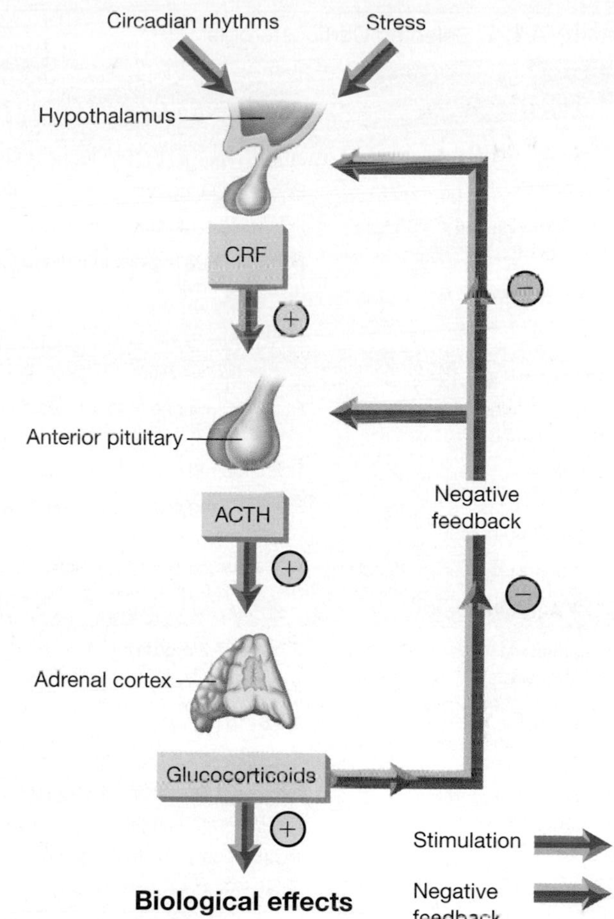

FIGURE 44.4 Feedback control of the adrenal cortex

44.9 Regulation of Corticosteroid Secretion

Control of corticosteroid levels in the blood begins with corticotropin-releasing factor (CRF), secreted by the hypothalamus. CRF travels to the pituitary where it causes the release of **adrenocorticotropic hormone (ACTH).** ACTH then travels through the blood to reach the adrenal cortex, causing it to release corticosteroids. When the level of cortisol in the blood rises, it provides negative feedback to the hypothalamus and the pituitary to shut off further release of corticosteroids. This negative feedback mechanism is shown in Figure 44.4.

Lack of adequate corticosteroid production, known as **adrenocortical insufficiency,** may be caused by either hyposecretion of the adrenal cortex or inadequate secretion of ACTH from the pituitary. Cosyntropin (Cortrosyn) closely resembles ACTH and is used to diagnose the cause of the adrenocortical insufficiency. After administration of a small dose of cosyntropin, plasma levels of cortisol are measured 30 to 60 minutes later. If the adrenal gland responds by secreting corticosteroids after the cosyntropin injection, the pathology lies at the level of the pituitary or hypothalamus (secondary adrenocortical insufficiency). If plasma cortisol levels fail to rise after the injection, the pathology is at the level of the adrenal gland (primary adrenocortical insufficiency).

ADRENAL DRUGS

Corticosteroids

The corticosteroids are used as replacement therapy for patients with adrenocortical insufficiency and to dampen inflammatory and immune responses. The corticosteroids, listed in Table 44.4, are one of the most widely prescribed drug classes.

44.10 Pharmacotherapy With Corticosteroids

Symptoms of adrenocortical insufficiency include hypoglycemia, fatigue, hypotension, increased skin pigmentation, and GI disturbances such as anorexia, vomiting, and diarrhea. Low plasma cortisol, accompanied by high plasma ACTH levels, is diagnostic, because this indicates that the adrenal gland is not responding to ACTH stimulation. *Primary* adrenocortical insufficiency, known as **Addison's disease,** is quite rare and includes a deficiency of both corticosteroids and

Table 44.4 Selected Corticosteroids

Drug	Route and Adult Dose (max dose where indicated)	Adverse Effects
SHORT ACTING		
cortisone	PO: 20–300 mg/day	*Sodium/fluid retention, nausea, acne, anxiety, insomnia, mood swings, increased appetite, weight gain, facial flushing*
hydrocortisone (Cortef, Solu-Cortef)	PO: 10–320 mg/day in three to four divided doses IV/IM: 15–800 mg/day in three to four divided doses (max: 2 g/day)	<u>Impaired wound healing, masking of infections, adrenal atrophy, hypokalemia, peptic ulcers, glaucoma, osteoporosis, muscle wasting/weakness, heart failure, edema, worsening of psychoses</u>
INTERMEDIATE ACTING		
methylprednisolone (Dep-Medrol, Medrol, others)	PO: 2–60 mg one to four times/day	
prednisolone	PO: 5–60 mg one to four times/day	
prednisone (see page 508 for the Prototype Drug box)	PO: 5–60 mg one to four times/day	
triamcinolone (Aristospan, Kenalog)	PO: 4–48 mg one to two times/day	
LONG ACTING		
betamethasone (Celestone, Diprolene, others)	PO: 0.6–7.2 mg/day IM: 0.5–9 mg/day	
dexamethasone	IM: 8–16 mg bid–qid PO: 0.25–4 mg bid–qid	
budesonide (Entocort EC, Pulmicort, Rhinocort, Ulceris)	Intranasal (Rhinocort): 1–2 sprays in each nostril/day (each spray: 32 mcg) PO (Entocort EC): 6–9 mg/day Inhalation (Pulmicort): 360–720 mcg bid	

Note: *Italics* indicate common adverse effects; <u>underlining</u> indicates serious adverse effects.

mineralocorticoids. Autoimmune destruction of both adrenal glands is the most common cause of Addison's disease. *Secondary* adrenocortical insufficiency is more common than primary and can occur when corticosteroids are suddenly withdrawn during pharmacotherapy.

When corticosteroids are taken as medications for prolonged periods, they provide negative feedback to the pituitary to stop secreting ACTH. Without stimulation by ACTH, the adrenal cortex shrinks and stops secreting *endogenous* corticosteroids, a condition known as *adrenal atrophy*. If the corticosteroid medication is abruptly discontinued, the shrunken adrenal glands will not be able to secrete sufficient corticosteroids, and symptoms of acute adrenocortical insufficiency will appear. Symptoms include nausea, vomiting, lethargy, confusion, and coma. Immediate administration of IV therapy with hydrocortisone is essential, because shock may quickly result if symptoms remain untreated. Acute adrenocortical insufficiency can be prevented by discontinuing corticosteroids gradually. Other possible causes of acute adrenocortical insufficiency include infection, trauma, and cancer. The development of adrenal atrophy following corticosteroid administration is shown in Pharmacotherapy Illustrated 44.1.

For chronic adrenocortical insufficiency, replacement therapy with corticosteroids is indicated. The goal of replacement therapy is to achieve the same physiological level of hormones in the blood that would be present if the adrenal glands were functioning properly. Patients requiring replacement therapy usually must take corticosteroids their entire lifetime, and concurrent therapy with a mineralocorticoid such as fludrocortisone (Florinef) is necessary.

In addition to treating adrenal insufficiency, corticosteroids are prescribed for a large number of nonendocrine disorders. Their ability to quickly and effectively suppress the inflammatory and immune responses gives them tremendous therapeutic utility to treat a diverse set of conditions. Indeed, no other drug class is used for so many different indications. Following are nonendocrine indications for pharmacotherapy with corticosteroids:

- Allergies, including allergic rhinitis (see chapter 39)
- Asthma (see chapter 40)
- Cancer, including Hodgkin's disease, leukemias, and lymphomas (see chapter 38)
- Edema associated with hepatic, neurologic, and renal disorders
- Inflammatory bowel disease, including ulcerative colitis and Crohn's disease (see chapter 42)
- Rheumatic disorders, including rheumatoid arthritis, ankylosing spondylitis, and bursitis (see chapter 48)
- Shock (see chapter 29)

Pharmacotherapy Illustrated

44.1 | Corticosteroids (Glucocorticoids) and Adrenal Atrophy

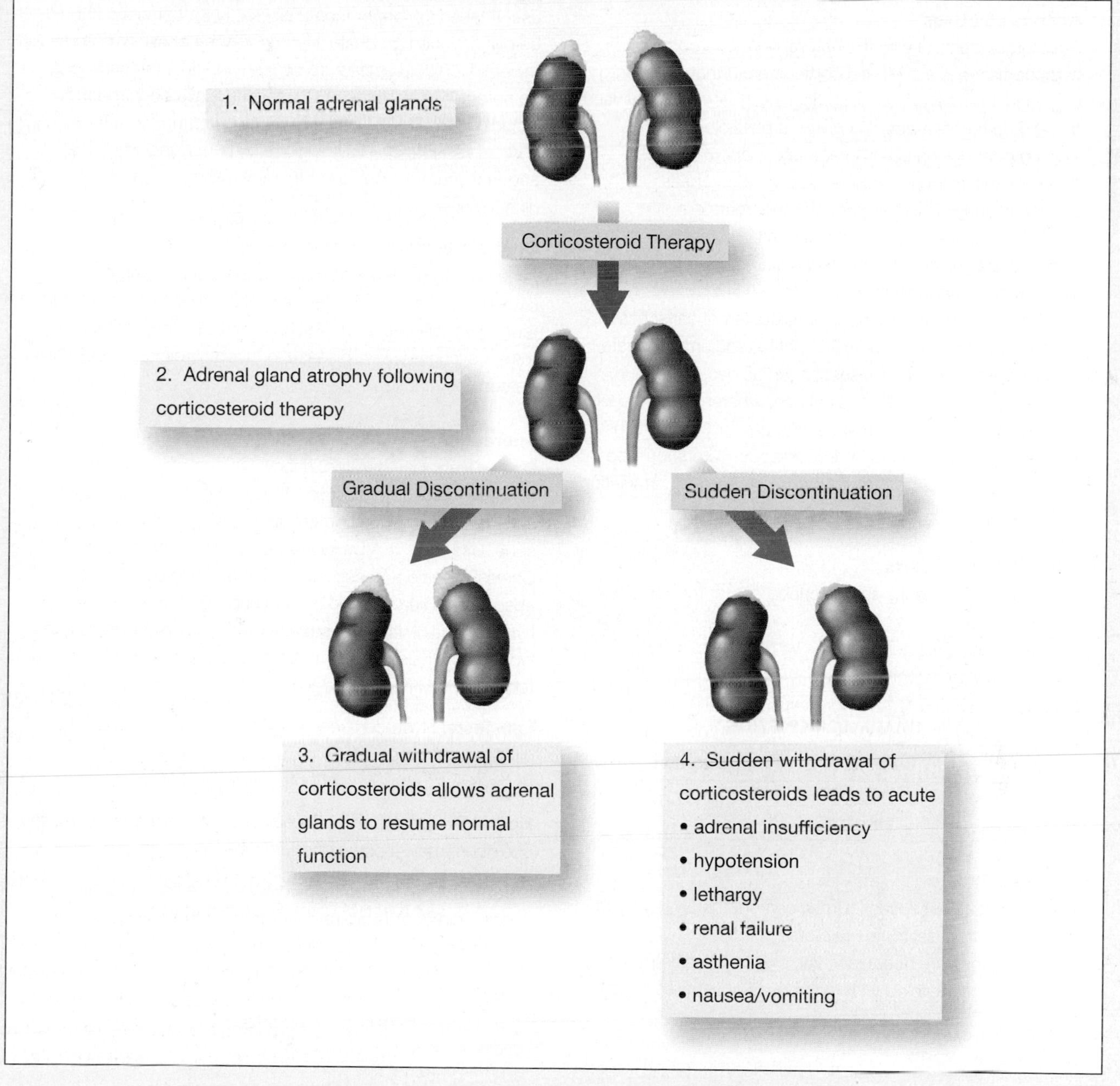
1. Normal adrenal glands
Corticosteroid Therapy
2. Adrenal gland atrophy following corticosteroid therapy
Gradual Discontinuation
Sudden Discontinuation
3. Gradual withdrawal of corticosteroids allows adrenal glands to resume normal function
4. Sudden withdrawal of corticosteroids leads to acute
• adrenal insufficiency
• hypotension
• lethargy
• renal failure
• asthenia
• nausea/vomiting

- Skin disorders, including contact dermatitis and rashes (see chapter 49)
- Transplant rejection prophylaxis (see chapter 34).

More than 20 corticosteroids are available as medications, and choice of a particular agent depends primarily on the pharmacokinetic properties of the drug. The duration of action, which is often used to classify these agents, ranges from short to long acting. Some, such as hydrocortisone, have mineralocorticoid activity that causes sodium and fluid retention; others, such as prednisone, have no such effect. Some corticosteroids are available by only one route: for example, topical for dermal conditions or intranasal for allergic rhinitis.

Corticosteroids interact with many drugs. Their hyperglycemic effects may decrease the effectiveness of antidiabetic drugs. Combining corticosteroids with other ulcer-promoting drugs such as aspirin and other NSAIDs markedly increases the risk of peptic ulcer disease. Administration with non–potassium-sparing diuretics may lead to hypocalcemia and hypokalemia.

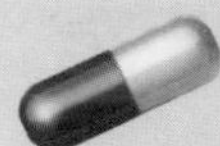

Prototype Drug | Hydrocortisone *(Cortef, Hydrocortone, others)*

Therapeutic Class: Adrenal hormone **Pharmacologic Class:** Corticosteroid

Actions and Uses

Structurally identical with the natural hormone cortisol, hydrocortisone is a synthetic corticosteroid that is the drug of choice for treating adrenocortical insufficiency. When used for replacement therapy, it is given at physiological doses. Once proper dosing is achieved, its therapeutic effects should mimic those of endogenous corticosteroids. Hydrocortisone is also available for the treatment of inflammation, allergic disorders, and many other conditions. Intra-articular injections may be given to decrease severe inflammation in affected joints.

Hydrocortisone is available in six different salts: base, acetate, cypionate, sodium phosphate, sodium succinate, and valerate. Some of the salts, such as hydrocortisone acetate, are designed for topical use, whereas others such as hydrocortisone sodium succinate are for parenteral use only. When administering hydrocortisone, care should be taken to use the correct route for the prescribed formulation of this drug.

Administration Alerts

- Administer exactly as prescribed and at the same time every day.
- Administer oral formulations with food.
- Pregnancy category C.

PHARMACOKINETICS

Onset	Peak	Duration
1–2 h PO; 20 min IM	1 h PO; 4–8 h IM	1–1.5 days PO or IM

Adverse Effects

When used at low doses for replacement therapy, or by the topical or intranasal routes, adverse effects of hydrocortisone are rare. However, signs of Cushing's syndrome can develop with high doses or with prolonged use. If taken for longer than 2 weeks, hydrocortisone should be discontinued gradually. Hydrocortisone possesses some mineralocorticoid activity, so sodium and fluid retention may be noted. A wide range of CNS effects have been reported, including insomnia, anxiety, headache, vertigo, confusion, and depression. Cardiovascular effects may include HTN and tachycardia. Long-term therapy may result in peptic ulcer disease.

Contraindications: Hydrocortisone is contraindicated in patients who are hypersensitive to the drug or who have known infections, unless the patient is being treated concurrently with anti-infectives. Patients with diabetes, osteoporosis, psychoses, liver disease, or hypothyroidism should be treated with caution.

Interactions

Drug–Drug: Barbiturates, phenytoin, and rifampin may increase hepatic metabolism, thus decreasing hydrocortisone levels. Estrogens potentiate the effects of hydrocortisone. Use with NSAIDs increases the risk of peptic ulcers. Cholestyramine and colestipol decrease hydrocortisone absorption. Diuretics and amphotericin B increase the risk of hypokalemia. Anticholinesterase drugs may produce severe weakness. Hydrocortisone may cause a decrease in immune response to vaccines and toxoids.

Lab Tests: Hydrocortisone may increase serum values for glucose, cholesterol, sodium, uric acid, or calcium. It may decrease serum values of potassium and T_3/T_4.

Herbal/Food: Use of hydrocortisone with senna, cascara, or buckthorn may cause potassium deficiency with chronic use.

Treatment of Overdose: Hydrocortisone has no acute toxicity and deaths are rare. No specific therapy is available and patients are treated symptomatically.

High doses of corticosteroids taken for prolonged periods offer a significant risk for serious adverse effects. These adverse effects, shown in Table 44.5, can affect nearly any body system. The following strategies are used to limit the incidence of serious adverse effects from corticosteroids:

- Keep doses to the lowest possible amount that will achieve a therapeutic effect.
- Administer corticosteroids every other day (alternate-day dosing) to limit adrenal atrophy.
- For acute conditions, give patients large amounts for a few days and then gradually decrease the drug dose until it is discontinued.

Give the drugs locally by inhalation, intra-articular injections, or topical applications to the skin, eyes, or ears, when feasible, to diminish the possibility of systemic effects.

Table 44.5 Adverse Effects of Long-Term Corticosteroid Therapy

Type of Adverse Event	Description
Behavioral changes	Psychological changes may be minor, such as nervousness or moodiness, or may involve hallucinations and increased suicidal tendencies.
Eye changes	Cataracts and open-angle glaucoma are associated with long term therapy.
Immune response	Suppression of the immune and inflammatory responses increases patients' susceptibility to infections. Their anti inflammatory actions may mask the signs of an existing infection.
Metabolic changes	Their hyperglycemic effect raises serum glucose and can cause glucose intolerance. Mobilization of lipids may cause hyperlipidemia and abnormal fat deposits. Electrolyte changes include hypocalcemia, hypokalemia, and hypernatremia. Fluid retention, weight gain, HTN, and edema are common.
Myopathy	Muscle wasting causes weakness and fatigue; may involve ocular or respiratory muscles.
Osteoporosis	Up to 50% of patients on long-term therapy will suffer a fracture due to osteoporosis.
Peptic ulcers	Development of peptic ulcers may occur, especially when combined with NSAIDs.

ANTIADRENAL AGENTS

44.11 Pharmacotherapy of Cushing's Syndrome

Cushing's syndrome occurs when high levels of corticosteroids are present in the body over a prolonged period. If the hypersecretion is caused by a pituitary gland tumor producing excess amounts of ACTH, the condition is called Cushing's disease. The most common cause of Cushing's syndrome is long-term therapy with high doses of systemic corticosteroids used as medications. Signs and symptoms include adrenal atrophy, osteoporosis, HTN, increased risk of infections, delayed wound healing, acne, peptic ulcers, general obesity, and a redistribution of fat around the face (moon face), shoulders, and neck (buffalo hump). Mood and personality changes may occur, and the patient may become psychologically dependent on the drug. Some of these drugs, including hydrocortisone, also have mineralocorticoid activity and can cause retention of sodium and water. Because of their anti-inflammatory properties, corticosteroids may mask signs of infection, and a resulting delay in antibiotic therapy may result.

Because Cushing's syndrome has a high mortality rate, the primary therapeutic goal is to identify and treat the cause of the excess corticosteroid secretion. If the patient is receiving high doses of a corticosteroid medication, gradual discontinuation of the drug is often sufficient to reverse the syndrome. When the cause of the hypersecretion is an adrenal tumor or perhaps an ectopic tumor secreting ACTH, surgical removal is indicated.

The antifungal drug ketoconazole (Nizoral) has become a preferred drug for patients with Cushing's syndrome who need long-term therapy. This drug rapidly blocks the synthesis of corticosteroids, lowering serum levels. Unfortunately, patients often develop tolerance to the drug and corticosteroids eventually return to abnormally high levels. Ketoconazole should not be used during pregnancy because it has been shown to be teratogenic in animals.

A newer approach to treating Cushing's syndrome is the drug pasireotide (Signifor), which was approved in 2012. Pasireotide is closely related to somatostatin (also known as GH-inhibiting hormone). Pasireotide causes inhibition of ACTH secretion by the pituitary and subsequently corticosteroid secretion from the adrenals. Given by the subcutaneous route, several weeks or months of therapy may be needed for optimal suppression of corticosteroid secretion. Signifor LAR is a depot form of this drug that is given IM once every 4 weeks for the management of acromegaly

Mitotane (Lysodren) is an antineoplastic drug, specific for cells of the adrenal cortex, that is approved to treat inoperable tumors of the adrenal gland. Although not specifically approved for Cushing's syndrome, it will reduce symptoms of this disorder if they were caused by adrenal cancer. GI symptoms such as anorexia, nausea, and vomiting will occur in 80% of patients. CNS adverse effects, including depression, lethargy, and dizziness, occur in 40% of patients.

Metyrapone (Metopirone) is an antiadrenal drug used for diagnostic purposes. A single dose is administered PO at midnight, and blood samples are taken 8 hours later. Levels of ACTH and corticosteroids are measured to determine if the adrenal glands responded to the inhibiting action of metyrapone. The drug may also be used off-label to treat Cushing's syndrome.

None of the preceding drug therapies cure Cushing's disease. Their use is temporary until the tumor can be removed or otherwise treated with radiation or antineoplastics.

Nursing Practice Application
Pharmacotherapy With Systemic Corticosteroids

ASSESSMENT	POTENTIAL NURSING DIAGNOSES*
Baseline assessment prior to administration: • Obtain a complete health history including cardiovascular, respiratory, neurologic, hepatic, or renal disease; pregnancy; or breast-feeding. Obtain a drug history including allergies, current prescription and OTC drugs, herbal preparations, caffeine, nicotine, and alcohol use. Be alert to possible drug interactions. • Obtain baseline vital signs and weight. • Evaluate appropriate laboratory findings (e.g., CBC, platelets, electrolytes, glucose, lipid profile, hepatic or renal function studies).	• *Deficient Knowledge (drug therapy)* • *Risk for Fluid Volume Excess,* related to fluid retention properties of corticosteroids • *Risk for Electrolyte Imbalance,* related to adverse drug effects • *Risk for Unstable Blood Glucose Level,* related to adverse drug effects • *Risk for Injury,* related to adverse drug effects • *Risk for Infection,* related to adverse drug effects • *Risk for Impaired Skin Integrity,* related to adverse drug effects *NANDA I © 2014
Assessment throughout administration: • Assess for desired therapeutic effects (e.g., signs and symptoms of inflammation such as redness or swelling are decreased). • Continue periodic monitoring of CBC, platelets, electrolytes, glucose, lipid profile, and hepatic or renal function studies. • Assess vital signs and weight periodically or if symptoms warrant. Obtain the weight daily and report any weight gain over 1 kg (2 lb) in a 24-hour period or more than 2 kg (5 lb) in 1 week. **Lifespan:** Obtain height and weight in children on long-term corticosteroid therapy. • Assess for and promptly report adverse effects: nausea, vomiting, symptoms of GI bleeding (dark or "tarry" stools, hematemesis or coffee-ground emesis, blood in the stool), abdominal pain, dizziness, confusion, agitation, euphoria or depression, palpitations, tachycardia, HTN, increased respiratory rate and depth, pulmonary congestion, significant weight gain, edema, blurred vision, fever, and infections.	

IMPLEMENTATION

Interventions and (Rationales)	Patient-Centered Care
Ensuring therapeutic effects: • Continue assessments as described earlier for therapeutic effects. (Diminished inflammation, allergic response, and increased feelings of wellness should begin after taking the first dose and continue to improve.)	• Teach the patient to report any return of original symptoms or increase in inflammation, allergic response, or generalized malaise to the health care provider.
Minimizing adverse effects: • Continue to monitor vital signs, especially blood pressure and pulse. Immediately report tachycardia or blood pressure over 140/90 mmHg, or per parameters as ordered, to the health care provider. (Corticosteroids may cause increased blood pressure and tachycardia due to the increased retention of fluids.)	• Teach the patient how to monitor the pulse and blood pressure. Ensure the proper use and functioning of any home equipment obtained. Immediately report tachycardia, palpitations, or increased blood pressure to the health care provider.
• Continue to monitor periodic laboratory work: CBC, electrolytes, glucose, lipid levels, and hepatic and renal function tests. (Corticosteroids affect the CBC and may cause hyperglycemia, hypernatremia, hyperlipidemia, and hypokalemia. Patients with diabetes may require a change in their antidiabetic medication if the blood glucose remains elevated.)	• Instruct the patient on the need to return periodically for laboratory work. • Advise the patient who is taking corticosteroids long term to carry a wallet identification card or wear medical identification jewelry indicating corticosteroid therapy. • Teach the patient with diabetes to test the blood glucose more frequently, notifying the health care provider if a consistent elevation is noted.

Nursing Practice Application *continued*

IMPLEMENTATION	
Interventions and (Rationales)	**Patient-Centered Care**
• Monitor for abdominal pain, black or tarry stools, blood in the stool, hematemesis or coffee-ground emesis, dizziness, and hypotension, especially if associated with tachycardia. (GI bleeding is an adverse drug effect.)	• Instruct the patient to immediately report any signs or symptoms of GI bleeding. • Teach the patient to take the drug with food or milk to decrease GI irritation. Alcohol use should be avoided or eliminated.
• Monitor for signs and symptoms of infection. (Corticosteroids suppress the immune and inflammatory responses and may mask the signs of infection.)	• Instruct the patient to immediately report any signs or symptoms of infections (e.g., increasing temperature or fever, sore throat, redness or swelling at the site of injury, white patches in the mouth, vesicular rash).
• Monitor for osteoporosis (e.g., bone density testing) periodically in patients on long-term corticosteroids. Encourage adequate calcium intake, avoidance of carbonated sodas, and weight-bearing exercise. (Corticosteroids affect bone metabolism and may cause osteoporosis and fractures. Weight-bearing exercise stresses bone and encourages normal bone remodeling. Excessive or long-term consumption of carbonated sodas has been linked to an increased risk of osteoporosis.)	• Teach the patient to maintain adequate calcium in the diet and to do weight-bearing exercises at least three to four times per week. • **Lifespan:** Teach the postmenopausal woman and older adult men to consult with the provider about the need for additional drug therapy (e.g., bisphosphonates) for osteoporosis.
• Monitor for unusual changes in mood or affect. (Corticosteroids may cause an increased or decreased mood, euphoria, depression, or severe mental instability.)	• Teach the patient, family, or caregiver to promptly report excessive mood swings or unusual changes in mood.
• Weigh the patient daily and report weight gain or increasing peripheral edema. Measure the intake and output in the hospitalized patient. (Daily weight is an accurate measure of fluid status and takes into account intake, output, and insensible losses.)	• Instruct the patient to weigh self daily, ideally at the same time of day. The patient should report a weight gain of more than 1 kg (2 lb) in a 24-hour period or more than 2 kg (5 lb) per week, or increasing peripheral edema.
• **Lifespan:** Monitor height and weight in children. (Children receiving long-term corticosteroid therapy should continue to display normal growth and development curves.)	• Teach the parents or caregivers to weigh the child periodically at home and record. Bring the record to each health care visit. • Encourage the parents or caregivers to discuss concerns or any unusual findings that would suggest developmental or growth delays with the health care provider if they are noted in the child between health care visits.
• Monitor vision periodically in patients on corticosteroids. (Corticosteroids may cause increased intraocular pressure and an increased risk or glaucoma and may cause cataracts.)	• Teach the patient to maintain eye exams twice yearly or more frequently as instructed by the provider. Immediately report any eye pain, rainbow halos around lights, diminished vision, or blurring and inability to focus.
• Do not stop the drug abruptly. The drug must be tapered off if used longer than 1 or 2 weeks. (Adrenal insufficiency and crisis may occur with profound hypotension, tachycardia, and other adverse effects if the drug is stopped abruptly.)	• Teach the patient to not stop corticosteroids abruptly and to notify the health care provider if unable to take the medication for more than 1 day due to illness.
Patient understanding of drug therapy:	
• Use opportunities during administration of medications and during assessments to provide patient education. (Using time during nursing care helps to optimize and reinforce key teaching areas.)	• The patient, family, or caregiver should be able to state the reason for the drug; appropriate dose and scheduling; what adverse effects to observe for and when to report; and the anticipated length of medication therapy.
Patient self-administration of drug therapy:	
• When administering the medication, instruct the patient, family, or caregiver in the proper self-administration of the drug (e.g., with food or milk). (Proper administration will increase the effectiveness of the drug.)	• The patient and family or caregiver are able to discuss appropriate dosing and administration needs, including: • Take the drug at the same time each day. • Take the drug with food, milk, or a meal to prevent GI upset. • Household measuring devices such as teaspoons differ significantly in size and should not be used for pediatric or liquid doses. Use dosage devices (e.g., syringe, medication spoon, or dropper) for all doses.

See Table 44.4 for a list of drugs to which these nursing actions apply.

Chapter Review

KEY Concepts

The numbered key concepts provide a succinct summary of the important points from the corresponding numbered section within the chapter. If any of these points are not clear, refer to the numbered section within the chapter for review.

44.1 The endocrine system maintains homeostasis by using hormones as chemical messengers that are secreted in response to changes in the internal environment. Negative feedback prevents overresponses by the endocrine system.

44.2 Hormones are used in replacement therapy, as antineoplastics, and for their natural therapeutic effects, such as their suppression of body defenses. Hormone blockers are used to inhibit actions of certain hormones.

44.3 The hypothalamus secretes releasing hormones, which direct the anterior pituitary gland to release specific hormones. The posterior pituitary releases its hormones in response to nerve signals from the hypothalamus.

44.4 Only a few pituitary and hypothalamic hormones have clinical applications as drugs. Growth hormone and ADH are examples of pituitary hormones used as drugs for replacement therapy.

44.5 The thyroid gland secretes thyroxine (T_4) and triiodothyronine (T_3), which control the basal metabolic rate and affect every cell in the body.

44.6 Hypothyroidism may be treated by administering thyroid hormone agents, especially levothyroxine (T_4).

44.7 Hyperthyroidism is treated by administering medications such as propylthiouracil that decrease the activity of the thyroid gland or by using radioactive iodide, which kills overactive thyroid cells.

44.8 The adrenal cortex secretes gonadocorticoids, mineralocorticoids, and glucocorticoids. The glucocorticoids mobilize the body for long-term stress and influence carbohydrate, protein, and lipid metabolism in most cells.

44.9 Corticosteroid release is stimulated by ACTH secreted by the pituitary. Adrenocortical insufficiency my be caused by hyposecretion of the adrenal cortex or inadequate ACTH secretion from the pituitary.

44.10 Corticosteroids are prescribed for acute and chronic adrenocortical insufficiency, allergies, cancer, and a wide variety of other conditions.

44.11 Antiadrenal drugs may be used to treat severe Cushing's syndrome by inhibiting corticosteroid synthesis. They are used temporarily until the cause of the excess corticosteroid secretion can be identified and treated.

REVIEW Questions

1. A nurse is preparing the teaching plan for a patient who will be discharged on methylprednisolone (Medrol Dosepak) after a significant response to poison ivy. The nurse will include instruction on reporting adverse effects to the health care provider. Which of the following should the patient report? (Select all that apply.)

1. Tinnitus
2. Edema
3. Eye pain or visual changes
4. Abdominal pain
5. Dizziness upon standing

2. The nurse is assisting a patient with chronic adrenal insufficiency to plan for medication consistency while on a family vacation trip. He is taking hydrocortisone (Cortef) and fludrocortisones (Florinef) as replacement therapy. What essential detail does this patient need to remember to do?

1. Take his blood pressure once or twice daily.
2. Avoid crowded indoor areas to avoid infections.
3. Have his vision checked before he leaves.
4. Carry an oral and injectable form of both drugs with him on his trip.

3. A patient is being treated with propylthiouracil (PTU) for hyperthyroidism, pending thyroidectomy. While the patient is taking this drug, what symptoms will the nurse teach the patient to report to the health care provider?
   1. Tinnitus, altered taste, thickened saliva
   2. Insomnia, nightmares, night sweats
   3. Sore throat, chills, low-grade fever
   4. Dry eyes, decreased blinking, reddened conjunctiva
4. Which of the following assessment findings would cause the nurse to withhold the patient's regularly scheduled dose of levothyroxine (Synthroid)?
   1. A 1-kg (2-lb) weight gain
   2. A blood pressure reading of 90/62 mmHg
   3. A heart rate of 110 beats/minute
   4. A temperature of 37.9°C (100.2°F)
5. A patient will be started on desmospressin (DDAVP) for treatment of diabetes insipidus. Which instruction should the nurse include in the teaching plan?
   1. Drink plenty of fluids, especially those high in calcium.
   2. Avoid close contact with children or pregnant women for 1 week after administration of the drug.
   3. Obtain and record your weight daily.
   4. Wear a mask if around children and pregnant women.
6. The nurse is talking with the parents of a child who will receive somatropin (Nutropin) about the drug therapy. Which important detail will the nurse include in the teaching for these parents?
   1. The drug must be given by injection.
   2. The drug must be given regularly to prevent mental retardation.
   3. If the drug therapy is given throughout adolescence, it could add 6 (15 cm) to 8 inches (20 cm) to the child's height.
   4. Daily laboratory monitoring will be required during the first weeks of therapy.

PATIENT-FOCUSED Case Study

Brandon Folleck, is a 17-year-old adolescent with a history of severe asthma who has been admitted to the intensive care unit. He is comatose, appears much younger than his listed age, and has short stature. The nurse notes that the asthma had been managed with prednisone for 15 days until 3 days ago. The patient's father is extremely anxious and says that he was unable to refill his son's prescription for medicine until he got his paycheck.

1. What is a potential cause for Brandon's condition?
2. As the nurse, what will you discuss with, or teach the father?

CRITICAL THINKING Questions

1. A 5-year-old girl requires treatment for diabetes insipidus acquired following a case of meningitis. Her DI is being treated with intranasal desmopressin, and the child's mother has been asked to help evaluate the drug's effectiveness using urine volumes and urine specific gravity. Discuss the changes that would indicate that the drug is effective.
2. A 42-year-old mother of two children is assessed by her health care provider after complaining of extreme fatigue, weight gain, and feelings of cold regardless of room temperature. Based on laboratory studies, she is diagnosed with hypothyroidism and started on levothyroxine (Synthroid). What teaching will she need about this drug?

Visit www.pearsonhighered.com/nursingresources for answers and rationales for all activities.

REFERENCES

Fruzza, A. G., Demeterco-Berggren, C., & Jones, K. L. (2012). Unawareness of the effects of soy intake on the management of congenital hypothyroidism. *Pediatrics, 130*, e699–e702. doi:10.1542/peds.2011-3350

Herdman, T. H., & Kamitsuru, S. (Eds.). (2014). *NANDA International nursing diagnoses: Definitions and classification, 2015—2017*. Oxford, United Kingdom: Wiley-Blackwell.

SELECTED BIBLIOGRAPHY

Adler, G. K. (2014). *Cushing syndrome*. Retrieved from http://emedicine.medscape.com/article/117365-overview

Almandoz, J. P., & Gharib, H. (2012). Hypothyroidism: Etiology, diagnosis, and management. *Medical Clinics of North America, 96*, 203–221. doi:10.1016/j.mcna.2012.01.005

Bahn, R. S., Burch, H. B., Cooper, D. S., Garber, J. R., Greenlee, M. C., Klein, I., . . . Stan, M. N. (2011). Hyperthyroidism and other causes of thyrotoxicosis: Management guidelines of the American Thyroid Association and American Association of Clinical Endocrinologists. *Thyroid, 21*, 593–646. doi:10.1089/thy.2010.0417

Crawford, A., & Harris, H. (2013). Tipping the scales: Understanding thyroid imbalances. *Nursing 2013 Critical Care, 8*(1), 23–28. doi:10.1097/01.CCN.0000418818.21604.22

Davenport, M. L. (2012). Growth hormone therapy in Turner syndrome. *Pediatric Endocrinology Reviews, 9*(Suppl. 2), 723–724.

Donangelo, I., & Braunstein, G. D. (2011). Update on subclinical hyperthyroidism. *American Family Physician, 83*, 933–938.

Falorni, A., Minarelli, V., & Morelli, S. (2013). Therapy of adrenal insufficiency: An update. *Endocrine, 43*, 514–528. doi:10.1007/s12020-012-9835-4

Fatourechi, V. (2014). Hyperthyroidism and thyrotoxicosis. In F. Bandier, H. Gharib, A. Golbert, L. Griz, and M. Faria (Eds.), *Endocrinology and diabetes: A problem-oriented approach* (pp. 9–21). New York, NY: Springer. doi:10.1007/978-1-4614-8684-8_2

Feelders, R. A., & Hofland, L. J. (2013). Medical treatment of Cushing's disease. *The Journal of Clinical Endocrinology & Metabolism, 98*(2), 425–438. doi:10.1210/jc.2012-3126

Ferguson, L. A. (2011). Growth hormone use in children: Necessary or designer therapy? *Journal of Pediatric Health Care, 25*, 24–30. doi:10.1016/j.pedhc.2010.03.005

Gorman, L. S. (2012). The adrenal gland: Common disease states and suspected new applications. *Clinical Laboratory Science: Journal of the American Society for Medical Technology, 26*(2), 118–125.

Griffing, G. T. (2015). *Addison disease clinical presentation*. Retrieved from http://emedicine.medscape.com/article/116467-clinical

Khardori, R. (2014). *Diabetes insipidus*. Retrieved from http://emedicine.medscape.com/article/117648-overview

Krogh, D. (2011). *Biology: A guide to the natural world* (5th ed.). San Francisco, CA: Benjamin Cummings.

Levitsky, L. L. (2013). *Pediatric Graves' disease*. Retrieved from http://emedicine.medscape.com/article/920283-overview

Marieb, E. N., & Hoehn, K. (2013). *Human anatomy and physiology* (9th ed.). San Francisco, CA: Benjamin Cummings.

Orlander, P. R. (2015). *Hypothyroidism*. Retrieved from http://emedicine.medscape.com/article/122393-overview

Silverthorn, D. U. (2013). *Human physiology: An integrated approach* (6th ed.). San Francisco, CA: Benjamin Cummings.

Sundaresh, V., Brito, J. P., Wang, Z., Prokop, L. J., Stan, M. N., Murad, M. H., & Bahn, R. S. (2013). Comparative effectiveness of therapies for Graves' hyperthyroidism: A systematic review and network meta-analysis. *The Journal of Clinical Endocrinology and Metabolism, 98*(9), 3671–3677. doi:10.1210/jc.2013-1954

Chapter 45

Drugs for Diabetes Mellitus

Drugs at a Glance

▶ **INSULIN** page 766
human regular insulin (Humulin R, Novolin R) page 768

▶ **ANTIDIABETIC DRUGS FOR TYPE 2 DIABETES** page 772
metformin (Fortamet, Glucophage, Glumetza, others) page 775

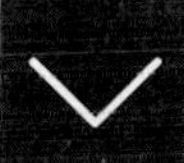

Learning Outcomes

After reading this chapter, the student should be able to:

1. Explain how blood glucose levels are maintained within narrow limits by insulin and glucagon.
2. Explain the etiology of type 1 diabetes mellitus.
3. Compare and contrast types of insulin.
4. Describe the signs and symptoms of insulin overdose and underdose.
5. Explain the etiology of type 2 diabetes mellitus.
6. Compare and contrast the drug classes used to treat type 2 diabetes mellitus.
7. For each of the drug classes listed in Drugs at a Glance, know representative drug examples, and explain the mechanisms of drug action, primary actions, and important adverse effects.
8. Use the nursing process to care for patients receiving pharmacotherapy for diabetes mellitus.

indicates a prototype drug, each of which is featured in a Prototype Drug box.

Diabetes is a leading cause of death in the United States. Mortality due to diabetes has been steadily increasing, causing some public health officials to refer to it as an epidemic. Worldwide, over 170 million people are believed to have diabetes mellitus (DM); by 2030, this number is expected to increase to 366 million. Diabetes can lead to serious acute and chronic complications, including heart disease, stroke, blindness, kidney failure, and amputations. Because nurses frequently care for patients with diabetes, it is imperative that the disorder, its treatment, and possible complications are well understood.

DIABETES MELLITUS

45.1 Regulation of Blood Glucose Levels

Located behind the stomach and between the duodenum and spleen, the pancreas is an organ essential to both the digestive and endocrine systems. It is responsible for the secretion of several enzymes into the duodenum that assist in the chemical digestion of nutrients. This is its exocrine function. Clusters of cells in the pancreas, called **islets of Langerhans,** are responsible for its endocrine function: the secretion of glucagon and insulin.

Glucose is one of the body's most essential molecules. The body prefers to use glucose as its primary energy source. The brain relies almost exclusively on glucose for its energy needs. Because of this need, blood levels of glucose must remain relatively constant throughout the day. Although many factors contribute to maintaining a stable serum glucose level, the two pancreatic hormones play major roles: **insulin** acts to *decrease* blood glucose levels, and **glucagon** acts to *increase* blood glucose levels (Figure 45.1).

Following a meal, the pancreas recognizes the rising serum glucose level and releases insulin. Without insulin, glucose stays in the bloodstream and is not able to enter cells of the body. Cells may be virtually surrounded by glucose but they are unable to use it until insulin arrives. It may be helpful to visualize insulin as a transporter or "gatekeeper." When present, insulin swings open the gate, transporting glucose inside cells: no insulin, no entry. Thus, insulin is said to have a **hypoglycemic effect,** because its presence causes glucose to *leave* the blood and serum glucose to *fall*. The physiological actions of insulin can be summarized as follows:

- Promotes the entry of glucose into cells
- Provides for the storage of glucose, as glycogen in skeletal muscle and the liver
- Inhibits the breakdown of fat and glycogen
- Increases protein synthesis and inhibits **gluconeogenesis:** the production of new glucose from noncarbohydrate molecules (protein and lipid).

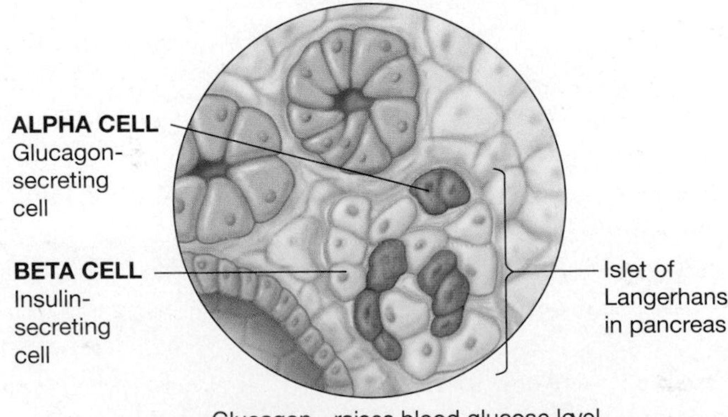

FIGURE 45.1 Glucagon- and insulin-secreting cells in the islets of Langerhans

The pancreas also secretes glucagon, which has actions *opposite* those of insulin. When levels of blood glucose fall, glucagon is secreted. Its primary function is to maintain adequate serum levels of glucose between meals. Thus, glucagon has a **hyperglycemic effect,** because its presence causes blood glucose to *rise*. Figure 45.2 illustrates the relationships among blood glucose, insulin, and glucagon.

Blood glucose levels are usually kept within a normal range by insulin and glucagon; however, other hormones and drugs can affect glucose metabolism. *Hyperglycemic* hormones include epinephrine, thyroid hormone, growth hormone, and glucocorticoids. Common drugs that can raise the level of blood glucose include corticosteroids, nonsteroidal anti-inflammatory drugs (NSAIDs), and diuretics. Drugs with a *hypoglycemic* effect include alcohol, lithium, angiotensin-converting enzyme (ACE) inhibitors, and beta-adrenergic blockers. It is important that serum glucose be periodically monitored in patients who are receiving medications who exhibit hypoglycemia or hypoglycemic effects. DM is a metabolic disorder in which there is deficient insulin secretion or decreased sensitivity of insulin receptors on target cells, resulting in hyperglycemia. The etiology of DM includes a combination of genetic and environmental factors. The recent increase in the frequency of the disease is probably the result of trends toward more sedentary and stressful lifestyles, increasing consumption of highly caloric foods with resultant obesity, and increased longevity.

TYPE 1 DIABETES MELLITUS

45.2 Etiology and Characteristics of Type 1 Diabetes Mellitus

Type 1 diabetes mellitus accounts for 5% to 10% of all cases of DM and is one of the most common diseases of childhood. Type 1 DM was previously called juvenile-onset diabetes, because it is often diagnosed between the ages of 11 and 13. Because approximately 25% of patients with type 1 DM develop the disease in adulthood, this is not the most

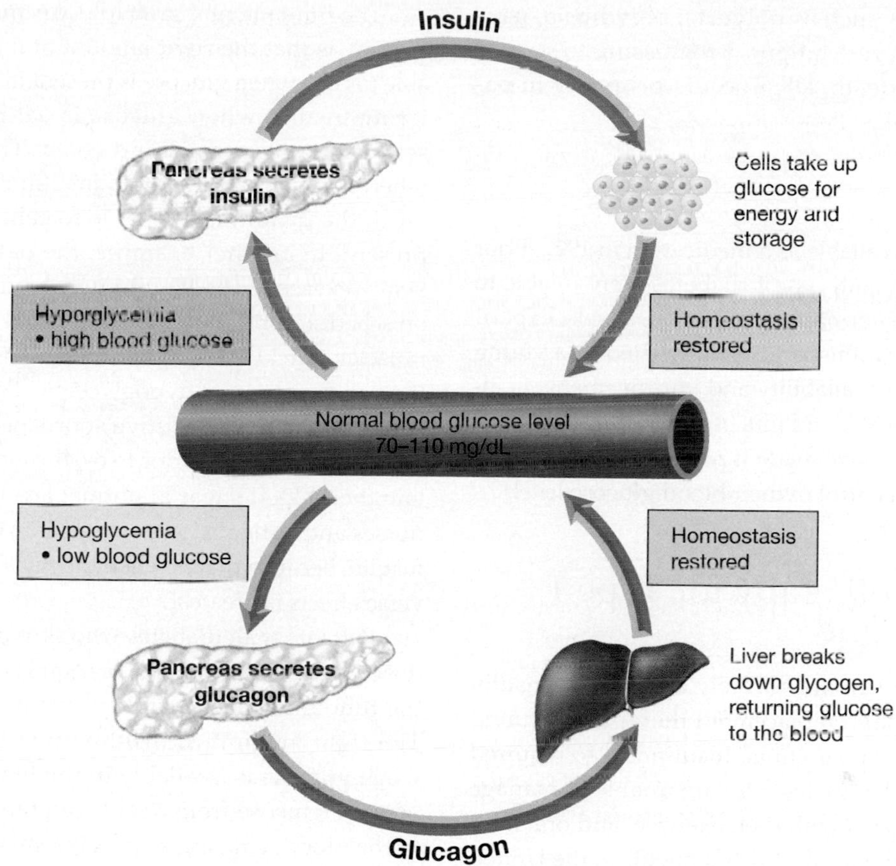

FIGURE 45.2 Glucose metabolism during periods of hyperglycemia (top) and hypoglycemia (bottom).

accurate name for this disorder. This type of diabetes is also referred to as insulin-dependent diabetes mellitus.

Type 1 DM is caused by the autoimmune destruction of pancreatic beta cells, resulting in lack of insulin secretion. The disease is thought to be an interaction of genetic, immunologic, and environmental factors. Because children and siblings of those with DM have a higher risk of acquiring the disorder, there is an obvious genetic component to the disease.

The signs and symptoms of type 1 DM are consistent from patient to patient, with the most diagnostic sign being sustained hyperglycemia. Following are the typical signs and symptoms:

- Hyperglycemia—fasting blood glucose greater than 126 mg/dL on at least two separate occasions
- Polyuria—excessive urination
- Polyphagia—increased hunger
- Polydipsia—increased thirst
- Glucosuria—high levels of glucose in the urine
- Weight loss
- Fatigue.

Although symptomology is important for recognizing the possibility of diabetes, many patients with the disease have no symptoms. Laboratory tests are required for proper diagnosis. The primary blood tests for diagnosing diabetes include the following:

- Hemoglobin A1C (HbA1C): HbA1C: As serum glucose increases, more glucose becomes bound to hemoglobin. A value of 6.5% or higher indicates diabetes. The advantage of HbA1C is that it does not require fasting, and it provides an average measure of glucose control over the 8 to 12 weeks prior to the test.
- Fasting plasma glucose (FPG): obtained following a fast of at least 8 hours. A value of 126 mg/dL or higher indicates diabetes.
- Oral glucose tolerance test (OGTT): A loading dose of 75 g of glucose is ingested and the plasma glucose level is obtained 2 hours later. A value of 200 mg/dL or higher indicates diabetes.

Untreated DM produces long-term damage to arteries, which leads to heart disease, stroke, kidney disease, and blindness. Lack of adequate circulation to the feet may cause gangrene of the toes, requiring amputation. Nerve degeneration, or neuropathy, is common, with symptoms ranging from tingling in the fingers or toes to complete loss of sensation of a limb. Because glucose is unable to enter cells, lipids are used as an energy source and ketones, also called **ketoacids,** are produced as waste products. These ketoacids can give the patient's breath an acetone-like, fruity odor. More important, high levels of ketoacids lower the pH of the blood, causing **diabetic ketoacidosis (DKA).** DKA typically develops over several days with symptoms such as polyuria, polydipsia, nausea, vomiting, and severe fatigue, progressing to stupor, coma, and possibly death. DKA occurs primarily in patients with type 1 DM.

Insulin

Insulin first became available as a medication in 1922. Prior to that time, patients with type 1 diabetes were unable to adequately maintain normal blood glucose levels, experienced many complications, and usually died at a young age. Increased insulin availability and improvements in insulin products, personal blood glucose monitoring devices, and the insulin pump have made it possible for patients to maintain more exact control of their blood glucose level.

45.3 Pharmacotherapy for Type 1 Diabetes Mellitus

Patients with type 1 DM are severely deficient in insulin production; thus, insulin replacement therapy is required in normal physiological amounts. Insulin is also required for those with type 2 diabetes who are unable to manage their blood glucose level with diet, exercise, and oral antidiabetic drugs. Among adults with diabetes in the United States, 14% take insulin only, 15% take insulin with oral drugs, 57% take oral drugs only, and 14% take no medication (Centers for Disease Control and Prevention, 2014).

Because normal insulin secretion varies greatly in response to daily activities such as eating and exercise, insulin administration must be carefully planned in conjunction with proper meal planning and lifestyle habits. The desired outcome of insulin therapy is to prevent the long-term consequences of the disorder by strictly maintaining blood glucose levels within the normal range.

PharmFacts

DIABETES MELLITUS

- Of the 29 million Americans who have diabetes, about 8 million are unaware that they have the disease.
- Gestational diabetes affects about 5–10% of all pregnant women in the United States each year.
- Diabetes is the seventh leading cause of death. The risk of death among people with diabetes is 1.5 times that of people of similar age without diabetes.
- Diabetes is the leading cause of blindness in adults.
- Diabetes is responsible for 60% of nontraumatic lower-limb amputations; over 73,000 amputations are performed each year on patients with diabetes.
- Diabetes is the leading cause of kidney failure, accounting for over 44% of new cases.

The fundamental principle to remember about insulin therapy is that the right amount of insulin must be available to cells when glucose is present in the blood. Administering insulin when glucose is *not* present can lead to serious hypoglycemia and coma. This situation occurs when a patient administers insulin correctly but skips a meal; the insulin is available to cells, but glucose is not present. In another example, the patient participates in heavy exercise. The insulin may have been administered on schedule, and food may have been eaten, but the active muscles quickly use up all the glucose in the blood, and the patient becomes hypoglycemic. Patients with diabetes who engage in competitive sports need to consume food or sports drinks just prior to or during the activity to maintain their blood sugar at normal levels. It is important for nurses and patients to know the time of peak action of any insulin, because that is when the risk for hypoglycemic adverse effects is greatest.

Patients with diabetes who skip or forget their insulin dose face equally serious consequences. Again, remember the fundamental principle of insulin pharmacotherapy: The right amount of insulin must be available to cells when glucose is available in the blood. Without insulin present, glucose from a meal can build up to a high level in the blood, causing hyperglycemia and possible coma. Proper teaching and planning by nurses is essential to successful outcomes and patient compliance with therapy.

Many types of insulin are available, differing in their source, time of onset and peak effect, and duration of action. Until the 1980s, the source of all insulin was beef or pork pancreas. Almost all insulin today, however, is human insulin obtained through recombinant DNA technology because it is more effective, causes fewer allergies, and has a lower incidence of resistance. Pharmacologists have modified human insulin to create certain pharmacokinetic advantages, such as a more rapid onset of action (Humalog) or a more prolonged duration of action (Lantus). These modified forms are called **insulin analogs.** The different types of insulin available are listed in Table 45.1.

Doses of insulin are highly individualized for the precise control of blood glucose levels in each patient. Some patients require two or more injections daily for proper diabetes management. For ease of administration, two different compatible types of insulin may be mixed, using a standard method, to obtain the desired therapeutic effects. A long-acting insulin may be taken daily to provide a basal blood level and supplemented with rapid-acting insulin given shortly before a meal. Some of these combinations are marketed in cartridges containing premixed solutions. Examples of premixed insulin combinations include the following:

Table 45.1 Types of Insulin: Actions and Administration

Drug	Action	Onset	Peak	Duration	Administration and Timing	Compatibility
insulin aspart (NovoLog)	Rapid	15 min	1–3 h	3–5 h	Subcutaneous; 5–10 min before a meal	Can give with NPH; draw aspart up first and give immediately
insulin lispro (Humalog)	Rapid	5–15 min	0.5–1 h	3–4 h	Subcutaneous; 5–10 min before a meal	Can give with NPH; draw lispro up first and give immediately
insulin glulisine (Apidra)	Rapid	15–30 min	1 h	3–4 h	Subcutaneous; 15 min before a meal or within 20 min after starting meal	Can give with NPH; draw glulisine up first and give immediately
insulin regular (Humulin R, Novolin R)	Short	30–60 min	2–4 h	5–7 h	Subcutaneous; 30–60 min before a meal; IV	Can mix with NPH, sterile water, or normal saline; do not mix with glargine
insulin isophane (NPH, Humulin N, Novolin N, ReliOn N)	Intermediate	1–2 h	4–12 h	18–24 h	Subcutaneous; 30 min before first meal of the day, and 30 min before supper, if necessary	Can mix with aspart, lispro, or regular; do not mix with glargine
insulin detemir (Levemir)	Long	Gradual: over 24 h	6–8 h	To 24 h	Subcutaneous; with evening meal or at bedtime	Do not mix with any other insulin
insulin glargine (Lantus)	Long	Gradual: begins at 1.1 h	No peak	To 24 h	Subcutaneous; once daily, given at the same time each day	Do not mix with any other insulin

- Humulin 70/30 and Novolin 70/30: contain 70% NPH insulin and 30% regular insulin
- Humulin 50/50: contains 50% NPH insulin and 50% regular insulin
- Novolog Mix 70/30: contains 70% insulin aspart protamine and 30% insulin aspart
- Humalog Mix 75/25: contains 75% insulin lispro protamine and 25% insulin lispro.

Because the gastrointestinal (GI) tract destroys insulin, it cannot be given PO. Some patients have an insulin pump (Figure 45.3). This pump is usually abdominally anchored and is programmed to release small subcutaneous doses of insulin into the abdomen at predetermined intervals, with larger boluses administered manually at mealtime if necessary. Most pumps contain an alarm that sounds to remind patients to take their insulin.

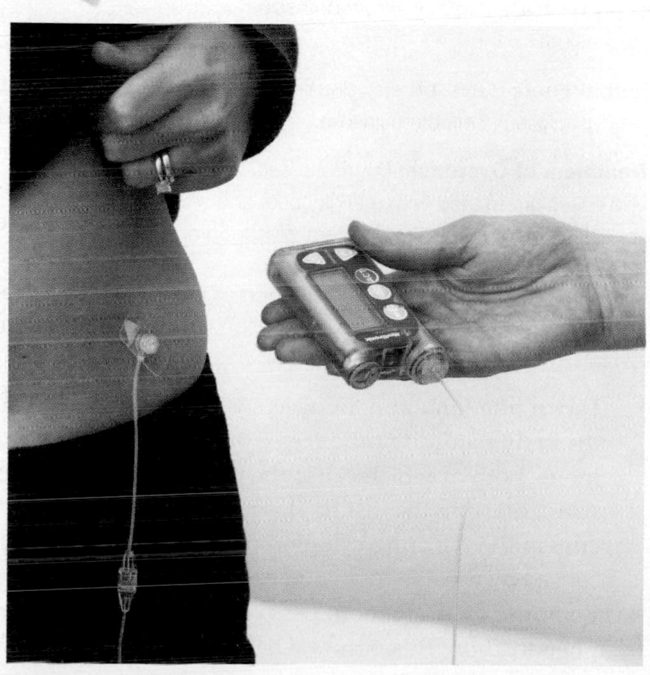

FIGURE 45.3 Insulin pump
ACE STOCK LIMITED/Alamy.

A common clinical problem occurring during insulin therapy is administering too much insulin relative to what the body needs. Excess insulin may remove too much glucose from the blood, resulting in hypoglycemia. This occurs when a patient with type 1 DM has more insulin in the blood than is needed to balance the amount of circulating blood glucose. Hypoglycemia may occur when the insulin level peaks, during exercise, when the patient receives too much insulin due to a medication error, or if the patient skips a meal. Some of the symptoms of hypoglycemia are the same as those of DKA. Those that differ and help in determining that a patient is hypoglycemic include pale, cool, moist skin, confusion, lightheadedness, weakness, and anxiety, with blood glucose less than 50 mg/dL. Symptoms have a sudden onset. Left untreated, severe hypoglycemia may result in death.

If the hypoglycemia is mild to moderate, symptoms can be reversed by consuming food or drinks that contain glucose, such as honey, regular soda, hard candies, or fruit juice. The quickest way to reverse serious hypoglycemia is to give intravenous (IV) glucose in a dextrose solution. The hormone glucagon is also used for the emergency treatment of severe hypoglycemia in patients who are unable to take IV glucose. Glucagon (1 mg) can be given IV, intramuscularly (IM), or subcutaneously to reverse hypoglycemic symptoms in 20 minutes or less, depending on the route.

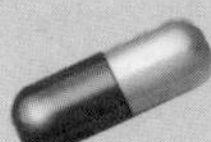

Prototype Drug | Human Regular Insulin *(Humulin R, Novolin R)*

Therapeutic Class: Parenteral drug for diabetes; pancreatic hormone
Pharmacologic Class: Short-acting hypoglycemic drug

Actions and Uses

Human regular insulin is used to help maintain blood glucose levels within normal limits. The primary effects of human regular insulin are: to promote cellular uptake of glucose, amino acids, and potassium; to promote protein synthesis, glycogen formation and storage, and fatty acid storage as triglycerides; and to conserve energy stores by promoting the utilization of glucose for energy needs and inhibiting gluconeogenesis. Because regular insulin is short acting, it is most often used in combination with intermediate or long-acting insulin to achieve 24-hour glucose control. Indications for insulin include the following:

- As monotherapy to lower blood glucose levels in patients with type 1 diabetes
- In combination with oral antidiabetic drugs in patients with type 2 diabetes
- For the emergency treatment of DKA
- For gestational diabetes

Administration Alerts

- Ensure that the patient has sufficient food and is not hypoglycemic before administering regular insulin.
- Regular insulin is the only type of insulin that may be used for IV injection.
- Rotate injection sites. When the patient is hospitalized, use sites not normally used by the patient when at home.
- Administer approximately 30 minutes before meals so insulin will be absorbed and available when the patient begins to eat.
- Pregnancy category B.

PHARMACOKINETICS

Onset	Peak	Duration
30–60 min subcutaneous; 15 min IV	4–12 h subcutaneous; 30–60 min IV	5–7 h subcutaneous; 30–60 min IV

Adverse Effects

The most common adverse effect of insulin therapy is hypoglycemia. Hypoglycemia may result from taking too much insulin, not properly timing the insulin injection with food intake, or skipping a meal. Signs of hypoglycemia include tachycardia, confusion, sweating, and drowsiness. Irritation at injection sites may occur, including lipohypertrophy, the accumulation of fat in the area of injection. This effect is lessened with rotation of injection sites. Weight gain is a possible side effect.

Contraindications: Insulin is used with caution in pregnancy, renal impairment or failure, fever, thyroid disease, and among older adults, children, or infants. Insulin should not be administered to patients with hypoglycemia. Patients with hypokalemia should be monitored carefully because insulin may worsen this condition.

Interactions

Drug–Drug: The following substances may potentiate hypoglycemic effects: alcohol, salicylates, monoamine oxidase inhibitors (MAOIs), anabolic steroids, and ACE inhibitors. The following substances may antagonize hypoglycemic effects: corticosteroids, thyroid hormone, and epinephrine. Serum glucose levels may be increased with furosemide or thiazide diuretics. Symptoms of hypoglycemic reaction may be masked with beta-adrenergic blockers.

Lab Tests: Insulin may increase urinary vanillylmandelic acid (VMA) and interfere with liver tests and thyroid function tests. It may decrease levels of serum potassium, calcium, and magnesium.

Herbal/Food: Garlic, bilberry, and ginseng may potentiate the hypoglycemic effects of insulin.

Treatment of Overdose: Overdose causes hypoglycemia. Mild cases are treated with oral glucose, and severe episodes are treated with parenteral glucagon or IV glucose.

Although it would seem logical that blood glucose would be lowest upon awakening, following 8 hours of not eating, this is not always the case. Morning hyperglycemia can occur in patients due to several mechanisms.

- **Waning insulin:** The amount of insulin in the blood may decline during the night, causing blood glucose levels to rise by morning. Adjusting the type or frequency of insulin dosing can manage this issue.
- **Dawn phenomenon:** Between 4:00 a.m. and 8:00 a.m. the body naturally produces cortisol and growth hormone, both of which cause the blood glucose level to rise. Adjusting the insulin dose so that peak action occurs in the morning can help prevent hyperglycemia caused by the dawn phenomenon.
- **Somogyi phenomenon:** Less common than the dawn phenomenon, this occurs when the patient has taken excessive insulin, drunk too much alcohol, or missed a meal, which cause a rebound fall in blood glucose.

During the night the body releases hormones that elevate blood glucose (epinephrine, cortisol, and glucagon), resulting in a high morning blood glucose level. This may be managed by having a protein snack before bedtime or reducing the evening insulin dose.

Other adverse effects of insulin include localized allergic reactions at the injection site, generalized urticaria, and swollen lymph glands.

Insulin Adjunct

Pramlintide (Symlin) is an antihyperglycemic drug that may be used along with insulin in persons with type 1 or type 2 diabetes who are not able to achieve glucose control by the use of insulin alone. The drug is a synthetic analog of amylin, a natural hormone released by the beta cells of the pancreas at the same time as insulin. The therapeutic actions of pramlintide are to slow gastric emptying time and increase satiety, thereby leading to reduced calorie intake. Pramlintide is administered subcutaneously immediately prior to each meal. When initiating treatment, rapid- or short-acting insulin doses are usually reduced by 50%. Adverse effects include nausea, vomiting, abdominal pain, headache, dizziness, fatigue, coughing, allergic reaction, or arthralgia. The drug carries a black box warning that severe hypoglycemia may occur during therapy.

Nursing Practice Application

Pharmacotherapy With Insulin

ASSESSMENT	POTENTIAL NURSING DIAGNOSES*
Baseline assessment prior to administration: • Obtain a complete health history including endocrine, cardiovascular, hepatic, or renal disease; pregnancy; or breast-feeding. Obtain a drug history including allergies, current prescription and over-the-counter (OTC) drugs, herbal preparations, caffeine, nicotine, and alcohol use. Be alert to possible drug interactions. • Obtain a history of current symptoms, duration and severity, and other related signs or symptoms (e.g., paresthesias of hands or feet). Assess the feet and lower extremities for possible ulcerations. • Obtain a dietary history including caloric intake if on an American Diabetes Association (ADA) diet, and the number of meals and snacks per day. Assess fluid intake and the type of fluids consumed. • Obtain baseline vital signs, height, and weight. • Evaluate appropriate laboratory findings (e.g., complete blood count (CBC), electrolytes, glucose, HbA1C level, lipid profile, osmolality, hepatic and renal function studies).	• *Imbalanced Nutrition, Less Than Body Requirements (type 1 diabetes)* • *Overweight (type 2 diabetes)* • *Obesity (type 2 diabetes)* • *Ineffective Health Management* • *Deficient Knowledge* (drug therapy) • *Risk for Unstable Blood Glucose* • *Risk for Deficient Fluid Volume* • *Risk for Injury*, related to adverse drug effects • *Risk for Infection* *NANDA I © 2014
Assessment throughout administration: • Assess for desired therapeutic effects depending on the reason the drug is given (e.g., glucose levels, electrolytes and osmolality remain within normal limits, HbA1C levels demonstrate adequate control of glucose). • Assess for and promptly report any adverse effects: signs of hypoglycemia (e.g., nausea, paleness, sweating, diaphoretic, tremors, irritability, headache, light-headedness, anxiety, decreased level of consciousness) and hyperglycemia (e.g., flushed, dry skin, polyuria, polyphagia, polydipsia, drowsiness, glycosuria, ketonuria, acetone breath), lipodystrophy, and infection.	

IMPLEMENTATION

Interventions and (Rationales)	Patient-Centered Care
Ensuring therapeutic effects: • Continue assessments as described earlier for therapeutic effects. (Depending on the severity of hyperglycemia, blood glucose levels should gradually return to normal.)	• Teach the patient to report any return of original symptoms. • Teach the patient the symptoms of hyper- and hypoglycemia to observe for and instruct the patient to check the capillary glucose level routinely and if symptoms are present. Promptly report any noticeable symptoms and concurrent capillary glucose level to the health care provider.

continued

Nursing Practice Application *continued*

IMPLEMENTATION	
Interventions and (Rationales)	**Patient-Centered Care**
• Administer insulin correctly and per the schedule ordered (e.g., routine dosing with or without sliding-scale coverage), planning insulin administration and peak times around meal times. (Maintaining a steady level of insulin with meal times arranged to match peak insulin activity will assist in maintaining a stable blood glucose level.)	• Teach the patient, family, or caregiver appropriate administration techniques for all types of insulin used, followed by teach-back until the patient, family, or caregiver is comfortable with the technique and is able to perform it correctly. • Teach the patient, family, or caregiver the importance of peak insulin levels and the need to ensure that adequate food sources are consumed to avoid hypoglycemia. Provide written materials for future reference whenever possible.
• Ensure that dietary needs are met based on the need to lose, gain, or maintain current weight and glucose levels. **Collaboration:** Consult with a dietitian as needed. Limit or eliminate alcohol use. (Adequate caloric amounts of protein, carbohydrates, and fats support the insulin regimen for glucose control. Activity and lifestyle will also be factored into dietary management. Alcohol can raise and then precipitously lower blood glucose as it is metabolized, raising the risk of hypoglycemia.)	• Review current diet, lifestyle, and activity level with the patient. Arrange a dietitian consult based on the need to alter diet or food choices. Teach the patient to limit or eliminate alcohol use. If alcoholic beverages are consumed, limit to one per day and take along with a complete meal to ensure that intake balances alcohol metabolism.
Minimizing adverse effects: • Continue to monitor capillary glucose levels. Hold insulin dose if the blood glucose level is less than 70 mg/dL or per parameters as ordered by the health care provider. (Daily glucose levels, especially before meals, will assist in maintaining stable blood glucose and will aid in assessing the appropriateness of the current insulin regimen.)	• Instruct the patient on blood glucose monitoring appropriate techniques to obtain capillary blood glucose levels, followed by teach-back, and when to contact the health care provider (e.g., glucose less than 70 mg/dL). Monitor use and ensure the proper functioning of all equipment to be used at home.
• Continue to monitor periodic laboratory work: CBC, electrolytes, glucose, HbA1C level, lipid profile, osmolality, and hepatic and renal function studies. (Periodic monitoring of laboratory work assists in determining glucose control, determines the need for any change in insulin needs, and assesses for complications. A1C levels provide a measure of glucose control over several months' time.)	• Instruct the patient on the need to return periodically for laboratory work.
• Assess for symptoms of hypoglycemia, especially around the time of insulin peak activity. If symptoms of hypoglycemia are noted, provide a quick-acting carbohydrate source (e.g., juice or other simple sugar), and then check capillary glucose level. Report to the health care provider if the glucose level is less than 70 mg/dL or as ordered. If meal time is not immediate, provide a longer-acting protein source to ensure that hypoglycemia does not recur. (Hypoglycemia is especially likely to occur around peak insulin activity, especially if food sources are inadequate. **Lifespan:** Age-related physiological differences may place the older adult at greater risk for hypoglycemia. Providing a quick-acting carbohydrate source and then checking the capillary glucose level will ensure that glucose does not decrease further while locating the glucose testing equipment. When in doubt, treating symptoms for suspected hypoglycemia is safer than allowing further decreases in glucose and possible loss of consciousness with adverse effects. Small additional amounts of carbohydrates will not dramatically increase blood sugar if testing shows a hyperglycemic episode.)	• Teach the patient to always carry a quick-acting carbohydrate source in case symptoms of hypoglycemia occur. If unsure whether symptoms indicate hypo- or hyperglycemia, treat as hypoglycemia and then check capillary glucose. If symptoms are not relieved in 10 to 15 minutes, or if blood sugar is below 70 mg/dL (or parameters as ordered), instruct the patient to notify the health care provider immediately.
• Monitor blood glucose more frequently during periods of illness or stress. (Insulin needs may increase or decrease during periods of illness or stress. Frequent monitoring during these times helps to ensure adequate glucose control.)	• Instruct the patient to check glucose levels more frequently when ill or under stress. Illness, especially associated with anorexia, nausea, or vomiting may decrease insulin needs. Instruct the patient to notify the health care provider if unable to eat normal meals during periods of illness or stress for a possible change in insulin dose.

Nursing Practice Application *continued*

IMPLEMENTATION	
Interventions and (Rationales)	**Patient-Centered Care**
• Encourage increased physical activity but monitor blood glucose before and after exercise and begin any new or increased exercise routine gradually. Continue to monitor for hypoglycemia up to 48 hours after exercise. (Exercise assists muscles to use glucose more efficiently and increases insulin receptor sites in the tissues, lowering blood glucose. Benefits of exercise and lowered blood sugar may continue for up to 48 hours, increasing the risk of hypoglycemia during this time.)	• Teach the patient the benefits of increased activity but to begin any new routine or increase in exercise gradually. Exercise should occur 1 hour after a meal or after a 10- or 15-g carbohydrate snack to prevent hypoglycemia. If exercise is prolonged, small, frequent carbohydrate snacks can be consumed every 30 minutes during exercise to maintain blood sugar. • Instruct the patient to check glucose levels more frequently before and after exercise.
• Rotate insulin administration sites weekly. If hospitalized, use sites that are less used or difficult to reach by the patient. Insulin pump subcutaneous catheters should be changed every 2 to 3 days. (Rotating injection sites weekly helps to prevent lipodystrophy. Use caution if using a new site, especially if the previous site used by the patient exhibits signs of lipodystrophy. Insulin in an unused site may be absorbed more quickly than a site with lipodystrophy, resulting in hypoglycemia. Insulin pump subcutaneous catheters should be changed to prevent infections at the site of insertion.)	• Instruct the patient on the need to rotate insulin injection sites on a weekly basis to prevent tissue damage or to rotate subcutaneous catheter sites (insulin pumps).
• Ensure the proper storage of insulin to maintain maximum potency. (Unopened insulin may be stored at room temperature but avoid direct sunlight and excessive heat. Opened insulin vials may be stored at room temperature for up to 1 month. If a noticeable change in solution occurs or if precipitate forms, discard the vial.)	• Teach the patient methods for proper storage of insulin and for storage during travel.
Patient understanding of drug therapy:	
• Use opportunities during administration of medications and during assessments to provide patient education. (Using time during nursing care helps to optimize and reinforce key teaching areas.)	• The patient, family, or caregiver should be able to state the reason for the drug; appropriate dose and scheduling; what adverse effects to observe for and when to report; and any special requirements of medication therapy (e.g., insulin needs during exercise, illness). • Instruct the patient to carry a wallet identification card or wear medical identification jewelry indicating diabetes.
Patient self-administration of drug therapy:	
• When administering the medication, instruct the patient, family, or caregiver in the proper self-administration of the drug. (Proper administration increases the effectiveness of the drug.)	• The patient, family, or caregiver is able to discuss appropriate dosing and administration needs, including: • Proper preparation of insulin: Rotate vials gently and do not shake; if insulins are mixed, draw up the quickest acting insulin and then longer-acting insulin if the insulins are compatible. Insulin glargine or insulin detemir should not be mixed with any other type of insulin. Use the appropriate syringe (100 unit) unless small amounts of insulin are ordered, then obtain syringes with smaller volumes to ensure accurate dosing. • Proper subcutaneous injection techniques: Select and cleanse the site with rotation every week. Inject at a 90-degree angle, applying a pad to the site after injection, but do not massage. • Proper use of all equipment, including blood glucose monitoring device and insulin pump.

See Table 45.1 for a list of drugs to which these nursing actions apply.

TYPE 2 DIABETES MELLITUS

45.4 Etiology and Characteristics of Type 2 Diabetes Mellitus

Type 2 diabetes mellitus is the more prevalent form of the disorder, representing 90% to 95% of people with diabetes. Because type 2 DM first appears in middle-aged adults, it has been referred to as age-onset diabetes or maturity-onset diabetes. These are inaccurate descriptions of this disorder, however, because increasing numbers of children and adolescents are being diagnosed with type 2 DM. Patients with type 2 DM are often asymptomatic and may have the condition for years before their diagnosis.

The primary physiological characteristic of type 2 DM is **insulin resistance;** target cells become unresponsive to insulin due to a defect in insulin receptor function. Essentially, the pancreas produces sufficient amounts of insulin but target cells do not recognize it.

As cells become more resistant to insulin, blood glucose levels rise and the pancreas responds by secreting even more insulin. Eventually, the hypersecretion of insulin causes beta cell exhaustion and ultimately leads to beta cell death. As type 2 DM progresses, it becomes a disorder characterized by insufficient insulin levels as well as insulin resistance. The activity of insulin receptors can be increased by physical exercise and lowering the level of circulating insulin. In fact, adhering to a healthy diet and a regular exercise program has been shown to reverse insulin resistance, and delay or prevent the development of type 2 DM.

The majority of people with type 2 DM are obese, have dyslipidemias, and will need a medically supervised plan to reduce weight gradually and exercise safely. Losing weight and exercising are important lifestyle changes for such patients; they will need to maintain these healthy habits for their lifetime. Patients with poorly managed type 2 DM suffer from the same complications as patients with type 1 DM (e.g., retinopathy, neuropathy, and nephropathy).

Hyperosmolar hyperglycemic state (HHS) is a serious, acute condition with a mortality rate of 20% to 40% that occurs in persons with type 2 DM. HHS is caused by insufficient circulating insulin. The onset of HHS is gradual and is sometimes mistaken for a stroke. Seen most often in older adults, the skin appears flushed, dry, and warm. Blood glucose levels may be extreme and rise above 600 mg/dL. Treatment consists of fluid replacement, correction of electrolyte imbalances, and low-dose insulin given by slow IV infusion to lower glucose levels to 250 to 300 mg/dL. Although less common, HHS has a higher mortality rate than DKA.

ANTIDIABETIC DRUGS FOR TYPE 2 DIABETES

Type 2 DM is usually controlled with noninsulin antidiabetic drugs, which are prescribed after diet and exercise have failed to reduce blood glucose to normal levels. As the disease progresses, insulin may become necessary or it may be required temporarily during times of stress such as illness or loss. These drugs are sometimes referred to as oral hypoglycemic drugs. However, this is an inaccurate name because some are given by the subcutaneous route and some do not cause hypoglycemia.

45.5 Pharmacotherapy for Type 2 Diabetes Mellitus

The six primary groups of antidiabetic drugs for type 2 DM are classified by their chemical structures and their mechanisms of action. These are alpha-glucosidase inhibitors, biguanides, incretin enhancers, meglitinides, sulfonylureas, and thiazolidinediones (or glitazones). Therapy with type 2 antidiabetic drugs is not effective for persons with type 1 DM. Doses for these drugs are listed in Table 45.2.

Treating the Diverse Patient: Diabetes Worldwide: The Role of a Changing Diet

Many factors are known to contribute to the development of type 2 diabetes, including a sedentary lifestyle, obesity, and aging. As rates of diabetes increase worldwide, changing nutritional patterns have been implicated for the increase.

Weeratunga, Jayasinghe, Perera, Jayasena, and Jayasinghe (2014) studied global sugar consumption and the prevalence of diabetes. There was a strong association between sugar consumption and diabetes, particularly in Asian countries. Basu, Stuckler, McKee, and Galea (2013) studied the effects of changing food markets in 173 countries worldwide and the incidence of diabetes in those countries. The researchers found that as a population's income increased, the importation, availability, and overall use of processed foods containing greater proportions of sugars and sweeteners increased. Increased consumption of sugars and related sweeteners was significantly correlated with rising rates of diabetes, independent of the presence of obesity.

In the United States, sugar-sweetened beverages are the largest source of added sugar, and the consumption of only one or two of these beverages daily increases the risk of type 2 diabetes by 29% (Hu, 2013). Whereas rising income can improve dietary choices and nutrition, nurses should be aware that sound nutritional practices may not always follow a rise in income or food choices.

Table 45.2 Antidiabetic Drugs

Drug	Route and Adult Dose (max dose where indicated)	Adverse Effects
ALPHA-GLUCOSIDASE INHIBITORS		
acarbose (Precose)	PO: 25–100 mg tid (max: 300 mg/day)	*Flatulence, diarrhea, abdominal distention*
miglitol (Glyset)	PO: 25–100 mg tid (max: 300 mg/day)	Hypoglycemia when used with other antidiabetic drugs (tremors, palpitations, sweating)
BIGUANIDE		
metformin immediate release (Glucophage, Riomet)	PO: 500 mg bid or 850 mg once daily; increase to 1,000–2,550 mg in two to three divided doses/day (max: 2.55 g/day)	*Flatulence, diarrhea, nausea, anorexia, abdominal pain, bitter or metallic taste*
Extended release (Fortamet, Glucophage XR, Glumetza)	Fortamet: 1,000 mg once daily (max: 2.5 g/day) Glumetza: 1,000–2,000 mg once daily (max: 2 g/day) Glucophage XR: 500 mg once daily (max: 2 g/day)	Lactic acidosis
INCRETIN ENHANCERS (GLP-1 AGONISTS)		
albiglutide (Tanzeum)	Subcutaneous: 30–50 mg once weekly	*Nausea, vomiting, diarrhea, nervousness, injection site reactions*
exenatide (Byetta, Bydureon)	Subcutaneous: 5–10 mcg q12h (Byetta) or 2 mg once weekly (Bydureon)	Antibody formation, pancreatitis (exenatide), renal impairment (exenatide), thyroid tumors
dulaglutide (Trulicity)	Subcutaneous: 0.75–1.5 mg once weekly	
liraglutide (Victoza)	Subcutaneous: 0.6–1.8 mg once daily	
INCRETIN ENHANCERS (DPP-4 INHBITORS)		
alogliptin (Nesina)	PO: 25 mg once daily	*Flulike symptoms, upper respiratory infection, back pain*
linagliptin (Tradjenta)	PO: 5 mg once daily	
saxagliptin (Onglyza)	PO: 2.5–5 mg once daily	Hypoglycemia when used with other antidiabetic drugs, hepatic impairment, anaphylaxis, pancreatitis
sitagliptin (Januvia)	PO: 100 mg once daily	
MEGLITINIDES		
nateglinide (Starlix)	PO: 60–120 mg tid, 1–30 min prior to meals (max: 360 mg/day)	*Flulike symptoms, upper respiratory infection, back pain*
repaglinide (Prandin)	PO: 0.5–4 mg bid–qid, 1–30 min prior to meals (max: 16 mg/day)	Hypoglycemia (tremors, palpitations, sweating), anaphylaxis, pancreatitis
SULFONYLUREAS, FIRST GENERATION		
chlorpropamide (Diabinese)	PO: 100–250 mg/day (max: 750 mg/day)	*Nausea, heartburn, dizziness, headache, drowsiness*
tolazamide (Tolinase)	PO: 100–500 mg one to two times/day (max: 1 g/day)	Hypoglycemia (tremors, palpitations, sweating), cholestatic jaundice, blood dyscrasias
tolbutamide (Orinase)	PO: 250–1,500 mg one to two times/day (max: 3 g/day)	
SULFONYLUREAS, SECOND GENERATION		
glimepiride (Amaryl)	PO: 1–4 mg/day (max: 8 mg/day)	*Nausea, heartburn, dizziness, headache, drowsiness*
glipizide (Glucotrol)	PO: 2.5–20 mg one to two times/day (max: 40 mg/day)	Hypoglycemia (tremors, palpitations, sweating), cholestatic jaundice, blood dyscrasias
glyburide (DiaBeta, Micronase)	PO: 1.25–10 mg one to two times/day (max: 20 mg/day)	
glyburide micronized (Glynase)	PO: 0.75–12 mg one to two times/day (max: 12 mg/day)	
THIAZOLIDINEDIONES		
pioglitazone (Actos)	PO: 15–30 mg/day (max: 45 mg/day)	*Upper respiratory infection, myalgia, headache, edema, weight gain*
rosiglitazone (Avandia)	PO: 2–4 mg one to two times/day (max: 8 mg/day)	Hypoglycemia (tremors, palpitations, sweating), hepatotoxicity, bone fractures, heart failure, myocardial infarction
MISCELLANEOUS DRUGS		
bromocriptine (Cycloset)	PO: 0.8–4.8 mg/day upon awakening	*Nausea, fatigue, dizziness, vomiting, headache* Confusion, agitation, hallucinations
colesevelam (WeChol)	PO: 1.875 g (3 tablets) q12h or 3.75 g (6 tablets) once daily	*Constipation, dyspepsia, and nausea* Increased seizure activity, reduced International normalized ratio (with concurrent warfarin), elevated thyroid stimulating hormone (with concurrent thyroid hormone)
canagliflozin (Invokana)	PO: 100 mg once daily (max: 300 mg/day) taken before first meal	*Female genital mycotic infections, urinary tract infection, and nasopharyngitis*
dapagliflozin (Farxiga)	PO: 5–10 mg once daily in the morning with or without food	
empagliflozin (Jardiance)	PO: 10–25 mg once daily in the morning, with or without food	Hypotension, renal impairment, hyperkalemia, hypoglycemia

Treatment goals recommended by the American Association of Clinical Endocrinologists (Handelsman et al., 2015) are designed to target an HbA1C level of 6.5% or less with a fasting plasma glucose level less than 110 g/dL. Treatment goals are optimized for each individual patient, based on comorbid conditions and severity of diabetic signs and symptoms. In general, all of the antidiabetic drugs are similar in their ability to lower HbA1C levels in the short term. There are some differences, however, in long-term control. For example, drugs in the thiazolidinedione class appear to maintain glycemic control for 5 to 6 years, whereas the sulfonylureas peak at 6 months and slowly decline in efficacy. The adverse effects observed for each class differ: Some cause hypoglycemia, whereas others cause weight gain or GI complaints such as diarrhea. Because there is no single perfect drug for type 2 diabetes, choice of therapy is guided by the experiences of the prescriber and the results achieved by the individual patient.

Therapy of type 2 DM is generally initiated with a single drug, usually metformin. Metformin is inexpensive, safe, and has been shown to reduce the incidence of cardiovascular events associated with diabetes. If glycemic control is not achieved with monotherapy, then a second drug is added to the therapeutic regimen. Choice of the second drug depends upon the experience of the prescriber and patient preference. Failure to achieve glycemic control with two antidiabetic drugs suggests the need for insulin to be added to the regimen, though some clinicians may add a third noninsulin drug rather than insulin.

Many fixed-dose combination products are available for the treatment of people with type 2 diabetes. The main advantage of taking a combination drug is that it is more convenient than taking two separate drugs and may improve compliance with the therapeutic regimen. Combination products are indicated for patients who fail to adequately control glucose levels with the use of a single drug. Doses for selected combination products are listed in Table 45.3.

☑ Check Your Understanding 45.1

As type 2 DM progresses, supplemental insulin is often required. What is the pathophysiology associated with this progression? *Visit www.pearsonhighered.com/nursingresources for the answer.*

Sulfonylureas

The first oral hypoglycemics available, sulfonylureas are divided into first- and second-generation categories. Although drugs from both generations are equally effective at lowering blood glucose, the second-generation drugs exhibit fewer drug–drug interactions.

The sulfonylureas act by stimulating the release of insulin from pancreatic islet cells and by increasing the

Table 45.3 Selected Combination Oral Antidiabetic Drugs

Brand Name Drug	Generic Drug Combination	Route and Adult Dose (maximum dose where indicated)
Actoplus Met	pioglitazone/metformin	PO: 15 mg/500–850 mg once or twice daily. Starting dose depends if patient was previously treated with metformin or pioglitazone combination or had an inadequate response with either drug alone (max: 45 mg/2,550 mg daily)
Avandamet	rosiglitazone/metformin	Patients with no prior treatment: PO: 2 mg/500 mg once or twice daily Previously treated patients: PO: 2–4 mg/500–1,000 mg bid (max: 8 mg/2,000 mg daily)
Avandaryl	rosiglitazone/glimepiride	PO: Start with 4 mg/2 mg once daily with the first meal of the day (max: 8 mg/4 mg daily)
Duetact	pioglitazone/glimepiride	PO: Start with 30 mg/2 mg once daily (max: 45 mg/8 mg daily)
Glucovance	glyburide/metformin	Patients with no prior treatment: PO: 1.25 mg/250 mg once or twice daily Previously treated patients: PO: 2.5 mg/500 mg to 5 mg/500 mg bid (max: 20 mg/2,000 mg daily)
Invokamet	canagliflozin/metformin	PO: 50 mg/500 mg bid with meals (max: 300 mg/2,000 mg)
Janumet	sitagliptin/metformin	PO: starting dose 50 mg/500 mg bid with meals (max: 100 mg/2,000 mg/day)
Jentadueto	linagliptin/metformin	PO: 2.5 mg/1,000 mg bid with meals
Juvisync	sitagliptin/simvastatin	PO: Start with 100 mg/40 mg once daily in the evening
Kazano	alogliptin/metformin	PO: 12.5 mg/500 mg bid with food
Metaglip	glipizide/metformin	PO: 2.5 mg/500 mg or 5 mg/500 mg bid (max: 20 mg/2,000 mg daily)
Oseni	alogliptin/pioglitazone	PO: 25 mg/15 mg once daily
PrandiMet	repaglinide/metformin	PO: start with 1 mg/500 mg given bid, 15 min before meals (max: 10 mg/2,500 mg daily)
Xigduo XR	dapagliflozin/metformin	PO: 5 mg/500 mg extended release once daily in the morning (max: 10 mg/2,000 mg extended release)

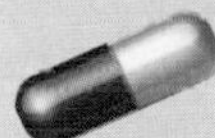

Prototype Drug | Metformin *(Fortamet, Glucophage, Glumetza, others)*

Therapeutic Class: Antidiabetic drug **Pharmacologic Class:** Hypoglycemic drug; biguanide

Actions and Uses

Metformin is a preferred oral antidiabetic drug for managing type 2 DM because of its effectiveness and safety. It is used alone or in combination with other antidiabetic medications or insulin. It is approved for use in children age 10 years or older. It is available as regular-release tablets, solution (Riomet), and sustained-release forms (Fortamet, Glucophage XR, and Glumetza).

Metformin reduces fasting and postprandial glucose levels by decreasing the hepatic production of glucose (gluconeogenesis) and reducing insulin resistance. It does not promote insulin release from the pancreas. A major advantage of the drug is that it does not cause hypoglycemia. The drug's actions do not depend on stimulating insulin release, so it is able to lower glucose levels in patients who no longer secrete insulin. In addition to lowering blood glucose levels, it lowers triglyceride and total and low-density lipoprotein (LDL) cholesterol levels, and it promotes weight loss.

Metformin is used off-label to treat women with polycystic ovary syndrome. Women with this syndrome have insulin resistance and high serum insulin levels. Metformin reduces insulin resistance, which in turn lowers insulin and androgen levels, thus restoring normal menstrual cycles and ovulation.

Administration Alerts

- Sustained-release tablets must be swallowed whole and not crushed or chewed.
- Fasting blood glucose levels should be obtained every 3 months, and the dose adjusted accordingly.
- Discontinue the medication immediately if signs of acidosis are present.
- Pregnancy category B.

PHARMACOKINETICS

Onset	Peak	Duration
Less than 1 h	1–3 h (regular release); 4–8 h (extended release)	12 h (regular release); 24 h (extended release)

Adverse Effects

The most common adverse effects are GI related and include nausea, vomiting, abdominal discomfort, metallic taste, diarrhea, and anorexia. It may also cause headache, dizziness, agitation, and fatigue. Unlike the sulfonylureas, metformin rarely causes hypoglycemia or weight gain.

Black Box Warning: Lactic acidosis is a rare, though potentially fatal, adverse effect. The risk for lactic acidosis is increased in patients with renal insufficiency or any condition that puts them at risk for increased lactic acid production, such as liver disease, severe infection, excessive alcohol intake, shock, or hypoxemia. Another drug in this class, phenformin, was withdrawn from the market in 1977 due to fatal cases of lactic acidosis.

Contraindications: Metformin is contraindicated in patients with impaired renal function, because the drug can rise to toxic levels. It is also contraindicated in patients with heart failure, liver failure, history of lactic acidosis, or concurrent serious infection. It is contraindicated for 2 days prior to and 2 days after receiving IV radiographic contrast. Metformin is used with caution in patients with anemia, diarrhea, vomiting or dehydration, fever, gastroparesis, GI obstruction, hyperthyroidism, pituitary insufficiency, trauma, pregnancy and lactation, and in older adults.

Interactions

Drug–Drug: Alcohol increases the risk for lactic acidosis. Captopril, furosemide, and nifedipine may increase the risk for hypoglycemia. Use with IV radiographic contrast may cause lactic acidosis and acute renal failure. The following drugs may decrease renal excretion of metformin: amiloride, cimetidine, digoxin, dofetilide, midodrine, morphine, procainamide, quinidine, ranitidine, triamterene, trimethoprim, and vancomycin. Acarbose may decrease blood levels of metformin. Use with other antidiabetic drugs potentiates hypoglycemic effects.

Lab Tests: Metformin may cause false-positive results for urinary ketones.

Herbal/Food: Metformin decreases the absorption of vitamin B_{12} and folic acid. Garlic and ginseng may increase hypoglycemic effects.

Treatment of Overdose: For overdose or development of lactic acidosis, hemodialysis can be used to correct the acidosis and remove excess metformin.

sensitivity of insulin receptors on target cells. The most common adverse effect of sulfonylureas is hypoglycemia, which is usually caused by taking too much medication or not eating enough food. Persistent hypoglycemia from these drugs may be prolonged and require administration of dextrose to return glucose to normal levels. Other adverse effects include weight gain, hypersensitivity reactions, GI distress, and hepatotoxicity. When alcohol is taken with these sulfonylureas, some patients experience a disulfiram-like reaction that includes flushing, palpitations, and nausea.

Biguanides

Metformin (Glucophage) is the only drug in this class. Information on this drug is presented in the prototype feature box in this chapter.

Alpha-Glucosidase Inhibitors

The alpha-glucosidase inhibitors, which include acarbose (Precose) and miglitol (Glyset), act by blocking enzymes in the small intestine that are responsible for breaking down complex carbohydrates into monosaccharides. Because carbohydrates must be in the monosaccharide form to be absorbed, digestion of glucose is delayed. These drugs are usually well tolerated and have minimal adverse effects that include abdominal cramping, diarrhea, and flatulence. Liver function should be monitored because a small incidence of liver impairment has been reported. Although alpha-glucosidase inhibitors do not produce hypoglycemia when used alone, hypoglycemia may occur when these drugs are combined with insulin or a sulfonylurea. If hypoglycemia does develop, it must be treated with glucose and not sucrose (table sugar), because the drug inhibits the absorption of sucrose. Concurrent use of garlic and ginseng may increase the hypoglycemic action of alpha-glucosidase inhibitors.

Thiazolidinediones

The thiazolidinediones, or glitazones, reduce blood glucose by decreasing insulin resistance and inhibiting hepatic gluconeogenesis. Optimal lowering of blood glucose may take 3 to 4 months of therapy. The most common adverse effects are fluid retention, headache, and weight gain. Hypoglycemia does not occur with drugs in this class. Liver function should be monitored, because thiazolidinediones may be hepatotoxic; in 2000, troglitazone (Rezulin) was withdrawn from the market because of drug-related deaths due to hepatic failure. Because of their tendency to promote fluid retention, thiazolidinediones are contraindicated in patients with serious heart failure or pulmonary edema. Both drugs in this class, rosiglitazone (Avandia) and pioglitazone (Actos), contain black box warnings for heart failure and for increased risk for myocardial ischemia. Using this drug class in patients with heart failure can increase fluid retention and exacerbate heart disease. These drugs are often combined with other antidiabetic drugs in the management of blood glucose (see Table 45.2).

Meglitinides

The meglitinides, repaglinide (Prandin) and nateglinide (Starlix), act by stimulating the release of insulin from pancreatic islet cells in a manner similar to that of the sulfonylureas. Both drugs in this class have short durations of action of 2 to 4 hours. Their efficacy is equal to that of the sulfonylureas, and they are well tolerated. Hypoglycemia is the most common adverse effect.

Incretin Enhancers and Miscellaneous Drugs

Several newer antidiabetic drugs act by affecting the incretin–glucose control mechanism. Incretins are hormones secreted by the mucosa of the small intestine following a meal, when blood glucose is elevated. Incretins signal the pancreas to increase insulin secretion and the liver to stop producing glucagon. Both of these actions lower blood glucose levels. In addition, these drugs decrease food intake by increasing the feeling of satiety in the patient, and they also slow gastric emptying, which delays glucose absorption. Drugs may be used to modify the incretin system in patients with diabetes in two ways: by mimicking the actions of incretins or by reducing their destruction.

Albiglutide (Tanzeum), exenatide (Byetta, Bydureon), and liraglutide (Victoza) are injectable drugs that *mimic* the effects of incretins. They accomplish their actions by activating a receptor called GLP-1. Activation of the GLP-1 receptor causes the same types of effects as the natural incretin hormone: lowering blood glucose by increasing the secretion of insulin, slowing the absorption of glucose, and reducing the action of glucagon. The drugs are approved as alternatives to metformin in patients who have not achieved adequate glycemic control during metformin or sulfonylurea monotherapy. A major disadvantage is that the drugs must be administered subcutaneously, sometimes twice a day, and they have a high incidence of nausea, vomiting, and diarrhea. They do not cause hypoglycemia.

The second group of incretin enhancers are the dipeptidyl peptidase-4 (DPP-4) inhibitors. Alogliptin (Nesina), linagliptin (Tradjenta), saxagliptin (Onglyza), and sitagliptin (Januvia) prevent the breakdown of natural incretins, allowing the hormone levels to rise and produce a greater response. These drugs are given orally and are effective at lowering blood glucose with few adverse effects. They work well with other antidiabetic drugs and do not cause hypoglycemia.

In 2013 the U.S. Food and Drug Administration (FDA) approved canagliflozin (Invokana), the first in a new class of drugs called the sodium-glucose co-transporter (SGLT) inhibitors. Inhibiting the SGLT in the kidney allows more glucose to leave the blood and be excreted via the urine. This drug has the advantage of promoting weight loss. Two additional drugs in this class, dapagliflozin (Farxiga) and empagliflozin, were approved in 2014 and have very similar actions and adverse effects. Recently approved fixed dose combinations include Invokamet (metformin with canagliflozin) and Xigduo XR (metformin with and dapagliflozin).

Two other miscellaneous drugs include bromocriptine and colesevelam. Bromocriptine (Parlodel) was originally approved in 1978 to treat Parkinson's disease, pituitary adenoma, acromegaly, and for women with amenorrhea and infertility caused by excessive prolactin secretion. The drug acts on the central nervous system to increase levels of the neurotransmitter dopamine. Approved for type 2 diabetes as Cycloset, the exact mechanism by which it improves glycemic control remains unclear. The most frequent adverse events associated with bromocriptine are nausea, fatigue, dizziness, vomiting, and headache.

More often used to treat hyperlipidemia, colesevelam (Welchol) is also indicated for type 2 diabetes. Being a nonabsorbed bile acid sequestrant, colesevelam can inhibit the absorption of other drugs, including fat-soluble vitamins.

Nursing Practice Application

Pharmacotherapy for Type 2 Diabetes

ASSESSMENT	POTENTIAL NURSING DIAGNOSES
Baseline assessment prior to administration: • *Refer to the Nursing Practice Application: Pharmacotherapy With Insulin for these items.*	
Assessment throughout administration: • *Refer to the Nursing Practice Application: Pharmacotherapy With Insulin for these items. Included here are assessment items unique to type 2 antidiabetic drugs.* • Continue periodic monitoring of hepatic function studies.	

IMPLEMENTATION

Interventions and (Rationales)	Patient-Centered Care
Ensuring therapeutic effects: • *Refer to the Nursing Practice Application: Pharmacotherapy With Insulin for these items. Included here are interventions unique to type 2 antidiabetic drugs.*	
• Ensure that dietary needs are met based on the need to lose, gain, or maintain current weight and glucose levels. **Collaboration:** Consult with a dietitian as needed. Limit or eliminate alcohol use. (Patients who are taking sulfonylureas should avoid or eliminate alcohol entirely to prevent a disulfiram-like reaction.)	• Instruct the patient on sulfonylureas (e.g., glyburide) to avoid or eliminate alcohol use.
Minimizing adverse effects: • *Refer to the Nursing Practice Application: Pharmacotherapy With Insulin for these items.* Included here are interventions unique to type 2 antidiabetic drugs.	
• Continue to monitor periodic laboratory work: CBC, electrolytes, glucose, HbA1C level, lipid profile, and hepatic and renal function studies. (Sulfonylureas may cause hepatic toxicity. Biguanides may cause lactic acidosis. **Lifespan:** Age-related physiological differences may place the older adult at greater risk for hepatic toxicity.)	• Instruct the patient on the need to return periodically for laboratory work. • Teach the patient on sulfonylureas to immediately report any nausea, vomiting, yellowing of the skin or sclera, abdominal pain, light or clay-colored stools, or darkening of urine to the health care provider. • Teach the patient on biguanides to immediately report any drowsiness, malaise, decreased respiratory rate, or general body aches to the health care provider.
• Assess for symptoms of hypoglycemia. (Hypoglycemia is especially likely to occur if the patient is taking sulfonylureas or meglitinides, although hypoglycemia may occur with other types of type 2 antidiabetic drugs, especially if food sources are inadequate. **Lifespan:** Age-related physiological differences may place the older adult at greater risk for hypoglycemia.)	• Teach the patient to always carry a quick-acting carbohydrate source in case symptoms of hypoglycemia occur.
• Monitor for hypersensitivity and allergic reactions. Continue to monitor the patient throughout therapy. (Anaphylactic reactions are possible although rare. As sensitivity occurs, reactions may continue to develop.)	• Teach the patient to immediately report any itching, rashes, or swelling, particularly of the face or tongue; urticaria; flushing; dizziness; syncope; wheezing; throat tightness; or difficulty breathing.

continued

Nursing Practice Application *continued*

IMPLEMENTATION	
Interventions and (Rationales)	**Patient-Centered Care**
• **Lifespan:** Assess for pregnancy. (Some type 2 antidiabetic drugs are category C and must be stopped during pregnancy. Due to the increasing metabolic needs of pregnancy, supplemental insulin, or switching to insulin, may be required.)	• Teach the female patient of childbearing age to alert the health care provider if pregnancy is suspected.
• Continue to monitor for edema, blood pressure, and lung sounds in patients who are taking thiazolidiones. (These drugs may cause edema and worsening of heart failure.)	• Instruct the patient to immediately report any edema of the hands or feet, dyspnea, or excessive fatigue to the provider.
• Monitor for hypoglycemia more frequently in patients on concurrent beta-blocker therapy. (Beta blockers may antagonize the action of some type 2 antidiabetic drugs and may mask the symptoms of a hypoglycemic episode, allowing the blood glucose to drop lower before it is perceived.)	• Teach the patient on concurrent beta-blocker therapy to monitor capillary blood glucose frequently and to check the blood glucose if minor changes in overall feeling are perceived (e.g., sweating, minor agitation or anxiety, slight tremors).
Patient understanding of drug therapy:	
• Use opportunities during administration of medications and during assessments to provide patient education. (Using time during nursing care helps to optimize and reinforce key teaching areas.)	• The patient, family, or caregiver should be able to state the reason for the drug; appropriate dose and scheduling; what adverse effects to observe for and when to report; and any special requirements of medication therapy (e.g., drug needs during exercise, illness). • Instruct the patient to carry a wallet identification card or wear medical identification jewelry indicating diabetes.
Patient self-administration of drug therapy:	
• When administering the medication, instruct the patient, family, or caregiver in the proper self-administration of the drug. (Using time during nurse-administration of these drugs helps to reinforce teaching.)	• The patient, family, or caregiver is able to discuss appropriate dosing and administration needs, including: • Timing of doses: For drugs given once a day, take approximately 30 minutes before the first meal of the day. Alpha-glucosidase inhibitors (e.g., acarbose) should be taken with meals. • Insulin requirements: While type 2 diabetics produce some insulin, insulin injections may be required in addition to the oral hypoglycemic drug on occasion. This does not necessarily signal a worsening of the disease condition, but may be a temporary need.

See Table 45.2 for a list of drugs to which these nursing actions apply.

Chapter Review

KEY Concepts

The numbered key concepts provide a succinct summary of the important points from the corresponding numbered section within the chapter. If any of these points are not clear, refer to the numbered section within the chapter for review.

45.1 The pancreas is both an endocrine and an exocrine gland. Insulin is released when blood glucose increases, and glucagon is released when blood glucose decreases.

45.2 Type 1 diabetes mellitus (DM) is caused by a lack of insulin secretion due to autoimmune destruction of pancreatic islet cells. If untreated, it results in serious, chronic conditions affecting the cardiovascular and nervous systems.

45.3 Type 1 DM is treated by dietary restrictions, exercise, and insulin therapy. The many types of insulin preparations vary as to their onset of action, time to peak effect, and duration.

45.4 Type 2 DM is caused by a lack of sensitivity of insulin receptors in the target cells and a deficiency in insulin secretion. If untreated, the same chronic conditions result as in type 1 DM.

45.5 More than six classes of drugs are available for the pharmacotherapy of type 2 DM. Type 2 DM is commonly treated by combining two drugs from different antidiabetic drug classes, which helps to better manage blood glucose levels.

REVIEW Questions

1. A patient receives NPH and regular insulin every morning. The nurse is verifying that the patient understands that there are two different peak times to be aware of for this insulin regimen. Why is this an important concept for the nurse to stress?

1. The patient needs to plan the next insulin injection around the peak times.
2. Additional insulin may be needed at peak times to avoid hyperglycemia.
3. It is best to plan exercise or other activities around peak insulin activity.
4. The risk for hypoglycemia is greatest around the peak of insulin activity.

2. The patient is scheduled to receive 5 units of Humalog and 25 units of NPH (Isophane) insulin prior to breakfast. Which nursing intervention is most appropriate for this patient?

1. Make sure the patient's breakfast is available to eat before administering this insulin.
2. Offer the patient a high-carbohydrate snack in 6 hours.
3. Hold the insulin if the blood glucose level is greater than 100 mg/dL.
4. Administer the medications in two separate syringes.

3. The nurse is initiating discharge teaching with the newly diagnosed patient with diabetes. Which of the following statements indicates that the patient needs additional teaching?

1. "If I am experiencing hypoglycemia, I should drink 1/2 cup of apple juice."
2. "My insulin needs may increase when I have an infection."
3. "I must draw the NPH insulin first if I am mixing it with regular insulin."
4. "If my blood glucose levels are less than 60 mg/dL, I should notify my health care provider."

4. What patient education should the nurse provide to the patient with diabetes who is planning an exercise program? (Select all that apply.)

1. Monitor blood glucose levels before and after exercise.
2. Eat a complex carbohydrate prior to strenuous exercise.
3. Exercise may increase insulin needs.
4. Withhold insulin prior to engaging in strenuous exercise.
5. Take extra insulin prior to exercise.

5. A patient with type 2 diabetes has been nothing by mouth (NPO) since midnight for surgery in the morning. He has been on a combination of oral type 2 antidiabetic drugs. What would be the *best* action for the nurse to take concerning the administration of his medications?
   1. Hold all medications as per the NPO order.
   2. Give him the medications with a sip of water.
   3. Give him half the original dose.
   4. Contact the health care provider for further orders.

6. A 63-year-old patient with type 2 diabetes is admitted to the nursing unit with an infected foot ulcer. Despite previous good control on glyburide (Micronase), his blood glucose has been elevated the past several days and he requires sliding-scale insulin. What is the most likely reason for the elevated glucose levels?
   1. It is a temporary condition related to the stress response with increased glucose release.
   2. He is converting to a type 1 diabetic.
   3. The oral antidiabetic drug is no longer working for him.
   4. Patients with diabetes who are admitted to the hospital are switched to insulin for safety and tighter control.

PATIENT-FOCUSED Case Study

Jorge Esperanza is a 35-year-old who has been on insulin therapy since he was diagnosed with type 1 diabetes at age 14. He had been taking twice daily doses of a combination of NPH and regular insulins. However, his provider has recently switched him to insulin glargine (Lantus) and regular insulin ordered for every morning.

1. How is insulin glargine (Lantus) different from other types of insulin?
2. As the nurse, how will you explain to Jorge the technique of administering these two types of insulins?

CRITICAL THINKING Questions

1. A 28-year-old woman who is pregnant with her first child is diagnosed with gestational DM. She is concerned about the fact that she might have to take "shots." She tells the nurse at the public health clinic that she does not think she can self-administer an injection and asks if there is a pill that will control her blood sugar. She has heard her grandfather talk about his pills to control his "sugar." What should the nurse explain to this patient?
2. A patient with type 2 diabetes on metformin (Glucophage) reports that he takes propranolol (Inderal) for his hypertension. What concerns would the nurse have about this combination of medications? What would the nurse teach the patient?

Visit www.pearsonhighered.com/nursingresources for answers and rationales for all activities.

REFERENCES

Basu, S., Stuckler, D., McKee, M., & Galea, G. (2013). Nutritional determinants of worldwide diabetes: An econometric study of food markets and diabetes prevalence in 173 countries. *Public Health Nutrition, 16*, 179–186. doi:10.1017/S1368980012002881

Centers for Disease Control and Prevention. (2014). *National diabetes statistics report: Estimates of diabetes and its burden in the United States.* Handelsman from the Bibliography Atlanta, GA: U.S. Department of Health and Human Services.

Handelsman, Y., Bloomgarden, Z. T., Grunberger, G. Umpierrez, G., Zimmerman, R. S., Bailey, T. S.,. . . . Zangeneh, F., (2015). American Association of Clinical Endocrinologists and American College of Endocrinology – Clinical practice guidelines for developing a diabetes mellitus comprehensive care plan – 2015—Executive summary. *Endocrine Practice, 21*(Suppl. 1), 1–53. doi:10.4158/EP15672.GL.

Herdman, T. H., & Kamitsuru, S. (Eds.). (2014). *NANDA International nursing diagnoses: Definitions and classification, 2015–2017.* Oxford, United Kingdom: Wiley-Blackwell.

Hu, F. B. (2013). Resolved: There is sufficient scientific evidence that decreasing sugar-sweetened beverage consumption will reduce the prevalence of obesity and obesity-related diseases. *Obesity Reviews, 14*, 606–619. doi:10.1111/obr.12040

Weeratunga, P., Jayasinghe, S., Perera, Y., Jayasena, G., & Jayasinghe, S. (2014). Per capita sugar consumption and prevalence of diabetes mellitus — global and regional associations. *BMC Public Health, 14*, 186. doi:10.1186/1471-2458-14-186

SELECTED BIBLIOGRAPHY

American Diabetes Association. (2014). Diabetes care in the school and day care setting. *Diabetes Care, 37*(Suppl. 1), S91–S96. doi:10.2337/dc14-S091

American Diabetes Association. (2015). *Standards of medical care in diabetes—2015.* Retrieved from http://professional.diabetes.org/ResourcesForProfessionals.aspx?typ=17&cid=84160&pcid=84160

Anguita, M. (2013). Next generation of diabetes drugs arriving, but approach with caution. *Nurse Prescribing, 11,* 59. doi:10.12968/npre.2013.11.2.58

Bennett, W. L., Maruthur, N. M., Singh, S., Segal, J. B., Wilson, L. M., Chatterjee, R., . . . Bolen, S. (2011). Comparative effectiveness and safety of medications for type 2 diabetes: An update including new drugs and 2-drug combinations. *Annals of Internal Medicine, 154,* 602–613. doi:10.7326/0003 4819-154-9-201105030-00336

Gates, B. J., & Walker, K. M. (2014). Physiological changes in older adults and their effect on diabetes treatment. *Diabetes Spectrum, 27,* 20–29. doi:10.2337/diaspect.27.1.20

Inzucchi, S. E., Bergenstal, R. M., Buse, J. B., Diamant, M., Ferrannini, E., Nauck, M., . . . Matthews, D. R. (2015). Management of hyperglycemia in type 2 diabetes, 2015: A patient-centered approach: Update to a position statement of the American Diabetes Association and the European Association for the Study of Diabetes. *Diabetes Care, 38,* 140–149. doi:10.2337/dc14-2441

Nathan, D. M. (2014). The diabetes control and complications trial/epidemiology of diabetes interventions and complications study at 30 years: Overview. *Diabetes Care, 37,* 9–16. doi:10.2337/dc13-2112

National Institute of Diabetes and Digestive and Kidney Diseases. (n.d.). *Complementary and alternative medical therapies for diabetes.* Retrieved from http://diabetes.niddk.nih.gov/dm/pubs/alternativetherapies

Powers, A. C., & D'Alessio, D. (2011). Endocrine pancreas and pharmacotherapy of diabetes mellitus and hypoglycemia. In L. L. Brunton, B. A. Chabner, & B. C. Knollman (Eds.), *Gordon and Gilman's the pharmacological basis of therapeutics* (12th ed., pp. 1237–1274). New York, NY: McGraw-Hill.

Rotenstein, L. S., Shivers, J. P., Yarchoan, M., Close, J., & Close, K. L. (2012). The ideal diabetes therapy: What will it look like? How close are we? *Clinical Diabetes, 30,* 44–53. doi:10.2337/diaclin.30.2.44

Wang, S. S. (2014). *Metabolic syndrome.* Retrieved from http://emedicine.medscape.com/article/165124-overview

Chapter 46

Drugs for Disorders and Conditions of the Female Reproductive System

Drugs at a Glance

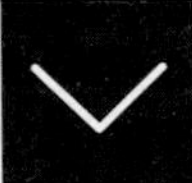

Learning Outcomes

After reading this chapter, the student should be able to:

1. Describe the roles of the hypothalamus, pituitary, and ovaries in maintaining female reproductive function.
2. Explain the mechanisms by which estrogens and progestins prevent conception.
3. Explain how drugs may be used to provide emergency contraception and to terminate early pregnancy.
4. Describe the role of drug therapy in the treatment of menopausal and postmenopausal symptoms.
5. Identify the role of the female sex hormones in the treatment of cancer.
6. Discuss the uses of progestins in the therapy of dysfunctional uterine bleeding.
7. Compare and contrast the use of uterine stimulants and relaxants in the treatment of antepartum and postpartum patients.
8. Explain how drug therapy may be used to treat female infertility.
9. Describe the nurse's role in the pharmacologic management of disorders and conditions of the female reproductive system.
10. For each of the classes shown in Drugs at a Glance, know representative drugs, and explain the mechanisms of drug action, primary actions, and important adverse effects.
11. Use the nursing process to care for patients who are receiving pharmacotherapy for disorders of the female reproductive system and for contraception.

indicates a prototype drug, each of which is featured in a Prototype Drug box.

Hormones from the pituitary gland and the ovaries provide for the growth and continued maintenance of the female reproductive organs. Although they are referred to as reproductive or sex hormones, these substances impact virtually every body system including effects on coagulation, blood vessels, bone, muscles, overall body metabolism, and behavior. Hormonal therapy of the female reproductive system is used to achieve a variety of therapeutic goals, ranging from increasing female fertility to prevention of pregnancy to promoting milk production. This chapter examines hormones and drugs used to treat conditions associated with the female reproductive system.

THE FEMALE REPRODUCTIVE SYSTEM

46.1 Hypothalamic and Pituitary Regulation of Female Reproductive Function

Regulation of the female reproductive system is achieved by hormones from the hypothalamus, pituitary gland, and ovary. The hypothalamus secretes **gonadotropin-releasing hormone (GnRH),** which travels a short distance to the pituitary to stimulate the secretion of **follicle-stimulating hormone (FSH)** and **luteinizing hormone (LH).** Both of these pituitary hormones act on the ovary and cause immature ovarian follicles to begin developing. The rising and falling levels of pituitary hormones create two interrelated cycles that occur on a periodic, monthly basis: the ovarian and uterine cycles. The hormonal changes that occur during the ovarian and uterine cycles are illustrated in Figure 46.1.

Under the influence of FSH and LH, several ovarian follicles begin the maturation process each month during a woman's reproductive years. On approximately day 14 of the ovarian cycle, a surge of LH secretion causes one follicle to expel its oocyte, a process called **ovulation.** The ruptured follicle, minus its oocyte, remains in the ovary and is transformed into the hormone-secreting **corpus luteum.** The oocyte, on the other hand, begins its journey through the uterine tube and eventually reaches the uterus. If conception does not occur, the outer lining of the uterus degenerates and is shed to the outside during menstruation.

PharmFacts

FEMALE REPRODUCTION

- There is a wide range of ages at which women reach menopause: 8 of 100 women will stop menstruating before age 40, and 5 of 100 women will continue to age 60 and beyond.
- About 90% of dysfunctional uterine bleeding occurs due to lack of ovulation.
- About 82% of women in the United States who have had sexual intercourse have used oral contraceptives at some time during their life.
- Over 10% of sexually experienced women aged 15 to 44 have used emergency contraception (Plan B). The percentage increases to about 25% for women age 20–24.
- Oral contraceptives confer benefits besides contraception, including the following:
  - Reduced symptoms of premenstrual syndrome (PMS).
  - Reduced risk for colorectal, ovarian, and endometrial cancer.
  - Decreased risk for benign breast disease, ovarian cysts, and endometriosis.
  - Improvement in acne and bone mineral density.

46.2 Ovarian Control of Female Reproductive Function

As ovarian follicles mature, they secrete the female sex hormones **estrogen** and **progesterone.** Estrogen is actually a general term for three different hormones: estradiol, estrone, and estriol. Estrogen is responsible for the maturation of the female reproductive organs and for the appearance of secondary sex characteristics. In addition, estrogen has numerous metabolic effects on nonreproductive tissues, including the brain, kidneys, blood vessels, and skin. For example, estrogen decreases the levels of low-density lipoprotein (LDL) and increases the amount of high-density lipoprotein (HDL) in the blood. These effects are cardioprotective and help lower the risk of myocardial infarction (MI) in premenopausal women. By blocking resorption of the bony matrix, estrogen causes bones to grow longer and stronger in younger women. When women enter menopause at about age 50 to 55, the ovaries stop secreting estrogen.

In the last half of the ovarian cycle, the corpus luteum secretes a class of hormones called progestins, the most abundant of which is progesterone. In combination with estrogen, progesterone promotes breast development and regulates the monthly changes of the uterine cycle. Under the influence of estrogen and progesterone, the uterine endometrium becomes vascular and thickens in preparation for receiving a fertilized egg. High progesterone and estrogen levels in the final third of the uterine cycle provide negative feedback to shut off GnRH, FSH, and LH secretion. This negative feedback loop is illustrated in Figure 46.2. Without stimulation from FSH and LH, estrogen and progesterone levels fall sharply, the endometrium is shed, and menstrual bleeding begins.

Estrogen and progesterone are used as drugs to achieve several therapeutic goals. The most widespread pharmacologic use of the female sex hormones is to prevent pregnancy. They are also prescribed to treat dysfunctional

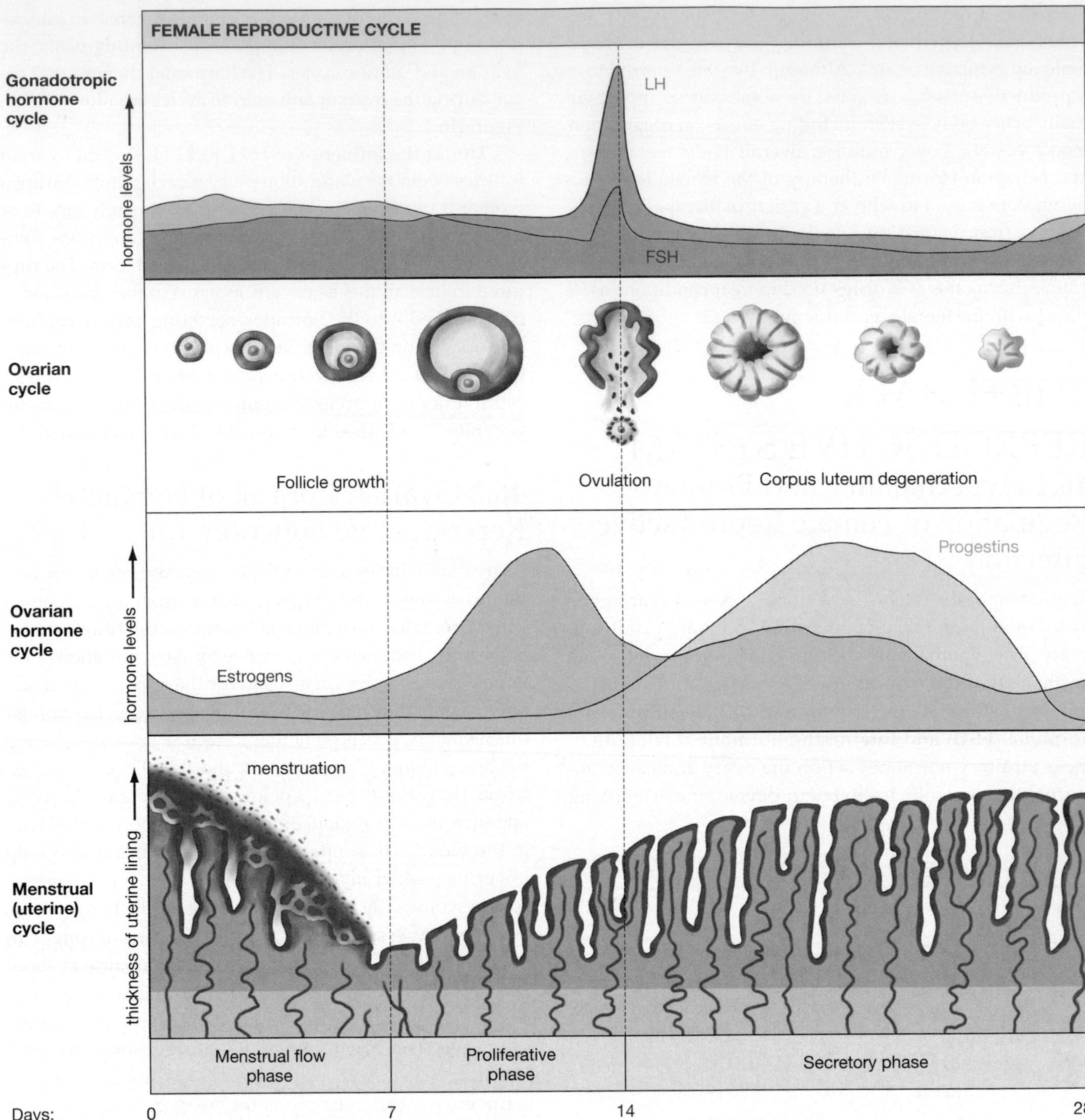

FIGURE 46.1 Hormonal changes during the ovarian and uterine cycles

uterine bleeding, severe symptoms of menopause, and certain neoplasms.

HORMONAL CONTRACEPTIVES

Hormonal contraceptives (HCs) are drugs used in low doses to prevent pregnancy. The oral formulations are commonly referred to as "the pill" or oral contraceptives. The HCs prevent fertilization by inhibiting ovulation. Selected HCs are listed in Table 46.1.

46.3 Estrogens and Progestins as Oral Contraceptives

Most HCs contain a combination of estrogen and progestin; a few preparations contain only progestin. The most common estrogen used for contraception is ethinyl estradiol, and the most common progestin is norethindrone. When used appropriately, hormonal contraception is nearly 100% effective.

A large number of HC drugs are available, differing in dose and by type of estrogen and progestin. Selection of a specific formulation is individualized to each patient and

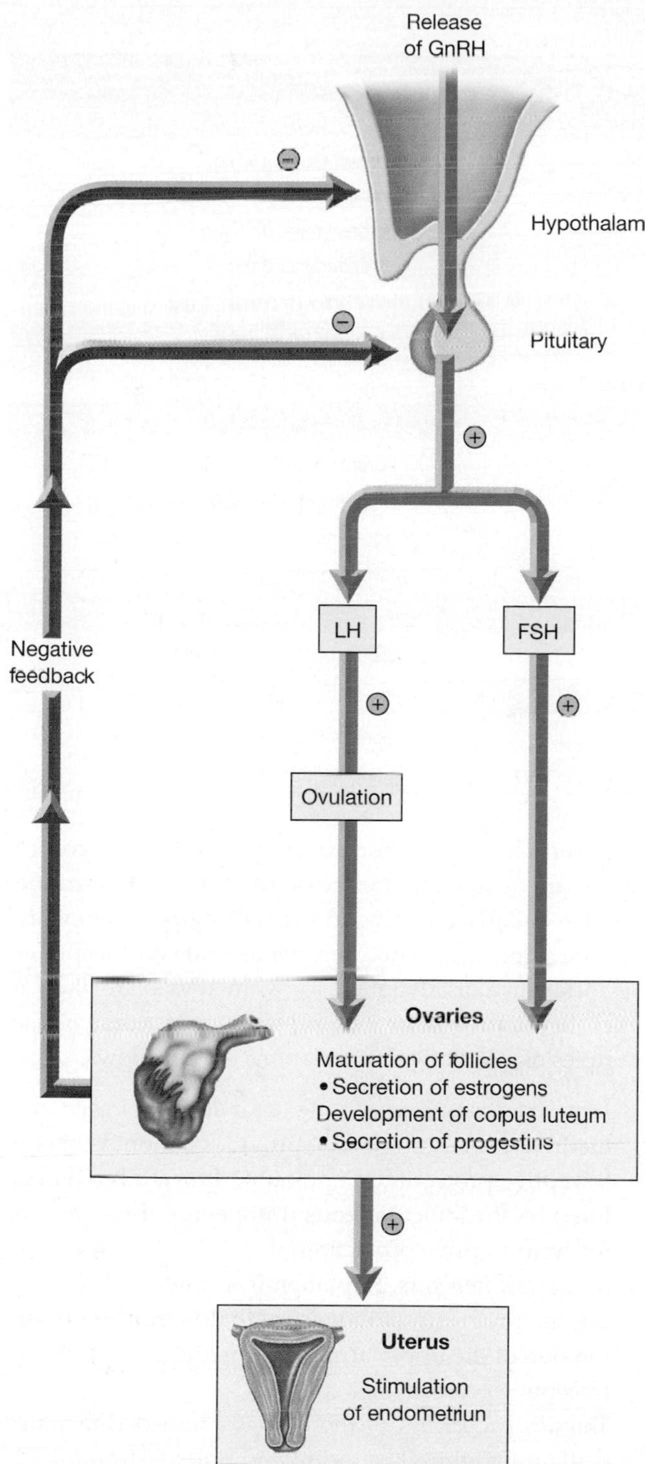

FIGURE 46.2 Negative feedback control of the female reproductive hormones

determined by which drug gives the best contraceptive protection with the fewest side effects. Daily doses of estrogen contained in oral contraceptives have declined from 150 mcg, 40 years ago, to 20–35 mcg in modern formulations. This reduction has resulted in a significant decrease in estrogen-related adverse effects.

Typically, administration of an oral contraceptive begins on day 5 of the menstrual cycle and continues for 21 days. During the final 7 days of the month, the woman

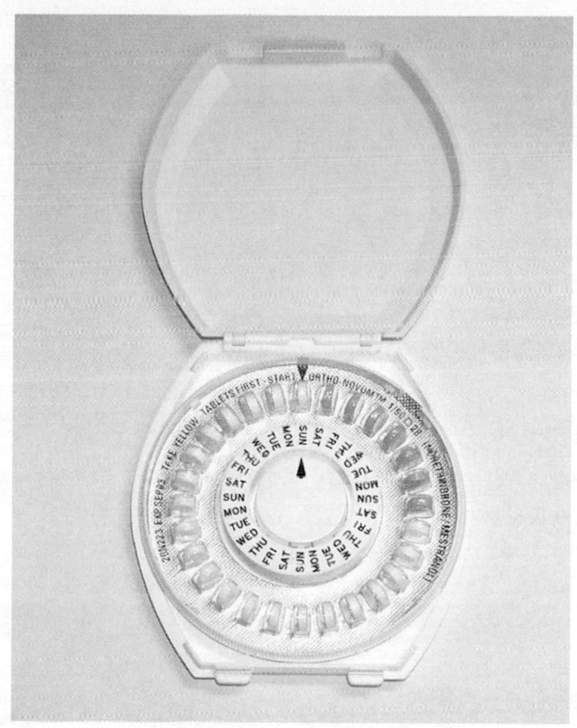

FIGURE 46.3 An oral contraceptive showing the daily doses and the different formulation taken in the last 7 days of the 28-day cycle

takes an inert tablet, which contains no hormone. Although the inert tablet serves no pharmacologic purpose, it does encourage the patient to take the pills on a daily basis. Some of these inert tablets contain iron, which replaces iron lost due to menstrual bleeding.

A common problem with oral contraceptives (OCs), and likely the most frequent reason for treatment failure (pregnancy), is forgetting to take the medication daily. If one dose is missed, two pills taken the following day around the usual time may provide adequate contraception. If two consecutive doses are missed, two tablets should be taken on the day the missed doses are remembered and again the following day. The regular schedule should then be continued, but a second method of contraception should be used for at least 7 days after restarting the pills. If 3 or more consecutive days are missed, the patient should implement other contraceptive precautions until the regimen can be restarted in the next monthly cycle. Figure 46.3 shows a typical monthly oral contraceptive packet with the 28 pills.

The estrogen–progestin combination contraceptives act by *preventing ovulation*. They accomplish this by providing negative feedback to the pituitary, which suppresses the secretion of LH and FSH. Without the influence of these pituitary hormones, the ovarian follicle cannot mature, and ovulation is prevented. The estrogen–progestin drugs also make the uterine endometrium less favorable to receive an embryo, thus reducing the likelihood of implantation. In addition to their contraceptive function, these drugs are sometimes prescribed to

Table 46.1 Selected Oral Contraceptives

Trade Name	Estrogen	Progestin
MONOPHASIC		
Desogen	ethinyl estradiol: 30 mcg	desogestrel: 0.15 mg
Loestrin 1.5/30 Fe	ethinyl estradiol: 30 mcg	norethindrone: 1.5 mg
Ortho-Cyclen-28	ethinyl estradiol: 35 mcg	norgestimate: 0.25 mg
Yasmin	ethinyl estradiol: 30 mcg	drospirenone: 3 mg
Zovia 1/50E-21 and 28	ethinyl estradiol: 50 mcg	ethynodiol diacetate: 1 mg
BIPHASIC		
Mircette	ethinyl estradiol: 20 mcg for 21 days; 10 mcg for 5 days	desogestrel: 0.15 mg for 21 days
TRIPHASIC		
Ortho-Novum 7/7/7-28	ethinyl estradiol: 35 mcg	norethindrone: 0.50, 0.75, 0.1 mg
Ortho Tri-Cyclen-28	ethinyl estradiol: 35 mcg	norgestimate: 0.18, 0.215, 0.25 mg
Tri-norinyl-28	ethinyl estradiol: 35 mcg	norethindrone: 0.50, 1, 0.5 mg
Trivora-28	ethinyl estradiol: 30, 40, 30 mcg	levonorgestrel: 0.05, 0.075, 0.125 mg
FOUR-PHASIC		
Natazia	ethinyl valerate: 3, 2, 2, 1 mg	dienogest: 0, 2, 2, 0 mg
PROGESTIN ONLY		
Micronor	None	norethindrone: 0.35 mg
Nor-Q.D.	None	norethindrone: 0.35 mg

promote timely and regular monthly cycles and to reduce the incidence of dysmenorrhea.

The four types of estrogen–progestin oral contraceptives are monophasic, biphasic, triphasic, and a quadriphasic (four-phase). The monophasic delivers a constant dose of estrogen and progestin throughout the 21-day treatment cycle. In biphasic agents, the amount of estrogen in each pill remains constant, but the amount of progestin is increased toward the end of the treatment cycle to better nourish the uterine lining. In triphasic formulations, the amounts of both estrogen and progestin vary in three distinct phases during the treatment cycle. The quadriphasic oral contraceptive (Natazia) contains estradiol valerate, a synthetic estrogen, and dienogest, a progestin. It is the first HC containing this specific combination. In 2012, Natazia became the first HC to be approved to treat heavy menstrual bleeding. All four types of OC formulations are equally effective.

The progestin-only oral contraceptives, sometimes called *minipills,* prevent pregnancy primarily by producing thick, viscous mucus at the entrance to the uterus that discourages penetration by sperm. They also tend to inhibit implantation of a fertilized egg. Minipills are less effective than estrogen–progestin combinations, having a failure rate of 1% to 4%. Their use also results in a higher incidence of menstrual irregularities such as amenorrhea, prolonged menstrual bleeding, or breakthrough spotting. They are generally reserved for patients who are at high risk for estrogen-related side effects. Unlike estrogens, progestins are not associated with a higher risk of thromboembolic events, and they have no effect on breast cancer. The progestin-only products are pregnancy category X.

Several long-term hormonal formulations of contraception are available. These extended-duration formulations are equally effective in preventing pregnancy and have the same basic safety profile as oral contraceptives. They offer a major advantage for women who are likely to forget their daily pill or who prefer a greater ease of use. Examples of alternative formulations are as follows:

- *Depot injections*. Depo-Provera is a deep IM injection of medroxyprogesterone that provides 3 months of contraceptive protection. Depo-SubQ-Provera is administered by the subcutaneous route every three months for contraceptive protection.
- *Subdermal implants*. Implanon is a single rod containing the progestin etonogestrel that is inserted under the skin of the upper arm that provides 3 years of contraceptive protection.
- *Transdermal patches*. Ortho-Evra is a transdermal patch containing ethinyl estradiol and norelgestromin. The patch is changed every 7 days for the first 3 weeks, followed by a patch-free week 4.
- *Vaginal route*. NuvaRing is a 2-inch-diameter ring containing estrogen and progestin that is inserted into the vagina to provide 3 weeks of contraceptive protection. The ring is removed during week 4, and a new ring is inserted during the first week of the next menstrual cycle.
- *Intrauterine route*. Mirena is a polyethylene cylinder that is placed in the uterus and releases levonorgestrel. About the size of a quarter and shaped like the letter *T*, Mirena acts locally to prevent conception for 5 years. Skyla is a newer intrauterine device, approved in

Table 46.2 Adverse Effects of Hormonal Contraceptives

Adverse Effect	Prevention
Breast milk reduction	Some studies suggest that HCs may reduce the quantity of breast milk. They should not be taken until 6 weeks postpartum.
Cancer	Women who test positive for the human papilloma virus have an increased risk of cervical cancer. These patients should have regular check-ups. Because estrogens promote the growth of certain types of breast cancer, patients with a history of this cancer should not take HCs.
Glucose elevation	HCs may cause slight increases in blood glucose. Patients with diabetes should monitor their serum glucose carefully during HC therapy.
Hypertension	Risk is increased with age, dose, and length of therapy. Blood pressure should be monitored periodically and antihypertensives prescribed as needed, or contraceptives re-evaluated.
Increased appetite, weight gain, fatigue, depression, acne, hirsutism	These are common effects often caused by high amounts of progestin. The dose of progestin may need to be lowered.
Lupus exacerbation	Lupus symptoms may become worse in some patients. A progestin-only HC may be an option for these patients.
Menstrual irregularities	Amenorrhea or hypermenorrhea are often caused by low amounts of progestin. The dose of progestin may need to be increased. Breakthrough bleeding and spotting are common with the low dose oral contraceptives. The patient may need a higher dose product.
Migraines	Estrogen may decrease or increase the incidence of migraines. Because migraines are a risk factor for stroke, patients with migraines should seek advice from their health care practitioner.
Nausea, edema, breast tenderness	These are common effects often caused by high amounts of estrogen. The dose of estrogen may need to be lowered.
Teratogenicity	Estrogens are pregnancy category X. Patients should be advised to discontinue HCs if pregnancy is confirmed.
Thromboembolic disorders	Estrogens promote blood clotting. HCs should not be prescribed for patients with a history of thromboembolic disorders, strokes, or coronary artery disease or who are heavy smokers.

2013. It contains the same progestin as Mirena, but it is smaller and can provide up to 3 years of contraception. While Mirena is recommended for women who have had at least one child, Skyla may be used for women who have not had children.

- *Extended-regimen OCs*. Seasonale consists of tablets containing levonorgestrel and ethinyl estradiol that are taken for 84 consecutive days, followed by 7 inert tablets. This allows for continuous contraceptive protection while extending the time between menses; only four menstrual periods are experienced per year. Seasonique is similar, but instead of inert tablets for 7 days, the patient takes low-dose estrogen tablets. The manufacturer claims that Seasonique has a lower incidence of bloating and breakthrough bleeding.

When discontinuing HCs it may take several months for ovulation to return to normal and for monthly menstrual periods to become regular. Some women can conceive in the first month, whereas others experience a delay for up to a year before fertility is restored. The length of HC use does not appear to affect fertility. The incidence of miscarriage is not increased in women who conceive after having taken HCs. Women taking extended-release forms of contraception, such as subdermal implants or depot injections should expect longer delays before fertility is restored.

Although hormonal contraceptives are safe for the large majority of women, they have some potentially serious adverse effects. As with other medications, the higher the dose of estrogen or progesterone, the greater will be the risk for adverse effects. With HCs, however, some effects are more prominent at lower doses. Thus, health care providers try to prescribe the combination with the lowest dose of hormones that will achieve the therapeutic goal of pregnancy prevention with minimal adverse effects. Table 46.2 summarizes the adverse effects of the OCs.

Numerous drug–drug interactions are possible with HCs. Certain anticonvulsants and antibiotics can reduce the effectiveness of the contraceptives, thus increasing a woman's risk of pregnancy. Because HCs can reduce the effectiveness of warfarin (Coumadin), insulin, and certain oral antidiabetic drugs, dosage adjustments may be necessary.

The incidence of cancer in women taking HCs has been studied for several decades in large numbers of women. Some studies have demonstrated that long term use may pose a slightly higher risk of breast cancer, whereas others have shown no relationship. The incidence of cervical cancer has also slightly increased, and this has been closely associated with human papilloma virus (HPV) infections. However, HCs appear to have a *protective* effect for ovarian and endometrial cancer that continues for many years after the drugs are discontinued. A protective effect has also been observed for colorectal cancer. Conclusions of these studies are that women who have a personal or close family history of breast cancer should explore nonhormonal means of contraception. All women taking these drugs should be instructed to perform breast self-exams and be

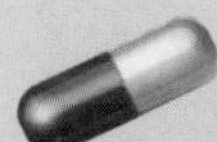

Prototype Drug | Estradiol and Norethindrone *(Ortho-Novum, others)*

Therapeutic Class: Combination oral contraceptive **Pharmacologic Class:** Estrogen/progestin

Actions and Uses

The primary use of Ortho-Novum is to prevent pregnancy, an indication for which it is nearly 100% effective. Ortho-Novum is available in monophasic, biphasic, and triphasic preparations. When an appropriate combination of estrogen and progestin is present in the bloodstream, the release of FSH and LH is inhibited, thus preventing ovulation. Off-label indications for the drug include acne vulgaris (in females who have achieved menarche), endometriosis, hypermenorrhea, and dysfunctional uterine bleeding. Noncontraceptive benefits of Ortho-Novum include improvement in menstrual cycle regularity and decreased incidence of dysmenorrhea.

Administration Alerts

- Tablets must be taken exactly as directed.
- If a dose is missed, take as soon as remembered, or take two tablets the next day.
- Pregnancy category X.

PHARMACOKINETICS

Onset	Peak	Duration
30–60 min (1 month for contraception)	1 month	Up to 27 h

Adverse Effects

The most frequent adverse effects of Ortho-Novum are nausea, breast tenderness, weight gain, and breakthrough bleeding. Less common effects include edema, changes in vision, gallbladder disease, nausea, abdominal cramps, changes in urinary function, dysmenorrhea, breast fullness, fatigue, skin rash, acne, headache, vaginal candidiasis, photosensitivity, and changes in urinary patterns. Cardiovascular adverse effects, the most serious of all, include HTN and thromboembolic disorders.

Black Box Warning: Cigarette smoking increases the risk of serious cardiovascular adverse effects in women who are taking hormonal contraceptives containing estrogen. This risk increases markedly with age (over age 35) and with heavy smoking (more than 15 cigarettes per day).

Contraindications: Hormonal contraceptives are contraindicated in women with the following conditions: current or past history of thromboembolic disorders, stroke, or coronary artery disease; hepatic tumors; known or suspected carcinoma of the breast, endometrium, or other estrogen-dependent tumor; abnormal uterine bleeding; cholestatic jaundice of pregnancy or jaundice with prior oral contraceptive use; known or suspected pregnancy.

Interactions

Drug–Drug: Estrogen-containing contraceptives should not be used concurrently with tranexamic acid due to an increased risk for thromboembolic events. Rifampin, some antibiotics, barbiturates, anticonvulsants, protease inhibitors, and antifungals decrease the efficacy of HCs, increasing the risk of breakthrough bleeding and the possibility of pregnancy. Ortho-Novum may decrease the effects of warfarin, heparin, and certain other anticoagulants leading to possible thromboembolic events.

Lab Tests: Values of the following may be increased: prothrombin time, certain coagulation factors, thyroid-binding globulin, protein bound iodine (PBI), T_4, platelet aggregation, and triglycerides. Values of the following may be decreased: antithrombin III, T_3, folate, and vitamin B_{12}.

Herbal/Food: Breakthrough bleeding has been reported with concurrent use of St. John's wort.

Treatment of Overdose: There is no specific treatment for overdose.

aware of the importance of routine scheduling of mammograms appropriate for their age range.

Hormonal contraceptives are associated with an increased risk of cardiovascular adverse effects such as hypertension (HTN) and thromboembolic disorders. The estrogen component of the pill can lead to venous and arterial thrombosis with resultant pulmonary embolism, MI, or thrombotic stroke. Other conditions associated with HCs are abnormal uterine bleeding, benign hepatic adenoma, multiple births, elevated plasma glucose, retinal disorders, and melanoderma, a patchy or generalized skin discoloration caused by increased production of melanin.

Certain pre-existing medical conditions are absolute contraindications for using HCs. These include current breast cancer, severe hepatic cirrhosis, major surgery with prolonged immobilization, migraines (with aura), impaired cardiac function, complicated valvular heart disease, HTN, smoking (over age 35 and 15 or more cigarettes/day), history of stroke, systemic lupus erythematosus, and high risk for thromboembolic disorders. These medications should be used with caution when there are pre-existing disorders such as depression, migraines (without aura), epilepsy, epilepsy therapy (with certain anticonvulsants), and diabetes.

☑ Check Your Understanding 46.1

What instruction should be given to a woman who has missed a dose of her oral contraceptive? *Visit www.pearsonhighered.com/nursingresources for the answer.*

Nursing Practice Application

Pharmacotherapy With Hormonal Contraceptives

ASSESSMENT	POTENTIAL NURSING DIAGNOSES*
Baseline assessment prior to administration: • Obtain a complete health history including cardiovascular, peripheral vascular, thyroid, hepatic, or renal disease; migraines; diabetes; pregnancy; or breast-feeding. Note personal or family history of thromboembolic disorders (e.g., MI, stroke, peripheral vascular disease) and of reproductive cancers (e.g., breast, uterine, or ovarian cancer). • Obtain a drug history including allergies, current prescription and over-the-counter (OTC) drugs, herbal preparations, alcohol use, and smoking. Be alert to possible drug interactions. • Evaluate appropriate laboratory findings (e.g., complete blood count [CBC], platelets, electrolytes, glucose, lipid, and thyroid function levels, Pap test). • Obtain baseline height, weight, and vital signs.	• *Decisional Conflict* • *Disturbed Body Image* • *Deficient Knowledge* (drug therapy) • *Risk for Excess Fluid Volume,* related to adverse drug effects • *Risk for Ineffective Peripheral Tissue Perfusion,* related to adverse drug effects • *Risk for Ineffective Cerebral Tissue Perfusion,* related to adverse drug effects • *Risk for Ineffective Cardiac Tissue Perfusion,* related to adverse drug effects *NANDA I © 2014
Assessment throughout administration: • Assess for desired therapeutic effects depending on the reason the drug is given (e.g., pregnancy prevention or hormone replacement). • Continue periodic monitoring of CBC, platelets, and glucose. • Monitor vital signs and weight at each health care visit. • Assess for adverse effects: nausea, vomiting, headache, weight gain, breast tenderness, skin rash, acne, fluid retention, changes in mood, and breakthrough bleeding. Immediately report tachycardia, palpitations, and HTN, especially associated with angina; severe headache; cramping in calves; chest pain; or dyspnea.	

IMPLEMENTATION

Interventions and (Rationales)	Patient-Centered Care
Ensuring therapeutic effects: • Monitor appropriate medication administration for optimal results. (Oral contraceptives are nearly 100% effective when taken as required. Skipping doses increases the risk of pregnancy. Other types of hormonal contraception such as transdermal patches or depot injections may be desirable for women who experience difficulty in adhering to oral contraceptives or for those who choose not to take daily medication.)	• Instruct the patient to take the drug at the same time daily to help remember to take the pill. Instruct the patient to not omit doses or increase or decrease the dose without consulting the health care provider. • Encourage women to discuss other available options (e.g., transdermal patches, depot injections, subdermal implants) with the health care provider as appropriate.

Minimizing adverse effects:
• Monitor for symptoms of thromboembolism. Monitor blood pressure at each clinical visit. (Thromboembolic events are an adverse effect of estrogen/progestin drugs. The risk increases with age over 35, in women with a previous history of cardiovascular disease, and in women who smoke.)
	• Instruct the patient to immediately report:
	  • Dyspnea, chest pain, or blood in sputum (possible pulmonary embolism)
	  • Heaviness, chest pain, or overwhelming feeling of fatigue and weakness accompanied by nausea and diaphoresis (possible MI)
	  • Sudden, severe headache, especially if associated with dizziness; difficulty with speech; numbness in the arm or leg; difficulty with vision (possible stroke)
	  • Warmth, redness, swelling, or tenderness in the calf or pain on walking (possible thrombophlebitis)
	• Teach the patient to monitor blood pressure periodically and report any reading above 140/90 mmHg or per parameters set by the health care provider.

• Encourage smoking cessation and provide information about smoking cessation programs. (Smoking greatly increases the risk of adverse effects of hormone therapy.)	• Advise the patient of the risk of smoking while using estrogens or progestins. Provide referral to appropriate support groups and literature on smoking cessation programs.

continued

Nursing Practice Application *continued*

IMPLEMENTATION	
Interventions and (Rationales)	**Patient-Centered Care**
• Monitor blood glucose levels in patients with diabetes more frequently. (Estrogens may affect carbohydrate metabolism, leading to increased glucose levels. Progestins may affect endogenous insulin levels.)	• Teach the woman with diabetes to monitor capillary blood glucose frequently while on drugs containing estrogen or progestin and to report consistent elevations to the health care provider.
• Monitor hepatic function tests and symptoms of liver dysfunction, lipid profile studies, and thyroid levels periodically. (Estrogens are associated with a rare risk of benign liver tumors and may adversely affect cholesterol synthesis, lipid levels, and thyroid function in sensitive patients.)	• Instruct the patient to return periodically for laboratory tests. • Teach the patient to immediately report any symptoms of abdominal or right upper quadrant discomfort or pain, yellowing of the skin or sclera, fatigue, anorexia, darkened urine, or clay-colored stools.
• Monitor concurrent drug therapy. (Many drugs decrease or alter the effectiveness of estrogens and progestins including drugs in the penicillin, barbiturate, antiseizure, antidepressant, and benzodiazepine classes. Check for drug interactions that may affect hormone effectiveness before any new prescription is started.)	• Teach the patient to advise all health care providers of the use of estrogens or progestins for contraception or for hormone replacement therapy before beginning any new prescription. If a prescription is required, discuss the need for alternative treatment or birth control measures as appropriate.
• Monitor routine Pap tests, HPV screening, and breast exams as ordered. (Routine screenings, including mammography as appropriate, will monitor for the development of breast tumors, cervical cancer, or HPV infection.)	• Teach the patient how to perform breast self-exams and encourage monthly exams. For women over 40, advise the patient on the need for follow-up mammography as per the health care provider. • Advise the patient on the need for regularly scheduled gynecologic exams to ensure continued health.
• Monitor the occurrence of any breakthrough bleeding. Report any continuous, unusual, or heavy bleeding. (Small amounts of "spotting" may occur at midcycle, especially with low-dose hormone therapy. Any continuous, unusual, or heavy bleeding may indicate adverse effects or disease and should be reported.)	• Teach the patient that slight spotting may occur midcycle while on hormone drugs but to report any unusual changes in the amount or if bleeding continues.
Patient understanding of drug therapy: • Use opportunities during administration of medications and during assessments to provide patient education. (Using time during nursing care helps to optimize and reinforce key teaching areas.)	• The patient should be able to state the reason for the drug, appropriate dose and scheduling, and what adverse effects to observe for and when to report them.

Patient self-administration of drug therapy:
• When administering the medication, instruct the patient, family, or caregiver in the proper self-administration of the drug (e.g., consistently at the same time each day to help remember the dose). (Proper administration increases the effectiveness of the drugs and helps to reinforce teaching.)
	• Teach the patient to take the drug following appropriate guidelines:
	  • Oral drugs should be taken at the same time each day to help remember the dose. If a dose is missed, follow the directions on the package insert specific to the type of OC taken.
	  • Intravaginal rings are placed in the vagina and removed after 3 weeks for 1 week before a new ring is inserted.
	  • Extended formulations (e.g., Seasonique or Seasonale) are taken for approximately 3 months (84 days) and then followed by 7 days of either inert pills or low-dose hormone pills.
	  • Transdermal patches (e.g., Ortho-Evra) are changed weekly for 3 weeks followed by no patch for 1 week.

See Table 46.1 for a list of drugs to which these nursing actions apply.

EMERGENCY CONTRACEPTION AND PHARMACOLOGIC ABORTION

Emergency contraception (EC) is the *prevention* of pregnancy following unprotected intercourse or contraceptive failure. Pharmacologic abortion is the *removal* of an embryo by the use of drugs after implantation has occurred. Drugs used for these purposes are listed in Table 46.3.

46.4 Drugs for Emergency Contraception and Termination of Early Pregnancy

Statistics suggest that more than half the pregnancies in the United States are unplanned. Some of these occur because of the inconsistent use or failure of contraceptive devices; even oral contraceptives have a failure rate of 0.3% to 1%. The treatment goal for EC is to provide effective and immediate contraception. Two different medications are approved for EC: Plan B and ulipristal (Ella). Table 46.3 lists drugs, routes, and dosages for EC. These drugs are not intended to replace regular methods of contraception.

Plan B is approved for purchase OTC. Dosing for Plan B involves taking 0.75 mg of levonorgestrel in two doses, 12 hours apart. Plan B One Step has largely replaced Plan B because it requires only a single 1.5-mg dose. The drug acts in a manner similar to HCs; it prevents ovulation and also alters the endometrium of the uterus so that implantation does not occur. If implantation has already occurred, Plan B will not terminate the pregnancy. It is important that the patient understand that Plan B will not induce an abortion.

Plan B must be administered as soon as possible after unprotected intercourse; if taken more than 120 hours later, it becomes less effective. By 7 days after intercourse, it is ineffective at preventing pregnancy. The normal rate of pregnancy from a single unprotected sex act is 8%; Plan B is estimated to lower this risk to 1% to 2%. Adverse effects are mild and may include nausea, vomiting, abdominal pain, fatigue, headache, heavy menstruation, diarrhea, and dizziness.

In 2010, ulipristal (Ella) was approved as a single-dose product for EC. This drug is a mixed progesterone agonist/antagonist that acts by preventing ovulation. Adverse effects are very similar to those of Plan B. Unlike Plan B, which is available OTC, ulipristal requires a prescription. Ulipristal retains its effectiveness for 5 days following unprotected sex, but it is most effective if taken within 24–72 hours.

Table 46.3 Drugs for Emergency Contraception and Pharmacologic Abortion

Drug	Route and Adult Dose (max dose where indicated)	Adverse Effects
EMERGENCY CONTRACEPTION		
levonorgestrel (Plan B, Plan B One Step)	PO: 1 tablet within 72 h of unprotected intercourse, followed by 1 tablet 12 h later (0.75 mg in each pill) Plan B One Step: 1.5 mg within 72 h of unprotected intercourse	*Nausea, vomiting, fatigue, headache, heavy menstrual bleeding, lower abdominal pain* Serious adverse effects are rare when only two doses are administered
ulipristal (Ella)	PO: 1 tablet (30 mg) within 5 days of unprotected intercourse or contraceptive failure	*Headache, abdominal pain, nausea, dysmenorrhea, fatigue, dizziness* Serious adverse effects are rare when only one dose is administered
PHARMACOLOGIC ABORTION		
carboprost (Hemabate)	IM: initial: 250 mcg (1 mL) repeated at 1 1/2–3 1/2-h intervals if indicated by uterine response Dosage may be increased to 500 mcg (2 mL) if uterine contractility is inadequate after several doses of 250 mcg (1 mL), not to exceed total dose of 12 mg or continuous administration for 1 month	*Nausea, vomiting, diarrhea, fever* Uterine laceration, rupture or hemorrhage
dinoprostone (Prostin E_2)	Intravaginal: insert suppository high in the vagina, repeat every 3–5 h until abortion occurs or membranes rupture (max: total dose 240 mg)	*Nausea, vomiting, diarrhea, fever* Uterine laceration, rupture, or hemorrhage
methotrexate with misoprostol	IM: methotrexate (50 mg/m^2) followed 5 days later by intravaginal 800 mcg of misoprostol	*Nausea, vomiting, diarrhea* Abdominal pain, uterine hemorrhage, respiratory arrest
mifepristone (Mifeprex) with misoprostol	PO: day 1: 600 mg of mifepristone; Day 3 (if abortion has not occurred): 400 mcg of misoprostol	*Nausea, vomiting, diarrhea* Abdominal pain, uterine hemorrhage

Note: *Italics* indicate common adverse effects; underlining indicates serious adverse effects.

Pharmacologic (medical) abortion is the removal of an embryo by the use of drugs *after* implantation has occurred. Drugs used to induce abortion are called abortifacients. A single dose of mifepristone (Mifeprex) followed 36 to 48 hours later by a single dose of misoprostol (Cytotec) is a frequently used regimen. Mifepristone is a synthetic steroid that blocks progesterone receptors in the uterus. If given within 3 days of intercourse, mifepristone alone is almost 100% effective at *preventing* pregnancy. Given up to 9 weeks after conception, mifepristone aborts the implanted embryo. Misoprostol is a prostaglandin that causes uterine contractions, thus increasing the effectiveness of the pharmacologic abortion. A **prostaglandin** is a hormone that acts directly at the site where it is secreted.

Although mifepristone–misoprostol should never be substituted for effective means of contraception such as abstinence or HCs, these medications do offer women a safer alternative to surgical abortion. The primary adverse effect is cramping that occurs soon after taking misoprostol. The most serious adverse effect is uterine bleeding, which may continue for 1 to 2 weeks after dosing. Pharmacologic abortion must always be conducted under the close supervision of a health care provider.

A few other drugs may be used to induce pharmacologic abortion. Methotrexate, an antineoplastic agent, combined with intravaginal misoprostol, usually induces abortion within 24 hours. Dinoprostone (Prostin E2) is a prostaglandin that, when given at high doses from week 12 through the second trimester, can induce strong uterine contractions resulting in a pharmacologic abortion. Also a prostaglandin, carboprost (Hemabate) is given by the intramuscular (IM) route to induce strong uterine contractions that can expel an implanted embryo between weeks 13 and 20 of pregnancy. Nausea, vomiting, fever, and diarrhea are common adverse effects of prostaglandins. Other uses of prostaglandins are discussed in Section 46.7.

Community-Oriented Practice

CHOICES FOR EMERGENCY CONTRACEPTION

Emergency contraception with levonorgestrel or "Plan B" and ulipristal (Ella) are highly effective when taken within 72 hours of unprotected intercourse. Estimates of pregnancy range from 0.9% to 3.1%, with greater effectiveness noted if the drug is taken within 24 hours of unprotected intercourse (Cleland, Raymond, Westley, & Trussel, 2014). Plan B's advantage is that it is available to women over the age of 17 without a prescription, whereas ulipristal requires a prescription. A nonpharmacologic option for EC, as well as long-term protection from pregnancy, is the copper IUD. It has been found to be almost twice as effective as oral EC and can be left in place for multiple years to prevent pregnancy (Turok et al., 2014). Disadvantages of the copper IUD include the need for insertion by the health care provider, as well as the cost of the office visit and the device.

MENOPAUSE

Menopause is characterized by a progressive decrease in estrogen secretion by the ovaries, resulting in the permanent cessation of menses. Menopause is neither a disease nor a disorder, but a natural consequence of aging that is often accompanied by unpleasant symptoms that include hot flashes, night sweats, irregular menstrual cycles, vaginal dryness, and bone mass loss.

46.5 Hormone Replacement Therapy

Over the past 50 years, health care providers have commonly prescribed **hormone replacement therapy (HRT)** for menopause. HRT supplies physiological doses of estrogen, sometimes combined with a progestin, to treat unpleasant symptoms of menopause and to prevent the long-term consequences of estrogen loss, listed in Table 46.4.

Two large studies have challenged the safety of using HRT during menopause: the Women's Health Initiative (WHI) and the Heart and Estrogen/Progestin Replacement Study (HERS). More than 26,000 women were enrolled in these studies, which were discontinued early when it became clear that the potential benefits of long-term HRT were not being realized. The results of the study depended on whether the HRT consisted of estrogen alone or an estrogen–progestin combination. Researchers reached the following conclusions:

- Women who are taking estrogen–progestin combination HRT experienced a statistically significant increased risk of MI, stroke, breast cancer, dementia, and venous thromboembolism. The risks were higher in women older than age 60; women aged 50 to 59 actually experienced a slight *decrease* in adverse cardiovascular events.

Table 46.4 Potential Consequences of Estrogen Loss Related to Menopause

Stage	Symptoms/Conditions
Early Menopause	Mood disturbances, depression, irritability
	Insomnia
	Hot flashes
	Irregular menstrual cycles
	Headaches
Midmenopause	Vaginal atrophy, increased infections, painful intercourse
	Skin atrophy
	Stress urinary incontinence
	Sexual disinterest
Postmenopause	Cardiovascular disease
	Osteoporosis
	Alzheimer's-like dementia
	Colon cancer

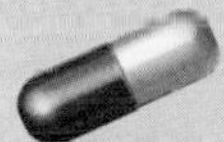

Prototype Drug | Conjugated Estrogens *(Cenestin, Enjuvia, Premarin)*

Therapeutic Class: Hormone **Pharmacologic Class:** Estrogen; hormone replacement therapy

Actions and Uses

Conjugated estrogens (Premarin) contain a mixture of different natural estrogens. Conjugated estrogen A (Cenestin) and conjugated estrogen B (Enjuvia) contain a mixture of 9–10 different synthetic plant estrogens. The primary indication for conjugated estrogens has been to treat moderate to severe symptoms of menopause caused by diminished estrogen secretion by the ovaries. Topical preparations may bring some benefit to menopausal women suffering from vulvar and vaginal atrophy. Other replacement therapies include treatment of female hypogonadism and use after oophorectomy. The drug is approved for the palliative treatment of prostate cancer and certain types of breast cancer.

Conjugated estrogens exert several positive metabolic effects, including an increase in bone density and a reduction in LDL cholesterol. It may also lower the risk of coronary artery disease and colon cancer in some patients. When used as postmenopausal replacement therapy, estrogen is typically combined with a progestin. Conjugated estrogens may be administered by the IM or intravenous (IV) route for dysfunctional uterine bleeding.

Administration Alerts

- Use a calibrated dosage applicator for administration of vaginal cream.
- For IM or IV administration of conjugated estrogens, reconstitute by first removing approximately 5 mL of air from the dry-powder vial, then slowly inject the diluent into the vial, aiming it at the side of the vial. Gently agitate to dissolve; do not shake.
- Administer IV push slowly, at a rate of 5 mg/min.
- Both are pregnancy category X.

PHARMACOKINETICS (PO)

Onset	Peak	Duration
Unknown	Unknown	Unknown

Adverse Effects

Adverse effects of conjugated estrogens include nausea, fluid retention, edema, breast tenderness, abdominal cramps and bloating, acute pancreatitis, appetite changes, acne, mental depression, decreased libido, headache, fatigue, nervousness, and weight gain. Adverse effects are dose dependent and increase in patients over age 35.

Black Box Warnings: Estrogens, when used alone, have been associated with a higher risk of endometrial cancer in postmenopausal women. Although adding a progestin may exert a protective effect by lowering the risk of uterine cancer, studies suggest that progestin may increase the risk of breast cancer following long-term use. When used alone, estrogens increase the risk of stroke, DVT, MI, and pulmonary emboli. Estrogens should not be used to prevent cardiovascular disease or to treat dementia.

Contraindications: Conjugated estrogens are contraindicated in pregnant patients and in women with known or suspected carcinoma of the breast or other estrogen-dependent tumor. Caution should be used when treating patients with a history of thromboembolic disease, hepatic impairment, or abnormal uterine bleeding.

Interactions

Drug–Drug: Drug interactions include a decreased effect of tamoxifen, enhanced corticosteroid effects, and decreased effects of anticoagulants, especially warfarin. The effects of estrogen may be decreased if taken with barbiturates or rifampin, and there is a possible increased effect of tricyclic antidepressants if taken with estrogens.

Lab Tests: Values of the following may be increased: prothrombin time, certain coagulation factors, thyroid-binding globulin, PBI, T_4, platelet aggregation, and triglycerides. Values of the following may be decreased: antithrombin III, T_3, folate, and vitamin B_{12}.

Herbal/Food: Red clover and black cohosh may interfere with estrogen therapy. Effects of estrogen may be enhanced if combined with ginseng.

Treatment of Overdose: There is no specific treatment for overdose.

- Women who are taking estrogen–progestin combination HRT experienced a decreased risk of hip fractures and colorectal cancer.
- Women who are taking *estrogen alone* experienced an increased risk of stroke and thromboembolic disorders.
- Women who are taking estrogen alone did not experience an increased risk for breast cancer or MI.

The potential adverse effects documented in the WHI and more recent studies suggest that the potential benefits of long-term HRT may not outweigh the risks for many women. However, the results of this study remain controversial. HRT does offer relief from the immediate, distressing menopausal symptoms, prevents osteoporosis-related fractures, and may offer some degree of protection from colorectal cancer. These are certainly significant and important benefits from HRT. The data from the WHI study and HERS are still being analyzed and follow-up studies are being conducted to determine which women benefit the most from HRT and which are at greatest risk. Until research provides more definitive answers, the choice of HRT to treat menopausal symptoms remains a highly individualized one, between the patient and her health care provider.

Several newer drugs have been marketed to treat symptoms of menopause while lowering the potential adverse effects of estrogen–progestin combinations. Duavee is a combination drug that contains conjugated estrogens with bazedoxifene, which belongs to a class of drugs called selective estrogen receptor modifiers (SERMs). Duavee offers the advantages of preventing intense hot flashes (the estrogen component) while reducing the risk of osteoporosis-related fractures that are common in postmenopausal women (the SERM component). Approved in 2013, Duavee is the first HRT that includes a SERM instead of a progestin. This drug carries the same black box warning as that for conjugated estrogens regarding an increased risk of endometrial cancer and deep vein thrombosis (DVT). Duavee is given by the oral (PO) route and is pregnancy category X.

Another SERM, ospemiphene (Osphema), was approved in 2013 to treat dyspareunia, a type of acute pain in postmenopausal women that may occur during intercourse. Ospemiphene acts by increasing the thickness of the vaginal epithelium. This drug carries the same black box warning as conjugated estrogens regarding an increased risk of endometrial cancer and DVT. Ospemiphene is given PO and is pregnancy category X.

In addition to their use in treating menopausal symptoms, estrogens are used for female hypogonadism, primary ovarian failure, and as replacement therapy following surgical removal of the ovaries, usually combined with a progestin. The purpose of the progestin is to counteract some of the adverse effects of estrogen on the uterus. When used alone, estrogen increases the risk of uterine cancer. Estrogen without progestin is considered appropriate only for patients who have had a hysterectomy.

High doses of estrogens are used to treat prostate and breast cancer. Prostate cancer is usually dependent on androgens for growth; administration of estrogens suppresses androgen secretion. In the treatment of cancer, estrogen is nearly always used in combination with other antineoplastic drugs, as discussed in chapter 38.

UTERINE ABNORMALITIES

Dysfunctional uterine bleeding is a condition in which hemorrhage occurs on a noncyclic basis or in abnormal amounts. It is the most frequent health care problem reported by women and is a common reason for hysterectomy. Progestins are the drugs of choice for treating uterine abnormalities.

46.6 Pharmacotherapy With Progestins

Secreted by the corpus luteum, endogenous progesterone prepares the uterus for implantation of the embryo and pregnancy. If implantation does not occur, levels of progesterone fall dramatically and menses begins. If pregnancy occurs, the ovary continues to secrete progesterone to maintain a healthy endometrium until the placenta develops sufficiently to begin producing the hormone. Whereas the function of estrogen is to cause proliferation of the endometrium, progesterone limits and stabilizes endometrial growth.

Dysfunctional uterine bleeding can have a number of causes, including early abortion, pelvic neoplasms, thyroid disorders, pregnancy, and infection. Types of dysfunctional uterine bleeding include the following:

- Amenorrhea—absence of menstruation
- Endometriosis—abnormal location of endometrial tissues
- Oligomenorrhea—infrequent menstruation

Complementary and Alternative Therapies

BLACK COHOSH FOR MENOPAUSE

Black cohosh (*Actaea racemosa*) is a perennial that grows in the eastern United States and parts of Canada. Use of the herb has been recorded by Native Americans for more than 100 years. Historically, black cohosh has been used in the management of menopausal hot flashes, vaginal dryness, and night sweats, and to induce labor (National Center for Complementary and Integrative Health, 2012). Doses of black cohosh are sometimes standardized by the amount of the chemical 27-deoxyactein, which is an active ingredient. A typical dose of black cohosh ranges from 40 to 80 mg of dried herb per day. (Approximately 1 mg of 27-deoxyactein is present in each 20-mg tablet or in 20 drops of the liquid formulation.)

Research regarding the effectiveness of black cohosh on relieving menopausal symptoms is mixed. A meta-analysis of 16 studies examining over 2,000 women found no significant difference between black cohosh and a placebo for reducing menopausal symptoms (Leach & Moore, 2012). However, several studies have confirmed its efficacy over placebo (Beer et al., 2013). Adverse effects include hypotension, uterine stimulation, and gastrointestinal (GI) complaints such as nausea. Black cohosh can increase the action of antihypertensives, so concurrent use should be avoided. Women with liver disorders should consult their health care provider before taking this herb.

- Menorrhagia—prolonged or excessive menstruation
- Breakthrough bleeding—hemorrhage between menstrual periods
- Premenstrual syndrome (PMS)—symptoms develop during the luteal phase
- Postmenopausal bleeding—hemorrhage following menopause
- Endometrial carcinoma—cancer of the endometrium.

Dysfunctional uterine bleeding is often caused by a hormonal imbalance between estrogen and progesterone. Although estrogen increases the thickness of the endometrium, bleeding occurs sporadically unless balanced by an adequate progesterone secretion. Administration of a progestin in a pattern starting 5 days after the onset of menses and continuing for the next 20 days can sometimes reestablish a normal, monthly cyclic pattern. HCs may also be prescribed for this disorder.

In cases of heavy bleeding, high doses of conjugated estrogens may be administered for 3 weeks prior to adding medroxyprogesterone for the last 10 days of therapy. Treatment with nonsteroidal anti-inflammatory drugs (NSAIDs) sometimes helps to reduce bleeding and ease painful menstrual flow. In 2009 tranexamic acid (Lysteda) was approved for the treatment of cyclic heavy menstrual bleeding. If aggressive hormonal therapy fails to stop the heavy bleeding, dilation and curettage (D & C) may be necessary.

Progestins are occasionally prescribed for the treatment of metastatic endometrial carcinoma. In these cases, they are used for palliation, usually in combination with other antineoplastics. Selected progestins and their dosages are listed in Table 46.5.

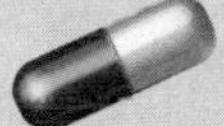

Prototype Drug | Medroxyprogesterone *(Depo-Provera, Depo-SubQ-Provera, Provera)*

Therapeutic Class: Hormone; drug for dysfunctional uterine bleeding **Pharmacologic Class:** Progestin

Actions and Uses

Medroxyprogesterone is a synthetic progestin with a prolonged duration of action. As with its natural counterpart, the primary target tissue for medroxyprogesterone is the endometrium of the uterus. It inhibits the effect of estrogen on the uterus, thus restoring normal hormonal balance. Indications include endometriosis, amenorrhea, uterine bleeding, and contraception.

Medroxyprogesterone may also be given by sustained release IM (Depo-Provera) or subcutaneous (Depo-SubQ-Provera) depot injection. This is available in two doses: a lower dose for contraception and a higher dose for the palliation of inoperable metastatic uterine or renal carcinoma.

Administration Alerts

- Give PO with meals to avoid gastric distress.
- Observe IM sites for abscess: presence of lump and discoloration of tissue.
- Pregnancy category X.

PHARMACOKINETICS (PO)

Onset	Peak	Duration
Unknown	2–4 h	Unknown

Adverse Effects

The most frequent adverse effects of medroxyprogesterone are breast tenderness, breakthrough bleeding, and other menstrual irregularities. Weight gain, depression, HTN, nausea, vomiting, dysmenorrhea, and vaginal candidiasis may also occur. The most serious adverse effect is an increased risk for thromboembolic events.

Black Box Warning: Progestins combined with conjugated estrogens may increase the risk of stroke, DVT, MI, pulmonary emboli, and invasive breast cancer. Women age 65 or older have an increased risk of dementia when treated with progestins. Women who are receiving injectable medroxyprogesterone are at significant risk for loss of bone mineral density.

Contraindications: Medroxyprogesterone is contraindicated during pregnancy and in women with known or suspected carcinoma of the breast. Caution should be used when treating patients with a history of thromboembolic disease, hepatic impairment, or undiagnosed vaginal bleeding. The drug should be used cautiously in patients with a history of depression, and the drug should be discontinued at the first sign of recurring depression.

Interactions

Drug–Drug: Serum levels of medroxyprogesterone are decreased by aminoglutethimide, barbiturates, primidone, rifampin, rifabutin, and topiramate.

Lab Tests: Medroxyprogesterone may increase values for alkaline phosphatase, glucose tolerance test (GTT), and HDL.

Herbal/Food: St. John's wort may decrease the effectiveness of medroxyprogesterone and cause abnormal menstrual bleeding.

Treatment of Overdose: There is no specific treatment for overdose.

Table 46.5 Drugs for Uterine Abnormalities and Hormone Replacement Therapy

Drug	Route and Adult Dose (max dose where indicated)	Adverse Effects
ESTROGENS		
estradiol (Alora, Climara, Divigel, Elestrin, Estraderm, Estrace, others)	PO (Estrace): 0.5–2 mg daily Transdermal patch: 1 patch either once weekly (Climara) or twice weekly (Alora, Estraderm, Minivelle) (0.025–0.1 mg/day) Topical gel (Divigel, Elestrin): 0.25–1 g/day applied to the skin of the upper thigh or arm Intravaginal cream (Estrace): Insert 2–4 g/day for 2 wk, then reduce to 1/2 the initial dose for 2 wk, then use 1 g one to three times/wk	*Breakthrough bleeding, spotting, breast tenderness, libido changes* HTN, gallbladder disease, thromboembolic disorders, increased endometrial cancer risk, hypercalcemia
estradiol valerate (Delestrogen)	IM: 10–20 mg every 4 wk	
estrogen, conjugated (Cenestin, Enjuvia, Premarin)	PO: 0.3–1.25 mg/day for 21 days each month	
estropipate (Ogen)	PO: 0.75–6 mg/day for 21 days each month Intravaginal cream (Ogen): Insert 2–4 g/day	
PROGESTINS		
medroxyprogesterone (Depo Provera, Depo-SubQ-Provera, Provera)	PO: 5–10 mg daily on days 1–12 of the menstrual cycle IM (Depo-Provera): 150 mg daily for 3 months. Give the first dose during the first 5 days of the menstrual period or within the first 5 days postpartum if not breast-feeding Subcutaneous (Depo-SubQ-Provera): 104 mg daily for 3 months. Give the first dose during the first 5 days of the menstrual period or at the 6th week postpartum if not breast-feeding	*Breakthrough bleeding, spotting, breast tenderness, weight gain* Amenorrhea, dysmenorrhea, depression, thromboembolic disorders
norethindrone (Micronor, Norlutin, Nor-Q.D.)	PO (for amenorrhea): 5–20 mg/day on days 5–25 of the menstrual cycle	
progesterone (Crinone, Endometrin, Prochieve, Prometrium)	IM (for amenorrhea or uterine bleeding): 5–10 mg/day Intravaginal (for assisted reproductive technology): 90 mg gel once daily or 100-mg inserted bid to tid	
ESTROGEN–PROGESTIN COMBINATIONS		
conjugated estrogens with medroxyprogesterone (Premphase, Prempro)	PO: Premphase: estrogen 0.625 mg/daily on days 1–28; add 5 mg medroxyprogesterone daily on days 15–28 PO: Prempro: estrogen 0.3 mg and medroxyprogesterone 1.5 mg daily Intravaginal cream: insert 1/2 to 2 g daily for 3–6 months	See above for adverse effects of estrogens and progestins
estradiol with norgestimate (Prefest)	PO: 1 tablet of 1-mg estradiol for 3 days, followed by 1 tablet of 1-mg estradiol combined with 0.09-mg norgestimate for 3 days. Regimen is repeated continuously without interruption	
ethinyl estradiol with norethindrone acetate (Activella)	PO: 1 tablet daily, which contains 0.5–0.1 mg of estradiol and 0.5–1 mg norethindrone Transdermal patch: 1 patch, twice weekly	

Note: *Italics* indicate common adverse effects; underlining indicates serious adverse effects.

LABOR AND BREAST-FEEDING

Several drugs are used to manage uterine contractions and to stimulate lactation. **Oxytocics** are drugs that *stimulate* uterine contractions to promote the induction of labor. **Tocolytics** are used to *inhibit* uterine contractions during premature labor. These medications are listed in Table 46.6.

46.7 Pharmacologic Management of Uterine Contractions

The most widely used oxytocic is the natural hormone oxytocin, which is secreted by the posterior portion of the pituitary gland. The target organs for oxytocin are the uterus and the breast. As the growing fetus distends the uterus, oxytocin is secreted in increasingly larger amounts. The rising blood levels of oxytocin provide a steadily increasing stimulus to the uterus to contract, thus promoting labor and the delivery of the baby and the placenta. As pregnancy progresses, the number of oxytocin receptors in the uterus increases, making it even more sensitive to the effects of the hormone. When used as a drug, oxytocin rapidly causes uterine contractions and induces labor.

In postpartum women, oxytocin is released in response to suckling, which causes milk to be *ejected* (let down) from the mammary glands. Oxytocin does not

Table 46.6 Uterine Stimulants and Relaxants

Drug	Route and Adult Dose (max dose where indicated)	Adverse Effects
OXYTOCIC		
oxytocin (Pitocin)	IV (to control postpartum bleeding): 10–40 units per infusion pump in 1,000 mL of IV fluid IV (to induce labor): 0.5–2 milliunits/min, gradually increasing the dose no greater than 1–2 milliunits/min at 30- to 60-min intervals until contraction pattern is established	*Nausea, vomiting, maternal dysrhythmias* Fetal bradycardia, uterine rupture, fetal intracranial hemorrhage, water intoxication, fetal brain hemorrhage
ERGOT ALKALOID		
methylergonovine (Methergine)	PO: 0.2–0.4 mg bid–qid	*Nausea, vomiting, uterine cramping* Shock, severe HTN, dysrhythmias
PROSTAGLANDINS		
carboprost (Hemabate)	IM: initial: 250 mcg (1 mL) repeated at 1 1/2–3 1/2-h intervals if indicated by uterine response	*Nausea, vomiting, diarrhea, headache, chills, uterine cramping*
dinoprostone (Cervidil, Prepidil)	Intravaginal; 10 mg	Uterine lacerations or perforation due to intense contractions
TOCOLYTICS		
magnesium sulfate (see page 725 for the Prototype Drug box)	IV: 1–4 g in 5% dextrose by slow infusion (initial max dose = 10–14 g/day, then no more than 30–40 g/day at a max rate of 1–2 g/h)	*Flushing, sweating, muscle weakness* Complete heart block, circulatory collapse, respiratory paralysis
hydroxyprogesterone (Makena)	IM: 250 mg once weekly, beginning at 16 wk gestation and continuing until wk 37	*Injection site pain and swelling, urticaria* Thromboembolic disorders, clinical depression
nifedipine (Adalat, Procardia) (see page 385 for the Prototype Drug box)	PO: Initial dosage of 20 mg, followed by 20 mg after 30 min If contractions persist, therapy can be continued with 20 mg q3–8h for 48–72 h with a maximum dose of 160 mg/day After 72 hours, if maintenance is still required, long-acting nifedipine 30–60 mg daily can be used	*Flushing, sweating, muscle weakness* Complete heart block, circulatory collapse, respiratory paralysis
terbutaline (Brethine)	IV: 2.5–10 mcg/min; increase every 10–20 min; duration of infusion: 12 h (max: 17.5–30 mcg/min) PO (maintenance dose): 2.5–10 mg q4–6h	*Nervousness, tremor, drowsiness* Bronchoconstriction, dysrhythmias, altered maternal and fetal heart rate

Note: *Italics* indicate common adverse effects; underlining indicates serious adverse effects.

increase the *volume* of milk production. This function is provided by the pituitary hormone prolactin, which increases the synthesis of milk. The actions of oxytocin during breast-feeding are illustrated in Figure 46.4.

Several prostaglandins are also used as uterine stimulants. Although the body makes dozens of different prostaglandins, only a few have clinical utility. In the uterus, prostaglandins cause intense smooth muscle contractions. Carboprost (Hemabate) is used to control serious postpartum hemorrhage that has not responded to more conventional means of treatment such as oxytocin. Dinoprostone is administered as a vaginal suppository (Cervidil) or gel (Prepidil) to promote cervical ripening, a softening and dilation of the cervix that must occur just prior to vaginal delivery. When used in high doses, the prostaglandins can induce pharmacologic abortion.

It is important to note that oxytocin and other uterine stimulants are indicated only when there are demonstrated risks to the mother or fetus in continuing the pregnancy. Because of potential adverse effects, they should never be used for elective induction of labor.

Some women enter labor before the baby has reached a normal stage of development. If the organ systems of the fetus are determined to be immature, attempts may be

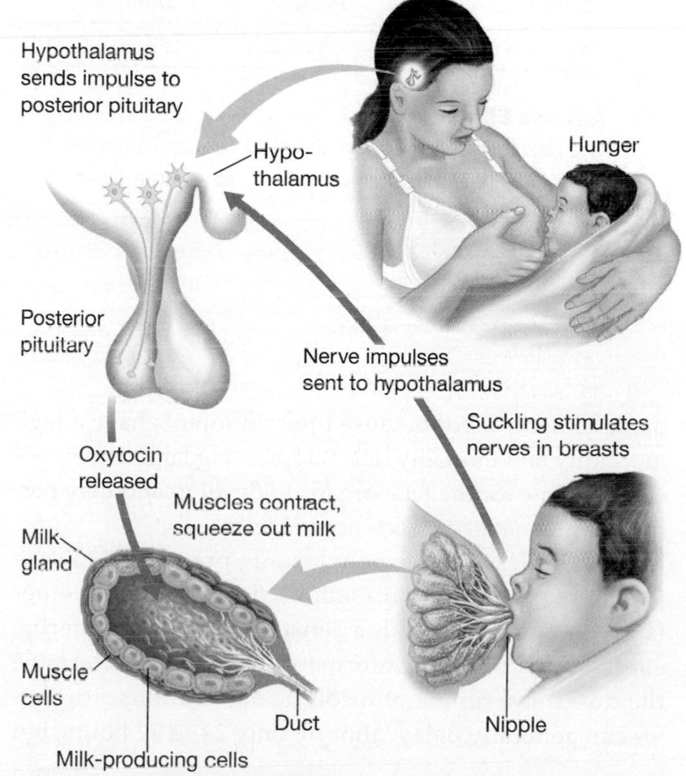

FIGURE 46.4 Oxytocin and breast-feeding

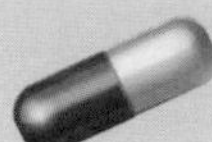

Prototype Drug | Oxytocin (*Pitocin*)

Therapeutic Class: Drug to induce labor; uterine stimulant **Pharmacologic Class:** Hormone; oxytocic

Actions and Uses

Oxytocin (Pitocin), identical to the natural hormone secreted by the posterior pituitary gland, is a preferred drug for inducing labor. Oxytocin is given by different routes depending on its intended action. Given antepartum by IV infusion, oxytocin induces labor by increasing the frequency and force of uterine contractions. It is timed to the final stage of pregnancy, after the cervix has dilated, membranes have ruptured, and presentation of the fetus has occurred. Doses in an IV infusion are increased gradually, every 15–60 minutes, until a normal labor pattern is established.

Oxytocin may also be administered postpartum to reduce hemorrhage after expulsion of the placenta and to aid in returning normal muscular tone to the uterus. This drug is approved at higher doses for the adjunct management of incomplete or inevitable abortion. Intranasal forms once used to promote milk letdown are no longer available in the United States.

Administration Alerts

- Dilute 10 units of oxytocin in 1,000 mL IV fluid prior to administration. For postpartum administration, may add up to 40 units in 1,000 mL IV fluid.
- Incidence of allergic reactions is higher when given IM or by IV injection, rather than IV infusion.
- Pregnancy category X.

PHARMACOKINETICS

Onset	Peak	Duration
immediate IV; 3–5 min IM	Unknown	1 h

Adverse Effects

The most common adverse effects of oxytocin are rapid, painful uterine contractions and fetal tachycardia. When given IV, vital signs of the fetus and mother are monitored continuously to avoid complications in the fetus, such as dysrhythmias or intracranial hemorrhage. Serious complications in the mother may include uterine rupture, seizures, or coma. Risk of uterine rupture increases in women who have delivered five or more children.

Black Box Warning: Oxytocin is not indicated for the elective induction of labor (the initiation of labor in a pregnant patient who has no medical indications for induction).

Contraindications: Antepartum use is contraindicated in the following: significant cephalopelvic disproportion; unfavorable fetal positions that are undeliverable without conversion before delivery; obstetrical emergencies in which the benefit-to-risk ratio for the fetus or mother favors surgical intervention; fetal distress when delivery is not imminent; when adequate uterine activity fails to achieve satisfactory progress; when the uterus is already hyperactive or hypertonic; when vaginal delivery is contraindicated, such as invasive cervical carcinoma, active genital herpes, total placenta previa, vasa previa, and umbilical cord presentation or prolapse of the cord.

Interactions

Drug–Drug: Vasoconstrictors used concurrently with oxytocin may cause severe HTN.

Lab Tests: Unknown.

Herbal/Food: None known.

Treatment of Overdose: Overdose causes strong uterine contractions, which may lead to uterine lacerations or rupture. Immediate discontinuation of the drug is necessary, along with symptomatic treatment.

made to delay labor because preterm infants have a high morbidity and mortality rate. Suppressing labor allows additional time for the fetal organs to develop and may permit the pregnancy to reach normal term.

Tocolytics are uterine relaxants prescribed to suppress preterm labor contractions. Typically, the mother is given a monitor with a sensor that records uterine contractions, and this information is used to determine the doses and timing of tocolytic medications. Tocolytics can generally delay labor by only 24 to 72 hours, but this is often enough time for the fetus to develop normal lung function. The benefits of these drugs must be carefully weighed against their potential adverse effects, which include tachycardia in both the mother and the fetus.

Only a few drugs are available as tocolytics. For over 30 years, magnesium sulfate, given by continuous IV infusion, was the preferred drug for suppressing preterm labor. However, evidence suggests it may be ineffective and poses undue risks to the fetus and mother.

Hydoxyprogesterone (Makena) is approved for delaying preterm labor but carries a risk for thromboembolism. Calcium channel blockers such as nifedipine (Adalat, Procardia) and beta-adrenergic agonists such as terbutaline (Brethine) are effective and used off-label for this indication.

FEMALE INFERTILITY

Infertility is the inability to become pregnant after at least 1 year of frequent unprotected intercourse. **Sexual desire disorder (SDD)** is a condition in which a man or a woman experiences a low level of sexual libido or desire to have sexual relations.

Nursing Practice Application

Pharmacotherapy With Oxytocin

ASSESSMENT	POTENTIAL NURSING DIAGNOSES*
Baseline assessment prior to administration: • Obtain a complete health history including length of current pregnancy; presence of preeclampsia or eclampsia; recent labor; type of delivery; history of labors or caesarean sections; cardiovascular, neurologic, hepatic, or renal disease; diabetes; and breast-feeding. • Obtain a drug history including allergies, current prescription and OTC drugs, herbal preparations, alcohol use, and smoking. Be alert to possible drug interactions. • Evaluate appropriate laboratory findings (e.g., CBC, platelets, coagulation studies, electrolytes, glucose, magnesium level, hepatic and renal function studies). • Obtain baseline height, weight, and vital signs. • Obtain fetal heart rate and intrauterine positioning. • Check for the presence of cervical dilation and effacement. Monitor quality and duration of any existing contractions. Monitor fetal response to contractions, noting any sign of fetal distress. • Check for postpartum bleeding and note the number of pads saturated.	• *Acute Pain* • *Deficient Knowledge* (drug therapy) • *Risk for Injury,* patient or fetus, related to adverse drug effects • *Risk for Excess Fluid Volume,* related to adverse drug effects *NANDA I © 2014
Assessment throughout administration: • Assess for desired therapeutic effects depending on the reason the drug is given (e.g., strong, regular contractions supportive of labor). • Continuously monitor the timing, quality, and duration of contractions. Immediately report sustained uterine contractions to the health care provider. • Continuously monitor the fetal heart rate and response to contractions. Immediately report signs of fetal distress to the health care provider. • Continue periodic monitoring of CBC, platelets, electrolytes, glucose, and magnesium level. • Monitor vital signs frequently and immediately and report any blood pressure above 140/90 mmHg or less than 90/60 mmHg, especially if accompanied by tachycardia, or per parameters, to the health care provider. • Continue to monitor postpartum bleeding and pad count. Notify the health care provider if more than two full-size pads are saturated in 2 hours' time. • Assess for adverse effects: nausea, vomiting, and headache. Immediately report tachycardia, palpitations, and HTN, especially associated with angina, severe headache, or dyspnea. Immediately report any severe abdominal pain, sustained uterine contraction, diminished urine output, dizziness, drowsiness, confusion, changes in level of consciousness, or seizures.	

continued

Nursing Practice Application *continued*

IMPLEMENTATION	
Interventions and (Rationales)	**Patient-Centered Care**
Ensuring therapeutic effects: • Monitor appropriate medication administration for optimal results. IV oxytocin must be given via an infusion pump to allow for precise dosing. (Infusion pumps allow for rapid dosage adjustments to maintain uterine contractions supportive of labor and cervical dilation reaching approximately 5 to 6 cm.)	• Instruct the patient about the rationale for all IV and monitoring equipment and the need for frequent monitoring to allay anxiety. • Teach the patient that labor contractions will gradually increase and that the drug will be decreased or stopped once contractions reach an optimal level. • Encourage the patient in labor to use pain-control measures (e.g., therapeutic breathing) or use pain control drugs as needed and ordered.
Minimizing adverse effects: • Monitor the timing, quality, and duration of contractions continuously. Immediately report any sustained uterine contractions to the health care provider. Stop the infusion, infusing normal saline or solution as ordered, and place the patient on her side until follow-up orders are obtained if sustained contractions continue. (Oxytocin may cause sustained uterine muscle contraction with potential uterine rupture. Uterine contractions must be continuously monitored.)	• Teach the patient that labor contractions will increase in strength and duration and will be monitored throughout. Instruct the patient to immediately report any sustained contraction or any severe abdominal pain.
• Continuously monitor the fetal heart rate and response to contractions. Immediately report signs of fetal distress to the health care provider. (Uterine contractions can affect the amount of blood flow through the placenta with diminished oxygenation to the fetus. Changes in fetal heart rate may signal fetal distress and the patient should be placed on her side, oxygen administered, the infusion stopped, and the health care provider notified.)	• Teach the patient that the fetal heart rate will also be monitored along with uterine contractions. Explain the purpose for all monitoring equipment to allay anxiety.
• Monitor vital signs and urine output frequently and report any blood pressure above 140/90 mmHg or less than 90/60 mmHg, especially if accompanied by tachycardia or diminished urine output, to the health care provider immediately. (Oxytocin has vasoconstrictive properties and water-retention properties. Blood pressure or pulse rate exceeding parameters, increasing disorientation or confusion, and diminished urine output may signify adverse drug effects or possible complications.)	• Instruct the patient to immediately report any headache, dizziness, disorientation or confusion, palpitations, or chest pressure or pain.
• Monitor fundal firmness and location and postpartum bleeding and pad count. (Oxytocin may be given to control postpartum bleeding. Lochia (usual postpartum bleeding) that increases, or if two or more pads are saturated over a 2-hour period, should be reported to the health care provider immediately.)	• Instruct the patient to report any sudden increase in lochia, dizziness or light-headedness, or if more than two pads are saturated after 2 hours.
Patient understanding of drug therapy: • Use opportunities during administration of medications and during assessments to provide patient education. (Using time during nursing care helps to optimize and reinforce key teaching areas.)	• The patient should be able to state the reason for the drug, appropriate dose and scheduling, monitoring needs, and what adverse effects to observe for and when to report them.

See Table 46.6 for a list of drugs to which these nursing actions apply.

46.8 Pharmacotherapy of Female Fertility

Infertility is a common disorder, with as many as 25% of couples experiencing difficulty in conceiving children at some point during their reproductive lifetimes. It is estimated that females contribute to approximately 60% of the infertility disorders. Drugs used to treat infertility are listed in Table 46.7. The three primary causes of female infertility are pelvic infections, physical obstruction of the uterine tubes, and lack of ovulation. Extensive testing is often necessary to determine the exact cause and it is not uncommon to find multiple etiologies for the infertility. For women whose infertility has been determined to have an endocrine etiology, pharmacotherapy may be of value. Endocrine disruption of reproductive function can

Table 46.7 Drugs for Female Infertility and Endometriosis

Drug	Mechanism
bromocriptine (Parlodel)	Reduction of high prolactin levels
clomiphene (Clomid, Serophene)	Promotion of follicle maturation and ovulation
danazol (Danocrine)	Anabolic steroid; suppression of FSH control of endometriosis
FSH AND LH ENHANCING DRUGS	
chorionic gonadotropin-HCG (Novarel, Ovidrel, Pregnyl)	Promotion of follicle maturation and ovulation
follitropin alfa (Gonal F)	
follitropin beta (Follistim)	
menotropins (Menopur, Repronex)	
urofollitropin (Bravelle)	
GnRH ANTAGONISTS	
cetrorelix (Cetrotide)	Prevention of premature ovulation or control of endometriosis
Ganirelix	
GnRH ANALOGS/AGONISTS	
goserelin (Zoladex)	Suppression of FSH and control of endometriosis
leuprolide (Eligard, Lupron, Viadur)	
nafarelin (Synarel)	

occur at the level of the hypothalamus, pituitary, or ovary, and pharmacotherapy is targeted to the specific cause of the dysfunction.

Ovulation (and thus pregnancy) cannot occur unless the ovarian follicles receive a hormonal signal to mature each month. This signal is normally supplied by LH and FSH during the first few weeks of the menstrual cycle. Lack of regular ovulation is a cause of infertility that can be successfully treated with drug therapy. Clomiphene (Clomid, Serophene) is a preferred drug for female infertility because it stimulates the release of LH, resulting in the maturation of more ovarian follicles than would normally occur. The rise in LH level is sufficient to induce ovulation in about 80% of treated women. The pregnancy rate of patients taking clomiphene is high, and twins occur in about 5% of treated patients. If ovulation is not induced by clomiphene, chorionic gonadotropin (HCG) may be added to the regimen. Made by the placenta during pregnancy, HCG is similar to LH and can mimic the LH surge that normally causes ovulation.

If the infertility is a result of disruption at the pituitary level, therapy with human menopausal gonadotropin (HMG) or GnRH may be indicated. These therapies are generally indicated only after clomiphene has failed to induce ovulation. Also known as menotropins (Menopur, Repronex), HMG acts on the ovaries to increase follicle maturation and results in a 25% incidence of multiple pregnancies. Newer formulations use recombinant DNA technology to synthesize gonadotropins containing nearly pure FSH. Other medications used to stimulate ovulation are gonadorelin (Factrel), bromocriptine (Parlodel), and HCG.

Premature ovulation, the expulsion of an oocyte from the ovary before it has fully matured, is another cause of infertility. GnRH antagonists such as ganirelix and cetrorelix (Cetrotide) suppress LH surges, thus preventing ovulation until the follicles are mature.

Endometriosis, a common cause of infertility, is characterized by the presence of endometrial tissue that has implanted outside the uterus in locations such as the surface of pelvic organs or the ovaries. Being responsive to hormonal stimuli, this abnormal tissue can cause pain, dysfunctional bleeding, and dysmenorrhea.

Leuprolide (Lupron) and nafarelin (Synarel) are GnRH agonists that produce an initial release of LH and FSH, followed by suppression due to the negative feedback effect on the pituitary. Many women experience relief from the symptoms of endometriosis after 3 to 6 months of therapy. As an alternative choice, danazol (Danocrine) is an anabolic steroid that suppresses FSH production, which in turn shuts down both ectopic and normal endometrial activity. Whereas leuprolide is given only by the parenteral route, danazol is given orally. Estrogen–progestin OCs are also useful in treating endometriosis.

46.9 Pharmacotherapy of Female Sexual Desire Disorder

Sexual desire disorder (also called acquired, generalized hypoactive sexual desire disorder) is a condition marked by persistent lack of interest in sexual activity over a prolonged period. It occurs in both sexes, although it is more common in women. In some women SDD can cause marked distress, interpersonal difficulty, and negatively impact the quality of life.

In 2015 the U. S. Food and Drug Administration (FDA) approved the first drug for female SDD. Flibanserin (Addyi) is approved to treat SDD in premenopausal women who previously had no problems with sexual desire. The drug carries a black box warning that it can cause severe hypotension and syncope if taken concurrently with alcohol or moderate or strong inhibitors of CYP3A4, such as azole antifungals, telaprevir, ritonavir, or verapamil. Because of the potential for serious hypotension, the FDA requires prescribers to enroll in and complete special training. In addition, pharmacies must be certified to dispense the medication, and patients must sign an agreement that they understand the side effects. Common side effects include dizziness, sleepiness, nausea, fatigue, and dry mouth. The mechanism by which flibanserin increases sexual desire is not known.

Chapter Review

KEY Concepts

The numbered key concepts provide a succinct summary of the important points from the corresponding numbered section within the chapter. If any of these points are not clear, refer to the numbered section within the chapter for review.

46.1 Female reproductive function is controlled by the secretion of gonadotropin-releasing hormone (GnRH) from the hypothalamus, and follicle-stimulating hormone (FSH) and luteinizing hormone (LH) from the pituitary.

46.2 Estrogens are secreted by ovarian follicles and are responsible for maturation of the sex organs and the secondary sex characteristics of the female. Progestins are secreted by the corpus luteum and prepare the endometrium for implantation.

46.3 Low doses of estrogens and progestins prevent conception by blocking ovulation. Long-term formulations are available that offer greater convenience.

46.4 Drugs for emergency contraception may be administered within 72 hours after unprotected sex to prevent implantation of the fertilized egg. Other drugs may be given to stimulate uterine contractions to expel the implanted embryo.

46.5 Estrogen–progestin combinations are used for hormone replacement therapy during and after menopause; however, their long-term use may have serious adverse effects.

46.6 Progestins are prescribed for dysfunctional uterine bleeding. High doses of progestins are also used as antineoplastics.

46.7 Oxytocics are drugs that stimulate uterine contractions and induce labor. Tocolytics slow uterine contractions to delay labor.

46.8 Medications may be administered to stimulate ovulation, to increase female fertility. Some of these medications are used to treat symptoms of endometriosis.

46.9 Flibanserin is the first drug approved to treat female sexual desire disorder, a condition characterized by diminished libido that can decrease the quality of life in some women.

REVIEW Questions

1. Which of the following patients would have a higher risk for adverse effects from estradiol and norethindrone (Ortho-Novum)? (Select all that apply.)

1. An 18-year-old with a history of depression
2. A 16-year-old with chronic acne
3. A 33-year-old with obesity per her body mass index (BMI)
4. A 24-year-old who smokes one pack of cigarettes per day
5. A 41-year-old who has delivered two healthy children

2. A patient is interested in taking levonorgestrel and estradiol (Seasonique) and asks how it is taken. Which explanation by the nurse is correct?

1. "Seasonique is taken year-round without a break and without a period."
2. "Seasonique is taken for 84 days and then followed by 7 days of a lower dose contained in the same package."
3. "Seasonique is a vaginal ring that is inserted monthly."
4. "Seasonique is taken for 2 months then off for 1 month using regular oral contraceptives."

3. The nurse completes an assessment of a patient in labor who is receiving an intravenous infusion of oxytocin. Which of the following assessments indicates the need for prompt intervention?
   1. There is no vaginal bleeding noted.
   2. The patient is managing her pain through breathing techniques.
   3. Fetal heart rate remains at baseline parameters.
   4. Contractions are sustained for 2 minutes in duration.

4. A woman consults the nurse about Plan B (levonorgestrel) after unprotected intercourse that occurred 2 days earlier. Which of the following instructions will the nurse give to this patient?
   1. "You must wait 7 days before taking the pills for Plan B to be effective."
   2. "Plan B is effective only within 24 hours of unprotected intercourse."
   3. "You will take one pill of Plan B at first, followed by another pill 12 hours later."
   4. "You will need to obtain a prescription for Plan B."

5. A 43-year-old patient is receiving medroxyprogesterone (Depo-Provera) for treatment of dysfunctional uterine bleeding. Because of related adverse effects, which of the following may indicate a potential adverse effect?
   1. Breakthrough bleeding between periods
   2. Insomnia or difficulty falling asleep
   3. Eye, mouth, or vaginal dryness
   4. Joint pain or pain on ambulation

6. A patient has started taking clomiphene (Clomid, Serophene) after an infertility work-up and asks the nurse why she is not having in-vitro fertilization. Which of the following nursing statements would be most helpful in explaining the use of clomiphene to the patient?
   1. The patient's diagnostic work-up suggested that infrequent ovulation may be the cause for her infertility and clomiphene increases ovulation.
   2. In-vitro fertilization is expensive and because clomiphene is less expensive, it is always tried first.
   3. There is less risk of multiple births with clomiphene.
   4. The patient's past history of oral contraceptive use has prevented her from ovulating. Clomiphene is given to stimulate ovulation again in these conditions.

PATIENT-FOCUSED Case Study

Yolanda Clerik is 22 years old and has been taking estradiol and norethindrone (Ortho-Novum) for contraception. She has been seen her provider today for a recurrent throat infection and has been given a prescription for penicillin.

1. As the nurse, what instructions will you give Yolanda about her new prescription and the effect it may have on her estradiol and norethindrone (Ortho-Novum)?
2. While Yolanda is in the office, what additional education will you give her to minimize the risk of adverse effects from her estradiol and norethindrone (Ortho-Novum)?

CRITICAL THINKING Questions

1. A 28-year-old woman has tried for over a year to become pregnant. Her husband has a 4-year-old child from a previous marriage and a physical work-up suggests that clomiphene (Clomid) may be useful in promoting pregnancy. What information should be included in a teaching plan for a patient who is receiving this drug?
2. A 22-year-old patient has been taking ethinyl estradiol with drospirenone (Yasmin) but has just started penicillin for a recurrent throat infection. She asks the nurse if she should stop taking her Yasmin. What instructions should the nurse give to this patient?
3. A nurse is assessing a 32-year-old postpartum patient and notes 2+ pitting edema of the ankles and pretibial area. The patient denies having "swelling" prior to delivery. The nurse reviews the patient's chart and notes that she was induced with oxytocin (Pitocin) over a 23-hour period. What is the relationship between this drug regimen and the patient's current presentation? What additional assessments should be made?

Visit www.pearsonhighered.com/nursingresources for answers and rationales for all activities.

REFERENCES

Beer, A. M., Osmers, R., Schnitker, J., Bai, W., Mueck, A. O., & Meden, H. (2013). Efficacy of black cohosh (Cimicifuga racemosa) medicines for treatment of menopausal symptoms-comments on major statements of the Cochrane Collaboration report 2012 "black cohosh (Cimicifuga spp.) for menopausal symptoms (review)." *Gynecological Endocrinology, 29*, 1022–1025. doi:10.3109/09513590.2013.831836

Cleland, K., Raymond, E. G., Westley, E., & Trussel, J. (2014). Emergency contraception review: Evidence-based recommendations for clinicians. *Clinical Obstetrics and Gynecology, 57*, 741–750. doi:10.1097/GRF.0000000000000056

Herdman, T. H., & Kamitsuru, S. (Eds.). (2014). *NANDA International nursing diagnoses: Definitions and classification, 2015–2017*. Oxford, United Kingdom: Wiley-Blackwell.

Leach, M. J., & Moore, V. (2012). Black cohosh for menopausal symptoms. *Cochrane Database of Systematic Reviews, Issue 9*, Art. No.: CD007244. doi:10.1002/14651858.CD007244.pub2

National Center for Complementary and Integrative Health. (2012). *Black cohosh*. Retrieved from https://nccih.nih.gov/health/blackcohosh/ataglance.htm

Turok, D. K., Jacobson, J. C., Dermish, A. I., Simonsen, S. B., Gurtcheff, S., McFadden, M.,. . . Murphy, P. A. (2014). Emergency contraception with copper IUD or oral levonorgestrel: An observational study of 1-year pregnancy rates. *Contraception, 89*, 222–228. doi:10.1016/j.contraception.2013.11.010

SELECTED BIBLIOGRAPHY

Bedell, S., Nachtigall, M., & Naftolin, F. (2014). The pros and cons of plant estrogens for menopause. *The Journal of Steroid Biochemistry and Molecular Biology, 139*, 225–236. doi:10.1016/j.jsbmb.2012.12.004

Brown, A. (2010). Long-term contraceptives. *Best Practice & Research Clinical Obstetrics & Gynecology, 24*, 617–631. doi:10.1016/j.bpobgyn.2010.04.005

Centers for Disease Control and Prevention. (2015). *Contraceptive use*. Retrieved from http://www.cdc.gov/nchs/fastats/contraceptive.htm

Daniels, K., Jones, J., & Abma, J. (2013). *Use of emergency contraception among women aged 15–44: United States, 2006–2010*. Retrieved from http://www.cdc.gov/nchs/data/databriefs/db112.htm#x2013;44:%20United%20States,%202006–2010

Daniels, K., Mosher, W. D., & Jones. J. (2013). *National Health Statistics Reports: Contraceptive methods women have ever used, 1982–2010*. Retrieved from http://www.cdc.gov/nchs/data/nhsr/nhsr062.pdf#x2013;2010%20[PDF%20-%20251%20KB]

Davidson, M. R., London, M. L., & Ladewig, P. L. (2012). *Maternal newborn nursing and women's health across the lifespan* (9th ed.). Upper Saddle River, NJ: Pearson.

deVilliers, T. J., Gass, M. L., Haines, C. J., Hall, J. E., Lobo, R. A., Pierroz, D. D., & Rees, M. (2013). Global consensus statement on menopausal hormone therapy. *Climacteric, 16*, 203–204. doi:10.3109/13697137.2013.771520

Estephan, A. (2014). *Dysfunctional uterine bleeding in emergency medicine*. Retrieved from http://emedicine.medscape.com/article/795587-overview#a0104

Gemzell-Danielsson, K., Berger, C., & Lalitkumar, P. G. L. (2013). Emergency contraception—mechanisms of action. *Contraception, 87*, 300–308. doi:10.1016/j.contraception.2012.08.021

Levin, E. R., & Hammes, S. R. (2011). *Estrogens and progestins*. In L. L. Brunton, B. A. Chabner, & B. C. Knollman (Eds.), *Goodman & Gilman's the pharmacological basis of therapeutics* (12th ed., pp. 1163–1194). New York, NY: McGraw-Hill.

Mansour, D. (2012). The benefits and risks of using a levonorgestrel-releasing intrauterine system for contraception. *Contraception, 85*, 224–234. doi:10.1016/j.contraception.2011.08.003

Nappi, R. E., & Cucinella, L. (2015). Advances in pharmacotherapy for treating female sexual dysfunction. *Expert Opinion on Pharmacotherapy, 16*, 875-887. doi:10.1517/14656566.2015.1020791

Ray, A., Shah, A., Gudi, A., & Homburg, R. (2012). Unexplained infertility: An update and review of practice. *Reproductive Biomedicine Online, 24*, 591–602. doi.10.1016/j.rbmo.2012.02.021

Schimmer, B. P., & Parker, K. L. (2011). Contraception and the pharmacotherapy of obstetrical and gynecological disorders. In L. L. Brunton, B. A. Chabner, & B. C. Knollman (Eds.), *Gordon & Gilman's the pharmacological basis of therapeutics* (12th ed., pp. 1833–1852). New York, NY: McGraw-Hill.

Schindler, A. E. (2013). Non-contraceptive benefits of oral hormonal contraceptives. *International Journal of Endocrinology and Metabolism, 11*(1), 41. doi:10.5812/ijem.4158

Streuli, I., de Ziegler, D., Santulli, P., Marcellin, L., Borghese, B., Batteux, F., & Chapron, C. (2013). An update on the pharmacological management of endometriosis. *Expert Opinion on Pharmacotherapy, 14*, 291–305. doi:10.1517/14656566.2013.767334

Chapter 47

Drugs for Disorders and Conditions of the Male Reproductive System

Drugs at a Glance

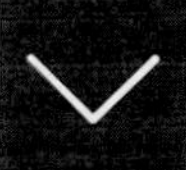

Learning Outcomes

After reading this chapter, the student should be able to:

1. Describe the roles of the hypothalamus, pituitary, and testes in regulating male reproductive function.
2. Identify indications for pharmacotherapy with androgens.
3. Describe the potential consequences associated with the use of anabolic steroids to enhance athletic performance.
4. Explain the role of medications in the treatment of male infertility.
5. Describe the etiology, pathogenesis, and pharmacotherapy of erectile dysfunction.
6. Describe the pathogenesis and pharmacotherapy of benign prostatic hyperplasia.
7. For each of the classes listed in Drugs at a Glance, know representative drugs, and explain the mechanism of drug action, primary actions, and important adverse effects.
8. Use the nursing process to care for patients who are receiving pharmacotherapy for disorders and conditions of the male reproductive system.

(prototype drug icon) indicates a prototype drug, each of which is featured in a Prototype Drug box.

As in women, reproductive function in men is regulated by a small number of hormones from the hypothalamus, pituitary, and gonads. Because hormonal secretion in men is relatively constant throughout the adult life span, the pharmacologic treatment of reproductive disorders in men is less complex, and more limited, than in women. This chapter examines drugs used to treat disorders and conditions of the male reproductive system.

THE MALE REPRODUCTIVE SYSTEM

47.1 Hypothalamic and Pituitary Regulation of Male Reproductive Function

The same pituitary hormones that control reproductive function in women also affect men. Although the name **follicle-stimulating hormone (FSH)** applies to its target in the female ovary, this hormone also regulates sperm production in men. **Luteinizing hormone (LH),** more accurately called interstitial cell–stimulating hormone (ICSH) in the male reproductive system, regulates the production of testosterone.

Although they are also secreted in small amounts by the adrenal glands in women, **androgens** are considered male sex hormones. The testes secrete **testosterone,** the primary androgen responsible for maturation of the male sex organs and the secondary sex characteristics of men. Unlike the 28-day cyclic secretion of estrogen and progesterone in women, testosterone secretion is relatively constant in adult men. Beginning in puberty, testosterone production increases rapidly and continues to be maintained at a high level until late adulthood, after which it slowly declines. If the level of testosterone in the blood rises above normal, negative feedback to the pituitary shuts off the secretion of LH and FSH. The relationship among the hypothalamus, pituitary, and the male reproductive hormones is illustrated in Figure 47.1.

Testosterone has profound metabolic effects in tissues outside the reproductive system. Of particular note is its ability to build muscle mass, which contributes to differences in muscle strength and body composition between men and women. Testosterone promotes the synthesis of erythropoietin, resulting in an increased production of red blood cells (RBCs) and accounting for the higher hemoglobin and hematocrit levels found in males.

HYPOGONADISM

Lack of sufficient testosterone secretion by the testes can result in male **hypogonadism.** Hypogonadism may be congenital or acquired later in life. When the condition is caused by a testicular disorder, it is called *primary* hypogonadism. Examples of disease states that may cause primary testicular failure include mumps, testicular trauma or inflammation, and certain autoimmune disorders.

Without sufficient FSH and LH secretion by the pituitary, the testes will lack their stimulus to produce testosterone. This condition is known as *secondary* hypogonadism. Lack of FSH and LH secretion may have a number of causes, including Cushing's syndrome, thyroid disorders, estrogen-secreting tumors, and therapy with gonadotropin-releasing hormone (GnRH) agonists such as leuprolide (Lupron).

Symptoms of male hypogonadism include a diminished appearance of the secondary sex characteristics of men: sparse axillary, facial, and pubic hair; increased subcutaneous fat; and small testicular size. In adult men, lack of testosterone can lead to erectile dysfunction, low sperm counts, and decreased **libido,** or interest in intercourse. Nonspecific complaints may include fatigue, depression, and reduced muscle mass. In young men, lack of sufficient testosterone secretion may lead to delayed puberty.

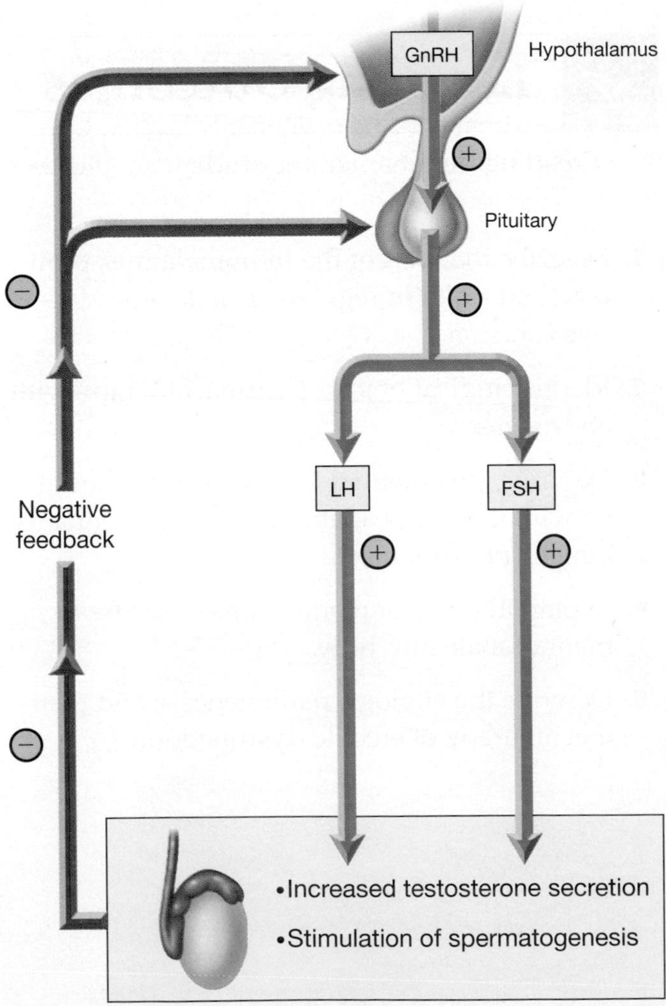

FIGURE 47.1 Hormonal control of the male reproductive hormones

PharmFacts

MALE REPRODUCTIVE CONDITIONS AND DISORDERS

- Erectile dysfunction affects 18 to 30 million American men—about one in four men older than 65 years.
- Smoking more than 20 cigarettes a day has been shown to produce a 60% higher risk of erectile dysfunction. Ten or fewer cigarettes daily still increases the risk by 16%.
- Approximately 50% of men with diabetes will experience erectile dysfunction.
- Benign prostatic hyperplasia (BPH) affects 50% of men older than 60 years and 90% of men by age 85.
- The estimated prevalence of male infertility is 12%; the incidence of infertility increases with age.

47.2 Pharmacotherapy With Androgens

Androgens include testosterone and related hormones that support male reproductive function. Other important androgens include androstenedione and dehydroepiandrosterone (DHEA). Therapeutically androgens are used to treat hypogonadism and certain cancers. These drugs are listed in Table 47.1.

Pharmacotherapy of hypogonadism includes replacement therapy with testosterone or other androgens at levels normally found in a healthy male. Within days or weeks of initiating therapy, androgens improve libido and correct erectile dysfunction caused by abnormally low testosterone levels. Male sex characteristics reappear, a condition called *masculinization* or **virilization.** Depression resolves and muscle strength rapidly improves. Therapy with androgens is targeted to return serum testosterone to normal levels. Above-normal levels serve no therapeutic purpose and increase the risk of adverse effects. Testosterone is available in a variety of different formulations, as listed in Table 47.2, to better meet the individual patient preferences and lifestyles.

Androgens have important physiological effects outside the reproductive system. Testosterone promotes the synthesis of erythropoietin, which explains why men usually have a slightly higher hematocrit than women. Testosterone has a profound anabolic effect on skeletal muscle, which is the rationale for giving this drug to debilitated patients who have muscle-wasting disease.

Anabolic steroids are testosterone-like compounds with hormonal activity that are taken inappropriately by athletes who hope to build muscle mass and strength, thereby obtaining a competitive edge. Use of steroids is high among teens, who sometimes take these drugs because they believe it improves their appearance. When taken in large doses for prolonged periods, anabolic steroids can produce significant adverse effects, some of which may persist for months after discontinuing the drugs. These drugs tend to raise cholesterol levels and may cause low sperm counts and impotence in men. In female athletes, menstrual irregularities are likely with an obvious increase in masculine appearance. Oral androgens are hepatotoxic, and permanent liver damage may result with prolonged use. Behavioral changes include aggression and psychological dependence. The use of anabolic steroids to improve athletic performance is illegal and strongly discouraged by health care providers and athletic associations. Most androgens are classified as Schedule III drugs because of their abuse potential.

Table 47.1 Selected Androgens and Anabolic Steroids

Drug	Route and Adult Dose (max dose where indicated)	Adverse Effects
fluoxymesterone (Halotestin)	PO: 5 mg one to four times/day	*Acne, gynecomastia, hirsutism and male sex characteristics (in women), sodium and water retention, hypercholesterolemia* <u>Anaphylaxis, testicular atrophy and oligospermia at high doses</u>
methyltestosterone (Android, Methitest, Testred)	PO: 10–50 mg/day Buccal; 5–25 mg/day	
nandrolone	IM; 50–200 mg/wk	
oxandrolone (Oxandrin)	PO: 2.5–20 mg/day divided bid–qid for 2–4 wk	
oxymetholone (Anadrol-50)	PO: 1–5 mg/kg/day	
testosterone (buccal: Striant); (transdermal patch: Androderm); (topical gels: Androgel, Fortesta, Testim, Vogelxo); (implantable pellets: Testopel); (nasal spray: Natesto)	Buccal: 30 mg q12h Transdermal: apply 1–2, 2.5 mg patches daily (max: 5 mg/day) Gel: apply 5–50 g daily Pellets: 150–450 mg every 6 months (each pellet is 75 mg) Nasal spray: 1 spray in each nostril tid (total daily dose: 33 mg)	
testosterone cypionate (Depo-Testosterone)	IM: 50–400 mg every 2–4 wk	
testosterone enanthate (Delatestryl)	IM: 50–400 mg every 2–4 wk	
testosterone undecanoate (Aveed)	IM: 750 mg initially, followed by the same dose at 4 weeks and every 10 weeks thereafter	

Note: *Italics* indicate common adverse effects; <u>underlining</u> indicates serious adverse effects.

Table 47.2 Androgen Formulations

Route	Drug	Advantages	Disadvantages
Implantable pellets (subcutaneous)	Testopel: 1–6 pellets are implanted on the anterior abdominal wall depending on the dose required	Doses last 3–4 months	Inflammation or infection may occur around the insertion site
Intramuscular (IM)	Testosterone cypionate (Depo-Testosterone) and testosterone enanthate (Delatestryl)	Doses last 2–4 wk	Serum testosterone levels may vary widely after administration, causing fluctuations in libido, energy and mood swings; soreness at the site of injection
testosterone intranasal	testosterone undecanoate (Aveed)	Easy to use	May require 3 doses/day; can cause nasal side effects such as nasopharyngitis, epistaxis, and rhinorrhea
Testosterone buccal system	Striant tablet is applied to the gum area just above the incisor	Produces a continuous supply of testosterone in the blood	May require twice-daily dosing; local irritation to the buccal mucosa
Transdermal testosterone gel	AndroGel, Fortesta, and Testim are applied once daily to the upper arms, shoulders, or abdomen	The drug is absorbed into the skin in about 30 minutes and released slowly to the blood; causes less skin irritation than patches	Gel can be transferred to another person by skin-to-skin contact, causing virilization of female contacts and fetal harm
Transdermal testosterone patch	Androderm patch is applied daily to the upper arm, thigh, back, or abdomen, rotating application sites	Easy to use	Rash may occur at the site of patch application

High doses of androgens are occasionally used as a palliative measure to treat certain types of breast cancer in combination with other antineoplastics. At the high doses required for breast cancer treatment, some virilization will occur in most patients. Because the growth of most prostate carcinomas is testosterone dependent, androgens should not be prescribed for older men unless the possibility of prostate cancer has been ruled out. Patients with prostate carcinoma are sometimes given a GnRH agonist such as leuprolide (Lupron) to reduce circulating testosterone levels.

MALE INFERTILITY

It is estimated that 30% to 40% of infertility among couples is caused by difficulties with the male reproductive system. Male infertility may have a psychological etiology, which should be ruled out before pharmacotherapy is considered.

47.3 Pharmacotherapy of Male Infertility

Like female infertility, male infertility may have a number of complex causes. The most obvious etiology is lack of sufficient sperm production. **Oligospermia,** the presence of fewer than 20 million sperm/mL of ejaculate, is considered abnormal and can lower reproductive success. **Azoospermia,** the complete absence of sperm in an ejaculate, may indicate an obstruction of the vas deferens or ejaculatory duct that can be corrected surgically. Infections such as mumps, chronic tuberculosis, and sexually transmitted infections can contribute to infertility. The possibility of erectile dysfunction must be considered and treated, as discussed in section 47.4. Infertility may occur with or without signs of hypogonadism.

The goal of endocrine pharmacotherapy of male infertility is to increase sperm production. Therapy often begins with IM injections of human chorionic gonadotropin (HCG) three times per week over 1 year. Although HCG is secreted by the placenta, its effects in men are identical to those of LH: increased testosterone secretion and spermatogenesis. Sperm counts are conducted periodically to assess therapeutic progress. If HCG is unsuccessful, therapy with menotropins (Menopur, Repronex) may be attempted. Menotropin consists of a mixture of purified FSH and LH. For infertile patients exhibiting signs of hypogonadism, testosterone therapy also may be indicated.

Other pharmacologic approaches to treating male infertility have been attempted. Antiestrogens such as tamoxifen (Nolvadex) and clomiphene (Clomid) have been used to block the negative feedback of estrogen (from the adrenal glands) to the pituitary and hypothalamus, thus increasing the levels of FSH and LH. Testolactone (Teslac), an aromatase inhibitor, has been administered to block the metabolic conversion of testosterone to estrogen. Various nutritional supplements have been tested, such as zinc to improve sperm production, L-arginine to improve sperm motility, and vitamins C and E as antioxidants to reduce reactive intermediates. Unfortunately, these and other therapies have not conclusively been shown to have any positive effect on male infertility.

Drug therapy of male infertility is not as successful as fertility pharmacotherapy in women, because only

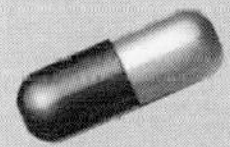

Prototype Drug | Testosterone

Therapeutic Class: Male sex hormone **Pharmacologic Class:** Androgen; anabolic steroid; antineoplastic

Actions and Uses

The primary therapeutic uses of testosterone are for the treatment of delayed puberty and hypogonadism in males. The drug promotes virilization, including enlargement of the sexual organs, growth of facial hair, and deepening of the voice. In adult males, testosterone administration will increase libido and restore masculine characteristics that may be deficient. Testosterone is approved to treat erectile dysfunction that is caused by low androgen levels. The drug is also approved for the palliative treatment of inoperable breast cancer in women.

Testosterone acts by stimulating ribonucleic acid (RNA) synthesis and protein metabolism. High doses may suppress spermatogenesis. Testosterone base is administered by the IM route, although other salts are available for the transdermal, implantable pellet, and buccal routes.

Administration Alerts

- If using a patch, place on hair-free, dry skin of the abdomen, back, thigh, upper arm, or as directed.
- Alternate patch site daily, rotating sites every 7 days.
- Give IM injection into gluteal muscles.
- Pregnancy category X.

PHARMACOKINETICS

Onset	Peak	Duration
Unknown PO; 2–4 wk IM, pellet	Unknown	1–3 days PO; 2–4 wk IM, pellet

Adverse Effects

Androgens may cause either increased or decreased libido. Salt and water are often retained, causing edema, and a diuretic may be indicated. Liver damage is rare, although it is a potentially serious adverse effect with high doses. Acne and skin irritation are common during therapy. Extreme doses in men (anabolic steroid abuse) may cause feminization rather than virilization because excess testosterone is metabolized to estrogen.

Black Box Warning: Virilization in children and women may occur following secondary exposure. Children and women should avoid the application sites in men using testosterone gel. Signs of virilization may include any of the following: suppression of ovulation, lactation, or menstruation; deepening of the voice; hirsutism; oily skin; clitoral enlargement; regression of breasts; and male-pattern baldness.

Contraindications: Testosterone is contraindicated in men with known or suspected breast or prostatic carcinomas and in women who are or may become pregnant (category X). The drug should be used with caution in patients with pre-existing prostatic enlargement or renal or hepatic disease.

Interactions

Drug–Drug: Testosterone may potentiate the effects of oral anticoagulants and increase the risk of severe bleeding. Concurrent use of testosterone with corticosteroids may cause additive edema, which can be a serious concern for those with heart failure. Hepatotoxic drugs should be avoided because use with testosterone can cause additive liver damage.

Lab Tests: Values of the following may be decreased: T_4, thyroxine-binding globulin, serum calcium, and clotting factors II, V, VII, and X. Creatinine may be increased, and cholesterol may be either increased or decreased.

Herbal/Food: The risk of hepatotoxicity may increase when testosterone is used with echinacea.

Treatment of Overdose: There is no specific treatment for overdose.

about 5% of infertile males have an endocrine etiology for their disorder. Many years of therapy may be required. Because of the expense of pharmacotherapy and the large number of injections needed, other means of conception may be explored, such as in vitro fertilization or intrauterine insemination.

ERECTILE DYSFUNCTION

Erectile dysfunction, or **impotence**, is a common disorder in men. The defining characteristic of this condition is the consistent inability to either obtain an erection or to sustain an erection long enough to achieve successful intercourse.

47.4 Pharmacotherapy of Erectile Dysfunction

The incidence of erectile dysfunction increases with age, although it may occur in an adult male of any age. Certain diseases, most notably atherosclerosis, diabetes, kidney disease, stroke, and hypertension, are associated with a higher incidence of the condition. Smoking increases the risk of erectile dysfunction by 30% to 60%, in a dose-dependent manner.

Nursing Practice Application

Pharmacotherapy With Androgens

ASSESSMENT	POTENTIAL NURSING DIAGNOSES*
Baseline assessment prior to administration: • Obtain a complete health history including cardiovascular, peripheral vascular, thyroid, hepatic, or renal disease; diabetes; BPH; or prostate or breast cancer. • Obtain a drug history including allergies, current prescription and over-the-counter (OTC) drugs, herbal preparations, alcohol use, and smoking. Be alert to possible drug interactions. • Evaluate appropriate laboratory findings (e.g., complete blood count [CBC], electrolytes, glucose, lipid levels, prostate-specific antigen [PSA]). • Obtain baseline height, weight, and vital signs.	• *Disturbed Body Image,* related to adverse drug effects • *Sexual Dysfunction,* related to adverse drug effects • *Fluid Volume Excess,* related to adverse drug effects • *Deficient Knowledge* (drug therapy) *NANDA I © 2014
Assessment throughout administration: • Assess for desired therapeutic effects depending on the reason the drug is given (e.g., hormone levels normalize, normal signs of masculinization are present). • Continue periodic monitoring of CBC, electrolytes, glucose, lipid levels, hepatic and renal function laboratory tests, and PSA levels. • Monitor vital signs, height, and weight at each health care visit. • Assess for adverse effects: nausea, vomiting, headache, weight gain, fluid retention, edema, increased blood pressure (BP), changes in mood, irritability, and agitation. Also assess for tachycardia, palpitations, or hypertension, especially associated with angina or dyspnea; abdominal pain; or signs of hepatotoxicity.	

IMPLEMENTATION

Interventions and (Rationales)	Patient-Centered Care
Ensuring therapeutic effects: • Monitor appropriate medication administration. (Appropriate administration, especially of gels or transdermal forms, will optimize drug absorption and therapeutic effects.)	• Teach the patient appropriate administration techniques.
Minimizing adverse effects: • Monitor BP at each clinical visit. Check body weight and for the presence of edema. (Androgens cause sodium and water retention with resulting increases in weight, BP, and possible edema.)	• Teach the patient to monitor BP on a weekly basis, ensuring proper functioning of any equipment used at home. Instruct the patient to report any BP over 140/90 mmHg or as directed by the health care provider; report any weight gain over 1 kg (2 lb) in 24 hours or 2 kg (5 lb) in 1 week; and report any peripheral edema.
• Continue to monitor electrolytes, lipid levels, and hepatic function laboratory tests periodically. (Androgens may increase cholesterol and calcium levels. Hepatotoxicity and hepatic neoplasms are rare but potential adverse effects. **Lifespan:** Age-related physiological differences may place the older adult at greater risk for hepatic toxicity.)	• Instruct the patient to return periodically for laboratory tests. • Teach the patient to immediately report any symptoms of abdominal or right upper quadrant discomfort or pain, yellowing of the skin or sclera, fatigue, anorexia, darkened urine or clay-colored stools, weakness, lethargy, nausea, or vomiting.
• Monitor blood glucose levels in patients with diabetes frequently. (Androgens may affect carbohydrate metabolism, leading to increased glucose levels.)	• Teach men with diabetes to monitor capillary blood glucose more frequently while on the drug and report consistent elevations to the health care provider.
• **Lifespan:** Monitor height and growth in children and adolescents. (Androgen administration may cause premature closure of epiphyses and loss of normal growth patterns.)	• Teach the patient, family, or caregiver to measure height once per month or as directed. Teach the patient to return for clinical assessments as needed, approximately every 6 months, to monitor bone growth.

Nursing Practice Application *continued*

IMPLEMENTATION

Interventions and (Rationales)	Patient-Centered Care
• **Lifespan:** Monitor use closely in adolescent patients. (Abuse of androgens and anabolic steroids may occur, along with resulting adverse effects.)	• Teach the adolescent patient to maintain daily dosing as instructed and not to increase dosage unless instructed to do so by the health care provider. The drug should never be shared with others.
Patient understanding of drug therapy:	
• Use opportunities during administration of medications and during assessments to provide patient education. (Using time during nursing care helps to optimize and reinforce key teaching areas.)	• The patient should be able to state the reason for the drug, appropriate dose and scheduling, and what adverse effects to observe for and when to report them.
Patient self-administration of drug therapy:	
• When administering the medication, instruct the patient, family, or caregiver in the proper self-administration of the drug (e.g., consistently at the same time each day to help remember the dose). (Proper administration will increase the effectiveness of the drug.)	• Teach the patient to take the drug following appropriate guidelines: • Oral drugs should be taken at the same time each day to maintain consistent drug levels. • Transdermal patches should be applied to the scrotal area after dry shaving; do not use depilatories. Change patch and rotate sites daily, and report any skin irritation. • Buccal tablets should be placed between the cheek and upper gum and held in place for 30 seconds. Rotate from side to side, avoiding areas of irritation. • Gels and creams should be applied to the upper torso, extremities, or abdomen. Swimming and showering should be avoided for several hours following administration. Do not allow women or children to come in contact with drug or application sites because the drug may rub off and cause adverse effects. • Transdermal pellets are implanted in the abdominal wall every 3 to 6 months. • Injections should be given into deep gluteal muscle. If the patient is to administer own injections, teach the appropriate technique, followed by teach-back until the patient is comfortable and demonstrates proper technique.

See Table 47.1 for a list of drugs to which these nursing actions apply.

Treating the Diverse Patient: Human Chorionic Gonadotropin (HCG) Abuse by Athletes

Most health care providers are familiar with the ongoing problem of anabolic steroid use by athletes and teens. Elite athletes have abused the placental hormone HCG since approximately the 1980s but its use has moved into the realm of everyday athletes and teenagers. HCG is not an anabolic steroid. Why would an athlete take a placental hormone? There are several reasons.

Men who are taking anabolic steroids experience a natural negative feedback phenomenon. The high levels of anabolic steroids provide feedback to the hypothalamus and pituitary to shut down production of testosterone by the testes. When the athlete stops taking the steroids the testes need several weeks to recover, and the man may suffer from loss of muscle strength, testicular atrophy, loss of libido, and impotence. Taking injectable HCG during this time immediately raises the man's testosterone level because HCG resembles LH, the natural stimulus for testosterone production. Thus, HCG is used to transition to regular (i.e., nonsteroid) training. HCG also masks steroid use by changing the types and amounts of steroids that show up on laboratory tests conducted by athletic organizations.

The World Anti-Doping Agency (WADA, 2015) includes both HCG and LH on its list of banned substances in competitive sports. Also included are multiple forms of growth hormone, including insulin-like growth factor 1 (IGF-1) and vascular-endothelial growth factor (VEGF). However, abuse of these hormones continues.

Because of the serious risks involved, particularly for young athletes who may not realize the long-term implications, nurses should include questions about use of HCG, anabolic steroids, and other performance enhancing drugs in the history for adolescents and athletes. If use is noted, a frank and nonjudgmental discussion of the adverse effects should be provided by the health care provider.

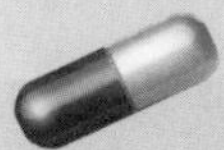

Prototype Drug | Finasteride *(Proscar)*

Therapeutic Class: Drug for BPH **Pharmacologic Class:** 5-alpha reductase inhibitor

Actions and Uses

Finasteride acts by inhibiting 5-alpha reductase, the enzyme responsible for converting testosterone to one of its metabolites, 5-alpha dihydrotestosterone. This active metabolite causes proliferation of prostate cells and promotes enlargement of the gland. Because it inhibits the metabolism of testosterone, finasteride is sometimes called an antiandrogen. Finasteride promotes shrinkage of enlarged prostates and subsequently helps restore urinary function. It is most effective in patients with larger prostates.

Finasteride is also marketed as Propecia, which is prescribed to promote hair regrowth in patients with male-pattern baldness. Doses of finasteride are five times higher when prescribed for BPH than when prescribed for baldness. Finasteride may be used off-label to treat hirsutism in women.

Administration Alerts

- Tablets may be crushed for oral administration.
- Pregnant nurses or pharmacists should avoid handling crushed medication, because it may be absorbed through the skin and cause harm to a male fetus.
- Patients who take finasteride should not donate blood while on drug therapy.

PHARMACOKINETICS

Onset	Peak	Duration
May take 3–6 months for maximum effect	1–2 h	5–7 days

Adverse Effects

Finasteride is well tolerated and side effects are generally mild and transient. Finasteride causes various types of sexual dysfunction in up to 16% of patients, including impotence, impaired fertility, diminished libido, and ejaculatory dysfunction. Other minor effects include headache, rash, dizziness, and asthenia.

Recent studies have suggested that finasteride can increase the risk for the development of high-grade prostate cancer. Men should be carefully screened to rule out the presence of prostate cancer prior to receiving 5-alpha reductase inhibitors. Increases in PSA values during finasteride therapy may indicate the presence of prostate cancer.

Contraindications: Contraindications include hypersensitivity to the drug, pregnancy, lactation, and use in children.

Interactions

Drug–Drug: Use with anticholinergics may decrease the effectiveness of finasteride. Use of finasteride with testosterone will result in a reduction in the effects of both drugs.

Lab Tests: Values for DHT and PSA may be decreased. Testosterone levels may be increased.

Herbal/Food: Saw palmetto may potentiate the actions of finasteride.

Treatment of Overdose: There is no specific treatment for overdose.

due to stimulation of baroreceptors is common with alpha blockers, and postural hypotension occurs when beginning therapy. Additional information on the alpha blockers and a prototype feature for doxazosin are presented in chapter 26.

Some patients are unable to tolerate the cardiovascular effects of the alpha$_1$-adrenergic blockers. For these patients, the 5-alpha reductase inhibitors offer an alternative. These drugs block an enzyme in the testosterone metabolic pathway, thus eliminating the hormonal signal for prostate growth. The most commonly prescribed drug in this class is finasteride (Proscar), which is featured as a prototype for BPH. These drugs may take several months to shrink the size of the prostate; thus, they are not appropriate for severe disease. The 5-alpha reductase inhibitors produce few adverse effects, although they can cause sexual dysfunction in some patients. An additional option for BPH pharmacotherapy is tadalafil (Cialis).

Drugs for BPH have limited effectiveness and have value only in treating mild-to-moderate disease as an alternative to surgery. Because pharmacotherapy alleviates the symptoms but does not cure the disease, these medications must be taken for the remainder of the patient's life, or until surgery is indicated.

Nursing Practice Application

Pharmacotherapy for Benign Prostatic Hyperplasia

ASSESSMENT	POTENTIAL NURSING DIAGNOSES*
Baseline assessment prior to administration: • Obtain a complete health history including cardiovascular, peripheral vascular, thyroid, hepatic, or renal disease; diabetes, BPH, or prostate cancer. • Obtain a drug history including allergies, current prescription and OTC drugs, herbal preparations, alcohol use, and smoking. Be alert to possible drug interactions. • Evaluate appropriate laboratory findings (e.g., CBC, hepatic and renal function, PSA). • Obtain baseline vital signs. • Assess the patient's ability to receive and understand instruction. Include the family or caregiver as needed.	• *Sexual Dysfunction,* related to adverse drug effects • *Deficient Knowledge* (drug therapy) • *Risk for Falls,* related to adverse drug effects (alpha-adrenergic blockers) *NANDA I © 2014
Assessment throughout administration: • Assess for desired therapeutic effects depending on the reason the drug is given (e.g., urinary stream increases, lessened urinary retention). • Continue periodic monitoring of CBC, hepatic and renal function laboratory tests. • Monitor vital signs at each health care visit. • Assess for adverse effects: nausea, headache, rash, dizziness, or sexual dysfunction.	

IMPLEMENTATION

Interventions and (Rationales)	Patient-Centered Care
Ensuring therapeutic effects:	
• Monitor appropriate medication administration for optimal results. (Full therapeutic effects from 5-alpha reductase inhibitors may take 3 to 6 months to be achieved.)	• Teach the patient to continue taking the medication consistently through the early months of therapy and that the drug may take several months for full effects.
Minimizing adverse effects:	
• Continue to monitor hepatic function laboratory tests periodically. (Hepatotoxicity is a potential adverse effect. **Lifespan:** Age-related physiological differences may place the older adult at greater risk for hepatic toxicity. **Diverse Patients:** Because finasteride metabolizes through the CYP 3A4 system pathways, monitor ethnically diverse patients to ensure optimal therapeutic effects and to minimize adverse effects.)	• Teach the patient to immediately report any increasing symptoms of urinary retention or slowing of the urinary stream. A prostate exam may be indicated. • Teach the patient to immediately report any symptoms of abdominal or right upper quadrant discomfort or pain, yellowing of the skin or sclera, fatigue, anorexia, darkened urine or clay-colored stools, weakness, lethargy, nausea, or vomiting.
• Monitor BP at each clinical visit. Check weight and for presence of edema. (Alpha-adrenergic blockers may trigger sodium and water retention with resulting increases in weight, BP, and possible edema. Immediately report any BP over 140/90 mmHg, peripheral edema, or weight gain.)	• Teach the patient who is taking alpha-adrenergic blockers to monitor BP on a weekly basis and to report any BP over 140/90 mmHg, or as directed, to the health care provider. Teach the patient to report any weight gain of 1 kg (2 lb) in 24 hours or 2 kg (5 lb) in 1 week to the health care provider and to report any peripheral edema. Ensure proper functioning of any equipment used at home.
• Monitor urine output and symptoms of dysuria such as hesitancy or nocturia. (5-alpha reductase inhibitors may cause urinary frequency, nocturia, or hesitancy.)	• Have the patient promptly report urinary hesitancy, frequency, or an increase in nocturia.
• Give the first dose of any alpha-adrenergic blocker at bedtime. (A first-dose response may result in a greater initial drop in BP than subsequent doses. This may also occur if the dose is increased. **Lifespan:** Be particularly cautious with the older adult who is a greater risk for falls.)	• **Safety:** Instruct the patient to take the first dose of medication at bedtime, immediately before going to bed, and to avoid driving for 12 to 24 hours after the first dose, or when the dosage is increased, until the effects are known. If dizziness occurs, the patient should sit or lie down and not attempt to stand or walk, until the sensation passes.

Nursing Practice Application *continued*

IMPLEMENTATION

Interventions and (Rationales)	Patient-Centered Care
• Do not abruptly stop alpha-adrenergic blockers used for BPH. (Rebound hypertension and tachycardia may occur.)	• **Safety:** Teach the patient not to stop the medication abruptly and to call the health care provider for instructions if unable to take the medication for more than 2 days due to illness.
• Protect against accidental exposure to 5-alpha reductase inhibitors by women of child-bearing age and children, including through handling of crushed or broken drugs. (The drug has teratogenic effects and handling by women of child-bearing age should be avoided. Men should wear condoms during sexual activity and should not donate blood while taking the drug and up to 1 month after stopping the drug.)	• Teach the patient to keep the drug in a secure location to guard against accidental exposure to women of child-bearing age or children. • Teach the patient to use condoms consistently for sexual activity to avoid exposing women of child-bearing age to semen, which may also contain the drug. • Instruct the patient not to donate blood during the time the drug is taken and up to 1 month after the drug is stopped.
Patient understanding of drug therapy: • Use opportunities during administration of medications and during assessments to provide patient education. (Using time during nursing care helps to optimize and reinforce key teaching areas.)	• The patient, family, or caregiver should be able to state the reason for the drug, appropriate dose and scheduling, what adverse effects to observe for, and when to report them.
Patient self-administration of drug therapy: • When administering the medication, instruct the patient or caregiver in proper self-administration of the drug (e.g., consistently over several months of therapy). (Using time during nurse-administration of these drugs helps to reinforce teaching.)	• The patient is able to discuss the appropriate dosing and administration needs.

See Table 47.4 for a list of drugs to which these nursing actions apply.

Chapter Review

KEY Concepts

The numbered key concepts provide a succinct summary of the important points from the corresponding numbered section within the chapter. If any of these points are not clear, refer to the numbered section within the chapter for review.

47.1 Follicle-stimulating hormone (FSH) and luteinizing hormone (LH) from the pituitary regulate the secretion of testosterone, the primary hormone contributing to the growth, health, and maintenance of the male reproductive system.

47.2 Androgens are used to treat hypogonadism in males and breast cancer in females. Anabolic steroids are frequently abused by athletes and can result in serious adverse effects with long-term use.

47.3 Male infertility is difficult to treat pharmacologically; medications include human chorionic gonadotropin, menotropins, testolactone, and antiestrogens.

47.4 Erectile dysfunction is a common disorder that may be successfully treated with sildenafil (Viagra), an inhibitor of the enzyme phosphodiesterase-5.

47.5 In its early stages, benign prostatic hyperplasia may be treated successfully with drug therapy, including $alpha_1$-adrenergic blockers and 5-alpha reductase inhibitors.

REVIEW Questions

1. Which of the following nursing assessments would be appropriate for the patient who is receiving testosterone? (Select all that apply.)
   1. Monitor for a decrease in hematocrit.
   2. Assess for signs of fluid retention.
   3. Assess for increased muscle mass and strength.
   4. Check for blood dyscrasias.
   5. Assess for muscle wasting.
2. The nurse is teaching a patient who has a new prescription for testosterone gel. Which of the following instructions should the nurse give to this patient?
   1. "Avoid exposing women to the gel or to areas of skin where the gel has been applied."
   2. "Report any weight gain over 2 kg (5 lb) in 1 month."
   3. "Avoid showering or swimming for at least 12 hours after applying the gel."
   4. "Apply the gel to the scrotal and perineal areas daily."
3. The nurse is teaching a patient about the use of tadalafil (Cialis). What will the nurse teach him about the effects of tadalafil?
   1. It should always result in a penile erection within 10 minutes.
   2. It may heighten female sexual response.
   3. It is not effective if sexual dysfunction is caused by psychological conditions.
   4. It will result in less intense sensation with prolonged use.
4. The patient with erectile dysfunction is being evaluated for the use of sildenafil (Viagra). Which of the following questions should the nurse ask before initiating therapy with sildenafil?
   1. "Are you currently taking medications for angina?"
   2. "Do you have a history of diabetes?"
   3. "Have you ever had an allergic reaction to dairy products?"
   4. "Have you ever been treated for migraines?"
5. A patient with a history of benign prostatic hyperplasia is complaining of feeling like he "cannot empty his bladder." He has been taking finasteride (Proscar) for the past 9 months. What should the nurse advise this patient to do?
   1. Continue to take the drug to achieve full therapeutic effects.
   2. Discuss the use of a low-dose diuretic with the health care provider.
   3. Decrease the intake of coffee, tea, and alcohol.
   4. Return to the health care provider for laboratory studies and a prostate exam.
6. A patient is given a prescription for finasteride (Proscar) for treatment of benign prostatic hyperplasia. Essential teaching for this patient includes which of the following? (Select all that apply.)
   1. Full therapeutic effects may take 3 to 6 months.
   2. Hair loss or male-pattern baldness may be an adverse effect.
   3. The drug should not be handled by pregnant women, especially if it is crushed.
   4. Blood donation should not occur while taking this drug.
   5. Report any weight gain of over 2 kg (5 lb) in 1 week.

PATIENT-FOCUSED Case Study

Michael Galvin is a 68-year-old who has been diagnosed with BPH. He has been given a prescription for finasteride (Proscar), but he says that he has been hearing about the benefits of saw palmetto, and is curious about it.

1. What is the action of finasteride (Proscar) and how will it be beneficial in treating Mr. Galvin's BPH?
2. How do the effects of saw palmetto compare to finasteride?

CRITICAL THINKING Questions

1. A 78-year-old widower has come to see his health care provider. The nurse practitioner interviews the patient about his past medical history and current health concerns. The patient states that he is planning to marry "a very nice lady" but is concerned about his sexual performance. He asks about a prescription for sildenafil (Viagra). What additional assessment data does the nurse need to collect given this patient's age?

2. A 16-year-old adolescent goes out for the football team. He is immediately impressed with the size of several junior and senior linemen. One older student offers to "hook him up" with a source for androstenedione (Andro). From a developmental perspective, explain why this young man may be susceptible to anabolic steroid abuse. Can anabolic steroid abuse affect his stature?

Visit www.pearsonhighered.com/nursingresources for answers and rationales for all activities.

REFERENCES

Avins, A. L., Lee, J. Y., Meyers, C. M., Barry, M. J., & CAMUS Study Group. (2013). Safety and toxicity of saw palmetto in the CAMUS trial. *The Journal of Urology, 189*, 1415–1420. doi:10.1016/j.juro.2012.10.002

Herdman, T. H., & Kamitsuru, S. (Eds.). (2014). *NANDA International nursing diagnoses: Definitions and classification, 2015–2017*. Oxford, United Kingdom: Wiley-Blackwell.

MacDonald, R., Tacklind, J. W., Rutks, I., & Wilt, T. J. (2012). *Serenoa repens* monotherapy for benign prostatic hyperplasia (BPH): An updated Cochrane systematic review. *BJU International, 109*, 1756–1761. doi:10.1111/j.1464-410X.2012.11172.x

World Anti-Doping Agency. (2015). *List of prohibited substances and methods*. Retrieved from http://list.wada-ama.org/

SELECTED BIBLIOGRAPHY

Albersen, M., Orabi, H., & Lue, T. F. (2012). Evaluation and treatment of erectile dysfunction in the aging male: A mini-review. *Gerontology, 58*, 3–14. doi:10.1159/000329598

Centers for Disease Control and Prevention. (2014). *Prostate cancer*. Retrieved from http://www.cdc.gov/cancer/prostate/

Corona, G., Mondaini, N., Ungar, A., Razzoli, E., Rossi, A., & Fusco, F. (2011). Phosphodiesterase type 5 (PDE5) inhibitors in erectile dysfunction: The proper drug for the proper patient. *Journal of Sexual Medicine, 8*, 3418–3432. doi:10.1111/j.1743-6109.2011.02473.x

Deters, L.A. (2014). *Benign prostatic hypertrophy*. Retrieved from http://emedicine.medscape.com/article/437359-overview

Kemp, S. (2014) *Hypogonadism*. Retrieved from http://emedicine.medscape.com/article/922038-overview

Kim, E. D. (2014). *Erectile dysfunction*. Retrieved from http://emedicine.medscape.com/article/444220-overview

Kring, D. (2012). Benign prostatic hyperplasia. *Nursing 2012, 42*(5), 37. doi:10.1097/01.NURSE.0000413610.36683.b3

Louis, J. F., Thoma, M. E., Sørensen, D. N., McLain, A. C., King, R. B., Sundaram, R., . . . Buck Louis, G. M. (2013). The prevalence of couple infertility in the United States from a male perspective: Evidence from a nationally representative sample. *Andrology, 1*, 741–748. doi:10.1111/j.2047-2927.2013.00110.x.

National Center for Complementary and Integrative Health. (2012). *Herbs at a glance: Saw palmetto*. Retrieved from https://nccih.nih.gov/health/palmetto/ataglance.htm

National Institute on Drug Abuse. (2012). *Drug facts: Anabolic steroids*. Retrieved from http://www.drugabuse.gov/infofacts/steroids.html

Porche, D. J., & Jeanfreau, S. G. (2010). Testosterone deficiency. Common in midlife and beyond. *Advanced Nurse Practitioner, 18*(6), 16.

Quallich, S. (2010). Male infertility: A primer for NPs. *Nurse Practitioner, 35*(12), 28–36. doi:10.1097/01.NPR.0000390435.13252.5a

Rittenberg, V., & El-Toukhy, T. (2010). Medical treatment of male infertility. *Human Fertility, 13*, 208–216. doi:10.3109/14647273.2010.534833

Roehrborn, C. G. (2011). Male lower urinary tract symptoms (LUTS) and benign prostatic hyperplasia (BPH). *Medical Clinics of North America, 95*, 87–100. doi:10.1016/j.mcna.2010.08.013

Surampudi, P. N., Wang, C., & Swerdloff, R. (2012). Hypogonadism in the aging male diagnosis, potential benefits, and risks of testosterone replacement therapy. *International Journal of Endocrinology, 2012*. doi:10.1155/2012/625434

Unit 9

The Integumentary System, Eyes, and Ears

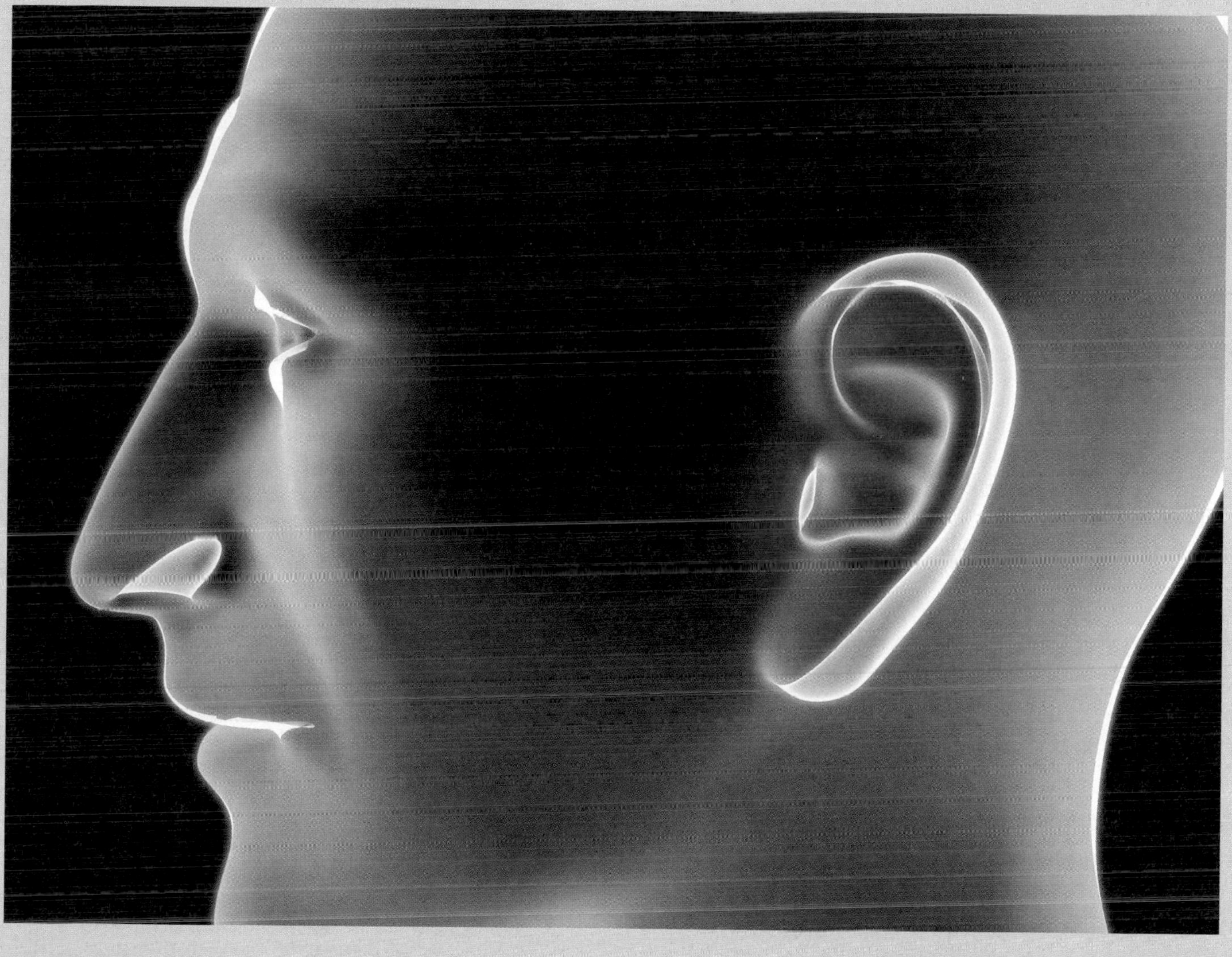

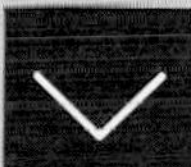

The Integumentary System, Eyes, and Ears

Chapter 48

Drugs for Bone and Joint Disorders

Drugs at a Glance

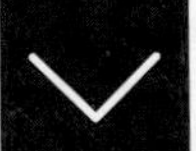

Learning Outcomes

After reading this chapter, the student should be able to:

1. Describe the role of calcium in the body in maintaining homeostasis in the nervous, muscular, and nervous systems.
2. Explain the roles of parathyroid hormone, calcitonin, and vitamin D in maintaining calcium balance.
3. Identify the types of calcium supplements used to correct hypocalcemia.
4. Explain the pharmacotherapy of metabolic bone diseases, including osteomalacia, osteoporosis, and Paget's disease.
5. Discuss drugs used to treat joint diseases, including osteoarthritis, rheumatoid arthritis, and gout.
6. Describe the nurse's role in the pharmacologic management of disorders related to bones and joints.
7. For each of the drug classes listed in Drugs at a Glance, know representative drugs, and explain their mechanisms of action, primary actions, and important adverse effects.
8. Use the nursing process to care for patients receiving pharmacotherapy for bone and joint disorders.

indicates a prototype drug, each of which is featured in a Prototype Drug box.

The bones and joints are at the core of body movement. Disorders associated with this system may affect a patient's ability to fulfill daily activities and lead to immobility. In addition, the skeletal system serves as the primary repository for calcium, one of the body's most important minerals.

This chapter focuses on the pharmacotherapy of important skeletal and joint disorders such as osteomalacia, osteoporosis, arthritis, and gout. The chapter stresses the importance of calcium balance and the action of vitamin D as they relate to the proper structure and function of bones.

CALCIUM BALANCE

48.1 Role of Calcium and Vitamin D in Bone Homeostasis

Calcium is the primary mineral responsible for bone formation and for maintaining bone health throughout the life span. This major mineral constitutes about 2% of our body weight and is critical to proper functioning of the nervous, muscular, and cardiovascular systems. To maintain homeostasis, calcium balance in the body is regulated by parathyroid hormone (PTH), calcitonin, and vitamin D, as shown in Figure 48.1. Acting together, these three substances

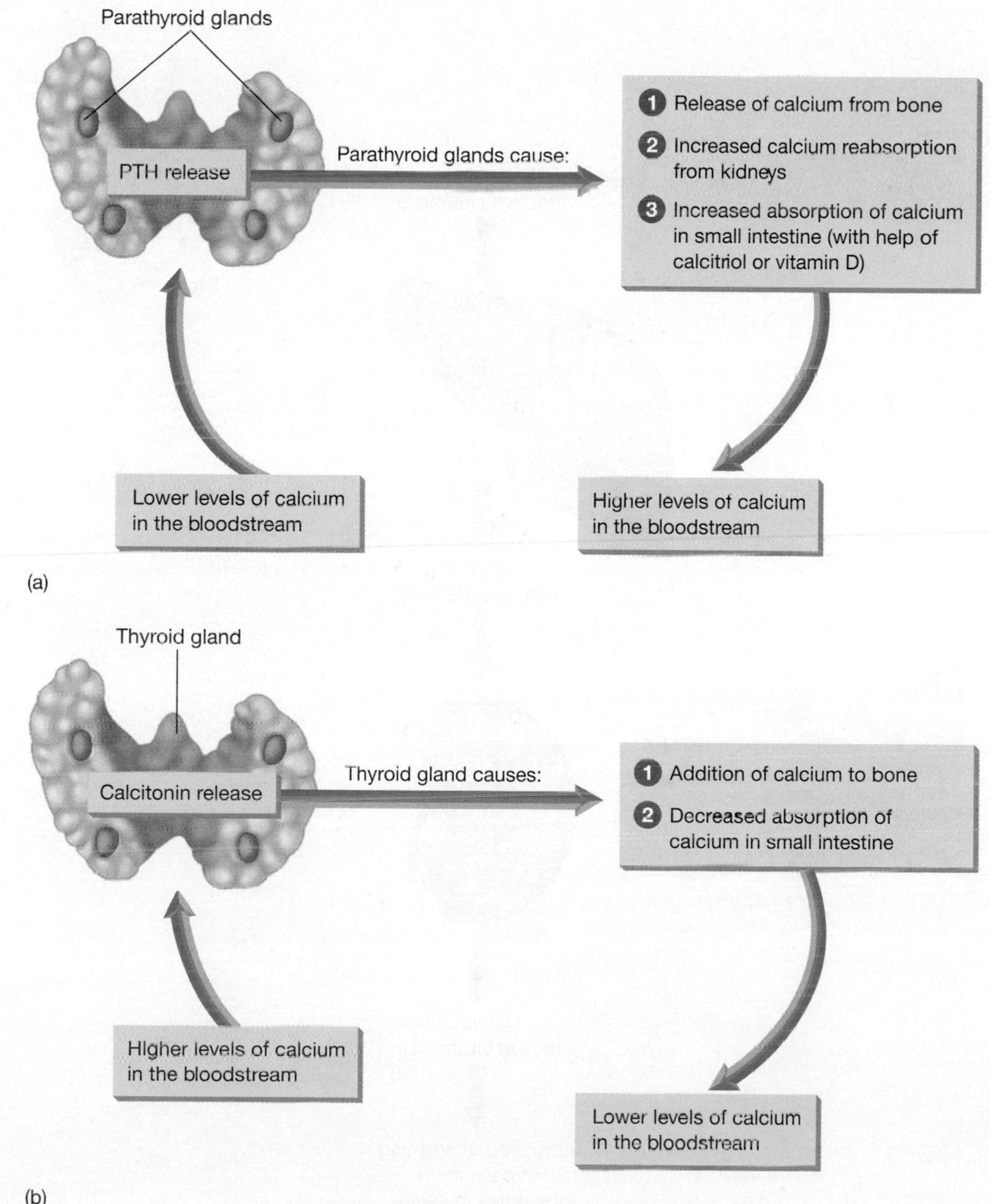

FIGURE 48.1 (a) Parathyroid hormone (PTH) and (b) calcitonin action

regulate the rate of absorption of calcium from the gastrointestinal (GI) tract, the excretion of calcium from the kidney, and the movement of calcium into and out of bone.

Secreted by the parathyroid glands, PTH stimulates bone cells called *osteoclasts*. These cells accelerate the process of **bone resorption,** demineralization that breaks down bone into its mineral components. Once bone is broken down (resorbed), calcium becomes available for transport to areas in the body where it is needed. The opposite of this process is **bone deposition,** or bone building, accomplished by cells called *osteoblasts*. This process, which removes calcium from the blood to be placed in bone, is stimulated by the hormone calcitonin. When serum calcium levels become elevated, calcitonin is released by the thyroid gland.

Vitamin D and calcium metabolism are intimately related: Absorption of calcium is increased in the presence of vitamin D, and inhibited by vitamin D deficiency. Thus, calcium disorders are often associated with vitamin D disorders.

Vitamin D is unique among vitamins because the body is able to synthesize it from precursor molecules. Several steps, however, are required before vitamin D can act on target tissues. The *inactive* form of vitamin D, **cholecalciferol,** is synthesized in the skin from cholesterol. Exposure of the skin to sunlight or ultraviolet light increases the level of cholecalciferol in the blood. Cholecalciferol can also be obtained from dietary products such as milk or other foods fortified with vitamin D. Figure 48.2 illustrates the metabolism of vitamin D.

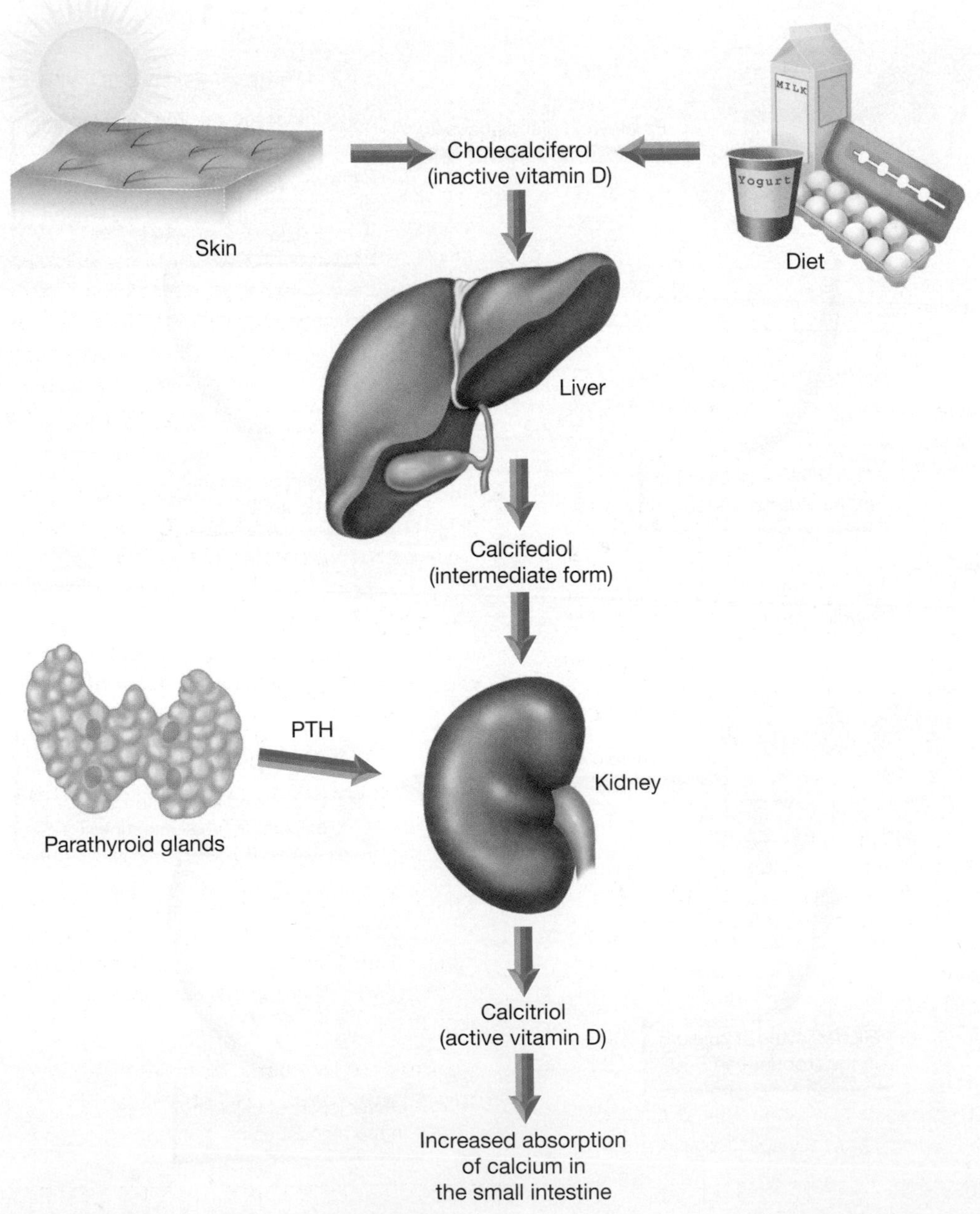

FIGURE 48.2 Pathway for vitamin D activation and action

Following its absorption from dietary sources or formation in the skin, cholecalciferol is converted to an intermediate vitamin form called **calcifediol.** Enzymes in the kidneys metabolize calcifediol to **calcitriol,** the *active* form of vitamin D. PTH stimulates the formation of calcitriol at the level of the kidneys. Patients with extensive kidney disease are unable to adequately synthesize calcitriol and thus frequently experience calcium and vitamin D abnormalities.

The primary function of calcitriol is to increase calcium absorption from the GI tract. Dietary calcium is absorbed more efficiently in the presence of active vitamin D and PTH, resulting in higher serum levels of calcium, which is then transported to bone, muscle, and other tissues.

The importance of proper calcium balance in the body cannot be overstated. Calcium ion influences the excitability of all neurons. When calcium concentrations are too high (hypercalcemia), sodium permeability decreases across cell membranes. This is a dangerous state, because nerve conduction depends on the proper influx of sodium into cells. When calcium levels in the bloodstream are too low (hypocalcemia), cell membranes become hyperexcitable. If this situation becomes severe, convulsions or muscle spasms may result. Calcium is also important for the normal functioning of other body processes such as blood coagulation and muscle contraction. It is, indeed, a critical mineral for life.

48.2 Pharmacotherapy of Hypocalcemia

Hypocalcemia is not a disease but a sign of underlying pathology; therefore, diagnosis of the cause of hypocalcemia is essential. Many factors can cause hypocalcemia. Lack of sufficient dietary calcium or vitamin D is a common cause, and one that can be easily reversed by nutritional therapy.

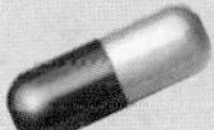

Prototype Drug | Calcium Salts

Therapeutic Class: Calcium supplement **Pharmacologic Class:** Hypocalcemia agent

Actions and Uses

For mild, chronic hypocalcemia, inexpensive calcium supplements are effective and readily available over the counter (OTC) in a variety of formulations. Calcium carbonate and calcium citrate are the two most common salts for routine supplementation. In addition to preventing or treating hypocalcemia, calcium salts are administered for osteoporosis, Paget's disease, osteomalacia, chronic hypoparathyroidism, rickets, pregnancy, lactation, and rapid childhood growth. Calcium carbonate is a common antacid used to treat heartburn. It may also be used to bind excessive dietary phosphate in patients with hyperphosphatemia due to end-stage renal disease.

For severe cases of hypocalcemia, multiple IV infusions of calcium salts may be necessary to return the serum calcium level to normal. Constant monitoring of serum calcium is required during IV administration to prevent the development of hypercalcemia.

Administration Alerts

- Give oral (PO) calcium supplements with meals or within 1 hour following meals.
- Administer intravenous (IV) supplements slowly to avoid hypotension, dysrhythmias, and cardiac arrest.
- Pregnancy category B.

Pharmacokinetics

The pharmacokinetics of calcium salts varies by the route of administration and the specific formulation.

Adverse Effects

Oral calcium products are safe when used as directed. The most common adverse effect is hypercalcemia, which is caused by taking too much of this supplement. Mild to moderate hypercalcemia may produces no symptoms. As calcium levels increase lethargy, weakness, anorexia, nausea, vomiting, confusion, renal stones, increased urination, and dehydration may occur. Acute hypercalcemia can cause serious symptoms such as syncope, coma, dysrhythmias, and cardiac arrest. If extravasation occurs during IV administration, severe necrosis and sloughing of the skin may result.

Contraindications: Calcium salts are contraindicated in patients with ventricular fibrillation, metastatic bone cancer, renal calculi, or hypercalcemia.

Interactions

Drug–Drug: Concurrent use with digoxin increases the risk of dysrhythmias. Magnesium may compete for GI absorption. Calcium decreases the absorption of tetracyclines. Calcium may antagonize the effects of calcium channel blockers.

Lab Tests: Calcium may increase values for blood pH and serum calcium. It may decrease serum phosphate and potassium levels and serum and urinary magnesium.

Herbal/Food: Zinc-rich foods may decrease the absorption of calcium. Alcohol, caffeine, and carbonated beverages affect the absorption of calcium. Oxalic acid in spinach, rhubarb, Swiss chard, and beets can suppress calcium absorption.

Treatment of Overdose: Measures may be taken to treat cardiac abnormalities caused by the resulting hypercalcemia.

If hypocalcemia occurs with normal dietary intake, GI causes must be examined, such as excessive vomiting or malabsorption disorders. Chronic kidney disease may cause excessive loss of calcium in the urine. Another etiology for hypocalcemia is decreased secretion of PTH, as occurs when the thyroid and parathyroid glands are diseased or surgically removed.

Drug therapy is occasionally a cause of hypocalcemia. Blood transfusions and certain anticonvulsants such as phenytoin can lower serum calcium levels. In addition, overtreatment with drugs used to *lower* serum calcium can result in "overshooting" normal levels. Some of these include furosemide (Lasix), phosphate therapy, or bisphosphonates (see section 48.4). Of special concern is long-term therapy with corticosteroids, which is a common cause of hypocalcemia and osteoporosis. To help prevent corticosteroid-induced osteoporosis, patients should receive daily supplements of calcium and vitamin D.

Minor to moderate hypocalcemia is often asymptomatic. Signs and symptoms of hypocalcemia are those of nerve and muscle excitability. Assessment may reveal muscle twitching, tremor, or abdominal cramping with hyperactive bowel sounds. Numbness and tingling of the extremities may occur, and convulsions are possible. Confusion and abnormal behavior may be observed. Hypocalcemia is associated with various types of cardiac dysrhythmias.

Unless the hypocalcemia is severe or life threatening, nutritional adjustments should be attempted prior to initiating therapy with calcium supplements. Increasing the consumption of calcium-rich foods, especially dairy products, fortified orange juice, cereals, and green leafy vegetables, is often sufficient to restore calcium balance.

If a change in diet is not practical or has not proved adequate for reversing the hypocalcemia, effective and inexpensive calcium supplements are readily available OTC in a variety of formulations. Calcium supplements often contain vitamin D. Severe hypocalcemia requires the IV administration of calcium salts.

In an adult, 99% of the body's calcium is bound as a hard matrix in bone. Although skeletal calcium is available for use by other tissues, turnover is relatively slow. When muscle, nerves or other tissues have an immediate need for calcium, it is taken from the plasma.

In the plasma, calcium occurs in the following forms:

- Ionized calcium: About 45% of calcium in the plasma is ionized or "free." Ionized calcium is considered its physiologically active form and is freely available for use by body tissues.
- Complexed calcium: About 10% of serum calcium is bonded to anions such as bicarbonate, lactate, and citrate. Like ionized calcium, complexed calcium is also able to diffuse into tissues.
- Bound calcium: About 45% of calcium is bound to albumin, the most abundant plasma protein. If bound to albumin, calcium is unable to diffuse into body tissues.

Calcium supplements consist of complexed calcium in salts such as carbonate, lactate, or phosphate. The amount of calcium in a tablet will differ, depending upon its salt. For example a 1,000 mg tablet of calcium carbonate contains 400 mg of calcium (the other 600 mg is carbonate). On the other hand a 1,000 mg tablet of calcium citrate only contains 200 mg calcium (the other 800 mg is citrate). As can be seen by this example, a 1,000 mg dose of a calcium salt will deliver a varied amount of calcium, depending upon the anion it is complexed with. This calcium dose is known as *elemental* calcium and is always listed on the product label. Table 48.1 lists example calcium supplements.

METABOLIC BONE DISEASES

48.3 Pathophysiology of Metabolic Bone Diseases

Metabolic bone disease (MBD) is a general term referring to a cluster of disorders that have in common defects in the structure of bone. MBDs are caused by abnormal amounts of the minerals or hormones required for proper bone homeostasis, such as calcium, phosphate, vitamin D, or PTH. Some MBDs have a genetic etiology, whereas others are caused by certain drugs and therapies. The three most common MBDs are osteoporosis, osteomalacia, and Paget's disease.

Osteoporosis, the most common MBD, is responsible for the majority of bone fractures in postmenopausal women. Osteoporosis occurs when bone is resorbed (lost) at a greater rate than it is deposited (gained). This disorder is usually asymptomatic until the bones become brittle enough to fracture or vertebrae to collapse. The following are risk factors for osteoporosis:

- Menopause
- Age over 60
- Family history of osteoporosis
- High alcohol consumption
- Anorexia nervosa
- Smoking history
- Physical inactivity
- Testosterone deficiency
- Low vitamin D or calcium in the diet
- Drugs such as corticosteroids, some anticonvulsants, and immunosuppressants that lower serum calcium levels.

The greatest risk factor associated with the development of osteoporosis is the onset of menopause. When women reach menopause, estrogen secretion declines, and bones become weak and fragile. One theory to explain this occurrence is that estrogen limits the life span of osteoclasts,

Table 48.1 Selected Calcium Salts and Vitamin D Therapies

Drug	Route and Adult Dose (max dose where indicated)	Adverse Effects
CALCIUM SUPPLEMENTS (DOSES ARE IN TERMS OF ELEMENTAL CALCIUM)		
calcium acetate (PhosLo)	PO: 2–4 tablets with each meal (each tablet contains 169 mg calcium)	*Constipation, nausea, vomiting, metallic taste*
calcium carbonate (Rolaids, Tums, others)	PO: 1–2 g bid–tid	
calcium chloride	IV: 0.5–1 g every 1-3 days	Serious adverse effects are observed only with IV administration. Hypercalcemia (drowsiness, lethargy, headache, anorexia, nausea and vomiting, increased urination, and thirst), dysrhythmias, cardiac arrest, confusion, delirium, stupor, coma
calcium citrate (Citracal)	PO: 1–2 g bid–tid	
calcium gluconate (Kalcinate)	PO: 0.5–2 g bid–tid IV: 0.5–4 g by slow infusions (1 g/h)	
calcium lactate (Cal-Lac)	PO: 325–650 mg tid before meals	
calcium phosphate tribasic (Posture)	PO: 1–2 g bid–tid	
VITAMIN D SUPPLEMENTS		
calcitriol (Calcijex, Rocaltrol)	PO: 0.25 mcg/day IV: 0.5 mcg three times/wk	*Side effects are not observed at normal doses.*
doxercalciferol (Hectorol)	PO: 10 mcg, three times/wk (max: 60 mcg/wk) IV: 4 mcg, three times/wk (max: 18 mcg/wk)	Overdose produces signs of hypercalcemia, bone pain, lethargy, anorexia, nausea and vomiting, increased urination, hallucinations, and dysrhythmias
ergocalciferol (Calciferol, Drisdol)	PO: 15–25 mcg/day	
paricalcitol (Zemplar)	IV: 0.04–0.1 mcg/kg, every other day (max: 24 mcg/kg) PO: 1–4 mcg every other day or three times per week	

Note: *Italics* indicate common adverse effects; underlining indicates serious adverse effects.

the bone cells that resorb bone. When estrogen levels fall, osteoclast activity is no longer controlled and bone demineralization is accelerated, resulting in loss of bone density. In women with osteoporosis, fractures often occur in the hips, wrists, forearms, or spine. The metabolism of calcium in osteoporosis is illustrated in Figure 48.3.

Osteomalacia is characterized by softening of bones due to demineralization. Worldwide, the most frequent cause of osteomalacia is a deficiency of vitamin D and calcium in the diet. This risk factor for the disease, however, is rare in the United States because many processed foods in this country are fortified with these vitamins. In the United States, osteomalacia is most prevalent in older adults, in premature infants, and in individuals on strict vegetarian or vegan diets. The term *osteomalacia* is usually used for adults with this MBD; if it occurs in children, it is called *rickets*.

Signs and symptoms of osteomalacia include hypocalcemia, muscle weakness, muscle spasms, and diffuse bone pain, especially in the hip area. Patients may also experience pain in the arms, legs, and spine. Classic signs of rickets in children include bowlegs and a pigeon breast. Children may also develop a slight fever and become restless at night. In extreme cases, surgical corrections of disfigured limbs may be required.

Paget's disease, or osteitis deformans, is a chronic condition characterized by accelerated remodeling of the skeleton, producing enlarged and softened bones. With this disorder, the processes of bone resorption and bone formation occur simultaneously but at a very high rate. The

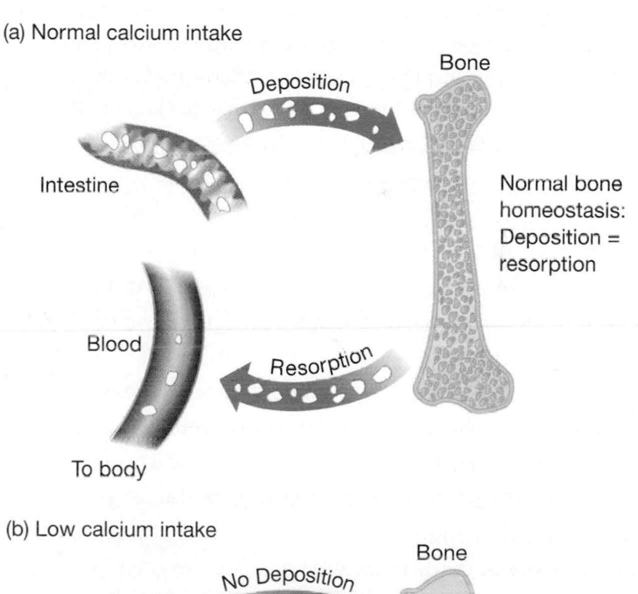

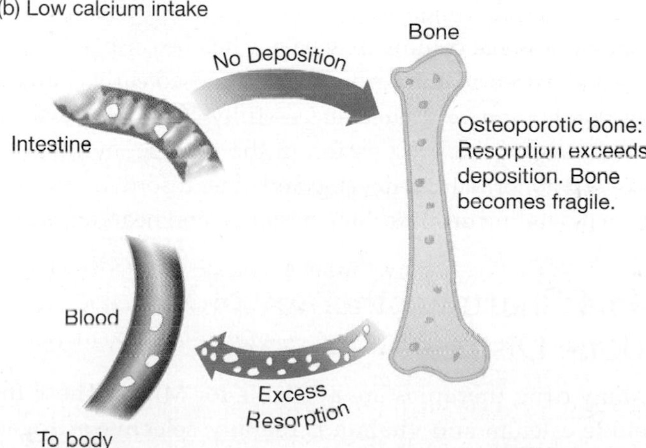

FIGURE 48.3 Calcium metabolism in osteoporosis: (a) normal calcium intake; (b) low calcium intake resulting in osteoporosis

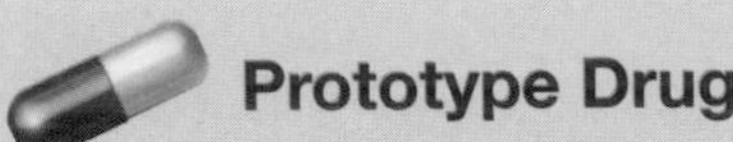

Prototype Drug | Calcitriol (*Calcijex, Rocaltrol*)

Therapeutic Class: Vitamin D **Pharmacologic Class:** Bone resorption inhibitor

Actions and Uses

Calcitriol is the active form of vitamin D. It promotes the intestinal absorption of calcium and elevates serum levels of calcium. This medication is indicated for patients with chronic kidney disease or hypoparathyroidism. Calcitriol reduces bone resorption and is used off-label to treat rickets. The effectiveness of calcitriol depends on an adequate amount of calcium; therefore, it is usually prescribed in combination with calcium supplements. It is available as oral tablets and solutions and by the IV route.

Administration Alerts

- Protect capsules from light and heat.
- Pregnancy category C.

PHARMACOKINETICS (PO)

Onset	Peak	Duration
2–6 h	10–12 h	3–5 days

Adverse Effects

Vitamin D therapy may cause symptoms of hypercalcemia. Early symptoms of hypercalcemia include weakness, confusion, anorexia, nausea, and vomiting. Later signs include increased urination, dysrhythmias, dehydration, and weight loss. At first sign of hypercalcemia, vitamin D therapy should be discontinued, and daily serum calcium levels should be obtained until the hypercalcemia is resolved.

Contraindications: This drug should not be given to patients with hypercalcemia or with evidence of vitamin D toxicity.

Interactions

Drug–Drug: Thiazide diuretics may enhance the effects of vitamin D, causing hypercalcemia. Too much vitamin D may cause dysrhythmias in patients who are receiving digoxin. Magnesium antacids or supplements should not be given concurrently due to the increased risk of hypermagnesemia.

Lab Tests: Vitamin D may increase serum cholesterol, phosphate, magnesium, or calcium values. It may decrease values for alkaline phosphatase.

Herbal/Food: Ingestion of large amounts of calcium-rich foods with vitamin D may cause hypercalcemia.

Treatment of Overdose: Vitamin D overdose results in hypercalcemia, hypercalciuria, and hyperphosphatemia. The patient is treated symptomatically and placed on a low-calcium diet until symptoms resolve.

rapid turnover causes new bone to be weak and brittle, resulting in deformities and fractures. The cause of Paget's disease is unknown.

Although many patients with Paget's disease are asymptomatic, approximately 10% experience vague, nonspecific complaints that include pain of the hips and femurs, joint inflammation, headaches, facial pain, and hearing loss if bones around the ear are affected. Nerves along the spinal column may be pinched because of the abnormal vertebral bone growth. If diagnosed early enough, symptoms can be treated successfully. If the diagnosis is made late in the progression of the disease, permanent skeletal abnormalities develop and other disorders may appear, including arthritis, kidney stones, and heart disease.

48.4 Pharmacotherapy of Metabolic Bone Diseases

Many drug therapies are available for MBDs. These include calcium and vitamin D therapy, selective estrogen receptor modulators, bisphosphonates, and calcitonin. A few miscellaneous drugs may be used if the primary drug classes fail to provide an adequate response. Some of the drug classes for MBD are also used for conditions unrelated to the skeletal system. Selected drugs for MBD are listed in Table 48.2.

Vitamin D Therapy

Drug therapy for children and adults consists of calcium supplements and vitamin D. Several forms of vitamin D are available for therapy. Three of those products—ergocalciferol, cholecalciferol, and calcitriol— are identical to the forms of vitamin D that occur in nature. Each vitamin D product has a slightly different potency and pharmacokinetics. These medications are summarized in Table 48.1.

The daily vitamin D needs of people vary depending on how much sunlight is received. After age 70, the average recommended intake of vitamin D increases from 400 units/day to 600 units/day. Patients with severe malabsorption disorders may receive 50,000 to 100,000 units/day. Because vitamin D is needed to absorb calcium from the GI tract, many supplements combine vitamin D and calcium into a single tablet.

Vitamin D is a fat-soluble vitamin that is stored by the body; therefore, it is possible to consume too much of this

Table 48.2 Selected Drugs for Osteoporosis and Other Bone Disorders

Drug	Route and Adult Dose (max dose where indicated)	Adverse Effects
BISPHOSPHONATES		
alendronate (Fosamax)	Osteoporosis: PO: 5–10 mg/day Paget's disease: PO: 40 mg/day for 6 months	*Nausea, dyspepsia, diarrhea, bone pain, back pain* Bone fractures, nephrotoxicity, hypocalcemia, hypophosphatemia, gastric ulcer, esophageal perforation, dysrhythmias, anemia, osteonecrosis of the jaw, atrial fibrillation
etidronate (Didronel)	PO: 5–10 mg/kg/day for 6 months or 11–20 mg/kg/day for 3 months	
ibandronate (Boniva)	PO: 2.5 mg/day or one 150-mg tablet per month, taken on the same date each month	
pamidronate (Aredia)	IV: 30–90 mg/day	
risedronate (Actonel, Atelvia)	PO (Actonel): 5 mg/day or 35 mg/wk at least 30 min before the first drink or meal of the day PO (Atelvia): 35 mg/wk taken immediately after the first meal of the day	
tiludronate (Skelid)	PO: 400 mg/day taken with 6–8 oz of water 2 h before or after food for 3 months	
zoledronate (Reclast, Zometa)	IV (Reclast): one 5-mg dose per year infused over at least 15 min IV (Zometa): 4-mg single dose infused over at least 15 min. May be repeated every 3–4 wk for cancer	
OTHER DRUGS		
bazedoxifene with conjugated estrogens (Duavee)	PO: 20 mg/0.45 mg (1 tablet)/day	*Muscle spasms, nausea, diarrhea, dyspepsia* From estrogen component: Stroke, deep vein thrombosis, endometrial hyperplasia
calcitonin—salmon (Fortical, Miacalcin)	Hypercalcemia: subcutaneous/IM: 4 international units/kg bid Osteoporosis: intranasal: 1 spray/day (200 international units) in one nostril, alternating nostrils each day	*Rhinitis, flushing of the face and hands, pain at the injection site* Anaphylaxis
cinacalcet (Sensipar)	PO: 30 mg once daily; may increase every 2–4 wk (max: 300 mg/day)	*Dizziness, noncardiac chest pain, hypertension, nausea, anorexia, hypocalcemia, myalgia* Hypocalcemia, seizures
denosumab (Prolia, Xgeva)	Subcutaneous (Prolia): 60 mg every 6 months Subcutaneous (Xgen): 120 mg every 4 wk	*Fatigue, asthenia, hypophosphatemia, nausea, hypercholesterolemia, musculoskeletal pain, and cystitis* Hypocalcemia, serious infections, osteonecrosis of jaw
raloxifene (Evista)	PO: 60 mg/day	*Hot flashes, sinusitis, flulike symptoms, nausea* Breast pain, vaginal bleeding, pneumonia, chest pain
teriparatide (Forteo)	Subcutaneous: 20 mcg/day	*Dizziness, depression, insomnia, vertigo, rhinitis, increased cough, leg cramps, nausea, arthralgia* Syncope, angina

Note: Italics indicate common adverse effects; underlining indicates serious adverse effects.

vitamin or to show signs of overdose from prescription or OTC medications. Excess vitamin D will cause calcium to leave bones and enter the blood. Signs and symptoms of hypercalcemia, such as anorexia, vomiting, excessive thirst, fatigue, and confusion, may become evident. Kidney stones may occur, and bones may fracture easily. The protoype medication for vitamin D is Calcitriol (Calcijex, Rocaltrol).

☑ Check Your Understanding 48.1

Is the amount of calcium available in a calcium supplement always the same? What is the difference? *Visit www.pearsonhighered.com/nursingresources for the answer.*

Bisphosphonates

The most frequently prescribed drug class for osteoporosis is the **bisphosphonates.** These drugs structurally resemble pyrophosphate, a natural substance that inhibits the

PharmFacts

OSTEOPOROSIS

- About 10 million Americans have osteoporosis and another 43 million have low bone density, which places them at risk for this disorder.
- Each year in the United States, about 2 million osteoporosis-related fractures occur, with about half being in the spine.
- Women are four times more likely to develop osteoporosis than men: 80% of all osteoporosis-related hip fractures occur in women.
- One of every two women and one of every four men over age 50 are likely to develop a fracture related to osteoporosis.

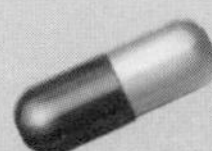

Prototype Drug | Alendronate *(Fosamax)*

Therapeutic Class: Drug for osteoporosis **Pharmacologic Class:** Bisphosphonate; bone resorption inhibitor

Actions and Uses

Alendronate lowers ALP, the enzyme associated with bone turnover. The most frequently prescribed drug in this class, it is approved for the following indications:

- Prevention and treatment of osteoporosis in postmenopausal women
- Treatment of corticosteroid-induced osteoporosis in both women and men
- Treatment to increase bone mass in men with osteoporosis
- Treatment of symptomatic Paget's disease in both women and men.

Several regimens for alendronate are available: once daily (10 mg), twice weekly (35 mg), or once weekly (70 mg). Although the once-weekly regimen is more convenient, higher doses can result in an increased incidence of GI-related side effects. All doses must be taken on an empty stomach, preferably in a fasting state 2 hours before breakfast. Therapeutic effects of alendronate may take 1 to 3 months to appear and may continue for several months after therapy is discontinued. Fosamax plus D combines alendronate and vitamin D into a single tablet.

Administration Alerts

- Take on an empty stomach with plain water, preferably 2 hours before breakfast.
- Remain in an upright position for at least 30 minutes after a dose and until after the first food of the day to reduce esophageal irritation.
- Pregnancy category C.

PHARMACOKINETICS

Onset	Peak	Duration
3–6 wks	3–6 months	12 wks after discontinuation

Adverse Effects

Adverse effects of alendronate are diarrhea, constipation, flatulence, nausea, vomiting, metallic taste, hypocalcemia, hypophosphatemia, abdominal pain, dyspepsia, arthralgia, myalgia, headache, and rash. Pathologic fractures may occur if the drug is taken longer than 3 months or in cases of chronic overdose.

Contraindications: Contraindications include patients with osteomalacia or abnormalities of the esophagus or who have hypersensitivity to the drug. Caution should be used in patients with renal impairment, heart failure, hyperphosphatemia, liver disease, fever or infection, active upper GI problems, and pregnancy.

Interactions

Drug–Drug: Calcium, iron, antacids containing aluminum or magnesium, and certain mineral supplements interfere with the absorption of alendronate and have the potential to decrease its effectiveness. Use with alcohol may increase the risk of osteoporosis and cause gastric irritation.

Lab Tests: Unknown.

Herbal/Food: The diet must have adequate amounts of vitamin D, calcium, and phosphates. Excessive amounts of calcium supplements or dairy products reduce alendronate absorption.

Treatment of Overdose: Hypocalcemia is an expected effect and may be treated with PO or IV calcium salts.

breakdown of bone. Bisphosphonates inhibit bone resorption by suppressing osteoclast activity, thus increasing bone density and reducing the incidence of fractures by about 50%. In addition to treating postmenopausal osteoporosis, some of the bisphosphonates are approved to treat corticosteroid-induced osteoporosis and osteoporosis in men.

The beneficial effects of bisphosphonates on bone mass density increase rapidly during the first year of therapy and plateau after 2 to 3 years. After discontinuation of therapy, bone density will remain increased for up to a year. For optimal effects, the patient must have adequate dietary consumption of calcium and vitamin D. Any deficiencies in this vitamin should be corrected prior to initiating bisphosphonate therapy. Research studies suggest that once-weekly dosing with bisphosphonates may give the same bone density benefits as daily dosing because of the extended duration of drug action.

Bisphosphonates are also preferred drugs for treating Paget's disease. Pharmacotherapy of this MBD is usually cyclic, with bisphosphonates administered until serum alkaline phosphatase (ALP) levels return to normal, followed by several months without the drugs. When the serum ALP level becomes elevated, therapy is begun again. The pharmacologic goals are to slow the rate of bone resorption and encourage the deposition of strong bone. Patients with Paget's disease should maintain adequate calcium and vitamin D in the diet or with supplements on a daily basis.

Several bisphosphonates are approved to treat bone metastases and the severe hypercalcemia that accompanies

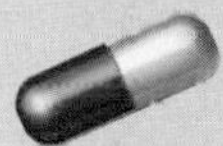

Prototype Drug | Raloxifene *(Evista)*

Therapeutic Class: Drug for osteoporosis prevention **Pharmacologic Class:** Selective estrogen receptor modulator

Actions and Uses

Raloxifene is a SERM. It decreases bone resorption and increases bone mass and density by acting through the estrogen receptor. Raloxifene is primarily used for the prevention of osteoporosis in postmenopausal women. Although the drug reduces vertebral fractures caused by osteoporosis of the spine, it does not appear to reduce the incidence of fractures at nonvertebral sites. This drug also reduces serum total cholesterol and low-density lipoprotein (LDL) without lowering high-density lipoprotein (HDL) or triglycerides.

In 2007, raloxifene was approved for invasive breast cancer prophylaxis in postmenopausal women at high risk for breast cancer. It is important for nurses and their patients to understand that this drug is for the prevention, not treatment, of breast carcinoma.

Administration Alerts

- Give with or without food.
- Pregnancy category X.

PHARMACOKINETICS

Onset	Peak	Duration
8 wk	Unknown	Unknown

Adverse Effects

The most common adverse effects of raloxifene therapy are hot flashes, leg cramps, and weight gain. Less common effects include fever, arthralgia, depression, insomnia, chest pain, peripheral edema, decreased serum cholesterol, nausea, vomiting, flatulence, cystitis, migraines, flulike symptoms, endometrial disorder, breast pain, and vaginal bleeding.

Black Box Warning: Raloxifene increases the risk of venous thromboembolism and death from strokes. Women with a history of venous thromboembolism should not take this drug.

Contraindications: This drug is contraindicated during lactation and pregnancy and in women who may become pregnant. Patients with a history of venous thromboembolism and those who are hypersensitive to raloxifene should not take this drug.

Interactions

Drug–Drug: Concurrent use with warfarin may decrease prothrombin time. Decreased raloxifene absorption will result from concurrent use with ampicillin or cholestyramine. Use of raloxifene with other highly protein-bound drugs (ibuprofen, indomethacin, diazepam, etc.) may interfere with binding sites. Cholestyramine decreases the absorption of raloxifene. Raloxifene should be used with caution in patients receiving concurrent treatment with estrogen-containing drugs.

Lab Tests: Raloxifene increases values of apolipoprotein A_1, corticosteroid-binding globulin, and thyroxine-binding globulin. It may decrease values of cholesterol, fibrinogen, apolipoprotein B, and lipoprotein (a), calcium, phosphate, total protein, and albumin.

Herbal/Food: Black cohosh has estrogenic effects and may interfere with the actions of raloxifene.

Treatment of Overdose: There is no specific treatment for overdose.

some bone cancers. Zoledronate and pamidronate are used in patients who have bone metastases. By inhibiting the resorption of bone by osteoclasts, these drugs prevent skeletal-related events such as acute pain and fractures that often accompany bony metastases. They also prevent the severe hypercalcemia of malignancy that sometimes occurs when large amounts of calcium are released from bone due to excessive osteoclast activity. Zoledronate (Zometa) is also approved for the management of multiple myeloma.

The most frequent adverse effects of bisphosphonates include GI problems such as nausea, vomiting, abdominal pain, and esophageal irritation. One unusual adverse effect that may occur during bisphosphonate therapy is osteonecrosis of the jaw, which can result in jaw pain and swelling, loosening of teeth, and infection at the site of the lesion. Because they are poorly absorbed, most drugs in this class should be taken on an empty stomach as tolerated by the patient. To avoid esophageal irritation, the patient should stay in an upright position for at least 30 minutes following the dose.

Selective Estrogen Receptor Modulators

Selective estrogen receptor modulators (SERMs) are drugs that are used in the prevention and treatment of osteoporosis. When SERMs bind to estrogen receptors, they may activate or inhibit them. Thus, SERMs may be estrogen agonists or antagonists, depending on the specific drug and the tissue involved. For example, raloxifene (Evista) blocks estrogen receptors in the uterus and breast; it has no estrogen-like proliferative effects on these tissues that might promote cancer. Raloxifene does, however,

Nursing Practice Application
Pharmacotherapy for Osteoporosis

ASSESSMENT	POTENTIAL NURSING DIAGNOSES*
Baseline assessment prior to administration: • Obtain a complete health history including musculoskeletal, GI, cardiovascular, neurologic, endocrine, hepatic, or renal disease. Obtain a drug history including allergies, current prescription and OTC drugs, herbal preparations, alcohol use, or smoking. Be alert to possible drug interactions. • Obtain a history of any current symptoms and effect on activities of daily living (ADLs). Assess muscle strength and gait, and note any pain or discomfort on movement or at rest. Obtain bone density studies as ordered. • Obtain a dietary history, noting adequacy of essential vitamins, minerals, and nutrients obtained through food sources, particularly calcium, vitamin D, and magnesium. Note the amount of daily soda and other nondairy beverage intake. • Note sunscreen use and the amount of sun exposure. • Obtain baseline height, weight, and vital signs. • Evaluate appropriate laboratory findings (e.g., complete blood count [CBC]; electrolytes; calcium, phosphorus, and magnesium levels; hepatic and renal function studies).	• *Acute or Chronic Pain* (bone or joints) • *Deficient Knowledge* (drug therapy) • *Risk for Injury,* related to adverse drug effects • *Risk for Falls,* related to adverse drug effects *NANDA I © 2014
Assessment throughout administration: • Assess for desired therapeutic effects (e.g., calcium, phosphate, and magnesium levels are within normal limits; bone density studies show improvement). • Continue monitoring laboratory values as appropriate, especially calcium, phosphorus, and magnesium. • Assess for and promptly report adverse effects: nausea, vomiting, abdominal pain, esophageal irritation, constipation or diarrhea, and electrolyte imbalances. Immediately report any severe GI irritation or pain.	

IMPLEMENTATION

Interventions and (Rationales)	Patient-Centered Care
Ensuring therapeutic effects: • Review the dietary history with the patient and discuss food source options for correcting any calcium or vitamin D deficiencies. Encourage the patient to adopt a healthy lifestyle. (Adequate amounts of calcium, vitamin D, and magnesium are needed for bone health. Any deficiencies should be corrected before bisphosphonates are started. Adequate sun exposure may assist in vitamin D formation. Excessive soda, caffeine, or other nondairy beverage intake may increase the risk of osteoporosis.)	• Encourage adequate amounts of calcium, vitamin D, and magnesium from food sources. Provide educational pamphlets or Web-based references to reputable sources. **Collaboration:** Provide dietitian referral as needed. • Encourage limited amounts of sun exposure daily without sunscreens, approximately 15 to 20 minutes. Discourage prolonged sun exposure. • Teach the patient to avoid excessive soda intake which may take the place of healthier beverages with milk or dairy. Excessive caffeine consumption may diminish the absorption of dietary calcium. • Encourage adequate activity, especially weight-bearing exercise, three to five times per week.
• Follow administration guidelines for optimal results. (Calcium supplements and vitamin D should be taken with meals or within 1 hour after meals. Bisphosphonates should be taken on an empty stomach with a full glass of water and the patient should remain upright for 30 minutes to 1 hour. Bisphosphonates and calcium preparations should be taken 2 hours apart.)	• Teach the patient appropriate administration guidelines. Ensure that the patient is able to remain upright after administration if bisphosphonates are used.
Minimizing adverse effects: • Monitor for GI irritation or abdominal pain. (Bisphosphonates may cause esophageal irritation and erosion. Increasing nausea and gastric or abdominal pain should be reported immediately.)	• Instruct the patient to immediately report any new onset of nausea or any increasing or severe chest or abdominal discomfort or pain.

Nursing Practice Application *continued*

IMPLEMENTATION	
Interventions and (Rationales)	**Patient-Centered Care**
• Continue to monitor periodic laboratory work, especially calcium, magnesium, phosphorus levels, and creatinine as needed. Assess for signs or symptoms of hypo- or hypercalcemia. (Calcium, magnesium, and phosphorus levels should return to, and remain within normal limits. Increased creatinine levels may require discontinuation of medications.)	• Instruct the patient on the need to return periodically for laboratory work. • Instruct the patient to immediately report symptoms of hypocalcemia (muscle spasms, facial grimacing, irritability, hyper-reflexes) or hypercalcemia (increased bone pain, anorexia, nausea, vomiting, constipation, thirst, lethargy, fatigue).
• Increase fluid intake, avoiding caffeine, soda, and alcohol. (Increased fluid intake decreases the risk of renal calculi formation.)	• Encourage the patient to increase fluid intake to 2 L (2 qt) of fluid per day, divided throughout the day, but avoid highly caffeinated beverages and excessive soda intake. Limit or eliminate alcohol use.
• Monitor the use of vitamin D. Excessive intake may lead to toxic effects. (Fat-soluble vitamins are stored in the body and may accumulate and result in toxic levels. Monitor liver function studies and for symptoms such as nausea, vomiting, headache, fatigue, dry and itchy skin, blurred vision, or palpitations. Report any symptoms immediately.)	• Instruct the patient not to take additional or large amounts of vitamin D unless instructed by the provider. • Encourage the patient to obtain fat-soluble vitamins from natural sources through a balanced diet whenever possible.
• Note and promptly report any new-onset thigh or groin pain, unilaterally or bilaterally. (An increased incidence of atypical fractures has been noted in some patients taking bisphosphonates, particularly with long-term use or with concurrent corticosteroid use. Thigh or groin pain has been noted to occur prior to fracture and should be reported to the provider for assessment.)	• Teach the patient to promptly report any new onset of groin or thigh pain, either unilaterally or bilaterally. • Advise the patient to review the need for continued bisphosphonate use with the health care provider based on bone density studies on a regular basis.
• Monitor compliance with the recommended regimen. (Bone remodeling occurs over several months' time. The patient may discontinue the drug because of perceived lack of response.)	• Teach the patient to continue taking the drug therapy regularly to ensure full effects. Therapeutic response may take 1 to 3 months, and effects continue after the drug has been discontinued.
Patient understanding of drug therapy:	
• Use opportunities during administration of medications and during assessments to provide patient education. (Using time during nursing care helps to optimize and reinforce key teaching areas.)	• The patient should be able to state the reason for the drug; appropriate dose and scheduling; what adverse effects to observe for and when to report; and the anticipated length of medication therapy.
Patient self-administration of drug therapy:	
• When administering the medication, instruct the patient, family, or caregiver in the proper self-administration of the drug (e.g., taken with additional fluids). (Proper administration increases the effectiveness of the drugs.)	• The patient is able to discuss appropriate dosing and administration needs.

See Tables 48.1 and 48.2 for a list of drugs to which these nursing actions apply.

decrease bone resorption; thus, it increases bone density and reduces the likelihood of fractures. It is most effective at preventing vertebral fractures. The newest drug in this class is bazedoxifene, which is combined with conjugated estrogens and marketed as Duavee. Duavee was approved in 2013 to prevent postmenopausal osteoporosis and vasomotor symptoms associated with menopause. The two other SERMs, tamoxifen and toremifene (Fareston), are used to treat estrogen receptor-positive metastatic breast cancer (see chapter 38).

Calcitonin

Calcitonin is a hormone secreted by the thyroid gland when serum calcium is elevated. It acts in direct opposition to PTH and vitamin D to lower serum calcium levels. As a drug, it is approved for the treatment of osteoporosis in women who are more than 5 years postmenopausal. It is available by nasal spray (Fortical) or subcutaneous injection (Miacalcin). Calcitonin increases bone density and reduces the risk of vertebral fractures. Adverse effects are generally minor; the nasal formulation may irritate the nasal mucosa, and allergies are possible. Because the parenteral form causes nausea and vomiting, it is less commonly used than the intranasal form. In addition to treating osteoporosis, calcitonin is indicated for Paget's disease and hypercalcemia. For osteoporosis, calcitonin is less effective than other therapies and is considered a second-line treatment.

Other Drugs for Metabolic Bone Disease

Cinacalcet (Sensipar) is an oral calcium modifier approved to treat hypercalcemia caused by parathyroid gland cancer or for hyperparathyroidism due to chronic kidney disease. Cinacalcet is a calcium mimic; the drug is recognized as calcium by the parathyroid glands. When the drug is present, the parathyroid glands shut down the production of PTH, serum calcium falls, and bone resorption diminishes. Nausea, vomiting, and diarrhea are common during therapy.

Denosumab (Prolia, Xgen) is one of the newer drugs to treat MBD. It is approved for the treatment of postmenopausal women at high risk for fracture (Prolia) and for the prevention of skeletal-related events in patients with bone metastases with solid tumors. This drug is a monoclonal antibody, given by subcutaneous injection. Common adverse effects include fatigue, asthenia, hypophosphatemia, nausea, hypercholesterolemia, musculoskeletal pain, and cystitis. Because the drug can cause severe hypocalcemia, serum calcium levels should be monitored regularly and calcium supplements and vitamin D administered as necessary.

Teriparatide (Forteo) is human PTH, produced by recombinant DNA technology. The actions of teriparatide are identical to those of endogenous PTH. It is the only drug available that will increase bone formation. It is approved for the treatment of osteoporosis in men and postmenopausal women. The drug is usually reserved for patients with a high risk of bone fractures. A disadvantage of the drug is that it must be given daily by the subcutaneous route. The drug is well tolerated with dizziness and leg cramps being the most frequent adverse effects.

PharmFacts

ARTHRITIS

- Over 20 million Americans are affected by osteoarthritis.
- About 80–90% of people over the age of 65 have osteoarthritis.
- Of the world's population, 1% have rheumatoid arthritis, which most often affects patients between 30 and 50 years of age. Women are three times more likely to develop rheumatoid arthritis than men.
- Although gout affects less than 1% of the general population, the rate increases to 20% in those with a family history of the disorder.

JOINT DISORDERS

Joint conditions such as osteoarthritis, rheumatoid arthritis, and gout are frequent indications for pharmacotherapy. Because joint pain is common to all three disorders, analgesics and anti-inflammatory drugs are important components of pharmacotherapy. Pharmacotherapy Illustrated 48.1 shows the pathophysiology and pharmacotherapy of these disorders.

Depending on the cause of the pain, nonpharmacologic therapies are sometimes effective at relieving joint pain. The use of nonimpact and passive range-of-motion (ROM) exercises to maintain flexibility along with adequate rest is encouraged. Splinting may help keep joints positioned correctly and relieve pain. Other therapies commonly used to relieve pain and discomfort include thermal therapies, meditation, visualization, distraction techniques, and massage. Knowledge of proper body mechanics and posture may offer some benefit. Surgical procedures such as joint replacement and reconstructive surgery may become necessary when other methods are ineffective.

48.5 Pharmacotherapy of Osteoarthritis

Osteoarthritis (OA) is a progressive, degenerative joint disease caused by the breakdown of articular cartilage. As cartilage thins in the affected joints, there is less padding and, eventually, the underlying bone is affected. The bone thickens in the damaged areas, forming bone spurs that narrow the joint space. As these growths enlarge, small pieces may break off, leading to inflammation and

---

Complementary and Alternative Therapies

GLUCOSAMINE AND CHONDROITIN FOR OSTEOARTHRITIS

Glucosamine is a natural substance that is an important building block of cartilage. With aging, glucosamine is lost with the natural thinning of cartilage. As cartilage wears down, joints lose their normal cushioning ability, resulting in the pain and inflammation of OA. Glucosamine sulfate is available as an OTC dietary supplement. Some studies have shown it to be more effective than a placebo in reducing mild arthritis and joint pain. It is claimed to promote cartilage repair in the joints. A typical dose is 500 to 10,000 mg/day.

Chondroitin is another dietary supplement purported to promote cartilage repair. It is a natural substance that forms part of the matrix between cartilage cells. Chondroitin is safe and almost free of side effects. A typical dose is 400 to 1,500 mg/day for 1–2 months. Chondroitin is usually combined with glucosamine in specific arthritis formulas. Reviews of the research show that glucosamine and chondroitin may be effective for OA pain and prevent joint space narrowing, but the evidence is inconclusive (Fransen et al., 2015; Reginster, Neuprez, Lecart, Sarlet, & Bruyere, 2012).

Pharmacotherapy Illustrated

48.1 | Joint Disorders

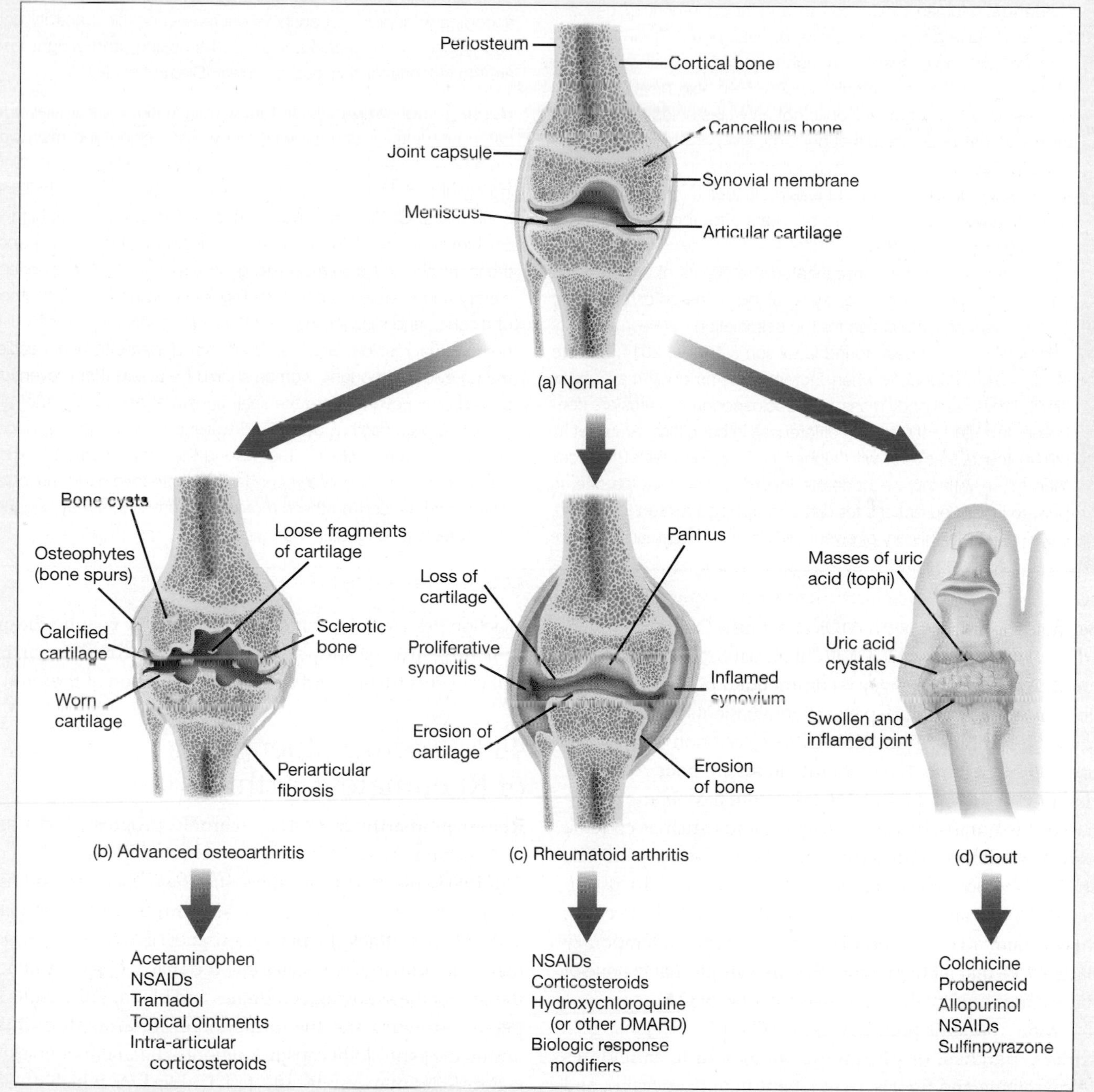

destruction of the synovial membrane lining the joint. The affected joint becomes unstable and more susceptible to injury, and partial joint dislocations and other deformities may occur.

Osteoarthritis is the most common type of joint disease. Weight-bearing joints such as the knee, spine, and hip are most frequently affected. Symptoms include localized pain and stiffness, joint and bone enlargement, and reduced range of movement. OA is not accompanied by the severe degree of inflammation associated with other forms of arthritis. Many consider this condition to be a normal part of the aging process.

The goals of pharmacotherapy for OA include reduction of pain and inflammation. The initial treatment of choice is acetaminophen because it is inexpensive and relatively safe. For patients whose pain is unrelieved by acetaminophen, nonsteroidal anti-inflammatory drugs (NSAIDs), including naproxen and ibuprofen-like drugs, are usually given.

Evidence-Based Practice: Predicting Bone Loss

Clinical Question: Does ethnicity influence bone loss or do other factors have effects?

Evidence: Women of Caucasian and Asian American descent appear to have a higher incidence of osteoporosis than those of African American descent, although postmenopausal women are at the highest risk in all ethnic groups. Men also develop osteoporosis, although the condition is not as well-studied in men as in women. It has been noted that bone mineral density (BMD) decline begins to accelerate in women approximately one year before the final menstrual period, and that loss continues to remain at a peak until it stabilizes around four to six years after the final menstrual period (Sowers et al., 2013).

Several studies have investigated the effects of ethnicity and other factors on the development of bone loss. For both men and women, no clear cause for the association between ethnicity and bone loss has been found (Jackson & Mysiw, 2014; Sowers et al., 2013), especially when factors such as body mass index (BMI), fat vs. lean body mass, and socioeconomic status are controlled. In a study of men and differences in bone loss, Araujo et al. (2014) found that men with higher incomes had less BMD loss than those with low or moderate incomes. This may be due, in part, to increased options for diet and exercise related to income. Physical activity, history of or current smoking habit, and BMI are also risk factors that predict fracture risk (Jackson & Mysiw, 2014). Finally, it appears that depression may increase the rate of bone loss, although whether depression itself, or the symptoms that accompany depression such as decreased physical activity and neuromuscular functioning, increased smoking, and weight loss are the reasons for this loss is unclear (Diem et al., 2013).

Nursing Implications: Even though medications are available to halt bone deterioration, prevention by establishing and maintaining a healthy lifestyle is the key to conquering osteoporosis. During childhood and adolescence, the focus should be on building bone mass. Children should be encouraged to eat foods high in calcium and vitamin D and to exercise regularly. During adulthood, the focus should be on maintaining bone mass, continuing healthy dietary and exercise habits, avoiding smoking and excessive use of alcohol, and maintaining treatment for conditions such as diabetes or depression. Because bone loss appears to begin earlier than previously thought, women should be aware that prevention should begin even before the final menstrual period. Diem et al., (2013) also found that decreased walking speed and the longer time to rise from a chair without using the arms seemed to suggest decreased bone loss secondary to decreased neuromuscular functioning. Observing these motor skills in patients may suggest further testing, such as BMD screening.

Because high doses of NSAIDs can cause GI bleeding and affect platelet aggregation, patients must be carefully monitored. Aspirin is no longer recommended because the high doses needed to produce pain relief in patients with OA may cause GI bleeding. Tramadol (Ultram) is a non-NSAID option for the treatment of moderate to severe pain. Although classified as an opioid, tramadol does not have abuse potential and is not a scheduled drug. Opioids such as codeine may be combined with acetaminophen for severe pain. The student should refer to chapter 18 for a complete discussion of the actions and side effects of analgesics. In acute cases, intra-articular corticosteroids may be used on a temporary basis. Note that all these therapies are symptomatic; none of these drugs modify the progressive course of OA.

Many patients with OA use OTC topical creams, gels, sprays, patches, or ointments that include salicylates (Aspercreme and Sportscreme), capsaicin (Capzasin), and counterirritants (Ben-Gay and Icy Hot). These therapies are well tolerated and have few side effects. Pennsaid is a prescription, topical form of the NSAID diclofenac that is rubbed on the knee for symptoms of OA.

For patients with moderate OA who do not respond adequately to analgesics, sodium hyaluronate (Hyalgan) is an option. This medication is a natural chemical found in high amounts within synovial fluid. Administered by injection directly into the knee joint, this drug replaces or supplements the body's natural hyaluronic acid that deteriorated because of the inflammation of OA. Treatment consists of one injection per week for three to five weeks. By coating the articulating cartilage surface, Hyalgan helps provide a barrier that prevents friction and further inflammation of the joint.

48.6 Pharmacotherapy of Rheumatoid Arthritis

Rheumatoid arthritis (RA) is a chronic, progressive disease that is characterized by disfigurement and inflammation of multiple joints. RA occurs at an earlier age than OA and has an autoimmune etiology. In RA, **autoantibodies** called *rheumatoid factors* attack the person's tissues, activating complement and drawing leukocytes into the area, where they attack the cells of the synovial membranes and blood. This results in persistent injury and the formation of inflammatory fluid within the joints. Joint capsules, tendons, ligaments, and skeletal muscles may also be affected. Unlike OA, which causes local pain in affected joints, RA may produce systemic manifestations that include infections, pulmonary disease, pericarditis, abnormal numbers of blood cells, and symptoms of metabolic dysfunction such as fatigue, fever, and anorexia.

The primary goals of RA pharmacotherapy are to control inflammation, reduce pain, and minimize physical disability. Pharmacotherapy for the relief of pain associated with RA is begun with NSAIDs, because these medications relieve both pain and inflammation. NSAIDs for patients with RA are usually given in higher doses than those for patients with OA. Aspirin is not recommended for long-term

Table 48.3 Selected Disease-Modifying Antirheumatic Drugs (DMARDs)

Drug	Route and Adult Dose (max dose where indicated)	Adverse Effects
BIOLOGIC THERAPIES		
abatacept (Orencia)	IV: 500–1,000 mg given on 0, 2, and 4 wk, then every 4 wk thereafter	*Local reactions at the injection site (pain, erythema, myalgia), headache, nasopharyngitis*
adalimumab (Humira)	Subcutaneous: 40 mg every other wk	Opportunistic infections (including tuberculosis [TB], sepsis, hepatitis B reactivation, and invasive fungal infections), lupus-like syndrome, tumor lysis syndrome (rituximab), worsening of heart failure (certolizumab, infliximab), Stevens–Johnson syndrome, hepatotoxicity (leflunomide, infliximab), malignancies (especially lymphomas)
anakinra (Kineret)	Subcutaneous: 100 mg/day	
certolizumab pegol (Cimzia)	Subcutaneous: 400 mg initially and at weeks 2 and 4, followed by 200 mg every other wk	
etanercept (Enbrel)	Subcutaneous: 25 mg twice weekly; or 0.08 mg/kg or 50 mg once weekly	
golimumab (Simponi)	Subcutaneous: 50 mg once monthly	
infliximab (Remicade)	IV: 3 mg/kg at weeks 0, 2, and 6, then every 8 wk	
rituximab (Rituxan)	IV: 1,000 mg every 2 wk for a total of two doses	
tocilizumab (Actemra)	IV: 4–8 mg/kg every other week Subcutaneous; 162 mg every other week	
tofacitinib (Xeljanz)	PO: 5 mg bid	
NONBIOLOGIC THERAPIES		
azathioprine (Azasan, Imuran)	PO: 1 mg/kg/day once or in divided doses bid for 6–8 wk (max: 2.5 mg/kg/day); Maintenance dose: 1–2.5 mg/kg/day as a single dose or divided	*Chills, fever, malaise, myalgia* Myelosuppression, hepatotoxicity, lymphoproliferative disorders
hydroxychloroquine (Plaquenil)	PO: 400–600 mg/day for 4–12 wk, then 200–400 mg once daily	*Anorexia, nausea, vomiting, headache, personality changes* Retinopathy, agranulocytosis, aplastic anemia, seizures
leflunomide (Arava)	PO: 100 mg loading dose for 3 days, then 20 mg/day	*Diarrhea, elevated hepatic enzymes, alopecia and rash* Hepatotoxicity, immunosuppression
methotrexate (Rheumatrex, Trexall) (see page 622 for the Prototype Drug box)	PO: 7.5 mg once/wk or 2.5 mg q12h for three doses once/wk (max: 20 mg/wk)	*Headache, glossitis, gingivitis, mild leukopenia, nausea* Ulcerative stomatitis, myelosuppression, aplastic anemia, hepatic cirrhosis, nephrotoxicity, sudden death, pulmonary fibrosis, agranulocytosis, hemolytic anemia, aplastic anemia, renal failure, teratogenicity
sulfasalazine (Azulfidine) (see page 701 for the Prototype Drug box)	PO: 1–2 g/day in four divided doses (max: 8 g/day)	*Headache, anorexia, nausea, vomiting* Anaphylaxis, Stevens–Johnson syndrome, agranulocytosis, leukopenia, reversible oligospermia

Note: *Italics* indicate common adverse effects; underlining indicates serious adverse effects.

therapy due to its adverse effects on the GI system and platelet aggregation. Acetaminophen is effective at relieving pain and fever but has no anti-inflammatory actions. Although these analgesics relieve symptomatic pain, they have little effect on disease progression. Because of their potent anti-inflammatory action, corticosteroids may be used for RA flare-ups but are not used for long-term therapy because of potential adverse effects such as increased susceptibility to infections, poor wound healing, and osteoporosis.

The progression of tissue damage caused by RA can be slowed or modified with a diverse group of drugs called **disease-modifying antirheumatic drugs (DMARDs).** Research has shown that these drugs improve symptoms, reduce mortality rates, and enhance the quality of life in patients with RA. Early therapy with DMARDs has become the standard of care in treating RA. Early treatment will result in better outcomes and can prevent joint damage that would otherwise be irreversible in the latter stages of RA. DMARDs are classified as biologic therapies or nonbiologic therapies. These medications and their adverse effects are listed in Table 48.3.

Therapy of RA occurs in a stepwise manner. Pharmacotherapy of patients with mild to moderate disease is begun as monotherapy with a nonbiologic DMARD, usually hydroxychloroquine (Plaquenil), methotrexate (Rheumatrex, Trexall), leflunomide (Arava), or sulfasalazine (Azulfidine). If symptoms have not improved or have worsened after 3 months of monotherapy, a second DMARD is added to the regimen. A third DMARD may be added for patients with persistent disease.

In patients with severe RA or those who have not responded to nonbiologic therapies, biologic therapies may be implemented. These biologic agents, most of which are

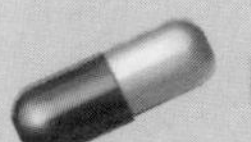

Prototype Drug | Hydroxychloroquine *(Plaquenil)*

Therapeutic Class: Antirheumatic drug; antimalarial **Pharmacologic Class:** Disease-modifying antirheumatic drug

Actions and Uses

Hydroxychloroquine is an older drug that is prescribed for RA and lupus erythematosus in patients who have not responded well to other anti-inflammatory drugs. This drug is also used for prophylaxis and treatment of malaria, but chloroquine (Aralen) is the preferred drug for this parasitic infection (see chapter 36). Hydroxychloroquine relieves the severe inflammation characteristic of these disorders, although its mechanism of action is not known. For full effectiveness, hydroxychloroquine is often prescribed with salicylates and corticosteroids.

Administration Alerts

- Take at the same time every day.
- Administer with milk to decrease GI upset.
- Store the drug in a safe place because it is very toxic to children.
- Pregnancy category C.

PHARMACOKINETICS

Onset	Peak	Duration
4–6 wk for antirheumatic response	1–2 h	Unknown

Adverse Effects

Adverse effects include anorexia, GI disturbances, loss of hair, headache, and mood and mental changes. Possible ocular effects include blurred vision, photophobia, diminished ability to read, and blacked-out areas in the visual field. With high doses or prolonged therapy, these retinal changes may be irreversible in some patients.

Contraindications: Patients who are hypersensitive to the drug or who exhibit retinal or visual field changes associated with quinoline drugs should not receive hydroxychloroquine.

Interactions

Drug–Drug: Antacids containing aluminum or magnesium may prevent absorption of hydroxychloroquine. Hydroxychloroquine may increase the risk of liver toxicity when administered with hepatotoxic drugs; alcohol use should be eliminated during therapy. This drug also may lead to increased digoxin levels and may interfere with the patient's response to rabies vaccine.

Lab Tests: Unknown.

Herbal/Food: Unknown.

Treatment of Overdose: Overdose may be life threatening, especially in children. Therapy with anticonvulsants, vasopressors, and antidysrhythmics may be necessary.

monoclonal antibodies, block steps in the inflammatory cascade, reduce joint inflammation, and slow the progression of joint damage. Adalimumab (Humira), etanercept (Enbrel), certolizumab (Cimzia), golimumab (Simponi), and infliximab (Remicade) are tumor necrosis factor (TNF) antagonists. TNF is a naturally occurring cytokine produced by macrophages and activated T cells that mediates inflammation and modulates cellular immune responses. The biologic agents are effective and relatively nontoxic but they are expensive and are not prescribed until conventional therapy has been attempted and failed. Combinations of biologic and nonbiologic agents may be necessary for some patients.

48.7 Pharmacotherapy of Gout

Gout is a form of acute arthritis caused by an accumulation of uric acid (urate) crystals in the joints and other body tissues, causing inflammation. Uric acid is a waste product created by the metabolic breakdown of DNA and RNA. Uric acid can accumulate in the body when there is increased metabolism of nucleic acids or when the kidneys cannot adequately excrete all the uric acid formed in the body. Xanthine oxidase is an important enzyme responsible for the formation of uric acid.

In patients with gout, uric acid accumulates and **hyperuricemia,** an elevated blood level of uric acid, occurs. Patients with mild hyperuricemia may be asymptomatic for many years. When serum uric acid rises to supersaturated levels, needlelike urate crystals form and symptoms appear, usually with a sudden onset. Acute symptoms most often occur in a lower extremity joint, especially the metatarsophalangeal joint of the big toe.

Gout is classified as primary or secondary. *Primary* gout is caused by a hereditary defect in uric acid metabolism that causes uric acid to be produced faster than it can be excreted by the kidneys. *Secondary* gout is caused by diseases or drugs that increase the metabolic turnover of nucleic acids or that interfere with uric acid excretion. Examples of drugs that may cause gout include thiazide diuretics, aspirin, cyclosporine, and alcohol when ingested on a chronic basis. Conditions that can cause secondary gout include diabetic ketoacidosis, kidney failure, and diseases associated with a rapid cell turnover such as leukemia and hemolytic anemia.

Acute gouty arthritis occurs when needlelike uric acid crystals accumulate in joints, resulting in extremely painful, red, and inflamed tissue. Attacks have a sudden onset, often occur at night, and may be triggered by ingestion of alcohol, dehydration, stress, injury to the joint, or fever. Of patients with gout, 90% are men. Kidney stones occur in 10% to 25% of patients with gout.

Treatment of Acute Gout

NSAIDs are the preferred drugs for treating the pain and inflammation associated with acute gout attacks. Indomethacin (Indocin) and naproxen (Naprosyn) are NSAIDs that have been widely used for acute gout. Corticosteroids may be used to treat exacerbations of acute gout, particularly when the symptoms are in a single joint, and the medication can be delivered intra-articularly.

Colchicine was the mainstay for treating acute gout attacks from the 1930s until the 1980s. Although it has important anti-inflammatory effects, the drug has a narrow therapeutic index and GI-related adverse effects occur in the majority of patients. At high doses, colchicine can cause bone marrow toxicity and aplastic anemia, leucopenia, thrombocytopenia, or agranulocytosis. The use of colchicine has declined, although it may still be prescribed for patients whose symptoms cannot be controlled with NSAIDs. Low doses may be prescribed for gout prophylaxis.

Treatment of Chronic Gout and Prophylaxis

Most patients with acute gout will experience subsequent attacks within 1 to 2 years after the first attack. Thus, long-term prophylactic therapy with drugs that lower serum

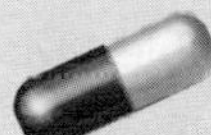

Prototype Drug | Allopurinol *(Lopurin, Zyloprim)*

Therapeutic Class: Drug for gout **Pharmacologic Class:** Xanthine oxidase inhibitor

Actions and Uses

Allopurinol is an older drug used to control the hyperuricemia that causes severe gout and to reduce the risk of acute gout attacks. It is also approved to prevent recurrent kidney stones in patients with elevated uric acid levels. It may be used prophylactically to reduce the severity of the hyperuricemia associated with antineoplastic and radiation therapies, both of which increase serum uric acid levels by promoting nucleic acid degradation. This drug takes 1 to 3 weeks to bring serum uric acid levels to within the normal range.

Allopurinol is available by the PO and IV routes. IV administration is usually reserved for patients with high uric acid levels resulting from cancer chemotherapy.

Administration Alerts

- Give with or after meals. Tablets may be crushed and mixed with food or fluids.
- Pregnancy category C.

PHARMACOKINETICS

Onset	Peak	Duration
12 h	30–120 min	Unknown

Adverse Effects

The most frequent and serious adverse effects are dermatologic. They include micropapular rash and rare cases of fatal toxic epidermal necrolysis and Stevens–Johnson syndrome. A rare, sometimes fatal, hypersensitivity syndrome may occur which includes a skin rash, fever, hepatitis, leukocytosis, and progressive renal failure. Other possible adverse effects include drowsiness, headache, vertigo, nausea, vomiting, abdominal discomfort, malaise, diarrhea, retinopathy, and thrombocytopenia.

Contraindications: Contraindications include hypersensitivity to allopurinol and idiopathic hemochromatosis. Use cautiously in patients with impaired hepatic or renal function, history of peptic ulcers, lower GI tract disease, bone marrow depression, and pregnancy.

Interactions

Drug–Drug: Alcohol may inhibit the renal excretion of uric acid. Ampicillin and amoxicillin may increase the risk of skin rashes. An enhanced anticoagulant effect may be seen with the use of warfarin, and toxicity risks increase for azathioprine, mercaptopurine, cyclophosphamide, and cyclosporine. The risk of ototoxicity is increased when allopurinol is used with thiazides and angiotensin-converting enzyme (ACE) inhibitors. Aluminum antacids taken concurrently with allopurinol may decrease its effects. An increased effect may be seen with phenytoin and anticancer drugs, necessitating the need for altered doses of these medications.

Lab Tests: Allopurinol may increase serum levels of ALP and serum transaminases. Hematocrit, hemoglobin, and leukocyte values may be decreased.

Herbal/Food: High purine foods may lower the effectiveness of allopurinol.

Treatment of Overdose: There is no specific therapy for overdose.

uric acid is often initiated. This can be accomplished through three strategies.

One strategy to prevent hyperuricemia is to use **uricosurics,** drugs that increase the excretion of uric acid by blocking its reabsorption in the kidney. The uricosuric drugs used for gout prophylaxis include probenecid (Probalan) and sulfinpyrazone (Anturane). These medications are effective in preventing hyperuricemia but they are not used to treat acute attacks of gouty arthritis because they have no analgesic or anti-inflammatory properties. These drugs may precipitate acute gout during the period of initial therapy because they mobilize the uric acid that has been stored in the tissues. The mobilization of uric acid may cause or worsen kidney stones due to the heavy burden of uric acid being excreted by the kidneys. To prevent these adverse effects of early therapy, the uricosurics are started at low doses and increased gradually over several weeks.

A second strategy for preventing hyperuricemia is to inhibit the formation of uric acid. The traditional drug for gout prophylaxis, allopurinol (Lopurin, Zyloprim), blocks the enzyme xanthine oxidase, thus inhibiting the formation of uric acid. A newer antigout drug, febuxostat (Uloric), acts by the same mechanism as allopurinol but is safer for patients with renal impairment because it is not excreted by the kidneys.

A third strategy for preventing hyperuricemia is to convert uric acid to a less toxic form. Two drugs are available that act by this mechanism. Rasburicase (Elitek) is an enzyme produced through recombinant DNA technology that is used to reduce uric acid levels in patients who are receiving cancer chemotherapy. The lysis of certain tumors sometimes releases large amounts of uric acid. Rasburicase is given IV for up to 5 days and carries a black box warning that severe hypersensitivity reactions, methemoglobinemia, and hemolysis may occur during therapy. Approved in 2010, pegloticase (Krystexxa) is a synthetic enzyme that metabolizes uric acid to an inert substance. It is used to lower uric acid levels in patients with chronic gout who have not responded to conventional therapies. The drug is administered by IV infusion once every 2 weeks and it carries a black box warning that anaphylaxis may occur during and after the infusion. Other common adverse effects include gout flares at the initiation of therapy, infusion reactions, nausea, ecchymosis, nasopharyngitis, and worsening of heart failure. Drugs for gout are listed in Table 48.4.

A plan for gout management should include dietary changes and avoidance of drugs that worsen the condition in addition to treatment with antigout medications. Patients should avoid high-purine foods such as meat, legumes, alcoholic beverages, mushrooms, and oatmeal, because nucleic acids will be formed when they are metabolized.

Table 48.4 Drugs for Gout

Drug	Route and Adult Dose (max dose where indicated)	Adverse Effects
allopurinol (Lopurin, Zyloprim)	PO: 100–800 mg/day	*Drowsiness, skin rash, diarrhea* Severe skin reactions, bone marrow depression, hepatotoxicity, renal failure
colchicine (Colcrys)	PO (gout flare): 1.2 mg at first sign of flare, followed by 0.6 mg q1–2h until pain is relieved PO (prophylaxis): 0.6 mg q12h (max: 1.2 mg/day)	*Nausea, vomiting, diarrhea, GI upset* Bone marrow depression, aplastic anemia, leukopenia, thrombocytopenia and agranulocytosis, severe diarrhea, nephrotoxicity
febuxostat (Uloric)	PO: 40–80 mg once daily	*Nausea, rash* Liver function abnormalities
pegloticase (Krystexxa)	IV: 8 mg every 2 wk by IV infusion	*Gout flare, nausea, ecchymosis, nasopharyngitis* Anaphylaxis, infusion reaction, worsening heart failure
probenecid (Probalan)	PO: 250 mg bid for 1 wk, then 500 mg bid (max: 3 g/day)	*Nausea, vomiting, headache, anorexia, flushed face* Anaphylaxis, severe skin reactions, hepatotoxicity
rasburicase (Elitek)	IV: 0.2 mg/kg over 30 min for up to 5 days	*Vomiting, nausea, pyrexia, peripheral edema, anxiety, headache, abdominal pain, constipation, diarrhea* Anaphylaxis, hemolysis, methemoglobinemia
sulfinpyrazone (Anturane)	PO: 100–200 mg bid for 1 wk, then increase to 200–400 mg bid	*GI distress, rash* Blood dyscrasias, nephrolithiasis

Note: Italics indicate common adverse effects; underlining indicates serious adverse effects.

Nursing Practice Application

Pharmacotherapy for Gout

ASSESSMENT	POTENTIAL NURSING DIAGNOSES*
Baseline assessment prior to administration: • Obtain a complete health history including musculoskeletal, GI, cardiovascular, neurologic, endocrine, hepatic, or renal disease. Obtain a drug history including allergies, current prescription and OTC drugs, herbal preparations, alcohol use, or smoking. Be alert to possible drug interactions. • Obtain a history of any current symptoms and effect on ADLs. Assess for inflammation and location, and note any pain or discomfort on movement or at rest. • Obtain a dietary history, noting correlations between food intake and increase in symptoms. Assess fluid intake. • Obtain baseline weight and vital signs. • Evaluate appropriate laboratory findings (e.g., uric acid level, CBC, hepatic and renal function studies, urinalysis).	• *Acute Pain* • *Activity Intolerance* • *Disturbed Body Image* • *Deficient Knowledge* (drug therapy) • *Risk for Injury*, related to adverse drug effects *NANDA I © 2014
Assessment throughout administration: • Assess for desired therapeutic effects depending on the reason for the drug (e.g., symptoms of acute inflammation are diminished or absent, no return of symptoms). • Continue monitoring of vital signs and urine output. • Continue to monitor uric acid level, CBC, and hepatic and renal studies. • Assess for and promptly report adverse effects: nausea, vomiting, abdominal pain, skin rash, pruritus, paresthesias, diminished urine output, fever, and infections.	

IMPLEMENTATION

Interventions and (Rationales)	Patient-Centered Care
Ensuring therapeutic effects:	
• Review the dietary history, noting any correlation between diet and symptoms, especially after ingestion of purine-containing foods. Avoid large doses of vitamin C. (Correlating symptoms to intake of high-purine foods assists in determining the most effective drug therapy. Large doses of vitamin C may acidify the urine, leading to formation of uric acid stones.)	• Encourage the patient to keep a food diary, noting any occurrence or increasing of symptoms related to food or beverage intake. • Teach the patient to limit intake of high-purine foods (e.g., salmon, sardines, organ meats, alcohol, mushrooms, legumes, oatmeal) and to limit or eliminate alcohol consumption.
• Increase fluid intake to 2 to 4 L (2 to 4 qt) per day. Monitor urine output and obtain periodic urinalysis. (Increased fluid intake increases uric acid excretion and prevents urinary uric acid crystal formation or renal calculi.)	• Teach the patient to increase fluid intake to 2 to 4 L (2 to 4 qt) per day, taken throughout the day.
• Continue to monitor serum and urinary uric acid levels and note improvement in symptoms of acute inflammation, gouty tophi, and improved movement with less pain of affected joints. (As uric acid levels decrease, inflammation due to uric acid crystals should improve.)	• Encourage the patient to maintain consistent drug dosing to ensure that uric acid levels are diminishing. • Instruct the patient on the need to return for periodic laboratory testing and urinalysis.
Minimizing adverse effects:	
• Monitor serum and urinary uric acid levels and symptoms associated with acute inflammatory period. (Continued or increasing inflammation may indicate the need for additional medication.)	• Instruct the patient to report any continued inflammation, pain, increased joint involvement, or general worsening of symptoms promptly.
• Monitor daily weight and urinary output. (Uric acid excretion may cause urate crystal formation in the kidneys with resulting renal impairment. Daily weight is an accurate measure of overall body fluid volume.)	• Instruct the patient to report any diminished urine output, changes in urine appearance, or flank pain, and to return periodically for urinalysis. • Have the patient weigh self daily at the same time each day and report any weight gain of over 1 kg (2 lb) in a 24-hour period to the health care provider.

continued

Nursing Practice Application *continued*

IMPLEMENTATION	
Interventions and (Rationales)	**Patient-Centered Care**
• Decrease the intake of purine-containing foods. Avoid large doses of vitamin C. (Intake of high-purine foods and alcohol may increase production of uric acid. Large doses of vitamin C may increase the formation of uric acid stones.)	• Teach the patient to avoid foods with a high purine content, decrease or eliminate alcohol consumption, and avoid increased vitamin C intake or supplementation. Provide a dietitian consult as needed.
• Observe for skin rashes, fever, stomatitis, flulike symptoms, or general malaise. (Bone marrow suppression may occur with antigout drugs and result in leukopenia and an increased risk of infection. Severe dermatologic reactions are possible and any skin rashes, especially with the appearance of blisters and discoloration, should be reported immediately.)	• Teach the patient to immediately report any flulike symptoms, fever, mouth irritation or soreness, or skin rashes.
Patient understanding of drug therapy: • Use opportunities during administration of medications and during assessments to provide patient education. (Using time during nursing care helps to optimize and reinforce key teaching areas.)	• The patient should be able to state the reason for the drug; appropriate dose and scheduling; what adverse effects to observe for and when to report; and the anticipated length of medication therapy.
Patient self-administration of drug therapy: • When administering the medication, instruct the patient, family, or caregiver in the proper self-administration of the drug (e.g., taken on an empty stomach or with meals, with additional fluids). (Proper administration increases the effectiveness of the drugs.)	• The patient is able to discuss appropriate dosing and administration needs, including taking medications at the first sign of gout attack. • Colchicine should be taken on an empty stomach. Other antigout medications should be taken with food or meals.

See Table 48.4 for a list of drugs to which these nursing actions apply.

Chapter Review

KEY Concepts

The numbered key concepts provide a succinct summary of the important points from the corresponding numbered section within the chapter. If any of these points are not clear, refer to the numbered section within the chapter for review.

48.1 Adequate levels of calcium in the body are necessary to properly transmit nerve impulses, prevent muscle spasms, and provide stability and movement. Adequate levels of vitamin D, parathyroid hormone, and calcitonin are also necessary for these functions.

48.2 Hypocalcemia is a serious condition that requires immediate therapy with calcium supplements, often concurrently with vitamin D.

48.3 Metabolic bone diseases (MBDs) occur when there is an imbalance of nutrients or hormones responsible for bone deposition and turnover. Three common MBDs include osteoporosis, osteomalacia, and Paget's disease.

48.4 Pharmacotherapy of MBD includes vitamin D, bisphosphonates, SERMs, calcitonin, and several miscellaneous medications.

48.5 For osteoarthritis, the main drug therapy is pain medication that includes acetaminophen, NSAIDs, or stronger analgesics.

48.6 Drug therapy for rheumatoid arthritis includes disease-modifying antirheumatic drugs (DMARDS). Therapy is begun with nonbiologic DMARDS and may progress to biologic therapies if the disease worsens.

48.7 Gout is characterized by a buildup of uric acid in either the blood or the joint cavities. Drug therapy includes agents that inhibit uric acid buildup or enhance its excretion.

REVIEW Questions

1. Which of the following teaching points will the nurse provide to a patient with a new prescription for alendronate (Fosamax)?
   1. Take the medication with a full glass of water 30 minutes before breakfast.
   2. Take the medication with a small snack or meal containing dairy.
   3. Take the medication immediately before bed.
   4. Take the medication with a calcium supplement.
2. Which assessment findings in a patient who is receiving calcitriol (Calcijex, Rocaltrol) should the nurse immediately report to the health care provider?
   1. Muscle aches, fever, dry mouth
   2. Tremor, abdominal cramping, hyperactive bowel sounds
   3. Bone pain, lethargy, anorexia
   4. Muscle twitching, numbness, and tingling of the extremities
3. The patient who is receiving allopurinol (Lopurin) for treatment of gout asks why he should avoid the consumption of alcohol. The nurse's response is based on the knowledge that the use of alcohol along with allopurinol may result in which of the following?
   1. It significantly increases the drug levels of allopurinol.
   2. It interferes with the absorption of antigout medications.
   3. It raises uric acid levels.
   4. It causes the urine to become more alkaline.
4. A patient has been taking hydroxychloroquine (Plaquenil) for rheumatoid arthritis. Which of the following symptoms may alert the nurse to a possible toxic effect?
   1. Cardiac dysrhythmias
   2. Joint stiffness or effusions
   3. Blurred vision or diminished ability to read
   4. Decreased muscle strength
5. The nurse is explaining to a student nurse the physiological principle for how colchicine (Colcrys) achieves its effect. What response will the nurse give to the student?
   1. It decreases the deposits of uric acid in the joint spaces.
   2. It reduces the pain associated with joint inflammation by uric acid crystals.
   3. It increases renal excretion of uric acid.
   4. It prevents the formation of uric acid in the liver.
6. A 62-year-old female has received a prescription for alendronate (Fosamax) for treatment of osteoporosis. The nurse would be concerned about this order if the patient reported which condition? (Select all that apply.)
   1. She enjoys milk, yogurt, and other dairy products and tries to consume some with each meal.
   2. She is unable to sit upright for prolonged periods because of severe back pain.
   3. She is lactose intolerant and rarely consumes dairy products.
   4. She has had trouble swallowing and has been told she has "problems with her esophagus."
   5. She has a cup of green tea every night before bed.

PATIENT-FOCUSED Case Study

A woman calls the health care provider's office, worried about her 82-year-old mother, Basanthi Singh. Mrs. Singh had a stroke 6 years ago and requires help with most ADLs. Since her husband's death 18 months ago, she rarely leaves home. She has lost 11 kg (25 lb) because she "just can't get interested" in her meals. She has never liked milk and now refuses to drink milk or eat dairy products. Mrs. Singh's daughter has been prescribed bisphosphonates, and wonders if her mother should also be on them.

1. What risk factors does Mrs. Singh have for osteoporosis and hypocalcemia?
2. What other factors should be considered before making a recommendation for an appointment to discuss a bisphosphonate prescription?

CRITICAL THINKING Questions

1. A young woman calls the triage nurse in her mother's health care provider's office with questions concerning her mother's medication. The mother, age 76, has been taking alendronate (Fosamax) after a bone density study revealed a decrease in bone mass. The daughter is worried that her mother may not be taking the drug correctly and asks for information to minimize the potential for drug adverse effects. What information should the triage nurse incorporate in a teaching plan regarding the oral administration of alendronate?

2. A 36-year-old man comes to the emergency department complaining of severe pain in the first joint of his right big toe. The triage nurse inspects the toe and notes that the joint is red, swollen, and extremely tender. Recognizing this as a typical presentation for acute gouty arthritis, what historical data should the nurse obtain relevant to this disease process?

Visit www.pearsonhighered.com/nursingresources for answers and rationales for all activities.

REFERENCES

Araujo, A. B., Yang, M., Suarez, E. A., Dagincourt, N., Chiu, G., Holick, M. F., . . . Zmuda, J. M. (2014). Racial/ethnic and socioeconomic differences in bone loss among men. *Journal of Bone and Mineral Research, 29,* 2552–2560. doi:10.1002/jbmr.2305

Diem, S. J., Harrison, S. L., Haney, E., Cauley, J. A., Stone, K. L., Orwoll, E., & Ensrud, K. E. (2013). Depressive symptoms and rates of bone loss at the hip in older men. *Osteoporosis International, 24,* 111–119. doi:10.1007/s00198-012-1975-0

Fransen, M., Agaliotis, M., Nairn, L., Votrubec, M., Bridgett, L., Su, S., . . . Day, R. (2015). Glucosamine and chondroitin for knee osteoarthritis: A double-blind randomized placebo-controlled clinical trial evaluating single and combination remedies. *Annals of the Rheumatic Diseases, 74,* 851–858. doi:10.1136/annrheumdis-2013-203954

Herdman, T. H., & Kamitsuru, S. (2014). *NANDA International nursing diagnoses: Definitions and classification, 2015–2017.* Oxford, United Kingdom: Wiley-Blackwell.

Jackson, R. D., & Mysiw, W. J. (2014). Insights into the epidemiology of postmenopausal osteoporosis: The Women's Health Initiative. *Seminars in Reproductive Medicine, 32,* 454–462. doi:10.1055/s-0034-1384629

Reginster, J., Neuprez, A., Lecart, M., Sarlet, N., & Bruyere, O. (2012). Role of glucosamine in the treatment for osteoarthritis. *Rheumatology International, 32,* 2959–2967. doi:10.1007/s00296-012-2416-2

Sowers, M. R., Zheng, H., Greendale, G. A., Neer, R. M., Cauley, J. A., Ellis, J., . . . Finkelstein, J. S. (2013). Changes in bone resorption across the menopausal transition: Effects of reproductive hormones, body size, and ethnicity. *Journal of Clinical Endocrinology and Metabolism, 98,* 2854–2863. doi:10.1210/jc.2012-4113

SELECTED BIBLIOGRAPHY

American College of Rheumatology. (2013). *Calcium pyrophosphate deposition disease (CPPD).* Retrieved from http://www.rheumatology.org/I-Am-A/Patient-Caregiver/Diseases-Conditions/Calcium-Pyrophosphate-Deposition-CPPD

Anderson, J., Caplan, L., Yazdany, J., Robbins, M. L., Neogi, T., Michaud, K., . . . Kazi, S. (2012). Rheumatoid arthritis disease activity measures: American College of Rheumatology recommendations for use in clinical practice. *Arthritis Care & Research, 64,* 640–647. doi:10.1002/acr.21649

Bethel, M. (2015). *Osteoporosis.* Retrieved from http://emedicine.medscape.com/article/330598-overview

Duque, G. (2013). Osteoporosis in older persons: Current pharmacotherapy and future directions. *Expert Opinion on Pharmacotherapy, 14,* 1949–1958. doi:10.1517/14656566.2013.822861

Gennari, L., Merlotti, D., Rendina, D., Gianfrancesco, F., Esposito, T., & Nuti, R. (2014). Paget's disease of bone: Epidemiology, pathogenesis and pharmacotherapy. *Expert Opinion on Orphan Drugs, 2,* 591–603. doi:10.1517/21678707.2014.904225

Islam, M. J., Yusuf, M. A., Hossain, M. S., & Ahmed, M. (2015). Updated management of osteoarthritis: A review. *Journal of Science Foundation, 11*(2), 49–55. doi:10.3329/jsf.v11i2.21597

Kumar, P., & Banik, S. (2013). Pharmacotherapy options in rheumatoid arthritis. *Clinical Medicine Insights: Arthritis and Musculoskeletal Disorders, 6,* 35. doi:10.4137/CMAMD.S5558

Lozada, C. J. (2014). *Osteoarthritis.* Retrieved from http://emedicine.medscape.com/article/330487-overview#a0156

Reid, M. C., Shengelia, R., & Parker, S. J. (2012). Pharmacologic management of osteoarthritis-related pain in older adults. *American Journal of Nursing, 112*(3), S38–S43. doi:10.1097/01.NAJ.0000412650.02926.e3

Rosman, Z., Shoenfeld, Y., & Zandman-Goddard, G. (2013). Biologic therapy for autoimmune diseases: An update. *BMC Medicine, 11,* 88. doi:10.1186/1741-7015-11-88

Ross, A. C., Manson, J. E., Abrams, S. A., Aloia, J. F., Brannon, P. M., Clinton, S. K., . . . Shapses, S. A. (2011). The 2011 report on dietary reference intakes for calcium and vitamin D from the Institute of Medicine: What clinicians need to know. *The Journal of Clinical Endocrinology & Metabolism, 96,* 53–58.

Rothschild, B. M. (2015). *Gout and pseudogout.* Retrieved from http://emedicine.medscape.com/article/329958-overview

Temprano, K. K. (2015). *Rheumatoid arthritis.* Retrieved from http://emedicine.medscape.com/article/331715-overview

Chapter 49

Drugs for Skin Disorders

Drugs at a Glance

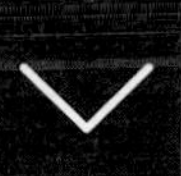

Learning Outcomes

After reading this chapter, the student should be able to:

1. Identify the structure and functions of the skin and associated structures.
2. Explain the process by which superficial skin cells are replaced.
3. Describe drug therapies for skin infections, mite and lice infestations, acne vulgaris, rosacea, dermatitis, and psoriasis.
4. Describe the prevention and management of minor burns.
5. Describe the nurse's role in the pharmacologic management of skin disorders.
6. For each of the classes listed in Drugs at a Glance, know representative drugs, and explain the mechanisms of drug action, primary actions, and important adverse effects.
7. Use the nursing process to care for patients who are receiving pharmacotherapy for skin disorders.

indicates a prototype drug, each of which is featured in a Prototype Drug box.

The integumentary system consists of the skin, hair, nails, sweat glands, and oil glands. The largest and most visible of all organs, skin provides an effective barrier between the outside environment and the body's internal tissues, helps to regulate body temperature, and assists in maintaining fluid and electrolyte balance. At times, however, environmental conditions damage the skin, or conditions within the body change, resulting in unhealthy skin. Some of these changes can even lead to systemic changes that affect tissues outside the integumentary system. The purpose of this chapter is to examine the broad scope of skin disorders and the drugs used for skin pharmacotherapy.

THE SKIN

49.1 Structure and Function of the Skin

To understand the actions of dermatologic drugs, it is necessary to have a thorough knowledge of skin structure. The skin comprises three primary layers: the epidermis, dermis, and subcutaneous layer. Each layer of skin is distinct in form and function and provides the basis for how drugs are injected or topically applied. The anatomy of the skin and associated structures is shown in Figure 49.1.

Epidermis

The epidermis is the visible, outermost layer that constitutes about 5% of the skin depth. The epidermis has either four or five sublayers depending on its thickness. The five layers from the innermost to outermost are the stratum basale (also referred to as the stratum germinativum), stratum spinosum, stratum granulosum, stratum lucidum, and the strongest layer, the stratum corneum. The stratum corneum contains an abundance of the protein keratin, which forms an effective barrier that repels bacteria and foreign matter: Most substances cannot penetrate this barrier.

The deepest epidermal sublayer, the stratum basale, supplies the epidermis with new cells after older superficial cells have been damaged or lost through normal wear. Over time, these newly created cells migrate from the stratum basale to the outermost layers of the skin. As these cells are pushed to the surface they are flattened and covered with a water-insoluble material, forming a protective seal. On average, it takes a cell about 3 weeks to move from the stratum basale to the body surface. Specialized cells within the deeper layers of the epidermis, called melanocytes, secrete the dark pigment melanin, which offers a degree of protection from the sun's ultraviolet rays. The number and type of melanocytes determine the overall pigment of the skin. The more melanin, the darker the skin color.

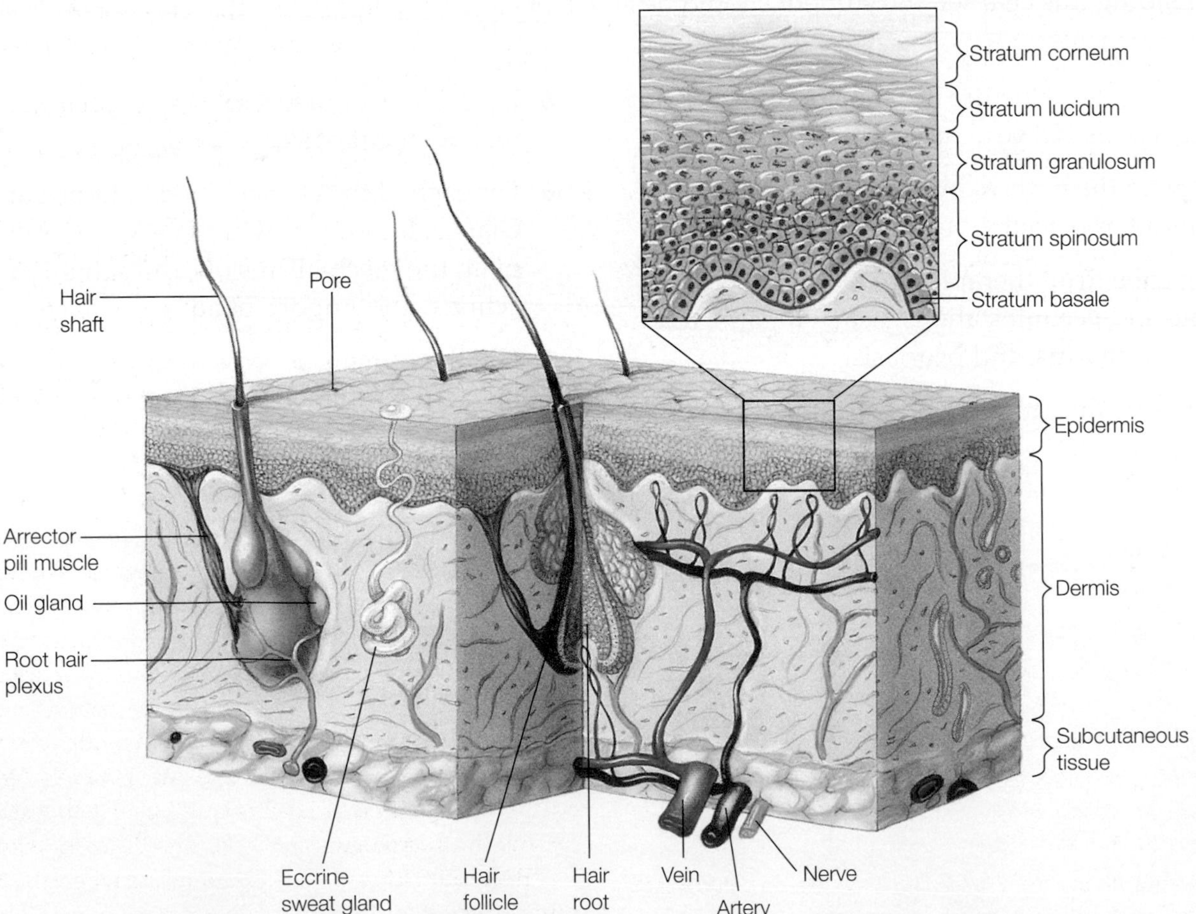

FIGURE 49.1 Anatomy of the skin

Dermis

The middle layer of the skin is the dermis, which accounts for about 95% of the skin thickness. The dermis provides a foundation for the epidermis and accessory structures such as hair and nails. Most sensory nerves that transmit the sensations of touch, pressure, temperature, pain, and itch are located within the dermis as well as the oil glands and sweat glands.

Subcutaneous Tissue

Beneath the dermis is the subcutaneous layer, or *hypodermis*, consisting mainly of adipose tissue, which cushions, insulates, and provides a source of energy for the body. The amount of subcutaneous tissue varies in an individual and is determined by nutritional status and heredity. Some sources consider the subcutaneous layer as being separate from the skin and not one of its layers.

49.2 Classification of Skin Disorders

Of the many types of skin disorders, some have vague, generalized signs and symptoms, and others have specific and easily identifiable symptoms. **Urticaria** is a hypersensitivity response characterized by hives, often accompanied by pruritus, or itching. Allergies to foods often manifest as urticaria. **Pruritus** is a general condition associated with dry, scaly skin, or a parasite infestation. Pruritus may also be a sign of *systemic* pathology, such as serious hepatic or renal impairment. A substantial number of drugs have urticaria or pruritus listed as potential adverse effects. **Erythema** or redness of the skin accompanies inflammation and many other skin disorders. Inflammation is a characteristic of burns and trauma to the skin.

One simple method of classifying skin disorders is to group them as infectious, inflammatory, or neoplastic. Skin disorders, however, are diverse and difficult to classify because they frequently have overlapping symptoms and causes. For example, lesions characteristic of acne may become inflamed and infected. Characteristics of these three classes of skin disorders are summarized in Table 49.1.

PharmFacts

SKIN DISORDERS

- An estimated 6 to 12 million children ages 3–11 years are infested with lice each year in the United States.
- Acne is not limited to adolescence. Twelve percent of women and 5% of men at aged 25 years still have acne.
- Atopic dermatitis is the most common inflammatory dermatologic condition in children, affecting 7% to 17% of American children.
- Psoriasis affects over 2% of the U.S. population and is slightly more common in women.

Table 49.1 Classification of Skin Disorders

Type	Examples
Infectious	Bacterial infections: boils, impetigo, and infected hair follicles
	Fungal infections: ringworm, athlete's foot, jock itch, and nail infection
	Parasitic infections: ticks, mites, and lice
	Viral infections: cold sores, fever blisters (herpes simplex), chickenpox, warts, shingles (herpes zoster), measles (rubeola), and German measles (rubella)
Inflammatory	Injury and exposure to the sun
	Combination of overactive glands, increased hormone production, or infection such as acne and rosacea
	Disorders with itching, cracking, and discomfort such as atopic dermatitis, contact dermatitis, seborrheic dermatitis, stasis dermatitis, and psoriasis
Neoplastic	Skin cancers: squamous cell carcinoma, basal cell carcinoma, and malignant melanoma
	Benign neoplasms include keratosis and keratoacanthoma

Dermatologic signs and symptoms often result from disease processes occurring in other body systems. Skin abnormalities such as changes in skin turgor and in the color, size, types, and character of surface lesions may have systemic causes such as liver or renal impairment, cardiovascular insufficiency, metastatic tumors, recent injury, and poor nutritional status. The relationship between the integumentary system and other body systems is illustrated in Figure 49.2.

The pharmacotherapy of skin disorders may be conducted with oral, parenteral, or topical drugs. In general, topical drugs are preferred because this route delivers the medication directly to the site of pathology and systemic adverse effects are rare. If the skin condition involves deeper skin layers or is extensive, oral or parenteral drug therapy may be indicated. Some conditions such as lice infestation or sunburn with minor irritation warrant only short-term pharmacotherapy. Prolonged and extensive therapy is sometimes required of eczema, dermatitis, and psoriasis.

SKIN INFECTIONS

Normal skin is populated with microorganisms or flora that include a diverse collection of viruses, fungi, and bacteria. As long as the skin remains healthy and intact, it provides an effective barrier against infection from these organisms. The skin is very dry, and keratin is a poor energy source for microbes. Although perspiration often provides a wet environment, its high salt content discourages microbial growth. Furthermore, the outer layer is continually being sloughed off, and the microorganisms leave with the dead skin.

Bacterial skin infections can occur when the skin is punctured or cut or when the outer layer is abraded through trauma or removed through severe burns. Some

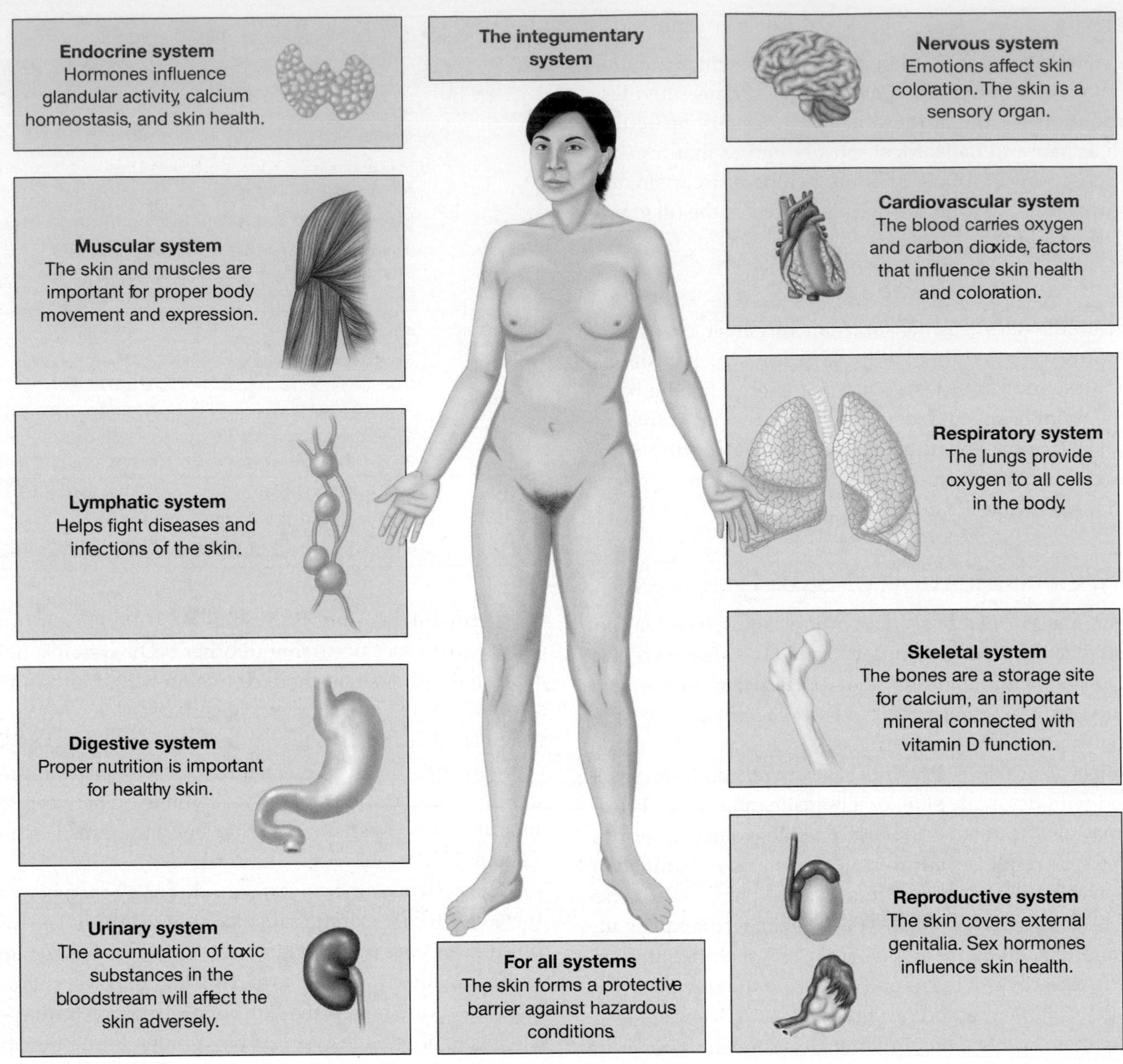

The integumentary system
Endocrine system
Hormones influence glandular activity, calcium homeostasis, and skin health.
Nervous system
Emotions affect skin coloration. The skin is a sensory organ.
Muscular system
The skin and muscles are important for proper body movement and expression.
Cardiovascular system
The blood carries oxygen and carbon dioxide, factors that influence skin health and coloration.
Lymphatic system
Helps fight diseases and infections of the skin.
Respiratory system
The lungs provide oxygen to all cells in the body.
Skeletal system
The bones are a storage site for calcium, an important mineral connected with vitamin D function.
Digestive system
Proper nutrition is important for healthy skin.
Reproductive system
The skin covers external genitalia. Sex hormones influence skin health.
Urinary system
The accumulation of toxic substances in the bloodstream will affect the skin adversely.
For all systems
The skin forms a protective barrier against hazardous conditions.

FIGURE 49.2 Interrelationships of the integumentary system with other body systems

bacteria also infect hair follicles. The two most common bacterial infections of the skin are caused by *Staphylococcus* and *Streptococcus,* which are also normal skin inhabitants. *Staphylococcus aureus* is responsible for furuncles (boils), carbuncles (abscesses), and other pus-containing lesions of the skin. Both *S. aureus* and *Streptococcus pyogenes* can cause impetigo, a skin disorder commonly occurring in school-age children. Cellulitis is an acute skin and subcutaneous tissue infection caused by *Staphylococcus* and *Streptococcus.*

49.3 Pharmacotherapy of Bacterial, Fungal, and Viral Skin Infections

Although many skin bacterial infections are self-limiting, others may be serious enough to require pharmacotherapy. Topical anti-infectives are safe, and many are available over the counter (OTC) for self-treatment. If the infection is deep within the skin, affects large regions of the body, or has the potential to become systemic, then oral or parenteral therapy is indicated. Furthermore, the incidence of methicillin-resistant *S. aureus* (MRSA) skin infections is increasing, which often requires pharmacotherapy with two or more antibiotics. Some of the more common topical antibiotics include the following:

- Bacitracin ointment
- Erythromycin ointment (Eryderm, others)
- Gentamicin cream and ointment
- Metronidazole cream and lotion
- Mupirocin (Bactroban)
- Neomycin with polymyxin B (Neosporin), cream and ointment
- Tetracycline.

Fungal infections of the skin or nails such as tinea pedis (athlete's foot) and tinea cruris (jock itch) commonly occur in warm, moist areas of the skin covered by clothing. Tinea capitis (ringworm of the scalp) and tinea unguium (nails) are also common. These pathogens are responsive to therapy with topical OTC antifungal drugs such as undecylenic acid (Cruex, Desenex, others). More serious fungal infections of the skin and mucous membranes, such as *Candida albicans* infections that occur in immunocompromised patients, require systemic antifungals (see chapter 36). Clotrimazole (Lotrimin, Mycelex, others) and miconazole (Micatin) are common antifungals available as creams or ointments that are used for a variety of dermatologic mycoses. Oral fluconazole (Diflucan) is indicated for more serious fungal infections of the skin and associated structures.

Certain viral infections can manifest with skin lesions, including varicella (chickenpox), rubeola (measles), and rubella (German measles). Usually, these infections are self-limiting and nonspecific, so treatment is directed at controlling the extent of skin lesions. Viral infections of the skin in adults include herpes zoster (shingles) and herpes simplex (cold sores and genital lesions). Pharmacotherapy of severe or persistent viral skin lesions may include topical or oral antiviral therapy with acyclovir (Zovirax), as discussed in chapter 37.

SKIN PARASITES

Common skin parasites include mites and lice. Scabies is an eruption of the skin caused by the female mite, *Sarcoptes scabiei*, which burrows into the skin to lay eggs that hatch after about 5 days. Scabies mites are barely visible without magnification and are smaller than lice. Scabies lesions most commonly occur between the fingers, on the extremities, in axillary and gluteal folds, around the trunk, and in the pubic area. The major symptom is intense itching; vigorous scratching may lead to secondary infections. Scabies is readily spread through contact with upholstery and shared bed and bath linens.

Lice are larger than mites, measuring from 1 to 4 mm in length. They are readily spread by infected clothing or close personal contact. These parasites require human blood for survival and die within 24 hours without the blood of a human host. Lice (singular: louse) often infest the pubic area or the scalp and lay eggs, referred to as **nits,** which attach to body hairs. Head lice are referred to as *Pediculus capitis*, body lice as *P. corpus*, and pubic lice as *Phthirus pubis*. The pubic louse is referred to as a crab louse, because it looks like a tiny crab when viewed under the microscope. Individuals with pubic lice will sometimes say that they have "crabs." Pubic lice may produce

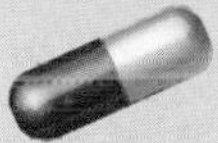

Prototype Drug | Permethrin *(Acticin, Elimite, Nix)*

Therapeutic Class: Antiparasitic **Pharmacologic Class:** Scabicide; pediculicide

Actions and Uses

Nix is marketed as a cream, lotion, or shampoo to kill head and crab lice and mites and to eradicate their ova. A 1% lotion is approved for lice and a 5% lotion for mites. The medication should be allowed to remain on the hair and scalp 10 minutes before removal. Patients should be aware that penetration of the skin with mites causes itching, which lasts up to 2 or 3 weeks even after the parasites have been killed.

Successful elimination of parasite infections should include removing nits with a nit comb, washing bedding, and cleaning or removing objects that have been in contact with the head or hair.

Administration Alerts

- Do not use on premature infants and children younger than 2 years.
- Do not use on areas of skin that have abrasions, rash, or inflammation.
- Pregnancy category B.

PHARMACOKINETICS

Onset	Peak	Duration
10 min	Unknown	3 h

Adverse Effects

Permethrin causes few systemic effects because almost none is absorbed across the skin. Local reactions may occur and include pruritus, rash, transient tingling, burning, stinging, erythema, and edema of the affected area.

Contraindications: Contraindications include hypersensitivity to pyrethrins, chrysanthemums, sulfites, or other preservatives. Permethrin should be used cautiously over inflamed skin, in those with asthma, or in lactating women.

Interactions

Drug–Drug: No clinically significant interactions have been documented.

Lab Tests: Unknown.

Herbal/Food: Unknown.

Treatment of Overdose: No specific treatment for overdose is available.

sky-blue macules on the inner thighs or lower abdomen. The bite of the louse and the release of saliva into the wound lead to intense itching followed by vigorous scratching. Secondary infections can result from scratching.

49.4 Pharmacotherapy With Scabicides and Pediculicides

Scabicides are drugs that kill mites, and **pediculicides** are drugs that kill lice. Some drugs are effective against both types of parasites. The choice of drug depends on where the infestation is located as well as factors such as age, pregnancy, or breast-feeding.

The preferred drug for lice infestation is permethrin, a chemical derived from chrysanthemum flowers and formulated as a 1% liquid (Nix). This drug is considered the safest agent, especially for infants and children. Pyrethrin (RID, others) is a related product also obtained from the chrysanthemum plant. Permethrin and pyrethrins, which are also widely used as insecticides on crops and livestock, kill lice and their eggs on contact. These medications are effective in about 90% to 99% of patients, although a repeat application may be needed. Side effects are generally minor and include stinging, itching, or tingling. Malathion (Ovide) is an alternative for resistant organisms. Approved in 2012, ivermectin (Sklice) is a lotion that is left on the scalp for 10 minutes and does not require a nit comb following treatment.

Permethrin is also a preferred drug for scabies. The 5% permethrin cream (Elimite) is applied to the entire skin surface and allowed to remain for 8 to 14 hours before bathing. A single application cures 95% of the patients, although itching may continue for several weeks as the dead mites are removed from the skin. Crotamiton (Eurax) is an alternative scabicide available by prescription as a 10% cream.

The traditional drug of choice for many decades for both mites and lice was lindane (Kwell). Because lindane has the potential to cause serious nervous system toxicity, it is now prescribed only after other less toxic drugs have failed to produce a therapeutic response.

All scabicides and pediculicides must be used strictly as directed, because excessive use has the potential to cause serious systemic effects and skin irritation. Drugs for the treatment of lice or mites must not be applied to the mouth, open skin lesions, or eyes, because this will cause severe irritation.

Nursing Practice Application

Pharmacotherapy for Lice or Mite Infestation

ASSESSMENT	POTENTIAL NURSING DIAGNOSES*
Baseline assessment prior to administration: • Obtain a complete health history including dermatologic and social history of recent exposure. • Obtain a drug history including allergies, current prescription and OTC drugs, herbal preparations, alcohol use, and smoking. Be alert to possible drug interactions. • Assess the skin areas to be treated for signs of infestation (e.g., lice or nits in hair, reddened track areas between webs of the fingers, around the belt or elastic lines), irritation, excoriation, or drainage. • Obtain baseline height, weight, and vital signs.	• *Disturbed Body Image* • *Impaired Skin Integrity* • *Deficient Knowledge* (drug therapy) • *Risk for Poisoning,* related to adverse drug effects *NANDA I © 2014
Assessment throughout administration: • Assess for desired therapeutic effects depending on the reason the drug is given (e.g., visible infestation is gone, nits are removed, skin healing is visible). • Assess for adverse effects: localized tingling, pruritus, stinging, or burning. Severe skin reactions or edema should be reported promptly.	

IMPLEMENTATION

Interventions and (Rationales)	Patient-Centered Care
Ensuring therapeutic effects: • Monitor appropriate medication administration for optimal results. Monitor the affected area after treatment over the following 1 to 2 weeks to ensure that the infestation has been eliminated. (Appropriate administration will optimize therapeutic effects and limit the need for retreatment.)	• Teach the patient appropriate administration techniques.

Nursing Practice Application *continued*

IMPLEMENTATION	
Interventions and (Rationales)	**Patient-Centered Care**
Minimizing adverse effects:	
• Monitor the area of infestation over the next 1 to 2 weeks. Reinfestations may appear within 1 week and need to be retreated at that time. (Most treatments are highly effective when administered correctly. Retreatment may be needed depending on the type of infestation.)	• Instruct the patient, family, or caregiver to continue to assess the area daily for 1 to 2 weeks and contact the health care provider for a second prescription if reinfestation is noted.
• Monitor family members, those in close care of the patient, or sexual contacts for infestation. Bedding and personal objects should be cleansed before reuse. (Reinfestation may recur if those in close contact with the patient are infested. Close contacts should be treated at the same time as the patient.)	• Instruct the patient, family, or caregiver to wash bedding, clothing used currently, and combs and brushes in soapy water and dry thoroughly. Advise the patient to vacuum furniture or fabric that cannot be cleaned to remove any errant vermin; dry clean hats or caps that cannot be washed; and seal children's toys in plastic bags for 2 weeks if they cannot be washed.
• Monitor skin in areas that have been treated. Promptly report any irritation, broken skin, erythema, rashes, or edema. (Skin reactions are relatively uncommon but may occur. Allergic reactions should be reported promptly.)	• Teach the patient, family, or caregiver to report any redness, swelling, itching, excoriation, or complaints of burning to the health care provider.
Patient understanding of drug therapy:	
• Use opportunities during administration of medications and during assessments to provide patient education. (Using time during nursing care helps to optimize and reinforce key teaching areas.)	• The patient should be able to state the reason for the drug, appropriate dose and scheduling, and what adverse effects to observe for and when to report them.
Patient self-administration of drug therapy:	
• When administering the medication, instruct the patient, family, or caregiver in the proper self-administration of the drug (e.g., use exactly as directed or per package directions). (Proper administration increases the effectiveness of the drugs.)	• Teach the patient to take the drug following appropriate guidelines: • Apply the drug per package directions and allow the drug to remain in the hair or on the skin for the prescribed length of time (usually approximately 10 minutes). Most packages contain enough drug for one treatment, although a second package may be required if the hair is long. • Dry thoroughly after showering or shampooing the drug out of the hair or skin. • Comb through hair with the fine-toothed comb provided to remove any remaining dead lice, nits, or nit casings. • If eyelashes are infested, apply a thin coat of petroleum jelly to them once a day for 1 week. Comb through using the fine-tooth comb. • Check hair, webbings of the fingers and toes, and belt or elastic lines for signs of reinfestation over the next week. If needed, a second application of the drug can be used after 1 week.

ACNE AND ROSACEA

Acne vulgaris and rosacea are two disorders that produce similar-appearing lesions on the face. Although the two conditions have some visual similarities and share a few common treatments, the pharmacotherapy of the disorders is very different.

Medications used for acne and related disorders are available OTC and by prescription. Because of their increased toxicity, prescription agents are reserved for more severe, persistent cases. These drugs are listed in Table 49.2.

49.5 Pharmacotherapy of Acne

Acne vulgaris is a disorder of the hair and sebaceous glands that affects up to 80% of adolescents. Although acne occurs most often in teenagers, it is not unusual to find patients with acne who are older than 30 years, a condition referred to as mature acne or acne tardive. Acne vulgaris is more common in men but tends to persist longer in women.

Although the precise cause of acne is unknown, several factors associated with acne vulgaris include

Table 49.2 Drugs for Acne and Rosacea

Drug	Remarks
adapalene (Differin)	Retinoid-like compound used to treat acne formation
azelaic acid (Azelex, Finacea)	For mild to moderate inflammatory acne
benzoyl peroxide (Clearasil, Fostex, others)	Keratinolytic available OTC: sometimes combined with erythromycin (Benzamycin) or clindamycin (BenzaClin) for acne caused by *P. acnes*
clindamycin and tretinoin (Veltin, Ziana)	Combination product with an antibiotic and a retinoid in a gel base; for mild to moderate acne
ethinyl estradiol and norgestimate	Oral contraceptives are sometimes used for acne; example: ethinyl estradiol plus norgestimate (Ortho Tri-Cyclen-28)
ivermectin (Soolantra)	For inflammatory lesions of rosacea
isotretinoin	For severe acne with cysts or acne formed in small, rounded masses; pregnancy category X
metronidazole (MetroCream, MetroGel)	For inflammatory papules and pustules of rosacea
sulfacetamide (Cetamide, Klaron, others)	For sensitive skin; sometimes combined with sulfur to promote peeling, as in the condition rosacea; also used for conjunctivitis
tazarotene (Avage, Tazorac)	A retinoid drug that may also be used for plaque psoriasis; has antiproliferative and anti-inflammatory effects
tetracyclines	Antibiotics; refer to chapter 35
tretinoin (Avita, Retin-A, others)	To prevent clogging of pore follicles; also used for the treatment of acute promyelocytic leukemia and wrinkles

abnormal formation of keratin that blocks oil glands and **seborrhea,** the overproduction of sebum by oil glands. The bacterium *Propionibacterium acnes* grows within oil gland openings and changes sebum to an acidic and irritating substance. As a result, small inflamed bumps appear on the surface of the skin. Other factors associated with acne include androgens, which stimulate the sebaceous glands to produce more sebum. This is clearly evident in teenage boys and in patients who are administered testosterone.

Acne lesions include open and closed comedones. Blackheads, or open **comedones,** occur when sebum has plugged the oil gland, causing it to become black because of the presence of melanin granules. Whiteheads, or closed comedones, develop just beneath the surface of the skin and appear white rather than black. Some closed comedones may rupture, resulting in papules, inflammatory pustules, and cysts. Mild papules and cysts drain on their own without treatment. Deeper lesions can cause scarring of the skin. Acne is graded as mild, moderate, or severe, depending on the number and type of lesions present.

The goals of acne therapy are to treat existing lesions and to prevent or lessen the severity of future recurrences. The regimen used depends on the extent and severity of the acne. Mechanisms of action of antiacne medications include the following:

- Inhibit sebaceous gland overactivity.
- Reduce bacterial colonization.
- Prevent follicles from becoming plugged with keratin.
- Reduce inflammation of lesions.

Benzoyl peroxide (Clearasil, Triaz, others) is the most common topical OTC medication for acne. Benzoyl peroxide has a **keratolytic** effect, which helps dry out and shed the outer layer of the epidermis. In addition, this drug suppresses sebum production and exhibits antibacterial effects against *P. acnes*. Benzoyl peroxide is available as a topical lotion, cream, or gel in various percent concentrations. Typically, the patient applies benzoyl peroxide once daily and in many instances this is the only treatment needed. The drug is very safe, with local redness, irritation, and drying being the most common side effects. Another keratolytic agent commonly used in OTC acne products is salicylic acid, which gives the same side effects as benzoyl peroxide.

In June of 2014 the U.S. Food and Drug Administration (FDA) issued a drug safety communication regarding the use of OTC acne products containing benzoyl peroxide and salicylic acid (FDA, 2014). The communication warns that these drugs may cause rare, but potentially life-threatening allergic reactions. Symptoms of this reaction include throat tightness; difficulty breathing; feeling faint; or swelling of the eyes, face, lips, or tongue. The allergic reaction may occur immediately or several days after initiating therapy. New users are urged to test the product on a small patch of skin for 3 days. If no discomfort occurs, the drug may be safely applied.

Retinoids are a class of drug closely related to vitamin A that are used in the treatment of inflammatory skin conditions, dermatologic malignancies, and acne. The topical formulations are often drugs of choice for patients with mild to moderate acne, particularly those with the presence of inflammatory cysts. Tretinoin (Avita, Retin-A, others) is an older drug with an irritant action that decreases comedone formation and increases extrusion of comedones from the skin. Tretinoin also has the ability to improve photodamaged skin and is used for wrinkle removal. Other retinoids include isotretinoin, an oral vitamin A metabolite medication that aids in reducing the size of sebaceous glands, thereby decreasing oil production and the occurrence of clogged pores. Although extremely effective, isotretinoin is rarely used due to the potential for birth defects (pregnancy category X) and the fact it has been associated with a risk of suicidal ideation. Therapy with retinoids may require 8 to 12 weeks to achieve maximum effectiveness.

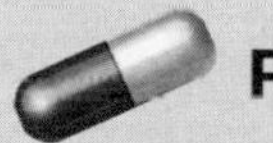

Prototype Drug | Tretinoin *(Avita, Retin-A, others)*

Therapeutic Class: Antiacne drug **Pharmacologic Class:** Retinoid

Actions and Uses

Tretinoin is a natural derivative of vitamin A that is indicated for the early treatment and control of mild to moderate acne vulgaris. Renova is a topical form of tretinoin approved to treat fine facial wrinkles and hyperpigmentation associated with photodamaged skin. Tretinoin has antineoplastic actions; an oral form (Vesanoid) is approved to treat acute promyelocytic leukemia (APL) and may be prescribed off-label for skin malignancies.

Acne symptoms take 4–8 weeks to improve, and maximum therapeutic benefit may take 5–6 months. Because of potentially serious adverse effects, this drug is most often reserved for cystic acne or severe keratinization disorders.

Administration Alerts

- Avoid administering OTC acne medications and using skin products that cause excessive drying of the skin during therapy.
- Avoid direct exposure to sunlight or UV lamps.
- Do not administer to patients who are allergic to fish (the product contains fish proteins).
- Pregnancy category C (topical) or D (oral [PO]).

PHARMACOKINETICS (TOPICAL)

Onset	Peak	Duration
Unknown	1–2 h	Unknown

Adverse Effects

Nearly all patients using topical tretinoin will experience redness, scaling, erythema, crusting, and peeling of the skin. Skin irritation can be severe and cause discontinuation of therapy; a lower strength solution may be necessary. Dermatologic adverse effects resolve once therapy is discontinued. Oral therapy can also cause skin adverse effects.

Very high oral doses used to treat APL can result in serious adverse effects, including bone pain, fever, headache, nausea, vomiting, rash, stomatitis, pruritus, sweating, and ocular disorders.

Black Box Warning: Patients with APL are at high risk for serious adverse effects. About 25% of patients develop retinoic acid-APL syndrome, which is a serious condition characterized by fever, weakness, fatigue, dyspnea, weight gain, peripheral edema, respiratory insufficiency, and pneumonia. About 40% of patients develop a rapidly evolving leukocytosis, which is associated with a high risk of life threatening complications. There is a high risk that infants will be severely deformed if this drug is administered during pregnancy.

Contraindications: Contraindications for topical administration include eczema, exposure to sunlight or UV rays, sunburn, hypersensitivity to the drug or vitamin A preparation, and children less than 12 years of age. This drug is contraindicated during lactation or pregnancy. Oral tretinoin is contraindicated in patients who have hepatic disease, leukopenia, or neutropenia or who are hypersensitive to the drug.

Interactions

Drug–Drug: Topical acne keratinolytics (benzoyl peroxide and salicylic acid) may increase inflammation and peeling; topical products containing alcohol or menthol may cause stinging. Additive phototoxicity can occur if tretinoin is used concurrently with other phototoxic drugs such as tetracyclines, fluoroquinolones, or sulfonamides.

Lab Tests: None known.

Herbal/Food: Excessive amounts of vitamin A or St. John's wort may result in photosensitivity.

Treatment of Overdose: Overuse of the topical drug will lead to excessive skin drying and peeling. Symptoms of oral overdose are nonspecific and resolve with symptomatic treatment.

Common reactions to retinoids include burning, stinging, and sensitivity to sunlight. Adapalene (Differin) is a third-generation retinoid that causes less irritation than the older agents. Epiduo is a topical drug that contains both adapalene and benzoyl peroxide. Additional retinoid-like drugs and related compounds used to treat acne are listed in Table 49.2.

Antibiotics are sometimes used in combination with acne medications to lessen the severe redness and inflammation associated with the disorder, especially when the acne is inflammatory and results in cysts and pustules. Doxycycline (Vibramycin, others), minocycline, and tetracycline, administered in small doses over a long period, have been the traditional antibiotics used in acne therapy. Erythromycin and clindamycin are frequently used topically and have a low incidence of adverse effects. Benzamycin is a presciption product that contains benzoyl peroxide with erythromycin.

Oral contraceptives containing ethinyl estradiol and norgestimate may be used to help clear the skin of acne by suppressing sebum production and reducing skin oiliness.

The agents are reserved for women who are unable to take oral antibiotics or when antibiotic therapy has proved ineffective. For the actions and contraindications of oral contraceptives, see chapter 46.

49.6 Pharmacotherapy of Rosacea

Rosacea is an inflammatory skin disorder of unknown etiology with lesions affecting mainly the face. Unlike acne, which most commonly affects teenagers, rosacea is a progressive disorder with an onset between 30 and 50 years of age. Rosacea is characterized by small papules or inflammatory bumps without pus that swell, thicken, and become painful. The face takes on a reddened or flushed appearance, particularly around the nose and cheek area. With time, the redness becomes more permanent, and lesions resembling acne appear. The soft tissues of the nose may thicken, giving the nose a reddened, bullous, irregular swelling called **rhinophyma.**

Rosacea is exacerbated by factors such as sunlight, stress, increased temperature, and agents that dilate facial blood vessels including alcohol, spicy foods, skin care products, and warm beverages. It affects more women than men, although men more often develop rhinophyma. The two most effective treatments for rosacea are topical metronidazole (MetroGel, MetroCream) and azelaic acid (Azelex, Finacea). Benzoyl peroxide may be applied as needed. Alternative medications include topical clindamycin (Cleocin-T, ClindaMax) and sulfacetamide. Tetracycline antibiotics are of benefit to patients with rosacea with multiple pustules or with ocular involvement. Severe, resistant cases may respond to isotretinoin. Newer topical therapies include brimonidine (Mirvaso) and ivermectin (Soolantra) which are approved to reduce the persistent redness and inflammation of rosacea. Another formulation of ivermectin (Sklice) is used to treat lice: Sklice and Soolantra are not interchangeable.

Complementary and Alternative Therapies

ALOE VERA

Aloe vera is derived from the gel inside the leaf of the aloe plant, which is a member of the lily family. Used medicinally for thousands of years, aloe vera contains over 70 active substances including amino acids, minerals, vitamins, and enzymes. Aloe vera is best known for its moisturizing and wound healing properties when applied topically. There are numerous aloe products available, including soaps, lotions, creams, and sunblocks.

The effectiveness of topical aloe vera in wound healing has been clearly demonstrated. Wounds heal faster, perhaps due to the ability of the herb to influence the expression of collagen and the rapid appearance of angiogenesis at the injury site (Yadav et al., 2012). There have been few standardized clinical research studies examining the effectiveness of aloe vera gel in treating acne vulgaris. One controlled study found that combining aloe vera gel with tretinoin resulted in significantly better outcomes than tretinoin alone when applied for acne vulgaris (Hajheydari, Saeedi, Morteza-Semnani, and Soltani, 2014).

Check Your Understanding 49.1

Why are antibiotics used in the treatment of some acne conditions? *Visit www.pearsonhighered.com/nursingresources for the answer.*

Nursing Practice Application

Pharmacotherapy for Acne and Related Skin Conditions

ASSESSMENT	POTENTIAL NURSING DIAGNOSES*
Baseline assessment prior to administration: • Obtain a complete health history including dermatologic, hepatic, or renal disease; psychiatric disorders; pregnancy; and breast-feeding. • Obtain a drug history including allergies, current prescription and OTC drugs, herbal preparations, alcohol use, and smoking. Be alert to possible drug interactions. • Evaluate appropriate laboratory findings (e.g., complete blood count [CBC], lipid profiles, hepatic or renal function laboratory tests). • Obtain baseline vital signs.	• *Disturbed Body Image* • *Impaired Skin Integrity,* related to skin condition or adverse drug effects • *Deficient Knowledge* (drug therapy) • *Risk for Injury,* related to adverse drug effects *NANDA I © 2014

Nursing Practice Application *continued*

ASSESSMENT	POTENTIAL NURSING DIAGNOSES*
Assessment throughout administration: • Assess for desired therapeutic effects (e.g., skin is clearing of acne lesions). • Continue periodic monitoring of CBC, lipid profile, glucose, and hepatic function tests if on oral drug therapy. • Monitor vital signs at each health care visit. • Monitor eye health periodically with eye examinations every 6 months while on oral drug therapy. • Assess for adverse effects: Localized skin irritation, erythema, pruritus, or dry or peeling skin, dry mouth, eyes, or nose may occur. Changes in mood, especially depression or suicidal thoughts, should be reported immediately in patients on oral isotretinoin.	

IMPLEMENTATION

Interventions and (Rationales)	Patient-Centered Care
Ensuring therapeutic effects:	
• Monitor appropriate medication administration for optimal results. (Topical treatment areas should show signs of improvement within 2–4 weeks. Oral treatment is usually successful within one course, and a second course may be delayed for several weeks to monitor continuing improvement.)	• Teach the patient appropriate administration techniques. • Advise the patient that whereas significant improvement may take several weeks, some improvement should be noticed within a few days of treatment.
Minimizing adverse effects:	
• Monitor the area under topical treatment for excessive dryness and irritation. (Overcleansing or overdrying of the skin may make the condition worse.)	• Teach the patient to gently cleanse the skin using a nonoily soap and avoiding vigorous scrubbing. If excessive dryness occurs, advise the patient to use a nonoily lotion to areas of dryness.
• Monitor patients on isotretinoin for emotional health or changes in mood. (Depression, including with suicidal ideation, has been noted as an adverse effect.)	• Instruct the patient, family, or caregiver to immediately report any signs of decreased mood, affect, depression, or expressed suicidal thoughts to the health care provider.
• Monitor CBC, lipid levels, and hepatic function periodically for patients on oral medication. (Lipid levels may increase in up to 70% of patients on oral acne therapy. Hepatotoxicity is an adverse effect of oral drugs.)	• Instruct the patient to return periodically for laboratory tests. • Teach the patient to report any symptoms of abdominal or right upper quadrant discomfort or pain, yellowing of the skin or sclera, fatigue, anorexia, darkened urine or clay-colored stools immediately.
• Monitor for vision changes. (Corneal opacities or cataracts are an adverse effect of oral antiacne medications. Dryness of eyes during treatment is common. Night vision may be diminished during treatment.)	• Instruct the patient to maintain regular eye exams and to report any changes in visual acuity, especially with night driving. • Teach the patient that artificial tear solutions may assist in relieving eye dryness.
• Monitor the patient's exposure to the sun and UV light. (Drying, skin sensitivity, and peeling skin are possible adverse effects, especially for patients on tretinoin. Protection from sun exposure is essential.)	• Teach the patient to use sunscreens of SPF 15 or higher and to wear protective clothing to avoid sun exposure to areas under treatment. • Teach the patient that UV light therapy from a health care provider is monitored and tanning beds are not a substitute and should be avoided.
• Monitor compliance with "iPledge" requirements for patients on isotretinoin. (iPledge is required of all patients on isotretinoin before receiving a prescription or refills of the drug. It requires the patient to ensure that all requirements to prevent teratogenic effects have been met.)	• Instruct the patient on isotretinoin of the requirements of the iPledge mandatory program to ensure continued prescriptions, including: • **Lifespan:** Females of child-bearing age must use two methods of birth control while on the drug and not donate blood while on the drug. • **Lifespan:** Females of child-bearing age must have two negative pregnancy tests one month before, during, and after drug therapy, conducted at certified laboratories. • **Lifespan:** Male patients must verify that they will use a barrier method of birth control and not donate blood while on the drug.

continued

Nursing Practice Application *continued*

IMPLEMENTATION	
Interventions and (Rationales)	**Patient-Centered Care**
Patient understanding of drug therapy:	
• Use opportunities during administration of medications and during assessments to provide patient education. (Using time during nursing care helps to optimize and reinforce key teaching areas.)	• The patient should be able to state the reason for the drug, appropriate dose and scheduling, and what adverse effects to observe for and when to report them.
Patient self-administration of drug therapy:	
• When administering the medication, instruct the patient, family, or caregiver in the proper self-administration of the drug (e.g., topical drug is used appropriately, iPledge program is followed). (Proper administration will increase the effectiveness of the drug.)	• Teach the patient to take the drug following appropriate guidelines: • Gently cleanse the affected skin twice daily with nonoily soap, avoiding excessive or vigorous scrubbing. • Apply a thin layer of topical drug after cleansing the skin. Allow to dry and avoid contact with clothing, towels, or bedding to avoid staining or bleaching. • For oral medications, take in the morning and if twice-a-day dosing is ordered, take the second dose approximately 8 hours after the first.

See Table 49.2 for a list of drugs to which these nursing actions apply.

DERMATITIS

Dermatitis is a general term that refers to superficial inflammatory disorders of the skin. General symptoms include local redness, pain, and pruritus. Intense scratching may lead to **excoriation**, which are scratches that break the skin surface and fill with blood or serous fluid to form crusty scales.

49.7 Pharmacotherapy of Dermatitis

A large number of factors can cause dermatitis, and symptoms may differ depending on the causative agent. The three most common types of dermatitis that respond to topical pharmacotherapy are atopic, contact, and seborrheic.

Atopic dermatitis, or **eczema,** is a chronic, inflammatory skin disorder with a genetic predisposition. Patients presenting with eczema often have a family history of asthma and hay fever as well as allergies to a variety of irritants such as cosmetics, lotions, soaps, pollens, food, pet dander, and dust. About 75% of patients with atopic dermatitis have had an initial onset before 1 year of age. In those babies predisposed to eczema, breast-feeding seems to offer protection, because it is rare for a breast-fed child to develop eczema before the introduction of other foods. In infants and small children, lesions usually begin on the face and scalp, and then progress to other parts of the body.

Contact dermatitis can be caused by a hypersensitivity response, resulting from exposure to allergens such as plants, chemicals, latex, drugs, metals, or foreign proteins. Accompanying the allergic reaction may be various degrees of cracking, bleeding, or small blisters. See Figure 49.3).

Seborrheic dermatitis is a form of eczema that can affect patients at any age. The exact cause of seborrheic dermatitis is unknown, but hormone levels, coexisting fungal infections, nutritional deficiencies, and immunodeficiency

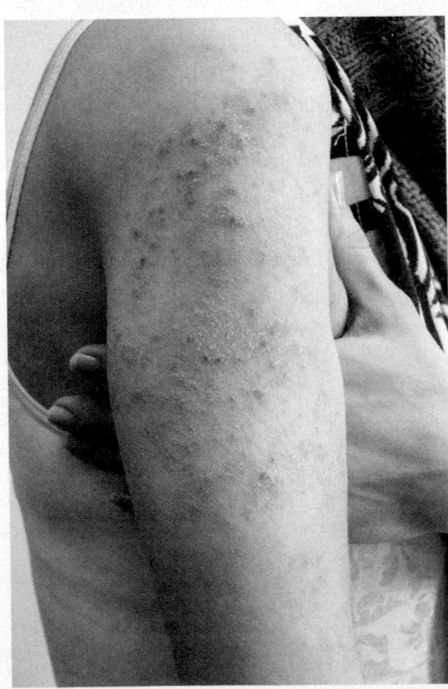

FIGURE 49.3 Inflamed skin and blisters characteristic of allergic or atopic dermatitis
Source: Serbia/Fotolia.

states are associated with the disease. Seborrheic dermatitis presents as greasy, not dry, scales that affect the scalp, central face, and anterior chest, often presenting as scalp scaling, or dandruff. Other symptoms may include redness of the nasolabial fold, particularly during times of stress, blepharitis, otitis externa, and acne vulgaris.

Pharmacotherapy of dermatitis is symptomatic and involves lotions and ointments to control itching and skin flaking. Antihistamines may be used to control inflammation and reduce itching, and analgesics or topical anesthetics may be prescribed for pain relief. Atopic dermatitis can be controlled, but not cured, by medications. Part of the management plan must include the identification and elimination of allergic triggers that cause flare-ups.

Topical corticosteroids (glucocorticoids) are the most effective treatment for controlling the inflammation and itching of dermatitis. Creams, lotions, solutions, gels, and pads containing these drugs are specially formulated to penetrate deep into the skin layers. Topical corticosteroids are classified by potency, as listed in Table 49.3. The high-potency agents are used to treat acute flare-ups and are limited to 2 to 3 weeks of therapy. The moderate-potency formulations are for more prolonged therapy of chronic dermatitis. The low-potency glucocorticoids are prescribed for children.

Long-term corticosteroid use may cause irritation, redness, hypopigmentation, and thinning of the skin. High-potency formulations are not advised for the head or neck regions because of potential adverse effects. If absorption occurs, topical corticosteroids may produce undesirable systemic effects including adrenal insufficiency, mood changes, serum imbalances, and loss of bone mass, as discussed in chapter 44. To avoid serious adverse effects, careful attention must be given to the amount of glucocorticoid applied, the frequency of application, and how long it has been used.

Several alternatives to corticosteroids are available. Patients with persistent atopic dermatitis who are not responsive to corticosteroids may benefit from oral immunosuppressive drugs, such as cyclosporine. This drug is generally used for the short-term treatment of severe disease. The topical calcineurin inhibitors pimecrolimus (Elidel) and tacrolimus (Protopic) are available for patients older than 2 years of age. These medications may be used over all skin surfaces (including face and neck) because they have fewer adverse effects than the topical corticosteroids. Adverse effects include burning and stinging on broken skin. Pimecrolimus and tacrolimus carry black box warnings that they should not be used for long term therapy because of a small risk of skin cancer and lymphoma. They are reserved for patients who have not responded to topical corticosteroids.

Another alternative to corticosteroids for atopic dermatitis is doxepin (Zonalon). When given PO, this drug is used to treat depression; however, Zonalon cream is indicated for atopic dermatitis. Some of the drug is absorbed across the skin, causing drowsiness in about 20% of patients.

Topical therapy for seborrheic dermatitis primarily consists of antifungal drugs and low-dose topical corticosteroids, depending on the location affected. The first-line therapy for seborrheic dermatitis that affects the scalp is topical corticosteroids, administered as a shampoo, topical solution, or a lotion applied to the scalp. Shampoos that contain selenium sulfide (Selsun), salicylic acid, zinc pyrithione, or an antifungal azole are sometimes used. Fluconazole (Diflucan), ketoconazole (Nizoral), or ciclopirox (Loprox) combined with 2 weeks of desonide (DesOwen) is recommended for seborrheic dermatitis of the face and ears.

Table 49.3 Topical Corticosteroids

Generic Name	Trade Names
VERY HIGH POTENCY	
betamethasone dipropionate, augmented	Diprolene
clobetasol propionate	Temovate
diflorasone diacetate	Maxiflor
halobetasol	Ultravate
HIGH POTENCY	
amcinonide	Cyclocort
fluocinonide	Lidex
halcinonide	Halog
MEDIUM POTENCY	
betamethasone benzoate	Uticort
betamethasone valerate	Valisone
clocortolone	Cloderm
desoximetasone, cream	Topicort
fluocinolone acetonide	Synalar
flurandrenolide, cream	Cordran
fluticasone propionate, cream	Cutivate
hydrocortisone valerate	Westcort
mometasone furoate	Elocon
prednicarbate	Dermatop
triamcinolone acetonide	Aristocort, Kenalog
LOW POTENCY	
alclometasone dipropionate	Aclovate
desonide	Desonate, DesOwen, Verdeso
dexamethasone	Decaspray
hydrocortisone	Cortizone, Hycort

PSORIASIS

Psoriasis is a chronic, noninfectious, inflammatory skin disorder that affects 1% to 2% of the population and

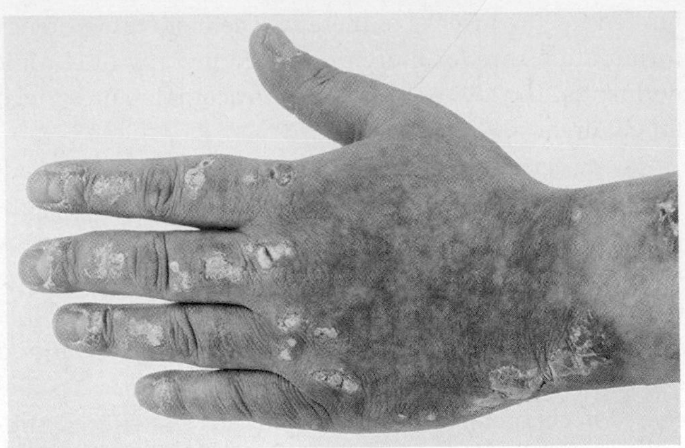

FIGURE 49.4 Psoriasis
Source: Casi/Fotolia.

appears with greater frequency in people of European ancestry. The onset of psoriasis is generally established by 20 years of age, although it may occur throughout the life span.

Psoriasis is characterized by red, raised patches of skin covered with flaky, thick, silver scales called plaques, as shown in Figure 49.4. These plaques shed the scales, which are sometimes grayish. The reason for the appearance of plaques is an extremely fast skin turnover rate, with skin cells reaching the surface in 4 to 7 days instead of the usual 14 days. Plaques are ultimately shed from the surface, while the underlying skin becomes inflamed and irritated. Lesion size varies, and the shape tends to be round. Lesions are usually discovered on the scalp, elbows, knees, and extensor surfaces of the arms and legs, sacrum, and occasionally around the nails. The various forms of psoriasis are described in Table 49.4.

Although the etiology of psoriasis is incompletely understood, it appears to have both genetic and autoimmune components. About 50% of the cases have a genetic basis, with a close family member also having the disorder. One theory of causation is that psoriasis is an autoimmune condition, because overactive immune cells release cytokines that increase the production of skin cells. There is also a strong environmental component to the disease: factors such as stress, smoking, alcohol, climate changes, and infections can trigger flare-ups. In addition, certain drugs act as triggers, including angiotensin-converting enzyme (ACE) inhibitors, beta-adrenergic blockers, tetracyclines, and nonsteroidal anti-inflammatory drugs (NSAIDs).

49.8 Pharmacotherapy of Psoriasis

The goal of psoriasis pharmacotherapy is to reduce skin reddening, plaques, and scales to improve the cosmetic appearance of the skin. This is accomplished by reducing epidermal cell turnover and promoting healing of the psoriatic lesions. Choice of therapy depends on the type and extent of the disease and the history of response to previous psoriasis treatment. A number of prescription and OTC drugs are available for the treatment of psoriasis and are listed in Table 49.5. Therapy is often conducted in a stepwise manner. Psoriasis is a lifelong disease, and there is no pharmacologic cure.

Topical Therapies

Topical corticosteroids are the primary, initial treatment for psoriasis. These drugs are effective, inexpensive, and relatively safe. Examples include betamethasone

Table 49.4 Types of Psoriasis

Form of Psoriasis	Description	Most Common Location of Lesions	Comments
Guttate (droplike) or eruptive psoriasis	Lesions smaller than those of psoriasis vulgaris	Upper trunk and extremities	More common in early-onset psoriasis; can appear and resolve spontaneously a few weeks following a streptococcal respiratory infection
Psoriasis vulgaris	Lesions are papules that form into erythematous plaques with thick, silver, or gray plaques that bleed when removed; plaques in dark-skinned individuals often appear purple	Skin over scalp, elbows, and knees; lesions possible anywhere on the body	Most common form; requires long-term specialized management
Psoriatic arthritis	Resembles rheumatoid arthritis	Fingers and toes at distal interphalangeal joints; can affect skin and nails	About 20% of patients with psoriasis also have arthritis
Psoriatic erythroderma or exfoliative dermatitis	Generalized scaling; erythema without lesions	All body surfaces	Least common form
Pustular psoriasis	Eruption of pustules; presence of fever	Trunk and extremities; can appear on palms, soles, and nail beds	Average age of onset is 50 years

Table 49.5 Selected Drugs for Psoriasis and Related Disorders

Drug	Route and Adult Dose (max dose where indicated)	Adverse Effects
TOPICAL MEDICATIONS*		
calcipotriene (Dovonex, Sorilux)	Topical: apply a thin layer to lesions one to two times/day	*Burning, stinging, folliculitis, itching* <u>No serious adverse effects</u>
coal tar (Balnetar, Cutar, others)	Topical: apply to affected areas qid	*Folliculitis, irritation, photosensitivity* <u>No serious adverse effects</u>
salicylic acid (Salex, Neutrogena, others)	Topical: apply to affected areas tid–qid in concentrations ranging from 2% to 10%	*Erythema, pruritus, stinging of the skin* <u>No serious adverse effects</u>
tazarotene (Tazorac)	Topical: apply a thin film daily in the evening	*Pruritus, burning, stinging, skin irritation, transient worsening of psoriasis, photosensitivity* <u>Hypersensitivity, teratogenicity</u>
SYSTEMIC MEDICATIONS		
acitretin (Soriatane)	PO: 25–50 mg/day with the main meal	*Dry mouth, alopecia, cheilitis, dry skin, dry mucous membranes, elevated triglycerides* <u>Paresthesia, rigors, arthralgia, skin peeling, pseudotumor cerebri, depression, elevated liver function tests, teratogenicity</u>
adalimumab (Humira)	Subcutaneous: 40–80 mg every other week	*Upper respiratory infection, injection site reactions, headache, rash* <u>Malignancies, serious infections</u>
alefacept (Amevive)	IM: 15 mg once weekly for 12 wk	*Pharyngitis, dizziness, cough, nausea, pruritus, myalgia, chills, injection site reactions* <u>Malignancies, serious infections, hepatotoxicity, lymphopenia</u>
apremilast (Otezia)	PO: Begin with 10 mg/day and increase over a 6 day period to 30 mg bid	*Diarrhea, nausea, headache* <u>Depression, weight loss</u>
cyclosporine (Sandimmune, Neoral) (see page 530 for the Prototype Drug box)	PO: 1.25 mg/kg bid (max: 4 mg/kg/day)	*Hirsutism, tremor, vomiting, headache, pruritus, nausea, vomiting, diarrhea* <u>Hypertension, myocardial infarction (MI), nephrotoxicity, hyperkalemia, gingival enlargement, paresthesias, hepatotoxicity, infection</u>
etanercept (Enbrel)	Subcutaneous: 25 mg twice/wk or 0.08 mg/kg or 50 mg once/wk	*Local reactions at the injection site (pain, erythema, myalgia), abdominal pain, vomiting, headache* <u>Infections, pancytopenia, MI, heart failure</u>
infliximab (Remicade)	IV: 5 mg/kg with additional doses 2 and 6 wk after the initial infusion, then every 8 wk thereafter	*Rash, minor infections* <u>Infusion-related reactions, serious infections, malignancies, worsening of heart failure, hepatotoxicity</u>
methotrexate (Rheumatrex, Trexall) (see page 622 for the Prototype Drug box)	PO: 2.5–5 mg bid for three doses each week (max: 25–30 mg/wk) IM/IV: 10–25 mg/wk	*Headache, glossitis, gingivitis, mild leukopenia, nausea* <u>Ulcerative stomatitis, myelosuppression, aplastic anemia, hepatic cirrhosis, nephrotoxicity, sudden death, pulmonary fibrosis</u>
secukinumab (Cosentyl	Subcutaneous: 150–300 mg at weeks 0, 1, 2, 3 and 4 followed by 300 mg every 4 wk	*Nasopharyngitis, diarrhea, upper respiratory tract infection* <u>Serious infections, hypersensitivity reactions</u>
ustekinumab (Stelara)	Subcutaneous: 45–90 mg initially and 4 wk later, followed by 45–90 mg every 12 wk	*Nasopharyngitis, upper respiratory tract infection, headache, fatigue* <u>Serious infections, malignancies</u>

*See Table 49.3 for topical corticosteroids for psoriasis.

Note: *Italics* indicate common adverse effects; <u>underlining</u> indicates serious adverse effects.

(Diprosone) ointment, lotion, or cream and hydrocortisone acetate (Cortaid, Caldecort, others) cream or ointment. Topical corticosteroids reduce the inflammation associated with fast skin turnover. Initial therapy may begin with a high-potency agent for 2 to 3 weeks to obtain rapid clearing of lesions or to treat acute flare-ups. The high-potency formulations are best applied to areas thickest with plaque, such as hands or feet, and should not be used on the face and genital areas. For chronic, maintenance therapy, the patient is switched to moderate- and low-potency corticosteroids because they have a lower potential for adverse effects.

Several other topical medications have been found to be effective when combined with corticosteroids or as monotherapy. Calcipotriene (Dovonex, Sorilux), a vitamin D analog, is effective in treating mild to moderate plaque psoriasis. Calcipotriene is combined with beclomethasone in Taclonex ointment. Tazarotene (Tazorac) is a retinoid-like drug that is approved to treat acne vulgaris and wrinkles, as well as plaque psoriasis. Although tazarotene is a first-line therapy, it is usually not prescribed for women with a potential for childbearing because it is pregnancy category X. Tacrolimus (Protopic) is a topical immunomodulator that is sometimes used off-label to treat severe plaque-type psoriasis.

Some other topical drugs may be effective in treating mild to moderate psoriasis. These include coal tar, salicylic acid and anthralin (Dithrocreme). Tar and anthralin inhibit DNA synthesis and arrest abnormal cell growth. These are considered second-line medications and are usually combined with corticosteroid therapy.

Systemic Therapies

Some patients have severe psoriasis that is resistant to topical therapy. Because systemic drugs have the potential to cause more serious adverse effects, they are generally used when topical drugs and phototherapy fail to produce an adequate response. In some cases, systemic drugs may be used for a few weeks to produce a rapid improvement in symptoms before beginning topical therapy.

The most frequently prescribed systemic drug for psoriasis is methotrexate. It is administered either once weekly or twice daily for 3 days each week. In 2013 a new formulation of the drug, Otrexup, was approved that permits a once-weekly subcutaneous injection for patients with severe psoriasis. Improvement requires several weeks to 2–3 months of therapy. Methotrexate (Rheumatrex, Trexall) is used for a variety of disorders, including carcinomas and rheumatoid arthritis, in addition to being used for the treatment of psoriasis. Methotrexate is presented as a prototype drug in chapter 38.

Acitretin (Soriatane) is taken PO to inhibit excessive skin cell growth. It is approved for severe, resistant psoriasis and is pregnancy category X. Cyclosporine (Sandimmune, Neoral), an immunosuppressant, may be used for severe conditions when other therapies fail. Approved in 2014, apremilast is used to treat psoriatic arthritis and plaque psoriasis that has not responded to other therapies. The drug inhibits the enzyme phosphodiesterase-4, which results in a reduction in several different pro-inflammatory mediators. It is the first drug approved for psoriasis that acts by this mechanism. Patients with a history of depression, suicidal behavior, or weight loss should be monitored regularly while on apremilast therapy.

The newest psoriasis treatments include biologic therapies such as alefacept (Amevive), adalimumab (Humira), ustekinumab (Stelara), etanercept (Enbrel), secukinumab (Cosentyx), and infliximab (Remicade). These drugs act by suppressing specific aspects of the inflammatory and immune responses. Because these medications induce general immunosuppression, patients are at an increased risk for infection, including reactivation of latent infections such as tuberculosis. Several are also used to treat rheumatoid arthritis (see chapter 48). A major disadvantage of these biologic drugs is that they are expensive and not available in oral formulations.

Nonpharmacologic Therapies

Phototherapy with ultraviolet-A (UVA) and ultraviolet-B (UVB) light is used in cases of severe debilitating psoriasis. Phototherapy with UVA is combined with methoxsalen, a

Evidence-Based Practice: The Efficacy of an Old-Fashioned Remedy: Coal Tar for Psoriasis

Clinical Question: Is coal tar still an effective treatment for psoriasis?

Evidence: The combination of coal tar and light therapy (phototherapy), also known as Goeckerman therapy, has been used since the early 1920s and probably longer. However, it fell out of favor as topical corticosteroids, methotrexate, biologic therapies, and other drugs became available. The use of coal tar and phototherapy, alone or combined with other drugs such as salicylates, still remains a useful therapy, especially for patients with psoriasis that has not responded well to other biologic treatments (Fitzmaurice, Bhutani, & Koo, 2013).

Khandpur and Sahni (2014) found that coal tar combined with salicylic acid was found to be equally effective as the topical use of calcipotriol combined with betamethasone. The calcipotriol with betamethasone resulted in a more rapid decrease in psoriatic plaques; however, over time, there was no significant difference in improvement between the two treatments. Other studies have also supported the use of coal tar and phototherapy as a cost-effective treatment with relatively few adverse effects (Dennis, Bhutani, Koo, & Liao 2013; Moscaliuc, Heller, Lee, & Koo, 2013).

Because there are no long-term studies as to the safety or cellular-level effects from coal tar use, caution is warranted (Borska et al., 2014; Samarasekera, Sawyer, Wonderling, Tucker, & Smith, 2013). Other treatment modalities, especially those such as calcipotriol with a more rapid response, may be considered first as they may be better tolerated cosmetically (Singh, Gupta, Abidi, & Krishna, 2013). Because psoriasis requires long-term treatment and at this time, is not curable, Goeckerman therapy with coal tar may be a cost-effective treatment option.

Nursing Implications: Coal tar solutions are available OTC and on the Internet. However, they may not be appropriate for self-use by patients who are seeking the success of coal tar and phototherapy because they may not contain sufficient coal tar to treat the condition. In addition, prolonged exposure to UVB can cause sunburn and other side effects. Nurses should be aware of the efficacy of coal tar and phototherapy but recommend to patients and their families that the treatment is labor intensive and requires skilled practitioners to achieve optimal effects.

drug from a chemical family known as the **psoralens.** The concurrent use of UVA and the drug is called PUVA therapy. Psoralens are oral or topical agents that produce a photosensitive reaction when exposed to UV light. This reaction reduces the number of lesions, but unpleasant side effects such as headache, nausea, and skin sensitivity still occur, limiting the effectiveness of this therapy.

UVB therapy is less hazardous than UVA therapy. The wavelength of UVB is similar to sunlight, and it reduces lesions covering a large area of body that normally resist topical treatments. With close supervision, this type of phototherapy can be administered at home. Keratolytic pastes are often applied between treatments.

SUNBURN AND MINOR BURNS

Burns are a unique type of stress that may affect all layers of the skin. Minor, first-degree burns affect only the outer layers of the epidermis, are characterized by redness, and are analogous to sunburn. Sunburn results from overexposure of the skin to UV light and is associated with light skin complexions, prolonged exposure to the sun during the more hazardous hours of the day (10 a.m. until 3 p.m.), and lack of protective clothing when outdoors. Chronic sun exposure can result in serious conditions, including eye injury, cataracts, and skin cancer.

In addition to producing local skin damage, sun overexposure releases toxins that may produce systemic effects. The signs and symptoms of sunburn include erythema, intense pain, nausea, vomiting, chills, edema, and headache. These symptoms usually resolve within a matter of hours or days, depending on the severity of the exposure. Once sunburn has occurred, medications can only alleviate the symptoms; they do not speed recovery time.

49.9 Pharmacotherapy of Sunburn and Minor Skin Irritation

The best treatment for sunburn is *prevention*. Sunscreens are liquids or lotions applied for chemical or physical protection. *Chemical* sunscreens absorb the spectrum of UV light that is responsible for most sunburns. Chemical sunscreens include those that contain benzophenone for protection against UVA rays; those that work against UVB rays include cinnamates, paminobenzoic acid (PABA), and salicylates. *Physical* sunscreens such as zinc oxide, talc, and titanium dioxide reflect or scatter light to prevent the penetration of both UVA and UVB rays. Parsol is another sunscreen product that is being used more frequently as a key ingredient in lip balm.

Treatment for sunburn consists of addressing symptoms with soothing lotions, rest, prevention of dehydration, and topical anesthetics if needed. Treatment is usually done on an outpatient basis. Topical anesthetics for minor burns include benzocaine (Solarcaine), dibucaine (Nupercainal), lidocaine (Xylocaine), and tetracaine HCl (Pontocaine). Aloe vera is a popular natural therapy for minor skin irritations and burns. These same drugs may also provide relief from minor pain due to insect bites and pruritus. In more severe cases, oral analgesics such as aspirin or ibuprofen may be indicated.

Chapter Review

KEY Concepts

The numbered key concepts provide a succinct summary of the important points from the corresponding numbered section within the chapter. If any of these points are not clear, refer to the numbered section within the chapter for review.

49.1 Three layers of skin—epidermis, dermis, and subcutaneous layer—provide effective barrier defenses for the body.

49.2 Skin disorders may be classified as infectious, inflammatory, or neoplastic. Skin disorders that may benefit from pharmacotherapy include acne, sunburn, infections, eczema, dermatitis, and psoriasis.

49.3 When the skin integrity is compromised, bacteria, viruses, and fungi can gain entrance and cause infections. Anti-infective therapy may be indicated.

49.4 Scabicides and pediculicides are used to treat parasitic mite and lice infestations, respectively. Permethrin is a preferred drug for these infections.

49.5 The pharmacotherapy of acne includes treatment with benzoyl peroxide, retinoids, and antibiotics.

49.6 Therapies for rosacea include metronidazole and azelaic acid.

49.7 The most effective treatment for dermatitis is topical corticosteroids, which are classified by their potency.

49.8 Both topical and systemic drugs, including corticosteroids, immunomodulators, and methotrexate, are used to treat psoriasis.

49.9 The pharmacotherapy of sunburn and minor skin irritations includes the symptomatic relief of pain using soothing lotions, topical anesthetics, and analgesics.

REVIEW Questions

1. The patient is treated for head lice with permethrin (Nix). Following treatment, the nurse will reinforce which of the following instructions?
   1. Remain isolated for 48 hours.
   2. Inspect the hair shafts, checking for nits daily for 1 week following treatment.
   3. Shampoo with permethrin three times per day.
   4. Wash linens with cold water and bleach.
2. The nurse is planning teaching for a patient prescribed desoximetasone (Topicort) for atopic dermatitis. The nurse will teach the patient to anticipate which possible adverse effects?
   1. Localized pruritis and hives
   2. Hair loss in the application area
   3. Worsening of acne
   4. Burning and stinging of the skin in the affected area
3. The nurse evaluates the patient's understanding of the procedure for application of triamcinolone (Kenalog, Aristocort) cream for acute contact dermatitis of the neck, secondary to a reaction to perfume. The patient asks why she can't just use up some fluocinonide (Lidex) cream she has left over from a poison ivy dermatitis last month. The nurse's response will be based on which of the following?
   1. High-potency corticosteroid creams should be avoided on the neck or face because of the possibility of additional adverse effects.
   2. All creams should be discarded after the initial condition has resolved.
   3. Fluocinonide cream is too low potency to use for contact dermatitis.
   4. Contact dermatitis from perfume is harder to treat than poison ivy dermatitis.
4. The teaching plan for a 24-year-old female who is receiving tretinoin (Avita, Retin-A, Trentin-X) for treatment of acne should include which of the following instructions? (Select all that apply.)
   1. Obtain 20 to 30 minutes of sun exposure per day to help dry the skin and prevent breakouts.
   2. Wash the face with a mild soap, avoiding scrubbing, twice a day.
   3. Use oil-free sunscreens, sun hats, and protective clothing to avoid sun exposure.
   4. Expect some dryness, redness, and peeling while on the drug but report severe skin irritation.
   5. Cover the area with a light dressing covered in plastic wrap to prevent the cream from rubbing off.
5. A 15-year-old patient started using topical benzoyl peroxide (Benzaclin, Fostex) 1 week ago for treatment of acne and is discouraged that her acne is still visible. What is the nurse's best response?
   1. "The cream should have started working by now. Check with your provider about switching to a different type."
   2. "Some improvement will be noticed quickly, but full effects may take several weeks to a month or longer."
   3. "Acne is very difficult to treat. It may be several months before you notice any effects."
   4. "If your acne is not gone by now, you may need an antibiotic too. Ask your provider."
6. After trying many other treatments, a 28-year-old female is started on isotretinoin for treatment of severe acne. While she is on this medication, what explicit instructions must be followed? (Select all that apply.)
   1. She must use two forms of birth control and have pregnancy tests before beginning, during, and after she is on the therapy.
   2. She must have vision checks performed every 6 months.
   3. She must increase intake of vitamin A–rich foods.
   4. She must return every 2 to 3 months for laboratory tests.
   5. She must delay any future pregnancies for a period of 5 years.

PATIENT-FOCUSED Case Study

Ryan Keogh is an 18-year-old high school student in his senior year and a catcher for the varsity baseball team. He has had acne for several years, but lately it has worsened. He has been using topical benzoyl peroxide but is becoming discouraged at the increase in breakouts. He feels it has started to affect his social life and his parents make an appointment for him with a dermatologist. The dermatologist diagnoses Ryan's skin condition as acne vulgaris and prescribes tretinoin (Retin-A).

1. What are some potential reasons why Ryan's acne outbreaks may have increased at this time?
2. As the nurse, what will you teach Ryan about the application of tretinoin and adverse effects that may occur?

CRITICAL THINKING Questions

1. A senior nursing student is participating in well-baby screenings at a public health clinic. While examining a 4-month-old infant, the student notes an extensive, confluent diaper rash. The baby's mother is upset and asks the student nurse about the use of OTC corticosteroid ointment and wonders how she should apply the cream. How should the student nurse respond?
2. A 36-year-old woman is seen by her health care provider for scaling patches on her forearms, elbows, and lower legs. She is diagnosed with psoriasis vulgaris and the provider prescribes betamethasone cream (Diprosone). After six months of therapy, her psoriasis has not been responsive to betamethasone and she is prescribed calcipotriene (Dovonex). What effect does betamethasone have in the treatment of psoriasis? What teaching should the patient receive about this new prescription for calcipotriene?

Visit www.pearsonhighered.com/nursingresources for answers and rationales for all activities.

REFERENCES

Borska, L., Andrys, C., Krejsek, J., Palicka, V., Chmelarova, M., Hamakova, K., . . . Fiala, Z. (2014). Oxidative damage to nucleic acids and benzo(a)pyrene-7, 8-diol-9, 10-epoxide-DNA adducts and chromosomal aberration in children with psoriasis repeatedly exposed to crude coal tar ointment and UV radiation. *Oxidative Medicine and Cellular Longevity, 2014*, Art. No.: 302528, 10 pages. doi:10.1155/2014/302528

Dennis, M., Bhutani, T., Koo, J., & Liao, W. (2013). Goeckerman therapy for treatment of eczema: A practical guide and review of efficacy. *Journal of Dermatological Treatment, 24*, 2–6. doi:10.3109/09546634.2011.607794

Fitzmaurice, S., Bhutani, T., & Koo, J. (2013). Goeckerman regimen for management of psoriasis refractory to biologic therapy: University of California San Francisco experience. *Journal of the American Academy of Dermatology, 69*, 648–649. doi:10.1016/j.jaad.2010.08.030

Hajheydari, Z., Saeedi, M., Morteza-Semnani, K., & Soltani, A. (2014). Effect of aloe vera topical gel combined with tretinoin in treatment of mild and moderate acne vulgaris: A randomized, double-blind, prospective trial. *Journal of Dermatological Treatment, 25*, 123–129. doi:10.3109/09546634.2013.768328

Herdman, T. H., & Kamitsuru, S. (2014). *NANDA International nursing diagnoses: Definitions and classification, 2015–2017*. Oxford, United Kingdom: Wiley Blackwell.

Khandpur, S., & Sahni, K., (2014). An open label prospective randomized trial to compare the efficacy of coal tar-salicylic acid ointment versus calipotriol/betamethasone dipropionate ointment in the treatment of limited chronic plaque psoriasis. *Indian Journal of Dermatology, 59*, 579–583. doi:10.4103/0019-5154.143523

Moscaliuc, M. L., Heller, M. M., Lee, E. S., & Koo, J. (2013). Goeckerman therapy: A very effective, yet often forgotten treatment for severe generalized psoriasis. *Journal of Dermatologic Treatment, 24*, 34–37. doi:10.3109/09546634.2012.658014

Samarasekera, E. J., Sawyer, L., Wonderling, D., Tucker, R., & Smith, C. H. (2013). Topical therapies for the treatment of plaque psoriasis: Systematic review and network meta-analyses. *British Journal of Dermatology, 168*, 954–967. doi:10.1111/bjd.12276

Singh, P., Gupta, S., Abidi, A., & Krishna, A. (2013). Comparative evaluation of topical calcipotriol versus coal tar and salicylic acid ointment in chronic plaque psoriasis. *Journal of Drugs in Dermatology, 12*(8), 868–873.

U.S. Food and Drug Administration. (2014). *FDA Drug Safety Communication: FDA warns of rare but serious hypersensitivity reactions with certain over-the-counter topical acne products*. Retrieved from http://www.fda.gov/Drugs/DrugSafety/ucm400923.htm

Yadav, K. H., Kumar, J. R., Basha, S. I., Deshmukh, G. R., Gujjula, R. A. V. I., & Santhamma, B. (2012). Wound healing activity of topical application of aloe vera gel in experimental animal models. *International Journal of Pharma and Bio Sciences, 3*(2), 63–72.

SELECTED BIBLIOGRAPHY

American Academy of Dermatology. (n.d.). *Psoriasis?* Retrieved from https://www.aad.org/dermatology-a-to-z/diseases-and-treatments/m---p/psoriasis

Bradby, C. (2014). *Atopic dermatitis in emergency medicine*. Retrieved from http://emedicine.medscape.com/article/762045-overview

Guenther, L. (2015). *Pediculosis and pthiriasis (lice infestation)*. Retrieved from http://emedicine.medscape.com/article/225013-overview

Hall, B. J., & Hall, J. C. (2010). *Sauer's manual of skin diseases* (10th ed.). Philadelphia, PA: Lippincott, Williams & Wilkins.

Meffert, J. (2015). *Psoriasis.* Retrieved from http://emedicine.medscape.com/article/1943419-overview

Radtke, M. A., Reich, K., Spehr, C., & Augustin, M. (2015). Treatment goals in psoriasis routine care. *Archives of Dermatological Research*, 307, 445–449. doi:10.1007/s00403-014-1534-y

Rao, J. (2015). *Acne vulgaris*. Retrieved from http://emedicine.medscape.com/article/1069804-overview

Roebuck, H. (2011). Treatment options for rosacea with concomitant conditions. *Nurse Practitioner, 36*(2), 24–31. doi:10.1097/01.NPR.0000392794.17007.36

Tüzün, Y., Wolf, R., Kutlubay, Z., Karakuş, Ö., & Engin, B. (2014). Rosacea and rhinophyma. *Clinics in Dermatology*, 32, 35–46. doi:10.1016/j.clindermatol.2013.05.024

Chapter 50

Drugs for Eye and Ear Disorders

Drugs at a Glance

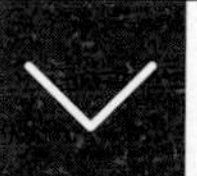

Learning Outcomes

After reading this chapter, the student should be able to:

1. Identify the basic anatomy of the eye.
2. Compare and contrast open-angle and closed-angle glaucoma.
3. Explain the two primary mechanisms by which drugs reduce intraocular pressure.
4. Identify drug classes for treating glaucoma and explain their basic actions and adverse effects.
5. Identify drugs that dilate or constrict pupils, relax ciliary muscles, constrict ocular blood vessels, or moisten eye membranes.
6. Identify drugs for treating ear conditions.
7. For each of the classes listed in Drugs at a Glance, know representative drugs, and explain the mechanisms of drug action, primary actions, and important adverse effects.
8. Use the nursing process to care for patients who are receiving pharmacotherapy for eye and ear disorders.

indicates a prototype drug, each of which is featured in a Prototype Drug box.

The senses of vision and hearing provide the primary means for us to communicate with the world around us. Disorders affecting the eye and ear can result in problems with self-care, mobility, safety, and communication. The eye is vulnerable to a variety of conditions, many of which can be prevented, controlled, or reversed with proper pharmacotherapy. The first part of this chapter covers drugs used for the treatment of glaucoma and those used routinely by ophthalmic health care providers. The remaining part of the chapter presents drugs used for treatment of common ear disorders, including infections, inflammation, and the buildup of earwax.

THE EYES

50.1 Anatomy of the Eye

A firm knowledge of basic ocular anatomy is required to understand eye disorders and their pharmacotherapy. Important structures of the eye are shown in Figures 50.1 and 50.2.

The interior of the eye is divided into the anterior and posterior cavities. The larger of the two, the posterior cavity, is filled with a gel-like substance called vitreous humor that helps the eyeball maintain its shape and keep the retina in place.

The anterior cavity contains a thin fluid called **aqueous humor** and has two divisions. The anterior chamber extends from the cornea to the anterior iris; the posterior chamber lies between the posterior iris and the lens. The aqueous humor is secreted by the ciliary body, a muscular structure in the posterior chamber.

Aqueous humor slowly circulates to bring nutrients to the area and remove wastes. From its origin in the ciliary body, the aqueous humor flows from the posterior chamber through the pupil and into the anterior chamber. Within the anterior chamber and around the periphery is a network of spongy connective tissue, or trabecular meshwork that contains an opening called the scleral venous sinus, or canal of Schlemm. The aqueous humor drains into the canal of Schlemm and out of the anterior chamber

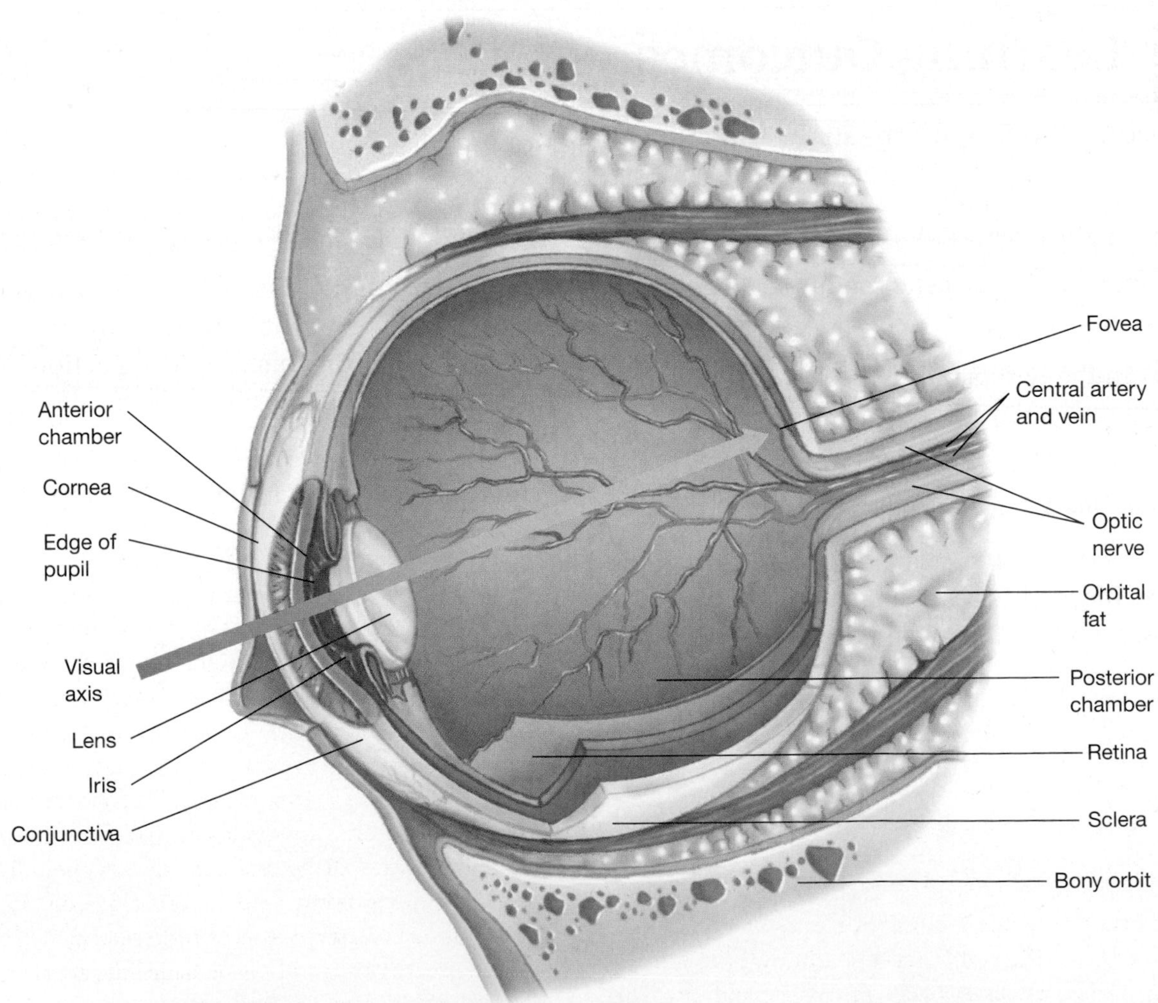

FIGURE 50.1 Internal structures of the eye

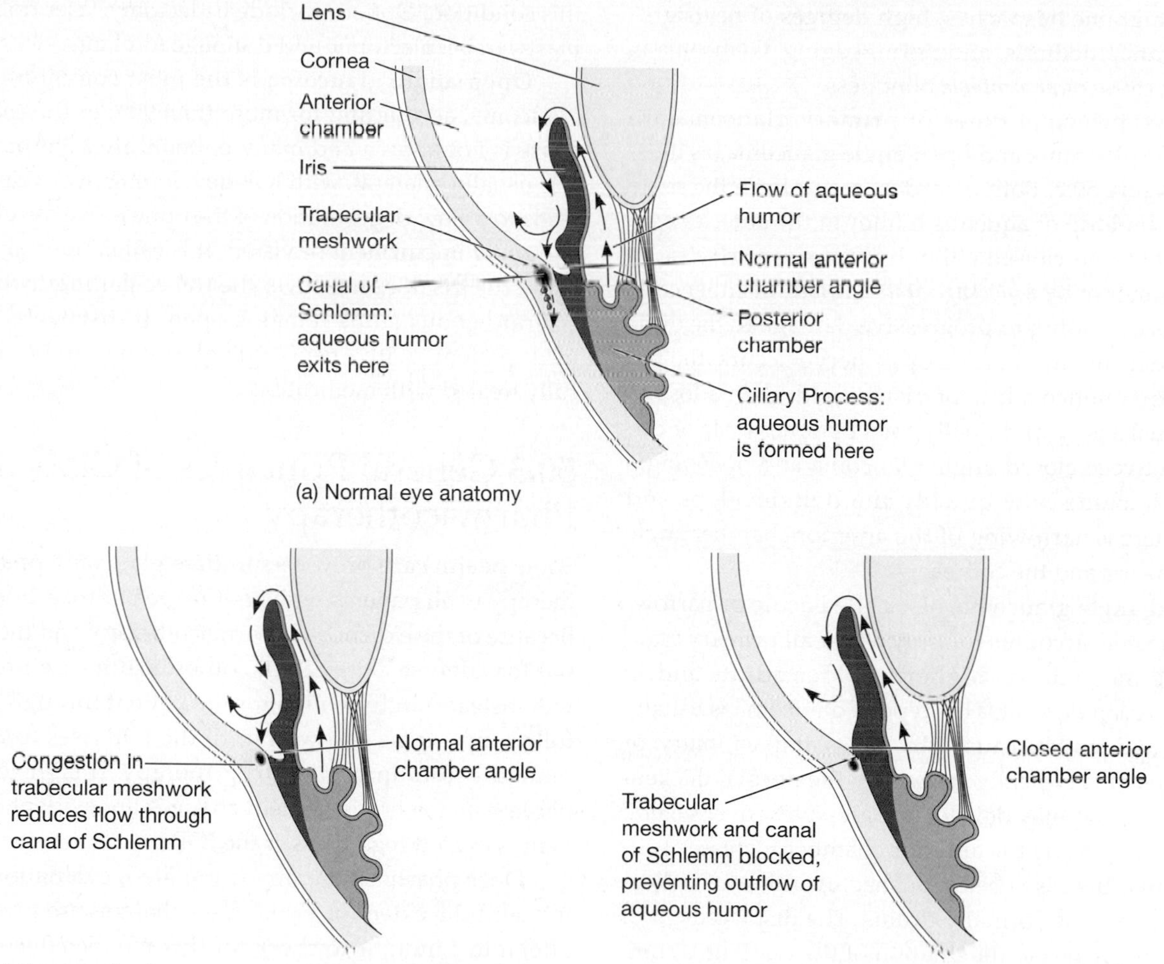

FIGURE 50.2 Forms of primary adult glaucoma: (a) Normal eye anatomy; (b) in chronic open-angle glaucoma, the anterior chamber angle remains open, but drainage of aqueous humor through the canal of Schlemm is impaired; (c) in acute closed-angle glaucoma, the angle of the iris and anterior chamber narrows, obstructing the outflow of aqueous humor

into the venous system, thus completing its circulation. Under normal circumstances, the rate of aqueous humor production (inflow) is equal to its outflow. This helps maintain intraocular pressure (IOP) within a normal range. Interference with either the inflow or outflow of aqueous humor, however, can lead to an increase in IOP.

GLAUCOMA

Glaucoma is an eye disease that is characterized by gradual loss of peripheral vision, possibly advancing to blindness. It is usually accompanied by increased IOP. Glaucoma may occur so gradually that patients do not seek medical intervention until late in the disease process.

50.2 Types of Glaucoma

Glaucoma occurs when the IOP becomes so high that it causes damage to the optic nerve. Although the median IOP in the population is 15 to 16 mmHg, normal pressure varies greatly with age, daily activities, and even time of day. As a rule, IOPs consistently above 21 mmHg are considered abnormal and place the patient at risk for glaucoma. Some patients, however, are able to tolerate IOPs in the mid to high 20s without damage to the optic nerve. IOPs above 30 mmHg require treatment because they are associated with permanent vision changes. Some patients of Asian descent may experience glaucoma at IOP values below 21 mmHg. In addition, patients who have had Lasik surgery, which removes corneal tissue to correct myopia, may appear to have normal IOPs yet have glaucoma.

Glaucoma usually occurs as a *primary* condition without an identifiable cause and is most frequently found in persons older than 60 years. In some cases, glaucoma is associated with genetic factors; it can be congenital and occur in young children. Glaucoma can also be *secondary* to eye trauma, infection, diabetes, inflammation, hemorrhage, tumor, or cataracts. Some medications may contribute to the development or progression of glaucoma, including the long-term use of topical corticosteroids, some antihypertensives, antihistamines, and antidepressants. Other major risk factors associated with glaucoma include high blood pressure, migraine headaches, high degrees of nearsightedness or farsightedness, and normal aging. Glaucoma is the leading cause of *preventable* blindness.

The two principal types of primary glaucoma are closed-angle glaucoma and open-angle glaucoma, as illustrated in Figure 50.2. Both disorders result from the same problem: a buildup of aqueous humor in the anterior cavity. This buildup is caused either by *excessive production* of aqueous humor or by a *blockage of its outflow*. In either case, IOP increases, leading to progressive damage to the optic nerve. As degeneration of the optic nerve occurs, the patient will first notice a loss of visual field, then a loss of central visual acuity, and finally total blindness. Major differences between closed-angle glaucoma and open-angle glaucoma include how quickly the IOP develops and whether there is narrowing of the anterior chamber angle between the iris and the cornea.

Closed-angle glaucoma, also called acute or narrow-angle glaucoma, accounts for only 5% of all primary glaucoma. The incidence is higher in older adults and in persons of Asian descent. This type of glaucoma is usually unilateral and may be caused by stress, impact injury, or medications. It is typically caused by the normal thickening of the lens and may develop progressively over several years. Pressure inside the anterior chamber increases suddenly because the iris is being pushed over the area where the aqueous humor normally drains. The displacement of the iris is due in part to the dilation of the pupil or accommodation of the lens, causing the angle between the posterior cornea and the anterior iris to narrow or close. Signs and symptoms, caused by acute obstruction of the outflow of aqueous humor from the eye, include dull to severe eye pain, headaches, bloodshot eyes, foggy vision with halos around bright lights, and a bulging iris. Ocular pain may be so severe that it causes vomiting. Once the outflow is totally closed, closed-angle glaucoma constitutes a medical emergency. Laser or conventional surgery is indicated for this condition. Options include iridectomy, laser trabeculoplasty, trabeculectomy, and drainage implants.

Open-angle glaucoma is the most common type of glaucoma, accounting for more than 90% of the cases. Its cause is not known and many patients are asymptomatic. It is usually bilateral, with IOP developing over years. This leads to a slow degeneration of the optic nerve, resulting in a gradual impairment of vision. It is called open angle because the iris does not cover the trabecular meshwork; the scleral venous sinus remains open. If discovered early, most patients with open-angle glaucoma can be successfully treated with medications.

PharmFacts

GLAUCOMA

- Worldwide, glaucoma is the second leading cause of blindness; cataracts are the number one cause.
- About 3–6 million Americans have glaucoma; this includes 4–10% of the population over age 40.
- The incidence of glaucoma in people of African heritage is three to four times higher than in Caucasians.
- Glaucoma is most common in people older than 60 years, in those with diabetes, and in those who have severe nearsightedness.
- Medical marijuana lowers IOP in patients with glaucoma but it has a shorter duration of action than most antiglaucoma medications.

50.3 General Principles of Glaucoma Pharmacotherapy

Some health care providers initiate glaucoma pharmacotherapy in all patients with an IOP greater than 21 mmHg. Because of the expense of pharmacotherapy and the potential for adverse drug effects, other health care providers will instead carefully monitor the patient through regular follow-up exams and wait until the IOP rises to 28 to 30 mmHg before initiating drug therapy. If signs of optic nerve damage or visual field changes are evident, the patient is treated regardless of the IOP.

Once pharmacotherapy is initiated, evaluation of the IOP and the extent of visual field changes are performed after 2 to 4 months to check for therapeutic effectiveness. Some antiglaucoma drugs take 6 to 8 weeks to reach peak effect. If the therapeutic goals are not achieved with a single medication, it is common to add a second drug from a different class to the regimen to produce an additive decrease in IOP. Some of the antiglaucoma medications continue to affect the eye for 2 to 4 weeks after they are discontinued.

Drugs for glaucoma work by one of two mechanisms: increasing the outflow of aqueous humor at the canal of Schlemm or decreasing the formation of aqueous humor at the ciliary body. Many drugs for glaucoma act by affecting the autonomic nervous system (see chapters 12 and 13).

ANTIGLAUCOMA DRUGS

50.4 Pharmacotherapy of Glaucoma

Many drugs are available to treat glaucoma. Although topical drugs are most frequently prescribed, oral medications are prescribed for severe disease. Drugs for glaucoma, listed in Table 50.1, include the following classes:

- Prostaglandin analogs
- Autonomic drugs, including beta-adrenergic blockers, nonselective sympathomimetics, $alpha_2$-adrenergic agonists, and cholinergic agonists
- Carbonic anhydrase inhibitors
- Osmotic diuretics.

Table 50.1 Selected Drugs for Glaucoma

Drug	Route and Adult Dose (max dose where indicated)	Adverse Effects
PROSTAGLANDIN ANALOGS		
bimatoprost (Lumigan)	1 drop of 0.03% solution in the evening	*Increased length and thickness of eyelashes, darkening of iris, sensation of foreign body in the eye*
latanoprost (Xalatan)	1 drop of 0.005% solution in the evening	With systemic absorption: respiratory infection, flu, angina, muscle or joint pain
tafluprost (Zioptan)	1 drop of 0.0015% solution in the evening	
travoprost (Travatan)	1 drop of 0.004% solution in the evening	
BETA-ADRENERGIC BLOCKERS		
betaxolol (Betoptic)	1 drop of 0.5% solution bid	*Local burning and stinging, blurred vision, headache*
carteolol (Ocupress)	1 drop of 1% solution bid	With systemic absorption: angina, anxiety, bronchoconstriction, hypertension, dysrhythmias
levobunolol (Betagan)	1–2 drops of 0.25–0.5% solution one to two times/day	
metipranolol (OptiPranolol)	1 drop of 0.3% solution bid	
timolol (Betimol, Timoptic, others)	1–2 drops of 0.25–0.5% solution one to two times/day or 1 drop of solution-forming gel daily	
ALPHA$_2$-ADRENERGIC AGONISTS		
apraclonidine (Iopidine)	1 drop of 0.5% solution bid	*Local itching and burning, blurred vision, dry mouth*
brimonidine (Alphagan)	1 drop of 0.2% solution tid	Allergic conjunctivitis, conjunctival hyperemia, hypertension
CARBONIC ANHYDRASE INHIBITORS		
acetazolamide (Diamox)	PO: 250 mg one to four times/day	*For topical drugs: blurred vision, bitter taste, dry eye, blepharitis, local itching, sensation of foreign body in the eye, headache*
brinzolamide (Azopt)	1 drop of 1% solution tid	For oral route: diuresis, electrolyte imbalances, blood dyscrasias, flaccid paralysis, hepatic impairment
dorzolamide (Trusopt)	1 drop of 2% solution in affected eye(s) tid	
methazolamide (Neptazane)	PO: 50–100 mg bid–tid	
CHOLINERGIC AGONISTS		
carbachol (Miostat)	1–2 drops of 0.75–3% solution in lower conjunctival sac q4h tid	*Induced myopia, reduced visual acuity in low light, eye redness, headache*
echothiophate iodide (Phospholine Iodide)	1 drop of 0.03–0.25% solution one to two times/day	With systemic absorption: salivation, tachycardia, hypertension, bronchospasm, sweating, nausea, vomiting
pilocarpine (Isopto Carpine, Pilopine)	Acute glaucoma: 1 drop of 1–2% solution q5–10 min for three to six doses Chronic glaucoma: 1 drop of 0.5–4% solution q4–12h	
NONSELECTIVE SYMPATHOMIMETIC		
dipivefrin HCl (Propine)	1 drop of 0.1% solution bid	*Local burning and stinging, blurred vision, headache, photosensitivity* Tachycardia, hypertension
OSMOTIC DIURETICS		
isosorbide (Ismotic)	PO: 1–3 g/kg one to two times/day	*Orthostatic hypotension, facial flushing, headache, palpitations, anxiety, nausea*
mannitol (Osmitrol)	IV: 1.5–2 mg/kg as a 15–25% solution over 30–60 min	Severe headache, electrolyte imbalances, edema

Note: Italics indicate common adverse effects; underlining indicates serious adverse effects.

Prostaglandin Analogs

Prostaglandin analogs are preferred drugs for glaucoma therapy because they have long durations of action and produce fewer adverse effects than other antiglaucoma drugs. They may be used as monotherapy or combined with drugs from other classes to produce an additive reduction in IOP in patients with resistant glaucoma.

Prostaglandin analogs lower IOP by enhancing the out flow of aqueous humor. Latanoprost (Xalatan), available as an eyedrop solution, is one of the most frequently prescribed prostaglandin analogs and is a prototype drug in this chapter. Other ocular prostaglandins include bimatoprost (Lumigan), tafluprost (Zioptan), and travoprost (Travatan). An occasional adverse effect of these medications is heightened pigmentation, which turns a blue iris to brown. This change may be irreversible. Many patients experience thicker and longer eyelashes. These drugs may cause local irritation, stinging of the eyes, and redness during the first month of therapy. Because of these effects, prostaglandins are normally administered just before bedtime.

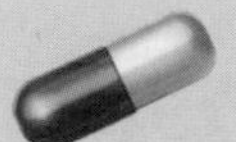

Prototype Drug | Latanoprost *(Xalatan)*

Therapeutic Class: Antiglaucoma drug **Pharmacologic Class:** Prostaglandin analog

Actions and Uses

Latanoprost is a prostaglandin analog that reduces IOP by increasing the outflow of aqueous humor. It is used to treat open-angle glaucoma. The recommended dose is one drop in the affected eye(s) in the evening. It is metabolized to its active form in the cornea, reaching its peak effect in about 12 hours.

Administration Alerts

- Remove contact lens before instilling eyedrops. Do not reinsert contact lens for 15 minutes.
- Avoid touching the eye or eyelashes with any part of the eyedropper to avoid cross-contamination.
- Wait 5 minutes before or after instillation of a different eye prescription to administer eyedrop(s).
- Pregnancy category C.

PHARMACOKINETICS

Onset	Peak	Duration
3–4 h	8–12 h	Unknown

Adverse Effects

Adverse effects include ocular symptoms such as conjunctival edema, tearing, dryness, burning, pain, irritation, itching, sensation of foreign body in the eye, photophobia, and visual disturbances. The eyelashes on the treated eye may grow thicker and darker. Changes may occur in pigmentation of the iris of the treated eye and in the periocular skin.

Contraindications: Contraindications include hypersensitivity to the drug or another component in the solution, pregnancy, lactation, intraocular infection, or conjunctivitis. It should not be administered to patients with closed-angle glaucoma.

Interactions

Drug–Drug: Latanoprost interacts with the preservative thimerosal: If used concurrently with other eyedrops containing thimerosal, precipitation may occur.

Lab Tests: Unknown.

Herbal/Food: Unknown.

Treatment of Overdose: Overdose with ophthalmic solution is unlikely.

Autonomic Drugs

Several structures within the eye are activated by the sympathetic and parasympathetic divisions of the autonomic nervous system. As such, a significant number of autonomic medications have been used to treat glaucoma and to aid in ophthalmic examinations of the eye.

- *Beta-Adrenergic Blockers.* Before the discovery of the prostaglandin analogs, beta-adrenergic blockers were drugs of choice for open-angle glaucoma. These drugs act by decreasing the production of aqueous humor by the ciliary body and generally produce fewer ocular adverse effects than other autonomic drugs. In most patients, the topical administration of beta blockers does not result in significant systemic absorption. Should absorption occur, however, systemic adverse effects may include bronchoconstriction, dysrhythmias, and hypotension. Because of the potential for systemic effects, these drugs should be used with caution in patients with asthma or heart failure.
- *Alpha$_2$-Adrenergic Agonists.* Alpha$_2$-adrenergic agonists act by decreasing the production of aqueous humor. Only two alpha$_2$-adrenergic agonists are currently approved for open-angle glaucoma, and neither of them is frequently prescribed. Apraclonidine (Iopidine) is indicated for the reduction in IOP during or following eye surgery. Brimonidine (Alphagan) is used as an adjunct in combination with other antiglaucoma drugs. The most significant adverse effects are allergic reactions, headache, drowsiness, dry mucosal membranes, blurred vision, and irritated eyelids. Alpha$_2$-adrenergic agonists are contraindicated in closed-angle glaucoma because the pupil dilation that results would worsen the condition.
- *Cholinergic Agonists.* Cholinergic agonists are autonomic drugs that activate cholinergic receptors in the eye and produce **miosis,** constriction of the pupil, and contraction of the ciliary muscle. These actions physically stretch the trabecular meshwork to allow greater outflow of aqueous humor and a lowering of IOP. The cholinergic agonists are applied topically to the eye. Pilocarpine (Isopto-Carpine, Pilopine) is the most frequently prescribed cholinergic agonist. Adverse effects include headache, induced myopia, and decreased vision in low light. Because of their greater toxicity and more frequent dosing requirements, cholinergic agonists are used in patients with open-angle glaucoma who have not responded adequately to other medications.
- *Nonselective Sympathomimetics.* Nonselective sympathomimetics activate the sympathetic nervous system to produce **mydriasis** (pupil dilation), which increases

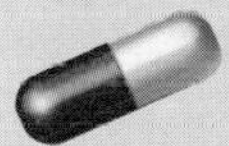

Prototype Drug | Timolol *(Betimol, Timoptic, others)*

Therapeutic Class: Antiglaucoma drug **Pharmacologic Class:** Miotic; beta-adrenergic antagonist

Actions and Uses

Timolol is a beta-adrenergic blocker available as 0.25% or 0.5% ophthalmic solutions taken twice daily. Timoptic XE is a long-acting solution that allows for once-daily dosing. Timolol lowers IOP in chronic open-angle glaucoma by reducing the formation of aqueous humor. The drug has no significant effects on visual acuity, pupil size, or accommodation. Treatment may require 2 to 4 weeks for maximum therapeutic effect. As an oral medication, timolol is prescribed to treat mild hypertension, stable angina, prophylaxis of myocardial infarction, and migraines. Cosopt is an antiglaucoma drug that combines timolol with dorzolamide, a carbonic anhydrase inhibitor. Combigan combines timolol and brimonidine.

Administration Alerts

- Proper administration lessens the danger that the drug will be absorbed systemically. Systemic absorption can mask symptoms of hypoglycemia.
- Pregnancy category C.

PHARMACOKINETICS

Onset	Peak	Duration
30 min	1–2 h	12 24 h

Adverse Effects

The most common adverse effects are local burning and stinging on instillation. Vision may become temporarily blurred. In most patients there is not enough absorption to cause systemic adverse effects as long as timolol is applied correctly. If absorption occurs, hypotension or dysrhythmias are possible.

Contraindications: Timolol is contraindicated in patients with asthma, severe chronic obstructive pulmonary disease (COPD), sinus bradycardia, second- or third-degree atrioventricular block, heart failure, cardiogenic shock, or hypersensitivity to the drug.

Interactions

Drug–Drug: Drug interactions may result when significant systemic absorption occurs. Timolol should be used with caution in patients who are taking other beta blockers due to additive cardiac effects. Concurrent use with anticholinergics, nitrates, reserpine, methyldopa, or verapamil could lead to hypotension and bradycardia. Epinephrine use could lead to hypertension followed by severe bradycardia.

Lab Tests: Unknown.

Herbal/Food: Unknown.

Treatment of Overdose: Overdose with ophthalmic solution is unlikely.

the outflow of aqueous humor, resulting in a lower IOP. They are less effective than the beta-adrenergic blockers or the prostaglandin analogs in treating open-angle glaucoma. Dipivefrin is converted to epinephrine in the eye; thus, its effects are identical to those of epinephrine. If epinephrine reaches the systemic circulation, it increases blood pressure and heart rate. Because of the potential for systemic adverse effects, these are rarely prescribed for glaucoma.

Carbonic Anhydrase Inhibitors

Carbonic anhydrase inhibitors (CAIs) may be administered topically or systemically to reduce IOP in patients with open-angle glaucoma. They act by decreasing the production of aqueous humor.

CAIs are grouped into topical or oral formulations. Dorzolamide (Trusopt) is used topically to treat open-angle glaucoma, either as monotherapy or in combination with other drugs. Dorzolamide and other topical CAIs are well tolerated and produce few significant adverse effects other than photosensitivity. Oral formulations such as brinzolamide (Azopt) are very effective at lowering IOP, but are rarely used because they produce more systemic adverse effects than drugs from other classes. Systemic effects include lethargy, nausea, vomiting, depression, paresthesias, and drowsiness. Patients must be cautioned when taking these medications because they contain sulfur and may cause an allergic reaction. Because the oral formulations are diuretics and can reduce IOP quickly, serum electrolytes should be monitored during treatment.

Osmotic Diuretics

Osmotic diuretics are occasionally used preoperatively and postoperatively with ocular surgery or as emergency treatment for acute closed-angle glaucoma attacks. Examples include isosorbide (Ismotic), urea, and mannitol (Osmitrol). Because they have the ability to quickly reduce plasma volume (see chapter 31), these drugs are effective in reducing the formation of aqueous humor. Adverse effects include headache, tremors, dizziness, dry mouth, fluid and electrolyte imbalances, and thrombophlebitis or venous clot formation near the site of intravenous (IV) administration.

Nursing Practice Application

Pharmacotherapy for Glaucoma

ASSESSMENT	POTENTIAL NURSING DIAGNOSES*
Baseline assessment prior to administration: • Obtain a complete health history including ophthalmologic, respiratory, cardiovascular, and endocrine disease. • Assess visual acuity and visual fields. Assess for the presence of eye pain, visual disturbances such as halos around lights, diminished "foggy" vision, or loss of peripheral vision. • Assess for history of recent eye trauma or infection. • Obtain a drug history including allergies, current prescription and over-the-counter (OTC) drugs, herbal preparations, alcohol use, and smoking. Be alert to possible drug interactions. • Obtain baseline vital signs.	• *Anxiety* • *Acute Pain* • *Deficient Knowledge* (drug therapy) • *Risk for Injury,* related to condition or adverse drug effects *NANDA I © 2014
Assessment throughout administration: • Assess for desired therapeutic effects depending on the reason the drug is given (e.g., IOP remains below 20 mmHg or at target value, improvement in visual acuity or fields). • Assess for adverse effects: conjunctival edema, tearing, dryness, burning, pain, irritation, itching, sensation of foreign body in the eye, or photophobia. Severe visual disturbances or eye pain should be promptly reported to the health care provider.	

IMPLEMENTATION

Interventions and (Rationales)	Patient-Centered Care
Ensuring therapeutic effects:	
• Monitor visual acuity, vision fields, and IOP. (Eye pressure should remain less than 21 mmHg or per parameters set by the health care provider. Visual acuity and fields remain intact.)	• Instruct the patient to immediately report changes in vision, eye pain, light sensitivity, halos around lights, or headache to the health care provider.
Minimizing adverse effects:	
• Monitor appropriate administration of the drug to avoid extra-ocular effects. (Eyedrops should be instilled into the conjunctival sac and the lacrimal duct area, and held with gentle pressure for 1 full minute to prevent drug leakage into the nasopharynx with possible systemic effects.)	• Teach the patient proper administration techniques for eyedrops. Oral medications should be taken as regularly throughout the day as possible and with consistent dosing.
• Monitor IOP periodically. (Consistent readings above the target value may indicate worsening disease or improper use of drug therapy.)	• Instruct the patient of the importance of returning for regular eye exams.
• Monitor for increasing eye redness, pain, light sensitivity, or changes in visual acuity. (Eye changes or pain may indicate worsening disease, infection, or adverse drug effects.)	• Instruct the patient to avoid touching the eyedrop tip to the conjunctival sac when instilling eyedrops. Instruct the patient to immediately report any increasing redness, eye pain, eye drainage, or changes in vision.
• Remove contact lenses before administering ophthalmic solutions. (Contact lenses may hinder the eye solution from fully reaching all eye surfaces or may absorb the solution, resulting in higher than expected amounts in the eye over time.)	• Instruct the patient to remove contact lenses prior to administering eyedrops and to wait at least 15 minutes before reinserting them.
• Monitor vital signs periodically for signs of systemic absorption of topical preparations. (Ophthalmic drugs such as beta blockers or cholinergic drugs may result in hypotension or bradycardia if the drug is absorbed systemically. Ensure that the patient is administering drops appropriately if changes in blood pressure are noted. **Lifespan:** Monitor older adults frequently for hypotension related to systemic absorption to prevent falls.)	• Teach the patient to return to the health care provider periodically for monitoring. Assess blood pressure once per week and report any values less than 90/60 mmHg or per provider parameters. Immediately report any dizziness, headache, palpitations, or syncope.
• Provide for eye comfort such as an adequately lighted room. (Ophthalmic drugs such as beta blockers used in the treatment of glaucoma can cause miosis and difficulty seeing in low-light levels.)	• **Safety:** Caution the patient about driving or other activities in low-light conditions or at night until the effects of the drug are known.

Nursing Practice Application *continued*

IMPLEMENTATION	
Interventions and (Rationales)	**Patient-Centered Care**
• Monitor compliance with the treatment regimen. (Noncompliance may result in the total loss of vision.)	• Teach the patient the importance in adhering to the medication schedule as prescribed. • **Collaboration:** Address any concerns the patient may have about cost and discomfort related to drug therapy, and provide appropriate referrals (e.g., social service agency) as needed.
Patient understanding of drug therapy:	
• Use opportunities during administration of medications and during assessments to provide patient education. (Using time during nursing care helps to optimize and reinforce key teaching areas.)	• The patient should be able to state the reason for the drug, appropriate dose and scheduling, and adverse effects to observe for and when to report them.
Patient self-administration of drug therapy:	
• When administering the medication, instruct the patient, family, or caregiver in the proper self-administration of the drug (e.g., appropriate instillation of eyedrops). (Proper administration increases the effectiveness of the drug.)	• Teach the patient to take the drug, following the guidelines provided by the health care provider.

See Table 50.1 for a list of drugs to which these nursing actions apply.

Check Your Understanding 50.1

Patients are taught to put gentle pressure on the lacrimal duct for one minute after instilling eye drops. What is the purpose of this technique? *Visit www.pearsonhighered.com/nursingresources for the answer.*

50.5 Pharmacotherapy for Eye Exams and Minor Eye Conditions

Various drugs are used to enhance diagnostic eye examinations. **Mydriatic drugs** dilate the pupil to allow better assessment of the retina. **Cycloplegic drugs** not only dilate the pupil but also paralyze the ciliary muscle and prevent the lens from moving during assessment. Drugs used for eye examinations include anticholinergics such as atropine (Isopto Atropine) and tropicamide (Mydriacyl), and sympathomimetics such as phenylephrine (Mydfrin).

Mydriatics cause intense photophobia and pain in response to bright light. Mydriatics can worsen glaucoma by impairing aqueous humor outflow and thereby increasing IOP. Cycloplegics cause severe blurred vision and loss of near vision. The response to mydriatics and cycloplegics can last 3 hours up to several days. The patient needs to be taught to wear sunglasses and that the ability to drive, read, and perform visual tasks will be affected during treatment.

Drugs for minor irritation and dryness come from a broad range of classes. Some agents lubricate only the eye's surface, whereas others are designed to penetrate and affect a specific area of the eye. Vasoconstrictors are commonly used to treat minor eye irritation. Common vasoconstrictors include phenylephrine (Neo-Synephrine), naphazoline (ClearEyes), and tetrahydrozoline (Murine Plus, Visine). Adverse effects of the vasoconstrictors are usually minor and include blurred vision, tearing, headache, and rebound vasodilation with redness. Examples of cycloplegic, mydriatic, and lubricant drugs are listed in Table 50.2.

Conjunctivitis is an inflammation or infection of the lining of the eyelids. Topical corticosteroids and nonsteroidal anti-inflammatory drugs (NSAIDs), such as ketorolac (Acular), can be used to treat conjunctivitis and other inflammatory conditions. Several medications, including antihistamines and mast cell stabilizers, are used to decrease the redness and itching associated with allergic conjunctivitis. Topical mast cell stabilizers, with or without an antihistamine, are the preferred treatment for allergic conjunctivitis because they do not cause excessive drying of the eyes. Two more recent drugs, olopatadine (Patanol) and pemirolast (Alamast), provide for daily dosed treatments for allergic conjunctivitis. Azelastine (Optivar) and epinastine (Elestat) are combination antihistamine–mast cell stabilizers, indicated for twice-daily dosing. Bepotastine (Bepreve) is an antihistamine approved for itching that is often associated with allergic conjunctivitis.

Infectious conjunctivitis, commonly referred to as "pink eye," is most commonly caused by bacteria, but may also result from viruses or fungi. The mainstay for treatment is topical antibiotic therapy. The anti-infectives are the same agents used to treat infections of other areas of the body. Commonly prescribed drugs include gentamicin, tobramycin, neomycin, ciprofloxacin, and erythromycin.

Table 50.2 Drugs for Mydriasis, Cycloplegia, and Lubrication of the Eye

Drug	Route and Adult Dose (max dose where indicated)	Adverse Effects
MYDRIATICS: SYMPATHOMIMETICS		
phenylephrine (Mydfrin, Neo-Synephrine) (see page 152 for the Prototype Drug box)	1 drop 2.5% or 10% solution before eye exam	*Eye pain, photosensitivity, eye irritation, headache* Hypertension, tremor, dysrhythmias
CYCLOPLEGICS: ANTICHOLINERGICS		
atropine (Isopto Atropine, others) (see page 140 for the Prototype Drug box)	1 drop of 0.5% solution each day	*Eye irritation and redness, dry mouth, local burning or stinging, headache, blurred vision, photosensitivity, eczematoid dermatitis (scopolamine and tropicamide)* Somnolence, tachycardia, convulsions, mental changes, keratitis, increased IOP (homatropine)
cyclopentolate (Cyclogyl, Pentolair)	1 drop of 0.5–2% solution 40–50 min before eye exam	
homatropine (Isopto Homatropine, others)	1–2 drops of 2% or 5% solution before eye exam	
scopolamine hydrobromide (Isopto Hyoscine)	1–2 drops of 0.25% solution 1 h before eye exam	
tropicamide (Mydriacyl, Tropicacyl)	1–2 drops of 0.5–1% solution before eye exam	
LUBRICANTS AND VASOCONSTRICTORS		
lanolin alcohol (Lacri-lube)	Apply a thin film to the inside of the eyelid	*Temporary burning or stinging, eye itching or redness, headache* No serious adverse effects
naphazoline (Albalon, Allerest, ClearEyes, others)	1–3 drops of 0.1% solution q3–4h prn	
oxymetazoline (OcuClear, Visine LR)	1–2 drops of 0.025% solution qid	
polyvinyl alcohol (Liquifilm, others)	1–2 drops prn	
tetrahydrozoline (Murine Plus, Visine, others)	1–2 drops of 0.05% solution bid–tid	

Note: *Italics* indicate common adverse effects; underlining indicates serious adverse effects.

Complementary and Alternative Therapies

BILBERRY FOR EYE HEALTH

Bilberry (*Vaccinium myrtillus*), a plant whose leaves and fruit are used medicinally, is found in central and northern Europe, Asia, and North America. It has been shown in clinical studies to increase conjunctival capillary resistance in patients with diabetic retinopathy, thereby providing protection against hemorrhage of the retina. Bilberry is rich in anthocyanin, an antioxidant that may have a collagen-stabilizing effect. Increased synthesis of connective tissue (including collagen) is one of the contributing factors that may lead to blindness caused by diabetic retinopathy. Bilberry has also been shown to reduce eye inflammation characteristic of uveitis, in laboratory animals (Miyake et al., 2012). Bilberry may be taken as a tea to treat nonspecific diarrhea and topically to treat inflammation of the mucous membranes of the mouth and throat. Controlled research studies have yet to conclusively demonstrate benefits of bilberry, yet it remains a popular herbal supplement (National Center for Complementary and Integrative Health, 2012).

EAR CONDITIONS

The ear has two major sensory functions: hearing and maintenance of equilibrium and balance. As shown in Figure 50.3, three structural areas—the outer ear, middle ear, and inner ear—carry out these functions. The basic treatment for ear conditions is topical preparations in the form of eardrops.

Otitis, or inflammation of the ear, is a common indication for pharmacotherapy. **External otitis,** commonly called *swimmer's ear,* is inflammation of the outer ear that is most often associated with water exposure. **Otitis media,** inflammation of the middle ear, is most often associated with upper respiratory infections, allergies, or auditory tube irritation. Of all ear infections, the most difficult ones to treat are inner ear infections. **Mastoiditis,** or inflammation of the mastoid sinus, can be a serious problem because, if left untreated, it can result in hearing loss.

Patient Safety: Improper Eyedrop Administration

Most adults will use eyedrops on occasion to treat dry eyes or allergy conditions, or as a prescribed treatment for more serious eye conditions. In a study of post-cataract surgical patients who did not regularly use eyedrops, An, Kasner, Samek, and Lévesque (2014) found that less than 8% of patients self-administered eyedrops correctly. Despite only 31% of patients reporting difficulty with self-administration, the most common problems observed were failure to wash hands before self-administration (78%); contaminating the bottle tip (57.4%); missing the eye (31.5%); and instilling an incorrect number of drops (64%). The authors also found that self-administration improved significantly after the patients were provided instruction in the proper administration techniques. To improve therapeutic outcomes and improve patient safety, adequate patient education is vital.

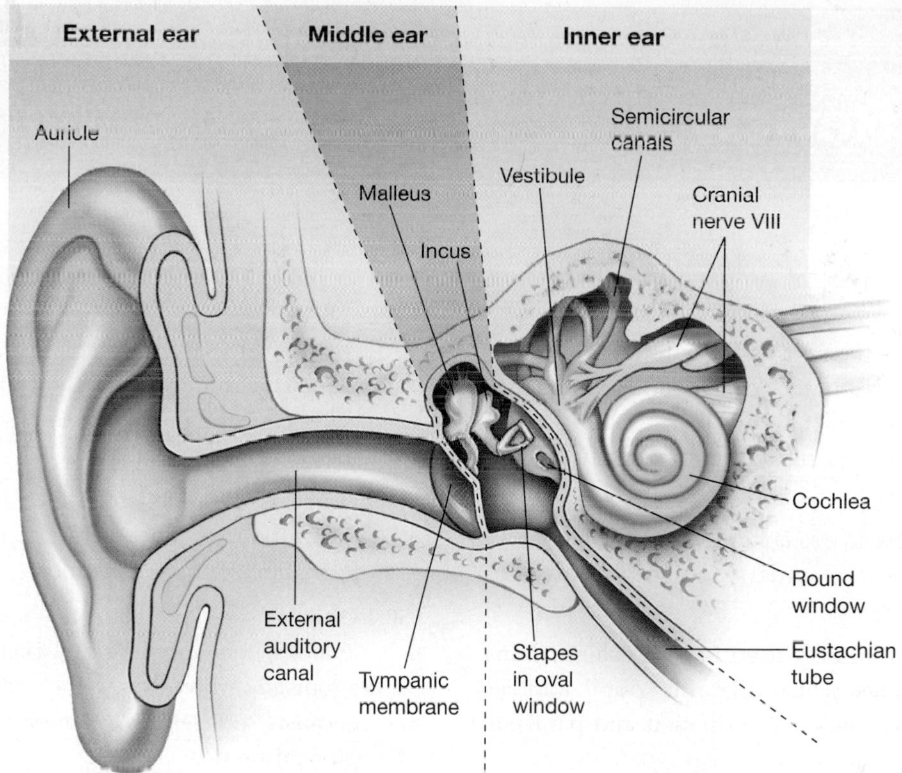

FIGURE 50.3 Structures of the external ear, middle ear, and inner ear

50.6 Pharmacotherapy With Otic Medications

Chloramphenicol (Chloromycetin, Pentamycetin) and ciprofloxacin (Cipro otic) are commonly used topical otic antibiotics. Otitis media is treated with a course of systemic rather than topical antibiotics. Amoxicillin, at a dose of 80 to 90 mg/kg/day, is prescribed for children.

In cases of otitis media, drugs for pain, edema, and itching may also be necessary. Topical corticosteroids are often combined with antibiotics or other drugs when inflammation is present. Examples of these drugs are listed in Table 50.3. Acetaminophen or NSAIDs such as ibuprofen are used to relieve pain and reduce fever.

Refer also to chapter 3 "Principles of Drug Administration," for proper administration technique for eardrops.

Mastoiditis is frequently the result of chronic or recurring bacterial otitis media. The infection moves into the bone and surrounding structures of the middle ear. The treatment of acute mastoiditis involves aggressive antibiotic therapy. IV gentamicin or ticarcillin may be used initially; therapy may be adjusted once culture and sensitivity results are obtained. Therapy is continued for at least 14 days. If the antibiotics are not effective and symptoms persist, surgery such as mastoidectomy or meatoplasty may be indicated.

Cerumen (earwax) softeners are also used for proper ear health. When cerumen accumulates, it narrows the ear canal and may interfere with hearing. This procedure usually involves instillation of an earwax softener and then a gentle lavage of the wax-impacted ear with tepid water using an asepto syringe to gently insert the water. An instrument called an ear loop may be used to help remove earwax, but should be used only by health care providers who are skilled in using it. Examples of earwax softeners include carbamide peroxide (Debrox) and triethanolamine.

Table 50.3 Otic Medications

Drug	Route and Adult Dose (max dose where indicated)	Adverse Effects
acetic acid and hydrocortisone (VoSoL HC)	3–5 drops q4h qid for 24 h, then 5 drops tid–qid	*Ear irritation, local stinging or burning, dizziness* Allergic reactions (antibiotics)
benzocaine and antipyrine (Auralgan)	Fill the ear canal with solution tid for 2–3 days	
carbamide peroxide (Debrox)	1–5 drops 6.5% solution bid for 4 days	
ciprofloxacin and dexamethasone (CiproDex)	4 drops in the affected ear bid for 7 days	
ciprofloxacin and hydrocortisone (Cipro)	3 drops of the suspension instilled into the ear bid for 7 days	
polymyxin B, neomycin, and hydrocortisone (Cortisporin)	4 drops in the ear tid–qid	

Note: Italics indicate common adverse effects; underlining indicates serious adverse effects.

Chapter Review

KEY Concepts

The numbered key concepts provide a succinct summary of the important points from the corresponding numbered section within the chapter. If any of these points are not clear, refer to the numbered section within the chapter for review.

50.1 Knowledge of basic eye anatomy is fundamental to understanding eye disorders and their pharmacotherapy.

50.5 Drugs that are routinely used for eye examinations include mydriatics, which dilate the pupil, and cycloplegics, which cause both dilation and paralysis of the ciliary muscle.

50.2 Glaucoma develops because the flow of aqueous humor in the anterior eye cavity becomes disrupted, leading to increased intraocular pressure (IOP). The two principal types of glaucoma are closed-angle glaucoma and open-angle glaucoma. Therapy of acute glaucoma may require laser surgery to correct the underlying pathology.

50.3 Drugs used for glaucoma decrease IOP by increasing the outflow of aqueous humor or by decreasing the formation of aqueous humor.

50.4 Drug classes for glaucoma include prostaglandin analogs, beta-adrenergic blockers, alpha$_2$-adrenergic agonists, carbonic anhydrase inhibitors, cholinergic agonists, nonselective sympathomimetics, and osmotic diuretics.

50.6 Otic medications treat infections and inflammations of the ear and earwax buildup.

REVIEW Questions

1. A patient with a history of glaucoma who has been taking latanoprost (Xalatan) eyedrops complains of severe pain in the eye, severe headache, and blurred vision. What should be the nurse's first response?
   1. Document the occurrence; this symptom is expected.
   2. Medicate the patient with a narcotic analgesic.
   3. Notify the health care provider immediately.
   4. Place the patient in a quiet darkened environment.
2. The nurse is planning health teaching for a patient who has been prescribed latanoprost (Xalatan) drops for open-angle glaucoma. The nurse should include which of the following in the teaching plan?
   1. The drops may cause darkening and thickening of the eyelashes and upper lid and darkening of the iris color.
   2. The drops may cause a temporary loss of eyelashes that will regrow once the drug is stopped.
   3. The drops will cause dilation of pupils, and darkened glasses should be worn in bright light.
   4. The drops will cause a permanent bluish tint to the conjunctiva that is harmless.
3. Timolol (Timoptic) drops have been ordered to treat glaucoma. Because of the possibility of systemic adverse effects, what essential instruction should the patient receive?
   1. Monitor urine output and daily weight. Promptly report any edema.
   2. Monitor blood glucose and alert the health care provider to any significant changes.
   3. Hold slight pressure on the inner canthus of the eye for 1 minute after instilling the drop.
   4. Monitor respiratory rate and for signs and symptoms of upper respiratory infection.
4. The nurse emphasizes to the patient with glaucoma the importance of notifying the health care provider performing an eye examination of a glaucoma diagnosis because of potential adverse reactions to which of the following drugs?
   1. Antibiotic drops
   2. Cycloplegic drops
   3. Anti-inflammatory drops
   4. Anticholinergic mydriatic drops

5. The patient is prescribed timolol (Timoptic) for treatment of glaucoma. During the history and physical, the nurse assesses for which of the following medical disorders that may be a contraindication to the use of this drug? (Select all that apply.)
   1. Heart block
   2. Heart failure
   3. Liver disease
   4. Chronic obstructive pulmonary disease
   5. Renal disease

6. Appropriate administration is key for patients who are taking eyedrops for the treatment of glaucoma to optimize therapeutic effects and reduce adverse effects. The nurse would be concerned if the patient reports administering the drops in which of the following manners?
   1. Into the conjunctival sac
   2. Holding slight pressure on the tear duct (lacrimal duct) for 1 minute after instilling the eyedrops
   3. Avoiding direct contact with the eye dropper tip and the eye
   4. Leaving contact lenses in to be sure the eyedrop is maintained in the eye

PATIENT-FOCUSED Case Study

Hazel Leonard is a 65-year-old African American woman who visits her ophthalmologist with reports of blurry vision and not being able to see well at night while driving. Her health history includes adult-onset diabetes for the past 10 years and osteoporosis since age 55. Her medical regimen includes diet control for the diabetes and Boniva monthly. She denies any injury to her eyes and last had an eye exam 1 year ago. Her provider diagnoses primary open-angle glaucoma.

1. What factors are present in Mrs. Leonard's health history that you identify as predisposing conditions for the development of primary open-angle glaucoma?
2. What would be possible effects from systemic absorption if the provider has prescribed beta-adrenergic drops (e.g., timolol, carteolol)? Prostaglandin drops (e.g., latanoprost, bimatoprost)? Cholinergic agonists (e.g., carbachol, pilocarpine)?

CRITICAL THINKING Questions

1. A 3-year-old girl is playing nurse with her dolls. She picks up her mother's flexible metal necklace and places the tips of the necklace in her ears for her "stethoscope." A few hours later, she cries to her mother that her "ears hurt." The child's mother takes her to see the health care provider at an after-hours clinic. An examination reveals abrasions in the outer ear canal and some dried blood. The health care provider prescribes corticosporin otic drops. What does the nurse need to teach the mother about instillation of this medication?
2. To determine a patient's ability to administer glaucoma medications, the nurse asks the 82-year-old woman to instill her own medications prior to discharge. The nurse notes that the patient is happy to cooperate and watches as the she quickly bends her head back, opens her eyes, and drops the medication directly onto her cornea. The patient blinks several times, smiles at the nurse, and says, "There, it is no problem at all!" What correction should the nurse make in the patient's technique?

Visit www.pearsonhighered.com/nursingresources for answers and rationales for all activities.

REFERENCES

An, J. A., Kasner, O., Samek, D. A., & Lévesque, V. (2014). Evaluation of eyedrop administration by inexperienced patients after cataract surgery. *Journal of Cataract and Refractive Surgery, 40*, 1857–1861. doi:10.1016/j.jcrs.2014.02.037

Herdman, T. H., & Kamitsuru, S. (2014). *NANDA International nursing diagnoses: Definitions and classification, 2015–2017*. Oxford, United Kingdom: Wiley-Blackwell.

Miyake, S., Takahashi, N., Sasakil, M., Kobayashi, S., Tsubota, K., & Ozawa, Y. (2012). Vision preservation during retinal inflammation by anthocyanin-rich bilberry extract: Cellular and molecular mechanism. *Laboratory Investigation, 92*, 102–109. doi:10.1038/labinvest.2011.132

National Center for Complementary and Integrative Health. (2012). *Bilberry*. Retrieved from https://nccih.nih.gov/health/bilberry

SELECTED BIBLIOGRAPHY

Gemenetzi, M., Yang, Y., & Lotery, A. J. (2012). Current concepts on primary open-angle glaucoma genetics: A contribution to disease pathophysiology and future treatment. *Eye, 26*, 355–369. doi:10.1038/eye.2011.309

Huber, M., Kölsch, M., Stahlmann, R., Hofmann, W., Bolbrinker, J., Dräger, D., & Kreutz, R. (2013). Ophthalmic drugs as part of polypharmacy in nursing home residents with glaucoma. *Drugs & Aging, 30*, 31–38. doi:10.1007/s40266-012-0036-x

Lieberthal, A. S., Carroll, A. E., Chonmaitree, T., Ganiats, T. G., Hoberman, A., Jackson, M. A., . . . Tunkel, D. E. (2013). The diagnosis and management of acute otitis media. *Pediatrics, 131*(3), e963–e999. doi:10.1542/peds.2012-3488

National Glaucoma Research. (2015). *Glaucoma facts and statistics.* Retrieved from http://www.ahaf.org/glaucoma/about/understanding/facts.html

Newman-Casey, P. A., Weizer, J. S., Heisler, M., Lee, P. P., & Stein, J. D. (2013, May). Systematic review of educational interventions to improve glaucoma medication adherence. *Seminars in Ophthalmology 28*, 191–201. doi:10.3109/08820538.2013.771198

Rhee, D. J. (2014). *Drug-induced glaucoma.* Retrieved from http://emedicine.medscape.com/article/1205298-overview

Saxby, C., Williams, R., & Hickey, S. (2013). Finding the most effective cerumenolytic. *The Journal of Laryngology & Otology, 127*, 1067–1070. doi.10.1017/S0022215113002375

Tehrani, S. (2015). Gender difference in the pathophysiology and treatment of glaucoma. *Current Eye Research, 40*, 191–200. doi:10.3109/02713683.2014.968935

Venekamp, R. P., Sanders, S., Glasziou, P. P., Del Mar, C. B., & Rovers, M. M. (2013). Antibiotics for acute otitis media in children. *Cochrane Database Systematic Reviews, Issue 1*, Art. No.: CD000219. doi:10.1002/14651858.CD000219.pub3

Yumori, J. W., & Cadogan, M. P. (2011). Primary open-angle glaucoma: Clinical update. *Journal of Gerontological Nursing, 37*(3), 10–15. doi:10.3928/00989134-20110210-01

Appendix A

Institute for Safe Medication Practices (ISMP)

ISMP List of *Error-Prone Abbreviations, Symbols,* and *Dose Designations*

The abbreviations, symbols, and dose designations found in this table have been reported to ISMP through the ISMP National Medication Errors Reporting Program (ISMP MERP) as being frequently misinterpreted and involved in harmful medication errors. They should **NEVER** be used when communicating medical information. This includes internal communications, telephone/verbal prescriptions, computer-generated labels, labels for drug storage bins, medication administration records, as well as pharmacy and prescriber computer order entry screens.

Abbreviations	Intended Meaning	Misinterpretation	Correction
µg	Microgram	Mistaken as "mg"	Use "mcg"
AD, AS, AU	Right ear, left ear, each ear	Mistaken as OD, OS, OU (right eye, left eye, each eye)	Use "right ear," "left ear," or "each ear"
OD, OS, OU	Right eye, left eye, each eye	Mistaken as AD, AS, AU (right ear, left ear, each ear)	Use "right eye," "left eye," or "each eye"
BT	Bedtime	Mistaken as "BID" (twice daily)	Use "bedtime"
cc	Cubic centimeters	Mistaken as "u" (units)	Use "mL"
D/C	Discharge or discontinue	Premature discontinuation of medications if D/C (intended to mean "discharge") has been misinterpreted as "discontinued" when followed by a list of discharge medications	Use "discharge" and "discontinue"
IJ	Injection	Mistaken as "IV" or "intrajugular"	Use "injection"
IN	Intranasal	Mistaken as "IM" or "IV"	Use "intranasal" or "NAS"
HS	Half-strength	Mistaken as bedtime	Use "half-strength" or "bedtime"
hs	At bedtime, hours of sleep	Mistaken as halfstrength	
IU**	International unit	Mistaken as IV (intravenous) or 10 (ten)	Use "units"
o.d. or OD	Once daily	Mistaken as "right eye" (OD-oculus dexter), leading to oral liquid medications administered in the eye	Use "daily"
OJ	Orange juice	Mistaken as OD or OS (right or left eye); drugs meant to be diluted in orange juice may be given in the eye	Use "orange juice"
Per os	By mouth, orally	The "os" can be mistaken as "left eye" (OS-oculus sinister)	Use "PO," "by mouth," or "orally"
q.d. or QD**	Every day	Mistaken as q.i.d., especially if the period after the "q" or the tail of the "q" is misunderstood as an "i"	Use "daily"
qhs	Nightly at bedtime	Mistaken as "qhr" or every hour	Use "nightly"
qn	Nightly or at bedtime	Mistaken as "qh" (every hour)	Use "nightly" or "at bedtime"
q.o.d. or QOD**	Every other day	Mistaken as "q.d." (daily) or "q.i.d. (four times daily) if the "o" is poorly written	Use "every other day"
q1d	Daily	Mistaken as q.i.d. (four times daily)	Use "daily"
q6PM, etc.	Every evening at 6 PM	Mistaken as every 6 hours	Use "daily at 6 PM" or "6 PM daily"
SC, SQ, sub q	Subcutaneous	SC mistaken as SL (sublingual); SQ mistaken as "5 every;" the "q" in "sub q" has been mistaken as "every" (e.g., a heparin dose ordered "sub q 2 hours before surgery" misunderstood as every 2 hours before surgery)	Use "subcut" or "subcutaneously"
ss	Sliding scale (insulin) or ½ (apothecary)	Mistaken as "55"	Spell out "sliding scale;" use "onehalf" or "½"
SSRI **SSI**	Sliding scale regular insulin Sliding scale insulin	Mistaken as selective-serotonin reuptake inhibitor Mistaken as Strong Solution of Iodine (Lugol's)	Spell out "sliding scale (insulin)"
i/d	One daily	Mistaken as "tid"	Use "1 daily"
TIW or tiw	3 times a week	Mistaken as "3 times a day" or "twice in a week"	Use "3 times weekly"
U or u**	Unit	Mistaken as the number 0 or 4, causing a 10-fold overdose or greater (e.g., 4U seen as "40" or 4u seen as "44"); mistaken as "cc" so dose given in volume instead of units (e.g., 4u seen as 4cc)	Use "unit"
UD	As directed ("ut dictum")	Mistaken as unit dose (e.g., diltiazem 125 mg IV infusion "UD" misinterpreted as meaning to give the entire infusion as a unit [bolus] dose)	Use "as directed"

Dose Designations and Other Information	Intended Meaning	Misinterpretation	Correction
Trailing zero after decimal point (e.g., 1.0 mg)**	1 mg	Mistaken as 10 mg if the decimal point is not seen	Do not use trailing zeros for doses expressed in whole numbers
"Naked" decimal point (e.g., .5 mg)**	0.5 mg	Mistaken as 5 mg if the decimal point is not seen	Use zero before a decimal point when the dose is less than a whole unit
Abbreviations such as mg. or mL. with a period following the abbreviation	mg mL	The period is unnecessary and could be mistaken as the number 1 if written poorly	Use mg, mL, etc. without a terminal period
Drug name and dose run together (especially problematic for drug names that end in "l" such as Inderal40 mg; Tegretol300 mg)	Inderal 40 mg Tegretol 300 mg	Mistaken as Inderal 140 mg Mistaken as Tegretol 1300 mg	Place adequate space between the drug name, dose, and unit of measure
Numerical dose and unit of measure run together (e.g., 10mg, 100mL)	10 mg 100 mL	The "m" is sometimes mistaken as a zero or two zeros, risking a 10- to 100-fold overdose	Place adequate space between the dose and unit of measure
Large doses without properly placed commas (e.g., 100000 units; 1000000 units)	100,000 units 1,000,000 units	100000 has been mistaken as 10,000 or 1,000,000; 1000000 has been mistaken as 100,000	Use commas for dosing units at or above 1,000, or use words such as 100 "thousand" or 1 "million" to improve readability

Drug Name Abbreviations	Intended Meaning	Misinterpretation	Correction
To avoid confusion, do not abbreviate drug names when communicating medical information. Examples of drug name abbreviations involved in medication errors include:			
APAP	acetaminophen	Not recognized as acetaminophen	Use complete drug name
ARA A	vidarabine	Mistaken as cytarabine (ARA C)	Use complete drug name
AZT	zidovudine (Retrovir)	Mistaken as azathioprine or aztreonam	Use complete drug name
CPZ	Compazine (prochlorperazine)	Mistaken as chlorpromazine	Use complete drug name
DPT	Demerol-Phenergan-Thorazine	Mistaken as diphtheria-pertussis-tetanus (vaccine)	Use complete drug name
DTO	Diluted tincture of opium, or deodorized tincture of opium (Paregoric)	Mistaken as tincture of opium	Use complete drug name
HCl	hydrochloric acid or hydrochloride	Mistaken as potassium chloride (The "H" is misinterpreted as "K")	Use complete drug name unless expressed as a salt of a drug
HCT	hydrocortisone	Mistaken as hydrochlorothiazide	Use complete drug name
HCTZ	hydrochlorothiazide	Mistaken as hydrocortisone (seen as HCT250 mg)	Use complete drug name
MgSO4**	magnesium sulfate	Mistaken as morphine sulfate	Use complete drug name
MS, MSO4**	morphine sulfate	Mistaken as magnesium sulfate	Use complete drug name
MTX	methotrexate	Mistaken as mitoxantrone	Use complete drug name
NoAC	novel/new oral anticoagulant	No anticoagulant	Use complete drug name
PCA	procainamide	Mistaken as patient controlled analgesia	Use complete drug name
PTU	propylthiouracil	Mistaken as mercaptopurine	Use complete drug name
T3	Tylenol with codeine No. 3	Mistaken as liothyronine	Use complete drug name
TAC	triamcinolone	Mistaken as tetracaine, Adrenalin, cocaine	Use complete drug name
TNK	TNKase	Mistaken as "TPA"	Use complete drug name
TPA or tPA	tissue plasminogen activator, Activase (alteplase)	Mistaken as TNKase (tenecteplase), or less often as another tissue plasminogen activator, Retavase (retaplase)	Use complete drug name
ZnSO4	zinc sulfate	Mistaken as morphine sulfate	Use complete drug name

Stemmed Drug Names	Intended Meaning	Misinterpretation	Correction
"Nitro" drip	nitroglycerin infusion	Mistaken as sodium nitroprusside infusion	Use complete drug name
"Norflox"	norfloxacin	Mistaken as Norflex	Use complete drug name
"IV Vanc"	intravenous vancomycin	Mistaken as Invanz	Use complete drug name
Symbols	**Intended Meaning**	**Misinterpretation**	**Correction**
ʒ	Dram	Symbol for dram mistaken as "3"	Use the metric system
♍	Minim	Symbol for minim mistaken as "mL"	
x3d	For three days	Mistaken as "3 doses"	Use "for three days"
> and <	More than and less than	Mistaken as opposite of intended; mistakenly use incorrect symbol; "<10" mistaken as "40"	Use "more than" or "less than"
/ (slash mark)	Separates two doses or indicates "per"	Mistaken as the number 1 (e.g., "25 units/10 units" misread as "25 units and 110" units)	Use "per" rather than a slash mark to separate doses
@	At	Mistaken as "2"	Use "at"
&	And	Mistaken as "2"	Use "and"
+	Plus or and	Mistaken as "4"	Use "and"
°	Hour	Mistaken as a zero (e.g., q2° seen as q 20)	Use "hr," "h," or "hour"
⦶ **or** ∅	zero, null sign	Mistaken as numerals 4, 6, 8, and 9	Use 0 or zero, or describe intent using whole words

**These abbreviations are included on The Joint Commission's "minimum list" of dangerous abbreviations, acronyms, and symbols that must be included on an organization's "Do Not Use" list, effective January 1, 2004. Visit www.jointcommission.org for more information about this Joint Commission requirement.

Appendix B

Institute for Safe Medication Practices (ISMP)

ISMP List of *High-Alert Medications in Acute Care Settings*

High-alert medications are drugs that bear a heightened risk of causing significant patient harm when they are used in error. Although mistakes may or may not be more common with these drugs, the consequences of an error are clearly more devastating to patients. We hope you will use this list to determine which medications require special safeguards to reduce the risk of errors. This may include strategies such as standardizing the ordering, storage, preparation, and administration of these products; improving access to information about these drugs; limiting access to high-alert medications; using auxiliary labels and automated alerts; and employing redundancies such as automated or independent doublechecks when necessary. (Note: manual independent double-checks are not always the optimal error-reduction strategy and may not be practical for all of the medications on the list.)

Classes/Categories of Medications
adrenergic agonists, IV (e.g., **EPINEPH**rine, phenylephrine, norepinephrine)
adrenergic antagonists, IV (e.g., propranolol, metoprolol, labetalol)
anesthetic agents, general, inhaled and IV (e.g., propofol, ketamine)
antiarrhythmics, IV (e.g., lidocaine, amiodarone)
antithrombotic agents, including: • anticoagulants (e.g., warfarin, low molecular weight heparin, IV unfractionated heparin) • Factor Xa inhibitors (e.g., fondaparinux, apixaban, rivaroxaban) • direct thrombin inhibitors (e.g., argatroban, bivalirudin, dabigatran etexilate) • thrombolytics (e.g., alteplase, reteplase, tenecteplase) • glycoprotein IIb/IIIa inhibitors (e.g., eptifibatide)
cardioplegic solutions
chemotherapeutic agents, parenteral and oral
dextrose, hypertonic, 20% or greater
dialysis solutions, peritoneal and hemodialysis
epidural or intrathecal medications
hypoglycemics, oral
inotropic medications, IV (e.g., digoxin, milrinone)
insulin, subcutaneous and IV
liposomal forms of drugs (e.g., liposomal amphotericin B) and conventional counterparts (e.g., amphotericin B desoxycholate)
moderate sedation agents, IV (e.g., dexmedetomidine, midazolam)
moderate sedation agents, oral, for children (e.g., chloral hydrate)
narcotics/opioids • IV • transdermal • oral (including liquid concentrates, immediate and sustained-release formulations)
neuromuscular blocking agents (e.g., succinylcholine, rocuronium, vecuronium)
parenteral nutrition preparations
radiocontrast agents, IV
sterile water for injection, inhalation, and irrigation (excluding pour bottles) in containers of 100 mL or more
sodium chloride for injection, hypertonic, greater than 0.9% concentration

Specific Medications
EPINEPHrine, subcutaneous
epoprostenol (Flolan), IV
insulin U-500 (special emphasis)*
magnesium sulfate injection
methotrexate, oral, non-oncologic use
opium tincture
oxytocin, IV
nitroprusside sodium for injection
potassium chloride for injection concentrate
potassium phosphates injection
promethazine, IV
vasopressin, IV or intraosseous

*All forms of insulin, subcutaneous and IV, are considered a class of high-alert medications. Insulin U-500 has been singled out for special emphasis to bring attention to the need for distinct strategies to prevent the types of errors that occur with this concentrated form of insulin.

Background

Based on error reports submitted to the ISMP National Medication Errors Reporting Program, reports of harmful errors in the literature, studies that identify the drugs most often involved in harmful errors, and input from practitioners and safety experts, ISMP created and periodically updates a list of potential high-alert medications. During May and June 2014, practitioners responded to an ISMP survey designed to identify which medications were most frequently considered high-alert drugs by individuals and organizations. Further, to assure relevance and completeness, the clinical staff at ISMP, members of the ISMP advisory board, and safety experts throughout the US were asked to review the potential list. This list of drugs and drug categories reflects the collective thinking of all who provided input.

Appendix C

Calculating Dosages

I. Calculating Dosage Using Ratios and Proportions

A. A *ratio* is used to express a relationship between two or more quantities. Ratios may be written using the following notations.

1:10 means 1 part of drug A to 10 parts of solution/solvent

In drug calculations, ratios are usually expressed as a fraction:

$$\frac{\text{1 part drug A}}{\text{10 parts solution}} = \frac{1}{10}$$

A *proportion* shows the relationship between two ratios. It is a simple and effective means for calculating certain types of doses.

$$\frac{\text{Dose on hand}}{\text{Quantity on hand}} = \frac{\text{Desired dose}}{\text{Quantity desired }(X)}$$

Using cross multiplication, we can write the same formula as follows:

Quantity desired (X) =

$$\frac{\text{Desired dose}}{\text{Dose on hand} \times \text{quantity on hand}}$$

Example 1: The health care provider orders erythromycin 500 mg. It is supplied in a liquid form containing 250 mg in 5 mL. How much drug should the nurse administer?

To calculate the dosage, use the formula:

$$\frac{\text{Dose on hand (250 mg)}}{\text{Quantity on hand (5 mL)}} = \frac{\text{Desired dose (500 mg)}}{\text{Quantity desired }(X)}$$

Then, cross-multiply:

$$250 \not{\text{mg}} \times X = 5 \text{ mL} \times 500 \not{\text{mg}}$$

Therefore, the dose to be administered is 10 mL.

B. The same proportion method can be used to solve solid dosage calculations.

Example 2: The health care provider orders methotrexate 20 mg/day. The methotrexate is available in 2.5-mg tablets. How many tablets should the nurse administer each day?

$$\frac{\text{Dose on hand (2.5 mg)}}{\text{1 tablet}} = \frac{\text{Desired dose (20 mg)}}{\text{Quantity desired (}X\text{ tablets)}}$$

Cross-multiplication gives:

$$2.5 \text{ mg } X = 20 \text{ mg} \times 1 \text{ tablet}$$

Therefore, the nurse should administer 8 tablets daily.

II. Calculating Dosage by Weight

Doses for pediatric patients are often calculated by using body weight. The nurse must use caution to convert between pounds and kilograms, as necessary (see Table 3.2 in chapter 3, page 25). Use the formula:

$$\text{Body weight} \times \text{amount/kg} = X \text{ mg of drug}$$

Example 3: The health care provider orders 10 mg/kg of methsuximide for a patient who weighs 90 kg. How much should be administered?

The patient should receive 900 mg of methsuximide.

Example 4: The health care provider orders 5 mg/kg/day of amiodarone. The patient weighs 110 pounds. How much of the drug should be administered daily?

Step 1: Convert pounds to kilograms.

$$110 \text{ lb} \times 1 \, kg/2.2 \text{ lb} = 50 \, kg$$

Step 2: Perform the drug calculation.

$$50 \not{\text{kg}} \text{ (body weight)} \times 5 \text{ mg}/\not{\text{kg}} = 250 \text{ mg}$$

The patient should receive 250 mg of amiodarone per day.

III. Calculating Dosage by Body Surface Area

Many antineoplastic drugs and most pediatric doses are calculated using body surface area (BSA).

The formula for BSA in metric units is:

$$\text{BSA} = \sqrt{\frac{\text{weight (kg)} \times \text{height (cm)}}{3600}}$$

The formula for BSA in household units is:

$$\text{BSA} = \sqrt{\frac{\text{weight (lb)} \times \text{height (inches)}}{3131}}$$

Example 5: The health care provider orders 10 mg/m^2 of an antibiotic for a child who is 2 feet tall and weighs 30 lb. How many milligrams should be administered?

Step 1: Calculate the BSA of the child.

$$\text{BSA} = \sqrt{\frac{30 \times 24}{3131}}$$

$$\text{BSA} = \sqrt{\frac{720}{3131}}$$

$$\text{BSA} = \sqrt{0.230} = 0.48 \text{ m}^2$$

Step 2: Calculate the drug amount.

$$10\ \text{mg/m}^2 \times 0.48\ \text{m}^2$$

The nurse should administer 4.8 mg of the antibiotic to the child.

IV. CaLculating IV Infusion Rates

Intravenous fluids are administered over time in units of mL/min or gtt/min (gtt = drops). The basic equation for IV drug calculations is as follows:

$$\frac{\text{mL of solution} \times \text{gtt/mL}}{\text{h of administration} \times 60\ \text{min/h}} = \frac{\text{gtt}}{\text{min}}$$

Example 6: The health care provider orders 1,000 mL of 5% normal saline to infuse over 6 hours. What is the flow rate?

$$\frac{1{,}000\ \cancel{\text{mL}} \times 10\ \text{gtt}/\cancel{\text{mL}}}{6\ \cancel{\text{h}} \times 60\ \text{min}/\cancel{\text{h}}} = \frac{28\ \text{gtt}}{\text{min}}$$

Other IV conversion formulas you may use include the following:

$$\text{mcg/kg/h} \rightarrow \text{mL/h}$$

$$\cancel{\text{kg}} \times \frac{\cancel{\text{mcg}}/\cancel{\text{kg}}}{\text{h}} \times \frac{\cancel{\text{mg}}}{1{,}000\ \cancel{\text{mcg}}} \times \frac{\text{mL}}{\cancel{\text{mg}}} = \frac{\text{mL}}{\text{h}}$$

$$\text{mcg/m}^2\text{/h} \rightarrow \text{mL/h}$$

$$\cancel{\text{m}^2} \times \frac{\cancel{\text{mcg}}/\cancel{\text{m}^2}}{\text{h}} \times \frac{\cancel{\text{mg}}}{1{,}000\ \cancel{\text{mcg}}} \times \frac{\text{mL}}{\cancel{\text{mg}}} = \frac{\text{mL}}{\text{h}}$$

$$\text{mcg/kg/min} \rightarrow \text{gtt/min}$$

$$\text{kg} \times \frac{\cancel{\text{mcg}}/\cancel{\text{kg}}}{\text{min}} \times \frac{\cancel{\text{mg}}}{1{,}000\ \cancel{\text{mcg}}} \times \frac{\cancel{\text{mL}}}{\cancel{\text{mg}}} \times \frac{10\ \text{gtt}}{\cancel{\text{mL}}} = \frac{\text{gtt}}{\text{min}}$$

Appendix D

NANDA-Approved Nursing Diagnoses 2015–2017

Activity, Deficient Diversional
Activity Intolerance
Activity Intolerance, Risk for
Activity Planning, Ineffective
Activity Planning, Risk for Ineffective
Adaptive Capacity: Intracranial, Decreased
Adverse Reaction to Iodinated Contrast Media, Risk for
Airway Clearance, Ineffective
Allergy Response, Risk for
Allergy Response, Latex
Allergy Response, Latex, Risk for
Anxiety
Anxiety, Death
Aspiration, Risk for
Attachment, Risk for Impaired
Bleeding, Risk for
Blood Glucose Level, Risk for Unstable
Body Image, Disturbed
Body Temperature: Imbalanced, Risk for
Bowel Incontinence
Breast Milk, Insufficient
Breastfeeding, Ineffective
Breastfeeding, Interrupted
Breastfeeding, Readiness for Enhanced
Breathing Pattern, Ineffective
Cardiac Output, Decreased
Cardiac Output, Decreased, Risk for
Cardiovascular Function, Impaired, Risk for
Caregiver Role Strain
Caregiver Role Strain, Risk for
Childbearing Process, Ineffective
Childbearing Process, Readiness for Enhanced
Childbearing Process, Risk for Ineffective
Chronic Pain Syndrome
Comfort, Impaired
Comfort, Readiness for Enhanced
Communication, Readiness for Enhanced
Communication: Verbal, Impaired
Confusion, Acute
Confusion, Chronic
Confusion, Risk for Acute
Constipation
Constipation, Perceived
Constipation, Risk for
Contamination
Contamination, Risk for
Coping: Community, Ineffective
Coping: Community, Readiness for Enhanced
Coping, Defensive
Coping: Family, Compromised
Coping: Family, Disabled
Coping: Family, Readiness for Enhanced
Coping: Readiness for Enhanced
Coping, Ineffective
Corneal Injury, Risk for
Decision Making, Readiness for Enhanced
Decisional Conflict (Specify)
Denial, Ineffective
Dentition, Impaired
Development: Delayed, Risk for
Diarrhea
Disuse Syndrome, Risk for
Dry Eye, Risk for
Dysreflexia, Autonomic
Dysreflexia, Autonomic, Risk for
Electrolyte Imbalance, Risk for
Emancipated Decision-Making, Impaired
Emancipated Decision-Making, Impaired, Risk for
Emancipated Decision-Making, Readiness for Enhanced
Emotional Control, Labile
Falls, Risk for
Family Processes, Dysfunctional
Family Processes, Interrupted
Family Processes, Readiness for Enhanced
Fatigue
Fear

Fluid Balance, Readiness for Enhanced
Fluid Volume: Deficient
Fluid Volume: Deficient, Risk for
Fluid Volume: Excess
Fluid Volume: Imbalanced, Risk for
Frail Elderly Syndrome
Frail Elderly Syndrome, Risk for
Functional Constipation, Chronic
Gas Exchange, Impaired
Gastrointestinal Motility, Risk for Dysfunctional
Gastrointestinal Motility, Dysfunctional
Grieving
Grieving, Complicated
Grieving, Risk for Complicated
Growth: Disproportionate, Risk for
Health: Community, Deficient
Health Behavior, Risk-Prone
Health Maintenance, Ineffective
Health Management, Family, Ineffective
Health Management, Ineffective
Health Management, Readiness for Enhanced
Home Maintenance, Impaired
Hope, Readiness for Enhanced
Hopelessness
Human Dignity, Risk for Compromised
Hyperthermia
Hypothermia
Hypothermia, Risk for
Impulse Control, Ineffective
Infant Behavior: Disorganized
Infant Behavior: Disorganized, Risk for
Infant Behavior: Organized, Readiness for Enhanced
Infant Feeding Pattern, Ineffective
Infection, Risk for
Injury, Risk for
Insomnia
Jaundice, Neonatal
Jaundice, Neonatal, Risk for
Knowledge, Deficient
Knowledge, Readiness for Enhanced
Labor Pain
Lifestyle, Sedentary
Liver Function, Risk for Impaired
Loneliness, Risk for
Maternal/Fetal Dyad, Risk for Disturbed
Memory, Impaired
Mobility: Bed, Impaired
Mobility: Physical, Impaired
Mobility: Wheelchair, Impaired
Mood Regulation, Impaired
Moral Distress
Nausea
Neglect, Unilateral
Neurovascular Dysfunction: Peripheral, Risk for
Noncompliance
Nutrition, Imbalanced: Less than Body Requirements
Nutrition, Readiness for Enhanced
Mucous Membrane: Oral, Impaired
Mucus Membrane: Oral, Impaired, Risk for
Obesity
Overweight
Overweight, Risk for
Pain, Acute
Pain, Chronic
Parenting, Impaired
Parenting, Readiness for Enhanced
Parenting, Risk for Impaired
Perfusion: Gastrointestinal, Risk for Ineffective
Perfusion: Renal, Risk for Ineffective
Perioperative Hypothermia, Risk for
Perioperative Positioning Injury, Risk for
Personal Identity: Disturbed
Personal Identity: Disturbed, Risk for
Poisoning, Risk for
Post-Trauma Syndrome
Post-Trauma Syndrome, Risk for
Power, Readiness for Enhanced
Powerlessness
Powerlessness, Risk for
Pressure Ulcer, Risk for
Protection, Ineffective
Rape-Trauma Syndrome
Relationship, Ineffective
Relationship, Risk for Ineffective
Relationship, Readiness for Enhanced
Religiosity, Impaired
Religiosity, Readiness for Enhanced
Religiosity, Risk for Impaired

Relocation Stress Syndrome
Relocation Stress Syndrome, Risk for
Resilience, Impaired
Resilience, Readiness for Enhanced
Resilience, Risk for Impaired
Role Conflict, Parental
Role Performance, Ineffective
Self-care, Readiness for Enhanced
Self-care Deficit: Bathing
Self-care Deficit: Dressing
Self-care Deficit: Feeding
Self-care Deficit: Toileting
Self-Concept, Readiness for Enhanced
Self-Esteem, Chronic Low
Self-Esteem, Chronic Low, Risk for
Self-Esteem, Situational Low
Self-Esteem, Situational Low, Risk for
Self-Mutilation
Self-Mutilation, Risk for
Self Neglect
Sexual Dysfunction
Sexuality Pattern, Ineffective
Shock, Risk for
Sitting, Impaired
Skin Integrity, Impaired
Skin Integrity, Risk for Impaired
Sleep Deprivation
Sleep Pattern, Disturbed
Sleep, Readiness for Enhanced
Social Interaction, Impaired
Social Isolation
Sorrow, Chronic
Spiritual Distress
Spiritual Distress, Risk for
Spiritual Well-Being, Readiness for Enhanced
Standing, Impaired
Sudden Infant Death Syndrome, Risk for
Stress Overload
Suffocation, Risk for
Suicide, Risk for
Surgical Recovery, Delayed
Surgical Recovery, Delayed, Risk for
Swallowing, Impaired
Thermal Injury, Risk for
Thermoregulation, Ineffective
Tissue Integrity, Impaired
Tissue Integrity, Impaired, Risk for
Tissue Perfusion: Cardiac, Risk for Decreased
Tissue Perfusion: Cerebral, Risk for Ineffective
Tissue Perfusion: Peripheral, Ineffective
Tissue Perfusion: Peripheral, Risk for Ineffective
Transfer Ability, Impaired
Trauma, Risk for
Trauma: Vascular, Risk for
Urinary Elimination, Impaired
Urinary Elimination, Readiness for Enhanced
Urinary Incontinence, Functional
Urinary Incontinence, Overflow
Urinary Incontinence, Reflex
Urinary Incontinence, Stress
Urinary Incontinence, Urge
Urinary Incontinence, Urge, Risk for
Urinary Retention
Urinary Tract Injury, Risk for
Ventilation: Spontaneous, Impaired
Ventilatory Weaning Response, Dysfunctional
Violence: Other-Directed, Risk for
Violence: Self-Directed, Risk for
Walking, Impaired
Wandering

Index

Note: Page numbers followed by *f* indicate figures and those followed by *t* indicate tables, boxes, or special features. Prototype drugs appear in **boldface**, drug classifications are in SMALL CAPS, and trade names are capitalized and cross-referenced to their generic names.

C

M

N

Q

R

S

U

V

Special Features

Community-Oriented Practice

Complementary and Alternative Therapies

Evidence-Based Practice

Lifespan Considerations

Nursing Practice Application

Patient Safety

Pharmacotherapy Illustrated

Pharmfacts

Prototype Drug

Treating the Diverse Patient